Critical Care Nursing: Body-Mind-Spirit

Critical Care Nursing:
Body-Mind-Spirit

Cornelia Vanderstaay Kenner, R.N., CCRN, M.S.
Director, Department of Surgical Critical Care
Nursing, The Hermann Hospital, Houston, Texas;
Instructor, Department of Surgery, Southwestern
Medical School, The University of Texas Health
Science Center at Dallas; Assistant Professor,
College of Nursing, The University of Texas at
Arlington

Cathie E. Guzzetta, R.N., CCRN, Ph.D.
Assistant Professor and Chairperson,
Cardiovascular Department, The Catholic University
of America School of Nursing; Staff Nurse, Coronary
Care Unit, Washington Hospital Center,
Washington, D.C.

Barbara Montgomery Dossey, R.N., CCRN, M.S.
Director, Holistic Nursing Consultants, Dallas; Staff
Nurse, Brookhaven Medical Center, Farmers
Branch; formerly Clinical Nursing Instructor, Texas
Woman's University, Dallas, Texas

Foreword by Frances Storlie

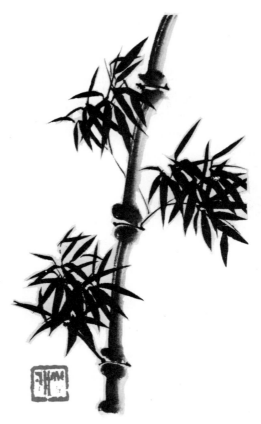

Little, Brown and Company
Boston

To our nursing colleagues
who never hesitate to ask who, where, when, why,
and how

To our husbands
Paul
Philip
Larry

Contents

Foreword

Critical Care Nursing: Body-Mind-Spirit is an attempt to integrate the *experience of being ill* with the assessment and management functions of critical care. Over the past decade there have been a number of such attempts; however, most have done little more than admonish the nurse to "treat the whole person" or to make nursing care "people oriented." Students have assimilated the content without questioning the clichés, and sadder yet, many have not recognized the lack of spiritual application in these discussions.

The authors do well, for into a fabric of physiological and pathological concepts, nursing assessment, and clinical inference they have threaded thoughts and "reflections" that make this book unique among textbooks. One finds oneself hurrying through the concrete, valuable though it is, to reach the mystique—the metaphysical—and to discover how it bears upon the content we have always assumed to be the *real* nursing.

Sparked, perhaps, by the unsettling events of the sixties, our profession has finally embraced social and ethical issues as a valid part of nursing. Yet the literature—the journals of critical care—remain strangely sterile, for their emphasis lies elsewhere, as though pure information has any value whatsoever apart from its application to human issues.

I have found no setting to compare with that of critical care; no better time to look inward. In so doing we will discover feelings within ourselves that are universally human and shared by each of our patients as well. Perhaps we can then understand better why in the ICU the banal so often seems lovely. No other nurses I know celebrate so genuinely the appearance of a few drops of urine. The nurse and patient understand without talking about it that hope lives on and on—if only the kidneys will cooperate. For 15 years I have nursed the critically ill. I know well what young nurses must ultimately learn: the case is not closed simply because a nurse's shift has ended. There will be reflections. There will be afterthoughts.

Think of moments, of minutes, or of hours. There are far too many that move too slowly for the patient. Yet the few there are pass too quickly for the nurse. There is so much more to do.

Think of pain. Is it possible for one human being to feel pain without another feeling compassion? We have been criticized by some who say that critical care nurses have ears too dulled to hear and eyes that will not see. I disagree. What can mere eyes and ears shut out from experience? The heart does not bend so easily to the dictates of the mind. That calmness in the nurse's voice, that poise that gives bearing, is but thin protection against the appearance of frailty. Nurses chose *this* place to work because they cared. Believe me, the patient's experience is shared!

Think of dying. Was there ever a measure devised that can tally the worth of a person? The death of a patient—the least of us—is felt as a loss to the whole of us. And who will define the threads that tie a life in transition with those who wait for the end to come? Stripped at the end of all possessions, with but one more job to be done, nurse and patient reach for the anchor that steadies the soul. With wonder they discover the foundation upon which all that matters rests.

Think of faith. Having set out in this direction, like a hiker intending a short walk in the woods, I would have gone farther. Surely faith—faith in One greater than ourselves—has a place in such a treatise. We are different from the dogs playing in the street. We have a capacity to hope beyond all hope, to expand our minds in order to weigh eternity, to see in the emptied hand the "substance of things hoped for—the evidence of things not seen."

The authors have honed out a solid text that will stand on its own merits. Concrete information is there in abundance. The learner will learn. But what makes this book different from other quality texts on critical care is the curious blend of metaphysical in its frequently interspersed Reflections and Scatterings.

This is the power, the poetry of nursing!

Frances Storlie

Preface

We are critical care nurses. We have been involved in the change, have participated in the expansion, and have experienced a need for a more holistic and interrelated approach to nursing. The current expansion of the practice of critical care nursing is providing the nurse with an exciting challenge and adventure never before available. As nurses in both the clinical and academic settings, we have worked to identify and impart standards of excellence in critical care and to explore complementary and unified approaches to practice.

We have spent many exciting hours of reading and discussion with Larry Dossey, M.D., and other colleagues trying to gain a greater insight into, and some degree of synthesis between, the traditional and nontraditional aspects of nursing, medicine, science, research, physics, and mysticism. Our understanding of humanity, consciousness, health, and disease was altered as a result of this experience, which led us to search for the relationships between the current biomedical model of practice and the power unleashed by the concepts identified in the mind-body interrelationships currently under investigation. As we attempted to encounter the interrelatedness of body-mind-spirit, we discovered *we* were changing: we were incorporating these concepts into our nursing practice and into our lives.

Our book presents an abundance of thought-provoking information clinically applicable to the practitioner and organized within the structure of actual patient situations. Although clinical judgment itself can only be learned at the bedside, the basis for such decision making must be synthesized from a well-constructed and educationally sound approach. The in-depth study of the psychobiological process forms a foundation for further theory and clinical development.

There is a continuing concern among students, critical care nurses, educators, and administrators as to what actually constitutes the basis of preparation, the level of learning, and the standards of practice for critical care nurses. In attempting to deal with this problem, we have drawn upon our own experiences and the pertinent literature.

Part I deals with the concept of psychobiological unity and provides the framework and philosophy of our text. It conveys the overall theme of body-mind-spirit relatedness and will assist the reader in the communication of this content. Because of the essential nature of this material, the authors strongly recommend reading this section before proceeding to other chapters of the book. These concepts are further developed in the Scatterings found at the beginning of each part, and in the Reflections that accompany each case study throughout the book. We have approached this subject of psychobiological unity with much enthusiasm and are confident that the reader will share our excitement.

The content of Parts II, III, and IV assumes a more traditional approach, which can be viewed as complementary to Part I. The information demands a commitment on the part of the critical care nurse that is mandatory to comprehensive and systematic patient care. As a means of dealing with this responsibility, we have constructed information responsive to many of the variables and constraints that confront the critical care nurse.

Parts V to X concentrate on a systems approach to patient care. Pertinent psychobiological ideas and problems are discussed there. The particular manner in which these parts are used will vary. The text is intended to be flexible. Each of the chapters begins with objectives, behavior needed to achieve these objectives, and approaches on how to proceed with the material. If these directions are used before reading the chapter, they can serve as a guide to informal or formal teaching and can be used to gauge one's progress. Each chapter contains a patient case study related to the problem. The case study, presented at the beginning of the chapter, can be used in a variety of ways depending on the needs of the learner. It may be read before proceeding with the chapter as a means of obtaining the overall picture of the problem; it may be read as a review and summary after finishing the chapter; it may be used in clinical conference as a teaching-learning tool. Parts V through X discuss pulmonary, cardiovascular, metabolic, neurological, renal, and special problems and include the relevant pathophysiology, clinical manifestations, physical findings, and diagnosis. The patient care objectives and nursing orders are presented to assist the nurse in assessing, planning, implementing, and evaluating care.

This book is addressed to all students, practitioners, educators, and researchers who are interested in updating, expanding, and refining their critical care practice and who are no longer satisfied with the duality of the current biomedical model of care. Our book only points the direction. You, the receptive student and teacher, will find a variety of ways to pursue the material. The ultimate goal of our book is to place you in control of your own learning process. A critical care nurse should never hesitate to delve deeply. Ask why. . . .

Have fun with our book!

C. V. K.
C. E. G.
B. M. D.

Contributing Authors

Carolyn Rea Atkins, R.N., B.S.
Renal Transplant Coordinator, Parkland Memorial Hospital, The University of Texas Health Science Center at Dallas

Donald A. Bille, R.N., Ph.D.
Associate Professor and Chairperson of Graduate Program, Department of Nursing, DePaul University, Chicago, Illinois

Carolyn Bascom Bilodeau, R.N., M.S.
Psychiatric Nursing Consultant, private practice, Stoughton, Massachusetts; formerly Psychiatric Nurse Clinician, Massachusetts General Hospital, Boston

Mary Blount, R.N., M.N.
Clinical Nurse Specialist of Neurology, University of Virginia Medical Center, Charlottesville

Angela Pruitt Clark, R.N., M.S.
Assistant Professor of Nursing, University of Texas at Austin; Clinical Nurse Specialist and Consultant to Diabetic Education Program, St. David's Hospital, Austin

Robert Berry Cook, Jr., J.D.
Legal Counsel, Baylor University Medical Center, Dallas, Texas

Barbara Montgomery Dossey, R.N., CCRN, M.S.
Director, Holistic Nursing Consultants, Dallas; Staff Nurse, Brookhaven Medical Center, Farmers Branch; formerly Clinical Nursing Instructor, Texas Woman's University, Dallas, Texas

Diane Turbin Ender, R.N., CNRN, M.S.
Executive Director of Learning Systems and Public Relations, Dallas Rehabilitation Institute, Dallas, Texas

Joan B. Fitzmaurice, R.N., M.S.N., F.A.A.N.
Assistant Professor, Department of Nursing, Boston College Graduate School of Arts and Sciences, Chestnut Hill; formerly Cardiovascular Clinical Specialist, Veterans Administration Hospital, West Roxbury, Massachusetts

Barbara Giordano, R.N., M.N.
Doctoral Candidate, Boston University, Boston; Nurse Clinician, Transplant Unit, Massachusetts General Hospital, Boston

Cathie E. Guzzetta, R.N., CCRN, Ph.D.
Assistant Professor and Chairperson, Cardiovascular Department, The Catholic University of America School of Nursing; Staff Nurse, Coronary Care Unit, Washington Hospital Center, Washington, D.C.

Cornelia Vanderstaay Kenner, R.N., CCRN, M.S.
Director, Department of Surgical Critical Care Nursing, The Hermann Hospital, Houston, Texas; Instructor, Department of Surgery, Southwestern Medical School, The University of Texas Health Science Center at Dallas; Assistant Professor, College of Nursing, The University of Texas at Arlington

Anna Belle Kinney, R.N., CNRN, F.A.A.N.
Clinical Nurse Specialist of Neurological Surgery, University of Virginia Medical Center, Charlottesville

Carol Lipin Speyerer, R.N., M.S.
Faculty, College of Nursing, El Centro College, Dallas, Texas; formerly Clinical Specialist, Stroke and Head Trauma Service, Mississippi Methodist Rehabilitation Center, Jackson

Martha L. Tyler, R.N., M.N., R.R.T.
Assistant Professor of Physiological Nursing and Adjunct Assistant Professor of Medicine, University of Washington, Seattle; Respiratory Nurse Specialist, Harborview Medical Center, Seattle

Yvonne Lawton Wagner, R.N., B.S.
Staff Development Coordinator, Nursing Service, Children's Medical Center, Dallas, Texas

Jay Warren, M.S.E.E.
Hospital Electrical Safety Consultant, Long Beach, California

Kathleen MacKay White, R.N., M.S.
Surgical Clinical Specialist, Methodist Hospital, Dallas, Texas

Reviewers

Judy Adams, R.N.
Critical Care Unit
Medical City Dallas Hospital
Dallas, Texas

James Atkins, M.D.
Department of Internal Medicine
The University of Texas Health Science
Center at Dallas

Kathleen Atwell, R.N., M.S.
Cardiovascular Clinical Specialist
Dallas Veterans Administration Hospital
Dallas, Texas

Chris Baker, R.N., M.S.
Cardiovascular Clinical Specialist
Medical City Dallas Hospital
Dallas, Texas

Charles R. Baxter, M.D., F.A.C.S.
Department of Surgery
The University of Texas Health Science
Center at Dallas

David Beesinger, M.D.
Department of Surgery
The University of Texas Health Science
Center at Houston

Delores Berkovsky, R.N., M.S.
Private practice
Fort Worth, Texas

Paula Bone, R.N., M.S.
Emergency Medical Services
The University of Texas Health Science
Center at Dallas

Lincoln Bynum, M.D.
Department of Internal Medicine
Presbyterian Hospital of Dallas
Dallas, Texas

Ned Cassem, M.D.
Department of Psychiatry
Massachusetts General Hospital
Boston

W. Kemp Clark, M.D.
Chairman, Division of Neurosurgery
The University of Texas Health Science
Center at Dallas

Zee Clark, R.N., B.S.
Neuro Clinical Specialist
Parkland Memorial Hospital
Dallas, Texas

Jo Cheek Cole, R.N., B.S.
Cardiac Rehabilitation Nurse
Parkland Memorial Hospital
Dallas, Texas

James R. Cotton, M.D.
Nephrology, private practice
Tyler, Texas

Donald S. Crumbo, M.D.
Cardiology
Dallas Diagnostic Association
Medical City Dallas Hospital
Dallas, Texas

Susan Davis, R.N.
Assistant Unit Coordinator, ICU/CCU
Northside Hospital
Atlanta, Georgia

Larry Dossey, M.D.
Internal Medicine, Director of Biofeedback
Laboratory
Dallas Diagnostic Association
Medical City Dallas Hospital
Dallas, Texas

Mary Gordon, R.N., M.S.
Department of Surgery
The University of Texas Health Science
Center at Dallas

Paul Guzzetta, M.D.
Department of Pulmonary Medicine
The University of Texas Health Science
Center at Dallas

Philip C. Guzzetta, M.D.
Department of Pediatric Surgery
Children's Hospital National Medical Center
Washington, D.C.

Tom L. Hampton, M.D.
Internal Medicine
Dallas Diagnostic Association
Medical City Dallas Hospital
Dallas, Texas

Kathy Hardin, R.N.
Critical Care Unit
Medical City Dallas Hospital
Dallas, Texas

David A. Haymes, M.D.
Internal Medicine
Dallas Diagnostic Association
Medical City Dallas Hospital
Dallas, Texas

Joe H. Sample, Jr., M.D.
Internal Medicine
Dallas Diagnostic Association
Medical City Dallas Hospital
Dallas, Texas

Jack Schwade, M.D.
Cardiology
Dallas Diagnostic Association
Medical City Dallas Hospital
Dallas, Texas

Charles L. Sledge, M.D.
Internal Medicine
Dallas Diagnostic Association
Medical City Dallas Hospital
Dallas, Texas

James W. Smith, M.D.
Department of Internal Medicine (Infectious Disease)
Dallas Veterans Administration Hospital
Dallas, Texas

Thomas C. Smitherman, M.D.
Chief, Coronary and Medical Intensive Care Units
Department of Cardiology
Dallas Veterans Administration Hospital
Dallas, Texas

Andy Sofranko, R.N.
Department of Hemodialysis
Dallas Veterans Administration Hospital
Dallas, Texas

Ralph Tompsett, M.D.
Chief of Internal Medicine
Baylor University Medical Center
Dallas, Texas

Molly Tyler, R.N., M.N.
Respiratory Disease Division
Harborview Medical Center
Seattle, Washington

Ronald H. Underwood, M.D.
Cardiology, private practice
Dallas, Texas

Charles S. White, M.D.
Hematology-Oncology
Dallas Diagnostic Association
Medical City Dallas Hospital
Dallas, Texas

Donald Whitener, M.D.
Pulmonary Medicine, private practice
Columbia, Missouri

Louise Miller Whitener, R.N., M.S.
College of Nursing
University of Missouri
Columbia

Grace Willard, R.N., M.S.
College of Nursing
The University of Texas at Austin

Elizabeth Winslow, R.N., M.S.
Doctoral Candidate
Texas Woman's University
Dallas, Texas

William Woodfin, M.D.
Texas Neurological Institute
Medical City Dallas Hospital
Dallas, Texas

I. Concepts of Psychobiological Unity

The critical care nurse must strive to be intellectually honest. This is a worthy goal not only for the nurse but for any human being. At the same time, it is necessary, as we deal with body-mind-spirit concepts, to be creative and adventuresome in our thinking and feeling. We can be logical to a fault. Our minds become sharpened only by narrowness if our thinking is restrictive and limiting.

If the critical care nurse is to know and feel body-mind-spirit concepts, she must be able to say with Hesse:

. . . I have begun to listen to the teachings
my blood whispers to me.

Hermann Hesse
Prologue to *Demian*

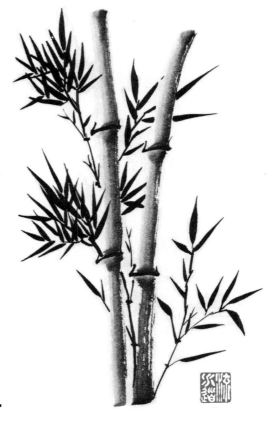

Body-Mind-Spirit

Barbara Montgomery Dossey
Cathie E. Guzzetta
Cornelia Vanderstaay Kenner

1

Body-Mind-Spirit: An Overview

Body-Mind-Spirit is a bold title for any book. It is perhaps more suggestive of an essay on mysticism than a textbook on critical care nursing.

Some readers of this book will be purists who will view the mixture of professionalism and concerns with body, mind, and spirit as inappropriate. Some readers will regard the introduction of these concerns as a retreat from today's scientific position to an era from the past when those concerns suggested superstition, quackery, and witchcraft.

Those of different persuasions may view the book in other ways. To someone with a less technically oriented way of thinking, a body-mind-spirit approach to critical care nursing may suggest that "at last someone feels the way I do. " Another person may be bewildered by the concept of body-mind-spirit—what does that concept mean and what does it have to do with critical care nursing?

Even someone who has a mechanistic orientation to nursing would agree that the patient who is critically ill has enormous psychological reactions to his illness and that it is the duty of the critical care nurse to help such a patient cope. The critical care nurse must not only understand the disease process, know how to operate sophisticated equipment (that often even the patient's physician may not understand), and render basic patient care, she must also cope with the patient's emotional responses to his illness.

As drawn up in almost all nursing and medical schools, the scenario follows familiar and predictable lines. On the one hand is the patient who is critically ill, who presents the nurse and the physician with physical derangements that must, if possible, be corrected. On the other hand are the "less substantial" problems—the patient's psychological responses to his disease—which may be almost a nuisance or a bother. They also must be dealt with, because they may become worse if neglected and thus may eventually interfere with recovery.

The patient's psychological responses to his illness are generally regarded as somehow less real than his so-called purely physical derangements. That fact can be verified by reviewing the literature on acute myocardial infarction. The most detailed discussions are generally of the physical complications of myocardial infarction, such as dysrhythmias, congestive heart failure, pulmonary embolism, and ventricular septal rupture. The psychological complications, such as fear, denial, rage, and depression, are mentioned, one feels, as a gesture toward completeness, the implication being that the psychological complications are distinct from the physical complications, which are somehow more real.

It has long been suggested that the distinctions between the psychological and physical aspects of illness are more artificial than real. Moreover, making those distinctions may hinder the development of more effective ways of treating critical illnesses. Making those distinctions may be like putting legs on a snake, as the ancient Chinese said; that is, they may create difficulties that might otherwise not exist.

The suggestion that mind and body are connected should strike no one in nursing as offensive. After all, today the concept of psychosomatic disease is hardly disputed. Most people agree that such illnesses as functional bowel diseases, tension headaches, and conversion reactions may reflect the patient's psychic distress.

However, what is suggested in this book goes far beyond the concept of psychosomatic illness. What is suggested is that the patient is a human being who is, in the words of Frank, a psychobiological unit [14].

As Frank has pointed out, the Cartesian view of the human being as divisible into two parts, mind and body, has been enormously beneficial for science. It has allowed scientists to investigate the human organism impartially, without having to consider the soul. It must be realized, however, that the Cartesian division of the human being into two parts is relatively recent in the history of the development of human thought and that substantial numbers of people do not hold that view.

Flirting with metaphor and myth can be treacherous, because what is consistently described as metaphor or myth may gradually come to be accepted as being real [19]. Ideas originally used on an "as if" basis may eventually acquire the status of scientific fact.

Consider, for example, LeShan's [19] discussion of the current use of the term vibrations. It may be that you and I affect each other's moods; for example, when you are sad, I may become sad. I may therefore choose to explain the interaction as your sending me "bad vibes." That is a perfectly legitimate way to communicate what I mean as long as you and I remain aware of the metaphorical quality of what I am saying. But what has occurred because of the widespread use of the term vibes is that the metaphor has gradually become elevated to the status of fact, and many people believe that an exchange of physical vibrations occurs.

The exchange may or may not occur. But for our purposes, whether it does is beside the point. Interpersonal exchanges of vibrations may occur, but since we cannot demonstrate that they do, it is best to allow them to retain their mythical status. To do otherwise results in the loss of our logical bearings; it becomes difficult to know where we have come from intellectually, as well as where we are going.

In the seventeenth century, confusion similar to that about vibrations arose in regard to Descartes's view of the human being as divisible into two parts, body and mind. Because that view permitted the astonishing growth of science, including medical science, science itself became the magic wand that transformed the metaphor into presumed fact. A human being could be regarded "as if" he were a body and a mind; and gradually the "as if–ness" of the mind-body duality was lost. So great was the impact of that transformation of metaphor into fact that today the tables are turned: it is the idea of the unity of the human being that seems mythical. We are the heirs of that gradual change in the way of thinking about the human being as being divisible into body and mind—an idea that before Descartes would have largely been regarded as mythical.

Let us for the moment admit that there is an "as if" quality to the ideas that man has a dual nature and

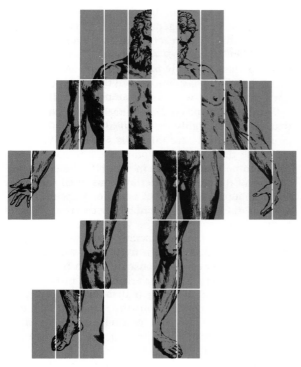

Figure 1-1
Lack of total-person concept. Separation of the person's body from his mind and spirit and subsequent division into a number of parts.

that the duality should be considered as a myth or metaphor. But why would we want to admit that since the idea of duality has been so beneficial for science? If the Cartesian view of the human being was so beneficial for medicine, why not continue to view man in that way? Why insist that the division of man into body and mind is wrong? Why demand a new view of man—as a psychobiological unity? What is wrong with the old way?

Let us look more closely at the old way.

The primary assumption guiding current nursing and medical care is that it is the patient's body that becomes sick (Fig. 1-1). His mind may, of course, be secondarily involved, but the mind is the prime cause of disease only in rather special cases. Medical therapies therefore are body oriented. Antibiotics are administered to infected bodies, hearts are defibrillated, and appendixes are removed. Those methods of therapy, compared to the methods of a century ago, are enormously successful, and are rightfully viewed

as monumental achievements. Unfortunately, however, what is obvious to anyone who has worked in a critical care setting for any length of time is that although bodily illnesses may be eradicated with body oriented therapy, the patient's psychological response to disease may impair his ability to return to full functioning. Or, as Frank has shown [14], psychological forces may actually interfere with healing. Conversely, patients with positive psychological attitudes may respond more positively than others to therapy. Often there seems to be a mind-body interaction affecting (positively or negatively) the patient's responses to what is done for him in the critical care setting.

There is a wealth of data from biofeedback research that bears on the concept that mind and body are connected [7]. Biofeedback is essentially the "feeding back" of physiological information to a person's conscious awareness. The person then uses the "feedback" to make further changes in whatever physiological phenomenon is being measured. To illustrate, temperature sensing devices may be attached to a person's hands. Information about his skin temperature is then given (fed back) to him by means of a monitor that he can see. He may then be told to make his skin warmer, and although unable to explain how he does it, he may be able to achieve this goal.

Biofeedback methods have been used to lower blood pressure in hypertensive people, to control migraine headaches, to reduce the incidence of certain supraventricular dysrhythmias, and to teach sphincter control to people with fecal incontinence—to name some of the clinical applications. But it is only fair to say that the clinical achievements from biofeedback research have been modest compared to early predictions. What is perhaps most important is that through biofeedback research something has been learned about the connectedness of body and mind, about their apparent inseparability.

The eventual impact of that knowledge on the traditional forms of critical care therapy cannot be predicted with certainty. But what is certain is that concepts of body-mind unity will continue to affect critical care therapy in ways that are even now astonishing. For example, Lown and his associates have described the successful treatment of recurrent ventricular fibrillation in a person who did not have coronary artery disease with both conventional drugs and transcendental meditation [23]. Most reports of such treatments are anecdotal and fragmentary, and few reports are as eloquent as Lown's. Another provocative study, one involving the use of Buddhist methods of meditation in treating a hypertensive population, was done by Stone and DeLeo [27].

Mind-body interactions can be demonstrated in the physiology laboratory in regard to blood pressure, heart rate, skin resistance, and skin temperature. With practice, most people can learn to make changes in those physiological phenomena. Theoretically, the application of the biofeedback techniques is quite extensive. The physiology involved has been described in some detail [3, 4, 32].

What is being challenged in this book is a view of man that has dominated our way of thinking for over 300 years. What this book suggests is not just a clever new way of dealing with certain illnesses. What it proposes is a "new" way of seeing the patient—as a unified being *not divisible* into the convenient compartments of mind and body.

But this way of seeing the patient is not new. It is an ancient view, one toward which the pendulum of Western thought may once again be swinging. In many ways, this view is more satisfying than the Cartesian view. The mind-body split has driven us to modes of therapy that approach the inhumane, in the opinion of many who are involved in critical care. The ethics of certain critical care procedures have been examined in the courts largely because of the questions: Are critical care techniques treating only bodies? And if we held the larger view of the patient—as a psychobiologically unified whole— would we apply certain standard critical care procedures so persistently and relentlessly?

It may be objected that it is not the purpose of a textbook on critical care nursing to raise questions of ethics. But the critical care nurse is a protagonist in the critical care drama. She is in a position to understand the psychological trauma that critical care patients undergo. Moreover, her psyche is also involved; and far too little attention has been paid to the psychological stress that critical care nurses undergo.

Getting rid of the old duality—of dividing the patient into mind and body and visualizing those entities as separate and disconnected—would go far toward improving the critical care process. But what is to be gained from adopting a unified view of the patient, of seeing him as "body-mind-spirit," as a psychobiological unity?

First, it might put the patient back into the healing process. From the view of unity, the patient is not simply a body that has become ill and a mind that has become involved in the illness secondarily—because in that view there is no body-mind split. There is no such thing as a physical derangement on the one hand and a psychological reaction to it on the other. Disease is seen as process—a process that involves the whole patient, the only patient there is. A part of the patient does not become ill. It is the whole patient, not a part of him, who is sick or who is well.

If nurses and physicians functioned according to that view, the highly technical and mechanistic approach to critical care might be softened. We might recognize that humanization of the critical care process is important not only in regard to the emotional support of the patient. After all, emotional support *is* physical support if we hold a unified view of the patient, if the idea of psychobiological unity guides our thinking.

In the psychobiological view, a soft, warm atmosphere in a patient's room may be as important in the healing process as the use of an electronic intravenous infusion pump. The critical care nurse's kindness, warmth, and caring may be as important as the use of an antiarrhythmia drug. Indeed, the autonomic-cardiovascular interactions are felt to be enormously responsive to emotional stimuli under certain situations [1, 13].

It is interesting that science may be revealing what mystics of diverse cultures and ages have suggested all along. As we have noted, the idea of psychobiological unity is as old as the history of ideas. But we are only now coming to feel as if we can legitimately adopt the psychobiological view since only recently has science been telling us it is all right to do so.

Somewhere the mystics must be smiling, having held those beliefs about unity long before modern science was born.

But there is a certain danger in a body-mind-spirit approach to illness and healing. When one reads reports, for example, of increased rates of healing and control of malignant dysrhythmias with biofeedback or meditation techniques, with or without the concomitant use of drugs, one is likely to become overly enthusiastic. One commonly feels exhilarated; after all, the idea of psychobiological unity offers people a new way of seeing themselves. That new way may feel more "right," more "whole," than the old way.

But uncontrolled enthusiasm for the new ideas has been damaging to their development. Enthusiastic investigators have made wild claims for the healing powers of meditation—for example, in the treatment of certain cardiovascular diseases. Some well-meaning investigators have even introduced psychic healing to critical care in their enthusiasm for the idea of body-mind relatedness.

Whether or not psychic healing will prove to be of value—or how efficacious the body-mind healing approaches in general will be—is not our concern here. For now we must be concerned that our enthusiasm does not outrun our judgment. We must keep our feet on the ground and not be carried away by the excitement that accompanies self-discovery and personal growth. We must remember that emotions unrestrained by logic can lead to disaster.

If there is benefit to the patient in a body-mind-spirit approach, the benefit will be demonstrable. We should demand the same kind of proof of efficacy of those new methods of care as we would demand of a new drug or surgical technique. And we can demand proofs that the ideas of body-mind relatedness can be applied to patient care. Studies such as those by Lown and his associates and by Stone and DeLeo proved that studies can be designed to investigate the interrelatedness of mind and body.

Enthusiasm about the new ways of seeing the patient often tempts one to discard critical care methods whose value has been proved. There is a trend away from the cold and technical toward the mystical—which is usually the sloppy and the irrational and not the truly mystical. We must not throw out the baby with the bath water. Even should we foresee that ideas about mind-body relatedness could one day be used to cure ventricular fibrillation without electroshock, at present we would do best to continue to use the existing forms of therapy. We must remember that our intellect is no less a part of us than is our spirit.

Mind-body relatedness has so far been discussed only in relation to the patient. We have stated that the patient is indivisible, and we have suggested that thinking about the patient as a unity is more fruitful than thinking about him as divided into mind and body. But does the idea of relatedness extend past the patient perhaps to the nurse-patient relationship?

The traditional nurse-patient relationship is familiar to most people. It is not different substantially from the physician-patient relationship. Traditionally the nurse is seen as standing apart from the patient. She helps the patient in familiar ways and occasionally in sophisticated, perhaps even heroic, ways. But whether the nurse is giving simple care (such as a bed bath) or sophisticated care (such as resuscitative measures), she stands apart from the patient, who is an *object* being treated, a person having things done

for him or *to* him. The patient has become, basically, an object of nursing care.

That way of viewing the patient is so commonsensical that we wonder why we should look for another way. And we wonder whether there are other ways of viewing the nurse-patient relationship.

The "patient-as-object" state of relatedness is more correctly a state of unrelatedness. But it seems accurate because that is the way patients see themselves in relation to the nurse. They see themselves as recipients: as people *to* whom and *for* whom things are done; for example, as people *into* whom medication is injected. They also view themselves as objects of critical care nursing. Indeed they are objectified in many ways. They are given a specific room with a number. They are given an arm band with another number. And, in change-of-shift jargon, they may be referred to impersonally as "the inferior M.I. in 4 with Mobitz I and rare PVCs."

Those kinds of objectification lead to an insidious disregard for a deeper kind of nurse-patient relationship. It becomes easy for the nurse to treat PVCs, forgetting that they happen to patients. Nurses fall into the trap of dividing patients into body and mind, forgetting the mind and concentrating on the body. They revert to seeing patients in the old way, the dual way, the fragmented way. After all, it is easier for nurses to function that way than to work a hectic eight-hour shift with the lofty notion of psycho-biological unity floating through their heads. And, really, who has time for grand and glorious concepts when the M.I. in 4 experiences ventricular tachycardia?

Those are some of the ways nurses rationalize their considering patients as objects.

But if there were no more to the nurse-patient relationship than practicality, nurses might as well be replaced by machines. Computers also could behave toward the patient as if he were only an object. But obviously, the nurse-patient relationship is much more subtle. It has been said that each time a nurse encounters a patient, something happens. The meeting is never a neutral event. It is the power of the nurse-patient relationship that makes nursing exciting blends of emotions and sophisticated skills, not a series of automatic performances. The blends are as varied as the nurses and patients themselves. The critical care nurse must understand that every patient encounter is meaningful, that it always has an impact, that it always affects both the patient and the nurse. The effect may be dramatic or it may be subtle;

but something—either positive or negative—always occurs.

Seen in the new way, the nurse is *in relation to* the patient. The patient is not a mere object. The nurse and patient are indispensable parts of a unit, just as an inside always has an outside. The nurse and patient are co-players of a single role and they have a single objective.

A "unitary" concept begins to emerge, one that involves nurse and patient. Just as we can describe the patient as a psychobiological unit, we can speak of a yet larger unit—that of patient and nurse.

How far does the unitary concept extend? Are there yet larger units involving the critical care staff and patients in general? Are there units that include the physician, other members of the health team, and the patient's family? One can see as much practicality or truth in those propositions as one's inclinations will allow. People who have a traditional turn of mind are likely to be content with the patient-as-object concept of the nurse-patient relationship. Others will not, we hope.

If the concepts of nurse-patient dynamics that have been discussed are valid, that will be most readily apparent to those critical care nurses who are willing to act on those concepts, who are adventuresome enough to use them to find their own personal truths, and who are willing to seek subjective evidence within their own professional life.

The disease entities that are frequently encountered in the critical care setting are discussed in the following pages. The discussions are accompanied by case presentations. We trust that the reader—whether student, staff nurse, or instructor—will use the concept of psychobiological unity in interpreting the case presentations. We believe that the ways of conceptualizing nurse-patient interactions that have been discussed in the preceding pages can lead to vivifying and growing experiences for both the patient and the nurse.

D. H. Lawrence spoke about human relationships in similar tones:

So that everything, even individuality itself, depends on relationship. . . . The light shines only when the circuit is completed. The light does not shine with one half of the current. Every light is some sort of completed circuit. And so is every life, if it is going to be a life.

We have our individuality in relationship. Let us swallow this important and prickly fact. Apart from our connections with other people, we are barely individuals, we amount, all of us, to next to nothing. It is in the living touch between us

and other people, other lives, other phenomena that we move and have our being. Strip us of our human contacts and of our contacts with the living earth and the sun, and we are almost bladders of emptiness [11].

A Body-Mind-Spirit Approach: Why and How

Why?

Why should critical care nurses consider changing their philosophy of patient care? Why are revisions in philosophy along body-mind-spirit lines, psychobiological lines, pertinent? Let us examine those questions, but before doing so, let us look again at what occurs in a nurse-patient encounter.

The Nurse-Patient Relationship

As discussed, the nurse-patient relationship can be described in subject-object terms; that is, the basic encounter involves an active subject (the nurse) who usually does something to or for an object (the patient). Even the patient may consider himself an object—perhaps a passive, dependent, and helpless one.

That view seems so natural that it is seldom questioned, and the distinctions between nurse and patient are therefore taken for granted. They seem to be valid explanations of the dynamics of the nurse-patient relationship. But the accuracy and effectiveness of that description of the nurse-patient relationship should be questioned. And the relationship may need to be revised if more effective means of interchange between nurse and patient are found to be possible.

The idea of separateness between nurse and patient is a function of consciousness. It reflects the ordinary way of conceiving reality. We usually feel that we exist quite apart from our surroundings. We live in a world of objects—and for the critical care nurse, some of those objects are patients. From the common sense feelings we derive from consciousness, there seems no alternative to that view.

Relatedness: An Alternative to the Subject-Object Approach

We learn from many sources, however, that there are other points of view. Those other points of view have diverse origins, and on the surface they appear distant and unrelated. But on closer examination, those sources are not so distant as they seem.

Healing methods used in many primitive cultures take a radically different approach from that of the traditional (subject-object) nurse-patient relationship [12, 24]. Descriptions of shamanistic healing, for example, suggest that a totally different approach is possible. The healer frequently identifies with the patient, in marked contrast to the Western approach of separateness.

The healer-patient interaction in psychic healing encounters has been examined closely by LeShan [20]. The interaction is difficult for most persons to understand, because it violates the commonsense ideas of the familiar subject-object world that we live in, the world that is most comfortable for us. LeShan describes a type of psychic healing encounter in which the healer attempts to achieve a psychological unity with the patient. He strives to become one with the patient. Through the attempted fusion the healer hopes to cure.

It is not clear what mechanisms are involved in that kind of approach. But it would be a mistake to dismiss the approach because it seems nonsensical or sensational or simply because one does not understand it. When one separates the good data from the bad, a solid residue of good remains, suggesting that positive physiological changes can occur when this approach to the patient is used [20].

Patients also sometimes have similar feelings of unity in the healing process. LeShan reports that patients have described a closeness with the healer [20]. Furthermore, the feeling of unity may extend beyond the healer, so that some patients who undergo psychic healing report a feeling of oneness with "all there is."

Those descriptions of unity suggest a way of viewing the world that is quite different from the usual subject-object way of everyday life. The sensation of fusion with the external world is an ancient one; it has been explicitly described in mystical literature. The striving for oneness, for unity with all there is, is the hallmark of the mystic. Descriptions of it come to us from mystical writings of diverse cultures, ones separated by geography and time. The idea of unity is central to the mystical traditions of the Orient, especially Buddhism and Taoism. The writings of Christian mystics abound with descriptions of a complete connectedness of the individual and the external world of objects [30, 31].

The artist and the poet also speak the language of unity. Many of the greatest poets, writers, and artists of our Western tradition are detailed in their descriptions of the feeling of oneness. The topic has been examined in detail by Durr [11].

The feeling of expansion beyond the individual, of interconnectedness and relatedness with all there is, is an experience commonly achieved by the use of certain drugs, among them marijuana, mescaline, LSD, and even alcohol. In no way, however, is that feeling always achieved by the use of drugs; nor should it be regarded as necessary to take drugs to attain the feeling. It is interesting that the descriptions of the feeling of oneness that is induced by drugs are virtually impossible to distinguish from the descriptions of the same feeling that arises naturally [11].

It should be emphasized that this way of "being in the world," this feeling of oneness and unity, is an extremely common occurrence. Since the advent of biofeedback techniques, the descriptions have become commonplace. Frequently those people most skilled in the use of biofeedback techniques report feelings of oneness and transcendence [7].

The popular use of meditation as a spiritual discipline and as a relaxation device has brought it almost to the level of the ordinary. Today it is virtually impossible not to know about the transcendent states, whether from personal experience, from the reports of friends and acquaintances, or from literature. Many readers will be able to attest to personal participation in this view of reality, in which the subject-object world vanishes, leaving feelings of unity in its place.

The Rational Basis for the Approach of Relatedness

The common occurrence of this kind of consciousness has led many to ask, "Is it rational to believe in this way of viewing reality?" That question has been discussed by LeShan, who bases his observations on modern physics [21]. LeShan discusses field theory, which is central to modern quantum physics [20].

Field theory, in its simplest expression, centers on relatedness. At the level of the atom, particles do not exist in isolation. To be fully described, a subatomic particle, such as an electron, must be described in terms of its relationship to other particles. Thus, relatedness is an essential quality of the microscopic world. Because particles behave as parts of a "field," not as discrete entities, the term field theory has arisen. The idea of the unity of the natural world underlies modern physics, and it is central to the Eastern disciplines of Hinduism, Buddhism, and Taoism. The philosophical similarities between modern quantum physical science and ancient Eastern traditions are astonishing. A detailed exploration of the subject has been made by Capra [8] and Zukav [39]. It is those ideas of unity that are finding yet another mode of expression in the concepts of psychobiological relatedness.

The idea that there is an inherent relatedness in the matter that makes up the physical world is difficult to conceptualize. How can things that we conceive of as individual particles, such as electrons and protons, behave as though they were not particles? How can those familiar particles exist as inseparable aspects of all other particles, defying the very definition of particle?

That "separate-but-not-separate" paradox is only one of the paradoxes in modern physics that defy our commonsense way of looking at the world. Another paradox is that of subject-object unity. That concept may be drawn from the observation that the experimenter (the subject) cannot stand apart from the experiment (the object). He is part of the experiment, unable to adopt a position of unrelatedness. His very performance of the experiment in some way affects the results he obtains. The subject becomes an integral part of the object.

The ideas of relatedness may indeed have a rational basis since we can demonstrate their validity through observations from modern physics. Could the principle of relatedness, which seems to be inherent in the physical world at the atomic level, extend to the macroscopic world of human-to-human interaction? If such an extension exists, could it possibly account for the feelings of unity, relatedness, and connectedness described by mystics, healers, poets, artists, biofeedback subjects, and meditators? Those questions are being studied by many investigators, among whom are physicists themselves [26, 28]. Through pursuing the answers to those questions, physicists have entered paths that on the surface seem distant from physics—psychology, parapsychology, and biology. The extension of physics into the paranormal (e.g., psychokinesis, clairvoyance, and telepathy) is itself remarkable. But the world of the quantum physicist is also nonordinary, strange, and paradoxical. Koestler suggests that physicists may be attracted to the paranormal because they feel somewhat at home there; they are used to dealing with the unusual paradox [16].

Practicality

As discussed, the ideas of unity and relatedness are commonplace in the experience of many kinds of people, and those ideas extend even into the quantum physics laboratory. We, therefore, need not consider them unusual. But, as we asked earlier, are they practical?

Practicality is relevant only to one who functions in a pure subject-object world. When one view of the world shifts from the subject-object way to a way of interrelatedness and unity, practicality ceases to be relevant. Practicality becomes apparent in terms of experience. One knows, one feels, and one senses the practicality of the approach.

The subject-object way of dealing with patients forces on the nurse a position of isolation, distance, and separateness from the patient. The nurse becomes the "doer," the patient becomes the "done to." The experience of different kinds of people, as we have seen, suggests that the position of isolation is unnatural, invalid, and illusory and that a more valid position is that of unity and relatedness. It may follow that the pursuit of an illusory world view will compromise not only the nurse's relatedness to the patient but also her effectiveness with the patient.

What are the consequences to the patient if the nurse relates to him in the familiar subject-object way? That question may be examined by asking another question: How does the patient benefit when he himself adopts a unified view, a position of relatedness? The answer to that second question may be found by examining the physiological changes that occur in the state of unity.

Profound alterations in cardiovascular and neuromuscular function have been described in persons during (for example) meditation [32]. Those alterations, which appear to be valid and reproducible, have been called "the relaxation response" by Benson [3]. Frank has compared the effects of anxiety and apprehension on the healing process with the effects of trust and confidence [14]. Patients demonstrating trust and confidence showed a more marked degree of healing than did apprehensive and anxious patients.

Anxiety, apprehension, and a sense of isolation and unrelatedness are often seen in patients who are dealt with in subject-object terms. If feelings of trust and confidence result from nurse-patient interrelatedness, it is reasonable to suspect that the patient responds better to treatment when the nurse uses an approach of unity.

The effectiveness of meditation in the treatment of

hypertension [27] may be a demonstration of that point. The successful use of biofeedback techniques in the treatment of various disorders may be due to their having similar mechanisms. In both biofeedback and meditation, the subjects have the same way of viewing the world—not in subject-object terms but in terms of unity and relatedness.

The effects the attitudes of the health care professional have on patient response have been studied. Torrey points out that the response of psychiatric patients depends primarily on the personal qualities of the health care professionals, such as warmth and caring, and that intellectuality, sophistication of theory, and "technique" are of secondary importance [10]. It has even been suggested that therapy given by a stern, distant psychiatrist may be worse than no therapy [10]. The negative effects of conveying negative feelings to patients should not be underestimated, particularly in the critical care area. Anxiety and despair have not only been related to poorer healing processes in general, but possibly they contribute to the development of life-threatening problems in the critical care unit, the most devastating of which may be dysrhythmias and sudden death [13, 23]. The practicality of the nurse-patient unity approach of relating to the patient can therefore be defended by noting improvement in the patient's therapeutic response when that approach is used. But is the implementation of the unity approach practical for the critical care nurse?

Those who have experienced transcendent feelings of unity and relatedness, those who know from experience the alternative to the subject-object world view, will find the question of practicality irrelevant. They will say that the value of a unified view of the world is self-evident, as well as imminently practical, for the nurse. And in this case, personal experience may be the most meaningful criterion of practicality.

A Dual Approach

It is likely, however, that effective nursing in the critical care setting will involve both ways of relating to patients. To use an analogy, if one sees that he is about to be run over by a car, it is highly practical for him to regard the car as a real object that is about to destroy him, a real subject. In the same way, if the critical care nurse witnesses an episode of ventricular fibrillation, it is highly useful for her to function in subject-object ways—for her to consider the ventricular fibrillation as a real object belonging to a pa-

tient (a real object) and to consider herself the subject and to reach for a defibrillator (another real object).

The idea that both ways of functioning can be used by the nurse is crucial. Seeing patients in subject-object terms and in unity-connectedness terms are *complementary* methods of nursing. *The methods are not mutually exclusive.* Each has its place in the total approach to the patient. They should not be seen in "either-or" terms, because one approach may be more applicable to a situation than the other. Both belong in the nurse's repertoire of responses [18].

How does the nurse know which response to use? There are no formulas, but there are certain guides, as discussed in the following paragraphs.

THE IMMEDIACY OF THE SITUATION

In situations like that of the patient with ventricular fibrillation, the nurse must act with immediacy and effectiveness. When there is little time for anything but emergency responses, the nurse is likely to be most effective if she acts in subject-object terms. In such cases, there seems to be no harm in the nurse's regarding herself (the subject) as the "doer" and the patient (the object) as the "done to." A Zen proverb is applicable: In sitting, sit; in walking, walk. But don't wobble.

THE RESPONSIVENESS AND ADAPTABILITY OF THE PATIENT

Critical care illnesses evoke a variety of emotional responses from patients. Many of those responses are beyond the ability of the critical care nurse to affect, and therefore the responses are frustrating to deal with. Many patients resist participating in exchanges with the nurse that take a psychobiological approach. Some patients will, for example, become withdrawn, isolated, or demanding. Their behavior demonstrates the way they see themselves—as objects to be cared for, as recipients of the nurse's efforts.

Many critically ill patients, however, deal with their illness in other ways. They may demonstrate a willingness to receive care in undemanding and grateful ways. They may exhibit an openness that symbolically says, "I am not an object; please regard me as more than that." That symbolic expression indicates that the patient understands psychobiological unity, his own body-mind-spirit continuum. It is an invitation to the nurse to take a view of relatedness and unity in her approach to that patient. If the patient is capable of seeing himself as more than an object of nursing care, should not the nurse be capable of responding?

THE CAPACITIES OF THE CRITICAL CARE NURSE

Observations from a variety of sources support the concept of psychobiological unity. We have examined reasons why it is valuable to view patients in a psychobiological way and why the usual subject-object approach to patient care is incomplete. In spite of rational argument, whether the critical care nurse adopts and implements those views is not likely to be determined by whether the views are intellectually valid. Rather, the nurse's response to the ideas is more likely to be affected by nonintellectual factors. The nurse's own personality and philosophy are the strongest determinants of her receptivity to ideas of psychobiological unity.

Personality and philosophy are individual matters. Consequently, all critical care nurses will not respond to body-mind-spirit ideas in the same way, no matter how valid the ideas may be. And because of the variation in receptivity to those ideas, critical care nurses will vary in their ability to respond to the patients who give the nurses opportunities to put those views into practice.

That observation is not a criticism of nurses who find body-mind-spirit ideas foreign or even harmful. One cannot be dogmatic and judgmental about the yet gray areas of body-mind-spirit concepts. A rejection of those ideas arrived at after careful consideration may be more honorable than a flimsy, noncritical acceptance of them.

The critical care nurse must realize her strengths and work from them. There is nothing to be gained from attempting to apply body-mind-spirit ideas to patient care if those ideas are not felt, or at least appreciated at an intellectual level. If the nurse feels more effective in the familiar subject-object world of patient care, she should remain there, at least temporarily. While functioning from her subjectively strongest position, she can experiment with new thoughts and new approaches to patient care.

On the other hand, psychobiological approaches to patient care will fit comfortably with the philosophy and beliefs of many critical care nurses. Those convictions can be strengthened by an examination of the evidence for the validity of those approaches. The critical care nurse can therefore add an element of rationality to what may already be deeply felt beliefs.

How?

Body-mind-spirit considerations will not be problems for those nurses who reject them outright or who accept them as compatible with their own experience and philosophy. It is the nurse who is undecided or confused, who feels that the psychobiological approaches are bewildering, who asks for help in understanding those approaches. How should she proceed? Are there practical ways of resolving doubts about those new approaches?

The methods of gaining understanding of the psychobiological approaches can be put in two broad categories: intellectual methods and nonintellectual methods.

INTELLECTUAL METHODS

Try to gain an understanding of the reason and logic underlying the idea of psychobiological unity. First become familiar with the literature in the field. Knowing that there are rational reasons for believing in psychobiological unity will make it easier to approach the nonrational and mystical literature on the subject.

Important readings on the rational side of those issues are listed in the bibliography at the end of the chapter. Particularly clearly written is *The Relaxation Response* [3]. *Stress and the Art of Biofeedback* [7] is a synthesis of observations from biofeedback research that are relevant to the concept of the body-mind-spirit continuum. Of particular interest is LeShan's *The Medium, the Mystic and the Physicist* [20]. It relates observations from the world of modern physics to the healing process in exciting ways, and it illustrates lucidly the ultimate fusion of science and mysticism. In *Alternate Realities* [18], LeShan explores vastly differing ways of viewing reality and examines in detail the idea of using complementary approaches to reality. The book is succinct and prophetic. The articles by Stone and DeLeo [27] and by Lown and his associates [23] show how techniques embodying body-mind-spirit ideas are used clinically. The recent volume *Psychiatry and Mysticism* [10] explores the state of research in many areas relating to psychobiology. It is a fascinating collection of essays that represent many points of view.

One reference leads to others. The reader will discover that both the elegant and the unsophisticated pose as "scientific." Be critical.

Become familiar with clinical attempts to employ

body-mind-spirit concepts. Of particular help might be a visit to a reputable biofeedback laboratory. Again, be critical. Quacks and charlatans abound in the field of biofeedback. However, biofeedback is a highly visible way to conceptualize psychobiological unity.

Lectures and seminars on psychobiology and body-mind-spirit unity are becoming more common. The lectures tend to be analytical and rational in their approach to those concepts, and they may be particularly helpful to the novice. Seminars may also offer chances for participation in workshops that demonstrate the body-mind-spirit continuum at a level that is observable, practical, and personal.

Generally, if one becomes convinced at an intellectual level of the validity of psychobiological considerations, one feels free to make excursions into the nonintellectual realms. How can that be done?

NONINTELLECTUAL METHODS

Again, the literature is impressive. It also seems inexhaustible. And what one reader finds exhilarating, another may find boring. Remember that one is in the realm of the nonintellectual, the subjective, where what one reads (like what one wears) is determined by personal taste.

One is drawn inevitably toward the mystical literature. To the unfamiliar, it can be a wasteland or it can be an oasis. Some of the most readable works by a Westerner are those of Watts, who is probably the best Western interpreter of Oriental mysticism, particularly Zen Buddhism and Taoism. Watts's writing is clear and entertaining. A starting point might be his *This Is It* [37] or *The Book* [35]. All Watts's books are worthwhile, but *Psychotherapy East and West* [34], *The Way of Zen* [36], and *Nature, Man, and Woman* [33] are particularly recommended. Watts is keenly human. *In My Own Way* [32], his autobiography, is a fascinating description of his personal encounter with mysticism. It brings mysticism into the down-to-earth realm.

Underhill has done for Christian mysticism what Watts has done for oriental mysticism. Her *Essentials of Mysticism* [30] is a treasure of elegance, brevity, simplicity, and fine literary style. Her *Mysticism* [29], written in 1911, is still the definitive work on Western mysticism. It is valuable for those who want to explore the subject further.

Herrigel's short classic, *Zen and the Art of Archery* [15], is captivating. Many have found Castaneda's

controversial books about Don Juan, the Yaqui Indian sorcerer, illuminating. Durr's *The Poetic Vision and the Psychedelic Experience* [11] is a scholarly and perceptive comparison of the unity of the views of the artist, the poet, and the user of hallucinogens. It has a valuable bibliography of mysticism in art and literature.

The personal experience of the nonintellectual approaches to body-mind-spirit considerations is possible. A myriad of approaches exist, but a word of caution is necessary. When one participates in the exercises with definite goals and results in mind, one may destroy the effectiveness and meaning of the experiences. As Watts said, just as one cannot smell smelling, one cannot experience experiencing. It is the smell and the experience that are real, not the representational ideas of them. Similarly, when one tries too hard to understand "what it's like" to experience a transcendent state, he may find that the experience eludes him. Abstractions are barriers to direct experience.

One approach is to read about the personal experience of others. Lilly describes well his personal experience of transcendent states (*The Center of the Cyclone* [22]), as does Durr [11].

To those not mystically inclined, some idea of transcendental experience can be easily gained by participating in biofeedback exercises. Again, one should choose carefully. Many biofeedback practitioners are little more than technicians and are not familiar with the deeper elements of the practice. Relaxation techniques can be helpful; again, Benson's *The Relaxation Response* [3] is recommended. With experience and practice, one finds that the boundaries between biofeedback techniques, relaxation techniques, and meditation are relatively thin. Meditation is a rigorous discipline, but it is perhaps the easiest way to experience directly the intrinsic and personal meaning of psychobiological unity. Advice about meditation abounds; LeShan's *How to Meditate* [19] is exceptionally brief and clear.

Both intellectual and nonintellectual methods of understanding body-mind-spirit concepts seem necessary. Unless at some point the nurse actually experiences those concepts, the concepts are likely to remain in the intellectual sphere, where they will forever be ineffective. The emphasis is not only on knowing but on feeling as well.

Any path is only a path, and there is no affront, to oneself or to others, in dropping it if that is what your heart tells you.

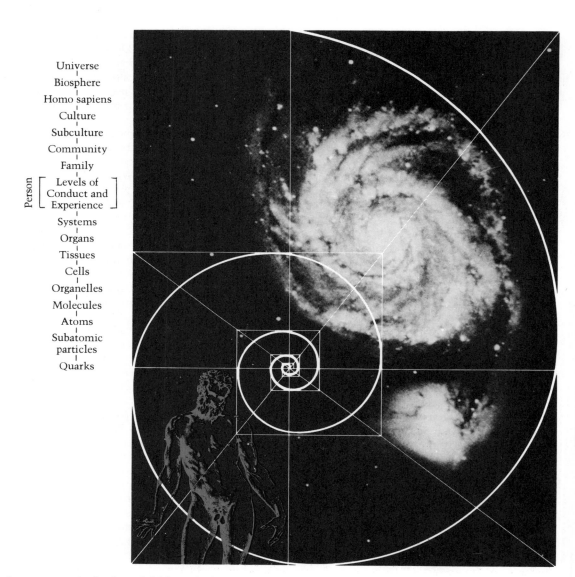

Universe
|
Biosphere
|
Homo sapiens
|
Culture
|
Subculture
|
Community
|
Family
|
Person [Levels of Conduct and Experience]
|
Systems
|
Organs
|
Tissues
|
Cells
|
Organelles
|
Molecules
|
Atoms
|
Subatomic particles
|
Quarks

Figure 1-2
The hierarchy of natural systems.

. . . Look at every path closely and deliberately. Try it as many times as you think necessary. Then ask yourself, and yourself alone, one question. . . . Does this path have a heart? If it does, the path is good; if it doesn't it is of no use [9].

Natural Systems: Another Approach to Psychobiological Unity

Quantum theory asserts that the world acts as a single indivisible unit, in which the very nature of each part depends on its relationship to the whole.

—David Bohm

We are deceived if we allow ourselves to believe that there is ever a pause in the flow of becoming, a resting place where positive existence is attained for even the briefest duration of time. It is only by shutting our eyes to the succession of events that we come to speak of things rather than processes.

—A. Coomaraswomy

Those comments—the first from a renowned quantum physicist, the second from a Hindu mystic of the twentieth century—reflect the same point of view: that all things are interrelated. It is the same concept of unity that is embodied by the psychobiological view of the patient.

The preceding diagram [6] illustrates that interrelatedness (Fig. 1-2).

Figure 1-2 provides a way of visualizing the interconnectedness of what have been called natural systems. In using the concept of natural systems, Laszlo has given a view of the interrelatedness of natural things [17]. That view can be enormously helpful in conceptualizing psychobiological unity.

The systems theory is complex, and a full description of it should be sought in other books [2]. In brief, natural structures of vastly different size can be viewed as natural systems, all possessing definite characteristics (described by Laszlo [17]). What is important to the nurse is that looking at the world through a natural systems approach provides her with a model of psychobiological unity.

An important characteristic of the natural systems that constitute man is that information may originate at any level of the hierarchy of natural systems and may flow to any other part. In other words, changes at the "small" end of the hierarchy (i.e., in the subatomic range) may be felt at the level of the "person" or even into the farthest reaches of the biosphere. (The atomic physicist would extend that interrelatedness even farther—to the farthest reaches of the universe, not stopping at the level of the biosphere, which is merely that part of the world in which life can exist.) Similarly, changes at the "large" end of the hierarchy of natural systems provide information or cause changes that can be felt at the smallest point in the subatomic realm.

According to Brody [6], health may be defined as the harmonious interaction of all the components of the hierarchy of natural systems, whereas disease is the result of a force that disturbs or disrupts the structure of the natural systems themselves. In comparison, the traditional ways of viewing disease usually do not extend above the "person" level on the diagram, and frequently they stop at the "organ" level. According to the natural systems approach, however, disease can result from a disturbance at *any* level, from the subatomic to the suprapersonal. In essence, that approach holds that it is necessary to adopt a comprehensive view of man if one is to define health and disease correctly.

The implications of that approach for nursing are profound. The natural systems approach is only an-

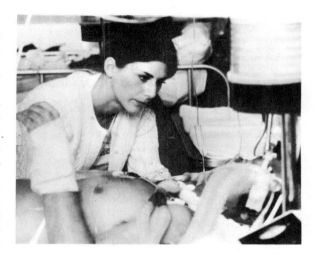

Figure 1-3
Even the simplest nursing act can never be a neutral event. (Photographer: Brian Anderson)

other psychobiological way of viewing the patient. To divide the patient is to disrupt the harmonious flow of information in the complex of systems that comprise man. When the critical care nurse regards the patient apart from the setting of "all there is," she concentrates on certain natural systems and disregards others. That is likely to lead to the fragmented subject-object methods of providing nursing care (discussed earlier) in which the nurse focuses on the disease process as though it were not a part of the patient, treating the renal disease, heart failure, and so on as though they could be abstracted from the patient, in disregard of his psychobiological unity.

The natural systems view shows the inaccuracy of that kind of nursing approach. The natural system view holds that the effects of every disease process are transmitted to all the natural systems that comprise man. Everyone—patient, nurse, or physician—is part of the collective entity and in some sense participates in every disease process; and in the same way, the effects of everyone's health are transmitted to all others.

"Sharing" is not, therefore, something the nurse "decides" to do in caring for critically ill patients. It is not something she can stop or start at will. Sharing is something that *occurs* at a fundamental level, even though one may not be aware of the occurrence. The natural systems approach holds that the simplest nursing act can never be a neutral event (Fig. 1-3).

References

1. Abboud, F. M. Relaxation, autonomic control and hypertension. *N. Engl. J. Med.* 294:107, 1976.
2. Ackoff, R. L. Views on General Systems Theory. In C. D. Mesarovic (ed.), *Proceedings from the Second Systems Symposium.* New York: Wiley, 1964.
3. Benson, H. *The Relaxation Response.* New York: Morrow, 1975.
4. Benson, H., Beary, J. F., and Carol, M. P. The relaxation response. *Psychiatry* 37:37, 1974.
5. Bohm, D., and Hiley, B. On the intuitive understanding of nonlocality as implied by quantum theory. *Foundations Physics* 5:93, 1975.
6. Brody, H. The systems view of man: Implications for medicine, science and ethics. *Perspect. Biol. Med.* Autumn, 1973. Pp. 71–92.
7. Brown, B. B. *Stress and the Art of Biofeedback.* New York: Harper & Row, 1978.
8. Capra, F. *The Tao of Physics.* Berkeley: Shambhala, 1975.
9. Castaneda, C. *The Teachings of Don Juan: A Yaqui Way of Knowledge.* New York: Ballantine, 1968.
10. Dean, S. R. (ed.). *Psychiatry and Mysticism.* Chicago: Nelson-Hall, 1975.
11. Durr, R. A. *The Poetic Vision and the Psychedelic Experience.* New York: Dell, 1970.
12. Elaide, M. *Shamanism: Archaic Techniques of Ecstasy.* Princeton, N.J.: Princeton University Press, 1964.
13. Engel, G. L. Psychological factors in instant cardiac death. *N. Engl. J. Med.* 294:664, 1976.
14. Frank, J. D. Mind-body relationships in illness and healing. *J. Int. Acad. Prev. Med.* 2:46, 1975.
15. Herrigel, E. *Zen and the Art of Archery.* New York: Vintage Books, 1971.
16. Koestler, A. *The Roots of Coincidence.* New York: Random House, 1972.
17. Laszlo, E. *The Systems View of the World.* New York: Braziller, 1972.
18. LeShan, L. *Alternate Realities.* New York: Evans, 1976.
19. LeShan, L. *How to Meditate: A Guide to Self-Discovery.* Boston: Little, Brown, 1974.
20. LeShan, L. *The Medium, the Mystic, and the Physicist: Toward a General Theory of the Paranormal.* New York: Viking, 1974.
21. LeShan, L. Physicists and mystics: Similarities in world view. *J. Transpers. Psychol.* 1:1, 1969.
22. Lilly, J. C. *The Center of the Cyclone: An Autobiography of Inner Spaces.* New York: Julian Press, 1972.
23. Lown, B., Temte, J. V., Reich, P., et al. Basis for recurring ventricular fibrillation in the absence of coronary heart disease and its management. *N. Engl. J. Med.* 294:623, 1976.
24. Middleton, J. *Magic, Witchcraft, and Curing.* New York: Natural History Press, 1967.
25. Murti, T. R. V. *The Central Philosophy of Buddhism.* London: Allen and Unwin, 1955.
26. Seminar on Quantum Psychology, Esalen Institute, Big Sur, California, October 8–10, 1976.
27. Stone, R. A., and DeLeo, J. Psychotherapeutic control of hypertension. *N. Engl. J. Med.* 294:80, 1976.
28. Toben, B. *Space—Time and Beyond.* New York: Dutton, 1975.
29. Underhill, E. *Mysticism.* New York: Dutton, 1961.
30. Underhill, E. *The Essentials of Mysticism.* New York: Dutton, 1960.
31. Wallace, R. K. Physiologic effects of transcendental meditation. *Science* 167:1751, 1970.
32. Watts, A. *In My Own Way.* New York: Pantheon Books, 1972.
33. Watts, A. *Nature, Man and Woman.* New York: Pantheon Books, 1958.
34. Watts, A. *Psychotherapy East and West.* New York: Pantheon Books, 1961.
35. Watts, A. *The Book: On the Taboo Against Knowing Who You Are.* New York: Pantheon Books, 1966.
36. Watts, A. *The Way of Zen.* New York: Vintage Books, 1957.
37. Watts, A. *This Is It.* New York: Macmillan, 1958.
38. Yogi, M. M. *The Science of Being and the Art of Living* (new ed.). London: International SRM Publications, 1966.
39. Zukav, G. *The Dancing Wu Li Masters.* New York: Morrow, 1979.

II. Critical Care Nursing Practice

For the critical care nurse to believe in body-mind-spirit concepts without a clear understanding of her beliefs is similar to saying, "I believe in defibrillation but I don't know how to turn on the defibrillator."

How is the critical care nurse to guide patients if she does not know where they are to be guided? Before guiding patients down any paths, she must become familiar with those paths, both *intellectually* and *experientially*. She must be able to say, "I understand with my mind the physiological bases of mind-body interrelations, and I feel with my spirit that these relationships are true."

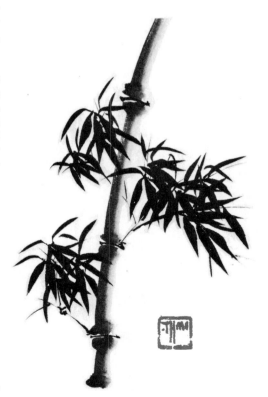

The Nursing Process

Barbara Montgomery Dossey

Commitment to the nursing process helps the critical care nurse interact with her patients and helps her stay in tune with the concept of the psychobiological unity of patients.

The critical care nurse is in a central position to understand the psychological and physiological changes that patients undergo in the critical care setting. Those changes occur frequently, and it is difficult for the nurses to escape involvement in them. As discussed in Chapter 1, nurse-patient interchanges are never neutral events. Being aware of the nursing process helps the nurse transform her technical skills into a blend of feeling states and sophisticated skills. In the process, every nurse-patient interchange is meaningful and never neutral.

The nursing process helps the nurse focus on human beings as whole persons. It helps the nurse to use her technical skills and apply her intellectual judgments and her feeling states in participating with patients in performing socially significant service for human beings.

The nursing process is a systematic way of determining a patient's problems, establishing the priority of those problems, making a plan to solve them, implementing that plan or assigning others to implement it, and evaluating and reassessing the extent to which the plan was effective in resolving the problems identified.

2

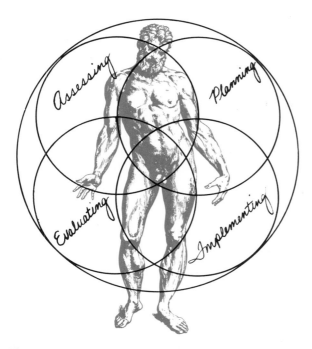

Figure 2-1
Components of the nursing process.

Component Phases

The nursing process is a *patient-centered* framework involving four component phases: (1) assessing, (2) planning, (3) implementing, and (4) evaluating (Fig. 2-1). The process is continuous. Once evaluation has taken place a new direction is established for the nurse and the patient. Problems are solved or they take on a new priority.

The nursing process is a specific adaptation of the organized problem-solving approach of other disciplines. Its fourfold approach (1) provides a systematic method of making an immediate assessment of the acutely ill patient on his admission to the hospital, (2) provides clues for a more comprehensive assessment to be done after the admission crisis, and (3) enables the nurse to outline the general aspects of the patient's problem areas and appropriate nursing actions for those areas.

When the critical care nurse uses a systematic approach, it implies that she has a framework for gathering a coherent body of knowledge and ideas. She carries out her design with thoroughness and reg-

ularity. The implication is that the nurse has the power to use her capabilities to comprehend and materialize all the information she has gathered from her patient, his family, his medical record, his physician, and her observations of the patient and to place the information into a practical framework.

Objective

The major objective of the nursing process is to identify factors that affect patient care. When a framework is used, the nurse is better able to organize information and provide the appropriate nursing care.

Purposes

When the nursing process is used, it fulfills the purposes of nursing, which are:

1. To maintain the patient's level of wellness
2. In illness or with changes in health, to provide the nursing care that will return the patient to as high a level of wellness as possible
3. When the patient's previous level of wellness cannot be achieved, to maximize his quality of life by improving his resources and making the appropriate referrals for community help

Health service agencies must encourage nurses to use the nursing process. Each nurse must become familiar with the nursing process and use it to provide the best possible care. The issue is not what forms are used in a particular facility. The written forms may differ, but the nursing process remains the best approach to good patient care.

The issue centers on the commitment of nurses to using a practical approach. At first, the nurses must be encouraged to use and record the nursing process. Soon success will provide the ongoing motivation.

The culmination of the work of nursing leaders in the midsixties was a definite concept of the nursing process [2–6]. Since 1975 significant advances have been made that contribute to the nursing process as a whole. The research includes work on nursing history, nursing diagnosis, nursing orders, and nursing care plans [7].

Nursing Diagnosis

Before the phases of the nursing process are discussed, the terms nursing diagnosis and nursing orders must be defined and discussed. For years the use of the term nursing diagnosis was forbidden. But with advances in nursing and medicine, it became obvious that the medical diagnosis and the nursing diagnosis are separate entities. For example, the medical diagnosis of the patient who has suffered a myocardial infarction may include arteriosclerosis, papillary muscle rupture, and angina. The nursing diagnosis may include chest pain, anxiety about hospitalization, and dyspnea. A nursing diagnosis is essential for the patient's welfare; it provides the basis for the nursing orders [1].

Nursing Orders

A nursing order is a written directive for a nursing action. It lists (1) what action is to be performed (a detailed description may be necessary), (2) who performs the action, and (3) when the action is to occur.

Nursing orders must be discussed with the nursing staff. Nursing orders (also called nursing treatments, nursing prescriptions, nursing therapies, nursing care plans) must be written and discussed with everyone involved in the patient's care, and they must be revised as necessary, according to the nursing diagnosis.

Therapeutic Plan—Medical and Nursing Diagnoses

The therapeutic plan for the patient comprises the medical diagnosis and the nursing diagnosis, as well as the medical orders and the nursing orders. The collaborative efforts of the physician and the nurse are complementary. The patient is the beneficiary. When the nurse realizes her responsibility for making a nursing diagnosis and writing nursing orders, exciting things occur. Patient care improves, and the nurse begins to use a systematic approach to her decisions and actions. The nurse must be aware of her responsibility for making a nursing diagnosis and writing nursing orders. During the entire course of patient care, the nurse must realize that her responsibility is not for making a medical diagnosis; her knowledge and energy must be directed toward the quality of nursing actions needed to resolve the patient's problems during the acute, intermediate, and convalescent phases of his illness.

The Steps in the Nursing Process

Several underlying factors determine the direction of the nursing process. The individuality of both the patient and the nurse are most important. Both those human beings bring their lifetime expectations and experiences together. The interpersonal relationship begins to form at the first contact and it continues thereafter. The patient has the right to expect something from each interview with the nurse. The nurse should make the patient feel that he is being understood. To achieve a relationship of mutual trust and respect, the nurse must communicate to the patient her sincere interest in him.

A second factor that affects the assessment of the patient's needs is the individual nurse's concept of herself and her role. The nurse must be alert to her own interests and concerns. Such a personal insight helps the nurse make a more complete assessment of her decisions and actions. It allows her to look objectively at her abilities and limitations, as well as at what areas she needs to know more about. By being aware of her self-concept, the nurse is in a better position to deal with problems of the patient and the patient's family.

Patient assessment is also affected by a third factor—the definition of health. Each nurse is responsible for developing her own philosophy of health; she must become consciously aware of her own philosophy. The awareness must include why she helps patients. Some patients can be helped to achieve a high level of wellness, whereas others, because of their illnesses, cannot return to their previous levels. Such patients must be helped to function to their maximum capability. And patients who are mortally ill must be helped to die a peaceful death.

In acute illnesses, the nurse must not succumb to the habit of stereotyping the patient and her care for that patient. Each patient must be viewed as a complex human being who has many mind-body-spirit interactions. The patient's psychological, physiological, and social needs must be recognized during and after his illness. The nurse must be geared to anticipate the possible events in the clinical course of the patient's illness.

Phases of the Nursing Process

Assessing

Assessing begins as soon as the nurse meets the critically ill patient. The assessment phase begins with the nurse's taking the history, and it ends with the making of the nursing diagnosis. During the assessment phase, problems must be identified with the use of the data collected. Information about the patient should be collected quickly on his arrival on the unit, and the ordered medical therapy should be started immediately. Timing is often crucial. The nurse should have a systematic approach to history taking and interviewing, which are used to provide:

1. Baseline information that will support specific nursing actions and the subsequent evaluations.
2. Comprehensive data about the location, duration, and severity of the patient's problems and the rate at which those problems are developing.
3. Insight into the patient's ability to express himself as independent or dependent or shy or evasive.
4. Insight into the patient's perception of his situation and his ability to cope with stress.

If the nurse uses a systematic approach, her organization will provide a broader base for planning, implementing, and evaluating nursing care. Assessment as the first phase will make her more aware of rapid changes in physical findings and of the patient's symptoms. Also, the reporting of physical findings is valuable to nurses, because it indicates to them whether to alter, expand, or discontinue the current treatment plans and when and how to discuss the patient's status with the physician.

Within three to four minutes of the patient's arrival on the unit, a brief history should be taken and a gross, systematic examination should be performed. A more complete history should be taken and a more complete examination should be performed after the crisis is under control. The purpose of the initial assessment is to collect data about the seriousness of the patient's major concerns and condition and about what body systems are involved so that the appropriate nursing actions can be taken. The nurse must interpret the data in terms of her knowledge and experience, and she must use the information to find out what are the immediate needs of the patient.

Communication is mandatory in the nursing process for data collection and for determining what the patient sees as his own needs. During the interview,

the nurse must keep in mind the focus and content level of the interview. If the patient starts to share his personal feelings while the factual information is being collected, time must be allowed for adequate expression by the patient. Often, if a patient is not allowed to express himself at the time he feels comfortable doing so, he may become anxious, and the interview could be blocked. The nurse should not probe. When the patient is ready to share more information, he will give clues.

Once the immediate crisis is resolved, a comprehensive assessment is in order. Assessment is a continuing process, never a completed one. A comprehensive assessment provides information that enables the nursing staff to provide completeness and continuity in their care for the patient. The assessment should include (1) information about the patient's personal data, present illness, past health, family health, personal and social history and (2) a systems review.

Weed [5] suggests that the following framework be used in determining what processes underlie the patient's symptoms.

Location:	Where is the symptom located?
Quality:	What is it like?
Quantity:	How intense is it?
Chronology:	When did the symptom begin and what has been its course?
Setting:	Under what circumstances does it occur?
Alleviating and aggravating factors:	What makes it better or worse?
Associated manifestations:	What other symptoms or other phenomena are associated with it?

Nurses gather information from the patient or from his family by observation and communication. Recorded observations are descriptions, not judgments, interpretations, or evaluations. Skill in observation can be increased only by systematic and regular practice. Observation involves seeing, hearing, touching, and smelling. The senses must be used to lay the foundation for patient assessment, and they should be used from the time of the patient's admission.

Physical assessment includes inspection, palpation, percussion, and auscultation. The nurse who delivers care to the critically ill adult must learn those four diagnostic skills. She must also understand the results of laboratory and other diagnostic tests, which reflect organ function and can determine what changes or alterations must be discussed with the physician and how the patient's plan of care must be changed. The nurse in the critical care setting is the person who is with the patient most. She must be able to distinguish normal from abnormal and to describe what is happening. Even if the nurse is not yet able to interpret laboratory values, she must know what needs to be reported to the physician for his interpretation. Nurses who are skilled are being given more and more responsibility.

Once the patient assessment has been done, the nurse must arrive at a nursing diagnosis based on the data collected. The assessment phase is over. A nursing diagnosis is always tentative since the condition of the acutely ill patient can change frequently. The nursing diagnosis should indicate the immediate needs or the high-priority needs of the patient. The nursing diagnosis is essential to professional nursing. It is needed to identify patient needs so that a plan of nursing care can be begun.

Planning

The first step in the planning phase of the nursing process is the nursing diagnosis. It is essential that the nurse involve the patient closely in the planning phase when appropriate. If the patient is in a critical state—for example, if he has an obstructed airway—he has a high-priority problem, and the nurse must intervene and correct the problem. When the patient is able to communicate effectively, he should be involved in his care and in decisions about the priority of his problems.

The essential reasons for the planning phase are that problems that have been diagnosed can be given a priority—high, medium, or low. The planning phase allows the nurse to decide what problems she must solve for the patient and what problems must be solved with the help of the patient, his family, and other health team members. Short-, intermediate-, and long-range goals are identified during the planning phase. The nursing care plan and nursing orders are also developed during the planning phase.

Many problems are multifaceted, and solutions must be decided on by the nurse with the help of the patient. If the patient understands the reasons for actions, success is more probable.

During the assessment and planning phases, the nurse uses her intellectual, interpersonal, and technical skills. At all times she must be aware of the need for safe judgment, observation, critical thinking, and decision making. Interpersonal skills help establish lines of communication and a trusting relationship between the nurse and the patient.

A written nursing care plan and nursing orders are sources of information about the patient and about the nursing actions that are appropriate for solving his problems. A clearly stated nursing care plan provides all the nurses involved with the patient's care with a written list of the patient's problems. It allows all the nurses to know the high-, medium-, and low-priority problems, what the short- and long-range goals are, how problems can be resolved, and how the patient's needs can be met. When nurses fail to assess and plan before they act, the patient suffers because the nurses' time and effort have been wasted.

The planning phase of the nursing process ends when the problems have been identified and the nursing care plan and nursing orders have been written. Nurses who use the nursing process become skilled at quickly identifying problems, and their nursing actions are meaningful and directed toward problem solving and decision making. In some critical care problems, certain actions must be taken before the nursing care plan and the nursing orders can be written. As soon as those problems are stabilized or solved the nurse must put her plan in writing. The nurse should remember that in critical care settings, the patient's problems and his nursing care plan may constantly change because the situation is a dynamic one.

Implementing

The implementing phase begins as soon as the nursing care plan is drawn up. The nursing diagnosis and the medical diagnosis are dealt with in this part of the nursing process. Each nursing diagnosis has specific nursing actions. Nursing actions are also needed to carry out the physician's orders; the physician writes the orders, and the nurse is responsible for performing the appropriate nursing actions. But the nurse does not blindly carry out the physician's orders. It is the nurse's responsibility to use critical thinking in carrying out medical and nursing orders. In making decisions, the nurse must use sound judgment and her knowledge base before deciding what action is to occur, when it is to occur, and how it is to occur.

The nursing actions during the implementation phase involve the nurse's intellectual, interpersonal, and technical skills. Data must continually be collected during that phase, because with each nursing action the patient's problems, feelings, and health status change. If a nursing care plan is developed and the priority of the problems and goals is clearly established, the nurse's actions will be meaningful and purposeful. Many times, highly technical skills are required to solve problems in the critical care area. Often nurses must work together to perform tasks requiring highly technical skills. Not only must communication exist between the nurses involved, but also the patient must be the focus. He must be seen as a total human being and not as a diseased organ system. When nurses make the patient the focus of their activities, the quality of nursing is at its highest.

The implementation phase ends when the nursing actions are completed and recorded. Nurses must record carefully the information about the nursing actions. The information that is recorded should be related to the identified problems, the results of the nursing actions, and any other data that are gathered. When only relevant information is recorded, all members of the health team have a clearer picture of the patient's status.

Evaluating

The fourth phase of the nursing process is evaluation. The nurse must keep in mind that she and the patient are the agents of evaluation. Other members of the health care team, as well as the patient's family, may also be involved. The evaluation phase of the nursing process looks at immediate, intermediate, and long-range goals. Those goals should be evaluated in terms of behavioral expectations of the patient relative to the established goals.

The nursing care plan should be periodically evaluated and reevaluated because of the dynamic nature of man himself as well as the frequent changes that may occur during an acute illness. The establishment of new objectives, identification of new patient needs, or alterations in the current diagnosis or problems must be assessed. Evaluation cannot be done by intuition. An effective evaluation is based on a set of standards or criteria that set up an ideal that is to be achieved. Evaluation identifies any omissions in the previous phases of the nursing process, as well as what was effective in each phase.

During the evaluation process, the nurse must ask herself what were the expected patient behaviors and what behaviors actually occurred. The subjective and objective data that were collected must be evaluated. Factors preventing solutions to problems, as well as factors helping attain goals, must be evaluated. The nurse must look at her nursing diagnosis, nursing care plan, and nursing orders to decide whether they were realistic or unrealistic for the patient. Once the evaluation is done, a new direction for the nurse and patient is established. Problems are either solved or they take on a new priority that requires the formulation of new goals and actions and specific patient education.

During all phases of patient education, it is most important that some form of written record be kept and that communication between the patient, his family, and the health team staff is a learning process. The nurse must be able to make judgments about what patients need to know, what they are capable of learning, how they can best be taught, and what they have learned. The nurse who teaches patients must be aware of the extent of evidence about the teaching-learning process. Knowledge of human behavior is at best tentative, particularly in regard to the learning process and motivation.

The quality of patient care must also be evaluated in regard to outcome criteria. The objective is to examine and evaluate the sum total of nursing care delivered in a specific setting by a group of nurses. The nursing audit, a review of patient records by nurses, is a means of improving and attaining quality care. It provides a systematic method of evaluating patient care and determining what can be done to improve patient care.

Nursing Research

It is not enough just to evaluate the effectiveness of the nursing care. New nursing approaches must be tried to improve existing practice. A continuous and thorough scrutiny of current nursing practice must be made as part of evaluating the nursing process. Stringent guidelines for clinical investigation should be used to draw up recommendations for the improvement of patient care. Nurse practitioners realize the need for clinical research. Research must be done for the development and refinement of the nursing process.

Nursing Process: A Problem-Solving Approach

The nursing process is problem solving because it designs a course of action. That course of action is aimed at changing an existing situation into a more desirable one. Inherent in problem solving are choices, decisions about choices, and decisions about decisions. Daily the nurse is faced with simple-to-complex problems. The more complex the problem, the more difficult it is to find a solution. Occasionally, several approaches are possible, and one must be chosen. Even though, in a sense, trial and error are inherent in the situation, the approach must be based on assessment, not on intuition. The built-in phase of evaluation in the nursing process demonstrates progress toward a goal.

When a problem is recognized and solved, the perception as well as the value system of the decision maker should be considered. Values determine the degree and nature of the action to be taken and give significance and meaning to the problem. The nursing process may then be recognized as a continuing dynamic process.

Case Study

Mr. R. S., aged 45, had an acute anterior wall myocardial infarction on a Sunday morning. His physician and nurse had told him about his acute myocardial infarction and the expected nursing and medical management in the coronary care unit over several days. All day Tuesday Mr. S. refused to eat or to move for fear of extending the infarction. By Tuesday evening, he was extremely depressed about his situation, and he cried often. When the nurse entered his room, Mr. S. tried to stop crying, but he became even more distressed and he cried harder.

The nursing process was utilized to determine the nurse's perception of the patient's behavior. The data gathered and the assessment quickly led to a nursing diagnosis of acute depression and anxiety caused by the myocardial infarction. The nurse's goals were to share with Mr. S. her perception of his state, to determine the validity of her perceptions, and to explore with Mr. S. what his experience meant to him. The nurse began the conversation by saying, "I know you are concerned about having had a heart attack." The patient replied, "I'm so young to have a heart attack. My brother had a heart attack last year, and he still is not over his heart attack. I don't want to be as helpless as he is."

Mr. S.'s responses gave the nurse validation for her nursing diagnosis, and she found out the reason for Mr. S.'s concern. He felt he was too young to have a heart attack, and he also had seen his brother in a similar state. The nurse communicated to Mr. S. her concern and interest in him as a human being. By permitting Mr. S. to express himself, the nurse communicated to him her availability and willingness to help. Appropriately phrased questions and silence and pauses during the conversation allowed a feeling of trust and open communication.

After the initial data were collected and during the initial conversation, the nurse decided on an action and made an assessment about Mr. S.'s most immediate need—help in coping with his depression and in decreasing his stress level so that cardiac rehabilitation could be effective.

The short range goals were to establish trust so that Mr. S. would feel capable of getting out of bed without making his condition worse and to explain the cardiac rehabilitation process to Mr. S.

During Mr. S.'s cardiac rehabilitation program and throughout his time in the unit and telemetry, the nursing staff encouraged him and continuously evaluated his progress. They continued to listen for any cues that might suggest regression in his progress or mental state. Prior to his discharge, Mr. S. again became severely depressed and wondered if he would be like his brother. In patient grand rounds, it was decided that Mr. S. would benefit from a psychological consultation. The cardiac rehabilitation continued and the nursing staff continued to evaluate Mr. S.'s activity and mental status. After 15 days of hospitalization, Mr. S. was discharged. He felt confident of his ability to recover from the myocardial infarction.

Analysis of Case Study

The nurse cannot overemphasize the importance of an accurate assessment. She must validate her observations with the patient and other medical team members. The nurse must openly communicate with the patient to confirm the assessment. Once the problem or problems are identified, a plan of care is developed from the data gathered. The plan of care will help the patient cope with the identified problems. When goals are established by the cooperative efforts of the nurse and the patient, the evaluation phase of the nursing process follows in a systematic manner.

Commitment

The successful nurse is the committed nurse. She must continue to develop her personal qualities, knowledge, skills and to have a systematic approach to problem solving. She must take into consideration at all times the many socially significant factors involved that are related to the problems she encounters. She must use her skills in her interactions with the patient at every stage of his illness. She must establish her own levels and guidelines for personal and professional growth.

References

1. Gebbie, K. M., and Lavin, M. A. *Classification of Nursing Diagnosis.* St. Louis: Mosby, 1975.
2. King, I. A conceptual frame of reference for nursing. *Nurs. Res.* 17:27, 1968.
3. Knowles, L. N. Decision Making in Nursing—a Necessity for Doing. In *ANA Clinical Sessions, 1966.* New York: Appleton-Century-Crofts, 1967. P. 248.
4. Orlando, I. J. *The Dynamic Nurse-Patient Relationship.* New York: Putnam, 1961.
5. Weed, L. L. *Medical Records, Medical Education and Patient Education: The Problem-Oriented Medical Record as a Basic Tool.* Cleveland: Case Western Reserve University Press, 1969.
6. Western Interstate Commission on Higher Education. *Defining Clinical Content, Graduate Nursing Programs, Medical and Surgical Nursing.* Boulder, Colo., 1967. P. 6.
7. Yura, H., and Walsh, M. *The Nursing Process* (3rd ed.). New York: Appleton-Century-Crofts, 1978.

Primary Care Nursing

Cathie E. Guzzetta

3

The Need for Primary Care Nursing

The concept of primary care has been in the developmental stages for many years. By definition primary care begins at the patient's point of entry into the health care system. Primary care was traditionally delivered by the family physician in his office or in the patient's home. Nurses, too, accepted the practice of primary care over five decades ago when they assumed the responsibility for patient care on a 24-hour basis in the home. Today, primary care is practiced in many settings outside the hospital. It can be found in outpatient departments, community health agencies, independent nurse practitioners' offices, and schools. Nurses are assuming major responsibilities for providing primary care in those settings [1]. A report from the Department of Health, Education, and Welfare committee that studied extended roles for nurses predicted that in the future nurses would take more responsibility for delivering primary health and nursing care, coordinating preventive services, initiating and participating in diagnostic screening, and referring to other professionals patients who require differential medical diagnosis and therapies [17].

The definition of primary care has recently been expanded to include a new organizational approach to nursing practice in the hospital or acute care setting. That approach is termed primary care nursing (primary nursing), and it includes primary nursing responsibility for the patient during all stages of his hospitalization. As our knowledge of the patient becomes more sophisticated, the role of the nurse becomes a more responsible one. In an attempt to deal with the responsibility, primary care nursing has become popular and gained acceptance. The acceptance has essentially come from a basic need to resolve some of the problems that have arisen from the traditional approaches to patient care, such as functional nursing and team nursing [11].

Functional nursing is viewed as an organizational pattern for the delivery of nursing care in which the delivery of care is determined by the technical aspects of the job to be done. In functional nursing, one nurse gives treatments, one nurse dispenses medications, another nurse changes beds, another nurse gives baths, and another nurse may pass out the meal trays. The delivery of functional nursing care requires that each nurse attend to her task with little time to focus on continuity of care for the individual patient. The system reduces the patient's humanism to a checklist of mechanical tasks that are done for the sake and efficiency of meeting the patient's physiological and technical needs.

The concept of team nursing was developed in an attempt to solve some of the problems of functional nursing. In team nursing, one nurse, or team leader, is responsible for supervising and coordinating care while the rest of the team performs assigned duties that are patient centered. Unfortunately, there are many problems associated with team nursing, and many of them are related to the concept of the team leader, who, in many cases, is regarded as "super nurse." She is expected to (1) be an expert clinician, (2) be knowledgeable about the patient's bio-psychosocial and medical histories and clinical status, (3) supervise the delivery of care given by all levels of nursing personnel, (4) know the principles of management, counseling, and administration, and (5) coordinate the services provided by the support departments. It is not surprising that problems arise from that approach; the responsibilities and demands placed on the team leader, the nurse who plays the essential role in the delivery of team nursing, are far too great for any one person. Also, although team nursing is said to be the method used for the delivery and coordination of care in many of our hospitals today, in reality, functional nursing is used with a team leader whose job it is to coordinate tasks and personnel. The concept of team nursing further implies that a group

of nurses share the responsibility for assessing, planning, implementing, and evaluating care for the individual patient. As a result, no one nurse is totally responsible or accountable for the care given to the patient. When a patient is the shared responsibility of a group of people, he is, in fact, no one's responsibility. For those and other reasons, team nursing has added to the fragmentation of care and has proved itself ineffective in achieving its desired level of patient-centered care.

In acute care settings, nursing has also begun to take on the "extended role," being responsible for the patient's 24-hour care and decision making. Too often, however, expanding the nurse's role simply means that the good "bedside nurses" are promoted to higher positions that take them away from the patient. Also, the health team itself has expanded within the hospital, and it now includes the physician, professional nurse, licensed vocational nurse, nursing assistant, respiratory therapist, occupational and recreational therapists, physical therapist, dietitian, social worker, chaplain, psychologist or psychiatrist, laboratory and x-ray technicians, and pharmacist. Patients, particularly in the critical care areas, are likely to come in contact with many members of the health team, thus adding to the fragmentation and confusion.

One must also consider that the current biomedical model of practice characteristically divides the patient (1) into physiological parts based on specialty areas (e.g., cardiology, obstetrics and gynecology, and neurology), (2) according to his age or developmental level, and (3) according to the type of treatment or the phase of care he requires (e.g., acute, chronic, or preventive) [11]. Health care agencies have tended to follow those divisions. Nursing education, nursing care, and nursing literature also conform to the model. The divisions arose from a need to advance scientific knowledge and to provide efficient and expert patient care. The divisions also succeeded in fragmenting the patient by developing an organizational pattern that promoted the duality of the model. The practice of nursing that views the patient in terms of his body-mind-spirit relatedness is not consistent with or supported by the biomedical model; it is also rarely visible. Such a system must be able to respond to the unity of the individual regardless of his diagnosis, physiological problem, plan of care, age, developmental level, or required phase of care. The concept of primary care nursing offers such an approach, and it appears to have the potential to help nursing face the challenge of redefining its role within the health team.

Concept of Primary Care Nursing

Primary care nursing may be defined as the nursing care provided to the patient by one member of the nursing staff who plans for the patient's total care from his hospital admission to his discharge. Primary care results from the nurse's collaboration with the primary physician and from her planning and coordination with people from other disciplines [9, 11, 16]. The primary care nurse is responsible and accountable for the nursing care delivered to her case load of patients. She is responsible for (1) assessing and identifying the patient's problems, (2) making nursing diagnoses, (3) defining, planning, and implementing the patient's care, (4) planning for the patient's educational and discharge needs, (5) coordinating the care with people from other disciplines, and (6) evaluating the effectiveness of the care.

It is obvious, however, that it is impossible for the primary care nurse to give physical care seven days a week, 24 hours a day. As a result, another type of nurse has also emerged, the associate nurse. The associate nurse is a staff nurse who is assigned to a primary care patient to provide total care when the primary care nurse is absent. Associate nurses discuss their ideas about patient care with the primary care nurse. They do not, however, make major changes in the patient's plan of care unless such action is warranted by a sudden change in the patient's condition or situation.

Purpose of Primary Care Nursing

The purpose of primary care nursing is to improve the quality of patient care and nursing practice. It establishes a care system that makes the patient the focus of the collective efforts of all the health team members. It transcends the duality of the current biomedical model because it promotes and supports concepts of body-mind-spirit relatedness. It includes prescriptions for the organization of nursing actions that are generated from experience and that can be systematically evaluated.

Primary care nursing has the potential to bridge the gap between education and practice. For example, even while they are students, nurses are assigned a specific case load of patients. As students, they are both responsible and accountable for total patient care. They learn to interact with a patient's family and with the staff members, physicians, and members of other departments in coordinating patient care. Primary care nursing is an extension of that process. It provides an approach to nursing practice the way "it ought to be." It incorporates the components of assessment, accountability, leadership, and management [12]. It is a flexible, creative, and innovative process that allows, even encourages, the nurse to achieve the highest professional level of practice.

Specifically, the objectives of primary care nursing are as follows:

1. To provide for the selection of primary patients, based on the abilities and interests of the nurse and on the needs of the patient and his family
2. To plan for comprehensive care through identification of the patient's physical needs, lifestyle, attitudes, feelings, and educational and discharge needs
3. To initiate and design a 24-hour plan of patient care
4. To give individualized and total patient care
5. To promote a multidisciplinary approach to the assessment, diagnosis, plan, implementation, and evaluation of patient care
6. To promote patient-centered nursing assignments
7. To promote and maintain better communication between and collaboration of health team members

Planning and Implementing Primary Care Nursing

The success of primary care nursing is greatly affected by careful, collaborative planning. The key organizational members must participate and support the process. The administrators must become thoroughly knowledgeable about the concept, understand the need for change, and be committed to the approach. Likewise, physicians must understand the concept, and they should be included in the planning and implementation phases. The support of the nursing director and the nursing service staff is essential. They must accept the responsibility for improving the quality of patient care and nursing practice. They must support and assist in the planning, educational, implementation, guidance, and evaluation phases of the primary care nursing model. Ideally, nursing personnel on the experimental unit should recognize the need for change. They must be included in the planning phase and guided in the development of the objectives, changes, and performance criteria.

Before the implementation of primary care nursing, the nursing staff, physicians, and members of the various departments should receive information and in-service education about the change. Nurses on the experimental unit should attend classes on the concepts of primary nursing, interviewing techniques, history taking, physical examination, problem identification, nursing diagnosis, 24-hour primary care plans, evaluation of care and outcome criteria, communication and teaching skills, discharge planning, and community referrals. They must understand how their role will change, what is expected of them, and how they will be evaluated.

The implementation of primary care nursing should be well defined. That goal may be accomplished by having a few staff members work as role models before the program is entirely implemented; or the program may be instituted by setting an appropriate date that marks the changeover to primary care nursing. The planning and implementation phases of the primary care model have been described in detail by Marram, Elpern, and others [2–4, 7, 11, 14].

The Primary Care Nurse in Assessment

Patient assignments are usually made by the head nurse based on the needs of the patient and the interests and abilities of the nurse [14]. Nurses, physicians, and other health team members are encouraged to specifically ask the patient's primary care nurse any questions they may have about problems and collaboration in patient care. The primary care nurse can be readily identified by the use of an assignment sheet that lists the names of each patient and his primary (and associate) care nurse. Also, the names of the primary care nurse and the associate nurse and their work schedules should be written on a label attached to the front of the patient's chart so that physicians and other hospital personnel can easily locate the information.

The primary care nurse admits the patient to the floor or critical care area. An explanation of primary care nursing is given to the patient and his family. The nurse explains her role as a primary care nurse and tells the patient about the associate nurse. The primary care nurse's initial responsibilities begin at the patient's admission interview, history taking, and physical examination. Basing her actions on the information gathered, the nurse assesses and lists the patient's problems in terms of nursing diagnoses. (Those topics are discussed more thoroughly in Chaps. 2, 4, 8, and 13.)

The Primary Care Nurse As Care Planner

The patient's care plan is one of the basic tools used in communicating with others about the patient's problems and plan of care [11]. The care plan is essential to the success of primary care nursing. All members of the health team should be told of its existence, location, and purpose.

The primary care nurse fills in the plan of care with pertinent information about the patient's past, present, and family histories, the patient's profile, the nursing diagnoses, and the nursing intervention. The plan should include criteria for measuring the effectiveness of predicted outcomes of care. As the specific outcomes are achieved, the primary care nurse updates the plan by summarizing what has been done and by checking off (initialing) or erasing the plan of action. It is essential that the care plan be kept current according to the patient's improved or otherwise changing status.

The associate nurse is responsible to the primary care nurse for contributing to and implementing the care plan. She should view the primary care nurse's judgments and decisions as being as authoritative as the physician's orders. In the absence of the primary care nurse, major changes in the care plan that are indicated by a sudden change in the patient's condition or needs are made by the associate nurse in keeping with good nursing and medical care [3]. Any changes are listed on the care plan and discussed with the primary care nurse on her return to duty.

The Primary Care Nurse As Collaborator and Coordinator

Implicit in the concept of primary care nursing are the factors of communication, collaboration, and coordination. The primary care nurse consults with the patient's primary physician and the other members of the health team concerned with the patient's care. She is responsible for planning, scheduling, and leading patient grand rounds. Patient grand rounds may be defined as planned, scheduled conferences attended by all members of the health team to discuss the patient's problems, assessment, solutions, and approaches to care. They are held as soon as possible after the patient's admission to establish and communicate to others the approaches to individualized care.

The primary care nurse is responsible for notifying all participants at least 24 hours in advance of the conference. The health team members who might be included are the physician, associate nurse, clinical supervisor, clinical nurse specialist, respiratory therapist, physical therapist, occupational or recreational therapist, dietitian, psychologist or psychiatrist, social worker, financial assistant, x-ray or laboratory technician, pharmacist, chaplain, public health nurse, and members of community agencies. When appropriate, the primary care nurse may wish to tell the patient about the conference to discover what problems or areas of concern the patient considers important, and she may wish to invite the patient and his family to part or all of the conference.

During the conference, the primary care nurse is responsible for presenting information about the patient's past and present histories, including the patient's physical and psychosocial problems. The patient's problems are identified, listed in the order of importance, and discussed with the health team members. The conference may also be used to comprehensively discuss the patient's medical diagnosis, surgical indications and techniques, the rationale for diagnostic tests, medical therapy, drugs, and treatments. Both the primary care nurse and the primary physician can share that part of the conference, giving the nursing and medical viewpoints. The length of the patient's hospitalization, prognosis, discharge planning, education, and possibilities for community referrals are also discussed during patient grand rounds. All members of the health team are encouraged to share their ideas with the group in planning specific approaches to patient care. The primary care nurse continues to guide and coordinate the conference while taking note of the suggestions offered by the group. She uses the suggestions to further develop the written plan of care.

Patient grand rounds provide a means for allowing the entire health team to view the patient and his problems as a whole. Because of the diversity in roles, each health team member is able to make a unique contribution to improve the quality of patient care. The collaborative effort results in greater communication, coordination, and respect among the members delivering patient care. Also, patient grand rounds are conducted in an environment that is conducive to the teaching-learning process and to the professional development of the health team members.

The Primary Care Nurse As Care Giver

The primary care nurse personally administers all aspects of care within her range of responsibility. She bathes her patients, administers medications, checks vital signs, gives treatments, makes rounds with the physicians, and teaches patients about procedures, medications, and hospital routines. She provides both technical and professional care. While giving care, the primary care nurse continues to gather information about changes in the patient's condition, and she evaluates his progress and his response to care.

The Primary Care Nurse As Teacher

I am strongly committed to the idea that patient education is an important responsibility for the primary care nurse. In this day of assignment-oriented nursing, one routinely sees that nurses are assigned the responsibility for a team of patients, for team medications, and for checking the crashcart, and are even assigned lunch and break times. But how often does one actually see patient education assigned as one of the responsibilities? Patient education and the teaching-learning process are discussed fully in Chapter 5. But it should be pointed out here that the concept of primary care nursing fosters consistent and comprehensive patient education [13]. The primary care nurse is responsible for developing, initiating, and evaluating the teaching plan. The primary care nurses may frequently become involved as a unit in developing formal patient education programs [5] and writing teaching booklets in collaboration with staff members, physicians, and members of the various departments. Such programs ensure the comprehensiveness of the content by clearly identifying the areas to be taught. The programs should incorporate a method of systematic documentation, evaluation, and follow-up to determine whether the program is meeting its goals and objectives.

Evaluation of Primary Care Nursing

Primary care nursing can be evaluated in a number of ways. The evaluation tools used to assess the primary care nurse should be developed from the objectives for primary care nursing. Performance criteria, which are generated from the objectives, reflect what nursing actions are to be taken to provide individualized patient care when the nurse is accountable for the patient's 24-hour plan of care and decision making. The criteria should be written in terms of behavioral objectives that lend themselves to observation and measurement of the nurse's performance.

Questionnaires can be given to staff members to identify their expectations for and satisfactions and problems with primary care nursing. Similar questionnaires may be given to primary care patients; the questionnaires can be completed during the patient's hospitalization or just before his discharge. Further evaluation tools can be designed to evaluate the nurse's ability to develop the written care plan and to conduct patient grand rounds. The nursing audit can serve as a means of evaluating primary care nursing. It assesses the quality of care and staff performance by developing standards of practice that are directly measurable in terms of the outcome criteria.

Some of the evaluation methods discussed have been used to assess primary care nursing. Many of the findings empirically document the superiority of primary care nursing to traditional approaches of nursing care. Primary care nurses have been found to have a higher rate of job satisfaction [10, 11, 13]. They report improved relationships with their patients [11, 16]. Primary care nurses tend to emphasize the importance of the emotional side of patient care and to place more importance on the quality of their performance than on getting the work done on time [11]. In support of those findings, Felton reported that the quality of nursing care as measured by the range of nursing competencies (evaluated by three outcome variables) on an experimental primary care unit was superior to that on controlled (traditional nursing) units [8]. Nurses from several experimental primary care units tended to feel more knowledgeable about their patients, and thus felt a greater sense of responsibility and accountability in their practice [10, 11, 15, 16]. As the primary care nurse's knowledge of the patient increased, her relationship with the physician seemed also to improve. Nurses and physicians tended to communicate more with each other, making patient rounds together, sharing staff conferences,

and planning more effective patient care together [6, 15]. The relationships among staff members were shown to change in regard to an increase in flexibility and cooperation in meeting patient needs. Respect and communication were also identified as changes observed in colleague relationships, as has a greater awareness of the strengths within the group for teaching and supporting one another [7, 11]. Primary care nursing was found to foster professional values. It appears to significantly change both the nurse's attitudes about work and her actual nursing performance and to promote professionalism in nursing [11, 16].

Patients also tend to view the concept of primary care nursing favorably. They think that their care is more personal and individual, and that they thus have more opportunities to express their problems and fears than they would on traditional nursing units [2, 4, 11]. Patients tend to be more satisfied with the nursing care on primary care units, to feel a greater sense of security about their care and to feel that it is more effective.

Continued evaluation of primary care nursing is mandatory. The research that has been done in that area has been encouraging. Additional prospective controlled studies are needed to:

1. Compare the quality of nursing care observed in primary care nursing with the quality of nursing care observed in team, functional, or "case method" nursing.
2. Evaluate the efficiency of primary care nursing from both the patient's and the nurse's viewpoints.
3. Evaluate the degree of satisfaction of primary care nursing from both the patient's and the nurse's viewpoints.
4. Evaluate the long-term transfer of function from conventional methods of care to primary care nursing. (The process involves analysis of the primary care unit after it has been tested and accepted and has become the permanent model of care.)
5. Investigate the long-term effects of primary care nursing to identify the benefits, disadvantages, and problems that could not be detected by evaluation of the short-term effects.

Additional research will undoubtedly help to identify a consistent body of knowledge related to primary care nursing and will provide essential information in regard to many of the questions, benefits, and problems not yet identified. Replication of those studies is strongly encouraged to ascertain the reliability and validity of the methods used in order to permit generalizations of the findings.

References

1. Aiken, L. H.   Primary care: The challenge for nursing. *Am. J. Nurs.* 77:1828, 1977.
2. Anderson, M.   Primary nursing in day-by-day practice. *Am. J. Nurs.* 76:802, 1976.
3. Bakke, K.   Primary nursing: Perception of a staff nurse. *Am. J. Nurs.* 74:1432, 1974.
4. Ciske, K. L.   Primary nursing: Evaluation. *Am. J. Nurs.* 74:1436, 1974.
5. Dahlen, A. L.   With primary nursing we have it all together. *Am. J. Nurs.* 78:426, 1978.
6. Donahue, M. W., Weiner, E., and Shirk, M.   Dreams and realities: A nurse, physician, and administrator view primary nursing. *Nurs. Clin. North Am.* 12:247, 1977.
7. Elpern, E. H.   Structural and organizational supports for primary nursing. *Nurs. Clin. North Am.* 12:205, 1977.
8. Felton, G.   Increasing the quality of nursing care by introducing the concept of primary nursing: A model project. *Nurs. Res.* 24:27, 1975.
9. Logsdon, A.   Why primary nursing? *Nurs. Clin. North Am.* 8:283, 1973.
10. Manthey, M.   Primary nursing is alive and well in the hospital. *Am. J. Nurs.* 73:83, 1973.
11. Marram, G. D., Schlegel, M. W., and Bevis, E. O.   *Primary Nursing: A Model for Individualized Care.* St. Louis: Mosby, 1974.
12. McGivern, D. O., Mezey, M. D., and Baer, E. D.   Teaching primary care in a baccalaureate program. *Am. J. Nurs.* 76:441, 1976.
13. Medaglia, M.   A coronary care unit implements primary nursing. *Can. Nurs.* 74:32, 1978.
14. Page, M.   Primary nursing: Perceptions of a head nurse. *Am. J. Nurs.* 74:1435, 1974.
15. Romero, M., and Lewis, G.   Patient and staff perception as a basis for change. *Nurs. Clin. North Am.* 12:197, 1977.
16. Spoth, J.   Primary nursing: The agony and the ecstasy. *Nurs. Clin. North Am.* 12:221, 1977.
17. U.S. Department of Health, Education, and Welfare.   Secretary's committee to study extended roles for nurses. Extending the scope of nursing practice. *Nurs. Outlook* 20:46, 1972.

The Problem Oriented System

Cornelia Vanderstaay Kenner

The problem oriented system (POS)—one method of achieving total patient care—is an orderly system of thinking based on an adequate collection of data that enables the interdisciplinary health team to move from understanding to intelligent actions [3]. In essence, the POS is a means of identifying the patient's problems and an organized analytical approach for solving those problems. It enables members of the health team from all disciplines to use the same logical system of patient care delivery and thus to work together in a unified approach toward a common goal. It enhances the competency of individual members of the team so that each one can learn as he cares for the patient. The quality of clinical judgment that can only be learned at the bedside and is the real result of our endeavors cannot help but be improved. The POS integrates both behavioral and cognitive learning approaches as the coordination of patient care is improved [3].

The nursing process and the POS are very similar. Both the nursing process and the POS are problem-solving approaches. Both are based on the systematic scientific method for collecting data, identifying problems, outlining plans, implementing those plans, and evaluating the outcomes. Thus their combined use provides the nurse with a framework in which she can analyze and revise both the process and content of the practice of nursing.

4

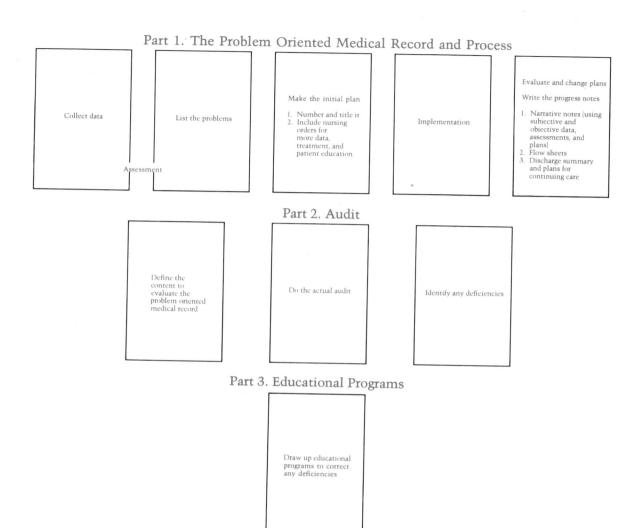

Part 1. The Problem Oriented Medical Record and Process

Collect data

List the problems

Make the initial plan
1. Number and title it
2. Include nursing orders for more data, treatment, and patient education

Implementation

Evaluate and change plans

Write the progress notes
1. Narrative notes (using subjective and objective data, assessments, and plans)
2. Flow sheets
3. Discharge summary and plans for continuing care

Assessment

Part 2. Audit

Define the content to evaluate the problem oriented medical record

Do the actual audit

Identify any deficiencies

Part 3. Educational Programs

Draw up educational programs to correct any deficiencies

Figure 4-1
The problem oriented system.

The three parts of the POS are (1) the problem oriented medical record (POMR), (2) the audit, and (3) the educational programs (Fig. 4-1). Each part is essential to the system. If one part is missing, the system is not complete.

The Problem Oriented Medical Record

The POMR is important because it documents the care the patient receives so that it can be evaluated and improved. With the POMR, corrections in care delivery can be made, and potential mistakes can be avoided. Discussion revolves more about the POMR than about any other part of the system since it is the written tool of the system and it is in daily use. The POMR is concise yet comprehensive, and it represents a logical approach to health care. It emphasizes problem solving and patient care management [4].

By the process of documentation, the ability of the health team to gather data, identify problems, plan patient care, implement the plan, and evaluate care delivery is revealed. Since all members of the health team help write up the POMR, the record becomes a vehicle for coordination.

The POMR has four major parts: (1) the data base, (2) the complete problem list, (3) the initial plan, and (4) the progress notes.

The Data Base

The first part of the nursing process, assessment, is the same as the first part of the POMR, collection of data. The data collected are written on the data base. The importance of the data base lies in the fact that the data base is defined; that is, it specifies precisely what data are to be obtained and it directs that the same data be gathered for every patient. Thus, the basic information necessary for planning and individualizing care is provided. Different types of data bases may be used; for example, one type may be used on the patient's admission to the critical care unit, another type may be used for a more detailed assessment of patients following trauma, and another type may be used for patients with cardiac disease.

What data are to be collected—and how—is determined by the circumstances in the particular critical care unit. For example, the nurse may take the health history while the physician does the physical examination and arranges for the laboratory work. Or, as in some coronary care units, the nurse may take the health history, do the physical examination, and arrange for the laboratory work on the patient's admission to the unit, with the physician verifying the information in the data base when he arrives.

The components of the data base (discussed also in Chaps. 8–12) are chief complaint, patient profile, history of present illness, past history, family history, review of systems, physical examination, and laboratory data.

The chief complaint is defined as the reason the patient is seeking health care. It often is placed on the chart in the patient's own words.

The patient profile is a short description of the patient's personal life and gives information about the patient as a person outside the medical setting. It helps the team to understand the patient better, so that care can be individualized. Three component parts form the basis of the profile: (1) background (occupational, educational, cultural, religious, and residence both past and present); (2) socioeconomic status (i.e., housing); and (3) habits and hobbies. Specific areas included are birthplace, marital status, education, religion, occupation, diet, stress, work habits, hobbies, personal habits, special interests, life-style, family and social relationships, basic temperament, impact of illness on the patient and family, and both his behavior during the assessment process and his ability to communicate and understand.

The history of the present illness is an in-depth description of the chief complaint as well as of the problem that has caused the patient to enter the health care setting. All signs and symptoms from the time of onset (including any that may no longer be present) should be documented. The examiner should ask for a detailed description of significant points, including chronology, quality, quantity, body location, aggravating or alleviating factors, and associated signs and symptoms.

The past history provides information about the past health status of the patient, and helps pinpoint factors that might influence the patient's response to treatment. Specific areas in the past history are pediatric and adult illnesses, allergies, hospitalizations, trauma, immunizations, transfusions, and habits.

The family history provides information about the age and health or manner of death of each member of the patient's family. In particular, hereditary predisposition to certain problems may be identified.

The review of systems provides information about the functioning of each body system. Any problems that initially may have escaped the patient's memory are identified with the rapid review.

The physical examination performed by the examiner provides information about how each part of the body functions (see Chaps. 8–12). The chief complaint and history of the present illness help identify for the examiner the focus of the physical examination. The extent of the initial physical examination depends on the patient's condition. Because of the extremely serious condition of any patient in the critical care unit, the physical examination there usually focuses on the respiratory, cardiac, and neurological systems. The particular body system affected by the patient's presenting problem is investigated thoroughly. The depth to which the other systems are examined is determined by a patient assessment. Later, following stabilization of the patient, a more thorough physical examination is conducted.

The laboratory data include studies pertinent to the patient's major problems and to the particular type of data base utilized. Usually, the complete blood count, baseline screening (SMA-12), urinalysis, ECG, and chest film are included.

The Problem List

The patient's problem list is drawn up from the analysis of the data base and subsequent investigation of findings. Drawing up the problem list requires disciplined thought. The facts must be interpreted if a meaningful problem list is to be synthesized. Problems that must be managed by the health team or that prevent attainment of a quality of life necessary to the patient are listed in a concise manner. The problems may be listed according to four categories: (1) pathophysiological (e.g., a physiological finding, a symptom, an abnormal laboratory finding, or a diagnosis, either nursing or medical), (2) social (e.g., the patient may have an alcoholic husband), (3) demographic, or increased risk factor (e.g., the patient may be a heavy smoker), or (4) psychological (e.g., the patient may be anxious about being hospitalized).

The problems are numbered and the list is placed at the front of the chart so that each member of the health team can immediately determine the patient's condition and progress. Thus fragmentation of care is avoided.

Each problem is stated at the best level of resolution or level of understanding that can be factually substantiated. If the diagnosis is not yet established, and the problem is best understood by a sign, a symptom, or combination of both, an arrow is put to the right of the particular problem to indicate that further data are needed. Investigation and management then follow. A specific diagnosis (e.g., anxiety about surgical procedure due to lack of information) is used only when the data are unequivocal. As new information is collected, the problem list is updated and refined. The problem may be called by the name of the specific diagnosis only when the parameters that define the condition are positive. Such a progression is extremely important since it eliminates making a false diagnosis or "jumping to conclusions." Additionally, it eliminates neglect of a problem that seems to be of little importance or that is poorly understood.

The problem list is a table of contents or an index to the patient's present illness and past history. Problems that are active are written on the left side of the problem list. They are considered active until they are resolved. Inactive problems are written on the right side of the problem list. When a problem is resolved, an arrow is drawn to the right side of the problem list under the list of inactive problems, and it is dated. If several problems turn out to be separate manifestations of the same condition, the first problem listed shows the diagnosis and the other problems are resolved in regard to the first problem. The number assigned to a particular problem cannot be used for another problem. If the data base has not been completed, that is the first problem listed in the problem list since an accurate assessment cannot be made with an incomplete data base. A temporary or self-limiting problem may be followed as such in the progress notes; however, if the problem still exists after 72 hours, it is transferred to the active problem list. Thus the completed problem list is an accurate, up-to-date summary of the patient's status.

Further classification of nursing diagnoses will help in planning, synthesizing, and completing the problem list. Once research has determined what the legitimate nursing diagnoses are, specific nursing interventions can be identified. The classification will center on areas unique to the practice of nursing that significantly affect overall patient care, such as sleep deprivation, confusion, and depersonalization. A nursing diagnosis is the focus for determining nursing plans and interventions, and describes the state of the patient. It does not describe patient needs or nursing interventions. Essentially, a nursing diagnosis is a judgment, and involves a synthesis of the data derived from the assessment. Nursing uses a holistic model that focuses on the body-mind-spirit of the person to define patient problems (or the patient's inability to function), while medicine tends to use the Descartes model that divides the body from the mind to define identifiable syndromes into disease entities. Although nursing has not yet systematically classified diagnoses, there is general agreement that the diagnosis should contain three parts: (1) the state of the patient or the health problem, (2) the cause or etiology of the problem, and (3) the signs and symptoms of the problem. As nurses gain skill, they will be increasingly able to identify the preexisting conditions of a problem and thus establish the relationship between the antecedents and the consequences. The critical care nurse will be much better able to exercise independent nursing action when she hears the diagnosis of altered state of consciousness due to sleeplessness caused by multiple environmental stimuli during the normal sleep cycle, than when she hears the diagnosis of uncooperative and combative.

Thoroughness in formulating the problem list is essential to the POS approach. Before planning is begun, the problems must be reviewed in relation to one another. The POS may have to be modified since the needs of the individual patient are always considered.

The precision with which plans for care are made and implemented is directly related to accuracy in defining problems.

The Initial Plan

The initial plan is the written framework of care for each patient. It is based on (1) the need for more data, (2) patient care management, and (3) patient education. The patient profile and problem list should be reviewed before the plan is made since the manner in which the problem interfaces with the entire problem list and the patient's life-style is important.

It may be necessary to collect more data to complete the data base, to determine a particular nursing diagnosis, and to prevent, monitor, or control any potential complications.

Patient care management comprises directives for the implementation and evaluation of patient care. Patient expected outcomes or patient care objectives are listed for each problem and implemented through the nursing orders. Under each objective are written the specific nursing orders to be used to attain the objective. In that way, everyone caring for the patient can easily determine what orders are associated with what problem and with what objective, thus enhancing both care delivery and staff education. A nursing order is a specific directive for nursing action. It tells (1) who performs the action, (2) what action is to be performed, and (3) when the action is to be performed (e.g., Staff Nurse: Assist patient with drinking high calorie protein supplement, 240 ml, at 2:30 P.M.). The implementation of the nursing order is known as the nursing intervention.

The plan for patient education is vital to the POS and, unfortunately, is often neglected in nursing practice. If the patient and his family understand what has and will happen to him and what they can do to help the situation, they are more likely to be active participants in care delivery (see Chap. 5).

The Progress Notes

The progress notes are continuing descriptions and analysis of the patient's condition and provide information concerning the stage of problem resolution. They are the most important part of the POMR. In a feedback mechanism, the problem list and the plan are evaluated and modified as needed. Initial inaccu-

rate problem solving can be understood, but subsequent follow-ups that do not identify the discrepancies and deficiencies and thus fail to rectify the situation cannot be understood. Only by careful monitoring, analysis, and recording of patient data can inaccuracies be identified and new plans formulated [4].

As new problems are identified, they are added to the problem list, dated, and numbered. There are three types of progress notes: narrative notes, flow sheets, and the discharge summary.

Example

Mr. M., a 66-year-old retired schoolteacher who has been transferred to the critical care unit following a urinary tract surgical procedure

Date: May 8	
Time: 8:00 P.M.	
Problem:	Hypothermia
Subjective data:	"I don't feel good, I'm cold."
Objective data:	Rectal temperature 96°F, pulse 116, respirations 26, blood pressure 94/66; weak, thready pulse, patient confused, extremities cold, abdomen distended, ST segment elevated on ECG
Assessment:	Clinical picture is indicative of low-flow state from a septic process. Patient is in high-risk group: he is over the age of 60, has had a surgical procedure involving instrumentation of the urinary system, and has signs of septic shock with hypovolemia
Plan:	Administer oxygen
	Notify physician
	Increase rate of intravenous infusion
	Monitor arterial blood gases, vital signs, and urinary output
	Institute protocol for hypothermia associated with low-flow state

Narratives notes are written for each problem according to a format that uses Subjective data, Objective data, Assessment, and Plan (SOAP). The subjective data are a description of symptoms gathered from what the patient says about his problem, care, feelings, and/or concerns. The objective data comprise factual information about phenomena observed (e.g., clinical signs or laboratory findings), the care given (e.g., elevation of the head of the bed or explanation of parenteral nutrition therapy), and the results of the care delivered. Any inconsistency between subjective data and objective data necessitates reexamination of the statement of the problem. Assessment is the

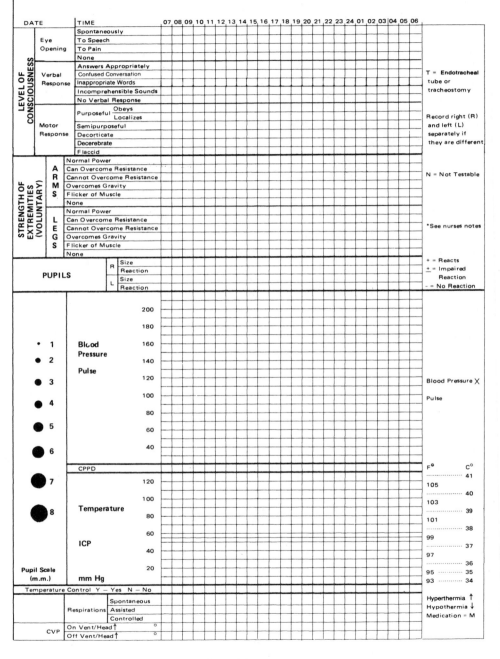

Figure 4-2
Sample flow sheet. (Courtesy Sarah Moody, R.N., Division of Neurosurgery, Department of Surgery, The University of Texas Health Science Center at Dallas.)

analysis and synthesis of the subjective and objective data in terms of what is happening to the patient on a particular day at a particular time in regard to a particular problem. Essentially, in the assessment, the nurse records the thought processes and interpretations that underlie her nursing interventions. Other nurses or other health team members may then share in her thinking. If others wish to make additional comments or disagree with her assessment, they place their assessment in the POMR, thus making the record a vehicle for communication. The plan notes any departures from the original plan, including additions, alterations, and deletions.

Flow sheets are instrumental in organizing and recording data needed repeatedly at different time periods to monitor the condition of the critically ill patient (Fig. 4-2). Usually the flow sheet remains at the patient's bedside so that the health team member may evaluate the data collected. Flow sheets contain the parameters representative of the patient's condition and are used to serially monitor the patient's condition in order to identify trends [1]. Because flow sheets are clear and efficient tools, most critical care units develop one or more types.

The discharge summary is usually not written when the patient is transferred from the critical care unit to the intermediate care unit but rather when he is discharged from the hospital. The discharge summary includes the information needed for the patient's continuing care. Each problem is summarized and discussed by number, title, and outcome. The salient aspects of resolved problems are summarized, and unresolved problems are thoroughly discussed. The patient care management that will be needed following discharge is outlined in the form of nursing orders.

Audit

The second part of the POS is the audit. Before an audit can be conducted, standards for care must be defined and validated. After the quality of care deemed acceptable has been defined, an audit is conducted to judge the quality of care delivery. There are two ways to judge the quality of nursing care: (1) direct regular observation by an expert nurse practitioner (however, such analysis is rarely feasible in the critical care unit), and (2) a systematic examination of the record to determine (a) whether information about the patient's course of illness, therapy, and response is readily available, and (b) to review the content and process of nursing care in accordance with the standards of nursing practice.

The audit may be general or specific [2]. In a general audit, the format of the POMR is reviewed. Sample questions include: Are all the data needed to complete the patient profile consistently collected? Is the family history consistently considered? In a specific audit, the relationship of problems and the quality of care delivered for patients with specific conditions (e.g., burns) are reviewed.

The quality of care can be determined from the POMR. Using the structure established for the POMR, the auditor can check the problem list, what was done for each problem, and the outcome. Adherence to the structure as well as quality of care can be audited. In reference to the nursing process, quality is the evaluative dimension of the elements and their interactions. Thus using the audit, the primary care nurse and other members of the health team can be evaluated for thoroughness, reliability, analytical sense, and efficiency.

Generally, the audit is done in three steps: (1) defining the quality of care, usually by identifying the components contained in the data base, the problem list, and the initial plan, (2) determining whether the individual factors are found in the record, and (3) identifying any deficiencies.

Educational Programs

The third component of the POS is educational programs to correct any deficiencies found during the audit. Educational programs must be based on an assessment of what the nurse knows. The audit of the POMR identifies what the nurse does not know and establishes a basis for orientation and other types of educational programs.

Summary

The POS is an excellent way to bring order and a rational approach to patient care. All members of the health team collaborate in order to optimize patient care. The POMR is central to the POS since it is a written record that documents what has happened to the patient and the problem solving approach used by the health team. The audit identifies the discrepancies in and deficiencies of the POMR. Educational programs are set up to rectify the problems. All three components of the POS—the POMR, the audit, and the educational programs—are essential to it. The POS will provide nursing with a structural framework by which the nursing process and nursing knowledge can be observed, analyzed, modified, and improved in a sound, systematic, and scientific manner.

References

1. Bjorn, C., and Cross, D. *The Problem-Oriented Private Practice of Medicine.* Chicago: Modern Hospital Press, 1970.
2. Hurst, J., and Walker, H. *The Problem-Oriented System.* New York: Medcom Press, 1972.
3. Weed, L. *Medical Records, Medical Education, and Patient Care.* Chicago: Year Book, 1971.
4. Weed, L. L. Medical records that guide and teach: Parts 1, 2. *N. Engl. J. Med.* 278:593, 652, 1968.

Bibliography

Abrams, K. S. Problem-oriented recordings of psychosocial problems. *Arch. Phys. Med. Rehabil.* 54:316, 1973.

Bloom, T. Problem-oriented charting. *Am. J. Nurs.* 71:2144, 1971.

Bryan, T., and Summers, R. How to start using the problem oriented medical record. *J. Iowa Med. Soc.* 60:183, 1972.

Cross, D. Educational needs as determined by the problem-oriented medical record. *J. Maine Med. Assoc.* 61:49, 1970.

Editorial. Ten reasons why Lawrence Weed is right. *N. Engl. J. Med.* 284:51, 1971.

Gardner, B. The problem-oriented record in critical care medicine. *Chest* 62:63, 1972.

Goldfinger, E. The problem-oriented record: A critique from a believer. *N. Engl. J. Med.* 288:606, 1973.

Gonnella, J. S. Evaluation of patient care. *J. Am. Med. Assoc.* 214:2040, 1970.

Hurst, J. How to implement the Weed system. *Arch. Intern. Med.* 128:456, 1971.

Hurst, J. The art and science of presenting a patient's problems. *Arch. Intern. Med.* 128:463, 1971.

Hurst, J. How to create a continuous learning system. *Am. J. Cardiol.* 29:889, 1972.

Phaneuf, M. A nursing audit method. *Nurs. Outlook* 12:42, 1968.

Phaneuf, M. Analysis of a nursing audit. *Nurs. Outlook* 16:57, 1978.

Schell, L., and Campbell, T. POMR—not just another way to chart. *Nurs. Outlook* 20:510, 1972.

Weed, L. L. New approach to medical teaching. *Med. Times* 94:1030, 1966.

Woody, M., and Mallison, M. The problem-oriented system for patient-centered care. *Am. J. Nurs.* 73:1168, 1973.

Vaughan-Wrobel, B., and Henderson, B. *The Problem-Oriented System in Nursing: A Workbook.* St. Louis: Mosby, 1976.

Promoting the Patient's Teaching-Learning Process

Donald A. Bille

Nurses in the critical care setting are responsible for helping their patients understand the information needed to reorder their lives. Few people entering a modern medical facility leave the facility without changes in life-style imposed by disease or injury. The changes may range from depending on medication to adapting to major structural changes in the body.

Objective

The overall objective of this chapter is to provide information that will help the critical care nurse draw up a teaching care plan for the critically ill patient.

Achieving the Objective

To achieve the objective, the nurse should be able to:

1. List four assumptions of adult education and explain their implications for patient teaching.
2. State her philosophy of patient teaching.
3. Explain the phases of the teaching-learning process and the importance of each phase.
4. Describe factors that hinder a nurse's teaching.
5. Describe factors that hinder the patient's ability to learn.

5

How to Proceed

To develop an approach to the patient's teaching-learning process, the nurse should first read the study questions at the end of the chapter. After reading the chapter, the nurse should try to answer the questions. After that, the nurse can best learn patient teaching activities by practicing them—by actually providing learning experiences for her patients.

Assumptions of Adult Education

In the past few years, a distinctive theory about how adults learn has begun to evolve. Educators have known for a long time that they cannot teach adults in the same way they teach children. Adults are nearly always voluntary participants in a learning experience, and they simply do not continue to participate in learning experiences that do not satisfy them. Even though the adult in a "captive audience" (such as a hospitalized patient) may be *physically* present in a learning environment, he will most likely tune out any instruction that he does not wish to participate in. Instruction given while the patient is tuned out will be a waste of time for the nurse and for the patient.

The theory of education that deals with the adult learner is known as "andragogy," which is based on the Greek stem *andr-*, meaning "man." Andragogy is the art and science of helping adults learn. Adult educators have identified at least four ways in which adult learners differ from child learners [5]: (1) the adult's self-concept has changed from that of a dependent person to that of a person who is capable of self-direction, (2) the adult has a large resource for learning based on his life experiences, (3) the adult's motivation to learn is more frequently oriented to problem solving than to learning for the sake of learning, and (4) the adult has changed his time perspective in that he desires immediate applicability of knowledge gained. In the following paragraphs, each of those differences in the adult learner is described briefly, and the implications for the nurse who is doing patient teaching are pointed out.

Self-Concept

The adult's self-concept may rule out certain teaching approaches, especially when a disease or injury is an added burden for the adult to deal with. Children have a self-concept of dependency, and they learn to act out the normal role of a child, that of a learner. The adult sees himself as a producer or doer—the breadwinner. He learns his adult role through conscious choice. He does not, however, choose to become sick, and therefore he does not choose the sick role; nor has he had any training in how to act in the sick role.

The adult's self-concept may also be based on early learning experiences (when he was a child) during which he was treated with less than optimum respect. He tends to avoid, resist, and resent any experiences in which he is again treated like a child—being told what to do, when to do it, and (even worse) judged or evaluated in regard to how well he did what he was told to do. Adult learners must be made to feel that they are treated with respect, and nurses must let the patients make their own decisions about their own lives.

Experience

Every adult has had a variety of experiences—good and bad—as a part of growing up. The adult becomes what he has done, and he therefore has a great investment in his accomplishments. Situations in which he does not get to use his experiences cause him to feel rejected. For the most part, serious illness is not a part of becoming an adult. Thus coping with illness is not something that the adult can readily call up from past experiences. In addition, adults have acquired a number of fixed habits, and therefore they may be less open minded about changing. Adults need a chance to plan and to practice how they are going to apply their learning to their activities of daily living.

Readiness to Learn

The adult passes through various phases of growth as he responds to the developmental tasks before him. The socially acceptable roles for adults include those of worker, mate, parent, homemaker, son or daughter of aging parents, citizen, friend, organization member, religious affiliate, and user of leisure time [4]. The sick role is not one of the "normal" developmental roles, and the adult who is ill needs time to adapt. The adult is ready to learn (the teachable moment occurs) only when he is made to recognize that a need to learn exists.

Orientation to Learning

Children tend to view education with a *subject-centered* frame of mind. That is, education is a process during which the child accumulates a reservoir of knowledge (and skills) that might be used in later life. The child is willing to postpone drawing on that reservoir until his later years.

Adults, on the other hand, need to be able to apply learned material immediately. They participate in the learning process more willingly when the learning activity responds to needs arising from pressures in their current life situation. Education to the adult patient, then, is a process of improving his ability to deal with life problems he is facing due to illness. He has a *problem-centered* frame of mind, and one that is oriented to the present.

Nursing Orders

The following nursing orders for patient teaching are derived from the assumptions of adult education:

1. Treat the adult learner with respect.
2. Allow the patient to make his own decisions about his life.
3. Allow the patient a chance to plan and to practice how he is going to apply his learning to his activities of daily living.
4. Help the patient to recognize that a need to learn exists.
5. Plan teaching sessions that solve *problems* in the patient's *current* life situation.

Philosophy of Patient Teaching

The overall objective of teaching done by professional nurses is to make changes in health-relevant behavior; ultimately it aims at adjustment to life-altering change with compliance to the medical regimen. Increasingly, nurse practitioners have come to realize that a philosophy for patient teaching cannot be separated from the practice of nursing. A recent survey, conducted by this author, indicated that because of the human element, nearly every nurse's philosophy,

or set of beliefs about how and why they teach patients, is different. Also, personal philosophy is not static; it changes as the nurse acquires new insights and skills.

Some of the more common beliefs about patient education include the following:

1. Patient education is an integral part of comprehensive patient care.
2. The patient, as a health care consumer, has a right to know what is being done to, for, and about him and his illness.
3. The patient has a need to have health care information in order to prevent disease and to improve and maintain his health.
4. Optimal health is the right of everyone. Inherent in that right is the person's responsibility to attain and/or maintain optimal health through his own actions.
5. Health care knowledge may be instrumental in decreasing the length of the patient's hospitalization and/or the number of times he has been rehospitalized for the same condition.

Nursing Orders

The following nursing orders for patient teaching are derived from the assumptions of patient teaching:

1. Examine your own feelings about patient teaching.
2. Decide whose responsibility it is to present information.
3. Decide whose responsibility it is to use the information presented.
4. Decide whose needs are being met by the patient teaching.

The Teaching-Learning Process

Introduction

The activities that comprise the relationship between the nurse and the patient who are engaged in teaching and/or learning are ongoing, not static; continuous, not intermittent; and interrelated, not compartmentalized. The teaching-learning process consists of five steps (assessment, planning, implementation, evaluation, and documentation). Even though in this chapter each step of the process is discussed individually, each of the steps may occur simultaneously and continuously.

Assessment

From the moment the patient is admitted to the hospital until he is discharged, different forms of assessment occur. During assessment for educational purposes, information relating to the patient's teaching program is gathered. This assessment is done for at least six reasons:

1. To elicit the patient's own perceived needs for learning. It is most important to begin at the point where the patient perceives his own needs before continuing with nurse-determined objectives for learning.
2. To determine the patient's present level of knowledge. The information the patient already has about his disease determines where the teaching begins.
3. To identify any special concerns (e.g., ethnic, cultural, religious, or financial ones). For instance, the male patient who is taking an anticoagulant drug would be safer if when he was discharged he shaved with an electric razor. It would do little good to tell that to a patient who cannot afford to buy an electric razor and who has no other way of getting one.
4. To identify any misconceptions and misinformation the patient has about his disease or condition. Many patients need to be "untaught" incorrect information before they are given the correct information.
5. To help identify concerns, limitations, and needs for learning in the patient's environment or in his family or significant others. Any patient teaching program that does not pay attention to the home environment (including relatives) may not be successful.
6. To help establish the success of the teaching-learning process by establishing a baseline of data for comparison. The nurse who is teaching patients cannot "prove" that the patient has learned from the *present* teaching-learning interactions unless she can show how much growth occurred during the present hospitalization.

Keeping those reasons in mind, the nurse does the assessment, which consists of interviewing the patient and obtaining answers to open-ended questions;

for example, "Have you ever had a heart condition?" (If the patient answers yes, the nurse should get him to explain further.) "What brings you to the hospital?" "Has your doctor told you what is wrong with you?" (Checking the answer with the patient's physician may uncover denial and/or lack of understanding of what the physician told the patient.) "What will your problems be because of your renal disease?" "What does your family think of your hospitalization? Renal disease? Colostomy?" At first, the questions should be general and not too personal. As the nurse builds rapport with the patient during the interview, the questions can be more specific and more personal (see Chap. 8).

By listening carefully and interpreting the patient's words, the nurse can clarify what the patient is saying. When the nurse is not sure what the patient means or does not understand what he said, she should seek clarification by saying something like, "I'm not sure I heard you." "I don't think I understand what you just said." Or, "Did you mean to say . . . ?" Seeking clarification not only helps the nurse understand puzzling information, but it also shows the patient that the nurse is paying attention to what he is saying.

Planning

Once the nurses who are responsible for the teaching-learning process have begun to get information from the patient, they can begin the next stage of the process, that of setting down (in writing) the teaching care plan. Realistically, the job is somewhat time consuming, especially until the nurse gains some practice in writing a teaching care plan. When it is written down, however, the teaching care plan can save time and promote an efficient teaching-learning experience in four ways. First, the teaching plan, when shared with the patient, outlines what both parties agreed was material to be learned (it organizes the learner's thinking). Second, it is a means of organizing the teaching content into a logical sequence. Third, it is a means of establishing continuity of everyone's teaching efforts since all health care team members involved in the patient's care will know what the plans for learning are without having to make a separate assessment or hold a planning session. And, finally, the carefully written teaching care plan helps in the evaluation and documentation of the learning outcomes.

The main component of the planning stage is the drawing up of objectives. The writing of objectives is considered the most difficult part of patient teaching. Writing objectives, however, is not as difficult as it seems. Each teaching-learning objective must have two components, a behavior and a content. The *behavior* tells what the nurse wants the patient to do to exhibit that he knows something. Sample behaviors are "To state," "To list," "To write," "To demonstrate." The *content* is the material to be learned, such as "symptoms of a recurring myocardial infarction," "signs of digoxin intoxication," "taking of his radial pulse." Thus when the behavior and the content are combined, the objective writing is nearly completed. The nurse wants the patient to be able (1) to state (or to list) the symptoms of a recurring myocardial infarction, (2) to write the signs and symptoms of digoxin intoxication, or (3) to demonstrate the taking of his radial pulse.

Once the nurse has written the behavior and content, she should evaluate each objective using three criteria before she begins to teach: Is the objective specific? Is it measurable? Is it realistic? For instance, the objective "To plan a diet for a cardiac patient" is neither specific nor measurable since the nurse does not know what kind of diet the patient is following or what criteria to use to demonstrate attainment of the objective. But the objectives "To plan a 2-gm low-salt diet," "To plan an 1800-calorie weight-reduction diet" are both specific and measurable. There is no doubt in anyone's mind what sorts of diets are to be planned, and measurement is in absolute terms (2 gm of salt, 1800 calories). Those same objectives might be realistic for an adult who is responsible for his own meals and who is alert although they would probably be unrealistic for someone who is senile or confused or someone who will receive long-term care in an institution.

Some sample objectives for a cardiac teaching program can be found in Table 5-1.

Implementation

The actual teaching probably begins at the time of the needs assessment since learning occurs constantly during human interactions. Teaching of patients can be accomplished by various techniques, but perhaps the single most important technique for the patient in a critical care setting is the one-to-one interpersonal relationship. A patient trying to adapt to his illness

Table 5-1
Life After a Heart Attack: Teaching-Learning Objectives

As a result of this program, the patient will be able to:
1. Distinguish between the functions of the right and left sides of the heart.
2. Describe the function of the coronary circulation.
3. Identify 11 of the most important factors that predispose humans to develop coronary artery disease.
4. Define the term heart attack (synonymous with coronary occlusion, coronary thrombosis, and myocardial infarction).
5. Describe the process of the development of collateral circulation.
6. List the "four Es" that may precipitate a myocardial infarction.
7. Identify the symptoms of an impending myocardial infarction.
8. List four actions to take when symptoms of an impending myocardial infarction occur.
9. Describe the heart's healing process after myocardial infarction.
10. State the goal of a rehabilitation program after myocardial infarction.
11. Describe the rationale of a progressive exercise program after a myocardial infarction.
12. Describe the rationale of a restrictive diet after a myocardial infarction.
13. Describe the rationale for decreasing coronary disease risk factors.

needs a one-to-one relationship. The relationship can include lectures, question and answer periods, demonstrations of procedures and techniques, and conversations.

Supplemental teaching techniques can be used along with the interpersonal relationship. Audiovisual aids, such as films, television, slides, audiotapes, and filmstrips, may be used. The teaching program that relies totally on audiovisual materials, however, will be neither too effective nor too wise since it is too impersonal.

Group discussions are effective and efficient ways for patients with similar conditions to learn. Participation should be voluntary, however, and patients who feel uncomfortable in a group setting should not be forced to participate. The patient should be told of the times and locations of group classes, and he should be expected to assume some responsibility for going to class. (If he needs a wheelchair or other help getting to the classroom, he may not be able to assume much responsibility for attending class.)

Evaluation

The hardest part of the evaluation process is finished once objectives for the teaching care plan have been written. A well-stated objective points out not only *what* is being evaluated but also *how* it is being evaluated. For instance, the patient's objective is "To state 11 risk factors in coronary artery disease." The nurse knows that the patient is to verbalize and that he can be expected to be able to verbally list 11 risk factors. If he cannot list all 11 risk factors, he has not attained the learning objective.

In evaluating the patient's attainment of the objective "To demonstrate taking his radial pulse accurately," the nurse counts the patient's pulse at the same time that he counts it. Besides evaluating the position of his fingers on the wrist, she evaluates his accuracy in counting the pulse.

When a patient fails to accomplish one or more of his objectives, it must be decided whether the material is to be retaught or the objective is to be changed. When the objective itself is not realistic (and thus responsible for the patient's not learning), it must be changed.

Documentation

Once a teaching-learning interaction has taken place, the interaction and its outcomes must be documented in the patient's medical records. The documentation is used for at least three purposes: communication, nursing audit, and medical-legal defense.

First, and perhaps most important, documentation promotes multidisciplinary communication of the patient's progress (in treatment as well as in learning). Teaching-learning interactions may occur anytime during the patient's day, and the results need to be made known to everyone who has contact with the patient at any moment during each 24-hour period.

Documentation of various items (e.g., communication of material taught, the patient's perceptions and reactions, and the need for follow-up teaching) promotes continuity of teaching done by the entire health care team.

Second, documentation helps demonstrate the attainment of standards of care during the nursing audit. Teaching efforts may have been effective in getting the patient to change his health-related behaviors, but accomplishments will not appear on nursing audit results unless they are documented.

Documentation, then, helps to "prove" that the standards of nursing care are being met.

A third reason for documenting the teaching-learning interaction is to provide medical-legal defense in the event of litigation. All the material in the medical record can be used as evidence in a court of law. Documentation also helps the nurse remember a patient's case and care.

Documentation of the teaching-learning interaction may be done using the narrative summary, the problem oriented method, or the checklist–flow sheet. (The format of documentation is determined by local policy; the nurse should check with her nursing administration.) Each documentation of the teaching-learning process should include information on the following:

1. Content taught (i.e., learning objectives)
2. Evaluation of the patient's progress (attainment of learning objectives)
3. Patient's reaction to material taught (e.g., acceptance or animosity)
4. Effectiveness of teaching (e.g., approach used, language and learning levels)
5. Need for follow-up

The particular institution may have other requirements for documentation of the patient's teaching-learning outcomes; the nurse should become familiar with the requirements in her institution.

The steps of the teaching-learning process (assessment, planning, implementation, evaluation, and documentation) flow one from another, and they occur constantly and simultaneously.

Signs of Lack of Learning

Patient teaching cannot be separated from the practice of nursing. In spite of that fact, the behavior of patients after their discharge from the hospital often indicates lack of knowledge resulting from not learning or from not being taught. For instance, one patient behavior that may be due to lack of knowledge is noncompliance with the medical regimen. Several studies indicate that a high percentage of patients (30%–95%) do not comply with their medical regimens [1, 3, 7, 10].

Failure of patients to keep follow-up appointments after discharge from the hospital is another behavior that may indicate that patients do not have enough information to understand the importance of follow-up care.

Many critical care nurses feel frustrated by the "revolving door" syndrome, in which patients stop treatment only to be readmitted to the unit to be treated for the same health practices and conditions that originally made them sick or that injured them. Recidivism, then, is a third patient behavior that may be ascribed to lack of learning. The patient has a lack of learning in the affectional domain—the area of learning that deals with values, attitudes, and beliefs.

Finally, patients seen in follow-up visits may be suffering from the effects of drug abuse. For instance, cardiac patients who take too much or too little of their medications soon have symptoms. Drug abuse may be due to lack of understanding of the importance of taking medications on schedule and in the right amounts.

Lack of compliance, broken follow-up appointments, recidivism, and drug abuse are only a few of the more obvious results of deficient teaching-learning. Each nurse can probably easily recall other situations with their own patients that indicated a breakdown of the teaching-learning process. The breakdown may have occurred in the nurse's teaching, the patient's learning, or both. A number of factors hinder the teaching-learning process. In the pages that follow, each of those factors is described and possible solutions are offered.

Factors That Hinder Teaching

The factors that hinder the nurse's ability to teach have been put into eight categories. (They are listed in their order of importance.)

1. Faulty teaching objectives
2. Nurse's lack of time for teaching
3. Poor communication with physicians
4. Language barrier
5. Gaps in knowledge
6. Overzealous teaching
7. Decreased involvement of patient's family or significant others
8. Lack of evaluation of learning outcomes

Faulty Teaching Objectives

To ensure that the proper teaching objectives are being used, each teaching-learning process should be individualized, dealing first with the material that the patient thinks is important for him to learn. Once the patient has learned what he thinks is important, other (higher level) learning needs will become apparent *to him*. If the learning needs the patient perceives are not satisfied first, any teaching done by the nurse will be less effective and, certainly, less efficient.

Faulty teaching objectives may themselves interfere with learning. If a teaching program is not completely successful, it may be the fault not of the teacher or the learner but of the objectives.

Teaching objectives that are drawn up by nurses without regard to what the patient wants (or perceives he needs) to learn may seem to the patient not important, as the following example shows. Mr. W. was a 75-year-old, retired businessman who lived with his wife. He was an alert-appearing man, and he was often seen reading materials of different types and levels of difficulty (e.g., *Time*, the *Wall Street Journal*, novels, and nonfiction). He was given several teaching booklets, and he read all of them carefully and participated actively in nurse-initiated discussions. He stated that he had no questions about any of the booklets.

Before his discharge, Mr. W. was given a written evaluative test. He did poorly on it. In reviewing the test results with Mr. W., the nurse came to the conclusion that the objectives were the cause of his poor performance. Mr. W. asked for an explanation of the theory of the ECG and of the blood tests that physicians use to determine a patient's progress during convalescence. The result of Mr. W.'s line of questioning was a 45-minute discussion of the theory of ECGs, cardiac electrophysiology, and cardiac muscle enzyme theory. Mr. W.'s comments indicated that he understood the rather complex material almost perfectly. Since the learning objectives were his own, he learned quickly and easily.

Nurse's Time

Another factor that is perceived as a barrier to nurses' teaching efforts is their lack of time for teaching their patients. At first glance that seems to be a realistic barrier, especially in view of today's heavy work loads. Staffing patterns, rotation of shifts, cyclical scheduling of days off, and methods of patient care assignment frequently add up to a "task-oriented" role for the nurses. The nurse has a list, often unwritten, of work that must be done, observations that must be made, and physicians who must be consulted. When all her tasks are finished, they still must be recorded if standards of care are to be met.

The problem of time may or may not be easy to solve, depending on the individual nurse's definition and philosophy of teaching. If teaching is defined as a process, separate from any other activity, during which the nurse and patient sit facing each other (and the nurse recites information as though a substance were being poured into an empty receptacle), teaching will indeed take a great deal of time. Such a teaching style is likely to be ineffective since the patient is a passive recipient of information.

If, however, the teaching-learning process is seen as an active process for both nurse and patient, patient teaching can be done easily as part of the workday. The nurse must come to realize that "to nurse is to teach"; many of the things she does as a nurse *can be* and *are* educational. For instance, each time the nurse gives a medication to a patient, an active interchange of information can occur. Thus the patient can become familiar with his medications from the start. By the third or fourth time the medication is given, the nurse may be able to ask the patient about his medications as a means of evaluation of learning outcomes. When a meal tray is served to a burn patient, the nurse can give him a short explanation of the foods on his high-protein, high-calorie diet, pointing to a particular food as she discusses it. In that way, the patient receives visual, auditory (and, one hopes, gustatory) stimulation of his learning process. More than just one sense is involved in learning, and he is actively involved in the teaching-learning process.

Patient teaching is a part of nursing care. Learning will be more effective as well as more efficient (for both the nurse and the patient), the nurse will have time to teach, and the patient will be stimulated to learn if teaching is done *during* the pertinent nursing activity, such as medication administration, personal hygiene care, and meal planning.

The nurse's time available for teaching is also involved with two other problems in teaching patients, such as attempting to teach too much information and/or teaching information that the patient was not ready or willing to learn. (Those problems are discussed later in the chapter.)

Poor Communication with Physicians

The third most frequent barrier to the teaching-learning process is poor communication between nurses and physicians. Nurses find it difficult to teach patients about their disease, treatment, care, and follow-up if they do not have essential information about the patient's medical regimen. The physician may have been too busy to discuss his patient with the nurse, or he may have thought that the nurse should not teach his patient.

If a group of nurses (e.g., all the nurses on a nursing unit) arrange to meet with the physician in a conference, the physician is more likely to realize the importance of the nurse's role in patient teaching than he would if an individual nurse approached him. In hospitals in which the physicians subscribe to the patriarchal belief that they are in complete charge of their patients, the nurses will have to be persistent about getting their philosophies of patient teaching accepted.

Encouraging the physicians to begin discharge planning from the time of the patient's admission may also improve the kind of communication necessary to promote patient teaching. Encouraging the physician to participate in nursing rounds, team conferences, and patient care planning may also improve communication. When the physician sees the nurse as a facilitator in care (and teaching), rather than as a threat to his status, he may be more willing to discuss the care of his patients with her and to collaborate with her.

Language Barriers

Language barriers often hinder patient teaching. But the traditional modern foreign languages are not the only languages that hinder the teaching-learning process. Another language that is foreign to most patients is the language called "nursology." Every nurse learns a new language during her nursing education. That new language is designed to facilitate the nurses' communication with one another in the medical-nursing workday. The language also gives the nurse an identity that sets her apart from someone who has not devoted two, three, four, or more years to study, and it therefore gives the nurse a psychological boost.

Nursology facilitates the nurse's communication with other health care professionals, but it hinders the teaching-learning process between nurse and patient, as the following example shows. A middle-aged woman who had been injured in an automobile accident was having a pedicle skin graft formed on her abdomen that would eventually be moved to her face. Midpoint in her hospital stay, the pedicle was attached to her arm and her arm was restrained against her abdomen with elastic bandages so that the graft could establish a blood supply from the arm. A few days after surgery, a nurse caring for the patient inspected the skin around the surgical area. She told the patient that the area was beginning to look macerated. Later, a staff member found the patient sobbing; her mascara-stained cheeks showed that she had been crying for some time. When the patient's feelings were explored, it was found that she thought the nurse had said her skin graft looked like a massacre. When it was explained that the word macerated means having the appearance of "dishpan hands," the patient not only understood what the area looked like but could also explain how it got to look that way.

The language the nurse uses in teaching should reflect the patient's level of understanding, not the nurse's level of education. Terms should be chosen that do not have a double meaning. For instance, no doubt exists in a nurse's mind about the direction "hold medication." But the patient who has been told "hold your medication if your pulse is less than 60 beats per minute" may wonder how holding his digoxin in his hand instead of swallowing it will affect his pulse.

Gaps in Knowledge

Gaps in the nurse's knowledge may hinder the teaching-learning process. The knowledge explosion occurring within the nursing profession today prevents even the most avid reader from having completely up-to-date information on all diseases and their treatment. It must be realized, however, that regardless of the amount of knowledge the nurse may have, she still knows much more than the patient does (or perhaps more than the patient *needs* to know) about his disease. Since the nurse is rarely the only care giver, co-workers can "supplement" one another in regard to teaching.

Overzealous Teaching

The zealous teacher who wants the patient to know as much as possible may actually hinder the teaching-learning process, especially the conscientious nurse who attempts to teach the patient everything he "needs" to know to care for himself. In addition to teaching a drug's name, the zealous teacher may want the patient to know its pharmacological

action, side effects, and signs of intoxication, as well as dosage and frequency. Perhaps the most important thing a patient needs to know is that he must take one of his white pills each morning and one of his yellow capsules four times a day. If he can learn *only* that, but learn it well, he will at least be receiving optimum therapeutic benefits.

During the initial stages of the teaching-learning process, the nurse must attempt to arrive at a realistic view of how much the patient can learn; then she should be aware of his behavior during teaching that indicates his understanding or lack of it.

Decreased Involvement of Family or Significant Others

Failure to include the patient's family or significant others in the teaching care plan may have disastrous results on learning outcomes, and ultimately on the patient's compliance with the medical regimen, as the following example shows. Mr. Y., 32 years old, had been unemployed for over a year. Less than two months after he secured a job as a cement construction worker, he suffered an extensive myocardial infarction. An avid reader, he quickly learned all of the material used in the hospital's teaching program for myocardial infarction patients. Before his discharge from the hospital, he was given a written test, and he made a nearly perfect score—the highest score achieved by a patient in the history of the teaching program.

Mr. Y. was discharged from the hospital. When he got home, he stated later in an interview, his wife began nagging him about all the bills that were accumulating, his two children wanted to play, his neighbors came over to wish him well, he smoked heavily, drank two six-packs of beer, had only pizza for supper, and didn't get to sleep until about 3 A.M. the next morning. (It is not surprising that his rate of compliance with the medical regimen was the lowest in the history of the teaching program.)

Mr. Y. was readmitted to the hospital two days later with an extension of his myocardial infarction. During the admission interview, Mr. Y. said, "Life is not like it's portrayed on 'Ozzie and Harriet.'" His later comments made the staff realize that the patient's wife had not been included in his teaching program and that therefore she did not have the knowledge or skill necessary to participate in her husband's convalescence.

Before a patient's teaching care plan is drawn up,

the patient's family or significant others should be consulted. His home environment should be examined to see how the teaching plan needs to be adapted to the individual. When the patient and his family are committed to a plan of follow-up care, the patient benefits to a much greater extent.

Lack of Evaluation of Learning Outcomes

A majority of professional nurses educated within the past few decades, regardless of the type of program they were enrolled in, have never been given any formal education in the teaching-learning process. Therefore, most nurses do not know how to evaluate whether the patient has learned, and how much the patient has learned. Most nurses also have never drawn up any kind of written teaching care plan (that includes teaching objectives) for their patients. Since they have not established or written any goals or objectives for teaching, they cannot know the results of their teaching.

Once the teaching objectives have been drawn up, everyone who works with the patient knows not only what is to be taught but also how and what to evaluate. Furthermore, through the use of teaching objectives, the results of evaluation can easily be documented in the patient's progress notes.

Once the teaching-learning process has been evaluated, the documentation helps the nurse in planning further teaching sessions, as well as to identify the need for follow-up in the teaching-learning process.

Factors That Affect Learning

Even when the nurse pays attention to all the principles of the teaching-learning process that are within the realm of control, there are factors in the patient that hinder his ability to learn. Those factors are as follows:

1. Poor psychosocial adaptation to illness
2. Poor motivation to learn
3. Low self-esteem
4. Patient schedule too crowded
5. Lack of trust and rapport
6. Weak physical condition
7. Fear
8. Barriers to communication

Psychosocial Adaptation to Illness

The patient's psychosocial adaptation to illness is a phenomenon that has been studied by various investigators [2, 6, 11]. The patient's psychosocial adaptation to illness affects his motivation to learn, and his readiness to learn differs at the various stages of his psychosocial adaptation. The theorists agree on the general characteristics of the adaptation process, but they divide the process into different numbers of stages. Table 5-2 presents a summary of the stages of psychosocial adaptation to illness, as theorized by Crate [2] and suggests teaching-learning behaviors for use during each stage.

The first stage of adaptation is entited *disbelief.* When a patient is told, initially, that something is wrong with him, he is not able to believe what he hears. The disbelief turns into a protective denial, which has two purposes: (1) since it may be painful for the patient to think about how his body has been changed, denial helps to cushion him against the painful emotional impact of the disease, and (2) worry is hard work, and denial helps conserve energy by removing the subject of his worries from his conscious mind.

During the disbelief stage, the patient may deny his illness to the extent that he says, "I don't have it." Therefore, he also may be heard saying "I don't have to diet (stop smoking, take pills . . .) because there is nothing wrong with me."

If denial is present, teaching efforts that aim at self-care, and are thus *future* oriented, not only will be unsuccessful but also will be harmful and increase the patient's need for denial. Therefore teaching during the initial phase of illness *must* be oriented to the present, not to the future; that orientation will help the patient eventually adapt. For instance, the patient who is receiving Pronestyl for a cardiac dysrhythmia should be educated about the drug from the time it is first administered. The explanation that the patient will still need to take the medication after his discharge will more often than not be met with, "Oh, my heart is OK; I don't need this pill!", whereas the patient who is told that the pill will take away the uneasy feeling that he now has in his chest because it will help keep his heart from skipping beats, is more likely to understand what is being said.

A few days or so later, the patient progresses to the second stage of adaptation, known variously as development of awareness, or assumption of sick role. During that stage, the patient has an increased energy

Table 5-2
Teaching-Learning Process in Adaptation to Chronic Illness

Stages of Adaptation	Patient's Behavior	Nurse's Behavior	Nurse's Facilitation of the Teaching-Learning Process

Disbelief	Denial of threatening condition to protect self and conserve energy:
	   Refuses to accept diagnosis
	   May claim to have something else
	   May behave so as to avoid the issue
	   May seem to accept diagnosis but avoid feeling about it
		Allows patient to deny illness as he needs to. Functions as non-critical listener:
		   Accepts patient's statements of how he feels
		   Helps clarify patient's statements
		   Does not point out reality
			Orients all teaching to the present, not to tomorrow or next week. Teaches as she does other nursing activities. Assesses patient's level of anxiety. Assures patient that he is safe and being observed carefully. Explains all procedures and activities to the patient. Gives clear, concise explanations. Coordinates activities to include rest periods

Developing awareness	Uses anger as a defense against being dependent and against guilt about being sick	Listens to patient's expressions of anger and recognizes them for what they are. Explores own feelings about illness and helplessness. Does not argue with patient. Gives dependable care with an attitude that it is necessary	Does not give anxious patient long lists of facts. Continues development of trust and rapport through good physical care. Orients teaching to present. Explains symptoms, care, and treatment in terms of the fact that they are necessary *now*. Does not mention long-range care needs
Reorganization	Accepts increased dependence and reorganizes relationships with significant others. Patient's family may also use denial while they adapt to what patient's illness means to them	Establishes climate in which family and friends can express feelings about patient's illness. Does not solve patient's problems, but helps build communication so that patient and family can work together to solve problems	Assures family that patient is all right and safe. Uses clear, concise explanations. Does not argue about need for care
Resolution	Acknowledges changes seen in self. Identifies with others with same problem	Encourages expression of feelings, including crying. Understands own feelings of loss	Brings groups of patients with same illness together for group discussions. Has recovered patient visit patient. Teaches patient what he wants to learn (or perceives he needs to learn) first
Identity change	Defines self as an individual that has undergone change and is now different. "There are limits to my life because I have a disease"	Understands own feelings about patient's becoming independent again	Realizes that as patient's own perceived needs are met, more mature (more progressive) needs will surface. Is prepared to answer patient's questions as they arise
Successful adaptation	Can live comfortably or resignedly with himself as a person who has a specific condition	Initiates closure of nurse-patient relationship	Has helped develop a relationship with the patient in which the nurse is a guide that the patient can consult when he wishes

Adapted from M. A. Crate, Nursing functions in adaptation to chronic illness. *Am. J. Nurs.* 65:72–76, 1965.

reserve and can begin to do the work of worrying about what has happened to him. Assumption of the sick role allows the patient to become dependent on others for his care. Assumption of the sick role, however, is threatening to many patients, and they react with anger, an emotion that needs to be vented. Some comments heard from patients who are angry are, "They don't know what they're doing," "It's all their fault," "Why did this have to happen to me?", and "What did I do to deserve this?" The venting of anger helps relieve the patient's blame and guilt feelings. During this phase, the nurse should practice techniques of therapeutic communication by listening to the patient's expressions of anger and by recognizing them for what they are. To do so may require a careful examination of the nurse's own feelings since she must realize that the patient is reacting to factors within him, *not* within the nurse.

At this stage, the patient is too anxious to hear facts. To confront him with a long list of medical facts may reinforce his need to hear not much of anything. Teaching done during this stage should continue to be oriented to the present, but can be slightly more to the point that it was during the denial stage. Symptoms, care, and treatments can be explained in terms of what they mean *now* without reference to the day the patient is discharged. There will be time for that.

The patient gains more ground in the process of adaptation as he passes into the third stage—reorganization. He has usually worked through the guilt and anger he feels about becoming dependent, and now he has to reorganize his relationships with family and friends so that they can accept him as "sick." The family also goes through the stages of psychosocial adaptation to illness, and the nurse must understand that the family may not learn easily or hear too well either.

During the final stages of adaptation—resolution and identity change—the patient is much more receptive than he was to teaching about the diagnosis, treatment, and course of illness. Useful teaching devices at those stages are (1) bringing together patients with the same illness so that they may learn from one another and (2) having a patient in the convalescent stage of the illness visit the patient so that he may have a chance to identify with a recovering patient. Once adaptation has been completed, the patient has learned to live with himself—with comfort or with resignation—as a person who has a specific disease or condition.

In the stages of psychosocial adaptation to illness, the patient first uses denial as a protective mechanism. Denial helps him to allay anxiety but interferes (at least temporarily) with adjustment measures, such as learning. At this early stage of illness, the patient will probably greet attempts at teaching with anger and hostility since he believes that he does not have the disease. It is recommended that teaching be oriented to the present.

As the patient progresses towards accepting his illness, he often becomes angry at himself and at others, because he dislikes being dependent. During this time, the patient uses much of his energy to express anger. He may meet teaching efforts during this time with anger and renewed denial. The teaching must still be oriented to the present, and references to long-range care needs should be postponed for a short time.

During the last stages of acceptance the patient begins to use some of his energy for learning how to alter his life-style and activities of daily living. (This stage of adaptation has been shown to occur as late as the fifth or sixth week after a myocardial infarction [9].) Teaching efforts at this point are probably the most effective and most efficient since the patient is now motivated to learn how to deal with the future. Unless the patient is ready to learn, a learning experience will be inefficient or learning simply will not occur.

Motivation to Learn

Patients learn only what they want to learn or are motivated to learn. All mental processes are caused by some tension. A person's behavior is always determined by his intention to do one thing or another. In other words, all behavior is motivated.

Abraham Maslow [8] has described a hierarchy of human needs that he feels motivate human behavior. In Maslow's hierarchy (Fig. 5-1) physiological needs are the most basic ones. Safety, belongingness and love, esteem, and self-actualization are needs at the upper end of the hierarchy. Maslow theorizes that needs at the lower end of the hierarchy must be satisfied before the person can attend to those at the upper end.

When a person has suffered a life-threatening disease, his needs center on physiology and safety, the two lowest needs on Maslow's hierarchy. It may be difficult or impossible for the person to think of

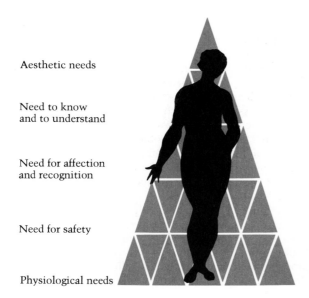

Aesthetic needs

Need to know
and to understand

Need for affection
and recognition

Need for safety

Physiological needs

Figure 5-1
The hierarchy of needs. (Adapted from Maslow [8].)

learning how to adjust to his illness since this activity is based on a much higher need in the hierarchy, such as the need to belong, the need for love, or the need for esteem. Teaching the patient who is afraid for his life and safety is nearly useless unless the nurse teaches the patient that he is in no immediate danger of dying and is safe. The person at this basic level of motivation is not likely to be able to absorb very much information, and teaching sessions should be kept short and the patient should be allowed to rest frequently.

Once the patient believes he is out of physical danger, such as death or worsening of his physical condition, he is ready to progress to a higher level of needs. He may now be able to devote time and energy to learning.

Self-esteem

Self-esteem is important at all stages of one's life, but when the patient is in a critical care setting, his self-esteem is in an even more precarious state of affairs. Many strangers are intruding on his territory or life space, to say nothing about intrusive procedures that probe, puncture, and persecute his physical being. Teaching efforts are seen as just another intrusion,

especially if the teaching objectives are those of the nursing staff and not at all those of the patient. Use of nurse-determined objectives may not only increase the patient's loss of self-esteem, but also detract from teaching-learning outcomes.

The patient's self-esteem can be enhanced (or at least not further injured) by including him in planning his own nursing care as well as in helping to determine his own teaching care plan. The patient will learn better, and he will feel better because he was respected and given some choice in his own care.

Patient's Schedule of Activities

The amount of activity scheduled may hinder the teaching-learning process; Mr. S., a 43-year-old married man with two teenaged children, is a patient whose case illustrates that point. Mr. S. had been a regularly employed businessman up to the time he suffered a myocardial infarction. During his hospitalization, Mr. S. stated that he had less time to rest than he had when he was working full time. His activities kept him rigorously busy throughout his hospitalization. He was awakened in the morning for a check of his vital signs. From that moment on, breakfast, physical therapy, lunch, medications, visitors, and visits from staff members kept him busy until bedtime at night. Midway in his 11-day hospitalization, he still had not read any of the materials given him, because he had been "too busy." When he did have a few moments of free time, he stated that he was either too tired or too sedated (on Valium) to pay attention to his booklets.

Patients who are participating in any teaching-learning process need time not only for physical rest but also to participate in learning activities. The nurse who is in charge of the patient must attempt to coordinate the patient's activities in order to provide rest periods and study periods. Those rest periods and study periods need to be explained to family members and/or significant others. Ideally, family members are included in the study periods to learn how best to help the patient care for himself.

Trust and Rapport

Trust and rapport affect the teaching-learning process. If a patient is not given a chance to develop a warm interpersonal relationship with his nurse, his learning may be hindered by a lack of trust in his caretaker-instructor. When skilled critical care nurses care for a patient, they quickly and easily meet his needs and also easily establish a trusting interpersonal relationship. The same relationship will carry through to any teaching effort the nurse makes for the patient. A nurse does not have to establish a trust relationship for teaching when such a relationship has already been established in nursing care.

If a nurse (such as a clinical specialist or a patient-education coordinator) is assigned patient teaching as one of her professional duties, she will have to spend some time getting acquainted, establishing a rapport, and building trust with the patient before an effective teaching-learning process can occur. The best person to do the teaching is the nurse who also gives the patient physical (and emotional and spiritual) care at his bedside. Trust and rapport in one realm of nursing care easily transfers to another realm.

Another aspect of trust evolves from the fact that patients may be aware that some physicians have reservations about how effective their recommendations are in preventing further disease. For instance, wide differences of opinion exist among physicians and nurses in regard to the effectiveness of the usual medical recommendations in reducing subsequent heart attacks. When that is the case, the patient may sense the physician's or nurse's reservations about the regimens they prescribe, and he may think, "If my doctor (nurse) doesn't really believe this, why should I?" An interesting research project would be an investigation of the extent to which patients are aware that their physicians have reservations about the regimens they prescribe.

Physical Condition

The extent of the patient's illness will hinder the teaching-learning process. Someone who is in pain will not have an attention span that is compatible with learning. The overtired or exhausted patient will not be able to maintain an attention span for learning. Electrolyte imbalances interfere with the teaching-learning process, as do fever and decreased cerebral perfusion.

The nurse must learn to be sensitive to the feelings her patients express, whether they express them verbally or otherwise.

Fear

Fear may be a motivating factor or a hindrance to learning. It will be motivating for high learning achievement only if the arousal of fear is accompanied by specific instructions for reducing the threat. When a patient realizes that his future is bleak unless he takes charge and does something about it, he will be more motivated to learn ways to solve the fear-inducing problems. If, however, the arousal of fear is not accompanied by specific instructions for reducing the threat, the threat may be reduced by denying its existence, as the following example shows.

Mr. T. was a married man, 62 years of age, whose children had grown up. He had suffered a mild myocardial infarction and was hospitalized. He was given booklets and other materials as part of his teaching program. He stated that while reading the first part of the materials given him, he became "scared to death" about the bleak picture the literature painted. Then, he said, he found the part of the pamphlet that said that the future was up to him, and he promised himself that he would do everything he was told to do as his part of his determination to live longer. A month after his discharge from the hospital, Mr. T.'s reported compliance with his medical regimen was the highest of any patient in the study. Fear became a motivation to learn, because the fear arousal was accompanied by specific instructions for reducing the threat.

Barriers to Communication

Barriers to communication probably exist in any interpersonal relationship, but a patient whose teaching program begins in a coronary care unit or intermediate care unit is subjected to a great many barriers to effective communication, including cardiac monitors that alarm constantly, mechanical ventilators that sigh monotonously, and a constant movement of busy physicians and nurses. The noise may hinder concentration and subsequent learning, even with ideal materials and an individualized teaching program.

When it is impossible to control noise and distractions and when the patient's ability to concentrate is limited by the distractions around him, the nurse will have to make explanations that are to the point, short, and clear.

The barriers to an effective teaching-learning process are legion, and teaching patients who are hospitalized because of disease or injury may, at times, pose frustrations for even an experienced teacher. It may even be true that the more serious the disease, the more difficulty there will be in accomplishing any teaching objectives.

Those observations may paint a gloomy picture for the nurse who wants (and feels the need) to teach patients. The nurse may say, "Why bother? There are too many barriers." And so it may seem to the person who is not familiar with a hospital and patients. The nurse is already armed with the most necessary weapon for patient teaching, even in the face of all the obstacles discussed. The weapon is simply an understanding of the human being and the recognition of the patient's dignity and value.

Nursing care delivered with understanding and a recognition of the patient's individuality will help to break down some of the barriers to the teaching-learning process. Further success in patient teaching is ensured if the nurse uses the principles of adult education (andragogy). (The theories of adult education can be used in teaching patients of any age.)

Nursing Orders

The following nursing orders for patient teaching are derived from the principles of patient teaching:

1. Identify what the patient perceives as his learning needs first.
2. Begin the teaching program at the patient's present level of knowledge.
3. Consider the patient's physical condition when determining what and how long to teach.
4. Provide the patient with an opportunity to practice what he is to learn.
5. Repeat the teaching to increase retention.
6. Give the patient a report on his progress in learning.
7. Adjust the material and the teaching rate to the individual patient.
8. Minimize distracting noises in the teaching-learning environment.
9. Allow time for an interpersonal relationship to develop before doing significant teaching.
10. Maintain trust between the patient and the nurse by being honest about one's own knowledge.

Summary

Patient teaching has been considered to be a role of the professional nurse for many years. Many nurses have philosophies of nursing care that include teaching as a direct or indirect function within patient care.

The steps of the teaching-learning process help to organize teaching and learning and provide for the assessment of knowledge, planning of teaching-learning, implementation of teaching, and evaluation and documentation of learning outcomes.

Despite the fact that patients need and want information about hospitalization and self-care after discharge, barriers exist that hinder the nurse's teaching and/or the patient's learning. Using the guidelines found in adult education research may help to break down some of the barriers to the teaching-learning process. By starting at the point where the patient perceives the need to learn, the nurse can promote a successful teaching-learning process for both the patient and herself.

Study Problems

1. What are your beliefs about patient teaching?
   a. What is the role of the nurse in patient teaching?
   b. What is the role of the patient in patient teaching?
2. Name the steps of the teaching-learning process.
   a. Do those steps occur separately and in sequence?
   b. Which step of the teaching-learning process helps the nurse not only to organize the teaching material but also to determine what and how to evaluate and what to chart?
3. Which of the barriers to the nurse's teaching are present in your own practice?
4. Recall the last patient you taught. Which of the barriers to the patient's learning were present in that situation?
5. List some important things to keep in mind when teaching according to adult education theory.
6. What are the differences between the way adults learn and the way children learn?

References

1. Bille, D. Patient's Knowledge and Compliance with Post-Hospitalization Prescriptions as Related to Body

Image and Teaching Format. Ph.D. dissertation, University of Wisconsin, 1975.

2. Crate, M. A. Nursing functions in adaptation to chronic illness. *Am. J. Nurs.* 65:72, 1965.

3. Davis, M. Variations in patients' compliance with doctors' orders: Analysis of congruence between survey responses and results of empirical investigations. *J. Med. Ed.* 41:1037, 1966.

4. Havighurst, R. J., and Orr, B. *Adult Education and Adult Needs.* Boston: Center for the Study of Liberal Education for Adults, 1956.

5. Knowles, M. *The Modern Practice of Adult Education.* New York: Association Press, 1970.

6. Lederer, H. D. How the sick view their world. *J. Soc. Issues* 8:4, 1952.

7. Marston, M. V. Compliance with Medical Regimens As a Form of Risk Taking in Patients with Myocardial Infarctions. Ph.D. dissertation, Boston University, 1969.

8. Maslow, A. *Motivation and Personality.* New York: Harper & Row, 1970.

9. Nite, G., and Willis, F. *The Coronary Patient: Hospital Care and Rehabilitation.* New York: Macmillan, 1964.

10. Stewart, R. B., and Cluff, L. E. A review of medication errors and compliance in ambulant patients. *Clinical Pharmacol. Ther.* 13:463, 1972.

11. Suchman, E. A. Stages of illness and medical care. *J. Health Hum. Behav.* 6:114, 1965.

Bibliography

Abdellah, F., and Levine, M. Polling patients and personnel, part I: What patients say about their nursing care. *Hospitals* 40:76, 1966.

Allendorf, E. E., et al. Teaching patients about nitroglycerine. *Am. J. Nurs.* 75:1168, 1975.

Alt, R. Patient education program answers many unanswered questions. *Hospitals* 40:76, 1966.

Bartlett, M. H. Patients receive current, concise health information by telephone. *Hospitals* 50:79, 1976.

Baum, S. S. A program for teaching cardiac surgery patients. *J. Assoc. Oper. Room Nurs.* 23:591, 1976.

Bergevin, P., et al. *Adult Education Procedures.* New York: Seabury Press, 1963.

Bille, D. Body image related to patients' knowledge and post-hospitalization prescriptions. *Heart Lung* January–February, 1977.

Bille, D. Patient's knowledge as related to teaching format and compliance. *Superv. Nurs.* March, 1977. Pp. 55.

Bird, R. H. Learner feedback and program change problems of parent education. *J. Contin. Ed. Nurs.* 6:50, 1975.

Borgman, M. F. Coronary rehabilitation—a comprehensive design. *Int. J. Nurs. Stud.* 12:13, 1975.

Bristow, O., et al. Discharge planning for continuity of care (321-1604). *National League of Nursing Publ. League Exchange* 112:143, 1976.

Cap, A. G. Pre-op classes produce more relaxed patients. *In-serv. Train. Educ.* 4:9, 1975.

Daniel, J. H. Working with high-risk families: Family advocacy and the parent education program. *Children Today* 4:23, 1975.

Davenport, R. R. Dietitians, nurses teach diabetic patients. *Hospitals* 48:81, 1974.

Deberry, P. Teaching cardiac patients to manage medications. *Am. J. Nurs.* 75:191, 1975.

Eddington, C. A home-centered program for parents. *Am. J. Nurs.* 75:59, 1975.

Engle, V. Diabetic teaching: How to win your patient's cooperation in his care. *Nurs. '75* 5:17, 1975.

Epstein, R., and Benson, D. J. The patient's right to know. *Hospitals* 47:47, 1973.

Friedland, G. M. Learning behaviors of a preadolescent with diabetes. *Am. J. Nurs.* 76:59, 1976.

Fylling, C. P. Health education. *Hospitals* 49:95, 1975.

Gibson, W. E. But who teaches the patient? *Arch. Dermatol.* 88:935, 1963.

Golodetz, A., et al. The right to know: Giving the patient his medical record. *Arch. Phys. Med. Rehabil.* 57:78, 1976.

Gusfa, A., et al. Patient teaching: One approach. *Superv. Nurs.* 6:17, 1975.

Haven, L. C. Reducing the patient's fear of the recovery room. *RN* 38:28, 1975.

Hayter, J. Fine points in diabetic care. *Am. J. Nurs.* 76:594, 1976.

Hecht, A. Improving medication compliance by teaching outpatients. *Nurs. Forum* 13:112, 1974.

Hegyvary, S. T., and Haussman, R. K. D. Monitoring nursing care quality. *J. Nurs. Admin.* 5:17, 1975.

Hicks, A. P., and Ashby, D. J. Teaching discharge planning. *Nurs. Outlook* 24:306, 1976.

Jamplis, R. W. The practicing physician and patient education. *Hosp. Pract.* 10:93, 1975.

Jenrich, J. A. Renal disease: A symposium. Some aspects of the nursing care for patients on hemodialysis. *Heart Lung* 4:885, 1975.

Johnson, B. L., et al. Eight steps to inpatient cardiac rehabilitation: The team effort—Methodology and preliminary results. *Heart Lung* 5:97, 1976.

Jorow, M. How to teach patients to catheterize themselves. *RN* 38:19, 1975.

Kelly, L. Y. The patient's right to know. *Nurs. Outlook* 24:26, 1976.

Laird, M. Techniques for teaching pre- and postoperative patients. *Am. J. Nurs.* 75:1338, 1975.

Lawless, C. A. Helping patients with endotracheal and tracheostomy tubes communicate. *Am. J. Nurs.* 75:2151, 1975.

Leahey, M. D., et al. Pediatric diabetes: A new teaching approach. *Can. Nurse* 71:18, 1975.

Long, M. L., et al. Hypertension: What patients need to know. *Am. J. Nurs.* 76:765, 1976.

Luciano, K., et al. Pediatric procedures—the explanation should always come first. *Nurs. '75* 5:49, 1975.

Marston, M. V. Compliance with medical regimens: A review of the literature. *Nurs. Res.* 19:310, 1970.

McGann, M. Group sessions for the families of postcoronary patients. *Superv. Nurs.* 7:17, 1976.

Murray, R. Guidelines for more effective health teaching. *Nurs. '76* 6:44, 1976.

Ostrow, L. S. Intensive respiratory care: From ICU to home. *Am. J. Nurs.* 76:111, 1976.

Pearson, B. Learning tool selection. *Superv. Nurs.* 6:30, 1975.

Prsala, H. Admission unit dispels fear of surgery. *Can. Nurse* 70:24, 1974.

Rahe, R., et al. Teaching the patient and the family. A teaching evaluation questionnaire for postmyocardial infarction patients. *Heart Lung* 4:759, 1975.

Rambousek, E. Teaching the Patient After Hospital Discharge. In F. Storlie (ed.), *Patient Teaching in Critical Care.* New York: Appleton-Century-Crofts, 1975.

Redman, B. K. *The Process of Patient Teaching in Nursing.* St. Louis: Mosby, 1972.

Redman, B. K. Client education therapy in treatment and prevention of cardiovascular diseases. *Nurs. Digest* 3:11, 1975.

Redman, B. K. Guidelines for quality of care in patient education. *Can. Nurse* 71:19, 1975.

Robinson, L. A. Patient's information base: A key to care. *Can. Nurse* 70:34, 1974.

Ryan, M. L. Patient educator teaches respiratory care patients. *Respir. Care* 21:36, 1976.

Salzer, J. E. Classes to improve diabetic self-care. *Am. J. Nurs.* 75:1324, 1975.

Scoggins, J. B. Communicate, dammit. *RN* 39:38, 1976.

Semmler, C., et al. Counseling the coronary patient. *Am. J. Occup. Ther.* 28:609, 1974.

Sexton, D. A nurse shows how to help the patient stop smoking. *Am. Lung Assoc. Bull.* 61:10, 1975.

Storlie, F. Some latent meanings of teaching of patients. *Heart Lung* 2:506, 1973.

Stufflet, S. K. If you want to do patient teaching, become a pulmonary nurse specialist. *Nurs. '76* 6:94, 1976.

Van Bree, N. S. Sexuality, nursing practice, and the person with cardiac disease. *Nurs. Forum* 14:397, 1975.

Visintainer, M. A., et al. Psychological preparation for surgical pediatric patients: The effect on children's and parents' stress responses and adjustment. *Pediatrics* 56:187, 1975.

Welford, W. Closing the communications gap. *Nurs. Times* 71:114, 1975.

Wenger, N. K. Patient and family education after myocardial infarction. *Postgrad. Med.* 57:129, 1975.

Wolf, Z. R. What patients awaiting kidney transplant want to know. *Am. J. Nurs.* 76:92, 1976.

Wootton, J. Prescription for error. *Nurs. Times* 71:884, 1975.

Nursing Malpractice Law

Robert Berry Cook, Jr.

The majority of medical malpractice lawsuits arise from incidents that occur during hospitalization. Since the critical care nurse works in the hospital environment, she should have a general understanding of medical malpractice law, and she should be aware of the fact that nursing is a "legally sensitive" profession. Nursing is legally sensitive because it is a people business; i.e., in nursing, people care for people. If the nurse dealt only with inanimate objects in her occupation (such as with merchandise in a retail store), her mistakes would not ordinarily result in a lawsuit. But because the nurse deals with people, her mistakes directly and perhaps immediately affect another person, the patient, who may well be in a bad mood because he is ill. An ill person may not be as forgiving as a well person. Many ill people are not, as indicated by the great increase in the number of medical malpractice lawsuits in recent years.

Approximately 90 percent of medical malpractice lawsuits ever filed have been filed since 1964. The average award in medical malpractice cases is rising at a rate of 14 percent a year. The increase in the number of suits filed is caused by several factors, as discussed in the following paragraphs.

1. This is the age of *consumerism*. Consumers are becoming increasingly litigious (prone to file lawsuits), resulting in an increase in all types of litigation, not just medical malpractice suits.

6

2. Specialization in medicine has resulted in some *loss of the traditional rapport between physician and patient,* the "family doctor"–type relationship. Busy specialists find it difficult to develop a close relationship with patients they may see only once or twice during hospitalization.

3. The contractual arrangement whereby an attorney is compensated on a *contingency fee* basis may contribute to the increase in the number of suits filed. Under that arrangement, the attorney representing the plaintiff receives a percentage of the settlement or court award, as opposed to being paid by the hour for his services. Of course, if the attorney is unable to settle the case out of court or loses the case in court, he gets nothing. The arrangement allows the complaining party to have a lawsuit filed on his behalf with little or no cost to him.

4. *Statutes of limitation* set forth the amount of time the complaining party has in which to file a lawsuit after the alleged negligence took place. If the lawsuit is not filed before the limitation period expires, it is barred by the statute of limitation. Courts in some states, however, have interpreted their statutes of limitation in such a way that a lawsuit can be brought after the limitation period has expired if the complaining party had not discovered within the limitation period—and with reasonable diligence could not have discovered within the limitation period—that he had been injured by allegedly negligent conduct. That interpretation allows a lawsuit to be brought 5, 10, 15, 20, or more years after the allegedly negligent conduct occurred. (In the insurance industry, such a lawsuit is called a "long tail" suit.) The "discovery" statutes of limitation have led to an increase in the number of lawsuits filed.

The increase in the dollar amount of settlements and court awards in medical malpractice cases can be attributed partly to general inflation, partly to the even greater increase in the cost of health care, and partly to an increase in the skill of the attorneys representing claimants in that type of lawsuit. Medical malpractice litigation is complex because the attorney not only must be educated in the law but also must educate himself in the area of medicine at issue in the lawsuit. As the plaintiffs' attorneys get more experience in medical malpractice litigation (as mentioned, 90 percent of the medical malpractice lawsuits ever filed have been filed since 1964), they learn more medicine and become better advocates for their clients.

A List of Terms Used in Personal Injury Law

Medical malpractice is included in the broad category of law called *personal injury law,* also referred to as *tort law.* Tort is derived from a Latin word that means "to twist." In our system of jurisprudence, tort means injury and tort law is subdivided into two broad fields: (1) personal injury law (injury to an individual) and (2) property damage law. Since in the conduct of their profession, nurses are primarily interested in personal injury law, the following list is that of terms commonly used in personal injury law.

1. *Plaintiff.* The plaintiff is the complaining party, the one who initiates the lawsuit. The plaintiff sues the defendant. In medical malpractice lawsuits, the patient is usually the plaintiff.

2. *Defendant.* The defendant is the person against whom the complaint is brought. The defendant is the party being sued by the plaintiff. In medical malpractice lawsuits, the nurse, physician and/or hospital may be the defendant(s).

3. *Pleadings.* The pleadings are the various allegations of the plaintiff and the defenses of the defendant contained in documents filed with the court by both parties to the suit.

4. *Plaintiff's petition or complaint.* The plaintiff's petition or complaint is the document filed with the court by the plaintiff that initiates the lawsuit. It names the defendant and sets forth the allegations of negligence on the part of the defendant. It also contains allegations of damages and asks for a sum of money to satisfy the damages. The petition is usually attached to the citation, and it is "served on" (delivered to) the defendant.

5. *Citation.* The citation is a document issued by the court and delivered to the defendant along with a copy of the petition. The citation is usually the defendant's first notice that he has been sued, and the petition gives the defendant notice of the allegations against him. The citation directs the defendant to file an answer to the suit with the court within a certain period of time.

6. *Defendant's answer.* The defendant's answer is the document filed with the court by the defendant in answer to the petition. It generally contains a denial of the allegations in the petition, and it may request that the plaintiff be required

to give more details of the alleged negligence and damages.

7. *Discovery.* Discovery is the phase of a lawsuit in which attorneys for both parties attempt to uncover or discover evidence for use in settlement negotiations and the trial. The tools of discovery are written interrogatories, requests for admissions, and depositions.

8. *Interrogatories.* An interrogatory is a document containing written questions that one party to the suit sends to the other party to answer. The party to whom the questions are directed must furnish written answers to the questions within a certain number of days after receiving the interrogatories.

9. *Request for admissions.* The request for admissions is a document sent by one party to another party asking that statements of fact concerning the case be admitted or denied. Facts that are admitted need not be proved at the trial; they are, in effect, agreed on by the parties.

10. *Deposition.* A deposition is testimony given by a party or a witness before the trial. The deposition is taken at the hospital or in the office of one of the attorneys. Attorneys for both parties are present, and the witness responds orally under oath to oral questions from the attorneys. A judge is not present. The questions and answers are recorded by a court reporter. The deposition may be used as evidence at the trial.

11. *Subpoena.* The subpoena is a document issued by the court that directs a witness to appear at a certain place at a certain time to give testimony in a lawsuit. A witness may be subpoenaed to give a deposition or to appear at the trial. A person disobeying a subpoena may be held to be in contempt of court and jailed until he agrees to obey the subpoena.

12. *Subpoena Duces Tecum.* The subpoena duces tecum is a document issued by the court directing a person to appear at a certain place at a certain time and to bring specified documents with him.

The Judicial Process

A lawsuit is initiated by the plaintiff's attorney by the filing of a petition with the clerk of the appropriate court. The petition names the defendant, contains allegations that the defendant has been negligent and that such negligence has harmed the plaintiff, and asks for a certain sum of money to compensate the plaintiff for the damages. The court then issues a citation with a copy of the petition attached. The citation and petition are delivered to the defendant by a sheriff's deputy or constable. The citation requires the defendant to file an answer to the lawsuit within a certain number of days after the day the citation is delivered to the defendant. A nurse or any other hospital employee who is served with a citation and petition involving his work at the hospital should notify the hospital administrator immediately. The citation and petition will be forwarded to an attorney, who will file an answer with the court on behalf of the defendant.

The next phase of the lawsuit is discovery. The attorney defending the lawsuit investigates the allegations with the assistance of hospital personnel. Both sides may use written interrogatories, requests for admissions, and depositions to discover facts to help them at the time of the trial or in settlement negotiations. Hospital employees should assist the defense attorney. They should not discuss the case with the plaintiff or the plaintiff's attorney unless advised to do so by the defense attorney.

Generally, a deposition is taken to discover what the witness knows about the incident that has given rise to the lawsuit. As mentioned, the deposition is taken at the hospital or in the office of one of the attorneys. The attorney representing the hospital will explain the details of giving a deposition to the hospital employee before the deposition is taken. A few general guidelines addressed to the employee are also given here.

1. If you do not know the answer to a question, simply state that you do not know the answer. Do not offer a guess and do not speculate about the correct answer. Even if you feel you should know the answer, do not be embarrassed to say you do not know the answer.

2. Your only objective in a deposition is to give the facts as you know them. You are not to give personal opinions unless your attorney instructs you to do so.

3. Do not ramble in answering a question. Be concise. Do not explain, do not try to justify, and do not elaborate on your answer. Do not volunteer additional information.

4. Your only duty is to give facts known to you. Do not ask your attorney or another witness that is

present for information needed to answer the question.

5. Do not let the opposing attorney make you angry. Anger will lessen the effectiveness of your testimony. Answer the opposing attorney's questions in an even tone of voice. Do not argue with him.

6. Take your time in answering a question. Pauses do not show on the typed transcript of the deposition. Try to answer questions in a direct and confident manner. Do not give wishy-washy answers.

If the parties to the lawsuit—the plaintiff and the defendant—do not settle the case, it will be tried in court, usually before a jury. If the nurse is to testify at the trial, the defense attorney will explain courtroom procedure to her before she testifies.

Negligence and the Standard of Care

To win the lawsuit, the plaintiff must prove that the defendant was negligent in her care of the plaintiff. Negligence is the failure to act as a reasonably prudent person would act in the same or similar situation. Negligence may result from omission or commission; that is, a person may omit doing something he should have done or a person may do something incorrectly. In medical malpractice lawsuits, the question of whether negligence was present in the care of a patient is determined by comparing the conduct of the allegedly negligent person to the standard of care in the profession. The standard of care is the care that is generally recognized in the profession as appropriate under the circumstances. A nurse's conduct is compared to the standard of care in the nursing profession. Thus an expert witness for the plaintiff might testify that the nurse's conduct did not meet the standard of care in the nursing profession, whereas an expert witness for the defendant might testify that the nurse's conduct met or exceeded the standard of care. The standard of care may be established by describing what is generally taught in nursing schools and what is customarily done in the clinical setting.

The Best Defense in a Medical Malpractice Lawsuit

The best defense in a medical malpractice lawsuit is, of course, competent nursing. If the patient has not been injured by the nurse's conduct, he cannot re-

cover money damages from the nurse. The problem lies in *proving* that the nursing care a patient received was competent. The statutes of limitation usually allow the aggrieved patient to file a lawsuit years after the alleged negligence took place. How many nurses can remember in detail the care they rendered to a patient last week, much less last year? How many patients does a nurse care for in a year? It is obvious that no nurse can rely on her memory to recall nursing care in the minute detail often required in medical malpractice lawsuits. Therefore, the only practical way for a nurse to prove that she rendered good nursing care to a patient is to *document the care rendered in the patient's medical record.* If good care was given and documented, the medical record is the nurse's best evidence in the courtroom. Even if the nursing care given was excellent, if it is not documented in the medical record, the nurse is at a distinct disadvantage in the lawsuit. Of course, good documentation of the care given is a vital part of good nursing care as well as good "legal nursing." The quality of documentation of care in nursing notes in the medical record should be subject to continual critical evaluation in the hospital setting.

To ensure that patient care is appropriately documented, the nurse must:

1. Record in the appropriate section of the medical record the dates *and times* of the physician's verbal or phone orders.

2. Record in the nurses' notes when physician's orders were carried out. Anyone reviewing the medical record should be able to look in the nurses' notes and verify both that the physician's orders were carried out and when they were carried out. The time the medications were administered should always be recorded.

3. Be familiar with hospital and critical care unit standing orders, and make sure that the medical record reflects that those orders were carried out when they were applicable to the patient care situation.

4. Record data about the patient's vital signs, fluid intake and output, the method of oxygen delivery, including the respirator settings, intravenous administration rates, and the observations of the patient's condition made according to standing orders, physician orders, and as needed.

5. Be sure that when a physician is notified of a change in the patient's condition, the following are recorded: the name of the physician, the time he was notified, and whether he gave orders.

6. Record the time of day a physician visits the patient.

Other Suggestions

Some medical malpractice lawsuits are instituted because the patient or a member of the patient's family overhears a health care professional criticizing the care given the patient by another health care professional. If a nurse believes the care rendered to a patient by another health care professional is substandard, she should report her concern to her immediate supervisor in such a manner as not to disturb the patient or the patient's family. Such a matter should never be discussed in the hallways, on elevators, or in other places where the conversation may be overheard.

The details of unusual events that occur during hospitalization that may result in injury to the patient should be documented separately from the patient's medical record, because the medical record is subject to subpoena, whereas a report setting forth the details of an unusual event may not be subject to subpoena. For instance, if a patient falls while walking from his bed to the bathroom, the nurse's notes in the medical record should state that the patient fell, should describe any injuries that resulted from the fall, and should document that the patient's attending physician was notified of the fall. Details of the fall, such as who found the patient on the floor, the condition of the floor (e.g., wet or dry), and whether the patient asked for help in walking to the bathroom, should be noted on a separate document that does not become a part of the patient's medical record.

Professional Liability Insurance and the Doctrine of *Respondeat Superior*

Nurses often ask whether they should buy liability insurance to cover the risk of being sued in connection with their work in the hospital. There is no clear-cut answer to this question. Some lawyers think that such insurance is mandatory for the professional nurse, and others advise against it on the basis of the doctrine *respondeat superior.*

Respondeat superior is a Latin phrase that means, "Let the master answer." In our system of jurisprudence, *respondeat superior* is the principle that an employer is responsible for the negligence of his employees. Thus a hospital is responsible for any negligence committed by a nurse or other hospital employee during the performance of the employee's duties. That is not to say the nurse is not also responsible for her negligent acts. She is responsible. The person who is negligent is legally responsible for the negligence, but when the negligence is committed by an employee in the course of performing duties as an employee, the employer is also legally responsible for the employee's negligence. Therefore, because of the doctrine of *respondeat superior*, most plaintiffs in medical malpractice lawsuits look to the employer hospital for payment of damages instead of to the allegedly negligent employee although the employee and hospital may both be named as defendants in the lawsuit. But if the plaintiff learns that the allegedly negligent employee has professional liability insurance, he may be encouraged to sue the employee as well as the hospital employer, whereas otherwise he would usually sue only the hospital.

Summary

This chapter has set forth for the nurse the basic principles and terminology of personal injury law and the judicial process. It should enable the nurse to understand the underlying causes of the medical malpractice crisis and to appreciate the importance of the patient's medical record in successfully defending medical malpractice lawsuits.

Provisions for Electrical Safety

Jay Warren

Considerable emphasis has recently been placed on electrical safety in the hospital. With the advent of sophisticated electronic patient-monitoring and assist equipment, critical care personnel need a basic understanding of electrical hazards and, more important, electrical safety. Increased understanding and the use of a few basic safety practices will help prevent a fatal electrical accident.

Physiological Effects of Electricity

In order for electricity to have any effect on the body, the body must become part of the electrical circuit itself. At least two connections must exist between the body and an external source of voltage to effect a current flow. The magnitude of the current flow is a function of both the voltage between the body connections and the resistance of the body. The electrical current can affect tissue in two different ways. First, the current flow can induce an action potential, causing the transmission of impulses through sensory and motor nerves. Stimulation of motor nerves in that manner can cause contraction of the muscle groups involved. A greater intensity of motor nerve or muscle stimulation can cause tetanus of the muscle. Stimulation of sensory nerves by small amounts of current flow can cause a tingling sensation, and greater amounts of current flow can cause extreme

7

pain. Second, electrical energy dissipated in the tissue resistance can cause a temperature increase, resulting in an electrical burn. That principle is used in electrosurgery, where concentrated electrical current from an electrical surgery unit (a radiofrequency generator with a frequency of 2.5 to 4 MHz) is used to cut tissue or coagulate small blood vessels.

The organ most susceptible to electric current is the heart. An electric current of sufficient magnitude can tetanize the myocardium, resulting in the cessation of circulation for the duration of the applied current. If a tetanizing current is applied for a long period of time, death can result from the lack of systemic circulation. A current of lower intensity, which stimulates only a localized section of the heart, can be considerably more dangerous than one sufficient to tetanize the entire heart. Local excitation of the myocardium can desynchronize the heart, causing random, ineffectual muscle activity known as fibrillation. Fibrillation in the ventricles can be fatal, and reversion to a normal rhythm usually does *not occur* when the electrical current is removed. To restore synchronous activity to the heart, the myocardium must be tetanized by a sufficiently strong current pulse from an external defibrillator.

Figure 7-1 shows the approximate current range for, and the resulting effects of, a one-second exposure to various levels of 60-cycle current applied externally to the body. Regarding the physiological effects that involve the heart or respiration, it is assumed that the current is introduced into the body by electrical contact with the extremities in such a way that the current path includes the chest region.

In the previous discussions, electrical intensity was described in terms of the electrical current. The magnitude of electrical current required to produce a certain physiological effect in a person is influenced by many factors. The voltage level required to effect a current flow is dependent on the resistance offered by the body. The skin offers the most body resistance. The skin provides a natural protection against electrical danger, but when it is permeated by a conductive fluid or when conductive objects such as hypodermic needles are introduced, the resistance of the skin is effectively bypassed. Once the skin resistance is bypassed, the resistance between the contacts is determined only by the resistance of the tissue in the current path, which in most cases is extremely low. Many medical procedures involve the introduction of conductive objects into the body, such as catheters and needles, or the use of electrode paste to measure

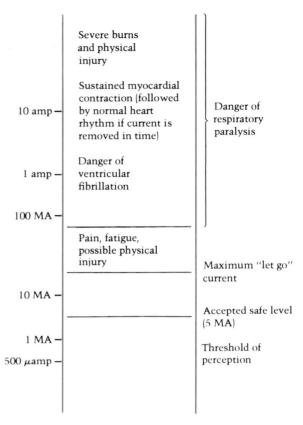

Figure 7-1
Physiological effects of electrical current from a 1-second external contact with the body (60 Hz A.C.).

bioelectric potentials, such as an EEG or ECG. In such procedures, the hospital patient is deprived of the natural protection against electrical hazards that his skin normally provides. With such a resulting low resistance, voltages of even small magnitude can result in a fatal electric current flow.

Macroshock Versus Microshock

In some specific procedures (e.g., cardiac catheterization and cardiac pacing) electrically conductive catheters are introduced directly into the heart. Those procedures pose unique problems. Introduction of an electrically conductive catheter into the heart can establish one of the two electrical contacts that can connect the heart directly to an external electric

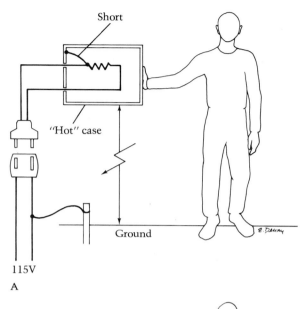

115V

A

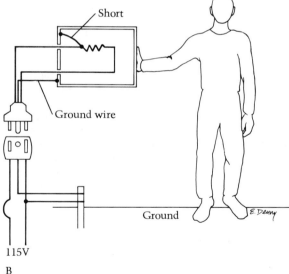

115V

B

Figure 7-2
A. Electrical power distribution with a simple two-wire system. B. Alternate pathway for electrical current flow.

source. In this situation, all the current introduced by the external electrical source flows directly through the heart itself. The current density in the heart can be several orders of magnitude higher than when the same current is applied to a contact more remote from the heart. As a result, a patient with any type of indwelling or cardiac catheter is much more sensitive to electric current than he would otherwise be. Such a patient is said to be "electrically susceptible." The effect of an electric current applied directly to the heart is known as *microshock*. In contrast, the effect of an electrical current applied when no direct connection to the heart exists is referred to as *macroshock*.

How much electrical current is required to induce ventricular fibrillation in humans has not been firmly established because of the obvious experimental difficulties. In a few measurements on humans whose hearts were intentionally fibrillated during open-heart surgery, currents of at least 180 μamp were required. In similar experiments on dogs, fibrillation could be achieved with as little as 20 μamp. For that reason, contemporary standards and specifications for medical equipment have set much lower limits than the 180 μamp found to be necessary to cause fibrillation in the limited number of cases referred to. For equipment to be used with electrically susceptible patients, a maximum leakage current of 10 μamp has been accepted by the majority of medical equipment manufacturers. That limit provides protection should the electrical current accidently flow into the patient.

Importance of the Equipment Ground

To understand any hazard presented by a piece of electrical equipment in the hospital environment, an understanding of the hospital's electrical power distribution system is necessary. Such a power system is illustrated in Figure 7-2A. Note that power distribution is taken care of by a simple two-wire system. In that type of system, one of the wall receptacle contacts is connected to the "hot" wire, and the other "neutral" wire is tied directly to an earth ground. "Earth ground" (or "ground") is a term used to denote any electrical conductor intimately in contact with the earth. Items typically connected to ground include water pipes, metallic room fixtures, or metallic building structures. To be exposed to an electrical macroshock hazard, a person must come in contact with both the hot and the neutral conductors. Remember that at least two connections are required to afford a path for electrical flow. However, because the neutral wire is connected to an earth ground, a shock hazard exists between the hot wire and any conductive object in any way in contact with ground. Great care is taken in the design of electrical equipment (by the use of insulating materials) to prevent accidental contact with the hot wire. However, through routine use, mechanical damage, or insulation breakdown, accidental contact between the equipment case and the hot wire can occur. In this simple "ungrounded" two-wire system, any person touching the equipment while in contact with a grounded object would be exposed to a severe shock hazard.

The purpose of the equipment ground contact on the wall receptacle and the third conductor in a power cord (Fig. 7-2B) is to provide an alternate path for electrical current flow should a short circuit occur. A short circuit, an accidental electrical connection (as illustrated in Fig. 7-2A and B), can occur between a hot wire within the instrument and the equipment case. If a short circuit should occur, the current can return to ground through the equipment ground connection, minimizing the shock hazard. If the resultant current flow in that alternate circuit is sufficiently large, it will trip the circuit breaker for the hot conductor, thus interrupting the current flow.

The benefits of the three-wire system can be realized only if the continuity of the equipment ground connection is always guaranteed. Any interruption of the circuit because of the use of a three-to-two prong adapter (cheater plug) or broken ground pin completely negates the system's protective value. Even if the ground connection is not completely interrupted but exhibits a resistance in excess of about 1 ohm, the resulting voltage developed across the resistance due to the flow of the fault current can be dangerous. If there is any contact with the instrument case exhibiting an elevated voltage, a macroshock hazard exists. For that reason, many hospitals have instituted a rigorous preventive maintenance schedule, checking various parameters of hospital equipment, including ground integrity, on a periodic basis.

Microshock, not macroshock, is a much larger concern in the modern hospital environment, since a microshock hazard can be created by equipment with perfectly intact insulation. This current leakage, which is frequently more than 10 μamp present-day manufacturers use as a guideline, can result from a phenomena known as "capacitive coupling." Much of

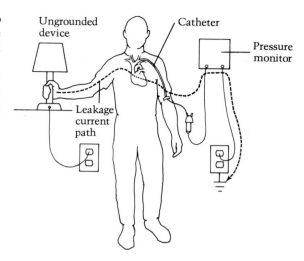

Figure 7-3
Patient directly touching hazardous object.

the patient-monitoring and therapeutic equipment found in the hospital, in household appliances, and in lamps have capacitive leakage in excess of 10 μamp. Although the leakage is of no particular concern for normal operation in places other than the hospital, it can present a true microshock hazard to the electrically susceptible patient. One way such a microshock hazard may occur is when a patient has an indwelling cardiac catheter to measure an intercavitary pressure, such as left or right atrial pressure. The catheter is part of an electronic line-powered monitoring system. The system establishes a path for current flow through the conductive fluid within the catheter, the pressure transducer, and the equipment ground lead in the line cord of the monitoring device. That arrangement establishes a ground connection directly to the patient's heart and more important, a direct path for current flow. Should that occur, a microshock hazard is created by any conductive connection between the patient and an ungrounded electrical device having an excessive leakage current. If that were to occur, the path of current leakage would include the heart of the patient, because it is at that point that the patient is grounded. Figure 7-3 shows the patient touching a hazardous piece of equipment directly. However, a similar conductive connection can be established by another person touching the device and the patient simultaneously. That is only one of the many ways a microshock accident can occur. What is important to note is that in every case a direct connection to the heart from outside the body is required. Therefore special care needs to be taken with a patient with such a connection.

Numerous measures have been taken by equipment manufacturers to reduce the possibility of a microshock accident as a result of patient monitoring. Ultimately, the critical care personnel are responsible for preventing accidental electrocution.

Caution must always be taken with patients who are electrically susceptible. Catheters used to measure pressure and bioelectric potentials should be connected only to monitors that are specially designed to limit current leakage. No steps should be taken intentionally to negate the equipment's inherent safety characteristics by using a three-to-two prong adapter (cheater) cord.

Patients with temporary or temporary-permanent pacing wires present a direct electrical connection to the heart. Care should be taken to ensure that no conductive portion of the pacing wire is exposed. No conductive portion of the wire should be touched by any person in contact with any piece of electrical equipment, including an electric bed, which is frequently found in critical care units.

In the United States, deaths from electricity account for about 1 percent of all accidental deaths. Since many hospital patients are more susceptible than others to danger from electrical current, it is the responsibility of all critical care personnel to not contribute to rising statistics.

III. Systematic Patient Assessment

The critical care nurse may say, "I 'feel' body-mind-spirit concepts, but I don't understand what I feel. What *is* it I feel, besides confusion?"

Ideas of body-mind relatedness are fairly concrete and easy to come to terms with. We can define these relations with what we know of physiology; we can experiment with them in the laboratory. It is when we move to the "spirit" of body-mind-spirit that we have trouble.

The spiritual side of the patient—of ourselves—confuses us as we grope for words because the concept is ineffable: It defies words. This should be expected. Such a discovery should neither surprise nor disappoint us.

If the Tao could be defined,
It would not be the Tao.*

Lao Tsu
c. 600 B.C.

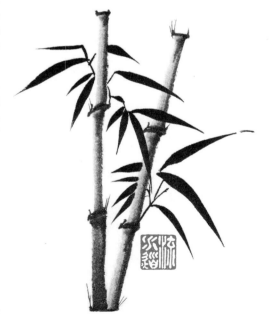

*The Tao is a Buddhist term meaning, roughly, "The Way."

A Practical Approach to the Nursing Assessment

Cathie E. Guzzetta
Cornelia Vanderstaay Kenner

The need for an ordered systematic approach to nursing assessment has become more apparent in recent years as the practice of nursing has expanded to require greater accountability and responsibility in nurse-related actions and care. Nursing assessment encompasses not only a method of identifying the patient's problems but also a method of gaining insight into the causes and/or precipitating factors of the patient's illness, complications, and coexisting abnormalities as they are related to the patient and to his biopsychosocial pattern of response. Nursing assessment as a part of the nursing process was discussed in Chapter 2. This chapter discusses two approaches to nursing assessment that may be used by the nurse in the critical care setting.

Objectives

The nurse should be able to (1) explain why nursing assessment is important, (2) identify the components of a nursing assessment, and (3) describe a systematic ordered approach to nursing assessment.

Achieving the Objectives

To achieve the objectives the nurse should be able to:

1. Describe the usefulness and methodology of a nursing assessment.

8

2. List interviewing techniques and give an example of each.
3. Identify strengths and weaknesses in interviewing techniques.
4. Describe the technique by which symptoms should be elicited and recorded.
5. Identify the specific information that should be elicited from the patient about his past history, medications, and family history.
6. Identify the information that should be looked for in the psychosocial history.
7. Compare and contrast the four techniques used in the physical examination.
8. Compare and contrast the head-to-toe approach and the major-body-systems approach to nursing assessment.
9. Identify the pertinent laboratory data needed for the data base.

How to Proceed

To develop an approach to nursing assessment, the nurse should:

1. Read the material in this chapter carefully.
2. Decide which method of assessment is preferred.
3. Commit herself to some form of systematic and ordered assessment approach as a method of improving skills and the quality of patient care.
4. Select a patient, enlist his cooperation, and use the techniques of interviewing and physical examination for assessment.

Developing an Approach to Nursing Assessment

In past years, nurses were inadequately prepared, both in attitude and by lack of knowledge and skills, to function as the primary care nurse who performs the nursing assessment. In recent years, the inadequacies of the health care system have become abundantly clear to practitioners of all health disciplines as well as to the consumer of health care, and remedies are being sought to improve the care delivery system. Thus, inclusion of the systematic assessment and expansion of the nursing role will be viewed as a significant advancement in health care.

A nursing assessment is a logical, systematic, and ordered collection of data used to evaluate the status of a patient. Developing and perfecting an ordered approach to patient assessment is not easy. The nurse must combine logical and disciplined thinking with deliberate action and methodology. She must develop her senses of touch, sight, hearing, smell and, most assuredly, her common sense. She must have an understanding of the behavioral, biological, social, nursing, and physical sciences. She must know what is normal before she attempts to understand the abnormal. She must know the anatomical, physiological, pathophysiological, and etiological aspects of disease processes, as well as their clinical manifestations. Assessment demands that the nurse have insight into human behavior, relationships, developmental processes, and reactions to stressors and that she be sensitive to human beings. It may also demand that the nurse learn new techniques, approaches, and procedures. Assessment is the analysis and synthesis of data derived from the assessment process. It may be an interpretation of the patient's condition, a determination about the status of a particular problem, or a nursing diagnosis. In short, nursing assessment helps to define the basis of nursing practice as developed and perfected within the framework of a body-mind-spirit approach.

Overlooking things that are, or appear to be, insignificant, is a common human failing [11]. Because critically ill patients tend to have multiple and complex problems, it is not improbable that the nurse may misinterpret or fail to identify clues to those problems. A subtle change in a physical sign or symptom could be the first indication of a serious problem. Early warning signs and/or slight changes in the patient's condition should alert the nurse to the possibility that the patient may have a general system malfunction.

Any change in the patient's condition must not be ignored. The cause of the change must be carefully explored. Every clue must be analyzed. Every unexpected sign must be fully understood before it is dismissed as unimportant. It is obvious that a systematic approach to patient assessment is essential in order to provide highly skilled, comprehensive care.

The initial nursing assessment is performed as soon as possible after the patient is admitted to the floor or unit. It is used to provide a basis for interpreting all future observations, plans, and evaluations. The baseline data include the information necessary to perform an assessment, to identify the nursing diagnoses, and to develop a plan of care. The nurse may then determine what other information is necessary.

The patient's status is reassessed as often as necessary after the initial assessment has been completed and after the patient's problem list and plan of care have been formulated. In that manner, priorities may be determined and nursing care individualized. Reassessment can help determine the acuteness and severity of a problem by comparing the findings to the baseline data. Consider the example of a patient who suddenly complains of a painful right hand 24 hours after his admission to the critical care unit. The nurse quickly assesses the patient and finds that he does not have a right radial pulse. She asks herself the following questions: Is the problem an acute one? Did the patient have a right radial pulse when he was admitted? Was the pulse present four hours ago, when the nurse came on duty? Did the patient's right radial pulse disappear a year ago, when he underwent cardiac catheterization? Did it disappear an hour ago, when his arterial blood was sampled? Should the nurse know the answers to those questions?

There are many useful and practical approaches to systematic assessment of the patient. The *head-to-toe assessment* (which begins with the patient's head and systematically and symmetrically continues to his feet) and the *major-body-systems assessment* (in which individual body systems are appraised; e.g., the respiratory, cardiovascular, and neurological systems etc.) are two popular approaches. At present, neither of those approaches is considered superior to the other (although an investigation to determine which approach is more effective might have interesting results). We ourselves have different opinions on the matter, and so we discuss both approaches in this chapter so that the reader can decide which method suits her better.

The following sections present a general outline that has been developed and used by nurses in the critical care setting. The information in the outline is an organizational tool that may be applied to the head-to-toe or major-body-systems approach or possibly a combination of those approaches. Those two approaches were developed, evaluated, and refined by hundreds of critical care nurses who believed it was important to have an organized approach to nursing assessment and who helped us create a useful, practical critical care assessment guide. The head-to-toe approach (see Chap. 21) and the major-body-systems approach (see Chap. 36) are illustrated in the case studies given in later chapters. (For detailed descriptions of the procedures and techniques related to the psychological and physical examination, the reader should consult the chapters on assessment—Chapters 9–13 and other texts [2, 4–10].)

Whatever approach is used, it should be one that the nurse finds flexible, comfortable, and efficient. But the approach chosen is not the essential factor. The essential factor is that the approach chosen be *systematic* and *ordered*. Adapting an approach to patient assessment implies that the critical care nurse is willing to accept a responsibility and a challenge. It implies *commitment*—commitment to *develop* the approach, to *practice* it, to *refine* it, and to *perfect* it.

To use either approach, the nurse must memorize and be able to immediately recall the components of the approach. She must discuss her findings with the appropriate members of the health care team and record the findings in an accurate concise manner. The initial assessment provides only the baseline data that can be used to evaluate later changes.

A thorough, complete assessment includes more than a systematic approach. If the nurse does not relate findings to pathophysiological and psychological causes, the findings can be of little value. Thus while analyzing the case studies throughout the text, the nurse should consider what pathophysiological phenomena might be related to the patient's chief complaint, history, physical findings and laboratory data. She should see how many things she can put together. In the critical care setting, the nurse has to think quickly and logically. It is impossible to give each body system equal attention, and usually, it is not necessary to do so. The nurse must focus on the patient's chief complaint, symptoms, signs, and diagnosis. That approach will frequently point to the organ system (or systems) involved. Almost all physical findings are related to pathophysiological processes or identified problems. The nurse must always consider those two domains together. By doing so, she is in a better position to alter, expand, or discontinue specific nursing acts. She can also be more aware of the direction for immediate and future observations of all plans and care delivered to her patients. When the nurse can correlate her assessment skills with her clinical knowledge and theoretical framework, she can experience the exhilaration that transforms patient care from a mundane chore to a transcendent, rewarding experience.

Collecting Data

The primary source of data for the nursing assessment is the patient. If the patient is unable to respond or if the patient is an unreliable source of information, the historical data can be supplemented through the use of secondary sources. Secondary sources are the patient's family and/or significant others, the health team members, people in the patient's immediate environment (i.e., other patients or people in the patient's community) and the patient's record.

Assessment Techniques

Five techniques are used in doing a nursing assessment: (1) interviewing, (2) inspection, (3) palpation, (4) percussion, and (5) auscultation. Those techniques will be outlined in the following sections. (Specific details for assessment of the patient's major body systems are contained in the following chapters.)

The Interview

The patient interview is conducted to gather specific information that can be used to develop a plan of patient care. In fact, it may provide more essential information than either the physical examination or the laboratory findings. The patient interview is also conducted to establish a trusting relationship between the patient and the nurse. The interview can help the professional nurse gain insight into the patient's ability to function, his behavior, and the severity of his illness.

During the interview, a psychosocial assessment is made of both the patient and his family. The nurse first attempts to identify any problems that may aggravate the patient's critical condition. Factors to be assessed include appearance, speech, behavior, thought processes, emotions, intellectual function, and judgment. The immediate critical care period is often filled with bewildering and painful treatments. If the patient has just been admitted to the hospital, the staff and the environment are new. Just how the experiences are handled by the nurse is important since a complex process of impressions and interrelationships is initiated. The event of hospitalization for each patient and his family has a potential for producing stress that will complicate treatments and affect future outcomes. Knowledge in many areas of physiological problems has progressed to the point of being able to predict high-risk factors and possible complications, but much less knowledge exists to predict possibilities of psychological problems. Illness

that requires hospitalization causes some disturbance in the patient's interpersonal and social functioning. Such disturbance arises out of the meaning that the illness has for the person, emotionally as well as intellectually. How he behaves will depend on his family, social, and cultural background. (Likewise, how others treat him when he is ill will depend on the meanings they attach to his illness and his behavior.) Social and cultural factors appear to be significantly related to the way the patient perceives and responds to happenings in his environment. The role of cultural and social patterns in human physiological processes may be commanding enough in certain situations to act against the direct biological needs of the patient.

Under normal circumstances, the patient may be viewed as part of a family system in which a change in one part of the system affects other parts of the system. The patient's return to a state of well-being enhances the family's well-being, and the family's ability to function in the stress situation enhances the patient's well-being. According to Lewis et al. [12], three major types of family systems are operant: the healthy, midrange, and pathological family systems. In the healthy family system, the family can examine, evaluate, and welcome new input into the system. The family structure is clear and flexible with a directional change viewed as nonthreatening. In the midrange family system, the structure is relatively clear, but the family members are rigid and adapt poorly to change. In the pathological family system, the individual family members lack autonomous functioning. The family operates as an ill-defined group in which the members are caught up together with no distinct ego boundaries. There is little vital interaction with the outside world. Importantly, independent estimates of the family system correlate with estimates of the degree of pathology of offspring from these families.

Interviewing involves communication between two individuals. Communication is the act of transmitting facts, feelings, and meanings by words, gestures, or other actions. Thus communication may be verbal or nonverbal. Facilitation of communication, as well as the provision of emotional support, involves paying close attention to the patient and determining what is going on inside the patient. The nurse must recognize the emotions or feelings that the patient may be having. Close attention must be paid to his facial expression, voice quality, body language, and other subjective and objective data. Once feelings are recognized, the nurse should respond to those feelings as accurately as possible and then remain silent for a few moments so the patient may respond.

Obtaining an informative interview depends on the nurse's approach and on the patient's response. The patient may be more motivated to respond if the nurse has an interested, accepting, and empathetic approach. The nurse must have a nonjudgmental attitude toward the philosophy, attitudes, and behavior of her patients. A calm, unhurried approach can convey a feeling of interest in the patient, and it is essential in facilitating the communication process. A pleasant, private, and unstressful setting for the interview is also essential. The critical care nurse must realize that interviewing is an art and that her techniques must be constantly practiced, reevaluated, and updated. To improve her skill, nurses should critically observe the interviewing techniques of other nurses, teachers, and physicians.

In the critical care unit, in-depth interviewing frequently cannot be implemented since the patient is seriously ill and since the interaction would seem artificial. The initial interview is limited to information essential for immediate care. Once the patient's condition has stabilized, support has been offered, and trust has been established, other important information such as dietary history and sleep patterns may be obtained. The nurse is at the patient's bedside many times during the day and selectively should employ appropriate interviewing techniques. A good time to communicate and obtain information is during the administration of physical care. It is important to record and communicate information accurately so the patient will not repeatedly be asked for the same information.

Factors that block communication should be considered. Those factors may be related to the patient's response, the nurse's attitude, the collection of data, the structure of the interview, and the validation of data. Using the following outline, nurses should reexamine their interviewing techniques in an attempt to identify problems that hinder an informative interview [1, 3, 5, 10].

PATIENT'S RESPONSE

1. Fear, anxiety, denial
2. Patient's inability to verbalize what he feels
3. Embarrassment
4. Ignorance

5. Shame
6. Poor memory

NURSE'S ATTITUDE

1. An inappropriately warm or cold attitude
2. Inattentive, disinterested, bored, or preoccupied
3. Lack of eye contact
4. Too much or too little interest in emotional factors
5. Unaware of patient's nonverbal communication and behavior
6. Inappropriate use of silence (e.g., teenagers are made uneasy by silences)
7. Failing to facilitate communication (e.g., too much or too little head nodding or rigid body and facial expression)

STRUCTURE

1. Beginning the interview too quickly, not allowing time to put the patient at ease
2. Allowing the patient to ramble
3. Needlessly repeating questions owing to forgetfulness or inattentive listening
4. Discussing emotional or embarrassing topics before gaining the patient's confidence and cooperation (e.g., sexual activities, alcohol, mental illness and/or illegal use of drugs)
5. Making poor transitions between topics
6. Failing to progress from the general to the specific or from the nonpersonal to the personal
7. Failing to use an organized approach

DATA COLLECTION

1. Failing to ask important questions
2. Failing to identify pertinent negatives
3. Failing to recognize time relationships
4. Failing to let the patient tell his own story
5. Failing to investigate important clues the patient gives

VALIDATION OF DATA

1. Using terms the patient does not understand (e.g., angina pectoris, epigastric pain); failing to adjust to the patient's vocabulary; failing to evaluate the patient's cultural and educational levels
2. Failing to give the patient time to complete his answers to questions

3. Overwhelming the patient with numerous, complicated, or long questions
4. Failing to consider various interpretations of the patient's symptoms
5. Failing to determine the patient's understanding of his illness and his expectations

Since one purpose of the interview is to obtain as much information as possible, it is essential that the nurse learn techniques that will both control the interview and facilitate communication. She must remember that the patient does not have a systematic, overall knowledge of his illness and, therefore, cannot be expected to give an organized history. Also, some patients need help in expressing their ideas, and others need help in directing their thoughts. Several types of statements and questions can be of help. Among them are the neutral question, the simple, direct question, the supplementary statement, the leading question, the open-ended question, the question that reflects content, and the loaded question. Depending on the patient and the situation, the skilled interviewer may use some or all of those statements and questions to gather, identify, explore, and clarify information [3, 5, 10].

1. *Neutral questions* are questions that are structurally unbiased and that do not prompt the patient to give a more acceptable or pleasing answer. Neutral questions should be used whenever possible. They may be either open or closed. "Tell me more about your chest pain" is an open neutral question. The closed neutral question is one that is structured to include several choices: "Would you say that your last episode of chest pain lasted for 5 minutes, 15 minutes, 30 minutes, or more?"
2. *Simple direct questions* are questions that require a direct answer, such as yes or no. It is important in gaining specific facts such as statistical data, and it helps the patient focus on a particular point of interest. Because the simple direct question demands a direct response, it is closed and generally it tends to discourage verbalization. It may be neutral, depending on the context. "Do you ever wake up at night with chest pain?" "Have any of your relatives had diabetes?" Although direct questions may be helpful in preventing the patient from discussing unimportant facts and in clarifying details, they should be used with moderation because they are self limiting.
3. *Supplementary statements* may encourage an open, neutral interview. The supplementary statement lets the patient know that the nurse is interested, and it stimulates him to continue verbalizing at his own pace. Statements such as "Yes," "Go on," or "Umm" and pauses allow the patient to verbalize as he wishes and help him remember what he wants to say.
4. *Leading questions* generate a bias and may put words in the patient's mouth. A patient may answer a leading question according to what he thinks the nurse wants to hear. However, leading questions may be useful for testing the validity of the patient's answers: "Would you say that your chest pain only develops several hours after eating a large meal?"
5. *Open-ended questions* may also help to generate free-flowing communication. Transitional phrases, such as, "You were saying?" and "And after that, you?" are often effective.
6. *Reflecting content* is a common communication technique. The nurse repeats the patient's feeling or interpretation of a particular subject.

Patient: I was pretty scared when I came to the hospital.
Nurse: You were pretty scared?
Patient: Yes, I thought I was going to die.

Reflecting content can be a difficult technique to develop because the nurse must determine what statements are likely to produce meaningful information when they are explored. But the technique provides a method of exploring emotionally charged subjects with the patient in a relatively neutral and unobjectionable manner.

7. *Loaded questions* may be used occasionally to assess the patient's reaction to a particular topic. Since a loaded question automatically generates a bias, the answer itself is not as important as the patient's reaction to it: "Do you think your wife is the cause of your nervousness?" Such a loaded question is used only after enough information has been gathered to make the nurse suspect that the patient is reacting to a marital problem. The "shock technique" is used to assess a specific problem and it should be used only when the interviewer has a specific objective in mind.

Inspection

Inspection (or observation) refers to the visual examination of the patient in which normal, unusual, and abnormal features are noted. Inspection is an extremely important technique, and it should never be neglected or hurried. One must learn not only to see but also to observe. The general appearance of the area is first observed, followed by inspection of the area for details and characteristics. The examiner observes for size, appearance, symmetry, normalcy, anatomical landmarks, color, movement, temperature, and abnormalities.

Palpation

After inspection, palpation is generally done. Palpation involves the use of the hands and fingers to determine texture, temperature, moisture, elasticity, position, pulsations, vibrations, consistency, and shape. It is also done to identify pain, tenderness, swelling, organ enlargement, muscular spasm, rigidity, or crepitus. In most situations, the examiner uses a light pressure technique and presses down on the area being examined several times rather than simply holding his fingertips in place. The fingertips are the most sensitive areas used for palpation for general purposes, with the back of the hands or fingers used for temperature sense and the palmar surface of the metacarpal joints used for vibratory sense. (Deep palpation and the bimanual technique are explained in Chapter 12.)

Percussion

Percussion is usually done after palpation. It involves striking the body surface with a finger or fingers to produce a sound. Percussion may be direct (the body surface is struck directly with the fingers) or indirect (the index or middle finger is placed firmly on the skin and the distal third of that finger is struck with the middle finger of the other hand). Percussion is used to determine size, density, organ boundaries, and location. The sounds heard on percussion may be tympanic, resonant, dull, or flat. A tympanic sound is clear and hollow, like the sound heard when a gas-filled stomach is percussed. A resonant sound is a clear, hollow sound that is heard when a normal lung is percussed. A dull sound is high pitched and thudding, like the sound heard over the heart. A flat sound is low pitched and abrupt; it can be produced by percussing a solid mass, such as an arm.

Auscultation

Auscultation, listening to sounds produced by various organs and tissues, generally involves the use of a stethoscope (see Chaps. 9, 10). The frequency, intensity, quality, and duration of each sound is considered. A well fitting, carefully selected stethoscope placed in the examiner's ears correctly is essential for effective auscultation [13].

Head-to-Toe Nursing Assessment: The History

History taking is essentially the same for both the head-to-toe nursing assessment and the major-body-systems nursing assessment. The two approaches differ mainly in the manner in which the recording of data is organized on the assessment sheet. The following outline has been specifically used for history taking in the head-to-toe nursing assessment (see Chap. 21).

Informant

A brief statement is generally made about the reliability of the person giving the history. In most cases, that person is the patient although under certain circumstances the informant may be a relative or friend (e.g., when the patient is unconscious, confused, or acutely ill).

Chief Complaint

The chief complaint is written up in a brief statement describing what the patient believes is his major problem. The chief complaint is not the diagnosis. It should reflect why the patient has sought medical help. The question, "What brought you to the hospital?" may elicit the patient's chief complaint. The chief complaint is frequently stated in the patient's own words and put in quotation marks.

History of Present Illness

The history of the present illness is a comprehensive description of the patient's current problems that he thinks are important. The history should describe, in the order in which they occurred, the patient's symptoms and problems. It includes information on medications, treatments, tests, surgical procedures, complications, attending physicians, and hospitals. The symptoms should be described in regard to:

1. Onset (time and date): Where and under what circumstances, gradual or sudden, and any previous history of the symptom
2. Location: Where it occurred (patient should point to the exact location)
3. Quality: How patient felt when it occurred
4. Quantity: Mild or severe; frequency
5. Duration: How long it lasts
6. Aggravating and alleviating factors: What makes it worse, what makes it better
7. Associated factors: Were any other phenomena associated with the symptom (ask about factors that one expects to be related to the symptom)
8. Course: How the sign/symptom progresses with time

It is important also to state pertinent negatives, the absence of certain signs or symptoms that might generally be involved with the problem or system being considered (e.g., absence of pedal edema, sudden weight gain, or dyspnea in a patient suspected of having heart failure). If the patient has more than one presenting complaint, it is important to identify each one separately and to develop it chronologically, using the outline and information just discussed, to determine its signs, symptoms, and characteristics (e.g., the patient whose chief presenting complaint is abdominal pain may also complain of night sweats and blurred vision).

Past Medical History

A summary of the patient's past medical history is meaningful in obtaining an overall picture of the patient's health history and prognosis. It should include information about:

1. All childhood illnesses
2. All major and minor adult illnesses (dates, treatment, complications)
3. All past hospitalizations (chronological dates and, if appropriate, attending physicians)
4. All past surgical procedures (chronological dates, attending physicians and complications if appropriate)

5. Injuries or accidents (dates, treatment, residual disability)
6. Previous blood transfusions (date of last blood transfusion, type of blood reaction if any)
7. Drug or food allergies (kind of reaction the patient has to each; e.g., diarrhea, dizziness, rash, nausea, vomiting)
8. Past pregnancies and deliveries (type of delivery, number of pregnancies, any abnormalities)
9. Foreign travel (dates, places)
10. Previous reactions and response to illness

Family History

A survey of the patient's family history is valuable in obtaining information about familial trends and in identifying genetic predisposition. It may also be used to grossly estimate life expectancy. The following information should be included in the family history:

1. Age, sex, and health status of living family members, including parents, siblings, children, and spouse
2. Age, sex, and cause of death of deceased family members
3. Any familial disease history related to the following:

Cancer	Hypertension
Heart disease	Kidney disease
Migraine headaches	Arthritic conditions
Tuberculosis	Hematological
Diabetes mellitus	abnormalities
Nervous or mental	Stroke
conditions	Rheumatic fever
Epilepsy	Sickle cell anemia

Current Drugs

A list of the medications taken (or omitted) by the patient on the day of admission should be recorded. If the patient has brought medications to the hospital, the names of the drugs, the dosages, and the frequency of administration should be identified before the drugs are taken from the patient's room. If the patient is not sure of the names of the medications, his family should bring the bottles to the hospital to be checked by the pharmacist. The patient should be questioned about his use of aspirin, laxatives, sleeping pills, diet pills, birth control pills, narcotics, insulin, digitalis, or steroid hormone replacements.

Alcohol and Tobacco Habits

Obtain the following information about the patient's alcohol and tobacco habits:

1. Alcohol (average daily, weekend, social consumption; type of alcohol: e.g., beer, gin, wine, whiskey; has alcohol consumption interfered with marriage, job, health)
2. Tobacco (type of tobacco: e.g., cigarettes, cigars, pipe, chewing tobacco; amount per day or per week; age began smoking; age smoking habit increased, decreased, ceased)

Dietary and Fluid Needs

A statement should be made about the patient's dietary and fluid habits (quantity, frequency, preference, or intolerance). Determine if the patient has difficulty chewing or swallowing. It may be helpful to ask the patient what he ate and drank the day before coming into the hospital. The patient may have been quite ill prior to his admission, and his oral intake the day before admission may not reflect his usual dietary and fluid habits. Also, the information may be helpful in determining specific nutritional and hydration problems that may have been precipitated by the acute illness. Record any fluid or dietary restrictions (low-sodium, low-fat, low-protein diets) or special diets due to cultural or religious preferences (vegetarian, kosher).

Sleep and Rest Patterns

Determine the amount of sleep the patient averages per night and what his normal sleeping times are (day or night). Does the patient have regular rest periods? Do his rest periods include sleep, relaxation, or meditation? What is the length, time, and reason for his rest periods? Does he have any problems with sleep and does he use any medications or other aids to induce sleep (warm shower, hot milk, alcohol, tranquilizers, hypnotics)?

Bowel and Bladder Habits

Bowel and bladder habits tend to be of major concern to the hospitalized patient. Note any problems the patient may have related to:

BOWEL HABITS

1. What is the patient's elimination pattern? (frequency, consistency, color, presence of blood, mucus)
2. Does the patient have trouble with elimination?
3. Does he use laxatives, suppositories, or enemas regularly? (type, amount, frequency)
4. Does he prefer one type of laxative?
5. When was his last bowel movement?
6. Does he have (or anticipate having) problems using a bedpan?
7. Does he have a colostomy or an ileostomy? If he does, how does he handle evacuation? What supplies does he need? Did he bring the supplies to the hospital? Does he need assistance? What are his teaching needs?

BLADDER HABITS

1. Does the patient have problems voiding?
2. Does he have nocturia?
3. Does he have (or anticipate having) problems using a urinal?
4. Did he have a Foley catheter in place when he came to the hospital? If he had, when was it last changed? Why was it placed?

Hygiene Needs

Knowing the patient's hygiene habits may help the nurse to plan the patient's care and make him more comfortable. What are the patient's bathing and hair-washing habits? How often and when does the patient generally bathe and wash his hair? Does he prefer a shower or a bath? Does the patient seem to have good hygiene? Does he have good oral hygiene?

Occupation and Education

Obtain information about the patient's job, including type of employment, number of hours he works every day and every week, whether he takes work home, the amount and type of strenuous physical or mental activity, the amount and type of stressful or pressured activity. Does he have a hazardous job (e.g., painting, working with radioactive substances, mining)? The information collected may alert the nurse to possible areas of patient education and/or job counseling referrals to be included in the plan of care. Important psychosocial problems, worries, and concerns that might affect the patient's hospital course and recovery are frequently uncovered in the history taking (e.g., loss of job, financial problems, an impending business deal, children at home unsupervised).

Find out about the patient's education. A point often overlooked is whether the patient can read or write. The patient's understanding of his condition and his ability to follow directions may be affected by his educational background.

Exercise Habits

Assess the patient's exercise habits. Ask about the amount, frequency, and type of exercise he gets in his job, in sports, and during household activities.

Spiritual Needs

Find out the patient's religious background and the depth of his involvement with his faith. Ask the patient whether he wishes the nurse to contact the hospital chaplain or his pastor about his hospitalization.

Personal Interest

Determine what the patient's interests and hobbies are (e.g., reading, watching television, listening to the radio). Too often critical care patients have nothing to do but dwell on their illness. When appropriate, allow the patient to engage in an unstressful pastime. A hobby can be extremely therapeutic, even in a critical care unit. Radios, magazines, novels, cards, checkers, and crossword puzzles can be kept on the critical care unit.

Family Member Interaction and Availability

The availability of family members, and what their interactions are, is important. Stress in the patient's family may be high, particularly right after the patient's admission, and their problem-solving abilities may be low.

Attitude Toward Illness and Hospitalization

Information should be obtained about the patient's perception of his illness and hospitalization. Does the patient seem anxious, depressed, withdrawn, or afraid? What experiences and coping mechanisms has the patient used in the past to deal with crises? Identify the patient's expectations in regard to his current illness. What does he expect from the health team members? From his family? From himself? What does the patient think is wrong with him? What has the patient been told about his hospitalization? What has the doctor told the patient about his illness and about methods of diagnosis and treatment? Information should also be obtained about the attitudes of the patient's spouse and other relatives, which may play an important role in determining how the patient will react and feel toward his current situation.

Head-to-Toe Nursing Assessment: Components of the Physical Examination

While performing the head-to-toe physical examination, the nurse first examines the patient's head and systematically continues the assessment to the patient's toes. Additionally, a systematic approach is used while examining each area. During examination of the patient's mouth, for example, the nurse begins with general observations. She reminds herself of the major functions of the mouth and she checks those functions for normalcy. She examines the external mouth and then the internal mouth, proceeding systematically with the buccal mucosa, gums, teeth, tongue, hard palate, and soft palate.

The components of the complete physical examination are outlined in the following sections. Frequently, in the critical care unit, however, only the most appropriate areas for examination are included in the initial assessment. The history will significantly help the nurse focus on the part of the physical examination to be emphasized. The following information can be used as an organizational guide during the head-to-toe physical assessment.

Vital Signs

The vital signs of each patient are routinely checked on his admission. The check provides a means of rapidly evaluating the condition of the patient. The vital signs are the temperature, apical and radial pulses, respirations, and blood pressure taken with the patient in the supine position in the right and left arm and in the sitting position. Also, the patient's height, weight, and ECG rhythm are recorded, and note is made of any evidence of atrial, junctional, or ventricular ectopic beats.

General Appearance

1. General observations: Age, race, weight, general state of health, nutritional status, development, personality, gross physical abnormalities, level of consciousness
2. Color: Pink, pale, redness, pallor, jaundiced, mottled, blanching, increased pigmentation, cyanosis (degree and location: eyes, ears, nose, mouth, tongue, neck, chest, legs, extremities, hands, fingers, toes)
3. Skin
   a. Pigmentation, color changes, vascularity, moistness, dryness, oiliness, temperature, elasticity, texture, turgor, mobility, thickness
   b. Lesions (type, color, distribution, size, shape, configuration): Macules (moles, petechiae, freckles), tumors, wheals, bullae, papules, blisters, pustules, vesicles, ulcerations, erosions, nodules, cysts, scales, crusts, fissures, calluses, bites, scars, keloids, hives, excoriations, plaques, bruises, bleeding, pruritus, dermatitis, edema
   c. Nails: Shape, color, thickness, texture, lesions, clubbing, splinter hemorrhages
   d. Hair: Color, distribution, quantity, texture, pattern of hair loss

Neurological (see also Neurological Assessment, Chapter 11)

1. Mental status: State of consciousness, behavior, mood, attitude, facial expression, emotional status (anxiety, fear, pain, restlessness, anger), affect, logic, coherence of thought, attention, concentration, recent memory, remote memory, intellectual performance, judgment, illusions, hallucinations, dress, grooming, speech (clarity, loudness, relevance, abnormalities)
2. Cranial nerves
3. Motor: Muscle size, tone, strength, symmetry, movement, atrophy, fasciculation, involuntary or other abnormal movements
4. Cerebellar: Posture and gait (use of cane, walker, wheelchair, crutches, prosthesis of extremity), balance, coordination, position, ability to perform rapid and alternating movement of upper and lower extremities, finger-to-nose-to-finger movement
5. Sensory: Perception of stimulus and symmetry; pain, light touch, temperature, vibratory, positional, and discriminative sensations
6. Deep tendon and superficial reflexes: Degree of response (4+ = very brisk, 3+ = brisker than normal, 2+ = average, 1+ = diminished, 0 = no response) and symmetry of stretch
7. Meningeal signs (not elicited routinely; elicited when inflammation of meninges suspected): Nucal rigidity (stiff neck); Brudzinski's sign (have patient flex his head on his chest and observe him for flexion of the hips and knees; Kernig's sign (have patient flex his leg at the hip and knee and observing him for resistance or pain while he straightens his knee)

Head and Face

1. Size, contour, symmetry, color, pain, tenderness, tumors, lesions, scars, discoloration, edema, involuntary or other abnormal movements
2. Scalp: Color, texture, scales, lumps, lesions, inflammation, swelling
3. Face: Movement, expression, pigmentation, acromegaly, moon facies, scleroderma, cachexia, myxedema, acne, facial tics, tremors, scars

Eyes

1. Visual acuity: Gross visual fields, visual loss, glasses, contact lenses, eye prosthesis, myopia, hyperopia, diplopia, photophobia, colored vision, pain, burning

2. Eyelids: Color, ptosis, periorbital edema, lesions, styes, xanthelasma (yellowish deposits), exophthalmos (prominence of eyes)
3. Extraocular movement: Ability to follow; position and alignment of eyes, strabismus, nystagmus (rapid, jerking motion of eyes), lid lag
4. Conjunctiva: Color, discharge, conjunctivitis, vascular changes, nodules, lesions, swelling
5. Iris: Color, markings
6. Sclera: Color, vascularity, nodules, lesions, jaundice
7. Cornea: Color, symmetry, abrasions, opacities, keratitis (inflammation), arcus senilis (grey-white ring around cornea)
8. Pupils: Size, shape, equality, reaction to light (direct pupillary reflex, or constriction, of lighted eye and consensual pupillary reflex, or constriction of unlighted eye)
9. Retina: Translucence, red reflex (orange glow in pupil), exudates, venous pulsations, arteriolar narrowing, arteriovenous nicking, hemorrhages, papilledema (swelling of optic nerve)

Ears

1. Auditory acuity: Hearing, lateralization and conduction of sound, hearing loss, hearing aid (attached to ear or glasses), pain, sensitivity to sound, tinnitus
2. External ear:
   a. Ear lobe: Size, shape, color, symmetry, deformities, ear lobe crease, sebaceous cysts, pain, tenderness
   b. Auricle (pinna): Size, shape, color, symmetry, deformities, sebaceous cysts, lumps, eczema, pain, tenderness, inflammation
   c. External auditory canal: Size, shape, color, deformities, cerumen (wax), foreign bodies, cysts, tumors, lesions, tophi (white uric acid deposits), calcification, discharge (serous, mucoid, sanguinous, purulent, malodorous), swelling, narrowing, pain
3. Tympanic membrane: Integrity (normal eardrum is oval, grey, and translucent), erythema, thickening, bulging (acute otitis media), retraction, flatness, perforation, scars, lesions, inflammation, redness, cholesteatomas

4. Inner ear: Signs and symptoms of vertigo and nystagmus

Nose

1. Sense of smell, size, symmetry, deformities, nasal flaring, sneezing
2. Nasal mucosa and vestibule: Color, size, shape, edema, exudate, bleeding, lesions, furuncles, pain, tenderness, narrowing, inflammation
3. Nasal septum: Shape, perforation, deviation, deformities, bleeding
4. Inferior and middle turbinates: Color, swelling, exudate, polyps
5. Sinus tenderness or pain

Mouth and Throat

1. Odor, pain, ability to bite, chew, taste, swallow, speak
2. Lips: Color, symmetry, hydration, lesions, fissures, crusting, fever blisters (herpes simplex), cracking, swelling, numbness, drooling, ulceration
3. Buccal mucosa: Color, pigmentation, moisture, parotid ducts, ulceration, nodules, white patches, plaques, dryness, excess saliva, hemorrhage
4. Gums: Color, edema, bleeding, lesions, inflammation, retraction, discoloration, pain
5. Teeth: Number, missing, dark, loose teeth, caries, bridges, dentures (should be removed for examination), pain, sensitivity to heat and cold
6. Tongue: Symmetry, color, mobility, size, hydration, markings, soreness, midline protrusion, ulcers, coating, nodules, tumors, burning, swelling, fasciculations, abnormal smoothness, tumors under tongue
7. Hard palate: Color, lesions, ulcers, cysts
8. Soft palate, uvula, anterior and posterior pillars, tonsils and posterior pharynx: Color, symmetry, edema, exudate, inflammation, swelling, ulceration, tonsillar enlargement, pain, tenderness. While patient says "Ah," note the rise of his soft palate and uvula.
9. Throat: Gag reflex, soreness, cough (productive, nonproductive, changing), sputum (character, color, consistency, amount, odor), hemoptysis

10. Voice: Hoarseness, decrease in loudness, loss of voice, change in pitch

Neck

1. Symmetry, movement, range of motion, contour, strength and tenderness of muscles, masses, scars, edema, pain, stiffness, paralysis
2. Trachea: Deviation, scars
3. Thyroid: Size, shape, symmetry, tenderness, enlargement, nodules, bruits, scars
4. Carotid arteries: Quality, strength and symmetry of pulsations, bruits (see Chap. 10)
5. Jugular veins: Internal jugular vein pulsations, jugular venous pressure, venous distention (see Chap. 10)
6. Lymph nodes: Size, shape, mobility, tenderness, enlargement

Chest

1. Size, shape, symmetry, anteroposterior (A-P) diameter, transverse diameter (should be smaller than A-P diameter), ribs (normal downward slope), deformities (pigeon chest, pectus excavatum, or inward depression of lower sternum), pain, tenderness, turgor, temperature, edema, crepitation
2. Skin: Color, rash, scars, hair distribution, spider nevi, muscular development, abnormal venous patterns
3. Intercostal spaces: Size, retraction, bulging

Breasts

1. Contour, symmetry, color, size, shape, inflammation, scars, masses (location, size, shape, mobility, tenderness), pain, dimpling, swelling
2. Nipples: Color, discharge, ulceration, bleeding, inversion, pain
3. Axilla: Axillary nodes, enlargement, tenderness, rash, infection

Respiratory (see also Respiratory Assessment, Chapter 9)

1. Inspection: Regularity, rate, depth, ease, sound, symmetry, abnormal breathing patterns (asymmetric, obstructive, restrictive), use of accessory (costal, abdominal) muscles for respiration
2. Palpation: Transmission of vocal or tactile fremitus (have patient say "99"; may be normal, increased, decreased, absent), respiratory excursion
3. Percussion: Intensity, pitch, quality, duration, equality of sound (percussion sounds may be flat, dull, resonant, hyperresonant, tympanic)
4. Auscultation: Normal vesicular, bronchovesicular, bronchial breath sounds; adventitious sounds (rales, rhonchi, wheezes, pleural friction rub); vocal resonance (bronchophony, egophony, pectoriloquy)

Cardiac (see also Cardiovascular Assessment, Chapter 10)

1. Inspection and palpation: Point of maximum impulse, or PMI (location, diameter, duration, amplitude), precordial lifts, heaves, thrills, implanted cardiac pacemaker
2. Percussion: Right and left cardiac borders
3. Auscultation: Cardiac rate, rhythm, intensity, regularity, skipped or extra beats; quality, intensity, and splitting of S_1 and S_2; extra sounds (S_3, S_4, clicks, snaps): location, time in cardiac cycle; murmurs (time in cardiac cycle, configuration, pitch, quality, intensity [grading], location, radiation, changes with respiration and position); pericardial friction rub (location, time in cardiac cycle, intensity, quality), clicking of ball-valve heart prosthesis

Abdomen (see also Abdominal Assessment, Chapter 12)

1. Inspection: Skin, color, size, symmetry, contour, fat, muscle tone, peristaltic activity, turgor, hair distribution, scars, umbilicus (contour, inflammation, herniation), striae, fetus, dilated vessels, tautness, rashes, lesions, distention, ascites, abnormal pulsations
2. Auscultation (done before palpation or percussion so that bowel sounds will not be altered): Bowel sounds (absent = 0, hypoactive = 1+, normal = 2+, hyperactive = 3+), bruits, liver or splenic friction rubs, venous hum

3. Percussion: Liver borders, gastric air bubble (left upper quadrant), splenic dullness, air, fluid, masses
4. Palpation: Liver edge, spleen, organ enlargement, muscle spasm or rigidity, ascites, masses (location, size, shape, mobility, tenderness, consistency, pulsations), involuntary guarding, tenderness, rebound tenderness, pain

Genitourinary

1. Renal: Urinary output (amount, color, odor, sediment, specific gravity, protein, sugar, acetone), frequency, urgency, hesitancy, burning, pain, dribbling, incontinence, hematuria, nocturia, oliguria, polyuria, anuria, bladder distention
2. Female genitalia: Inspection of labia majora, labia minora, clitoris, urethral and vaginal orifices; discharge (consistency, color, odor, amount), color, swelling, ulceration, lesions, nodules, inflammation, tenderness, pain
3. Male genitalia: (a) Penis: skin, prepuce, foreskin, glans, urethral orifice; size, contour, color, discharge, ulceration, lesions, nodules, inflammation, pain, (b) Scrotum: color, size, nodules, inflammation, swelling, ulceration, tenderness, pain, (c) Testes: size, shape, consistency, absence, atrophy, swelling, tenderness, pain, masses
4. Rectum: Pilonidal cysts, anal pigmentation, hemorrhoids, excoriation, rash, abscess, anal fissure, anorectal fistula, masses, lesions, inflammation, tenderness, pain, itching

Extremities

1. Size, shape, symmetry, range of motion, hair distribution, temperature, color, pigmentation, paralysis, numbness, prosthesis, scars, pain, nodules, lesions, ulceration, bruising, hematomas, rash, deformities, swelling, edema (pitting, nonpitting, dependent, positional)
2. Joints: Symmetry, active and passive mobility, deformities, stiffness, fixation, masses, inflammation, swelling, redness, heat, fluid in joint capsule, bogginess, crepitation, bony enlargement, pain, tenderness
3. Muscles: Symmetry, size, strength, tone, weakness, stiffness, cramps, rigidity, hypertrophy, atrophy, myotonia (inability to relax muscle con-

traction), spasm, tremor, fasciculation, pain, tenderness
4. Bones: Resistance, deformities, fractures, tenderness, pain
5. Arteries: Symmetry and strength of pulses (radial, brachial, axillary, femoral, popliteal, dorsalis pedis, posterior tibial), claudication
6. Veins: Venous filling, varicosities, phlebitis, superficial or deep thrombophlebitis

Back

Scars, sacral edema, spinal abnormalities, kyphosis (accentuation of convexity of thoracic spine), scoliosis (curvature of thoracic spine), spinal tenderness, scars

Major-Body-Systems Approach to Nursing Assessment

The written format of the major-body-systems approach is based on the problem oriented system and is particularly useful as an initial nursing assessment tool in coordination with the problem oriented medical record (see Chap. 4). Since the physician will obtain information primarily needed for medical care, it is the responsibility of the nurse to obtain information primarily needed for nursing care. Although the organization of the written document differs from the head-to-toe systematic assessment tool, the information to be obtained is essentially the same and has been previously described in this chapter.

In assessing the patient using the major-body-systems approach, the examiner evaluates one system and then another, rather than one part of the body and then another. With the major-body-systems approach, the examiner can think about and assess each system as she is proceeding with the examination. Thus she can evaluate one system more thoroughly than another if she needs to. The major-body-systems approach is a way of thinking.

In life-threatening situations or when the patient is unconscious, a rapid evaluation of the patient according to the ABCs of basic life support and a rapid head-to-toe assessment naturally take precedence over a major-body-systems assessment.

As the first part of the major-body-systems assessment, the examiner evaluates the pertinent historical findings and correlates these findings with the corresponding body system. The nurse thus knows which body systems should be emphasized. Depending on the patient's condition, the initial examination may be thorough or it may be quick with parts of the examination completed later. And when the patient is critically ill, a more detailed data base should always be completed later. The respiratory system is usually examined first, and then the cardiovascular and neurological systems. If the examiner prefers to do a regional examination, she thinks of body systems as she moves from region to region. The examination of one body system does not have to be completed before the examination of another body system is started. (Chapters 9–13 include the specific parameters for patient assessment according to major body systems.) Once the examiner has the components of the data base well in mind, she is able to obtain the necessary information. The data are recorded on the data base according to body systems.

Laboratory Tests

Laboratory tests are used to corroborate the information gathered in the interview and physical assessment. Laboratory tests are used by the physician and nurse to:

1. Support and establish a diagnosis by clinically measuring an abnormality.
2. Identify the body system involved in the condition.
3. Quantitate the severity of the abnormality.
4. Evaluate the effectiveness of treatments.
5. Screen for a specific illness.

The following points about laboratory tests should be kept in mind:

1. The purpose of the test
2. The specificity and reliability of the test
3. The need for the test
4. The cost to the patient
5. The benefit or risk aspects of the test
6. The normal values for the entity tested
7. The possibility of faulty techniques or other laboratory error
8. The limitations of the test

Laboratory tests are only as good as the person interpreting the results. The results of a single labora-

tory test are not definitive. If an accurate picture of the patient's condition is to emerge, all the observations must be considered in the clinical evaluation.

Machines and Tubes: A Word of Caution

The chapter thus far has discussed methods and techniques used in a nursing assessment. The reader may wonder why there has been no mention of machines or tubes. The omission is an intentional one on the part of the authors.

Students of critical care should consider the following question. Have you ever seen a professional nurse walk up to a patient's bedside and observe the intravenous flow rate, the amount of urine in the bag, or the ECG pattern *before* she looks at and assesses the patient?

In the past, critical care nurses have been criticized as being more interested and skillful in caring for complex and sophisticated machines and tubes than in caring for their patients. It cannot be disputed that complex equipment is essential not only in the moment-to-moment care of the patient but also in the prevention and early detection of complications. Furthermore, it cannot be disputed that the nurse's skill in using this equipment is important in making rapid assessments, administering lifesaving therapy, and prolonging human life.

But machines and tubes are only as good as the nurse using them. Thus the nurse must understand the indications and rationale for each piece of equipment she uses, as well as its complications and limitations. Monitoring equipment and other machines should be evaluated in regard to reliability, settings, alarm mechanisms, and electrical safety (see Chap. 7). All tubes should be assessed for placement, patency, proper attachment, and infection control. All tube drainage should be evaluated in regard to amount, color, consistency, and odor.

Quality nursing care, however, does not center on machines and tubes. If nursing is to be considered a practice profession, the delivery of health care must center on the patient. The machines and tubes can only serve to enhance the skill of the nurse delivering health care to her patient.

Problems That May Require Referral

The biopsychosocial needs and problems of the patient must be identified, assessed, and evaluated throughout his hospitalization. The nurse who cares for the total patient is aware of potential problems that require the expertise of people from other disciplines within the hospital and community settings. The nurse should be familiar with the services and know the availability and capabilities of the members of each department. Some of the people to whom a patient might need to be referred are the clinical nurse specialist, dietitian, physical therapist, occupational therapist, recreational therapist, respiratory therapist, social worker, psychiatrist, psychologist, chaplain, pharmacist, financial assistant, and vocational counselor, as well as people in community and health agencies.

Teaching Needs

As the nurse evaluates her patient, she must remain alert to the teaching the patient may need in regard to his illness, diet, medications, activity, and limitations. She should be aware of his short-term needs (what the patient should be taught in regard to his critical care needs) as well as his long-term needs (what the patient should be taught in regard to his illness, recovery, discharge, and preventive measures). (The patient's long-term needs are discussed more fully in Chapter 5.)

Problem List

All data are recorded on the appropriate data base assessment sheet regardless of which assessment approach is used. The assessment process is evaluated, and the data are synthesized. The patient problem list is then developed. The data for each problem on the list are written as nursing diagnoses to cover the physiological, psychological, social, cultural, educational, and developmental needs of the patient. The problem list then serves as a guideline and provides the primary focus by which the patient's plan of care may be developed.

A Challenge

For those nurses willing to accept the challenge and responsibility of refining and perfecting their assessment skills, the following suggestions are offered:

1. For several days or weeks, make it a goal to evaluate and improve your interviewing techniques. Become aware of your deficiencies, especially those that block communication.
2. After interviewing each patient, perform a physical assessment. Then reread the information in this chapter to see whether you missed anything. Did you organize your objectives, thoughts, and observations? Was your approach systematic and complete? What areas need more study and practice?
3. Write down your observations and findings, and organize your conclusions by using one of the assessment approaches discussed in this chapter. Can you express your thoughts and findings adequately and logically?
4. Make a resolution to look at machines and tubes only *after* assessing the patient.
5. Be more *aware* of everything in the patient's environment. *Listen* to your patient. While assessing the patient, try *not to overlook* even one minor point. Be sensitive to the patient and his surroundings. Smell, feel, hear, touch, and look at everything.

References

1. Barbee, R. A., Feldman, S., and Chosy, L. W. The quantitative evaluation of student performance in the medical interview. *J. Med. Ed.* 42: 238, 1967.
2. Bates, B. *A Guide to Physical Examination.* Philadelphia: Lippincott, 1974.
3. Buckingham, W. B. The Technique of History Taking. In W. B. Buckingham, M. Sparberg, and M. Brandfonbrener (eds.), *A Primer of Clinical Diagnosis.* New York: Harper & Row, 1971.
4. Buckingham, W. B., Sparberg, M., and Brandfonbrener, M. (eds.). *A Primer of Clinical Diagnosis.* New York: Harper & Row, 1971.
5. Fowkes, W. C., and Hunn, V. K. *Clinical Assessment for the Nurse Practitioner.* St. Louis: Mosby, 1973.
6. Froemming, P., and Quiring, J. Teaching health history and physical examination. *Nurs. Res.* 22:432, 1973.
7. Jarvis, C. M. Perfecting physical assessment, part I. *Nurs. '77* 7:28, 1977.
8. Jarvis, C. M. Perfecting physical assessment, part II. *Nurs. '77* 7:38, 1977.
9. Jarvis, C. M. Perfecting physical assessment, part III. *Nurs. '77* 7:44, 1977.
10. Judge, R. D., and Zuidema, G. D. (eds.). *Methods of Clinical Examination.* Boston: Little, Brown, 1974.
11. Lee, J. Y. *Sokdam: Capsules of Eastern Wisdom.* Korea: Folklore Research Institute, 1977.
12. Lewis, J., Beavers, R., Gossett, J., et al. *No Single Thread.* New York: Brunner and Mazel, 1976.
13. Littman, D. Stethoscopes and auscultation, *Am. J. Nurs.* 72:1232, 1972.

Respiratory Assessment

Cornelia Vanderstaay Kenner

The patients in critical care units collectively exhibit a gamut of respiratory problems. In some patients, the respiratory problem is the primary illness, and in others, it is secondary to another illness.

It is important for the nurse to know that most patients in critical care units have some degree of respiratory trouble. It is equally important (in the opinion of many authorities more important) to know what respiratory problems are likely to occur while patients are in critical care units. Even if no other respiratory trouble occurs, the supine position decreases the functional residual capacity of the patient's lung and contributes to the development of atelectasis.

The specific pulmonary problems exhibited by the critically ill patient are discussed elsewhere in the text. This chapter discusses both a method of systematically assessing the respiratory system of the critically ill patient and the tools needed for an accurate nursing assessment.

It is obvious that the nurse in the critical care unit does not make the entire patient assessment. Her responsibility varies according to the situation. It is the responsibility of the critical care team in each unit to decide what are the basic responsibilities and complementary roles of the physician, nurse, and respiratory therapist. What the nurse does depends a great deal on the availability of colleagues skilled in respiratory care. Thus if a patient has given a complete history to the physician, it would be redundant for the

9

nurse also to take his history. But if a complete history cannot be obtained when the patient is admitted, the physician might elicit from the patient information that is relevant to the patient's immediate care, and the nurse might later gather additional information for the history as she cares for the patient.

Objective

The nurse should be able to make an assessment based on the history, physical examination, and laboratory data relevant to the patient's pulmonary condition.

Achieving the Objective

To achieve the objective the nurse should be able to:

1. Integrate data obtained from the history, physical examination, and laboratory tests.
2. Use the equipment skillfully.
3. Perform the techniques of inspection, palpation, percussion, and auscultation systematically and accurately.
4. Calculate compliance.
5. Interpret selected spirometric data.

How to Proceed

To develop an approach to respiratory assessment the nurse should:

1. Review the anatomy and physiology of the respiratory system.
2. Study the material in the following pages and read some of the material listed in the references.
3. List the components of assessment.
4. Incorporating information learned from the review of anatomy and physiology, write a paragraph explaining the assessment techniques. Memorize the information in the paragraph.
5. Define the elements of the history that are essential to the respiratory assessment.
6. Practice interviewing skills while taking histories.
7. Practice techniques of physical examination in the learning laboratory.
8. Listen to recordings of breath sounds.
9. Listen to her own breath sounds.
10. In association with another nurse learn assessment. Evaluate one another's techniques.
11. Use videotape equipment to demonstrate the nurse's and a fellow learner's performance of the respiratory assessment.
12. Ask a person to act as a preceptor and review the nurse's physical examination techniques.
13. Observe the techniques the preceptor uses in the respiratory clinic and during patient rounds.
14. When she has learned the techniques thoroughly, perform selected techniques under the direct observation of the preceptor.
15. Validate her assessment of the patient by checking it against assessments performed by her preceptor and thus receive immediate feedback.
16. Strengthen her weak points. Review the patients' charts to determine what patients have the signs and symptoms pertinent to the weak points she wishes to strengthen. Explain to the patient what she is doing and ask his permission to do certain parts of the examination. Then she should reverse the process, reviewing the chart after assessing the patient. She should validate her findings when possible.
17. Make a complete respiratory assessment of at least 15 patients—or until she feels relatively proficient in each part of it.
18. Maintain her skills by practicing them and by taking continuing education courses.

History

Years ago at the Johns Hopkins Hospital, Sir William Osler taught that if one listens to a patient long enough the patient will tell him what's wrong. Unfortunately that truth is easily forgotten in the hustle and bustle of the modern day hospital. Another problem in today's mobile society is that patients do not always visit and revisit the same hospital. Thus a patient may be cared for by people who are unfamiliar with his history. The nurse must take the patient's history efficiently so she can individualize care.

The history clarifies why the patient has sought health care and how his problem has affected him and his family. It paints a picture within whose framework therapy may be instituted [2]. The history need not be long. Relevant questions can pinpoint parts of the physical examination to be stressed.

Chief Complaint

The chief complaint is the reason the patient has sought medical attention, and frequently is in his own words. The complaint needs to be further clarified by the patient. For example, a constricting feeling in his chest may be dyspnea or pain. Open-ended questions are useful in starting the history. If the patient gives several complaints, ask him which one is troubling him the most.

History of Present Illness

The history of the present illness dates from the time the patient noted a change. It is a chronologic review of the patient's immediate illness, including the initial symptoms and the development of the illness [9].

The cardinal symptoms of respiratory illness are carefully investigated and information about onset and progression, frequency and duration, severity, precipitating factors, and aggravating and alleviating factors is recorded. The patient's past and present use of medications is reviewed.

Information about general constitutional symptoms, such as anorexia, weight loss, weakness, tiredness, sweating, chills, and fever must be elicited [15]. Upper respiratory tract symptoms include (1) nasal discharge (onset, character, precipitating factors, sneezing), (2) obstruction of the nasal passages (pain or sinus tenderness), and (3) hoarseness. Sputum is evaluated in regard to amount, consistency, color, odor, and presence of blood.

If the person complains of shortness of breath, he should be asked to describe any other changes in his breathing. The subjective sensation of breathlessness may have various causes. Dyspnea needs to be differentiated from pressure sensations in the chest, weakness, and fatigability. For example, angina may be associated with a feeling of suffocation and may be mistaken for breathlessness. Also, patients with hyperventilation often say that they are unable to take in enough air [8]. The cause of chest pain is often difficult to determine. For example, the pain from cardiac ischemia and pulmonary embolism are similar. Usually the possibility of embolism is considered if hemoptysis or pleuritic pain is present.

The ongoing assessment in the critical care unit of subjective data considers the signs and symptoms the person has observed as well as any the medical team anticipates. For example, mental dullness or confu-sion may accompany hypoxemia or fluid volume depletion. Subjective data are essential for the total patient assessment, and they must be elicited and recorded.

Past Health History

The past health history includes the patient's illnesses since birth. Frequency of illness and the treatment are noted particularly with regard to pneumonia, pleurisy, fungal disease, tuberculosis, bronchiectasis, chronic obstructive lung disease, asthma, allergies, colds, sinus problems, and pneumothorax [5]. The patient's compliance with the various medical regimens, along with the dates of his last chest film, tuberculin skin test, and pulmonary function tests, is noted.

Family History

The family history includes information about the health status or causes of death of members of the patient's immediate family. If the patient has asthma or some other possibly hereditary disease, the family history should include a review of similar problems in other family members [23].

Review of Systems

The review of systems is a rapid check to ensure that the patient has mentioned all his signs and symptoms. Each body system is reviewed to obtain pertinent information. Any additional information uncovered may require further clarification [25].

Patient Profile

The patient profile not only gives personal information that describes the patient's life and helps to individualize his care, but it also gives clues to possible unidentified respiratory conditions [3, 4].

The patient's job history may point to past or present factors conducive to the development of respiratory disease, as the following example shows. A 40-year-old man was admitted to a coronary care unit with severe chest pain. The early test results were negative for cardiac disease, but a detailed history revealed that years ago the man had been an asbestos pipe fitter. Further study established the diagnosis of asbestosis.

Geography may also be an important factor in the patient's background. The patient may have lived in a part of the country where certain fungal diseases are endemic [12, 13].

The profile has three basic components:

1. Background (educational, occupational, cultural, religious, past and present places of residence)
2. Socioeconomic status; housing
3. Habits and hobbies (smoking, consumption of alcohol)

Physical Examination

The next step in the assessment of the patient's respiratory functioning is the physical examination. The techniques described in Chapter 8—inspection, palpation, percussion, and auscultation—are used. Since most people in the critical care unit are in bed most of the time and have little physical stamina, the usual systematic approach following evaluation of the head and neck is examination of first the anterior chest and then the lateral and posterior chest [21]. The complete physical examination is described here although the nurse in the critical care unit would rarely do the entire examination. Rather she would examine selected aspects determined by the patient's condition.

Inspection

The examination actually begins with the nurse's observation of the patient while she elicits historical data. General notations are made about the patient's overall condition. Then the nurse examines each area of the respiratory system and makes notes about normal and abnormal findings [6, 22]. Inspection and palpation are often done at the same time.

The nurse begins the inspection of the head and neck by noting any signs of respiratory distress: airway difficulty, gasping, cyanosis, open mouth, flared nostrils, and/or the use of accessory muscles. Bilateral jugular vein distention is indicative of elevated venous pressure. The inspiration-expiration ratio is noted. The forced vital capacity may be estimated roughly by having the patient forcefully blow on the

examiner's hand [10, 14]. The examiner notes the sputum and the odor of the breath.

The patient's chest is inspected in regard to respiratory rate (normal = 16 to 18 respirations per minute), amplitude or depth of expansion, and rhythm. Diaphragmatic breathing is more apparent in men and costal breathing is more apparent in women. Symmetry is ascertained, and any paradoxical movements are immediately assessed. Any other movements that denote labored inspirations, such as elevation of the clavicle and shoulder or retraction, are observed. Retraction on inspiration is indicative of airway obstruction. Increased use of expiratory muscles may also be seen on forced expiration in a patient with a severe asthma attack or respiratory failure with chronic obstructive lung disease [17, 28]. Observation is made of the contour and size of the chest, noting the anteroposterior diameter.

Examination of the extremities may reveal clubbing of the fingers or toes, thus verifying the presence of pulmonary disease. The evidence may be difficult to evaluate. Normally the angle at the nail bed is 160°, but early in pulmonary disease hypertrophy of the nail bed is such that the angle increases to 180° or more [16]. Eventually the nail has a characteristic bulbous blunted appearance as the pulp under the nail enlarges further. In some instances, the changes in the nails are accompanied by a painful arthritis of the wrists and ankles termed hypertrophic pulmonary osteoarthropathy.

Palpation

The chest is palpated with the heel of the examiner's hand held flat against the person's chest or with the ulnar aspect of the hand. Palpation combined with inspection is particularly effective in assessing whether the movements of each side of the chest during deep inspiration and expiration are equal in amplitude and are symmetrical.

In an effective way of comparing chest excursions, the examiner first has the patient sit and then he places his hands on the posterior aspects of the patient's chest, with his thumbs meeting in the midline. As the chest moves, the examiner's hands move so that he can assess the excursion of each side simultaneously. Any unilateral asymmetry may be indicative of a disease process in that region. Evaluation also includes noting any tenderness of the chest wall, muscle tone, swelling, and tactile (vocal) fremitus.

To assess tactile fremitus, the examiner palpates the patient's chest wall while the patient says phrases that produce relatively intense vibrations (e.g., "99"). The vibrations are transmitted from the larynx via the airways and can be palpated at the chest wall. The intensity of vibrations on both sides is compared. Stronger vibrations are felt over areas where there is consolidation of the underlying lung. Decreased tactile fremitus is usually associated with abnormalities that move the lung further from the chest wall, such as pleural effusion and pneumothorax.

Percussion

If the chest is tapped with the finger, the vibrations of the tissues, lung and chest wall produce an audible sound wave. Just as with all musical tones, those vibrations are described in regard to their acoustic properties of frequency, intensity, duration, and quality. Those four properties are then further evaluated and recorded as resonant, dull, flat, or tympanic.

Frequency, or pitch, refers to the number of vibrations per second. Intensity refers to the amplitude of the sound wave. Duration is the length of time the sound is present. Quality is the characteristic most difficult to describe since it comprises many subjective elements besides pitch, intensity, and harmonics [17].

Resonant sounds have a relatively low pitch (100 to 140 cycles per second), variable intensity, long duration, and nonmusical quality. Hyperresonant sounds have an even lower pitch and overtones that are somewhat musical. Dull sounds have a higher pitch (140 to 190 cycles per second), decreased intensity, short duration, and nonmusical quality. Flat sounds have a higher pitch (190 cycles per second), even less intensity, a very short duration, and a nonmusical quality. Tympanic sounds have an even higher pitch (200 to 350 cycles per second), a very loud intensity, a long duration, and a relatively rich (musical) quality.

Percussion usually begins at the apices and proceeds to the bases, moving from the anterior areas to the lateral areas and then to the posterior areas. Ideally, the patient is seated and percussion proceeds in an unhurried manner, with several points percussed in each intercostal space. If the patient is unable to sit up, he is examined first in one lateral decubitus position and then in the other. That procedure allows comparison of the two sides.

Changes in sound waves are produced by changes in the underlying structures. For example, increased air from emphysema or air in the pleural cavity produces a hyperresonant or even tympanic sound. Decreased air from consolidation in atelectasis or pneumonia produces a dull sound.

Auscultation

Auscultation, along with inspection, is the technique most frequently used in the critical care unit. By listening to the lungs with a stethoscope while the patient breathes with his mouth open, the examiner is able to assess three things: (1) the character of the breath sounds, (2) the character of the spoken and whispered voice, and (3) the presence of adventitious sounds [11, 30]. While the examiner listens, he must keep in mind the segmental pulmonary anatomy (Fig. 9-1) in order to determine what segment of the lung he is listening to.

The breath sounds heard result from the transmission of vibrations produced by the movement of air in the respiratory passages from the larynx to the alveoli. The voice sounds heard result from the transmission of vibrations produced by sound waves from the larynx. The airways to the area examined must be open to have transmission of voice sounds. Adventitious sounds are abnormal sounds (rales, rhonchi, and friction rubs) superimposed on the breath sounds.

BREATH SOUNDS

Breath sounds are termed vesicular, bronchial, and bronchovesicular (Fig. 9-2). Vesicular breath sounds are normal sounds. During inspiration, the sound is heard longer and louder than during expiration. The sound during inspiration is produced by air moving into the terminal bronchioles and alveoli. Since air flow is greater during the earlier phase of expiration, more sound is heard early in expiration. In general, expiration is described as very quiet to silent. The inspiration-expiration ratio in vesicular breathing is normally 3:1. Decreased breath sounds are heard when there is fluid, air, or increased tissue in the pleural space that interferes with the transfer of vibrations to the chest wall. Absent or diminished breath sounds are heard also in bronchial obstruction since there can be no air flow and thus no vibrations.

Bronchial breath sounds are produced by vibrations of air in larger airways. They are normally heard over the trachea and peristernal areas. No breath sounds

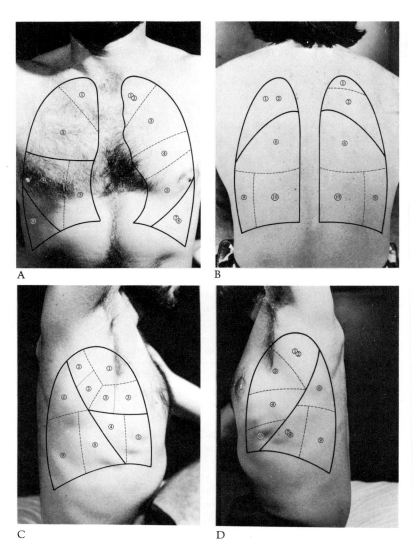

Figure 9-1
Location of the lung segments. A. Front chest. B. Dorsal chest. C. Right lateral chest. D. Left lateral chest. **Right lung:** *Upper lobe*—(1) Apical segment, (2) posterior segment and axillary subsegment, (3) anterior segment and axillary subsegment; *Middle lobe*—(4) Lateral segment, (5) medial segment; *Lower lobe*—(6) Superior segment, (7) medial basal segment, (8) anterior basal segment, (9) lateral basal segment, (10) posterior basal segment. **Left lung:** *Upper lobe*—Superior division: (1, 2) Apical-posterior segment, (3) anterior segment; Inferior division: (4) Superior lingular segment, (5) inferior lingular segment; *Lower lobe*—(6) Superior segment, (7, 8) anteromedial basal segment, (9) lateral basal segment, (10) posterior basal segment.

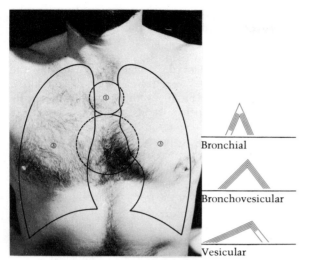

Figure 9-2
Sites of origin and graphic representations of various breath sounds. (1) Bronchial, (2) bronchovesicular, and (3) vesicular breath sounds.

are heard between inspiration and expiration since there is no air flow. In the area between the trachea and the peripheral lung areas, a mixture of bronchial and vesicular sounds are heard. Those sounds are called bronchovesicular sounds.

VOICE SOUNDS

Auscultation also includes assessment of the spoken and whispered voice. Sounds produced by speaking are transmitted from the larynx to the chest wall and may be heard with the stethoscope. In the normal lung, since most of the vibrations caused by the voice are absorbed by the lung tissue, the waves are not clear. A decrease in voice sounds can be caused by any factor that impairs the transmission of the vibrations, such as airway obstruction. Voice sounds are also evaluated by having the patient whisper. With whispering, resonance and vibrations are less than with normal speech. Therefore in the normal lung a weak sound is heard at the chest wall.

If consolidation develops, there is increased transmission of bronchial vibrations to the chest wall (since fluid is a better conductor of sound than is air). During the evaluation of bronchophony, vocal sounds are transmitted better and spoken words are clearer to the examiner. The patient's whisper is heard clearly and distinctly during the evaluation of whispered pectoriloquy. (Liquid in the airways caused by consolidation may also vibrate and cause rhonchi.) Another valuable clinical test to assess consolidation is the evaluation of egophony. If consolidation is present in the patient's lung, the letter E spoken by him is not heard as E by the examiner. Rather, the examiner, listening with a stethoscope, hears the sound as A.

ADVENTITIOUS SOUNDS

Adventitious sounds are abnormal sounds superimposed on normal sounds in the lung. They are classified as (1) rales, (2) rhonchi, or (3) pleural friction rubs (Fig. 9-3).

Rales
Rales are sounds produced when alveoli that are partially filled with fluid reinflate. Thus rales are produced from the combined effect of air flow and abnormal moisture. Rales have varying degrees of coarseness and are heard during early inspiration, particularly during a deep inspiration. Rales have a sound similar to the sound produced by placing the thumb and index finger next to one's ear and then pulling the fingers apart.

Rales are classified as fine, coarse, or medium. Fine rales (crepitant rales) have a fine, dry, crackling sound, and they are heard best over the lung periphery. Coughing does not clear the sound. Usually fine rales are indicative of inflammation or congestion in the terminal bronchioles or alveoli.

Coarse rales are produced when inspired air causes the secretions in the larger air passages to vibrate. The vibrations have loud, rough, bubbling, gurgling sounds. They are heard best at the beginning of inspiration. Usually clearing occurs after vigorous coughing or suctioning.

Medium rales are intermediate between fine rales and coarse rales. Medium rales are produced as a result of (1) air passing through secretions in the bronchioles or (2) separation of the bronchiolar walls that have become adherent. Medium rales have a midrange sound that is described as fine, moist, and rattling. Medium rales are heard earlier in inspiration than are fine rales and later in inspiration than are coarse rales. Clearing may occur with very vigorous coughing.

Rhonchi
Rhonchi are different from rales in that rhonchi have relatively musical sounds that are heard during inspi-

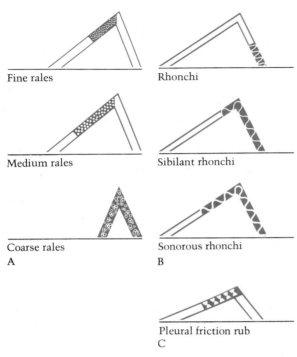

Fine rales

Rhonchi

Medium rales

Sibilant rhonchi

Coarse rales

Sonorous rhonchi

A

B

Pleural friction rub

C

Figure 9-3
Graphic representations of adventitious sounds. A. Fine, medium, and coarse rales. B. Sibilant and sonorous rhonchi. C. Pleural friction rub.

ration and expiration. The passage of air through fluid-filled narrowed air passages produces the sounds. Rhonchi have multiple causes, including: (1) extrinsic pressure, (2) mucosal spasm, (3) mucosal swelling, and (4) strands of adherent, tenacious mucus.

Rhonchi may be further described as sibilant (musical) or sonorous. Sibilant rhonchi are high pitched, musical, almost squeaky sounds. Sonorous rhonchi are low pitched, almost snoring sounds that are best heard over the sternum and trachea.

Wheezing is another sound produced by air flowing through airways that are narrowed or partially filled with fluid or mucus. Wheezing is the sound heard at the end of expiration in a normal person when he exhales forcefully.

Pleural Friction Rub
A pleural friction rub is produced from pleural inflammation. The cause may be pneumonia, pulmonary infarction, or pleurisy. The sound is described as rough, grating, and crackling, much like two pieces of leather being rubbed together. The pleural surfaces are roughened, and the normal lubrication between the visceral and parietal layers is lost. Usually those layers move noiselessly during inspiration and expiration but because of the roughness caused by the inflammation, the characteristic sound is produced. Since movement produces the sound, there is no sound when the person holds his breath. Timing of the sound in the respiratory cycle varies; it may be heard only during inspiration and expiration, or it may be heard in both phases. Usually increasing the pressure of the stethoscope on the chest wall increases the intensity of the sound. The rub is most commonly heard over the involved area.

Procedure

For the patient confined to bed, the physical assessment is done by using all four examination techniques for one body region, and then repositioning the patient and using the techniques for another body region. The findings are recorded separately for each region: for example, left lower lobe: increased tactile fremitus, dull to percussion, breath sounds bronchial, crepitant rales, bronchophony, and egophony [17].

ANTERIOR AND LATERAL CHEST

Inspection (combined with palpation)

1. Skin: Color, lesions, edema, dilated veins, physical characteristics
2. Chest: Size and shape, symmetry and deformity, muscular size
3. Respirations: Rate and rhythm, inspiration-expiration ratio, depth, equality, symmetry, labored respirations, use of accessory muscles, retractions, abdominal or thoracic respirations

Palpation

1. Tenderness in the skin, tissues, or bone
2. Muscle tone
3. Equal and synchronous movement
4. Tactile fremitus

Percussion

1. Bilateral corresponding areas for resonance, dullness, flatness, tympany
2. Note bases in particular

Auscultation

1. Bilateral corresponding areas for breath sounds, voice sounds, adventitious sounds

POSTERIOR AND LATERAL CHEST

(Patient may have to be turned and examination repeated for opposite posterior chest)

Inspection

1. Skin: Color, lesions, edema
2. Chest: Symmetry, anteroposterior diameter, scapular position
3. Respirations: Symmetry

Palpation

1. Tenderness
2. Muscle tone
3. Chest expansion

Percussion

1. Corresponding bilateral intercostal spaces. Note bases.
2. Diaphragmatic excursion after a deep inspiration and a deep expiration

Auscultation

1. Bilateral corresponding areas for breath sounds, voice sounds, and adventitious sounds

Additional Studies

Many other parameters may be used to evaluate the patient's respiratory status. The choice depends on the patient's disorder. If the findings are abnormal, further examination is indicated.

Chest Radiograph

The best chest examination tool is the chest film, but it is not sufficient. The history and physical examination are essential since the chest film gives a picture of only one moment in time. Also, in critical care units, most chest films are taken by a portable machine, and so the results vary in quality.

The chest film is systematically evaluated or read in regard first to the normal areas and then to the abnormal areas. The bony structures and the diaphragm are examined, then the heart shadow, tracheobronchial tree, and lung parenchyma. On a normal chest film, the lung is black. The volume may be roughly estimated by the size of the lung fields. Atelectasis, the most common complication in the critically ill patient, is seen on the film as a density. The fine, white, wispy, thin structures that fan out from the hili are the shadows of blood vessels. Those vascular markings are present over the entire lung field, and when they look enlarged and fuzzy they are abnormal [19].

Work of Breathing

Several mechanical properties of the chest and lung are involved in the work of breathing. Changes in lung volumes are affected by the (1) movement of thoracic and diaphragmatic muscles, (2) energy of elastic tissues, and (3) surfactant, the lipoprotein that decreases surface tension and maintains alveolar stability [18, 24].

Pulmonary Function Tests

Pulmonary function tests are frequently used for clinical evaluation and research. In most respiratory care units, spirometric measurements are the nurse's responsibility. The cooperation of the patient is essential for an accurate spirogram.

Lung capacities are composed of two or more lung volumes, which are more useful measurements in the clinical situation since lung capacities are static and relatively difficult to determine clinically. Total lung capacity (TLC) is composed of four volumes. It is the maximum lung volume following full inspiration (Fig. 9-4). At TLC, the force generated by a maximum contraction of the inspiratory muscles equals the recoil of the lung. Normal variations occur, depending on the person's age, sex, and height. Since TLC is dependent on the strength of the respiratory muscles and the elastic resistance of the lung and the chest wall, abnormalities in those limit the volume obtained. For example, a person with a restrictive disease (e.g., sarcoidosis) would have a decreased TLC.

The lung volumes that make up TLC are (1) residual volume, (2) tidal volume, (3) expiratory reserve

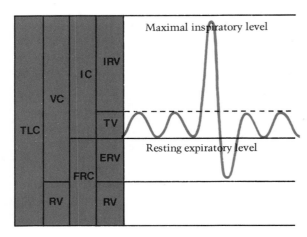

Figure 9-4
Lung volumes.

volume, and (4) inspiratory reserve volume. Residual volume (RV) is the amount of air remaining in the lungs after a maximal voluntary expiration. Residual volume is approximately 20 percent of total lung capacity in younger adults, and it increases with age or any abnormal condition that involves high airway resistance. Tidal volume (TV) is the amount of gas expired during normal ventilation. The expiratory reserve volume (ERV) is the volume of gas between the residual volume and the tidal volume. The inspiratory reserve volume (IRV) is the volume of gas between the tidal volume and the upper limits of total lung capacity. The expiratory reserve volume and the inspiratory reserve volume are available to increase the tidal volume, but they are not used under conditions of normal resting ventilation.

Functional residual capacity (FRC) is the volume of gas remaining in the lungs at the end of a normal expiration. It comprises the expiratory reserve volume and the residual volume. FRC is the volume at which the inward recoil of the lung is balanced by the outward recoil of the chest wall. Thus it is termed the resting level or the midposition. In addition to any existing pathophysiology, FRC is reduced in the supine patient because the weight of the abdominal contents forces his diaphragm upward. FRC is also reduced by ascites or increased lung recoil, as in the patient with sarcoidosis.

SPIROGRAM

Spirometry is the determination of lung volume that involves the forceful exhalation of air by the person

being tested. The time volume indices most frequently used are the forced vital capacity (FVC), the forced expiratory volume (FEVt), and the mean forced expiratory flow (forced midexpiratory flow, FEF 25–75). Results on any of those tests may be reduced because of poor cooperation, poor muscular effort, fatigue, or airway obstruction.

The FVC is the total volume that can be expired following a maximal inspiration; it is the sum of the tidal volume and the inspiratory-expiratory reserve volumes. The FVC is the maximum ventilatory volume or the maximum breathing ability of the patient. The patient makes the deepest possible inspiration and then expires as completely as possible. The exhalation is measured as the FVC. If the patient's FVC is less than 75% of his predicted normal vital capacity, he is said to have restrictive disease. In true restrictive disease, the forced vital capacity is small and the residual lung volume is unchanged, resulting in a decreased total lung capacity. The volume of gas in the lungs is also found to be small on posteroanterior and lateral chest film.

Example
Patient with restrictive disease from pulmonary fibrosis

FVC = 1.65 liters
Estimated normal = 3.02 liters
Percentage of normal = 55%

The FEV is the amount of gas exhaled over a given period of time (usually one second) during the performance of an FVC test. The volume is also expressed as a percentage of the FVC. The measurement is particularly indicative of obstruction of the larger airways, and it is one measurement that is responsive to bronchodilator therapy.

The FEF is the average rate of flow for a specified volume segment of the FVC. Usually a notation is made after the abbreviation to denote the volume segment in cubic centimeters or as a percentage. The middle segment of an FVC maneuver is often used as an index of disease of the small airways and as a means of evaluating the patient's response to bronchodilator therapy [1]. It is the FEF between 25% and 75% of the FVC (FEF25–75).

In obstructive disease the results of pulmonary function tests show the following. The residual volume is increased, and the total lung capacity is normal to increased. Chest film shows the volume of gas in the lungs to be increased [31]. The patient's FEV_1 is reduced because of the obstruction. If a person's FEV_1

is not 75% of his predicted normal value, he is said to have obstructive lung disease. An FEV_1/FVC ratio of less than 75% also documents airway obstruction. An even more sensitive indicator is the FEF25–75 test. That test (flow rate) is so sensitive that in the presence of early airway obstruction, the FEF25–75 may be reduced even though other measurements are normal. After bronchodilator therapy, the two tests are usually repeated to assess the reversibility of the obstruction.

Example
Patient with obstructive disease from asthma

	Predicted	Observed	
	Normal	Before Broncho-dilator Therapy	After Broncho-dilator Therapy
FVC	4.66 L	4.16 L (89%)	4.54 L (97%)
FEV_1	3.92 L	1.42 L (36%)	2.32 L (59%)
FEF25–75	4.33 L/sec	0.81 L/sec (19%)	1.01 L/sec (23%)

In some patients, expiratory airway obstruction becomes so severe that they also develop what appears to be a restrictive ventilatory defect. The residual volume in their lungs is so large that their FVC is decreased even though their TLC is normal to increased. On chest film, a large volume of gas is seen in their lungs and their FEV is more severely impaired than is their FVC.

Example
Patient with apparent restrictive lung disease from airway obstruction

	Predicted	Measured	Percent
FVC	3.88 L	2.18 L	56
FEV_1	3.26 L	0.69 L	21
FEF25–75	3.57 L/sec	0.25 L/sec	7

Compliance

Ventilation is ultimately determined by the interaction of volume, pressure, and resistance. Changes in airway resistance require that different pressures be exerted to maintain lung volumes and air flow.

What pressures must be exerted by the respiratory muscles is dependent on two factors: (1) the resistance to the movement of gas through the airways and (2) the elasticity or stiffness of the lungs. Thus while caring for critically ill patients, the nurse must remember that ventilation may be affected by changes in airway resistance or in the elasticity of the lungs [20].

Compliance is the change in volume divided by the change in pressure necessary to produce that volume change. It is a gross reflection of the forces required to cause air to move into the lungs. A lung with low compliance (an inelastic lung) is one that requires a high distending pressure and that is difficult to inflate.

A parameter that is useful in following the clinical course of critically ill patients undergoing mechanical ventilator therapy is effective compliance (dynamic effective compliance). Effective compliance is the ratio of tidal volume to peak airway pressure. It normally ranges from 35 to 50 ml/cm H_2O [29]. Unless high airway resistance is present, it may be used as an indicator of the total compliance of the chest wall and lungs.

It must be stressed that effective compliance is a measurement of both lung inelasticity and airway resistance. Patients with any change in effective compliance will, in all probability, be evaluated by a physician who specializes in pulmonary disorders. He will assess the patient's status by attempting to separate the effects of lung inelasticity from the effects of airway resistance.

Static compliance measures pertain only to the inelasticity of the lung since the measurements are made at the end of inspiration, when there is no airflow and therefore no airway resistance. With a patient using a ventilator, the lung is inflated, and the volume exhaled is noted during several inspirations. On a subsequent inspiration, the exhalation tube is occluded. Initially the peak pressure on the manometer of the ventilator is noted, and the pressure decrease is noted when air flow stops at the static pressure. To obtain static compliance, the static pressure is then divided into the average volume exhaled.

In normal people, the values for static compliance and dynamic compliance are approximately the same. However, in patients with airway obstruction, dynamic compliance decreases, and it may be less than static compliance.

For example:

Tidal volume	$= 1000$ ml
Dynamic pressure	$= 50$ cm H_2O
Static pressure	$= 20$ cm H_2O

$$\text{Dynamic compliance} = \frac{1000}{50} = 20$$

$$\text{Static compliance} = \frac{1000}{20} = 50$$

References

1. Abboud, R. T., and Morton, J. W. Comparison of maximal mid-expiratory flow, flow volume curves, and nitrogen closing volumes in patients with mild airway obstruction. *Am. Rev. Respir. Dis.* 111:405, 1975.
2. Barbee, R. A., Kettel, L. J., and Burrows, B. The medical history in evaluation of patients with pulmonary disease. *Basics Respir. Dis.* 2:1, 1974.
3. Bates, B. *Guide to Physical Examination.* Philadelphia: Lippincott, 1974.
4. Bates, D. V., Macklem, P. T., and Christie, R. V. *Respiratory Function in Disease* (2nd ed.). Philadelphia: Saunders, 1971.
5. Baum, G. L. *Textbook of Pulmonary Diseases* (2nd ed.). Boston: Little, Brown, 1974.
6. Broughton, J. O. Chest physical diagnosis for nurses and respiratory therapists. *Heart Lung* 1:200, 1972.
7. Canizaro, P. C., Nelson, J. L., Hennessy, J. L., et al. A technique for estimating the position of the oxyhemoglobin dissociation curve. *Ann. Surg.* 180:364, 1973.
8. Cherniack, R. M. *Pulmonary Function Testing.* Philadelphia: Saunders, 1977.
9. Cherniack, R. M., Cherniack, L., and Naimark, A. *Respiration in Health and Disease* (2nd ed.). Philadelphia: Saunders, 1972.
10. Comroe, J. H., Forster, R. E., Duboid, A. B., et al. *The Lung.* Chicago: Year Book, 1962.
11. Cregill, P. W. Use of tape recordings of respiratory sound and breathing pattern for instruction in pulmonary auscultation. *Am. Rev. Respir. Dis.* 104:948, 1971.
12. Crofton, J., and Douglas, A. *Respiratory Diseases.* Oxford: Blackwell, 1969.
13. DeGowin, E., and DeGowin, R. *Bedside Diagnostic Examination* (2nd ed.). New York: Macmillan, 1971.
14. Egan, D. F. *Fundamentals of Respiratory Therapy* (2nd ed.). St. Louis: Mosby, 1973.
15. Geschickter, C. F. *The Lung in Health and Disease.* Philadelphia: Lippincott, 1973.
16. Guyton, A. C. *Textbook of Medical Physiology* (3rd ed.). Philadelphia: Saunders, 1969.
17. Hockstein, E., and Rubin, A. *Physical Diagnosis.* New York: McGraw-Hill, 1964.
18. Lambertsen, C. J. The Atmosphere and Gas Exchanges with the Lungs and Blood. In V. B. Mountcastle (ed.), *Medical Physiology.* St. Louis: Mosby, 1974. P. 1372.
19. Laver, M. B., and Austen, W. G. Lung Function: Physiologic Considerations Applicable to Surgery. In D. C. Sabiston (ed.), *Textbook of Surgery.* Philadelphia: Saunders, 1972. P. 1744.
20. McConn, R. The oxyhemoglobin dissociation curve in acute disease. *Surg. Clin. North Am.* 55:627, 1975.
21. Morgan, W. L., and Engel, G. L. *Clinical Approach to the Patient.* Philadelphia: Saunders, 1969.
22. Murray, J. *The Normal Lung.* Philadelphia: Saunders, 1976.
23. Petty, T. L. A chest physician's perspective on asthma. *Heart Lung* 1:611, 1972.
24. Pontoppidan, H., Geffin, B., and Lowenstein, E. *Acute Respiratory Failure in the Adult.* Boston: Little, Brown, 1973.
25. Prior, J., and Silberstein, J. *Physical Diagnosis.* St. Louis: Mosby, 1973.
26. Ruppel, G. *Manual of Pulmonary Function Testing.* St. Louis: Mosby, 1975.
27. Shapiro, B. A., Harrison, R. A., and Trout, C. A. *Clinical Application of Respiratory Care.* Chicago: Year Book, 1975.
28. Sweetwood, H. Bedside Assessment of Respirations. *Nurs. '73* 3:50, 1973.
29. Tomashefski, J. F., and Abdullah, M. B. Blood Gas Exchange. In B. L. Gordon, R. A. Carleton, and L. P. Faber (eds.), *Clinical Cardiopulmonary Physiology.* New York: Grune & Stratton, 1969. P. 377.
30. Weiss, E. B., and Carlson, C. J. Recording of breath sounds. *Am. Rev. Respir. Dis.* 105:835, 1972.
31. Woolcock, A. J., Vincent, N. J., and Macklem, P. T. Frequency dependence of compliance as a test for obstruction in small airways. *J. Clin. Invest.* 48:1097, 1969.

Cardiovascular Assessment

Cathie E. Guzzetta
Barbara Montgomery Dossey

Assessment of the cardiovascular system is a unique process because it involves evaluation of not only the heart but also the peripheral arterial and venous circulation. Patient signs and symptoms may be subtle, and clinical findings can frequently be transient, making the assessment a challenging and exciting process. In the following discussions, a systematic approach to the history and physical examination is presented, along with a comprehensive discussion of the major cardiac diagnostic procedures and dysrhythmias.

Chief Complaint

The patient should be asked to describe his initial symptoms and his reason for seeking medical assistance. Additional complaints should be noted if they appear to be of major importance to the admission history.

History of Present Illness

The history of the present illness should be reviewed in a chronological order, recording changes in symptoms over a period of time, circumstances that predisposed, precipitated, aggravated, prolonged, or alleviated the problem, as well as the patient's response

10

to medical or drug therapy (for details, see also Chap. 8).

Past Medical History

The past health history includes a review of the patient's past health, as well as information pertinent to the origin of his heart disease. The history is explored to elicit information related to congenital abnormalities, heart murmurs acquired in infancy or childhood, cyanosis, arthritis, rheumatic fever, glomerulonephritis or hypertension. Bacterial, viral, and fungal infections should be identified, especially those associated with pneumonia, influenza, tuberculosis, mumps, chickenpox, venereal disease, dental extractions, or invasive genitourinary manipulations (e.g., cystoscopy).

Injuries and accidents should be recorded, particularly those involving chest trauma, thrombophlebitis, or arterial problems. Any history of cardiovascular disease, cardiovascular surgery or invasive cardiovascular tests should be elicited. Metabolic abnormalities, such as gout, diabetes mellitus and hypothyroidism or hyperthyroidism, should be investigated. Dietary habits specifically related to the intake of carbohydrates, cholesterol, or triglycerides, as well as known blood lipid abnormalities, should be noted. The use of alcohol, tobacco, and drugs is also recorded.

Family History

The nurse must elicit information about any family history of congenital heart disease, cardiac disease, hypertension, heart murmur, cerebrovascular disease, diabetes mellitus, gout, rheumatic fever, renal disease, and premature or sudden death due to cardiovascular disease.

Review of Systems

The review of systems involves gathering data that are particularly pertinent to the cardiovascular system, keeping in mind the cardinal symptoms: chest pain, dyspnea, palpitations, and fluid retention.

When information about *chest pain* is elicited from the patient it is necessary to categorize the quality of the pain as crushing, squeezing, aching, heavy, tight, dull, burning, pleuritic, or associated with a feeling of indigestion. The patient should be asked to describe the location and radiation of the pain. The "4E" signs that produce angina pectoris, or its classic precipitating factors, should be identified: (1) exertion, (2) eating, (3) exposure to cold, and (4) excitement. Any symptoms that occur during rest or sleep should be sought (e.g., orthopnea, nocturia, edema). The time of onset, duration, and frequency of the attacks should be determined, along with any associated symptoms, such as dizziness, syncope, diaphoresis, nausea, vomiting, or dyspnea. The patient should describe any factors that aggravate or precipitate the discomfort (e.g., breathing, lying down, walking, and eating) and any factors that alleviate it (e.g., resting, walking, eating, and sitting up).

Dyspnea is a symptom described by the patient as shortness of breath. The history should list the factors that precipitate or alleviate the dyspnea and should identify the body position associated with the phenomenon. Dyspnea is characterized according to type, degree, progression, and duration. Dyspnea may be associated with congestive heart failure and/or chronic lung disease. It is generally referred to as one of three types: dyspnea on exertion, orthopnea, or paroxysmal nocturnal dyspnea.

Exertional dyspnea, a common complaint, may be associated with both heart failure and lung disease. Common precipitating factors include climbing a hill or stairs, upper extremity exercise, and sexual intercourse. Exertional dyspnea, produced by either heart or lung disease, may also be accompanied by wheezes. It is important to determine the degree of activity in a normal day that is necessary to produce the symptom (e.g., the number of flights of stairs climbed or blocks walked) and the length of time it has increased in severity.

Orthopnea is a form of dyspnea that occurs within a few minutes of the patient's assuming the supine position and that is relieved when the patient sits, stands, or is propped up. The patient often sleeps elevated on two or three pillows to improve his breathing. Orthopnea is most frequently associated with congestive heart failure, but occasionally it is associated with severe lung disease.

Paroxysmal nocturnal dyspnea is generally specific for left ventricular failure. The patient characteristically has little difficulty going to sleep in the recumbent position, but he is awakened from sleep one to two hours later with severe shortness of breath. In contrast to orthopnea, paroxysmal nocturnal dyspnea is not relieved immediately when the patient assumes an upright position. It requires a number of minutes to subside.

Palpitation is the term sometimes used by patients to describe an unpleasant awareness of the heart beat. The phenomenon is commonly caused by anxiety although it may also be produced by changes in heart rate, rhythm, and hemodynamic states. Patients may use such terms as "stopping," "jumping," "skipping," "pounding," and "turning over" to describe their heart action. It is valuable to have the patient describe sensations of rhythm, rate, and forcefulness of the heart beat. He should describe his experiences at the times of onset and termination of the episode, as well as precipitating and terminating factors (e.g., coughing, gagging, and vomiting). The nurse should remember that emotional states often can cause dysrhythmias, and it is important to find out what the patient was doing at the onset of symptoms. Questions should be phrased to determine whether the patient experienced any associated congestion, cyanosis, dizziness, syncope, dyspnea, diaphoresis, or chest pain. Often it is helpful to ask relatives or others who witnessed the event to describe the details surrounding it.

Fluid retention often indicates cardiac failure. It is often caused by inadequate ventricular function. The history should note any lower extremity edema and/or weight gain of gradual onset. Any associated dyspnea, fatigue, or urinary frequency, particularly nocturia, should be documented.

Often important related cardiovascular signs and symptoms require further investigation. They include dizziness, syncope, cyanosis, cough, hemoptysis, varicosities, thrombophlebitis, claudication, Raynaud's phenomenon, vertigo, and convulsions.

Patient Profile

The patient's occupational history is obtained to determine his physical work load, the demands on his time, his satisfactions, disappointments, degree of stress, and emotional involvement, as well as his financial status.

A marital history is obtained to investigate such things as number of marriages, years married, age of spouse, number of children, sexual relationship, and other related information that may be important in determining whether his environment is stable or stressful.

The patient's habits and life patterns are examined in regard to relaxation time, physical exercise, vacations, diet, recent stressful life changes, the use of tobacco, alcohol, tea, or coffee, and exposure to toxins, chemicals, or fumes.

Physical Assessment

Inspection and Palpation

The cardiovascular examination initially is best done from the patient's right side with the patient lying first in a comfortable, supine position and then later with his head elevated at a 30 to 45-degree angle.

Starting with the head and face, the nurse observes the patient for cyanosis of the earlobes, tip of the nose, cheeks, chin, lips, mucous membranes, and tongue. The presence of facial pallor, exophthalmos, petechiae (especially conjunctival), or rhythmic nodding of the head (produced by hyperdynamic carotid artery pulsations) is also noted.

JUGULAR VENOUS PRESSURE DETERMINATION

The external (superficial) jugular veins and the internal (deep) jugular veins are inspected to estimate venous pressure, right atrial pressure, and right heart function. They are located just above the clavicle and the sternocleidomastoid muscle. Normally the right atrium is the zero point at which venous pressure is measured. During physical examination, however, that landmark is difficult to determine. Instead, the sternal angle of Louis is used because it maintains a fairly constant position 5 to 7 cm above the right atrium. When venous pressure is assessed at the bedside, the patient's head is placed at a 45-degree angle. The patient's head is turned to the side so that the neck veins can be observed tangentially. (The use of tangential lighting is helpful.) The venous pressure level is determined by finding the point above which the internal or the external jugular vein collapses. The venous pressure is recorded by measuring the vertical distance in centimeters from the collapsed jugular vein and the sternal angle. Normally, neck veins will become distended when the patient is lying down (Fig. 10-1A). When the patient is placed at a 45-degree angle, the neck veins should collapse or become visible only 1 to 2 cm above the clavicle. Pressures greater than 3 cm above the sternal angle are considered to be elevated (Fig. 10-1B). The venous

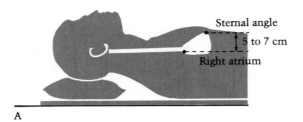

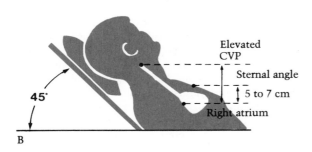

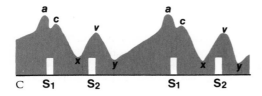

Figure 10-1

A. Neck veins are normally distended when the patient is in the supine position. B. Measurement of jugular venous pressure. C. Jugular venous pulsations illustrating *a*, *v*, and *c* waves, and the *x* and *y* descents.

pulses are affected by respiration; deep inspiration lowers the pulsation level, whereas deep expiration increases the pulsation. Increased jugular venous pressure is observed during inspiration in congestive heart failure, cardiac tamponade, and restrictive cardiomyopathies. Both the right and the left jugular veins should be inspected. Pressure elevation on only one side may indicate a local abnormality.

HEPATOJUGULAR REFLEX

The hepatojugular reflex (HJR) is also evaluated. It is demonstrated by positioning the patient at the point where the highest venous pulsation can be visualized in the middle of the patient's neck. Firm pressure is placed over the right upper quadrant of the patient's abdomen for 30 to 40 seconds. An increase in jugular venous pressure of more than 1 cm during this period is abnormal. A pulsating liver (with or without HJR) suggests triscuspid regurgitation, usually concomitant with right heart failure. If present, that sign reveals that the right heart is unable to accommodate an increased blood flow without a corresponding rise in venous pressure, and it suggests right heart failure. If the patient tenses his abdominal muscles or performs a Valsalva maneuver during the procedure, a false-positive response may be observed.

JUGULAR VENOUS PULSATIONS

Next, jugular venous pulsations are inspected bilaterally and at the base of the neck. Normally they are seen when the patient is supine; however, if the patient's venous pressure is elevated, his head must be raised so that the top of the blood column in the veins can be observed. The two pulsations that are visible are the *a* wave and the *v* wave (Fig. 10-1C). The *a* wave is produced by right atrial contraction that occurs just before ventricular systole. When the examiner palpates the carotid pulse on the opposite side of the neck, the *a* wave is seen to slightly precede the carotid pulsation. If the *a* wave is exaggerated, it indicates elevation of the right atrial pressure. The *a* wave disappears in the presence of atrial fibrillation because of the loss of coordinated atrial contractions.

The tricuspid valve then closes, and the atrium relaxes during the start of ventricular systole. As a result, right atrial pressure is reduced and can be observed as a fall in the height of the blood column in the jugular venous pulse, the *x* descent (Fig. 10-1C). The *v* wave is a consequence of continued atrial filling during the latter part of ventricular systole, when the tricuspid valve is closed. If the *v* wave is exaggerated, it suggests tricuspid insufficiency or right ventricular overloading. At the beginning of ventricular diastole, the tricuspid valve opens and rapidly empties blood into the right ventricle. As the right atrial pressure falls again, the *y* descent is formed. The *c* wave, not generally visible in the neck veins, is caused by a slightly backward deflection of the tricuspid valve during early ventricular systole.

ARTERIAL PULSES

The arterial pulses are palpated for rate, rhythm, amplitude, and equality. Each carotid pulse is palpated separately so that cerebral blood flow is not compromised. It is important to check for any impairment of the blood supply to the extremities. Absence of hair on the toes and feet implies arterial insufficiency. All peripheral pulses, which include the brachial, radial, femoral, popliteal, posterior tibial, and dorsalis pedis pulses, are assessed. During inspection and palpation of the extremities, any changes in color and temperature of the extremities, complaints of cramps, intermittent claudication, clubbing, edema, varicosities, and pain are noted.

CHEST

After inspecting and palpating the pulses, the examiner, standing at the right side of the patient, inspects the patient's chest. The examiner should first note the gross appearance of the chest, looking for distortions of the thoracic cage, bulges, lack of symmetry, skin lesions, scars, increased pigmentation, and petechiae. The following topographic areas are defined (Fig. 10-2):

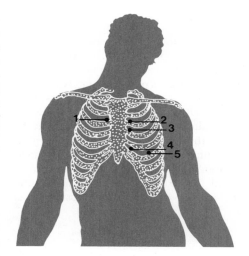

Figure 10-2
Topographic areas of the chest. (1) Aortic area, (2) pulmonic area, (3) Erb's point, (4) tricuspid area, (5) mitral area.

1. The primary aortic area, located in the second intercostal space at the right sternal border (2ICS, RSB).
2. The pulmonic area, located in the second intercostal space at the left sternal border (2ICS, LSB).
3. The secondary aortic area, or Erb's point, located in the third intercostal space at the left sternal border (3ICS, LSB).
4. The tricuspid area, located in the fifth intercostal space at the lower left sternal border (5ICS, LLSB). It is also called the septal or right ventricular area.
5. The mitral area, located in the fifth left intercostal space at the midclavicular line (5ICS, MCL). The mitral area is sometimes referred to as the apical or left ventricular area or the point of maximal impulse.

Inspection and palpation should proceed in an orderly manner, from the primary aortic, pulmonic, secondary aortic, tricuspid, and mitral areas. The examiner first locates the apical impulse and then examines the rest of the precordium for other pulsations or thrills.

The apical impulse is caused by the forward and rightward rotation of the heart at the onset of ventricular systole that brings the apex of the heart closer to the chest wall. The apical impulse, also known as the point of maximal impulse (PMI) is normally found near the fifth intercostal space, 7 to 9 cm from the midsternal line. It may, however, be absent in the normal person who is obese or muscular. Palpation is done by placing the hand over the anterior precordium and shifting the second and third fingers until the apical impulse is located. It is normally the size of a penny or a nickel. If the apical impulse is as large as a quarter, left ventricular enlargement is suspected.

The examiner continues inspecting and palpating the precordium for other pulsations or thrills. Thrills are vibratory sensations generally produced by the turbulent flow created by heart murmurs. (One palpates for thrills and listens for heart murmurs.) The flat portions of three fingers are used to systematically palpate the precordium for thrills. Palpable pulsations in the second or third intercostal space to the left or right of the sternum are abnormal findings; they suggest pulmonary hypertension, aortic aneurysm, or systematic hypertension. Palpation of a right ventricular lift (a diffuse impulse causing the palpating hand to rise) along the left sternal edge is indicative of possible right ventricular hypertrophy since the right ventricle normally does not produce a palpable pulsation. The examiner should also palpate for friction rubs. They also are located over the precordium and are caused by the two pericardial layers rubbing together (the visceral and parietal pericardium [and pleura]) (see Chap. 20).

Percussion

The third step of cardiovascular assessment is precordial percussion to define the cardiac borders. It is often not done because it is not always reliable. Furthermore, the cardiac size is more accurately assessed by means of a chest x ray. When percussion is used, the patient is placed in the supine position. The left border of cardiac dullness (LBCD) can be defined by percussing in the third, fourth, and fifth left intercostal spaces, beginning over resonant lung tissue near the axilla and moving medially until relative cardiac dullness is heard. Those distances usually are around 4, 7, and 10 cm in each of the three intercostal spaces respectively.

Auscultation

BLOOD PRESSURE

When evaluating the patient initially, the critical care nurse must listen carefully to hear more than just the appearance and disappearance of the arterial sounds below the blood pressure cuff. During the procedure of indirect blood pressure measurement, she should pay attention to the changes in sounds and be aware of using the equipment properly and doing the procedure correctly.

On the initial evaluation, the patient's blood pressure should be taken in both arms. There may normally be a 5 to 10 mm Hg difference between the two arms. For an accurate blood pressure recording, the patient should be comfortable, with his arms slightly flexed at the elbow and his brachial artery near heart level. The inflatable sphygmomanometer cuff should be applied snugly over the brachial artery, with the lower cuff border approximately 2.5 cm above the antecubital crease. The cuff is inflated to about 30 mm Hg above the level where the radial pulse disappears. As the cuff pressure is lowered, the radial pulse is palpated. When a mercury sphygmomanometer is used, the readings are noted with the meniscus at the operator's eye level. When the radial pulse is felt, it represents the palpable systolic pressure. At that point, the cuff is deflated. The same procedure is repeated after a pause by inflating the cuff to about 30 mm Hg above the palpable systolic pressure. The diaphragm of the stethoscope is placed firmly over the brachial artery in the antecubital space, avoiding contact with the cuff or clothing. The cuff is slowly deflated about 3 mm Hg per second. Blood pressure in

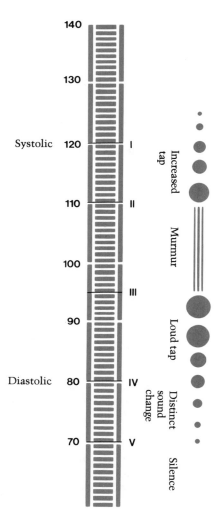

Figure 10-3
Korotkoff sounds.

the arterial system varies with the cardiac cycle. As the pressure falls, the examiner begins to hear Korotkoff sounds, which normally consist of five phases (Fig. 10-3), as discussed in the following paragraphs.

1. *Phase I.* Phase I is characterized by the appearance of faint, clear tapping sounds that gradually increase in intensity. The sounds are produced by the quick distention of the collapsed artery walls as the pulse wave becomes greater than the cuff pressure. Blood suddenly enters the collapsed ar-

tery. The force of blood determines the intensity of the tap. Phase I represents the systolic pressure.

2. *Phase II.* Phase II is marked by the beginning of a murmur sound. The murmur sound is thought to be due to blood flow produced from the narrowed artery under the blood pressure cuff into a wider artery distal to the inflated cuff. This change of artery width creates eddy currents that, in turn, cause the blood and vessel walls to vibrate. The examiner should keep in mind that the forearm and hand are cut off from the general circulation when the blood pressure cuff is inflated.

3. *Phase III.* Phase III is identified by a crisper and more intensified tapping sound than that of phase I. It is louder and higher pitched than the sound of phase II. During phase III, there is no audible murmur.

4. *Phase IV.* Phase IV is marked by a distinct change in sound that is muffled, less intense, and lower pitched than the sounds of the other phases. Phase IV represents the diastolic pressure.

5. *Phase V.* Phase V is the point at which the sound disappears.

Phase I is identified as the systolic pressure, or the greatest pressure of blood against the vessel wall following ventricular contraction. The cuff pressure should continue to be lowered until the muffled sound of phase IV is heard that denotes the diastolic pressure. The diastolic pressure is the lowest pressure following closure of the aortic valve. The cuff pressure is then completely released until no sounds are heard (phase V). All three points are recorded (e.g., 120/80/70). The difference between the systolic and diastolic pressure readings is called the pulse pressure; it represents the range of pressure in the arteries.

In some patients who are hypertensive, an auscultatory gap may be recognized. It is a silent gap between the systolic and diastolic pressures. If the gap is not recognized, incorrect systolic or diastolic pressures may be recorded. When phase I is heard and phase II is absent, the silent period is called an auscultatory gap. The usual length of this gap is 20 to 40 mm Hg. The complete recording of the blood pressure in this situation would be 210/110/100, with an auscultatory gap of 180 to 140 mm Hg.

The examiner taking a blood pressure reading may encounter one or more problems. If the patient's arm is obese, a wider cuff should be used for an accurate measurement. The width of the cuff should equal the diameter of the patient's arm. In obese patients, arte-rial sounds often are higher than the simultaneous intraarterial pressure. A normal-size cuff may give a false hypertensive reading because the force applied by the cuff is lost in the subcutaneous layers of the patient's arm.

On admission or during other phases of hospitalization, the patient may be apprehensive and anxious, and his blood pressure reading may be misleadingly high. In such a case, the pressure should be retaken after the patient has had time to relax. Because dysrhythmias may produce a variation in the systolic pressure, several readings should be taken and the average should be recorded.

On occasion, the nurse may have difficulty hearing the blood pressure sounds. The most severe problem causing an inaudible blood pressure is shock. Shock should be immediately recognized and treated. If the blood pressure cannot be heard by auscultation, then the systolic blood pressure can be evaluated by means of palpation. Since the diastolic pressure cannot be obtained by palpation, the pressure would be recorded as (for example) 90/p. The examiner must also be aware of the problems with techniques in taking indirect blood pressure measurements. If the blood pressure sounds are inaudible, the examiner must consider incorrect placement of the stethoscope or venous engorgement of an arm caused by repeated inflation of the blood pressure cuff. Three techniques can be used to increase the intensity of the sounds:

1. Rapid inflation of the cuff decreases the amount of blood that is trapped in the forearm. Inflating the cuff slowly causes an increased amount of blood to be trapped in the forearm with each beat.
2. The patient's arm can be raised before inflating the cuff. That permits venous blood to drain from the forearm before cuff inflation.
3. The patient can rapidly open and close his hand 8 or 10 times after inflation of the cuff above the systolic level. That technique increases the blood-holding capacity of forearm vessels and thus lowers the pressure in the forearm.

The examiner must not reinflate the cuff to take another systolic reading until the cuff has been fully deflated. Full deflation allows the forearm to fill with blood, affecting the intensity and quality of the sounds.

In some clinical situations, the leg pulses must be evaluated and an indirect blood pressure in the lower extremities must be assessed. If necessary, the volume

Table 10-1
Heart Sounds

Source	Cause	Stethoscope	Location
S_1 $(M_1 T_1)$	Closure of tricuspid and mitral valves	Diaphragm	Entire precordium (apex)
S_2 $(A_2 P_2)$	Closure of pulmonic and aortic valves	Diaphragm	A_2 heard at 2RICS; P_2 at 2LICS
S_3 Ventricular gallop	Rapid ventricular filling	Bell	Apex
S_4 Atrial gallop	Forceful atrial ejection into distended ventricle	Bell	Apex
Ejection clicks (ECs)	Distention of great vessels or opening of deformed aortic or pulmonic valve	Diaphragm	2RICS, 2LICS, or apex
Midsystolic clicks (MSCs)	Prolapse of mitral valve leaflet	Diaphragm	Apex
Opening snaps (OSs)	Abrupt recoil of stenotic mitral or tricuspid valve	Diaphragm	LLSB

and timing of the radial and femoral pulses should be determined and a comparison of arm and leg pressures should be made, especially when coarctation of the aorta is suspected. Normally an 18- to 20-cm blood pressure bladder and a wide cuff are used for the thigh recordings. The patient should lie on his abdomen, if possible. The compression bag of the blood pressure cuff should be placed over the posterior aspect of the patient's midthigh. The examiner then places the stethoscope in the popliteal fossa over the popliteal artery and uses the techniques used for measuring arm pressure. If the patient cannot lie on his abdomen, the examiner should have the patient lie in the supine position. The patient should flex his knee enough to permit the examiner to place the stethoscope in the correct position in the popliteal fossa. Thigh recordings usually reveal a systolic pressure from 10 to 40 mm Hg higher than that in the arm, but the diastolic pressure is approximately the same as that in the arm.

HEART SOUNDS

The final step of cardiovascular assessment is cardiac auscultation. Several theories attempt to explain the generation of heart sounds. Heart sounds may arise from energy sources within the heart and/or the great vessels; or they may be produced by the acceleration and deceleration of blood in the cardiac chambers. Cardiac sounds do occur after the closure of heart valves, however, and they are related to various pressure gradients within the heart and great vessels.

The point of maximum intensity in the chest wall may be closest to the points where the sounds are produced although those sounds can often be heard in other areas. Many heart sounds may be best heard over the auscultatory areas (the places where vibratory sounds radiate) rather than over the anatomic locations (the places where the sounds originate) (see Fig. 10-2).

Auscultation must proceed systematically. The listener should concentrate on one sound at a time rather than try to take in all the sounds at once. For example, the examiner should identify the first heart sound and then the second heart sound. She should count the heart rate. She should determine whether the rhythm is regular or irregular. If it is irregular—is it "regularly irregular," or is it totally irregular? Listen to the heart sounds by "inching" the stethoscope over the precordium from the aortic auscultatory area, to the pulmonic area, to Erb's point, and finally to the tricuspid and mitral areas. Individually identify the first and second heart sounds by appraising the intensity, pitch, splitting, and respiratory changes of each sound. Listen for extra systolic sounds, such as ejection clicks, and for extra diastolic sounds, such as the third heart sound, or the fourth heart sound, or a mitral opening snap. Finally, listen for murmurs or rubs and evaluate the timing, configuration, pitch, quality, intensity, location, and radiation.

The diaphragm of the stethoscope filters out low frequencies and should be used to identify high-pitched sounds, such as the first and second heart sounds and the murmurs of aortic and mitral insuffi-

Pitch	Respirations	Position	Variations
High	Softer on inspiration	Any position	Increased with excitement, exercise, amyl nitrite, epinephrine, atropine
High	Expiration produces fusion of A_2P_2; inspiration produces physiological split	Sitting or supine	Increased in thin chest walls and with exercise
Low	Increased on inspiration	Supine or left lateral	Increased with exercise, fast heart rate, elevation of legs, and increased venous return
Low	Increased on forced inspiration	Supine or left semilateral	Same as for S_3
High		Sitting or supine	
High	Increased on expiration	Sitting or supine	
High		Any position	May be confused with S_3

ciency, friction rubs, and clicks. The bell of the stethoscope is then used to identify low-pitched sounds, such as the third and fourth heart sounds and the murmurs of aortic and mitral stenosis.

First Heart Sound
The first heart sound (S_1) is associated with closure of the tricuspid and mitral valve at the time when ventricular pressures exceed atrial pressures. It corresponds to the onset of ventricular contraction and therefore indicates the beginning of systole (Table 10-1). It is heard shortly after the QRS complex on the ECG.

Right-sided events usually follow left-sided events because of the higher pressures found in the left heart. Accordingly, the mitral valve closes slightly before the tricuspid valve. The first heart sound is, therefore, split into two components—mitral (M_1) and tricuspid (T_1) (Fig. 10-4A). The louder M_1 is followed immediately by T_1. S_1 can be differentiated from other heart sounds because it closely corresponds to each carotid pulsation. Palpation of the carotid artery during auscultation helps the examiner to correctly identify the first heart sound, which may be particularly difficult to distinguish from other heart sounds when the patient has a fast heart rate. S_1 is usually a lower-pitched and longer sound than S_2. It is heard best with the diaphragm of the stethoscope over the entire precordium although it is generally loudest at the apex. The sounds may become softer during inspiration because expansion of the lungs increases the distance between the heart and the chest wall. In the presence of atrial

fibrillation, S_1 may assume a variable intensity. Exercise, excitement, or drugs, such as amyl nitrite, epinephrine, or atropine sulfate, intensify the sound. The split of S_1 into M_1T_1 may often be easy to hear in young children but difficult to hear in adults.

The first heart sound may be abnormally split and therefore audible in adults as a result of mechanical or electrical problems, causing the ventricles to contract at different times. In right bundle branch block, for example, right ventricular stimulation, tricuspid valve closure, and right ventricular contraction are abnormally delayed, producing a longer time period between M_1T_1. Mechanical delay problems, on the other hand, such as in mitral stenosis, may produce a reverse split of S_1 in which the tricuspid valve closes before the mitral valve (T_1M_1).

Second Heart Sound
The second heart sound (S_2) is associated with closure of the pulmonic and aortic valves when the pressures in the pulmonary artery and aorta exceed right and left ventricular pressures, respectively (Table 10-1). S_2 corresponds with the onset of ventricular relaxation and indicates the beginning of ventricular diastole. Because of the higher pressure on the left side of the heart, left-sided events precede those on the right. The phenomenon is accentuated during inspiration, when increased venous return to the right heart occurs as a result of a lowered negative intrathoracic pressure. During inspiration, the right ventricle needs a longer time to eject blood than does the left ventricle because of augmented right-sided

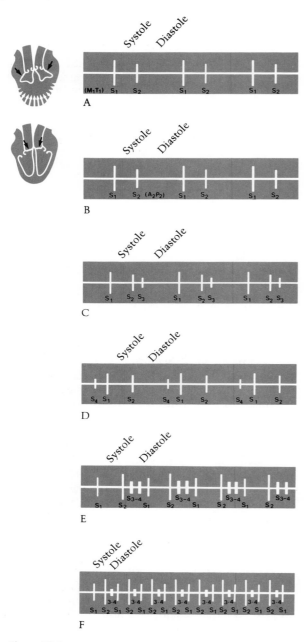

Figure 10-4

A. First heart sound (S_1). B. Second heart sound (S_2). C. Third heart sound (S_3). D. Fourth heart sound (S_4). E. Quadruple rhythm. F. Summation gallop.

volumes. That causes the pulmonic valve to close after the aortic valve closes, thereby producing a *physiological split* of S_2. The split may also be a result of a pooling of blood in the inflated lung during inspiration that causes a reduced flow of blood into the left atrium and earlier aortic valve closure. Physiological splitting of S_2, composed of a louder aortic component (A_2), followed by a softer pulmonic sound (P_2), is a normal event during inspiration in the adult (Fig. 10-4B). The disparity between right- and left-sided volumes is normally reversed during expiration, causing A_2 and P_2 to narrow and occur about the same time to produce a single sound. The physiological split is often accentuated in people with thin chest walls or during exercise.

S_2 is generally a higher-pitched sound and of shorter duration than S_1. It is best heard with the diaphragm of the stethoscope and with the patient in either the sitting or the supine position. The aortic component (A_2) is loudest over the second to third right intercostal space; the pulmonic component is heard best over the second to third left intercostal space.

An abnormal variation in the splitting pattern of the second heart sound is known as a *fixed S_2 split*. In that phenomenon, the split of the two components is unaffected by respiration or blood volume changes, causing A_2P_2 to be heard with equal intensity during both inspiration and expiration. Fixed splitting suggests problems related to pulmonary stenosis or atrial septal defect.

Other pathophysiological states may produce variations in the normal splitting pattern of S_2. *Paradoxical or reversed splitting* of S_2 occurs when left ventricular systole is delayed, causing the aortic valve closure to follow pulmonic valve closure instead of preceding it. As a result, the pulmonic sound occurs before the aortic sound during expiration (P_2A_2). (Normally, during expiration, the two components of the second heart sound fuse.) During inspiration, however, when pulmonic valve closure is normally delayed due to augmented right-sided filling, P_2 moves closer to the abnormally delayed aortic sound to produce a fusion of the two components. That produces a reversal of the normal splitting pattern and may be caused by patent ductus arteriosus, left bundle branch block, aortic stenosis, severe left ventricular disease or uncontrolled hypertension.

Third Heart Sound

A normal physiological third heart sound (S_3) is frequently heard in children and young adults, and it usually disappears completely if the patient stands or sits up. A pathological S_3 is synonymous with such terms as ventricular gallop, protodiastolic gallop, and an early diastolic ventricular filling sound. S_3 is caused by the vibrations of a noncompliant ventricle that occur during the period of rapid ventricular filling in early diastole after closure of the aortic and pulmonic valves and the opening of the mitral and tricuspid valves (Table 10-1).

S_3 is a low faint sound best heard with the bell of the stethoscope applied lightly to the apex and with the patient in the left lateral or supine position. It occurs immediately after S_2. The rhythm and pattern of S_1, S_2, and S_3 somewhat resemble the sounds produced by saying Ken–tuc–ky (Fig. 10-4C).

S_3 is an abnormal sound found in the adult, and it is associated with any condition that increases early diastolic pressures or rapid ventricular filling. S_3 is generally an early sign of congestive heart failure. A left-sided S_3 may be produced by mitral regurgitation or left ventricular failure caused by myocardial ischemia or infarction, hypertension, or aortic valvular disease. A right-sided S_3 may be the result of right heart failure, pulmonary embolism, or pulmonary hypertension. S_3 is accentuated by exercise, inspiration, elevation of the legs or any other factor that increases the rate of blood flow to the heart. Conversely, the sound is diminished by phenomena that decrease venous return, such as assuming an upright posture or using venous tourniquets.

Fourth Heart Sound

The fourth heart sound (S_4) is often referred to as an atrial gallop or a presystolic gallop. Generally, it is an abnormal finding in the adult, but it may be heard normally in infants or small children and it may occasionally be heard in the athlete and in the "normal" person. It is a soft, low-pitched diastolic sound heard best with the patient in the supine or the left semilateral position with the stethoscope bell placed at the apex (Table 10-1). S_4 closely precedes S_1 so that the cadence of S_4, S_1, and S_2 is similar to the sound produced by saying Ten–nes–see (Fig. 10-4D). S_4 may indicate increased resistance to ventricular filling; it is produced following atrial contraction as a result of the forceful ejection of blood into an overdistended ventricle. It is caused by any condition that impairs ventricular compliance, such as hypertensive cardiovascular disease, coronary artery disease, or aortic stenosis. S_4 becomes intensified and diminished by the same maneuvers that accentuate or diminish S_3.

Quadruple Rhythms

Quadruple rhythms refer to the cadence of the normal S_1 and S_2 plus S_3 and S_4. When the heart rate is slow, all four components may be heard separately, and they have been described as sounding like a cogwheel or a locomotive (Fig. 10-4E).

In the presence of tachycardia or delayed atrioventricular (AV) conduction time, S_3 and S_4 may fuse together in middiastole to form a single sound almost as loud as S_1 and S_2. Instead of a quadruple rhythm, a triple rhythm is heard to produce what is known as a *summation gallop* (Fig. 10-4F). That rhythm sounds much like a horse cantering on a dirt track.

Ejection Clicks

Ejection clicks (ECs) (early systolic ejection clicks) are sounds that occur during the onset of early ventricular systole (Table 10-1). The sound may be produced either by vibrations resulting from the sudden distention of the great vessels or by the movement of stiff and deformed valves. Ejection clicks are commonly heard in association with pulmonic or aortic stenosis and in pulmonary or systemic hypertension. They are sharp, high-pitched sounds heard immediately after S_1 (Fig. 10-5A) in the pulmonic or aortic auscultatory areas. They are best heard with the diaphragm of the stethoscope and with the patient in the sitting or supine position.

Midsystolic Clicks

Midsystolic clicks (MSCs), also known as middle or late systolic sounds, are most commonly associated with prolapse of the mitral leaflet into the left atrium (Table 10-1). They are sharp, high-pitched sounds heard during the midportion of ventricular systole (Fig. 10-5B). They are best heard during expiration, with the diaphragm of the stethoscope placed at the apex and with the patient in the sitting or supine position.

Opening Snaps

In the normal setting, the opening of the mitral and tricuspid valves is inaudible. In the presence of mitral and tricuspid stenosis, opening snaps (OSs) may be heard as a result of the abrupt recoil or cessation of opening movement of the valve during ventricular diastole (Table 10-1). The high-pitched, snapping sound is heard shortly after S_2 (Fig. 10-5C) with the diaphragm of the stethoscope over the mitral and tricuspid areas, and it is often followed by a rumble. The timing frequently overlaps with an S_3, making it

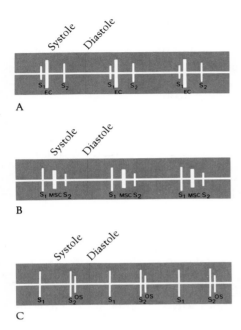

Figure 10-5
A. Ejection click (EC). B. Midsystolic click (MSC). C. Opening snap (OS).

difficult to distinguish without the aid of an apex ECG or phonocardiogram.

Murmurs

During auscultatory assessment of the heart, each area must be checked carefully for the presence of murmurs. Murmurs are audible vibratory sounds. There are several mechanisms that are responsible for heart murmurs. The to-and-fro flow of blood over diseased heart valves creates turbulence and eddy currents, producing vibrations and resultant murmurs. Other conditions, such as increased blood flow (the flow murmur of hyperthyroidism or of fever), an abnormal communication between intracardiac chambers, or blood flow in a dilated great vessel may also generate vibrations and produce murmurs. In some people with normal heart valves, a functional murmur may be heard that is caused by normal hemodynamic factors rather than disease states. Murmurs are identified and assessed in regard to their timing, configuration, pitch, quality, intensity, location, and radiation.

Timing in the Cardiac Cycle. Murmurs are classified according to their timing in the cardiac cycle as sys-

tolic, diastolic, or continuous. A systolic murmur begins with or after S_1 and ends at or before S_2. A diastolic murmur begins with or after S_2 and ends at or before S_1. A continuous murmur begins in systole and extends through S_2 into part or all of diastole.

Systolic murmurs may be further subdivided according to their time of onset and duration. An early systolic murmur begins with S_1 and ends about the middle of systole. A midsystolic ejection murmur begins in the middle of systole and ends before S_2. A late systolic murmur begins in the middle or late systole and ends with S_2. Likewise, diastolic murmurs may be subdivided into early, middle, and late diastolic murmurs.

Configuration. Murmurs frequently have an identifiable configuration. A crescendo murmur is one that progressively increases in loudness. A decrescendo murmur progressively decreases in sound (such as the murmur of aortic regurgitation). A crescendo-decrescendo, or diamond-shaped murmur (such as the murmur of aortic stenosis), is one that peaks to intensity and then progressively decreases in sound. A holosystolic (pansystolic, sustained, or plateau) murmur is one that remains constant throughout its duration.

Pitch and Quality. Murmurs may be classified as high, medium, or low pitched. A high- or medium-pitched murmur, such as that in aortic regurgitation, is heard best with the diaphragm of the stethoscope; it sounds much like the forceful expiration of air through an open mouth. A low-pitched murmur, such as that in mitral stenosis, makes a rumbling noise and it is best heard with the bell. Murmurs may be further identified by their quality of sound; they may be described as harsh, rumbling, blowing, or whooping.

Intensity (Grading). Murmurs are usually graded on a scale of one to six according to the intensity of sound. A grade 1 murmur is barely audible (it is sometimes thought that only the instructor can hear a grade 1/6 murmur!). A grade 2 murmur is faint but audible; a grade 3 murmur is moderately loud; a grade 4 murmur is a loud murmur associated with a thrill; a grade 5 murmur is the loudest murmur heard that requires the use of a stethoscope; a grade 6 murmur is so loud that it can be heard without a stethoscope.

Location and Radiation. Each murmur is generally heard the loudest at a specific area or location over the precordium (e.g., the aortic, pulmonic, mitral, and tricuspid locations), as discussed earlier. Radiation of a murmur refers to the transmission of the sound to the sites other than the primary anatomic location of the murmur. Sound may be transmitted through the vascular wall, soft tissues, bone, and blood stream. The radiation of sound is dependent on the quality and pitch of the murmur, as well as on its anatomic proximity to adjacent structures. The direction of radiation gives important information about the origin of the murmur. If a valve leaks, for example, the murmur may be best heard in the direction of the leak rather than in the auscultatory region.

Types of Murmurs. Using the characteristics of timing, configuration, pitch, quality, intensity, location, and radiation, murmurs associated with abnormalities of the AV and semilunar valves will be classified in the following paragraphs. (Aortic and mitral valvular disease, the most common abnormalities found in the adult, are discussed in detail in Chapter 21.)

Aortic Stenosis (Fig. 10-6A)
  Cause: Forward flow of blood from left ventricle to aorta through obstructed aortic valve
  Timing: Systole
  Configuration: Crescendo–decrescendo
  Quality and pitch: Harsh and low pitched
  Location: Aortic auscultatory area
  Radiation: Into the neck or carotid vessels

Aortic Regurgitation (Fig. 10-6B)
  Cause: Backward flow of blood from aorta to left ventricle through incompetent (leaky) aortic valve
  Timing: Diastole
  Configuration: Decrescendo
  Quality and pitch: Blowing and high pitched
  Location: Aortic auscultatory area
  Radiation: Left sternal border

Mitral Stenosis (Fig. 10-6C)
  Cause: Forward flow of blood from left atrium to left ventricle through obstructed mitral valve
  Timing: Diastole
  Configuration: Crescendo–decrescendo
  Quality and pitch: Rumbling and low pitched
  Location: Apex
  Radiation: Usually none

Mitral Regurgitation (Fig. 10-6D)
  Cause: Backward flow of blood from left ventricle to left atrium through incompetent mitral valve

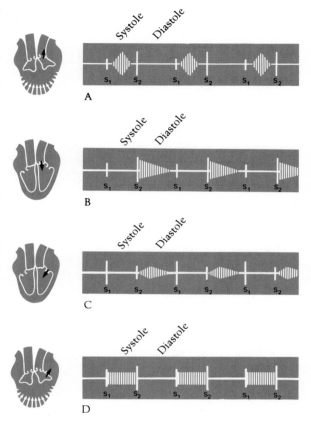

Figure 10-6
A. Aortic stenosis. B. Aortic regurgitation. C. Mitral stenosis. D. Mitral regurgitation.

  Timing: Systole
  Configuration: Holosystolic
  Quality and pitch: Blowing and high pitched
  Location: Apex
  Radiation: Left axillary line

Pulmonary Stenosis (Fig. 10-7A)
  Cause: Forward flow of blood from right ventricle to pulmonary artery through obstructed pulmonic valve
  Timing: Systole
  Configuration: Crescendo–decrescendo
  Quality and pitch: Harsh and medium pitched
  Location: Pulmonary auscultatory area
  Radiation: Usually none

Pulmonary Regurgitation (Fig. 10-7B)
  Cause: Backward flow of blood from pulmonary

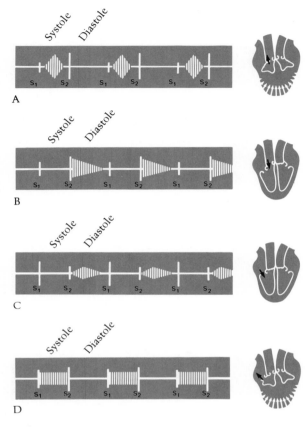

Figure 10-7
A. Pulmonary stenosis. B. Pulmonary regurgitation. C. Tricuspid stenosis. D. Tricuspid regurgitation.

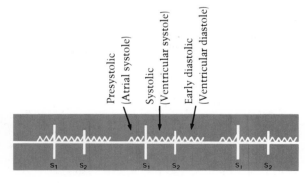

Figure 10-8
Pericardial friction rub.

artery to right ventricle through incompetent pulmonic valve
Timing: Diastole
Configuration: Decrescendo; increases in intensity with inspiration
Quality and pitch: Blowing and high (or low) pitched
Location: Third and fourth left intercostal spaces
Radiation: Usually none

Tricuspid Stenosis (Fig. 10-7C)
Cause: Forward flow of blood from right atrium to right ventricle through obstructed tricuspid valve
Timing: Diastole
Configuration: Crescendo–decrescendo
Quality and pitch: Rumbling and low pitched
Location: Lower left sternal border and tricuspid auscultatory area
Radiation: Usually none

Tricuspid Regurgitation (Fig. 10-7D)
Cause: Backward flow of blood from right ventricle to right atrium through an incompetent tricuspid valve
Timing: Systole
Configuration: Holosystolic; increases in intensity with inspiration
Quality and pitch: Blowing and high pitched
Location: Tricuspid auscultatory area
Radiation: Usually none

Pericardial Friction Rub (Fig. 10-8)
Pericardial friction rubs sound similar to and may be confused with heart murmurs. Rubs are characterized by the following:
Cause: Roughening and irritation of pericardial surface
Timing: Systole, diastole or both (may have systolic, early diastolic, and presystolic components)
Quality and pitch: Usually loud, leathery, scratchy, and high pitched
Location: Third intercostal space at left sternal border
Radiation: Usually none

Noninvasive Techniques of Assessment

Electrocardiogram

The ECG is a routine diagnostic procedure used to evaluate patients with possible cardiovascular disease. The ECG provides baseline data that may be used for comparison when a patient's condition changes. It can be used in the diagnosis of acute myocardial infarctions, dysrhythmias, conduction disturbances, atrial and ventricular hypertrophy, cardiac drug intoxication, and electrolyte or metabolic disturbances.

Chest X Ray

A chest x ray is also a routine part of the initial cardiovascular examination. It is more reliable than percussion for determining the exact size and contour of the heart. It can help to evaluate pulmonary congestion and pulmonary arterial blood flow and to arrive at certain cardiac diagnoses, such as coarctation of the aorta. In some situations, special overpenetrated films can be used for better visualization of particular abnormalities.

Echocardiogram

The echocardiogram, a noninvasive technique, may be used to help identify abnormalities of the mitral valve (e.g., mitral stenosis), idiopathic hypertrophic subaortic stenosis, left atrial tumors, pericardial effusions, left atrial thrombi, abnormal aortic size, abnormal tricuspid or prosthetic mitral valve motion, congenital cardiac lesions, and abnormal left ventricular function. During the procedure, the patient is awake and is in a recumbent position. An electromechanical transducer is placed on the patient's chest; it serves as both an emitter and a receiver of ultrasound. As the ultrasound echoes are received, they are amplified on an oscilloscope and recorded on paper. The procedure does not involve any risk or discomfort.

Phonocardiogram

The phonocardiogram simultaneously records the ECG (for a reference point) and heart sounds and murmurs, and it increases the assessment of auscultatory phenomena. It is of major value in identifying the timing of heart sounds, (splits, ejection sounds, and extra sounds). The patient is awake during the procedure. There is no risk or discomfort to the patient.

Vectorcardiogram

The vectorcardiogram is a technique that is useful in the diagnosis of myocardial infarction and minor intraventricular conduction defects and in confirming myocardial hypertrophy caused by intraventricular conduction defects. The procedure is done by placing a number of lead connections on the patient's body. Frontal, sagittal, and transverse loops are recorded and interpreted to make specific diagnoses.

Exercise Tolerance Test

A stress, or exercise, tolerance test (ETT) is an important means of evaluating the cardiovascular function of patients with or without known heart disease. ETT is generally accomplished by the use of one of three types of procedures: the Master's double two-step test, bicycle ergometry, and a multistage treadmill test. The Master's test, the oldest of the techniques, involves having the patient walk up and down a set of 9-inch steps. Bicycle ergometry measures the effects of dynamic leg or arm exercises applied against a calibrated amount of resistance. The treadmill test subjects the patient to graduated levels of exercise. The treadmill is adjusted by increasing the walking speed and the incline.

Ideally, ETT should be performed between 8:00 A.M. and 12:00 NOON to avoid fluctuations in the patient's circadian rhythms. The patient should not eat or drink anything except water or Sanka for three hours before the testing. Generally most medications are also withheld. Since physical work can alter the interpretations and results of the study, patients are instructed to avoid strenuous exercise 24 hours before the testing.

The nature of the test and the test procedures should be thoroughly explained to the patient. A tour of the exercise laboratory before the testing may help reduce the patient's anxiety. Since high levels of anxiety may alter the results of the test and/or produce serious complications during the procedure, the test should probably be postponed if the patient is anxious until the source of the patient's fear is identified and the fear reduced.

Before the ETT is done, a complete history must be taken and a complete physical examination done. Patients who are found to have new or changing chest pain, hypertension, thrombophlebitis, uncontrolled heart failure, serious dysrhythmias, severe valvular disease or other life-threatening cardiovascular dis-

Table 10-2
End Points for Exercise Tolerance Testing

Subjective End Points	Objective End Points
Chest pain	ST-segment elevation or depression
Severe fatigue	
Severe dyspnea	Supraventricular dysrhythmias
Leg pain	
Patient asks to stop (even if none of the above is present)	Frequent PVCs or other ventricular dysrhythmias
	Drop in blood pressure
	Elevation of blood pressure
	Signs of cerebral hypoxia
	Signs of circulatory insufficiency

ease are not candidates for stress testing. Patients who are severely limited by noncardiac illnesses, such as those that produce neurological, peripheral vascular, or musculoskeletal disease, also are generally not eligible for stress testing.

An ECG is done before and after the test. Continuous ECG monitoring and blood pressure determinations are done before, during, and 5 to 10 minutes after the test. Rhythm strips are made with the patient at rest and every two or three minutes during and after the exercise. The testing is continued until the patient reaches his maximum heart rate (determined by his sex and age) or until he reaches the subjective or the objective endpoints for ETT (Table 10-2). Emergency equipment, such as emergency drugs, intravenous fluids, and a direct current defibrillator, should be at hand in the exercise laboratory. Physicians and other staff members should be trained in both basic and advanced life support (see Chap. 18).

ETT can be used as an indicator of heart disease, in the differential diagnosis of chest pain, in objectively classifying the patient's functional ability and symptoms, and in advising a patient convalescing from an acute myocardial infarction about his physical rehabilitation.

Invasive Techniques of Assessment

Cardiac Catheterization

Cardiac catheterization is an important technique used to diagnose and quantify the extent of coronary atherosclerotic, valvular and congenital heart disease and to evaluate specific heart pressures. Before the catheterization is done, a complete history is taken, and a physical examination, an ECG, a chest x ray, an exercise tolerance test, and, possibly, a phonocardiogram and an echocardiogram are done. Generally cardiac catheterization is an elective procedure, and it is contraindicated in patients who are not clinically stable. It may be performed on an emergency basis to evaluate life-threatening illnesses that are potentially correctable by surgery. Since most of the contrast mediums contain iodine, the patient should be asked whether he is allergic to iodine.

The physician generally is responsible for explaining the procedure to the patient and informing him about the indications, benefits, and risks of the study. The nurse should be present during the explanation, and she should reinforce the information given by the physician, clarify the instructions, and answer the patient's questions. The patient should be made familiar with the laboratory, and he should practice the things that will be expected of him during the catheterization, such as holding his breath, coughing, and deep breathing. He should be told that he may experience a number of sensations, such as flushing, palpitations, nausea, and some minimal discomfort at the insertion site.

During the catheterization, the patient receives continuous cardiac monitoring. Cardiac catheterization may include a right heart study, a left heart study and/or a coronary artery angiogram. Depending on the procedure and the physician's preference, the catheter may be inserted into the right basilic vein and brachial artery or the femoral vein and artery. Right heart catheterization is done to evaluate right heart pressures, left-to-right shunts, and pulmonic, tricuspid, or mitral valve disease and to calculate cardiac output. Left heart catheterization is done to determine left heart pressures and to evaluate left ventricular function. Selective coronary angiography is done to visualize a suspected narrowing or obstruction of the coronary arteries.

A His bundle (HB) ECG may also be done by using the technique of a right heart catheterization to evaluate conduction abnormalities and to determine the origin of tachycardias and ectopic beats. The HB recording allows the PR interval to be divided into two components, the A-H interval and the H-V interval. The A-H interval represents the time segment from the onset of atrial depolarization to the HB depolarization, whereas the H-V interval represents the period of depolarization down the HB to the ventricles.

The common complications of cardiac catheterization include vessel spasm and dysrhythmias. Infrequently the procedure may also be associated with such serious complications as acute myocardial infarction, systemic or pulmonary embolism, severe allergic reactions, perforation of the heart, cerebral vascular accidents, and death.

After the procedure, the patient's vital signs are checked every 15 minutes for several hours. The distal pulse of the extremity used during the procedure is also checked for pulsation and for bleeding. The patient is generally instructed to stay in bed and not to move or bend the extremity until the time specified by the physician. Complications observed during the post–catheterization period include hemorrhage, hypotension, cerebral dysfunction, infection, vessel thrombosis, and fever.

Assessment of the Cardiac Rhythm

Properties of Cardiac Muscles

The three types of cardiac muscles are the atrial, the ventricular, and the noncontractile muscles. The primary characteristics of those muscles are automaticity, excitability, conductivity, and contractility.

Automaticity refers to the ability of the heart to initiate its own impulse. Excitability is the heart's ability to respond to an impulse. The ability of the heart to transmit electrical impulses to other areas of the heart is referred to as conductivity. Contractility may be defined as the heart's ability to achieve tension and muscle fiber shortening.

Autonomic Nervous System Control

The two divisions of the autonomic nervous system—the sympathetic system and parasympathetic system—control the visceral functions of the body and maintain a balance by their opposing forces.

The origin of the sympathetic nerves supplying the heart is at the level of the first thoracic through the second lumbar vertebrae of the spinal column. Sympathetic nerve endings are located in the atria and the ventricles. Stimulation of those nerve endings releases norepinephrine, producing an increase in the overall activity of the heart by (1) increasing the rate of discharge from the SA node, (2) increasing conduction through the AV node, (3) augmenting the force of atrial and ventricular contractility, and (4) increasing

the excitability of the heart. The system is referred to collectively as the adrenergic system.

Parasympathetic nerve endings, on the other hand, are found primarily in the atria, and they leave the central nervous system via the cranial and sacral spinal nerves. The vagi are the parasympathetic nerves of the heart. When stimulated, acetylcholine is released at the vagal nerve endings, producing (1) a reduction in the rate of discharge from the SA node, (2) a decrease in the excitability of the AV junctional fibers, and (3) a slowing of AV node conduction. The system is generally referred to as the cholinergic system.

Electromechanical Physiology

In the normal heart, electrical activity precedes mechanical activity. Electrical activity refers to the origin and transmission of an electrical impulse through the conduction system, which in turn comprises the various stages of cardiac stimulation as recorded on the ECG. Mechanical activity is the actual contraction and pump activity of the heart after it has been electrically stimulated.

Electrochemical Physiology

The electrical activity of the heart consists of depolarization (stimulation) and repolarization (relaxation). Those two events are the results of electrochemical events within the cell membrane. Fluid inside and outside the cell membranes is composed of electrolyte solutions made up of positive and negative charges. In the resting cell, there is an accumulation of positive ions (cations) on the outside surface of the cell membrane and an equal number of negative ions (anions) on the inner surface of the membrane (Fig. 10-9A). Likewise, a high concentration of potassium is found inside the cell, and a high concentration of sodium is found outside the cell.

MEMBRANE POTENTIAL

The difference in ionic concentration causes the development of a membrane potential. A membrane potential develops because the cell membrane is equipped with a sodium-potassium pump that allows sodium ions to be pumped to the exterior of the cell and potassium ions to be pumped to the interior of

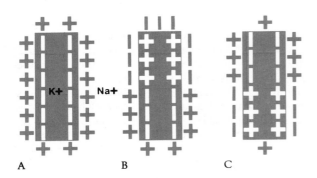

Figure 10-9
A. Polarized cell. B. Depolarization. C. Repolarization.

the cell. Those ions may also be exchanged by the process of diffusion. Since the membrane is 50 to 100 times more permeable to potassium than to sodium, potassium ions diffuse through the membrane with relative ease, whereas sodium ions and nondiffusible anions, such as phosphates, sulfates, and proteins, diffuse very poorly.

A current flows when there is a reversal in the polarity of the cell. In the normal resting cell, the ions of opposite polarity are lined up on either side of the semipermeable membrane. There is no current flow, and the cell is said to be polarized. As long as the membrane remains undisturbed, the cell remains in its resting state (Fig. 10-9A).

ACTION POTENTIAL

Any factor that suddenly changes the polarity of the membrane produces rapid changes in the membrane potential. The sequence of rapid changes is termed the action potential; it consists of two separate stages, depolarization and repolarization. Factors that can elicit an action potential are electrical or chemical stimulation, heat, cold, ischemia, injury, or any other phenomenon that temporarily disturbs the normal resting state of the cell.

DEPOLARIZATION

Pacemaker cells, however, do not rely on those factors to produce action potentials because they are capable of self-excitation. SA, atrial, junctional, and ventricular pacing cells do not maintain a constant resting membrane potential. The process of self-excitation is probably caused by a high degree of membrane permeability to sodium ions (slow diastolic depolarization) as soon as the cell returns to its resting state. That causes enough positively charged sodium ions to accumulate inside the cell to disturb the resting membrane potential and even to develop a positive state within the cell instead of the normal negative state. At that point, a threshold is reached. The action potential begins, and depolarization (stimulation) occurs.

An action potential produced at any point on a cell membrane can excite adjacent membranes, resulting in propagation (spread) of the action potential. Figure 10-9B illustrates a local circuit of current flow between the depolarized and resting membrane sections until all parts of the membrane and adjacent fibers have been stimulated. The transmission of depolarization is called an impulse.

REPOLARIZATION

As soon as the cell is depolarized, it quickly returns to its polarized, or resting, state as a result of the rapid diffusion of potassium out of the membrane. The positive ions again return to the outside of the cell, and the negative ions return to the inside due to the sodium-potassium pump. The phenomenon is called repolarization (Fig. 10-9C).

REFRACTORY PERIODS

Before the cells of the heart can be depolarized again, they must return to a resting state. Repolarization must be completed before the cell can accept another stimulus. If a cell is stimulated during repolarization before reaching its resting state, it will be refractory or not able to respond to the stimulus. Thus the cell is said to be in a refractory period.

Three refractory periods of the heart must be understood (Fig. 10-10). At the completion of depolarization, all cells are refractory and unable to accept a stimulus. That is the *absolute refractory period*. During the vulnerable phase, or the *relative refractory period* of the heart, some of the cells are repolarized and still others are depolarized. The repolarized cells are able to accept a stimulus because they are nonrefractory whereas the depolarized cells are still refractory. At that point (known as the vulnerable period), the heart is difficult to stimulate, but it may be excited by a strong stimulus that may produce various lethal dysrhythmias. A heart that is

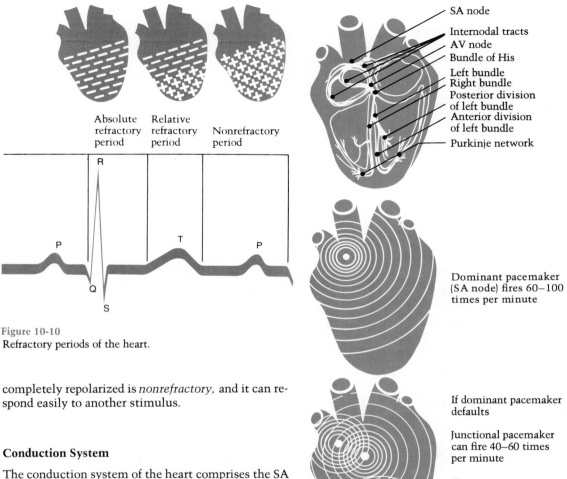

Figure 10-10
Refractory periods of the heart.

SA node
Internodal tracts
AV node
Bundle of His
Left bundle
Right bundle
Posterior division
of left bundle
Anterior division
of left bundle
Purkinje network

Dominant pacemaker
(SA node) fires 60–100
times per minute

If dominant pacemaker
defaults

Junctional pacemaker
can fire 40–60 times
per minute

or

Ventricular Purkinje
system can fire
30–40 times per minute

Figure 10-11
Conduction system of the heart.

completely repolarized is *nonrefractory*, and it can respond easily to another stimulus.

Conduction System

The conduction system of the heart comprises the SA node, the interatrial conduction pathways, the AV node, the bundle of His, the left and right bundle branches, and the Purkinje network (Fig. 10-11).

Those specialized portions of the myocardium initiate the sequence of events in the cardiac cycle and control the cycle's regularity.

The dominant pacemaker of the heart, the SA node, which normally fires 60 to 100 times per minute, is located in the right atrium near the superior vena cava. The characteristic of automaticity is found within the SA node, allowing it to initiate its own impulse. Cells located within the atrium, the AV node, and the Purkinje fibers also have automaticity and are potential pacemakers. The rate of impulse generation differs for each part of the heart. Since the SA node fires faster than other areas of the electrical conduction system, it overrides the lower slower pacemakers and is the primary pacemaker of the heart. If the SA node should fail as the primary pacemaker, one of the other components of the conduction system can act as a secondary pacemaker. If that occurs, the farther the secondary pacemaker is from the SA node, the slower the rate will be.

Once the impulse is fired from the SA node, it spreads through both atria in a wavelike manner, through the interatrial, and internodal pathways, as

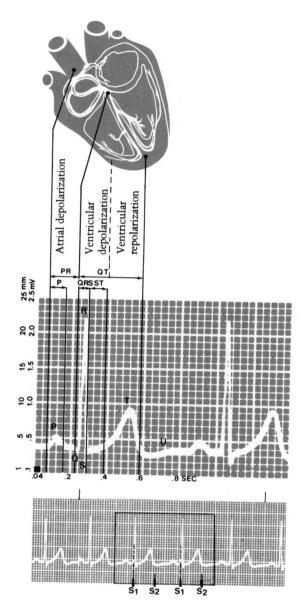

Figure 10-12
Electrical impulse formation and recording.

well as the atrial muscle itself. The internodal pathways are (1) the anterior internodal pathway with an interatrial branch (to the left atrium) called Bachmann's bundle, (2) the middle internodal pathway (Wenckebach's bundle), and (3) the posterior internodal pathway (Thorel's bundle). The last two internodal pathways have interatrial connections as well as internodal fibers.

The conduction tissue that connects the atria and the ventricles is referred to as AV junction. It is composed of the lower AV node and the proximal bundle of His. An intact, healthy pathway across the AV junction is needed for normal ventricular activation. Under abnormal circumstances, the AV junction can take over as a secondary pacemaker, firing at its inherent rate of 40 to 60 beats per minute. Such a rhythm is called an AV junctional rhythm.

The impulse travels from the SA node to the AV node located near the interventricular septum in the inferior wall of the right atrium near the tricuspid valve. At that point, the impulse is conducted more slowly than it is anywhere else in the conduction system, thereby allowing the atria to completely contract to fill the ventricles before the onset of ventricular contraction. Once it enters the bundle of His, the impulse moves rapidly into the right and left bundle branches. The right bundle branch is located on the right side of the interventricular septum and extends almost to the apex of the right ventricle, where it branches to all areas of the right ventricle through the Purkinje system. The left bundle crosses to the left side of the interventricular septum and immediately divides into the anterior and posterior branches. The left anterior branch (anterior fascicle) spreads superiorly and the left posterior branch (posterior fascicle) spreads inferiorly to the diaphragmatic wall of the left ventricle. Once the impulse has passed through the bundle branches, it quickly spreads through the Purkinje network found within the ventricular myocardium. If the SA node or AV junction default, the ventricular Purkinje system can fire at 30 to 40 beats per minute. Such a rhythm is called an idioventricular rhythm.

Record of Electrical Impulse

As the normal impulse travels through the conduction system, the ECG or oscilloscope records the electrical forces. Since the body acts as a conductor of electrical currents, any two points on the body can be connected to record the heart rhythm. A series of waves have been arbitrarily labeled on the ECG as the P, QRS, T, and U waves (Fig. 10-12).

The P wave represents depolarization of the atria. The P wave is generally upright and rounded in leads 1, 2, aVF, aVL, and V_3, V_4, V_5, and V_6, but it may be found to be peaked, diphasic, notched, flat, or inverted in those and other leads. The PR interval lasts from the beginning of the P wave to the beginning of the QRS complex; it represents the time period from atrial depolarization to the beginning of ventricular depolarization (Fig. 10-12). The PR interval, normally 0.12 to 0.20 second, represents normal conduction delay in the AV node.

The QRS complex represents ventricular depolarization. The initial downward deflection following the P wave is the Q wave. The first upward deflection of the QRS complex is the R wave. The S wave is the downward deflection following the R wave. Not every QRS complex, however, will show a Q or an R or an S wave. A QRS complex, for example, may consist only of an R wave (nevertheless, it is still referred to as the QRS complex). The duration of a normal QRS complex is 0.04 to 0.09 second. The T wave represents ventricular recovery or repolarization, and it is associated with the period of time known as the vulnerable period. Should a stimulus occur during the vulnerable refractory period, serious ventricular dysrhythmias may be precipitated. The T wave is generally upright although it may be peaked or inverted as a result of conduction disturbances or ischemic changes (see Chap. 19).

The ST segment is the time interval from the end of the QRS complex to the onset of the T wave. It represents the early phase of ventricular repolarization. Normally the ST segment is isoelectric (flat), but it may be elevated or depressed (above or below the isoelectric line) in some cardiac disease states or with certain drugs (e.g., digitalis).

The QT interval varies with the heart rate; it represents electrical systole. It lasts from the beginning of the QRS complex to the end of the T wave. Serial measurements may be important to determine the effects of certain medications on the QT interval. The significance of the U wave is still not understood. When present, the U wave follows the T wave and appears with a variety of phenomena, such as electrolyte shifts, digitalis, and premature ventricular contractions. It is more prominent in women than in men. The relationship between the cardiac cycle and the normal ECG impulses is shown in Figure 10-12.

Isoelectric Line

A baseline, known as the isoelectric line, may be seen to run through the length of the ECG tracing. It represents complete cardiac rest or electrical inactivity, and it is present whenever there is no flow of electrical current. The isoelectric line is determined by running an imaginary line across the ECG tracing from its origin at the TP interval (end of the T wave to the beginning of the next P wave).

The ECG Paper

Time is measured on the horizontal axis of the ECG paper. Each small square on the ECG paper represents 1 mm in length and 0.04 second in time. The larger square (or five small squares) represents 5 mm in length or 0.20 second in time (Fig. 10-12). The interval between the two vertical lines above the ECG grid represents 3 seconds.

Amplitude or voltage is measured on the vertical axis. The height or depth of a wave is measured from the isoelectric line. Twelve-lead ECGs are standardized so that 1 mv is equal to 10 mm, or two large vertical squares.

Calculation of Heart Rate

When the rhythm is regular, the single ECG tracing can be used to calculate the heart rate by several different methods. The first method involves finding a QRS complex that lands on and within the vertical line above the ECG grid. The number of cycles within six seconds (two 3-second intervals) multiplied by 10 gives the approximate number of beats per minute (Fig. 10-13A).

A second method of determining the rate when the rhythm is regular is to find a QRS complex that falls on a heavy line. Then count off the numbers 300, 150, 100, 75, 60, 50 for each line that follows. The next QRS complex determines the rate (Fig. 10-13B). The rationale for the counting system is that the distance between heavy lines is 1/300 minute. Therefore, the second method seen on Figure 10-13B shows that from a QRS complex on a heavy line to the next QRS complex (R to R interval) are six large squares. The rate is determined by dividing six into 300.

Other calculations and special rulers can also be used to determine the rate. It should be remembered

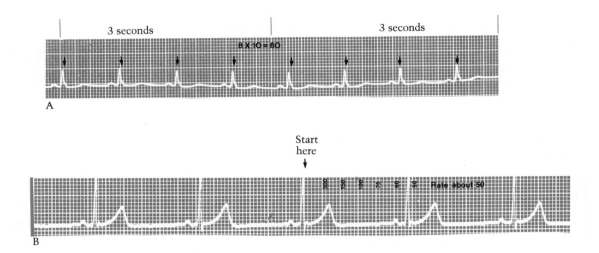

Figure 10-13
Two methods for calculation of heart rate. A. Count the number of QRS complexes within a 6-second strip and multiply by 10. B. Identify a QRS complex that falls on a heavy line. Count off the numbers 300, 150, 100, 75, 60, 50 for each heavy line that follows.

that *all* of the methods are used to get a rough estimate of the heart rate (i.e., to determine if the rate is normal, fast, or slow) and that they should not be used if the rhythm is irregular. None of those methods, however, is exact, and they should never replace the measurement of an apical-radial pulse by the nurse who is assessing the patient's condition at his bedside.

Standard Limb Leads

Monitor leads, or electrodes, are attached to the patient's extremities or chest by means of either self-adhering disposable disks or small metal plates or clamps with straps. The standard limb leads (e.g., 1, 2, and 3), which have been used for many years, are especially good for the recognition of dysrhythmias and heart blocks. The standard limb, or bipolar, leads are placed in pairs on the body to record the difference in electrical potentials between the two connected limbs. The third electrode, or ground lead, may be placed anywhere on the body. For monitoring purposes, it is actually more accurate to think of the potential as derived from the proximal respective limbs (shoulders and groin).

The axis of lead 1 extends from shoulder to shoulder, with the negative electrode on the right arm and the positive electrode on the left arm. The axis of lead 2 extends from the right shoulder (or the point just below the sternum) to the left leg, with the negative electrode on the right arm and the positive electrode on the left leg. Lead 3 extends from the left shoulder to

the left leg, with the negative electrode on the left arm and the positive electrode on the left leg (Fig. 10-14A). Remembering that placement, one can see that the axes of the three bipolar limb leads form a triangle around the area of the heart known as Einthoven's triangle (Fig. 10-14B). That is referred to as the triaxial reference system that is formed by the sides of Einthoven's triangle as they bisect one another (Fig. 10-14C). The sum of the potentials of those leads is zero. (The P waves in lead 2 should be the tallest, and the QRS complex in lead 2 should equal the sum of the corresponding complexes in leads 1 and 3.)

Augmented Leads

The augmented, or unipolar, extremity leads are leads aVR, aVL, and aVF (Fig. 10-14D). The letter *a* means augmented. A lead may be augmented by disconnecting the central terminal attached to the explored limb, thereby causing the amplitude of the deflection to be increased by 50 percent without changing the shape of the wave form. The *V* stands for vector, and the letters *R*, *L*, and *F* indicate the placement of the positive electrode (e.g., right arm, left arm, left leg

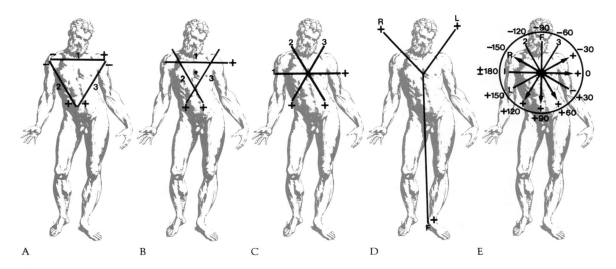

A   B   C   D   E

Figure 10-14
Intersection of standard limb leads and augmented leads. A. The three standard limb leads create Einthoven's triangle. B. The three limb leads come together to form a zero potential point. C. The triaxial reference system is formed by the sides of Einthoven's triangle as they bisect. D. The unipolar leads come toward the zero potential point. E. The hexaxial reference system consists of the six limb leads as they bisect each other.

[foot]). The other two electrodes are negative, and they are used as a common ground.

Those leads intersect at a 60-degree angle, and when they are superimposed on the standard limb leads, they intersect at 30-degree angles to form the frontal plane, which is referred to as the hexaxial reference system (Fig. 10-14E). The ECG records the same electrical activity in each lead, but the morphology of the waves is different because the activity is viewed from different positions.

Precordial Leads

The precordial (or chest) leads are unipolar, with each lead consisting of one positive electrode and a zero potential reference point. The axis of those leads is an imaginary line drawn from the positive electrode toward the center of the heart, and it identifies the horizontal plane. The precordial leads are placed at the following positions (Fig. 10-15):

V_1. Fourth intercostal space, at the right sternal border

V_2. Fourth intercostal space, at the left sternal border

V_3. Midway between positions 2 and 4

V_4. Fifth intercostal space, at the left midclavicular line

V_5. Fifth intercostal space, in the anterior axillary line

V_6. Fifth intercostal space, in the midaxillary line

V_7. (Not shown, not always used.) Fifth intercostal space, in the left posterior axillary line

V_8. (Not shown, not always used.) Fifth intercostal space, in the left midscapular line

Normal ECG

A normal ECG is composed of 12 leads: 3 standard leads, 3 augmented leads, and 6 precordial leads (Fig. 10-16). In a normal ECG, there are small q waves in leads 1, 2, aVL, aVF, V_4, and V_6 (0.02 second in duration; 0.1 to 0.2 mv in amplitude). The ST segments in all leads are isoelectric. Leads V_1 through V_6 show normal R wave progression.

MCL$_1$ Monitoring

A popular monitoring lead used frequently in coronary care units is the modified chest lead or MCL$_1$ (Fig. 10-17). A bipolar lead, it is similar to the unipolar precordial lead V_1. The positive electrode is placed in

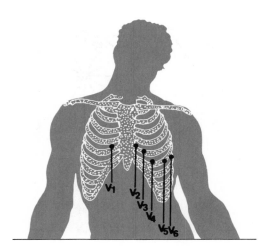

Figure 10-15
Precordial leads (unipolar leads).

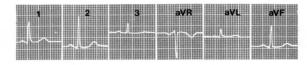

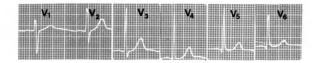

Figure 10-16
Normal ECG.

the fourth right intercostal space at the right sternal border, while the negative electrode is placed just below the left midclavicle. MCL_1 has diagnostic value as a monitoring lead because it is an extremely useful lead for recognizing and recording atrial activity and for distinguishing right from left bundle branch block and right from left ventricular ectopic beats.

Monitoring Tips

It is important to remember that a normal P wave configuration is observed when organized atrial activity is present. Lead placement is chosen so that P waves are prominently displayed. The amplitude of the QRS complex should be sufficient to trigger the

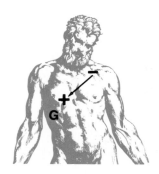

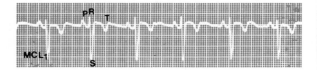

Figure 10-17
MCL_1 monitoring (bipolar lead). G = ground lead.

cardiac monitor rate meter properly. When possible, the patient's chest should be left loosely covered or exposed, and electrode pads should be carefully positioned so that defibrillation paddles may be easily placed if necessary.

Artifact

Frequently, artifacts are observed on the cardiac monitor. An artifact is any movement on the ECG that is not due to currents generated during the cardiac cycle. Artifacts may be due to muscle tremor, a wandering baseline, alternating current interference, standardization, and complexes produced during external cardiac massage.

When patients are tensing their muscles, electrical potentials are picked up by electrodes and recorded on the ECG. They may be recorded as irregular jerks or a grossly uneven baseline (Fig. 10-18A). A wandering baseline reveals easily identified complexes, but the baseline is undulating (see Fig. 10-18B). Alternating current interference that produces regular deflections at 60 cycles per second (Fig. 10-18C) is usually due to a leakage of electrical power during the recording of the ECG. A standardization artifact is deliberately introduced by the person recording the ECG. The artifact is generally a 10-mm deflection (two large squares) that is used to standardize the machine and

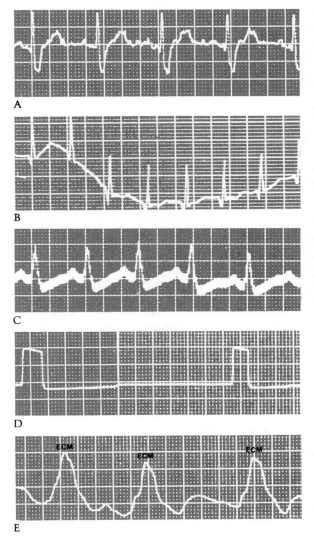

Figure 10-18
A. Muscle tremor. B. Wandering baseline. C. Alternating current interference. D. Standardization mark. E. Complexes during external cardiac massage (ECM).

to compare the size of the recorded cardiac complexes (Fig. 10-18D). Complexes produced during external cardiac massage (ECM) can easily be identified (Fig. 10-18E) and resemble regular, wide ventricular beats.

Similarly, the oscilloscope may show a straight line if one of the electrodes has lost contact with the skin. The authors remember only too vividly almost delivering a precordial thump to a patient who had straight lined on the cardiac monitor—and who was sleeping—with two electrodes loose. Regardless of the presumptive observation, the findings must always be correlated with the nurse's observation of the patient.

Evaluation of Cardiac Rhythm

When evaluating the patient's cardiac rhythm, the critical care nurse must combine her findings of the patient's clinical status with a systematic assessment of the rhythm strip. The following must be carefully assessed:

1. Atria
   a. What is the atrial rate? (P-P wave? Normal? Abnormal?)
   b. What is the atrial rhythm? (Regular? Irregular?)
2. Ventricle
   a. What is the ventricular rate? (QRS-QRS? Normal? Abnormal?)
   b. What is the ventricular rhythm? (Regular? Irregular?)
3. P wave
   a. Is it normal in configuration?
   b. Is it abnormal in configuration? (Peaked? Notched? Diphasic? Flat? Inverted? Missing?)
4. PR interval
   a. Is it normal? (0.12–0.20 second)
   b. Is it prolonged? (longer than 0.20 second)
   c. Is it consistent for each QRS complex?
5. QRS complex
   a. What is the contour of the complex? (Small r wave and large S wave–rS? Small q wave and large R and S wave–qRS?)
   b. Is there a P wave for every QRS complex?
6. QRS interval
   a. Is it normal? (0.04–0.09 second)
   b. Is it abnormal? (longer than 0.09 second)
7. ST segment
   a. Is it normal? (Isoelectric)
   b. Is it elevated above the isoelectric line?
   c. Is it depressed below the isoelectric line?

8. T wave
   a. Is it normal? (Upright)
   b. Is it abnormal? (Peaked? Inverted?)
9. Extra beats
   a. Are there any atrial, junctional, or ventricular premature beats?
   b. Are there any escape beats?
   c. Are there any aberrantly conducted beats?

If the PR interval is prolonged and not measured, for example, the rhythm strip may appear normal when a first-degree heart block is in fact present. We have found that once the nurse has acquired the basic knowledge, her success in recognizing dysrhythmias is dependent largely on her developing and using a consistent, systematic method of evaluation.

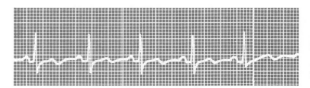

Figure 10-19
Normal sinus rhythm.

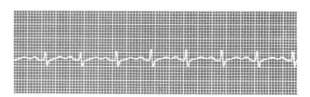

Figure 10-20
Sinus tachycardia.

Normal Sinus Rhythm

Because the sinus node normally maintains the fastest rate of impulse formation over other pacer sites, it is the dominant pacemaker of the heart. Normal sinus rhythm (NSR) (Fig. 10-19) is 60 to 100 beats per minute. The P waves are normal and upright in leads 1, 2, and V_3 and inverted in leads aVR, V_1 and V_2. The PR interval is 0.12 second to 0.20 second. The QRS complex is normal and ranges from 0.04 second to 0.09 second. If the cardiac cycle varies from those defined parameters, a dysrhythmia is present.

Dysrhythmias

Sinus Tachycardia

Sinus tachycardia results from sympathetic nervous system activity and the release of catecholamines due to fear, anxiety, tension, exercise, fever, myocardial disease, anemia, anoxia, hyperthyroidism, or from medications, such as atropine sulfate, isoproterenol, and epinephrine.

A sinus tachycardia is present when the rate of normally conducted beats that originate from the SA node exceeds 100 beats per minute. The atrial and ventricular response is 100 to 160 per minute (Fig. 10-20). The rhythm is regular, with a P wave preceding each QRS complex. The PR and QRS intervals are normal. With very rapid rates, the TP interval is shortened, causing the P wave to be superimposed on the preceding T wave. Sinus tachycardia reduces diastolic ventricular filling (and coronary artery filling) and may produce angina pectoris. The rapid rate may decrease cardiac output and precipitate congestive heart failure in the patient with myocardial disease or injury. The treatment depends on the underlying cause of the dysrhythmia.

Sinus Bradycardia

A sinus rhythm of less than 60 beats per minute is referred to as a sinus bradycardia. It is normally observed in healthy young athletes, and it can be caused by excessive vagal tone due to a variety of circumstances. It is seen in patients with severe pain, myxedema, atherosclerotic heart disease, and it may be produced by drugs, such as digitalis, reserpine, or propranolol. It is frequently observed during the first few hours after acute inferior myocardial infarction.

Sinus bradycardia is a regular rhythm that rarely falls below 45 beats per minute. A normal P wave precedes each QRS complex. The PR and QRS intervals are normal (Fig. 10-21). The slow rhythm may predispose the person to premature ectopic beats. If ventricular filling or stroke volume is significantly reduced, the slow rate may decrease cardiac output and play a major role in the development of congestive heart failure.

If the sinus bradycardia significantly reduces cardiac output, lowers the blood pressure, or predisposes

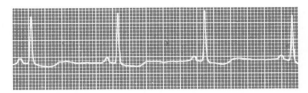

Figure 10-21
Sinus bradycardia.

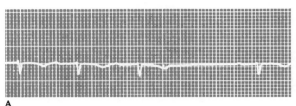

A

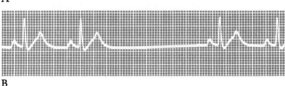

B

Figure 10-22
A. Sinus exit block. The pause is equal to a multiple of the sinus cycle. The sinus node rhythm is not reset. B. Sinus arrest. The pause is not equal to some multiple of the previous sinus rhythm.

the person to premature ventricular contractions, 0.5 to 1 mg of atropine sulfate may be diluted in 10 ml of normal saline solution and given slowly intravenously over several minutes (see Chap. 18).

Sinus Exit Block and Sinus Arrest

Sinus exit block (SA block) and sinus arrest may be caused by vagal stimulation, atherosclerotic disease involving the SA node, occlusion of the SA nodal artery, acute infections, and medications, such as digitalis, quinidine sulfate, and procainamide. SA block implies that the conduction pathway from the SA node to the atria is blocked. SA block is recognized by the absence of an expected P wave from the SA node. Because the sinus node is not able to release a rhythmic discharge, the entire cardiac cycle of P–QRS–T waves is missing. If a sinus beat is blocked, the resulting pause is exactly equal to some multiple

of the sinus cycle (i.e., the pause is equal to two sinus cycles or 2:1 SA block). That occurs because the timing cycle of the SA node has not been reset and the SA node continues to fire at the same rate whether or not the impulse is released or its exit is blocked (Fig. 10-22A). A sinus arrest or a sinus pause, on the other hand, exists when there is an abrupt failure of the SA node to send out a pacemaking stimulus. The resulting pause, however, is not equal to the same multiple of the sinus cycle (Fig. 10-22B). After the pause produced by SA block or arrest, there may be a resumption of the sinus rhythm; or a junctional or ventricular escape beat may occur, thereby replacing the sinus cycle. Sinus or atrial standstill is observed when there is a total absence of all P waves, indicating complete SA block or sinus arrest.

The most common clinical symptoms associated with those dysrhythmias result from the pause in rhythm and cardiac activity. The patient may be completely asymptomatic, or he may complain of angina pectoris, dizziness, or syncope. The treatment depends primarily on the cause of the SA block or arrest and on the clinical manifestations. Therapy may include the use of such medications as atropine sulfate, epinephrine, and isoproterenol. When pharmacological measures are not effective, artificial cardiac pacing is indicated.

Sick Sinus Syndrome

Diseases of the SA node have recently become the subject of much attention. The terms sick sinus syndrome (SSS), bradycardia-tachycardia syndrome (BTS), sluggish sinus node syndrome, and sinoatrial syncope have been used to describe a variety of dysrhythmias and associated clinical manifestations produced by some pathological process of the SA node.

Damage to the SA node may be caused by ischemic, rheumatic, inflammatory, sclerotic, or hypertensive disease [15]. SSS appears in about 5 percent of patients suffering from acute myocardial infarction. Many patients with inferior wall infarctions develop SA node dysfunction because the right coronary artery most often supplies the SA nodal artery. The term SSS is used to describe dysfunction of the SA node as manifested by one or more of the following [6]:

1. Severe sinus bradycardia
2. Sinus arrest with or without replacement by atrial or junctional escape rhythms

3. Sinus node exit block
4. Sinus or atrial standstill
5. Chronic atrial fibrillation with a slow ventricular response that is not related to drug therapy
6. Inability of the heart to resume a sinus rhythm following electrocardioversion
7. Bradycardia-tachycardia syndrome

In addition to those factors, a high incidence of AV block, intraventricular conduction defects, and inhibition of lower pacemakers is associated with the SSS.

Patients may be completely asymptomatic or may complain of syncope, dyspnea, angina pectoris, edema or other symptoms resulting from low cardiac output produced by the dysrhythmias associated with ·the SSS [18]. Symptomatic SSS is generally refractory to pharmacological therapy, such as atropine sulfate and isoproterenol, and it usually requires the insertion of a permanent artificial pacemaker. If the BTS syndrome is present, drugs are used to suppress the tachycardic phase.

Sinus Dysrhythmia

When all impulses originate from the SA node but the rate of discharge alternately increases and decreases with respiration, a sinus dysrhythmia is present. The dysrhythmia is generally a physiological variation of normal sinus rhythm, and it is not believed to indicate underlying heart disease. It is prominent from childhood through adolescence, but it may also be found in old age.

The heart rate is usually slightly irregular because of the variations in venous return, ventilation, and vagal tone. The heart speeds up slightly during inspiration as the right heart distends with an increased venous return, and it slows slightly during expiration. A sinus dysrhythmia is present when the difference in time between the two fastest continuous beats and the two slowest continuous beats exceeds 0.12 second (Fig. 10-23). To verify the rhythm, it is important to run a rhythm strip that includes the entire respiratory cycle. The patient is generally asymptomatic, and treatment is not necessary.

Atrial Tachycardia

Atrial tachycardia is a rapid, regular supraventricular rhythm that is usually faster than sinus tachycardia.

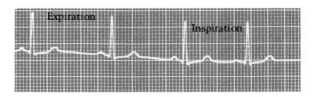

Figure 10-23
Sinus dysrhythmia. The rhythm slows with expiration and speeds up with inspiration. The time difference between the two fastest beats and the two slowest beats is .20 second.

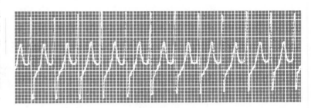

Figure 10-24
Paroxysmal atrial tachycardia clinically confirmed when carotid sinus massage abruptly converted the dysrhythmia back to NSR. The ventricular rate is 215. The P waves are buried in the T waves.

It occurs in both healthy and ill people. It may occur spontaneously, or it may be precipitated by excitement, fatigue, alcohol, tobacco, or exercise. It is also associated with rheumatic or ischemic heart disease and digitalis intoxication. Premature atrial contractions may predispose the person to atrial tachycardia.

The dysrhythmia occurs suddenly and ends abruptly. The paroxysms may last for a few minutes to several hours or days. The rate is from 120 to 220 beats per minute. The P waves are upright in leads 2, 3, and aVF, but they may be buried in the preceding T wave with extremely rapid rates. The QRS complex may be normal or distorted due to aberrant AV conduction (Fig. 10-24).

Atrial tachycardia does not generally produce severe hemodynamic impairment. Patients frequently complain of palpitations and lightheadedness. Rapid atrial tachycardias can reduce ventricular diastolic filling time and, together with the accelerated ventricular response, may be responsible for seriously lowering cardiac output. Patients with underlying heart disease may have symptoms of angina pectoris, dyspnea, or congestive heart failure. Vagal stimulation produced by carotid sinus massage, a Valsalva maneuver, or gagging can abruptly stop the paroxysm. The patient can be taught the two last procedures if he has the paroxysms often and if he finds them unpleasant. A vagal response may also be elicited by applying pressure to the eyeball, but that method is not recommended because of possible damage to the eye.

Short paroxysms of the heart rhythm may be common in the normal person, and they are usually not treated. Longer paroxysms may be controlled by the use of sedatives, tranquilizers, quinidine sulfate, or propranolol. In resistant cases, elevation of the systolic blood pressure by dilute intravenous infusions of phenylephrine, metaraminol, or norepinephrine may be used to terminate the dysrhythmia. Propranolol can be effective in terminating the dysrhythmia, especially when it is produced by digitalis intoxication. If the atrial tachycardia is responsible for producing severe heart failure or shock, electrical countershock is recommended.

Premature Atrial Contractions

Premature atrial contractions (PACs) occur during the cardiac cycle when an impulse or ectopic focus, located in either the right or left atrium, discharges the atrium earlier than the next expected impulse. PACs are common among all age groups, and they may result from the use of tobacco, caffeine, stress, alcohol, or from heart disease. Although isolated PACs are common in the normal person, frequent PACs may indicate organic heart disease and may predispose the person to other supraventricular dysrhythmias, such as atrial flutter, atrial fibrillation, and atrial tachycardias.

The ventricular rate will depend on the number of PACs while the rhythm is essentially irregular because of the premature beats. The P wave of the PAC often has a different contour and configuration than the P wave that originates from the SA node, or it may be buried in the preceding T wave (Fig. 10-25). The PR interval may be normal or prolonged, or the P wave may be completely blocked. A QRS complex follows each P wave. It is usually normal in contour, but it may appear distorted as a result of aberrant conduction, which may occur when the conduction pathway is still refractory.

The patient may experience a pause in the cardiac rhythm or a feeling of palpitation. The palpitation is due not directly to the PAC but to the beat following the ectopic one. Generally there is an incomplete compensatory pause associated with the PAC that

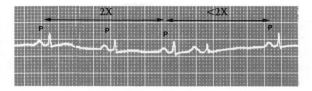

Figure 10-25
Normal sinus rhythm with PAC. The fourth beat is premature and the QRS complex is preceded by a P wave. An incomplete compensatory pause associated with the PAC is present (the interval between the P wave before and the P wave after the PAC is less than two normal P-P intervals).

allows greater ventricular filling time and stroke volume to be associated with the impulse following the PAC and thus produces a sensation of "jumping" or "skipping."

An *incomplete compensatory pause* is evaluated by measuring the distance between three consecutive normal P waves (or 2X; see Fig. 10-25) preceding the PAC. That distance is then compared to the distance between the P waves immediately preceding and immediately following the PAC. If the distance between the P waves preceding and following the PAC is less than the distance between the three consecutive normal P waves (<2X), an incomplete compensatory pause is present (see Fig. 10-25).

Treatment is rarely necessary. If the PACs are frequent, one should omit alcohol or stimulants, such as tobacco and caffeine. Occasionally, sedation may lower a patient's stress level and thus may reduce the number of PACs. In rare situations, digitalis, propranolol, quinidine sulfate, or procainamide may be used.

Atrial Flutter

Atrial flutter may be defined as an abnormally fast but regular atrial rhythm that originates from an accelerated atrial focus. Atrial flutter rarely occurs in a healthy person. It occurs most commonly in patients in their forties who have ischemic myocardial disease, but it may occur in (and complicate) any kind of heart disease. It is observed in 2 percent to 5 percent of patients with acute myocardial infarction [10, 12], and it may be precipitated by many kinds of acute illness (e.g., hypoxia and pericarditis).

The exact physiological mechanism involved in atrial flutter is not understood although several theories to explain it have been proposed. The circus movement theory hypothesizes activation of a primary focus whose impulse produces a circulating wave that goes around and around within the atrium. The unifocal theory proposes that all the impulses originate from a single ectopic focus. The multiple foci theory suggests the presence of several foci that are simultaneously activated to produce the atrial flutter. According to the multiple reentry theory, a sinus or ectopic impulse occurs during a vulnerable period, producing multiple reentry sites and multiple circulating waves. There is no evidence, however, that any one mechanism is responsible for all cases of the dysrhythmia.

Electrocardiographically, atrial flutter is identified by an atrial rate of 250 to 300 beats per minute, and it is characterized by flutter, or F, waves. The common flutter waves are regular and sawtooth in configuration, especially in leads V_1, 2, 3, and aVF. Other leads in the same ECG may not, however, reveal flutter waves. The PR interval is not measurable. The QRS complex is normal in configuration, except when aberrant conduction is present. A QRS complex does not usually follow every P wave, which results in some degree of AV block since the ventricles cannot respond to the rapid atrial rate.

The ventricular rate is usually a whole number fraction of the atrial rate (e.g., 3:1, 4:1, or 5:1), and the ratio 2:1 AV conduction is the most common one, generally resulting in a regular ventricular response (Fig. 10-26A, B). Frequently, the typical ECG pattern will reveal a sawtooth atrial rhythm of 280 to 300 beats per minute, and a ventricular response of 140 to 150 beats per minute. The ventricular response may, however, disclose an irregular rhythm because of an alternating variation in AV conduction (e.g., 2:1–4:1 conduction).

On physical examination, flutter *a* waves may be observed in the jugular venous pulse. Although atrial flutter may be suspected, it may be difficult to differentiate the rhythm from paroxysmal atrial tachycardia. Carotid sinus pressure is diagnostically helpful because it will characteristically and temporarily increase the degree of AV block, thereby halving the ventricular response and uncovering additional flutter waves (e.g., from a 2:1 atrial flutter with a ventricular response of 150 before carotid sinus pressure to a 4:1 atrial flutter with a ventricular response of 75 during massage). After the carotid stimulation has ceased, the former rate will reappear.

The patient may be totally unaware of his dysrhythmia, or he may complain of symptoms that are

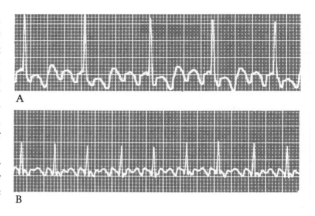

Figure 10-26
A. 4:1 atrial flutter with a normal ventricular response. B. 3:1 atrial flutter with a fast ventricular response.

primarily dependent on the rate and regularity of the ventricular response. If the ventricular response is normal and regular, the patient is not likely to have any symptoms. If, however, the ventricular response is rapid, as in 2:1 atrial flutter, or irregular, the patient may complain of palpitations, angina pectoris, dyspnea and/or symptoms of pulmonary edema and cerebrovascular insufficiency. Also, atrial flutter tends to be an unpredictable dysrhythmia, one in which the patient may be completely asymptomatic with 4:1 ventricular response and then suddenly becomes symptomatic if the response changes to 2:1.

Treatment of atrial flutter consists of converting the rhythm to normal or controlling the ventricular response. Elective cardioversion or countershock, usually using low voltage levels, is very effective in converting the dysrhythmia and is generally the treatment of choice (see Chap. 18). Digitalis is used in some situations, however, to slow the ventricular rate by increasing the degree of AV block. Quinidine sulfate is then frequently used to restore the rhythm to normal. Quinidine should not be given without digitalis because it may improve AV conduction and accelerate the ventricular response to dangerously rapid rates (e.g., converting a 2:1 AV conduction to a 1:1). When pharmacological cardioversion is effective, the patient will usually convert from atrial flutter to atrial fibrillation and, finally, to normal sinus rhythm.

Atrial Fibrillation

Atrial fibrillation is a rapid and uncoordinated atrial dysrhythmia. It is relatively common, and it may oc-

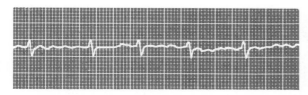

Figure 10-27
Atrial fibrillation with a normal ventricular response. Note the coarse *f* waves and the irregularly irregular ventricular response.

casionally be observed in the healthy person. Generally atrial fibrillation is a more stable dysrhythmia than is atrial flutter, and it is associated with such disease states as rheumatic mitral valvular disease, hypertension, ischemic heart disease, or thyrotoxicosis. It may also be seen in patients with acute myocardial infarction, atrial septal defects, chronic obstructive lung disease, pericarditis, and congestive heart failure, and it may be precipitated by PACs, as discussed.

The ECG characteristically reveals two important features of atrial fibrillation: (1) fibrillatory, or *f*, waves and (2) an "irregularly irregular" ventricular response. The fibrillatory atrial waves, which range in rate from 350 to 600 per minute, may vary in amplitude, spacing, and contour. The *f* waves may be coarse and irregular, resembling flutter waves, or they may be fine fibrillatory waves that look much like a wavy baseline or, occasionally, like a straight line. Fibrillatory waves are best identified in leads V_1, 2, 3, and aVF. The PR interval is not measurable (Fig. 10-27). The QRS complex is generally of normal configuration as a result of normal ventricular conduction. Because of the rapid atrial rate, some degree of AV block is usually present. The ventricular response, therefore, may be normal, rapid, or slow. The ventricular contractions are irregular in intensity and rhythm and are frequently described as having an irregular irregularity. Occasionally the QRS complex may be conducted aberrantly and may be mistaken for ventricular ectopic activity. Aberration is likely to develop when a long ventricular cycle (R-R interval) is immediately followed by a short cycle, with the beat ending the short cycle being aberrantly conducted (Fig. 10-28). This long–short sequence is termed *Ashman's phenomenon,* and it usually follows a right bundle branch pattern.

Because of the rapid atrial rate, the atrium does not depolarize or contract as a unit. The ventricles, therefore, do not receive the benefit of the atrial

"kick," or atrial contraction, which may augment ventricular filling by as much as 30 percent. As a result, the cardiac output can drop, especially in the patient with already acutely compromised circulation. Furthermore, because of the uncoordinated, passive, and dilated state of the atrium, thrombi can develop on the atrial walls to produce systemic or pulmonary embolism.

Patients in atrial fibrillation frequently complain of palpitations or symptoms consistent with heart failure or embolism. Atrial fibrillation is immediately suspected when an irregularly irregular pulse is discovered. With rapid ventricular rates, many of the audible apical impulses fail to produce a peripheral arterial pulse, thereby causing an apical-radial deficit to occur. The jugular neck veins may reveal a rippling from the fibrillatory waves, but more frequently it is found on inspection that *a* waves are missing from the jugular venous pulse. On auscultation, the first heart sound is found to vary in intensity from one beat to the next and to be louder at the end of shorter cycles.

Electrical countershock is successful in converting most acute cases of the dysrhythmia, and it is the treatment of choice for atrial fibrillation. When countershock is not successful and when the ventricular response is rapid, propranolol or digitalis may be used to slow the ventricular rate. Quinidine sulfate and/or procainamide may then be added to convert the rhythm back to normal. If the dysrhythmia has had a recent onset, treatment should also be directed toward correction of the underlying disturbance (e.g., heart failure, hyperthyroidism, or hypertension).

Elective cardioversion is generally ineffective for patients with long-term atrial fibrillation. When countershock is attempted and successful, the normal rhythm frequently reverts to atrial fibrillation. Thromboembolic complications can be reduced by the use of anticoagulation before cardioversion. The treatment for that type of patient, however, usually consists of controlling the ventricular response rather than converting the rhythm to normal.

AV Junctional Rhythms

If the SA node fails to fire or if atrial impulses are not transmitted through the AV node, the AV junction may take over as the primary pacemaker to produce a junctional rhythm. A junctional rhythm serves as a safety mechanism to prevent asystole. The term junctional rhythm has replaced the old term nodal

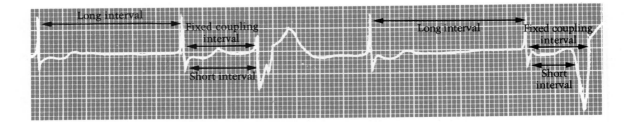

rhythm because physiologists have been unable to find pacemaking cells within the AV node itself but have been able to identify pacemaking cells around the AV junction and in the bundle of His. Any problem that suppresses SA node activity, such as sinus bradycardia, SA block, and digitalis-induced vagal stimulation, can result in a junctional rhythm. The rhythm may also be a result of any problem that enhances AV junctional automaticity, such as digitalis intoxication, acute inferior myocardial infarction, or rheumatic fever.

Impulses originating from the AV junction tend to produce an unreliable rhythm. When the sinus pacemaker has been suppressed, junctional pacemaker sites can assume the role of primary impulse formation, usually at a rate of 40 to 60 beats per minute, producing a *junctional rhythm* (Fig. 10-29A). When the junctional rhythm is a result of enhanced AV junctional activity, with a rate 60 to 100 beats per minute, an *accelerated* AV *junctional rhythm* is present. An AV *junctional tachycardia* exists when the rate exceeds 100 beats per minute (Fig. 10-29B). Impulses arising prematurely from the AV junction are known as *premature* AV *junctional contractions* (PJCs) (Fig. 10-29C).

Impulses arising from the AV junction can spread simultaneously upward to the atria and downward to the ventricles. The ECG displays a normally conducted QRS complex. The atria are usually, but not always, activated by retrograde conduction from the AV junction. The resulting P waves may be inverted in leads 2, 3, and aVF, and they may occur before, during, or after the QRS complex. When present, the PR interval is generally less than 0.12 second. The premature junctional beat may or may not be associated with a *complete compensatory pause*. A full compensatory pause is determined by measuring the distance between three normal consecutive sinus beats (QRS complexes) on the ECG (2X). That distance is then compared to the distance between the two beats on either side of the premature beat. If both

Figure 10-28

Ashman's phenomenon. Patient is in atrial fibrillation. The QRS complex ending the short cycle (which is immediately preceded by a long cycle) reveals aberrant ventricular conduction. The initial deflection of the first aberrantly conducted QRS complex is identical to that of the normally conducted beat.

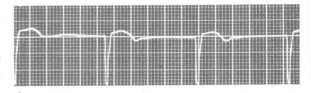

A

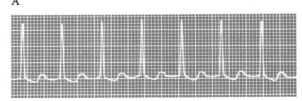

B

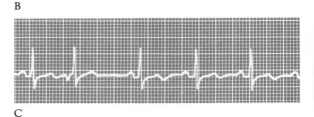

C

Figure 10-29

A. Junctional rhythm. The ventricular rate is 55. There are no P waves present. B. Junctional tachycardia. The ventricular rate is 125. C. Normal sinus rhythm with PJC. The second beat is a PJC with an inverted P wave.

distances are equal, a complete compensatory pause exists (≥ 2X) (see Fig. 10-29C).

The clinical signs and symptoms depend on the ventricular response and are similar to other types of bradydysrhythmias and tachydysrhythmias. The physical examination may be normal, or it may reveal cannon *a* waves in the jugular venous pulse with each heart beat (i.e., an atrial contraction that occurs with or follows a ventricular contraction), together with a loud S_1.

The treatment involves increasing the discharge rate of higher pacemakers, improving the AV conduction, or using artificial cardiac pacing. Premature junctional contractions are treated like premature atrial extrasystoles.

First-Degree AV Block

First-degree AV block most frequently has one of two primary causes: (1) ischemia of the AV node or (2) drug intoxication (primarily digitalis intoxication). Ischemic changes in the AV node result in a delayed transmission of impulses from the atria to the ventricles. First-degree heart block exists when the PR interval (in adults) exceeds 0.20 second (Fig. 10-30A). The patient usually has no symptoms. When first-degree heart block is noted in a patient who is receiving digitalis, digitalis intoxication should be suspected, and the physician should be consulted before the drug is given again. Usually the PR interval will revert to normal and not progress to a higher degree of AV block although the patient must be observed closely. If the patient has a slow heart rate and is symptomatic, atropine sulfate, 0.5 to 1 mg in 10 ml of saline solution, may be slowly administered intravenously to correct the problem.

Second-Degree AV Block

Second-degree AV block may be due to ischemia or injury of the AV node, drug intoxication, coronary artery disease, rheumatic fever, or various viral infections. Second-degree block is divided into two major types: (1) Mobitz type I (the Wenckebach phenomenon) and (2) Mobitz type II.

The Wenckebach phenomenon characteristically has a progressive lengthening of the PR interval for several successive beats until a P wave occurs that is not followed by a ventricular response. As the con-

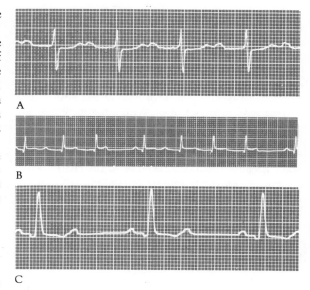

A

B

C

Figure 10-30

A. First-degree AV heart block. The PR interval is .36 second. B. 5:4 Wenckebach phenomenon (Mobitz type I AV block). The fourth beat begins the cycle. Note the progressive lengthening of the PR interval in the 4th, 5th, 6th, and 7th beats, but by decreasing increments, such that the ventricular cycle (R-R interval) shortens (particularly between the 4th and 5th beats, and the 5th and 6th beats). Note the blocked P wave resulting in no QRS complex (dropped beat) following the 7th beat. C. 2:1 Mobitz type II second-degree AV heart block. There are two P waves for each QRS complex—hence 2:1 AV block (every other sinus beat is blocked). Note that the atrial rate is 90 while the ventricular rate is 45.

duction velocity slows within the AV node, the refractory period lengthens. Thus P waves come closer to the refractory period of the AV node until a P wave inevitably becomes nonconducted (blocked). At the same time, each R-R interval is progressively shortened. The QRS complexes are narrow since the block occurs above the bundle of His (Fig. 10-30B). The patient is usually asymptomatic. If the Wenckebach phenomenon occurs while the patient is receiving digitalis, digitalis intoxication should be suspected and the physician notified before the drug is given again. The Wenckebach phenomenon, a transient form of heart block, usually does not advance to a higher degree of block. Generally it is not treated, but the patient should be observed closely.

Mobitz type II second-degree AV block is a more serious form of heart block. Characteristically, a sudden drop in AV conduction occurs in which only every second, third, or fourth impulse reaches the ventricles. That drop results in a ventricular rate that is one-half, one-third, or one-fourth of the atrial rate (i.e., the ratio is 2:1, 3:1, or 4:1) (Fig. 10-30C). The patient may or may not be symptomatic. When the ventricular rate becomes excessively slow, cardiac output falls and the patient may complain of dizziness or syncope. The QRS complexes are usually wide, because the block develops in the His-Purkinje system or below the bundle of His. Heart failure or hypotension associated with acute myocardial infarction should be corrected. Because Mobitz type II block may progress to complete AV block in the presence of acute myocardial infarction, a temporary demand cardiac pacemaker is always indicated (see Chap. 18).

Third-Degree AV Heart Block

Third-degree AV heart block can be caused by ischemia or injury to the AV node, bundle of His, or bundle branches, drug intoxication, trauma, or congenital abnormalities. Classically, in third-degree AV block, there are two active pacemakers within the heart, one in the atria and one in the ventricle, causing the atria and ventricles to depolarize and contract independently (Fig. 10-31). P waves and QRS complexes appear at regular intervals, but they are completely independent of each other. Typically the ventricular rate is slower than the atrial rate, ranging from 30 to 40 beats per minute. If the ventricular pacemaker is high in the region of the AV node, the QRS complexes will be narrow. When the pacemaker is lower in the ventricles, the QRS complexes will be wide (greater than 0.12 second).

If the rate becomes excessively slow and thus produces a drop in cardiac output, the patient may complain of dizziness and syncope (Stokes-Adams syndrome). Congestive heart failure may be precipitated or aggravated. If digitalis intoxication is suspected, the drug is discontinued. In symptomatic patients or in those who develop ventricular asystole, an emergency situation exists that requires external cardiac compression, the use of isoproterenol, and the insertion of a temporary demand cardiac pacemaker. If third-degree heart block persists, implantation of a permanent pacemaker is considered.

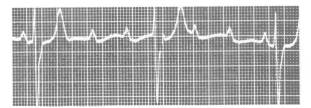

Figure 10-31
Third-degree (complete) AV heart block. Note the regular idioventricular rhythm at a rate of 36 and the regular atrial rhythm at a rate of 125. The atrial rhythm is completely independent of the ventricular rhythm as evidenced by the changing relationship of the P waves to the QRS complexes.

Bundle Branch Block

Bundle branch blocks are frequently caused by ischemia, rheumatic disease, aortic valvular disease, hypertension, and congenital abnormalities (specifically septal defects). Both the right and left bundles receive an excitatory impulse about the same time, depolarizing the entire ventricular muscle. Obstruction of impulse conduction from the AV node to the bundle of His or to the right or left bundle branch can cause one of the ventricles to depolarize and contract before the other. When impulse conduction is blocked, a bundle branch pattern is produced. The ECG reveals an incomplete bundle branch block when the QRS complex is 0.10 to 0.12 second. When the QRS complex is wider than 0.12 second, a complete bundle branch block is said to exist.

RIGHT BUNDLE BRANCH BLOCK

Right bundle branch block (RBBB) is present when the QRS interval is greater than 0.12 second and an rSR′ pattern is seen in V_1. Complete right bundle branch block also has a broad prominent S wave in lead 1 (Fig. 10-32). Patients with RBBB are usually asymptomatic and require no treatment.

LEFT BUNDLE BRANCH BLOCK

Left bundle branch block (LBBB) reveals ventricular deflections greater than 0.12 second that are of widest duration upward in leads 1, V_5, and V_6. Leads 3, V_1, and V_2 show ventricular deflections that are of widest duration downward, with upright T waves in V_1 and V_3. The left precordial leads, V_5 and V_6, show notched

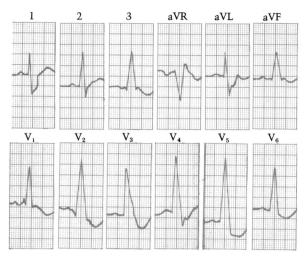

Figure 10-32
Right bundle branch block.

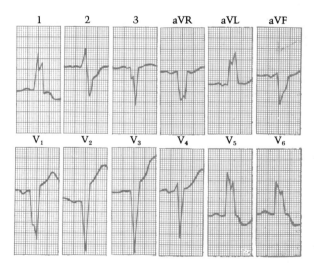

Figure 10-33
Left bundle branch block.

deflections (M slurred complex) (Fig. 10-33). Patients with RBBB and LBBB are usually asymptomatic. If the patient's ECG demonstrates RBBB or LBBB, the changes of acute myocardial infarction may be hidden.

The main left bundle branch divides into an anterior and posterior fascicle (see Fig. 10-11). When a block is observed on the ECG in only half of the left bundle, it is termed a *hemiblock*. The term *bifascicular block* describes an existing RBBB in combination with a left anterior or left posterior hemiblock. The term *trifascicular block* describes a block in the right bundle and in both the anterior and posterior branches of the left bundle or main left bundle. In the presence of acute myocardial infarction, the patient should be closely observed for the development of bifascicular block or complete heart block.

LEFT ANTERIOR HEMIBLOCK

Left anterior hemiblock (LAH) occurs more frequently than does left posterior hemiblock (LPH) because the area involved is a more vulnerable structure of the ventricular conduction system. LAH is seen with anteroseptal and anterolateral myocardial infarctions since the anterior division of left bundle branch receives its blood supply from the left coronary artery. ECG diagnosis of LAH is made when the frontal axis is negative more than −45°; lead 1 is positive; leads 2 and aVF are negative; lead 1 has a qR configuration and leads 2 and aVF have an rS configuration. The QRS duration usually does not exceed 0.10 to 0.12 second (Fig. 10-34A).

LEFT POSTERIOR HEMIBLOCK

Left posterior hemiblock (LPH) is seen with more extensive myocardial damage and is almost always associated with RBBB. LPH is less common than LAH since the posterior division of the left bundle branch has a dual blood supply—from the right and left coronary arteries. The ECG diagnosis of LPH is made when the frontal axis is positive and greater than +120°. The QRS is negative in lead 1 and positive in leads 2 and aVF. Lead 1 has an rS configuration and leads 3 and aVF have a qR configuration (Fig. 10-34B). Patients with bundle branch blocks and hemiblocks must be observed closely for the development of second- and third-degree AV blocks.

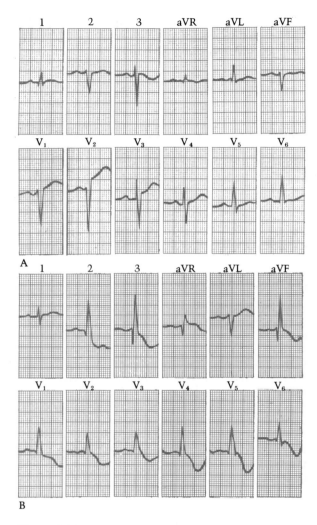

Figure 10-34
A. Left anterior hemiblock. B. Left posterior hemiblock.

Premature Ventricular Contractions

Even healthy people may develop premature ventricular contractions (PVCs), caused by coffee, tobacco, exercise, excitement, or slow heart rates. In the presence of cardiac disease, however, PVCs indicate ventricular irritability. PVCs are most frequently caused by ischemia, hypoxemia, heart failure, acute myocardial infarction, digitalis intoxication, or electrolyte imbalance. Characteristically, a PVC originates from an ectopic focus in the wall of the ventri-

cle. There are generally no P waves preceding the QRS complex. Because the impulse originates in an ectopic center in one of the ventricles and spreads anomalously, the QRS complex is distorted, bizarre, and prolonged. The PVC occurs prematurely in the cycle, and it is usually followed by a compensatory pause (Fig. 10-35A).

PVCs may have characteristic patterns. When every other beat is a PVC, the phenomenon is termed *bigeminy* (Fig. 10-35B); if every third beat is a PVC, the phenomenon is termed *trigeminy*; and if every fourth beat is a PVC, the phenomenon is termed *quadrigeminy*. If two or more PVCs are consecutive, they are referred to as *sequential* or paired PVCs (Fig. 10-35C). When the PVCs have different configurations, they are termed *multifocal* PVCs. The term indicates that the vector is different to the axis of the lead with each ectopic beat (i.e., the PVCs originate from different foci within the ventricle), and the phenomenon generally reflects a very sick and irritable heart (Fig. 10-35D).

The "R-on-T" phenomenon exists when a PVC occurs during the vulnerable phase of recovery. Actually the PVC (R wave) occurs during the relative refractory period (T wave). During that period of time, a dangerous ventricular dysrhythmia can occur since the heart is not yet ready to respond to the ectopic stimulus in a normal organized manner (Fig. 10-35E).

PVCs are considered dangerous, and they must be treated aggressively in the following situations:

1. When they occur frequently—more than six PVCs per minute
2. When they are sequential or paired
3. When they occur in short runs—"salvos"
4. When they are multifocal
5. When the R-on-T phenomenon is present (i.e., when the PVC occurs close to or on the peak of a T wave)

The drug therapy of choice is a bolus of lidocaine followed by a continuous lidocaine infusion (see Chap. 18). Some PVCs may be innocuous, but often, especially in the presence of acute myocardial infarction, they can be forerunners of ventricular tachycardia or ventricular fibrillation.

Interpolated PVC

One type of PVC that does not interrupt the regular basic rhythm is the interpolated PVC. The interpo-

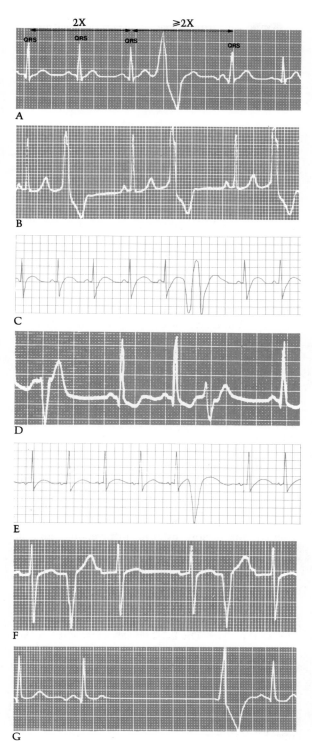

A

B

C

D

E

F

G

lated PVC does not have a compensatory pause, and it usually occurs with a slow rhythm. It falls between two normal sinus beats. The sinus node continues to discharge in a normal manner, and a normal ventricular response follows the discharge. The interpolated PVC can occur only when the normal rate is slow enough to find the myocardium physiologically nonrefractory for a period sufficient to complete the response to an ectopic stimulus and then return to a nonrefractory state before the next normal ventricular response (Fig. 10-35F).

Ventricular Escape Beat

When the sinus node fails to conduct impulses to the ventricle, a ventricular escape may occur. The ECG reveals a broad ventricular beat since the impulse originates below the bifurcation of the bundle of His (Fig. 10-35G). That is one situation in which lidocaine is not the drug of choice to treat the PVCs. If the patient is symptomatic, with a ventricular rate below 60 beats per minute and has frequent ventricular escape beats, the drug of choice is intravenous atropine sulfate, which speeds up the intrinsic heart rate and suppresses the ectopic rhythm.

Ventricular Tachycardia

Ventricular tachycardia is a dangerous dysrhythmia characterized by irritability of the ventricles. It may be caused by ischemia, hypoxemia, acidosis, acute myocardial infarction, or drug intoxication. The ECG reveals wide, bizarre ventricular complexes at a rate of 100 to 250 beats per minute. The rhythm is usually regular, but may be slightly irregular. The P waves are often lost in the QRS complexes; the QRS interval is greater than 0.12 second (Fig. 10-36A).

Presence of the following phenomena may help to

Figure 10-35
A. Normal sinus rhythm with premature ventricular contraction (PVC). The fourth QRS complex is wide, bizarre, and premature. A complete compensatory pause associated with the PVC is present (the distance between the QRS complex before and the QRS complex after the PVC is greater than or equal to the distance between two normal R-R intervals). B. Bigeminy of PVCs. C. Paired PVCs. D. Multifocal PVCs. E. R-on-T phenomenon. F. Interpolated PVCs. G. Ventricular escape.

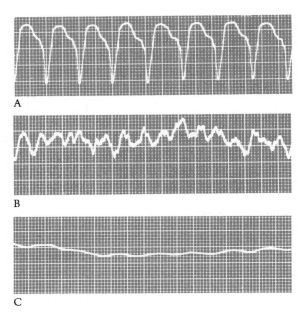

Figure 10-36
A. Ventricular tachycardia. B. Ventricular fibrillation. C. Cardiac standstill.

confirm the diagnosis of ventricular tachycardia: (1) a fusion beat, (2) AV dissociation, and (3) ventricular capture beats. A *ventricular fusion beat*, or Dressler's beat (a small narrow complex), frequently occurs when an irritable ectopic focus in the ventricle discharges about the same time that a normally conducted impulse begins at the AV junction. *AV dissociation* is a state in which the atria and ventricles are beating independently, a phenomenon that may result from: (1) a slowing (default) of the primary pacemaker, (2) acceleration of a secondary pacemaker, or (3) heart block. A *ventricular capture beat* is defined as an ectopic beat originating from the ventricle following a period of AV dissociation.

Ventricular tachycardia is extremely dangerous in the setting of acute myocardial infarction since it will cause mild-to-severe hemodynamic changes that can precipitate heart failure or shock and that may also be a precursor to ventricular fibrillation.

Treatment is aimed at quick recognition. If a patient is stable, first an intravenous bolus of lidocaine and then a lidocaine infusion are given (see Chap. 18). When ventricular tachycardia does not respond to lidocaine or when hypotension, heart failure, or a

change in sensorium have occurred, the treatment is electrical cardioversion. Ventricular tachycardia, associated with digitalis intoxication, may be converted to normal sinus rhythm by the slow intravenous administration of dyphenylhydantoin (Dilantin).

Ventricular Fibrillation

Ventricular fibrillation occurs when myocardial function is severely compromised by ischemia, drug intoxication, high-voltage electrical shock, or trauma. The ECG is characterized by a rapid, totally irregular rate and rhythm. No P waves are seen. The QRS complex is wide, bizarre, and irregular (Fig. 10-36B). Because ventricular depolarization and contraction are completely uncoordinated, there is an abrupt cessation in cardiac output. The patient becomes unconscious and is considered clinically dead. The immediate treatment of choice is direct current countershock. A precordial thump (see Chap. 18) may be delivered immediately after the onset of ventricular fibrillation if the cardiac arrest was witnessed and has been monitored in the hope of converting the dysrhythmia to a normal sinus rhythm. If the precordial thump is unsuccessful, basic life support should be instituted until defibrillation can be attempted.

If the patient reverts to ventricular fibrillation after a successful defibrillation attempt, lidocaine is given intravenously. Sodium bicarbonate is given according to the patient's body weight to correct metabolic acidosis, which develops as a result of anaerobic metabolism. In the presence of a fine ventricular fibrillation, defibrillation is generally more effective in converting the rhythm back to normal sinus if the fine fibrillatory pattern is first converted to a coarse ventricular fibrillation by the intravenous administration of epinephrine (see Chap. 18).

Cardiac Standstill

Cardiac standstill (literally, the only true arrhythmia) is the total absence of electrical activity and contraction of the heart. The ECG reveals a straight line, and the patient loses consciousness, pulse, and blood pressure (Fig. 10-36C). Death results unless treatment is immediate. External cardiac massage is the treatment of choice. Epinephrine, sodium bicarbonate, isoproterenol, and calcium chloride may also be used (see Chap. 18). Insertion of a transvenous pacemaker may be indicated.

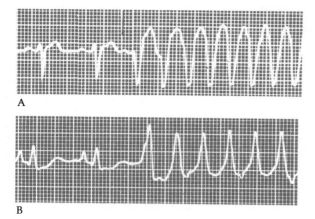

Figure 10-37
A. Aberrant ventricular conduction. B. Ventricular tachycardia.

Aberrant Ventricular Conduction

Aberrant ventricular conduction (AVC) is a term that applies only to a transient conduction defect. AVC occurs when one of the bundle branches (usually the right bundle branch) is still partially refractory at the time of the next stimulus. AVC frequently occurs with very premature atrial contractions, rapid rates, and changes in the length of the cycle. It may also be caused by a reduction in the membrane or action potential. The configuration of the abberant beat has a RBBB pattern because the RBB repolarizes relatively later than the LBB and is more liable to be caught in a refractory state by a premature beat. The patient is asymptomatic unless the tachycardia is extremely fast and causes hemodynamic changes.

PACs with aberrant ventricular conduction can be easily mistaken for—and inappropriately treated as—PVCs (Fig. 10-37A, B). Whenever there is a less than full compensatory pause, the beat should be closely examined for a P wave hidden in the preceding T wave. PACs with AVC should be recognized but not treated.

It is often difficult to differentiate supraventricular tachycardia with AVC from a ventricular tachycardia. There are some identifying signs, but they are not always seen. However, it is helpful to use the following procedures when considering the diagnosis of AVC.

1. Identify the start of the tachycardia. A PAC begins supraventricular tachycardia, and a PVC begins ventricular tachycardia.

2. Identify P waves. P waves associated with ventricular complexes are suggestive but not diagnostic of supraventricular tachycardia. P waves that are independent suggest AV dissociation and ventricular tachycardia.

3. Identify isolated extrasystoles in the same tracing or other tracings. A PAC with AVC that resembles the tachycardia indicates that the origin is supraventricular. A PVC that has the same configuration as the tachycardia indicates that the tachycardia is ventricular in origin.

4. Identify Dressler's (ventricular fusion) beats, which show partial or complete capture of the ventricles by the atria after a period of AV dissociation and suggest ventricular tachycardia.

When the tachycardia is supraventricular in origin and when hemodynamic changes occur, treatment is aimed at reducing the rate or cardioverting the rhythm.

Wolff-Parkinson-White (WPW) Syndrome

The Wolff-Parkinson-White (WPW) syndrome, a preexcitation syndrome, is produced when there is accelerated conduction between the atria and ventricles and abnormal excitation of the ventricles. An abnormal pathway between the atria to the ventricles exists that can bypass all or part of the AV node. The atrial rate, autonomic tone, and the refractory period of the anomalous pathway determine the degree of preexcitation.

The ECG reveals a PR interval of less than 0.12 second due to an accessory pathway rather than the normal conduction pathway. The QRS is 0.12 second or more. The upstroke of the QRS complex is slurred; it is termed the *delta wave*.

The WPW syndrome can be classified according to specific ECG patterns as type A or type B. In type A WPW syndrome (Fig. 10-38A), the left bundle of Kent connects the left atrium with the left posterior epicardium. The delta wave in leads 1, aVL, V_1, and V_6 will be positive, with a Q wave or QS wave in leads 3 and aVF. The preexcitation of the ventricular tissue causes vector forces to travel from epicardium (posterior) to endocardium (anterior), producing the characteristic deflections mentioned (RBBB pattern).

Type B WPW syndrome (Fig. 10-38B) involves the right bundle of Kent, which connects the right atrium with the right ventricle. The ECG will record V_1 as a QS,

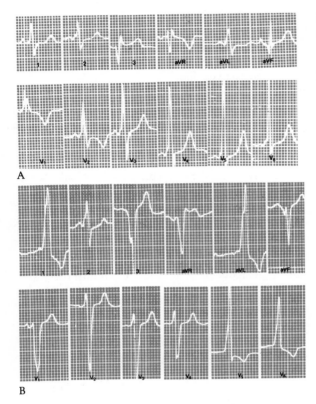

Figure 10-38
A. Type A of Wolff-Parkinson-White syndrome. B. Type B of Wolff-Parkinson-White syndrome.

rS, or a biphasic delta wave and V_6 as a positive delta wave and a tall R wave. Leads 3 and aVF frequently have a Q or QS wave. The bundle of Kent terminates in the epicardium of the anterolateral side of the right ventricle. Thus the right ventricle depolarizes first and the left ventricle follows in the expected fashion (LBBB pattern). Other accessory pathways, the James fibers (AV junctional bypass fibers) and fibers connecting the conducting bundles to the ventricular system, may also be present in type B WPW syndrome.

The patient is usually asymptomatic unless he develops a supraventricular or ventricular tachycardia. Those dysrhythmias can occur in patients with WPW syndrome and are thought to result from a retrograde atrial excitation. Those dysrhythmias are attributed to a circus movement of depolarization from the atrium across the AV junction and back again to the atrium via the accessory pathway. When the patient becomes symptomatic, treatment is directed toward slowing the ventricular response.

References

1. Castellanos, A., Spence, M. I., and Chapell, D. E. Hemiblock and bundle branch block: A nursing approach. *Heart Lung* 1:36, 1972.
2. Castellanos, A., Lemberg, L., Berkovits, E. E., et al. Vectorcardiography: General concepts. *Heart Lung* 4:697, 1975.
3. Coats, K. Techniques in cardiac diagnosis. *Nurs. Clin. North Am.* 2:259, 1976.
4. DeGowin, E. L., and DeGowin, R. L. *Bedside Diagnostic Examination* (3rd ed.). London: Macmillan, 1976.
5. Doyle, J. T., and Kinch, S. H. The prognosis of an abnormal electrocardiographic stress test. *Circulation* 41:545, 1970.
6. Ferrer, M. I. The sick sinus syndrome. *Circulation* 47:635, 1973.
7. Guyton, A. C. *Textbook of Medical Physiology* (5th ed.). Philadelphia: Saunders, 1976.
8. Hurst, J. W., and Logue, R. B. *The Heart, Arteries and Veins* (4th ed.). New York: McGraw-Hill, 1978.
9. Judge, R. D., and Zuidema, G. D. *Physical diagnosis: A Physiologic Approach to the Clinical Examination* (3rd ed.). Boston: Little, Brown, 1973.
10. Julian, D. G., Valentine, P. A., and Miller, G. G. Disturbances of rate, rhythm, and conduction in acute myocardial infarction. *Am. J. Med.* 37:915, 1964.
11. Marriott, H. J. L., and Gozensky, C. Analysis of arrhythmias in coronary care—A plea for precision. *Heart Lung* 1:51, 1972.
12. Meltzer, L. E., and Kitchell, J. B. The incidence of arrhythmias associated with acute myocardial infarction. *Prog. Cardiovasc. Dis.* 9:50, 1966.
13. Naggar, C. Z. Ultrasound in medical diagnosis. Part I: Application in cardiology. *Heart Lung* 5:895, 1976.
14. Rodbard, S. The clinical utility of the arterial pulses and sounds. *Heart Lung* 1:776, 1972.
15. Rubenstein, J. J., Schulman, C. L., Yurchak, P. M., et al. Clinical spectrum of the sick sinus syndrome. *Circulation* 46:5, 1972.
16. Schamroth, L. Some basic principles governing the electrophysiology and diagnosis of heart rhythms. *Heart Lung* 1:45, 1972.
17. Vinsant, M., Spence, M., and Chapell, D. *A Commonsense Approach to Coronary Care: A Program* (2nd ed.). St. Louis: Mosby, 1975.
18. Winslow, E. H., and Powell, A. H. Sick sinus syndrome. *Am. J. Nurs.* 76:1262, 1976.
19. Yu, P. N., and Goodwin, J. F. *Progress in Cardiology.* Philadelphia: Lea & Febiger, 1974.
20. Zalis, E. G., and Conover, M. H. *Understanding Electrocardiography.* St. Louis: Mosby, 1972.

Neurological Assessment

Cornelia Vanderstaay Kenner

The primary purposes of the neurological nursing assessment in the critical care unit are to identify life-threatening neurological changes, determine trends by serially monitoring the patient's status, and assess dysfunction that will affect the life-styles of the patient and his family. The nurse predicts potential problems and assesses how well the patient can care for himself.

Objective

After assimilating the information that follows, the nurse in the clinical situation should be able to perform an accurate screening neurological assessment involving interviewing and a physical examination. The nurse in the critical care unit will be able to identify the salient neurological findings and, in association with other members of the health team, perform ongoing clinical assessment.

Achieving the Objective

To achieve this objective the nurse should be able to:

1. List the tests for the functioning of the cranial nerves and reflexes, cerebellum, motor system, and sensory system.

11

2. Develop an assessment tool for the neurological examination of the eyes to be used for examining both the conscious patient and the unconscious patient.
3. Write a paragraph describing the major points in the assessment of consciousness.
4. Compare and contrast the possible respiratory patterns exhibited by the patient.
5. List the assessment findings in common pathophysiological, neurological, and neurosurgical conditions.
6. Differentiate decorticate from decerebrate posture.
7. Develop nursing orders for the patient for whom the neurologist or neurosurgeon has ordered diagnostic studies.
8. Compare and contrast the interviewing techniques used for two types of patients admitted to the critical care unit: (1) the patient with ascending paralysis and (2) the patient with head injuries.

How to Proceed

To develop an approach to neurological assessment the nurse should:

1. Study the material in the following pages.
2. Review the anatomy and physiology of the nervous system.
3. Establish a professional relationship with a preceptor whom she can observe in neurological and pain clinics. Then she should begin to perform patient assessments.
4. Observe and identify respiratory patterns, eye movements, and posture in unconscious patients.
5. Plan a continuing education program to maintain and update her skills (perhaps a program using audiovisual materials).

Interview

Chief Complaint

The chief complaint is a precise statement of the patient's subjective problem. The details may have to be elicited from others if the patient has a mental impairment.

Patient Profile

To assemble the patient profile a complete nursing history must be obtained. The history should include information about the patient's education, life-style, drug and alcohol intake, exposure to toxins, recent travel, and employment. It should be determined whether the patient finds his work interesting and enjoyable or strife laden. If possible, his relationship with his wife and other family members and his feelings, attitudes, goals, and frustrations should be assessed.

History of the Present Illness

The history of the present illness comprises an in-depth description of the problems of greatest concern. The patient's own evaluation should include strengths, deficiencies, what he thinks is happening, and what has helped his situation. The problems are described and recorded as follows:

1. Onset: Sudden or gradual
2. Progression of disease: (1) Disease steadily increases, (2) patient had periods of exacerbation and remission, or (3) symptoms reached plateau, stabilized for a time, and then progressed. Notation is made about whether the remissions were complete or incomplete and whether progression was rapid or slow, recording days, months, and years
3. Location
4. Quality and quantity: The description is carefully evaluated since some terms (e.g., numbness and dizziness) have different connotations
5. Duration
6. Precipitating factors
7. Alleviating and aggravating factors

Pain is an extremely important symptom. Notation should be made about its location, duration (intermittent or constant), intensity, nature, radiation, alleviating factors (e.g., heat, posture, movement, environment, and dosage of medication), and aggravating factors (e.g., posture, movement, environment, straining, and sneezing). In regard to headache, it must be determined whether the headache is (1) unilateral or bilateral, (2) frontal, temporal, or occipital, (3) focal or generalized, (4) throbbing or steady, and (5) associated with nausea, vomiting, or change in vision.

The term *dizziness* may refer to a simple feeling of faintness or to vertigo. Vertigo implies a sensation of motion. Notation should be made about whether the vertigo is accompanied by nausea, vomiting, or a change in hearing and gait. Particular attention must be paid to the patient's choice of words, and the patient's response must be validated so that there is no doubt that the communication has been understood.

Numbness is another term that is open to interpretation and that therefore must be clarified. The specific quality of the numbness or sensory alteration and the precise location and extent may be difficult for the patient to communicate and the examiner to pinpoint. The following question should be asked: Does the location indicate a lesion that interferes with the patient's ability to care for himself?

Convulsions or *seizures* must be accurately observed and described. Characteristics such as warning, sensory aura, alteration of consciousness, abnormal movements, including blinking, staring, lip smacking, tonic-clonic activity, and level of functioning after the acute episode are important. The patient is asked whether he fell, bit his tongue, or was incontinent. He is asked also about the onset and presumed cause. The origin, family history, relationship to any other condition, frequency, and whether there was an association with another event must be determined. The effectiveness of any medication that has been administered is assessed.

Blurred vision is another term that has different meanings to patients. The term may be used to refer to normal phenomena, such as awareness of the physiological blind spot, or to floaters. It may refer to double vision (diplopia) or to oscillopsia, the phenomenon sometimes associated with nystagmus in which objects seem to move. If there is true blurring of vision, is it monocular, or are both eyes involved? Is the entire visual field involved or only a portion of it? Is the blurring more to one side than to the other? Is it bitemporal? How long does it last, and what precipitates it? Is the patient able to function?

Past Medical History

The past medical history may be divided into perinatal, childhood, and adult history. Notation is made about any history of head trauma, meningitis, poliomyelitis, encephalitis, tuberculosis, otitis media, mastoiditis, venereal disease, viral infections, heavy alcohol consumption, and use of anticoagulants.

Family History

Many conditions have a familial incidence (e.g., migraine headaches, diabetes, epilepsy, tremor, spinocerebellar degenerations, hereditary spastic paralysis, Huntington's chorea, and familial periodic paralysis). Symptoms and signs (e.g., seizures or fits, sick headaches, and paralysis) rather than names of diseases are elicited since many illnesses may not have been diagnosed. Notation is also made about any history of psychiatric illness.

Review of Systems

In the review of systems and psychiatric problems, a quick determination is made of other problems. The patient is asked general questions, and if he answers in the affirmative, specific information is elicited.

1. Central nervous system: Headache, syncope, seizures, vertigo, amaurosis (loss of vision), diplopia, paralysis, paresis, muscle weakness, tremor, ataxia, dysesthesia, fainting, drowsiness, insomnia, speech, memory, concentration, disorientation
2. Eyes: Vision, scotomata, ptosis, reading difficulties, blinking
3. Ears: Tinnitus, loss of hearing
4. Nose, throat, and sinuses: Hoarseness
5. Cardiorespiratory system: Tightness in the chest, palpitations
6. Gastrointestinal system: Abnormalities of smell, taste, chewing, swallowing
7. Urinary tract: Impairment of sphincter control, polyuria
8. Reproductive system: Impotence, menstrual disturbances
9. Musculoskeletal system: Motor disturbances of the face, trunk, extremities; sensory disturbances of the face, trunk, extremities; muscle weakness, muscle wasting, rigidity; problems in walking, or sitting
10. Psychiatric: Hallucinations, hyperventilation, nervousness, depression, insomnia, nightmares, memory loss

Examination

The examination is divided into broad areas for testing integrated functions: level of consciousness, mentation, respiratory pattern, cranial nerves, motor system, sensory system, coordination, and reflexes.

Consciousness

Consciousness is assessed in regard to level of consciousness and content of consciousness. Level of consciousness is principally controlled by the reticular-activating system in the brainstem. That system is analogous to an "off-on" switch in regard to consciousness, and it is subtentorial in location. The content of consciousness is controlled by the cerebral hemispheres, which are above the cerebellar tentorium.

To compare the patient's level of consciousness at one examination period with his level of consciousness at another period, it is best to describe the behavior of the patient, including information about his spontaneous activity and his responsiveness. Even if the nurse does not totally understand the significance of the findings, an accurate description is needed to make serial determinations and identify trends in the patient's status. Critically ill people often lose their orientation first to time, then to place, then to persons—but the exceptions are many. The Glascow coma scale (see Chaps. 4 and 30) is extremely helpful in assessing and monitoring the level of consciousness. The following is a general description of the classic states of consciousness [18]. A precise delineation of each state is difficult.

1. The alert, wakeful state is characterized by much spontaneous activity and prompt, appropriate response to command.
2. Lethargy is a state of drowsiness characterized by some spontaneous activity.
3. Obtundation is a state of extreme drowsiness characterized by little spontaneous activity. The obtunded patient responds sluggishly and inconsistently to strong voice commands.
4. Stupor is a state of extreme drowsiness characterized by a complete lack of spontaneous motor activity. The stuporous patient is aroused only by strong stimuli. His responses tend to be stereotyped and simplified.
5. Deep coma is a state in which the patient cannot be aroused. It is not always easy to determine whether or not a person is in coma. An accurate description of his behavior is imperative.

It is important to determine whether the cause of the altered level of consciousness is structural or metabolic-toxic, the direction the disease process is taking, and what part of the brain might be the most affected. The phenomena assessed are the patient's state of consciousness, pattern of breathing, size and reactivity of the pupils, eye movements and oculovestibular responses, and skeletal muscle tone, posture, movement, and reflexes [1, 4, 9] (see Fig. 4-2).

Mentation

If an impairment in the content of consciousness is present, it must first be determined whether the cause is functional or organic. Bizarre thoughts and behavior with intact intellectual functioning point to a functional cause [22, 24]. The markedly depressed patient, however, may demonstrate problems with tests of mental status that mimic the signs of an organic disorder. If it is determined that the patient has a true organic encephalopathy, it must be determined whether it is generalized or represents focal hemispheric dysfunction (e.g., asphasia, unawareness of illness).

The person's alertness, ability to cooperate, educational level, and handedness are evaluated first. The person's general facial expression, level of consciousness, mood, and behavior are assessed. Next the person's general intellectual level is determined (based on the person's occupational history, activities, vocabulary, grammar, and knowledge of the subjects discussed) to help the examiner structure his questions and evaluate the patient's responses. Then the patient is asked whether he is lefthanded or righthanded. It is important to remember that some lefthanded people write with their right hands. Determining handedness is helpful in ascertaining hemispheric language dominance and thus in localization (see Chap. 29).

The mental status examination tests the patient's (1) immediate recall, (2) recent or short-term memory, (3) remote memory, (4) interpretation and use of previously gained knowledge, and (5) behavior [5, 7]. The test of the patient's immediate recall evaluates his attention span. The patient is told a series of numbers, and he is asked to repeat the numbers forward and backward. Normally a person is able to repeat five to seven numbers forward and four to five numbers backward. Short-term memory is evidenced by the ability (1) to recall information about dates, time, or current political happenings and (2) to learn information, such as the plot of a short story, and to tell the story in several minutes. Remote memory is evaluated by the patient's ability to remember information about his childhood or young adult life. For example, the patient may be asked about his confirmation or his wedding.

The ability to interpret and use previously gained knowledge is evaluated by a series of tests. Abstract thinking may be tested by the patient's ability to point out similarities between objects, such as between iron and silver or between a tree and a dog. Second, a slightly more difficult test involves proverb interpretation. For example, the person being tested is asked to explain a saying such as "A rolling stone gathers no moss." An even more difficult test involves problem solving, which requires the person to think through a problem and arrive at a solution. For example, a person's ability to calculate can be tested by asking the person to subtract by sevens from 100, to change inches to feet, to perform simple algebraic equations, or to make change from five dollars. The person should be asked to do a calculation of suitable difficulty. One would not expect a person with a Ph.D. in mathematics to have difficulty with a simple algebraic equation; however, someone with a third-grade education would normally have difficulty with an algebraic calculation.

Behavior is assessed by subjectively evaluating the person's affect and judgment. Essentially affect is the person's emotional status, and such factors as happiness, sadness, and irritability are noted. Also, the person is asked to evaluate himself in regard to his own feeling state and his perspective on his illness. The patient's judgment is assessed by the appropriateness of his behavior; often judgment is difficult to assess on the first interview. The family is frequently asked for their assessment of the patient's past behavior [2].

Factors that assess language include spontaneous speech, repetition, and comprehension (see Chap. 29).

Respiratory Patterns

Identification of respiratory patterns helps to identify the lesion site and to anticipate patient problems. Respiratory abnormalities may be listed as post–hyperventilation apnea, Cheyne-Stokes breathing, and central neurogenic hyperventilation (Fig. 11-1). It is important to recognize that a change from one pattern to another may herald a change in the patient's condition that allows little time for reversal. Change from a normal breathing pattern to Cheyne-Stokes breathing or to central neurogenic hyperventilation

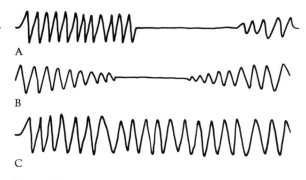

Figure 11-1

Abnormal respiratory patterns. A. Posthyperventilation apnea. B. Cheyne-Stokes respiration. C. Central neurogenic hyperventilation.

may be the first sign of impending central herniation, and death may rapidly ensue.

Post–hyperventilation apnea is a transient cessation of breathing after hyperventilation. Usually, hyperventilation causes a lowered partial pressure of arterial carbon dioxide and removes the major stimulus to the inspiratory stimulus in the medulla. A normal person would continue to breathe since control areas in the cerebral cortex have priority over respiratory medullary control. However, if the patient has a bilateral impairment of his cerebral functioning, the control is removed and he exhibits post–hyperventilation apnea.

Cheyne-Stokes breathing is a waxing and waning respiratory pattern. The respiration starts with apnea, increases to a maximum (crescendo), and then decreases to apnea (decrescendo). It is characterized by intermittent periods of hyperventilation followed by gradually decreasing breathing, then periodic apnea followed by gradually increasing breathing [3]. In Cheyne-Stokes breathing, an increased ventilatory response to arterial carbon dioxide levels exists in the medulla, resulting in hyperventilation. The hyperventilation is in addition to the loss of cortical influence on respiration, resulting in post–hyperventilation apnea. Cheyne-Stokes breathing is usually seen in patients with bilateral deep lesions of the cerebral hemispheres and basal ganglia that damage the internal capsule [9–10, 21].

Central neurogenic hyperventilation is sustained, regular, deep, rapid breathing. It results from a lowered threshold to respiratory stimulation and leads to decreased arterial carbon dioxide tension and respiratory alkalosis. The syndrome normally is caused by lesions involving the tegmentum of the lower midbrain or upper pons.

The other types of abnormal respirations (apneustic breathing and ataxic respirations) that have been described, do not correlate well with the site of damage.

Cranial Nerves

The *first cranial nerve,* the olfactory nerve, serves the sense of smell. Loss of smell (anosmia) may be unilateral or bilateral. The most common causes of anosmia are upper respiratory illness, fracture of the cribriform plate, and tumor of the olfactory groove or frontal lobe (especially meningioma). Although the test is frequently not included in the examination, it is included if anosmia, trauma, visual problems, intellectual deterioration, or other neurological problems are present. Defects in the olfactory bulb and tract or in the olfactory receptors in the nasal mucosa may interfere with smell. Familiar and mild odors, such as those of coffee, tea, vanilla, or peppermint, are used in testing, and volatile, irritating substances, such as ammonia or vinegar, are avoided. The ability to distinguish between odors is more important than the ability to identify odors exactly [6, 8].

OPTIC NERVE

The *second cranial nerve,* the optic nerve, is tested by direct examination of the optic nerve and in regard to visual acuity, visual fields, and pupillary response. On fundoscopic examination, the head of the optic nerve can be viewed directly. The examiner notes the color, size, and shape of the optic disk, presence of physiological cup, distinctness of the edges of optic disk, size, shape, and configuration of vessels, and presence of exudate, hemorrhage, or pigment. Swelling indicates inflammation or increased intracranial pressure. Pallor indicates chronic changes. Visual acuity may be tested by the use of a standardized chart, such as the Snellen chart; or the patient may be asked to read various sizes of print. If the patient usually wears glasses, he should wear them for the test. Visual fields may be roughly tested by the confrontation test. The patient, who is seated 2 to 3 feet from the examiner, fixes his gaze on the examiner's nose, and covers one eye with a piece of paper. The exam-

iner's finger is then brought in along the main axes (superior, inferior, nasal, and temporal) of the visual field to be examined. Normally, visual fields extend 60° on the nasal side, 100° on the temporal side, and 130° vertically [14]. Gross hemianopic field defects or scotomas may be detected by the examination, and a more accurate determination may be performed with a perimeter or tangent screen [13]. All quadrants must be tested separately and carefully. The particular areas impaired are often diagnostic. For example, a lesion of one optic tract results in blindness in the opposite half of both visual fields. A lesion in the temporal lobe results in blindness in the eye on the opposite side in both upper quadrants. (Pupillary response is considered in the discussion that follows of the third nerve.)

OCULOMOTOR, TROCHLEAR, AND ABDUCENS NERVES

The *oculomotor nerve* (third cranial nerve), *trochlear nerve* (fourth cranial nerve) and *abducens nerve* (sixth cranial nerve) are usually tested together since they supply the muscles that rotate the eyeball. The observer looks for strabismus, nystagmus, ptosis, and exophthalmos. The size of each pupil and, in particular, the size relative to the other is noted. The size is determined by the balance between the sympathetic and parasympathetic fibers. Next, the patient's direct light and consensual responses are evaluated [12]. The examiner should note whether the pupil is dilated or constricted and whether the abnormality is unilateral or bilateral. The response to light is tested by shining a focused bright light onto one pupil and then onto the other. Both pupils normally constrict when light is focused on one eye. The eye that receives the direct light shows the direct light response, and the other eye shows the consensual response. Accommodation and convergence are tested simultaneously. The patient focuses on a distant object, such as a penlight, and continues to look at it as it is brought to his nose. His eyes should begin to look at the penlight in a cross-eyed, or convergent, manner. At the same time, his pupils constrict, showing the accommodation response. Ocular movements are observed to note any defects in conjugate movements or nystagmus. The patient follows the movement of an object to the extremes of the lateral and vertical planes. Individual eye movements are tested by covering one eye and observing movement in all axes. If diplopia is present, one eye is covered with red glass, so that the patient can describe what area of the visual field has diplopia and where divergence between the two images is greater.

A lesion affecting the oculomotor nerve changes the pupillary reflexes and eye movements [11]. An expanding mass in one portion of the cerebral hemisphere may cause the uncal gyrus to herniate through the opening of the tentorium. As the uncus is pushed downward, the oculomotor nerve is compressed against the tentorium. The pupil is maximally dilated and unreactive. If the compression continues, ptosis ensues and the eye deviates laterally as oculomotor function is lost.

Observation of the direct light and consensual responses helps the examiner to pinpoint the problem to the optic or oculomotor nerve [16–17, 20]. The retina and the optic nerve form the afferent limb of the light reflex and carry sensory stimuli toward the brain. The oculomotor nerve, the efferent limb of the light reflex, carries motor stimuli away from the brain. If the optic nerve is injured, the pupil is dilated and the direct light response is lost. Since the consensual response, or motor pathway, remains intact, the pupil constricts when light is shown in the other eye. If the oculomotor nerve is impaired, both the direct light and consensual responses are absent in that eye.

It is of particular importance to observe the pupillary reflexes and eye movements of the patient with impaired consciousness. Formerly, the presence of the ciliospinal reflex—dilatation of an ipsilateral pupil secondary to noxious stimuli at the neck—was thought to reflect the structural integrity of the brainstem, but it is now thought to reflect only the integrity of the cervical spinal cord and the peripheral sympathetic fibers to the eye [23]. The following observations should be made in regard to each eye: (1) resting position, (2) spontaneous motion, and (3) the oculocephalic and oculovestibular reflexes. First each eye is observed in the resting position, noting conjugate or disconjugate positioning. That applies whether the eyes are in midposition or deviated in any direction. The direction of any deviation is particularly important. Notation is made of the eye(s) involved and whether the deviation is conjugate or disconjugate. A skew position is present when one eye is up and the other down (disconjugate vertical position) (Fig. 11-2).

The normal resting position of the eyes is midposition [15]. A forced, lateral, conjugate gaze results from lesions of the frontal lobes or pons. A unilateral destructive lesion in the frontal lobe produces a forced

Figure 11-2
Skew position.

lateral conjugate gaze toward the side of the lesion. A unilateral irritative lesion in the frontal lobe and a unilateral destructive lesion in the pons produces a forced lateral conjugate gaze away from the side of the lesion. A lesion of the third cranial nerve causes (1) the eye to deviate outward, (2) alterations in pupillary size and reflexes, and (3) ptosis. A lesion of the sixth cranial nerve causes the affected eye to deviate inward.

If the person has a unilateral destructive lesion in the frontal lobe, his eyes are deviated toward the side of the lesion and away from the side of the hemiparesis. If he has a unilateral destructive lesion in the pons, his eyes are deviated away from the lesion and toward the side of the hemiparesis. Skewing of the eyes is produced by brainstem lesions. Skewing cannot be used to further localize the lesion within the brainstem.

Next the presence of any spontaneous movement of the eyes is noted. A normal finding is (1) no spontaneous movement or (2) conjugate or disconjugate roving of the eyes (similar to that seen in a normal sleeping person). The four major types of abnormal spontaneous eye movements are shown in Figure 11-3. They must be differentiated from the normal roving, conjugate, or disconjugate eye movements. Retraction nystagmus is a conjugate, irregular, jerking movement that seems to pull both globes into the orbits. It results from simultaneous contraction of all the eye muscles. There is rapid retraction of the globes, followed by a slow return to normal position. It occurs with lesions in the midbrain tegmentum. Ocular bobbing consists of quick, downward, conjugate eye movements, followed by a slow return to neutral position; it occurs with lesions of the lower pons. Convergence nystagmus is a slow, drifting, divergent movement of each eye followed by a quick compensatory jerk of convergence. It sometimes is associated with retraction nystagmus, and it occurs with lesions of the midbrain. The fourth type of abnormal spontaneous eye movement is occasional jerking of only one eye in any direction; it occurs with large lesions of the pons.

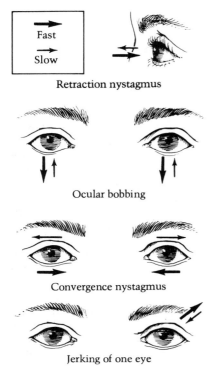

Figure 11-3
Four major types of abnormal spontaneous eye movements.

Additional tests can be performed by the physician to determine the integrity of the oculocephalic and oculovestibular reflexes. Those tests evaluate the integrity of the extraocular muscles and the vestibular system.

The test of the oculocephalic reflex (the doll's head maneuver) consists of rapidly and carefully turning the patient's head to one side or the other and up and down and noting how the patient's eyes follow his head movements. In the normal, awake person, the patient's eyes will follow his head unless the patient is fixing his gaze. Normally, in the unconscious patient, the eyes do not move with the head. Thus movement lags, and what is seen on rotating the head to one side is an apparent deviation of the eyes to the opposite side, followed by a slow return to midposition. Abnormalities consist of the eyes moving with the head or not deviating in certain directions—up, down, in, or out.

There are many reasons for an abnormal oculocephalic reflex. A large lesion in the brainstem will limit all eye movements, and the person's eyes will move with his head in all directions. A lesion in the cerebral cortex above the level of the nucleus of the third cranial nerve will cause the eyes to deviate to one side. The eyes will come to, but not cross, the midline. If the person has a unilateral lesion in the medial longitudinal fasciculus, the eye ipsilateral to the lesion will be unable to deviate toward the midline, and his opposite eye will deviate laterally. The condition is known as internuclear ophthalmoplegia, and the disconjugate lateral position is either unilateral or bilateral. If the person has a lesion in the midbrain pretectal area, his eyes cannot conjugately move upward.

If full range of eye movements cannot be elicited with the oculocephalic reflex, the oculovestibular reflex is tested [19]. The test employs the same reflex mechanisms as does the test of the oculocephalic reflex but it uses stronger stimulation. Approximately 100 to 200 ml of cold water or a puff of cold air is injected into the patient's external auditory canal. In the comatose patient, the test will usually elicit prolonged conjugate deviation to the same side if the oculovestibular pathways are intact.

TRIGEMINAL NERVE

The fifth cranial nerve, the *trigeminal nerve,* has both motor and sensory functions. In a test of the motor portion of the trigeminal nerve, the person clenches his teeth, and the examiner palpates the volume and firmness of the masseter and the temporal muscles. The patient then opens his mouth against resistance. While the patient's mouth is open, any deviation of the mandible to the weak side is more apparent. In a test of the sensory portion of the trigeminal nerve, pain is evaluated with a pin and light touch is evaluated by passing a piece of cotton over the patient's face and anterior half of scalp. Temperature may also be tested if indicated. Interestingly, if sensation is lost only in the patient's face and not in his scalp, the condition is probably psychogenic. Sensation on each side of the face is compared in each of the three divisions of the trigeminal nerve (ophthalmic, maxillary, and mandibular) (Fig. 11-4). Last, the corneal reflex is tested. A hair or piece of cotton so fine that it is invisible to the person is used. The patient's cornea is approached from the side and touched lightly with the hair or cotton. A normal reaction is a rapid forceful contraction of the eyelid. A contralateral blink is also common. If the patient has no reaction, he is

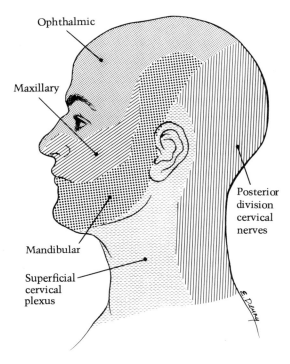

Ophthalmic

Maxillary

Mandibular

Superficial
cervical
plexus

Posterior
division
cervical
nerves

Figure 11-4
Ophthalmic, maxillary, and mandibular divisions of the
trigeminal nerve.

asked whether he felt the stimulus. (Care is taken not
to touch the eyelashes or conjunctiva since the response to such a touch would also be a forceful
blink.)

FACIAL NERVE

The seventh cranial nerve is the *facial nerve*. In tests
of the facial nerve, expression, symmetry, and mobility during speaking, smiling, and laughing are assessed. The patient performs all the voluntary
movements that can be done with the face. He frowns
or scowls, wrinkles his forehead, closes his eyelids
(the examiner attempts to forcibly open his eyes),
opens his mouth, retracts his mouth, blows out his
cheeks, puckers his lips, shows his teeth, whistles,
and screws up his nose. Careful observation is made
of any asymmetry of the nasolabial folds and of eye
blinking. Involvement of the low facial musculature,
called a lesion of the central seventh, occurs only in
upper motor neuron lesions. It is characterized by

weakness of movement of the lower portion of the
face on the side opposite the lesion. Involvement of
all the facial musculature on one side of the face occurs in lesions of the nucleus of the facial nerve; the
phenomenon is called a peripheral seventh. The lesion is ipsilateral to the paralysis. If a paralysis is
noted on one side of the facial musculature, taste
(which may be lost on the affected side) is tested on
the anterior two-thirds of the tongue with small
quantities of sweet (sugar), salt (saline), bitter
(quinine), and sour (lemon or vinegar) substances. The
person is asked to identify each substance without
putting his tongue back into his mouth.

AUDITORY NERVE

The eighth cranial nerve, the *auditory nerve,* is tested
in regard to its cochlear and vestibular portions. The
cochlear portion is tested in regard to the ability to
hear the spoken voice, a whisper, and/or a watch
ticking. The patient repeats a sentence whispered
from across the room, occluding each ear in turn. If
further assessment is needed, the Rinne test and the
Weber test may be performed. The Rinne test determines air and bone conduction. The vibrating tuning
fork is placed on the mastoid process until sound is
no longer heard, and it is moved in front of the patient's ear. Usually air conduction is greater than
bone conduction. In auditory or nerve deafness, there
may be a complete or partial inability to hear the vibrating tuning fork. In the Weber test, a vibrating
tuning fork is placed on a patient's forehead, and the
patient states where he hears sound. Normally sound
is heard equally well in both ears. In nerve deafness,
sound is not heard in the diseased ear, even with occlusion. If further testing is needed, an audiometer is
used. Next the vestibular portion is tested in three
ways. First the past-pointing test is performed by
having the patient bring the index finger of his outstretched arm down on the examiner's finger. He does
this vertically and horizontally with his eyes opened
and then with his eyes closed. In vestibular disease,
his finger past points to one side or the other consistently. Then the patient is tested for nystagmus. The
patient is told to look to one side. In true nystagmus,
a sustained movement with two components, there is
a fast jerk to the side of the deviation and a slow jerk
back to the midline. The nystagmus may be horizontal or vertical or rotary. The third test consists of
stimulation of the semicircular canal by injection of
cold water or a puff of cold air into the normal ear

canal with the patient sitting (if possible). To avoid nausea, in the conscious patient only a few drops are used. The normal reactions to such a test of the right ear are:

1. Vertigo within about two minutes of the injection.
2. Lateral and rotary nystagmus to the left. In unconscious patients, the normal response is deviation toward the irrigated ear.
3. Past pointing to the right.

GLOSSOPHARYNGEAL NERVE

The ninth cranial nerve, the *glossopharyngeal nerve,* is normally tested when the vagus nerve is tested. Its chief function is sensory; its motor function involves a minor muscle of the pharynx.

VAGUS NERVE

The tenth cranial nerve is the *vagus nerve.* The pharynx and larynx are assessed by noting swallowing and elevation of the uvula. While the patient says "Ah," his pharynx is observed. Normally the soft palate and uvula are pulled up in the midline. If the vagus nerve is weak, the affected side droops and the healthy side elevates. If the paralysis is bilateral, there is no palatal movement. The gag reflex is tested by touching the soft palate. Its absence is most significant if it is unilateral.

The character, sound, and volume of the patient's voice and his pulse and respirations are also noted. The nerve may be indirectly assessed by laryngoscopy.

SPINAL ACCESSORY NERVE

The eleventh nerve is the *spinal accessory nerve.* The innervation of the trapezius muscle is tested by asking the patient to shrug his shoulders against resistance. Then the opposite sternocleidomastoid muscle is tested by asking the patient to rotate his head against a resistance applied to the side of his chin. With nerve impairment, disability is evident when the chin turns away from the side of weakness. With hysteria, disability is likely to be evident when the chin turns toward the side of weakness. In the test of both sternocleidomastoid muscles the patient flexes his head forward against a resistance applied under his chin.

HYPOGLOSSAL NERVE

The twelfth cranial nerve, the *hypoglossal nerve,* is the motor nerve to the tongue. In the test of that nerve, the person protrudes his tongue and the observer looks for atrophy, involuntary movements, or fasciculations. A paralysis of the muscles on the left will produce a protrusion to the left. Strength is tested by having the person push his tongue against each cheek or by pushing against a tongue blade.

Motor System

The fourth major part of the physical examination is assessment of the motor system. The examination includes determination of muscle bulk, tone, strength, symmetry, and presence of abnormal muscle movements. Both sides are compared.

Any hypertrophy or atrophy of muscles should be noted. To check any suspected asymmetry, a tape measure is used to measure corresponding muscles at corresponding places on the limbs. Muscle tone is evaluated by passive range of motion exercises and active movement, noting any involuntary resistance, spasticity, flaccidity, or rigidity. Muscle strength is tested by having the patient push against resistance. Any abnormal movements, such as swift, jerking motions or slow, irregular movements, twistings, tics, tremors, or choreiform movements are noted.

The results may be graded as follows: 0 = no movement; 1 = flicker of movement; 2 = movement with gravity eliminated; 3 = movement against gravity; 4 = mild impairment of power; 5 = normal power.

The hands and arms are assessed by having the patient squeeze two of the examiner's fingers. The strength of the hand is estimated by the force the examiner must exert to withdraw his fingers. Next the person clenches his fist and fixes his wrist, and the examiner tries to overcome the dorsiflexion. The procedure is repeated to test for abduction of fingers and apposition of thumbs. Next the patient flexes and extends his arm against resistance. Last, arm abduction at the shoulders is tested. Assessment of the trunk may be done by having the patient rise from a lying to a sitting position. The lower extremities may be tested in several ways. First the patient flexes and extends his legs against resistance. He elevates one leg at a time and holds it for 10 to 20 seconds. The power of leg extension at the knee and at the hip is evalu-

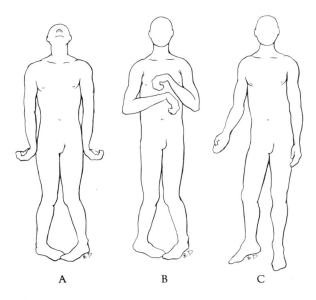

A   B   C

Figure 11-5
Abnormal posturing. A. Decerebrate position. B. Decorticate position. C. Position in early hemiplegia.

The patient with decerebrate posture exhibits extension, internal rotation, and wrist flexion in the upper extremities and extension, internal rotation, and plantar flexion in the lower extremities. His jaw may be clenched and his neck hyperextended. Decerebrate posture is symmetrical, and it is usually produced by lesions in the midbrain and pons. The patient with decorticate posture exhibits bilateral adduction of his shoulders, pronation and flexion of his elbows and wrists, and extension, internal rotation, and plantar flexion of his lower extremities.

In hemiplegia, the affected side and the normal side are not symmetrical. Initially, the affected extremities show an outward rotation and decreased muscle tone. A hemiplegic extremity lifted off the bed and allowed to fall drops abruptly, much like a dead weight. An extremity with normal muscle tone falls to the bed in a smooth motion. Later (the time varies) there is spasticity and resistance to passive movement. The upper extremity exhibits adduction of the shoulder and pronation with flexion of the elbow and wrist. The lower extremity exhibits extension, internal rotation, and plantar flexion.

ated. Then dorsiflexion is tested by having the patient push his partially flexed foot against the examiner's hand. Plantar flexion is tested by having the patient push down against the examiner's hand.

Subtle weakness due to an upper motor neuron (or "pyramidal") lesion may be evidenced by a downward drift in one of the patient's outstretched arms while he has his eyes closed. With pyramidal lesions, muscles that abduct and extend the joints in the upper extremities are weaker than their antagonists. In the lower extremities, the flexors of the hips and knees and the dorsiflexors of the feet are the weaker. Testing can be performed manually by having the patient exert maximum pressure against the examiner's resistance.

If the patient is unconscious, his motor system is assessed by observation of his resting posture, spontaneous movement, any asymmetry of position, and abnormal movement. In regard to localizing the lesion, posture, muscle tone, and the position of each limb are important for the nurse to observe. Posture may be decerebrate, decorticate, or hemiplegic (Fig. 11-5). Certain patients may consistently assume the first two postures, but mainly those postures are assumed in response to pain stimulation.

Sensory Assessment

There are three aspects of the sensory examination: (1) qualitative, to determine what elements of sensation are affected, (2) quantitative, to determine the degree of impaired sensation, and (3) regional, to determine the exact distribution of sensory impairment or loss.

The following terms are used in sensory testing:

1. Hypesthesia, hypoesthesia: Abnormally decreased sensitivity of the skin
2. Hypalgesia: Decreased pain
3. Analgesia: Loss of pain
4. Paresthesia: Unpleasant spontaneous cutaneous sensation (tingling, burning) resulting from contact with an object
5. Dysesthesia: Impairment in sensation; a state in which a disagreeable sensation is produced by ordinary stimuli
6. Anesthesia: Complete sensory loss

In testing for light touch, the skin surface is stroked with the tip of finger, a wisp of cotton, or a camel's hair brush. Care is taken to avoid tickling. Pain sense is tested by asking the patient to distinguish the sharp from the dull end of a pin in a side-to-side comparison. Temperature is tested by having the patient differentiate test tubes filled with hot water from those filled with ice.

Deep sensation assesses the posterior columns and pain. In vibration testing, a tuning fork (C128) is placed over elbows, wrists, ankles, shins, and other bony prominences. The patient is asked to identify sensation and then to determine when sensation ceases. The duration of the sensation may be timed. In testing position sense, many joints of the body are evaluated. Most commonly, the big toe is tested. The larger joints of the extremities are tested if any impairment is demonstrated in the digits. A digit is grasped on its sides, and the patient, with eyes closed, tries to determine whether the digit is moved upward or downward. In testing for deep pain, muscle pain is assessed by pressing on a muscle (usually the calf or shoulder muscle) to the point of pain. Tendon pain sense is tested by pressing on a tendon (usually the Achilles tendon). The tendon is compressed between the knuckle of the thumb and the tip of the index finger. Testicular pain sense is tested by squeezing the testicle gently between the thumb and finger.

There is a certain degree of localization in the spinal cord for transmission of the various types of sensation. Light touch has a rather diffuse representation. Pain and temperature are conveyed largely in the spinothalamic tracts, proprioception in the posterior columns, and vibration in the posterior and lateral columns. In the brain, the initial relay station for gross sensation is the thalamus. Functions such as two-point discrimination, stereognosis, and graphesthesia involve additional and higher centers located predominantly in the parietal lobes.

Tests of stereognosis evaluate the patient's ability to recognize objects placed in his hand. Familiar objects, such as a coin, key, or knife, are used. The patient closes his eyes, the object is placed in his hand, and he attempts to identify the object. In a test of graphesthesia, numbers or letters are traced on the patient's skin with a blunt object, and the patient tries to identify what has been drawn. In a test of two-point discrimination, the patient indicates whether he feels one point or two points pressed over various parts of his body with the use of a calibrated compass. (The shortest normal distances are fingertips = 0.3–0.6 cm; palms of hands and soles of feet = 1.5–2 cm; dorsum of hand = 3 cm; shin = 4 cm.) In a test of topognosis (tactile localization), the patient closes his eyes and the examiner touches a spot on the patient's body. The patient points to the spot. Corresponding areas of both sides of the body are tested. Normally, the patient is more accurate in regard to tests on his fingers and hands than in regard to tests on his arms.

Assessment of Coordination

The cerebellum functions primarily in balance and coordination. Incoordination is usually seen in attempted cooperative muscle movement; it results from involvement of the cerebellum or the nerve systems associated with the cerebellum. Most commonly, the movement is jerking and inaccurate.

Movement in the upper extremities is assessed by several tests. In the finger-to-nose test, the patient brings the tip of his index finger to the tip of his nose, first with his eyes open and then closed; first slowly and then rapidly. The test is considered positive if the movement to the nose is irregular or if the tip of the nose is consistently missed. In the finger-to-finger test, the same sequence is used but the examiner's finger is substituted for the patient's nose. In assessment of rapid alternating movements of the fingers, the patient is asked to flex and extend his fingers rapidly or to tap a table rapidly with his fingers extended. In the patting test, the patient rapidly pats his leg on the examiner's hand. Amplitude and rhythm are noted. In supination and pronation of the forearm, continuous rapid alternations using the elbows as a fulcrum are tested. A positive finding is the inability to perform the test quickly and smoothly (adiadokokinesia). In testing for the rebound phenomenon (Holmes' sign), the patient flexes his elbow and resists the examiner's attempt to extend his forearm. Then the patient's forearm is suddenly permitted to extend. Normally the patient's forearm will undergo a mild compensatory flexion. If cerebellar disease is present, the compensatory flexion will be great enough that the patient's hand will strike his own shoulder, neck, and face.

The same type of tests are used in the lower extremities. In the heel-to-knee test, the patient places one heel on his opposite knee and then slides the foot down his shin. The test is positive when the person has difficulty placing or holding the heel on the knee or cannot keep the heel firmly on the leg as the heel is moved downward. In the patting test, the patient pats his foot quickly on the floor. In the figure-of-eight test, the patient draws an 8 in the air with his big toe.

In the toe-finger test, the supine patient touches the examiner's finger with his big toe. Then the examiner moves his finger to a new position approximately 6 to 18 inches away, and the patient follows the finger with his toe.

Tests for gait and station to assess truncal coordination and dorsal column function are usually not performed in the critical care unit.

Reflexes

Reflexes are specific muscular responses to stimuli. They are usually evaluated with the cranial nerves in regard to functions served. The reflexes tend to be increased in upper motor neuron disease and decreased in lower motor neuron disease.

SUPERFICIAL REFLEXES

Two superficial reflexes are commonly evaluated: the abdominal reflex and the cremasteric reflex. The abdominal reflex is composed of abdominal muscle movements in all four quadrants. With the patient lying supine and his abdominal muscles relaxed, the skin of each quadrant is stroked with a pin, key, brush, or blunt end of an orangewood stick; the movement is from the periphery toward the umbilicus or in the shape of a diamond. A normal response consists of movement of the abdominal muscles and a pull of the umbilicus toward the quadrant that was stroked. (The response is difficult to elicit in patients who are overweight.) The cremasteric reflex is elicited by stroking the inner aspect of a man's thigh. The normal response is contraction of the scrotum on that side. Absence of an abdominal or cremasteric reflex may indicate a spinal cord lesion.

DEEP TENDON REFLEXES

The common deep tendon reflexes elicited are the biceps, triceps, radial, Achilles, and patellar reflexes. The biceps reflex tests the intactness of the innervation of C5–6. The patient flexes his elbow while the examiner presses his thumb against the patient's biceps tendon in the antecubital space. The patient's thumb is hit with the percussion hammer to produce a quick sharp contraction of the biceps tendon. The result is flexion of the arm.

The radial reflex also indicates the intactness of C5–6. With the patient's forearm midway between pronation and supination, the lower third of the radius is tapped. The result is flexion of the forearm on the arm with slight pronation and, usually, flexion of the fingers and hand. If there is a lesion at the fifth cervical segment, the radial response consists of flexion of the hand and fingers but not of the forearm.

The triceps reflex tests the intactness of C7–8. The tendon is put under slight tension by placing the forearm on a horizontal plane in front of the chest or by holding the upper arm straight out from the body and allowing the lower arm to dangle loosely. In the supine patient, the arm is drawn across the chest, and the forearm is slightly flexed. Directly striking the triceps tendon with the percussion hammer produces extension of the arm.

The patellar (knee) reflex tests the intactness of L3–4. The patient is sitting and his knees hang loosely over the side of the bed. In the supine position, (the more usual position in the critical care unit) several test methods are possible: (1) flex the patient's knees over the examiner's arm and have his heels resting lightly on the bed, (2) place a pillow under his knees, or (3) cross his legs. The reflex is elicited by striking the tendon immediately below the patella. The normal response is contraction of the quadriceps muscle and extension of the knee, much like a kick. If the response is difficult to elicit, it can be strengthened by having the patient lock the fingers of both hands and pull as hard as he is able in opposing directions.

The Achilles tendon (ankle) reflex, tests the intactness of L5–S2, particularly S1. The patient relaxes his foot and lies prone, kneels on a chair, or lies supine with his legs flexed and hip rotated outward. Gentle pressure is applied to the ball of the foot, and the Achilles tendon is tapped with the percussion hammer. The normal response is plantar extension of the foot.

ABNORMAL REFLEXES

The plantar reflex is elicited by stroking the sole of the foot with a blunt object from the heel up the lateral margin of the foot to the ball of the foot and then across the ball to the base of the big toe. The normal response is flexion of the toes. The abnormal (Babinski) response consists of extension of the big toe, flexion of the small toes, spreading of the small toes, and flexion of the leg. A Babinski response suggests an upper motor neuron lesion.

Chaddock's sign is elicited by stroking the lateral aspect of the dorsum of the foot and the external malleolus. The abnormal response is extension of the big toe. Oppenheim's sign is elicited by stroking the medial aspect of the tibia in a firm downward motion. The abnormal response is extension of the big toe. Gordon's sign is elicited by firm compression of the calf. The abnormal sign is extension of the big toe. Ankle clonus is elicited with the foot relaxed and the knee flexed. The foot is quickly pushed with a moderate force in a dorsal direction and held in that position. The abnormal response is a persistent clonic contraction of the posterior muscles of the leg.

Several similar abnormal flexion reflexes may be seen in the upper extremity. Those finger reflexes are common in the healthy person, and they do not have the importance of an abnormal plantar response. Hoffman's sign is indicative of increased reflex activity [22]. With the patient's wrist and fingers relaxed, his wrist is held in horizontal pronation. Two techniques are common: (1) light snapping of the nail of the middle finger or (2) flexing the distal phalanx of the middle finger over one of the examiner's fingers and quickly releasing the phalanx. The abnormal response is flexion of the fingers and thumb. Trömner's sign is elicited by tapping the patient's middle or index finger on the palmar surface. The abnormal re-

sponse is flexion of all five fingers. The grasp reflex is elicited by placing something in the patient's hand. The abnormal response is a strong grasp.

Three additional reflexes of the face are commonly noted. The sucking reflex is elicited by oral stimuli. The abnormal response is sucking or pursing of the lips; it is indicative of cerebral dysfunction. The snout reflex is elicited by tapping the middle of the mandible or maxilla. The abnormal response is a rooting movement; it is indicative of cerebral dysfunction. The jaw reflex is elicited by tapping the partially open mandible. The abnormal response is a very brisk upward movement of the jaw.

RECORDING

The response elicited after testing the reflex is graded and recorded from 0 to 4+; 0 = absent; tr = trace; 1+ = hypoactive; 2+ = normal; 3+ = hyperactive; and 4+ = sustained clonus.

Several different methods may be used for recording the results of testing the reflexes. If the data base does not include a printed method, the examiner may select the method she prefers. Three different examples commonly accepted for recording the reflexes are shown below.

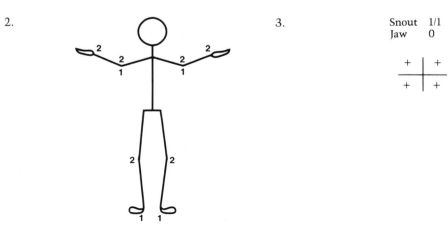

1.

	Bi	Tri	F	K	A	Plantar	Abdomen	Snout	Grasp	Jaw	Suck
R											
L											

2.

3.

Snout   1/1
Jaw   0

Diagnostic Studies

What diagnostic studies the neurologist or neurosurgeon chooses depends on the individual patient's pathophysiology. The studies most commonly ordered are skull and spinal films, lumbar puncture, angiography, brain scanning, electroencephalography, and computerized axial tomography (see Chap. 30).

Skull films are ordered as a screening procedure. In patients with trauma, the skull fracture may be outlined or a foreign body may be visualized. If the pineal gland is calcified, a shift in its position may indicate the side of the intracranial mass. Cervical, dorsal and/or lumbosacral spinal films are ordered whenever a disease process in the particular area is suspected.

The lumbar puncture is particularly valuable in patients with suspected subarachnoid hemorrhage or meningitis. It is sometimes deferred when the patient has increased intracranial pressure because of the possibility of uncal or cerebellar herniation. Normally, the spinal fluid pressure varies from 70 to 200 mm H_2O. Pressures over 200 mm H_2O are considered elevated, and they result from tumors, abscesses, cysts, subdural hematoma, infection, cerebral hemorrhage or thrombosis, subarachnoid hemorrhage, hydrocephalus, and pseudotumor cerebri. Pressures below 70 mm H_2O are considered decreased, and they result from inadequate technique, spinal cord tumor, dehydration, and dislocated vertebrae. Under normal circumstances, the cerebrospinal fluid is colorless and has a low blood cell count. A white blood cell count of more than six cells and any red blood cells are considered abnormal. The normal protein content is 15 to 45 mg/100 ml. Protein electrophoretic rather than colloidal gold reaction studies may be ordered to evaluate the patient for inflammatory disease, such as multiple sclerosis. The glucose content is 50 to 75 mg/100 ml, and it is normally 20 mg/100 ml less than that found in the blood.

Cerebral angiography is one of the most useful neurodiagnostic techniques available for the assessment of structural abnormalities, abnormal positioning of blood vessels, and alterations in flow patterns. Catheterization of the carotid, brachial, or femoral arteries enables the contrast material to be injected directly into the carotid or vertebral arteries or indirectly into the brachial vessels or aortic arch. Serial evaluation in the lateral and anteroposterior planes is then possible as the contrast material progresses through the arteries, capillaries, and veins [5]. The films are read by the neurologist or neurosurgeon and radiologist for size and placement, changes in the position of vessels, abnormal proliferation of vessels, and direction and velocity of blood flow. Angiography has replaced air studies as the procedure of choice in most situations.

Radioisotope brain scanning is used to identify abnormal areas of isotope concentration and to help in the diagnosis of abscesses, cerebral infarctions, subdural hematomas, and, especially, neoplasms.

Electroencephalography is used in the diagnosis of seizure disorders, focal and generalized encephalopathies, and brain death. The electrical activity of the brain is amplified, transmitted, and recorded by means of electrodes applied to the scalp. The waveform tracings are analyzed and interpreted by the neurologist according to the frequency, amplitude, form, and distribution of the wave activity.

References

1. Alpers, J., and Mancall, E. *Essentials of the Neurological Examination.* Philadelphia: Davis, 1971.
2. Baker, A. B. *An Outline of Applied Neurology.* Dubuque, Iowa: Kendal/Hunt, 1970.
3. Bates, B. *Guide to Physical Examination.* Philadelphia: Lippincott, 1974.
4. Bentley, W., Daly, D., and Vollmer, V. *Evaluation of the Comatose Patient.* Dallas: The University of Texas Health Science Center at Dallas, 1975.
5. Bickerstaff, E. R. *Neurological Examination in Clinical Practice.* Oxford: Blackwell, 1973.
6. Buckingham, W. B., Sparberg, M., and Brandfonbrener, M. *A Primer of Clinical Diagnosis.* Hagerstown, Md.: Harper & Row, 1971.
7. Chusid, J. G. *Correlative Neuroanatomy and Functional Neurology.* Los Altos, Calif.: Lange, 1973.
8. DeGowin, E. L., and DeGowin, R. L. *Bedside Diagnostic Examination* (2nd ed.). New York: Macmillan, 1969.
9. DeJong, R., Sahs, A. L., Aldrich, C. Knight, et al. *Essentials of the Neurological Examination.* Philadelphia: Smith, Kline & French Laboratories, 1968.
10. Erickson, R. Cranial check: A basic neurological check. *Nurs. '74,* 4:67, 1974.
11. Fisher, C. M. Some neuro-opthalmological observations. *J. Neurol. Neurosurg. Psychiatry* 30:383, 1967.
12. Fowkes, W. C., and Hunn, V. K. *Clinical Assessment for the Nurse Practitioner.* St. Louis: Mosby, 1973.
13. Gordan, D. M. *The Fundamentals of Ophthalmoscopy.* Kalamazoo, Mich.: The Upjohn Co., 1971.
14. Hochstein, E., and Rubin, A. L. *Physical Diagnosis.* New York: McGraw-Hill, 1964.
15. Jimm, L. R. Nursing assessment of patients for increased intracranial pressure. *J. Neurol. Nurs.* 6:27, 1974.

16. Judge, R. D., and Zuidema, G. *Physical Diagnosis: A Physiological Approach to Clinical Medicine.* Boston: Little, Brown, 1963.
17. Morgan, W. L., and Engel, G. *The Clinical Approach to the Patient.* Philadelphia: Saunders, 1969.
18. Plum, F., and Posner, J. B. *Diagnosis of Stupor and Coma.* Philadelphia: Davis, 1972.
19. Prior, J. A., and Silberstein, J. S. *Physical Diagnosis: The History and Examination of the Patient.* St. Louis: Mosby, 1973.
20. Sherman, J. L., and Fields, S. K. *Guide to Patient Evaluation.* Flushing, N.Y.: Medical Examination Publishing Co., 1974.
21. Sabin, T. D. The differential diagnosis of coma. *N. Engl. J. Med.* 290:1062, 1974.
22. Simpson, J. F., and Magee, K. R. *Clinical Evaluation of the Nervous System.* Boston: Little, Brown, 1973.
23. Raman, P. T., Reddy, P. R., and Sarasvaniv, R. Orbicularis oculi reflex and facial muscle electromyography: Pre- and post-operative evaluation of posterior fossa lesions. *J. Neurosurg.* 44:550, 1976.
24. Ross, E. Disorders of Higher Cortical Functions In Sanford, J. (ed.), *The Science and Practice of Clinical Medicine.* New York: Grune & Stratton, 1977.
25. Van Allen, M. W. *Pictorial Manual of Neurologic Tests.* Chicago: Year Book, 1969.

Abdominal Assessment

Barbara Montgomery Dossey

This chapter discusses techniques for the examination of the abdominal and renal system that is done by the nurse in the critical care setting. (Examination of the reproductive system and lower gastrointestinal system is not discussed.)

Location of the Abdominal Organs

To permit accurate description of the abdomen, the abdomen is divided anteriorly by imaginary lines into quadrants. A horizontal line passes through the umbilicus, and a vertical line extends from the ziphoid process to the symphysis pubis (Fig. 12-1A).

The abdomen is sometimes divided into nine sections (Fig. 12-1B). Two imaginary horizontal parallel lines cross at the lower costal margin border and the anterior superior spine of the iliac bones. Two vertical lines drop from the midclavicular lines to the approximate borders of the abdominal muscle.

Normally, the only areas that are palpable in the abdomen are the edge of the liver at the right costal margin, the lower pole of the right kidney (in a thin person), and the sigmoid colon in the left lower quadrant. The abdominal aorta is papable in some people, especially women. If the patient's bladder is full, it may be palpable in the lower midline area.

The renal system comprises the kidneys, the ureters, the urinary bladder, and the external male

12

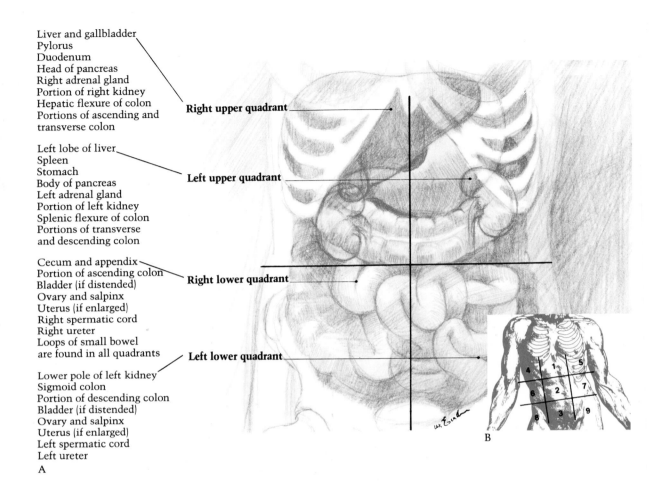

Liver and gallbladder
Pylorus
Duodenum
Head of pancreas
Right adrenal gland
Portion of right kidney
Hepatic flexure of colon
Portions of ascending and
transverse colon

Right upper quadrant

Left lobe of liver
Spleen
Stomach
Body of pancreas
Left adrenal gland
Portion of left kidney
Splenic flexure of colon
Portions of transverse
and descending colon

Left upper quadrant

Cecum and appendix
Portion of ascending colon
Bladder (if distended)
Ovary and salpinx
Uterus (if enlarged)
Right spermatic cord
Right ureter
Loops of small bowel
are found in all quadrants

Right lower quadrant

Lower pole of left kidney
Sigmoid colon
Portion of descending colon
Bladder (if distended)
Ovary and salpinx
Uterus (if enlarged)
Left spermatic cord
Left ureter

Left lower quadrant

A

B

genitalia. Except for the male genitalia, those organs are relatively inaccessible for palpation. Physical complaints and the medical history often provide the first clues to problems occurring in the abdomen or kidneys. Laboratory tests and special radiological studies are necessary to confirm the diagnosis.

Figure 12-1
A. The four regions of the abdomen identified are the right upper quadrant, left upper quadrant, right lower quadrant, and left lower quadrant. B. The nine areas of the abdomen are the (1) epigastric, (2) umbilical, (3) pubic, (4), (5) right and left hypochondriac, (6), (7) right and left lumbar, and (8), (9) right and left inguinal areas.

History of Present Illness

In regard to a patient's abdominal complaints, the nurse should ask the patient to describe the character, duration, frequency, location, and distribution of his discomfort in relation to food, drugs, activity, and defecation [4]. Abdominal pain is referred or perceived in different areas. Information about constipation, diarrhea, frequency of bowel movements, and

the use of enemas and laxatives must be obtained. The nurse should ask the patient about any problems with swallowing, nausea, and vomiting, as well as about the types of food and drinks (including alcoholic drinks) he consumes and any changes in his eating and drinking habits. Special attention should be given to complaints of weight loss.

Gastrointestinal symptoms frequently accompany genitourinary complaints. The right kidney lies in the

Posterior view

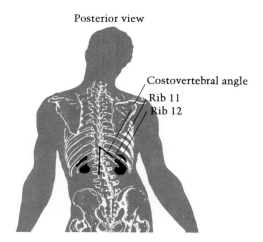

Costovertebral angle
Rib 11
Rib 12

Figure 12-2
Renal pain can be elicited in the area of the costovertebral angle formed by the vertebral column and the rib cage.

right quadrant with the liver, gallbladder, duodenum, and hepatic flexure of the colon. The left kidney lies in the left quadrant with the stomach, spleen, pancreas, and splenic flexure of the colon. Because those organs have a common autonomic sensory innervation, a patient with renal disease may present with gastrointestinal symptoms. Since the kidneys are surrounded by the peritoneum, inflammation of the kidneys frequently produces an irritation of the peritoneum. If it does, rebound tenderness and muscle rigidity mimicking peritonitis are present.

Most renal conditions are painless because distention of the renal capsule progresses slowly. Renal pain is usually a constant, dull ache in the costovertebral angle (Fig. 12-2). Ureteral pain due to spasm of smooth muscle and hyperperistalsis can be observed; or the patient may tell about expelling a foreign object (a kidney stone). Patients may complain of severe back pain—intermittent pain radiating from the midback to the lower anterior abdomen. Women may complain of pain in the vulva, whereas men may complain of pain in the testicles and scrotum. Overdistention of the bladder can cause severe suprapubic pain. When the examiner feels a suprapubic bulge, he suspects an overdistended bladder due to acute urinary retention.

Prostate pain is rare. Usually men complain of a feeling of fullness or discomfort in the perineal or rectal area. Discomfort from cystitis and referred pain to the lumbosacral area are not uncommon. Pain in the

testicles caused by trauma or infection is severe. Spermatic cord involvement usually causes referred lower abdominal pain. Infection involving the epididymis causes pain in the lower abdomen, groin, and, sometimes, the adjacent testicle. The pain can mimic that of a ureteral stone or appendicitis. Leg and back pain can be the result of more severe problems. The nurse should ask the patient about the quantity, quality, setting, and course of any renal pain.

Complaints of dysuria must be investigated. A burning sensation on urination usually indicates some kind of irritation. Spasm of the bladder and anal sphincter associated with pain and a desire to evacuate the bladder and bowel is referred to as tenesmus. Frequency of urination is usually a result of an inflamed mucosa, a decreased bladder capacity, or the loss of bladder elasticity. Nocturia (excessive urination that interrupts sleep) is common in obstructive conditions and renal diseases in which there is a loss of parenchymal concentrating power.

Patients may describe abnormalities that are characteristic of acute or chronic obstruction of the neck of the bladder or the prostate. Urinary hesitancy (a delay in initiating a urinary stream) and/or an increased physical effort in starting the flow of urine is the most common. Loss of force and caliber of the urinary stream are not the only phenomena associated with increased muscular effort. Terminal dribbling refers to the urine continuing to drip in spite of muscular effort to stop it. Abrupt interruption of the urinary flow can occur, and it may often be accompanied by suprapubic pain.

The nurse should investigate any complaints of incontinence. With stress incontinence, a patient urinates involuntarily during physical exertion. With urgency incontinence, urination occurs involuntarily after the patient experiences an urge to void. With true incontinence, urination occurs periodically without warning. In patients with renal disease, complaints of itching, nausea and vomiting, and changes in sensorium usually indicate advanced renal disease.

Nurses in the acute care setting must be aware of any abnormalities in urine volume. The amount of urine voided, as well as the amount of fluids lost through drainage and through daily insensible loss, must be compared to intake of fluids. Oliguria is present when a patient voids less than 400 ml per day. Anuria, the absence of urine, indicates a malfunction of the kidneys or a bilateral ureteral obstruction. Both phenomena are critically important and warrant immediate medical attention.

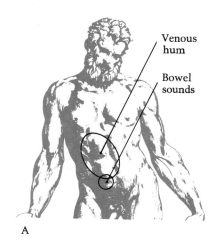

A

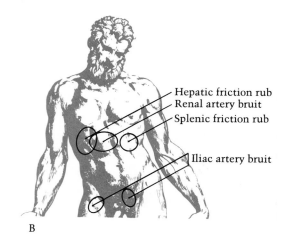

B

Systematic Assessment of the Abdomen

The physical examination of the abdomen should proceed in a systematic manner from quadrant to quadrant and in the sequence of inspection–auscultation–percussion–palpation. Auscultation is performed before percussion and palpation since percussion and palpation are apt to alter the frequency of bowel sounds [1].

Inspection

While inspecting the patient's abdomen, the nurse can put the patient at ease by talking with him and making him as comfortable as possible. While talking to the patient, the nurse should observe his facial expression and note any signs of anxiety, tension, or pain. The general inspection is best done from the patient's right side. It should include observation of the abdominal surface, striae, old or new scars, rashes, lesions, or dilated veins. Size, shape, contour, and symmetry should be noted. Peristalsis can be observed by watching the abdomen. Sometimes it may be several minutes before peristalsis can be seen.

Auscultation

Auscultation of the abdomen is performed in a systematic manner, with the examiner moving from quadrant to quadrant. The diaphragm of the stethoscope is kept in place long enough to determine the frequency, quality, and pitch of bowel sounds (Fig.

Figure 12-3

Abdominal auscultation. A. Bowel sounds are best heard over the area of the small circle. Listen for at least 1 to 2 minutes to determine whether they are present or absent. The venous hum may be heard over the area of the large circle. The venous hum is a systolic bruit heard sometimes over the patient with a cirrhotic liver; it is due to an increased flow through the portal and the systemic venous collaterals. B. The systolic bruit heard in the epigastrium or anterior lumbar region may be a sign of renal artery stenosis. The systolic bruit heard over the iliac region may be a sign of stenosis of the iliofemoral artery. Peritoneal friction rubs can be heard over the spleen in splenic infarction and over the liver in liver tumor.

12-3A). Most intestinal sounds originate in the small bowel; they are high-pitched and gurgling. The frequency of bowel sounds varies with meals. After listening to bowel sounds, the examiner should listen for bruits, which are vascular sounds (Fig. 12-3B). The examiner should listen in the midepigastrium for bruits that indicate stenosis of the renal arteries and in the iliac region for bruits that indicate stenosis of the iliofemoral artery. If splenic infarction or liver tumor is suspected, the examiner should listen over the spleen and liver for peritoneal friction rubs.

Percussion

Percussion is done to determine the degree of resonance, tympany, and dullness. Tympany usually is more dominant. The patient should be observed at all times for any tenderness or pain. Percussion of the

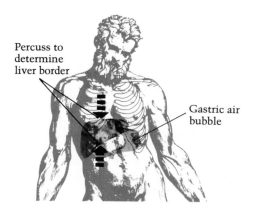

Percuss to determine liver border

Gastric air bubble

Figure 12-4
Percussion of the liver. A gross estimate of the liver size can be made by identification of the borders of the liver. The dark arrows show percussion from the level of the umbilicus upward and from lung resonance downward until liver dullness is elicited. The normal heights are 6 to 12 cm in the right midclavicular line and 4 to 8 cm in the midsternal line. Percussion of the stomach. The tympany sound of the gastric air bubble is in the left lower anterior rib cage.

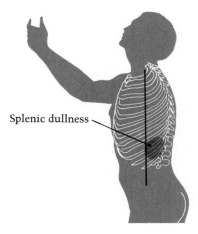

Splenic dullness

Figure 12-5
Percussion of the spleen. Splenic dullness can be elicited by percussion posterior to the left midaxillary line near the tenth rib.

liver provides only a good estimate of liver size [3, 8]. To percuss the liver, the examiner starts in the right midclavicular line below the umbilicus and percusses upward toward the liver (Fig. 12-4). The lower border of the liver can be found in the midclavicular line. Next the examiner percusses downward from lung resonance in the right midclavicular line until dullness is heard. The distance from the border of upper dullness and lower dullness indicates the height of the liver. Normal liver heights are 6 to 12 cm in the right midclavicular line and 4 to 8 cm in the midsternal line. Borders of liver dullness can be obscured by gas in the colon, by lung consolidation, or by right pleural effusion.

The stomach is percussed on the left side in the area of the left lower anterior rib cage (Fig. 12-4). The examiner can hear the tympany of a gastric air bubble. If abdominal distention is obvious and if the size of the gastric air bubble is increased, gastric dilatation is suspected.

The spleen is more difficult to percuss [2]. In the area of the left tenth rib posterior to the midaxillary line, a small oval area may be identified (Fig. 12-5). If it cannot be identified, the patient should take a deep breath, and the examiner should percuss in the lowest intercostal space in the left anterior axillary line. That area is usually tympanic.

Palpation

Both light palpation and deep palpation are done in the abdominal examination to give the examiner information about abdominal tenderness, muscular resistance, and masses. If the patient is sensitive to palpation and cannot relax, the examiner can have the patient place his own hand on his abdomen under the examiner's hand. Then as the patient relaxes, his hand can be moved to the side. Light palpation helps to relax and reassure the patient. In a light, gentle, rotating motion, the examiner places his fingertips together and palpates with his fingertips. Areas of tenderness, any masses, and organs are identified. Deep palpation is usually needed to detect abdominal masses and organs. If masses are palpated, their shape, size, consistency, mobility, tenderness, and pulsation are determined and recorded. It is possible to distinguish an abdominal wall mass from an abdominal cavity mass. A mass in the wall remains palpable when the patient tightens his abdominal muscles, whereas a mass in the abdominal cavity is obscured when the patient tightens his abdominal muscles.

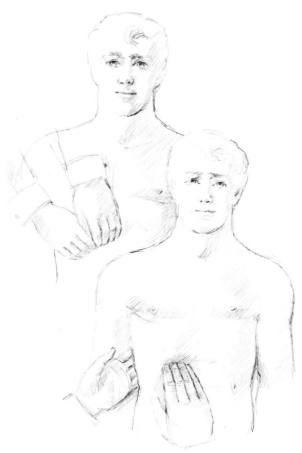

Figure 12-6
Palpation of the liver: two methods.

The liver is palpated by having the patient breathe with his abdominal muscles (Fig. 12-6). By placing his examining hand lateral to the rectus muscle, with the fingers pointing to the patient's head, the examiner should try to feel the liver as it comes down to meet his fingertips.

At the peak of inspiration, it may be necessary to release the pressure of the right hand and move up a little toward the costal margin. The edge of a normal liver is a firm, regular ridge with a smooth surface. If the liver is felt, its distance below the costal margin is recorded in centimeters. The liver may also be palpated by the hooking technique. (Fig. 12-6). The examiner should stand to the right of the patient and face the patient's feet. Next the examiner places both

hands side by side on the patient's right abdomen below the border of liver dullness. As the examiner asks the patient to take a deep breath, the examiner presses in with his fingers and up toward the costal margin.

If palpable, the spleen is felt by palpation in the left upper quadrant. The examiner remains on the right side of the patient and reaches across the abdomen with both hands. The examiner's right hand is placed below the left costal margin. His left hand is placed around the patient and used to press upward on the lower left rib cage for support. At this point, the right fingertips are pressed in toward the area of the spleen. An enlarged spleen is fragile, and it should only be percussed or palpated very gently by an experienced examiner.

Systematic Assessment of the Renal System

The examining techniques that are used for the renal system are inspection, palpation, percussion, and auscultation. (The discussion of auscultation of the abdomen lists some specifics that are appropriate to auscultation of the renal system.)

Inspection

With inspection, the examiner looks for any raised area, which may indicate a kidney mass. The ureters are not accessible for direct examination. The urinary bladder is inspected in the suprapubic area for any evidence of bulging. If urinary retention is present, the examiner can determine the level of the bladder by percussing and listening for a dull fluid sound. The outline of a distended bladder can be determined by palpation. The examiner will elicit pain if distention is present.

Palpation

The examiner palpates the kidneys by placing the fingertips of his upper hand at the costal margin in the midclavicular line and his lower hand posteriorly at the costovertebral angle (Fig. 12-7). At this point, the patient, who is supine, is instructed to take a deep breath. The examiner exerts firm upward pressure on the patient's right upper quadrant, with his upper

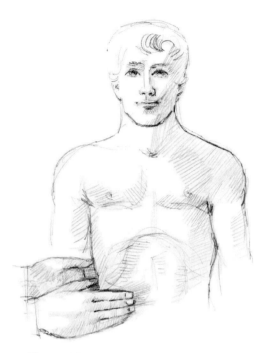

Figure 12-7
Palpation of the kidney.

Special Studies

A complete assessment requires many specific studies of the gastrointestinal and renal systems. It is of utmost importance that the nurse give the patient information about the tests. The patient whose anxiety has been relieved by the nurse's show of concern and by the information she has given him will be less anxious and better able to cooperate.

Following a thorough history taking and complete physical examination by the physician, all the data are gathered and tests are ordered that can support or provide the medical diagnosis [5].

The tests that are frequently done for gastrointestinal diagnosis are complete blood count, urinalysis, and examination of stool specimen. The stool specimen is examined by gross inspection and in specific laboratory and microscopic studies as indicated.

X-Ray Examination of Gastrointestinal System

Radiographic examination of the patient includes a gastrointestinal series to visualize the stomach and intestinal tract. Barium enema examination reveals information about the colon; barium double-contrast enema examination examines the colonic mucosa.

Fluoroscopy

Fluoroscopic examination shows shadows of all the organs from the esophagus to the anus. Gastric contents obtained via Levin drainage may be examined for gastric acidity. Or a fiberoptic gastroscope may be used for a biopsy study and photographs of any gastric lesions. Anoscopic, proctoscopic, and sigmoidoscopic examinations permit direct observation of the mucosa lining the colon [7]. Because of risks that are involved with those studies, the nurse must obtain the patient's signed consent for diagnostic procedures of the abdomen and renal system.

hand exerting slightly more pressure above than below. He may feel the right kidney. If the right kidney is palpable, the size, contour, and degree of tenderness should be discussed. The same maneuver is repeated for palpation of the left kidney. A normal left kidney is rarely palpable.

Percussion

While examining the patient's back, the examiner should check for kidney tenderness. He should place the palm of his left hand over each costovertebral angle and strike it with the ulnar surface of his right fist.

Auscultation

The examiner should auscultate in the costovertebral angles posteriorly and listen in the upper quadrants anteriorly for bruits. If bruits are present, they should be investigated further via diagnostic procedures.

Urinalysis

Special studies that are done for patients with renal problems involve frequent urinalysis. Urine is inspected for evidence of blood (hematuria), for cloudiness (due to phosphate constituents precipitated in an alkaline medium), leukocytes (pyuria), feces (fecaluria), red blood cells, and casts. The specific gravity of urine is checked. A diseased kidney is unable to dilute or concentrate urine normally. Urine is excreted with solute concentration equivalent to that of plasma. The pH of urine is measured for alkalinity or acidity. Urine is usually acidic, and its acidity is affected by food intake. Consistently alkaline urine is abnormal; it can result from an alkaline-producing organism such as *Proteus*, which causes a urinary tract infection; alkalinity may also indicate that the kidneys are unable to acidify urine. Urine is examined for the presence of protein, most commonly albumin. The presence of protein in the urine usually indicates an abnormality.

Hematology and Blood Chemistries

Hematological and electrolyte studies are routinely done. Other laboratory data that are significant in renal disease are the levels of serum calcium, creatinine, blood urea nitrogen (BUN), phosphorus, uric acid, and total protein.

Abnormalities in serum calcium levels may cause abnormalities in excretion. Since the urinary creatinine level is constant and is relative to a person's total body mass, determination of the creatinine level is a useful test to measure kidney function [5]. When renal function is reduced, the creatinine level is elevated. Urea, a by-product of protein, is filtered by the glomerulus and reabsorbed in the renal tubule. The BUN level rises in conditions that reduce renal function, such as acute and chronic renal failure, chronic glomerulonephritis, chronic pyelonephritis, nephrosclerosis, and obstructive uropathy. In conditions characterized by decreased renal perfusion, such as shock or congestive heart failure, the BUN level may rise.

Elevated serum phosphate and serum uric acid levels are observed in renal insufficiency. When serum uric acid and the total body pool of uric acid increases, deposition of uric acid may occur in the kidney and renal collecting system. Uric acid stones, which can disturb kidney function, are formed.

Total serum protein comprises albumin and globulin. Serum proteins have many functions, including normal clotting and distribution of water in the body due to their osmotic activity. When serum protein levels are reduced, the albumin fraction is most often affected by excessive loss from the kidney. Hypoalbuminemia is seen in the nephrotic syndrome.

X-Ray Examination and Special Studies of Renal System

If necessary, cystoscopic study is done for direct visualization of renal structures. Plain abdominal films are obtained when some abnormality of the urinary tract is suspected. Stones in the urinary tract can be identified when a patient has renal colic. Intravenous pyelograms, also referred to as excretory urograms, may be ordered with urinary tract abnormalities, such as hematuria, recurrent urinary tract infection, and pain of renal colic, and to investigate abdominal mass or to evaluate hypertension. Renal arteriography is done to look specifically at the circulation of the kidneys and for any cysts, tumors, or other renal diseases. Other special techniques can be done as indicated to study structures adjacent to or related to the urinary tract.

In patients who require both abdominal and renal contrast films, the intravenous pyelogram and cholecystogram are done before the barium studies. When both barium enema studies and upper gastrointestinal tract studies are to be done, the barium enema study is done before the upper gastrointestinal tract study, because barium from that study may be retained in the colon for a long period and may thus delay the barium enema test.

Renal Biopsy

A renal biopsy study is sometimes necessary to make a diagnosis in a patient with known or suspected renal disease. It is most helpful in any renal disease when the disease process is distributed evenly throughout the kidney tissue, affecting the glomeruli specifically and causing hematuria and proteinuria. Some examples of those diseases are the nephrotic syndrome and any form of glomerulonephritis. Other disease processes in which renal biopsy study may be helpful are the collagen diseases, unexplained acute oliguric renal failure, inflammatory and infectious diseases of the kidney, following healing in reversible conditions, determining early stages of renal disease that are not explained by other diagnostic studies. A renal biopsy study should be done only by an experienced physician. A dangerous invasive procedure, it is performed only after comprehensive evaluation of the patient. The patient's signed consent must be obtained. The most common complications are bleeding and hematuria, and the nurse must understand what nursing care is to follow the procedure. Firm pressure is applied to the biopsy site immediately, followed by application of a pressure dressing. The patient must remain prone for 30 minutes and then flat for one hour; bed rest should follow for 24 hours. The patient's condition is assessed; his vital signs are taken, and any patient complaint must be investigated, especially in regard to pain at the biopsy site or to frequent or urgent urination.

References

1. Bates, B.   *A Guide to Physical Examination* (2nd ed.). Philadelphia: Lippincott, 1979.

2. Castell, D. O.   The spleen percussion sign. A useful diagnostic technique. *Ann. Intern. Med.* 67:1265, 1967.

3. Castell, D. O., O'Brien, K. D., Muench, H., et al.   Estimation of liver size by percussion in normal individuals. *Ann. Intern. Med.* 70:1183, 1969.

4. Cope, Z.   *The Early Diagnosis of the Acute Abdomen* (14th ed.). London: Oxford University Press, 1972.

5. DeGowin, E. L., and DeGowin, R. L.   *Bedside Diagnostic Examination* (3rd ed.). London: Macmillan, 1976.

6. Guyton, A. C.   *Textbook of Medical Physiology* (5th ed.). Philadelphia: Saunders, 1976.

7. Judge, R. D., and Zuidema, G. D.   *Physical Diagnosis: The History and Examination of the Patient* (3rd ed.). St. Louis: Mosby, 1973.

8. Sullivan, S., Krasner, N., and Williams, R.   The clinical estimation of liver size; a comparison of techniques and an analysis of the source of error. *Br. Med. J.* 2:1042, 1976.

IV. Psychosocial Aspects of Nursing the Critically Ill Adult

For the critical care nurse to know and feel that patient experiences are *always,* in some measure, nurse experiences is to also understand the opposite: nurse experiences are always patient experiences.

When this is keenly felt, the critical care nurse knows that she can transmit more to the patient than mere drugs and bed baths.

Words, glances, touches become powerful tools of therapy.

As we live, we are transmitters of life.
And when we fail to transmit life, life fails to flow
   through us.

And if, as we work, we can transmit life into our work,
life, still more life, rushes into us to compensate, to
be ready and we ripple with life through the days.

Give, and it shall be given unto you
is still the truth about life.
But giving life is not so easy.
It doesn't mean handing it out to some mean fool, or letting the living dead eat you up.
It means kindling the life-quality where it was not,
even if it's only in the whiteness of a washed pocket-
   handkerchief.

D. H. Lawrence
"We Are Transmitters"

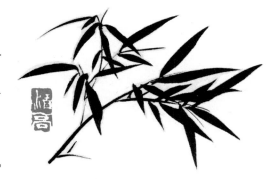

Psychosocial Aspects

Carolyn Bascom Bilodeau

Patients with myocardial infarction, burns, respiratory distress, and mitral valve disease have been cared for by nurses for many years. Yet, the nursing care of those and other critically ill adults has dramatically changed within the past few years. With the development of electronic monitoring equipment, cardiopulmonary resuscitative techniques, drugs to prevent and control dysrhythmias and hypotension, devices to assist and maintain ventilation, and specialized medical and surgical techniques, the era of critical care nursing as we know it today was born.

Although critical care nursing can be practiced wherever patients are critically ill, the bulk of the care is given to hospitalized patients in specialized intensive or critical care units. Nurses in those units, responding to the recent technological, pharmacological, medical, and surgical developments, have heightened their skills, increased their knowledge, and gained the expertise necessary to give specialized personalized care to the critically ill.

Increasing attention has also been paid in recent years to investigating, describing, and understanding the psychological aspects of the critical care setting; namely, factors that influence or contribute to the development, onset, or exacerbation of illness; factors that affect the seeking of medical attention; and the psychological responses of patients, families, and staff to illness, treatments, surgery, environment, and death [1–5, 7, 9–12, 14–23, 25–30, 32–37, 39–40,

42–44, 46–58, 60, 62–63, 66–74]. The nurse's heightened awareness of those aspects, her greater acceptance of their importance in the total management of the critically ill patient, and her planning and implementation of nursing intervention that considers those aspects can greatly enhance the quality of patient care [70].

This chapter focuses on (1) the patient and his responses to illness, (2) the factors that affect his responses, and (3) suggestions for nursing intervention. The psychological impact of illness on family and nursing staff is discussed briefly.

Objective

The nurse caring for a critically ill adult should be able to assess the psychological impact of the illness on the patient, his family, and the staff and employ appropriate nursing measures to lessen anxiety and enhance comfort.

Achieving the Objective

To achieve the objective, the nurse should be able to:

1. Identify seven of the most common mechanisms used by patients in critical care units to allay anxiety.
2. Determine the parameters used to assess the patient's mental status.
3. Outline factors that affect the patient's feeling responses and coping mechanisms.
4. Suggest nursing interventions that help the patient cope with denial, anxiety, depression, sexual aggression, suspicion, delirium, communication disability, and approaching death.
5. Identify common stress-related behaviors in critical care nurses.

How to Proceed

To develop an approach to psychosocial aspects, the nurse should:

1. Study the material and references that follow.
2. Evaluate each example in the chapter and look at each situation from the patient's point of view.
3. Role play interactions that are particularly difficult for her.

4. Learn to listen attentively, to determine what the patient is really saying, and to offer her interpretation for validation.
5. Identify ways family members can become members of the critical care team.
6. Compare her stress-related behaviors with those of her colleagues.

Responses to Illness

When we think of the critically ill adult, various patients come to mind. Although those patients may differ in regard to preparation for the critical illness, suddenness of onset of the illness, number of presenting problems, and the nature of the illness, they all have in common the here-and-now experience of being acutely ill. The presence of illness alters the individual's perception of his state of well-being, his physical integrity, and his ability to be independent and self-sufficient. Attached to equipment, filled with tubes, covered with dressings; experiencing nausea, pain, or loss of sensation; having problems with breathing, swallowing, or moving; he is now dependent on others to meet most of his needs. His altered perception of himself leads to a loss of self-esteem; the person no longer sees himself as he would like to be. Accompanying the loss of self-esteem are feelings of sadness over what has been lost or changed and feelings of anxiety over the uncertainty of the future.

Patients face the task of coping with their feelings not only about the illness or accident but also about being in a critical care unit. Admittance to a critical care unit marks a disruption in one's normal routine. Patients are no longer in familiar surroundings. Instead they see, hear, and smell unaccustomed sights, sounds, and odors. Interactions with family, friends, and employers have been temporarily suspended; patients do not know whether, when, or how they can resume any of their former activities and relationships.

It is no wonder, then, that patients in a critical care setting may feel sad, anxious, angry, frightened, dependent, frustrated, or helpless. Although some patients express those feelings directly through words, many others communicate those feelings only indirectly through words or behavior. Most patients use conscious or unconscious mechanisms of some kind to help allay anxiety [13]. Some of the ones more commonly seen in the critical care setting are:

1. Displacement: the unconscious transfer of feelings from one object, situation, or idea to another seen

as more acceptable (e.g., "You don't know how to change burn dressings; all of you are so darned incompetent, you make me sick").

2. Projection: the unconscious attribution of one's own ideas or impulses (usually unacceptable ones) to another (e.g., "The doctors don't think I'm going to pull through; in fact, none of you do").

3. Suppression: the conscious and deliberate putting out of one's mind thoughts that can be anxiety producing (e.g., "I don't want to talk about the accident right now. I would get too upset").

4. Repression: the involuntary blocking of painful thoughts or memories from consciousness (e.g., "I don't remember being in the fire").

5. Rationalization: the justification of behavior or decisions that are not necessarily rational or logical (e.g., the patient with severe burns who says, "I pulled off the dressings because they were not put on straight").

6. Regression: the process of returning to an earlier level of emotional development or adaptation (e.g., the previously independent patient who becomes childlike, clinging, dependent, and helpless following a tracheostomy).

7. Denial: the "conscious or unconscious repudiation of all or a portion of the total available meaning of an illness in order to allay anxiety and to minimize emotional stress" [33] (e.g., "Who me?—A heart attack? Ha, you've got the wrong man, Doc.").

Assessment of Patient's Responses

One tool the nurse in the critical care setting can use to help her identify the patient's feelings and responses to illness is the mental status evaluation. The evaluation consists of a systematic observation of the patient's behavior so that the observable aspects of a patient's psychological functioning can be objectively determined and recorded [45]. The following paragraphs discuss the components of the mental status evaluation.

General Appearance and Attitude

In a critical care setting, the nurse cannot accurately assess the patient's grooming, dress, posture, and gait. But she can observe the patient's

1. Facial expression (e.g., wide-eyed, tense, sad, no expression).

2. Unique mannerisms (e.g., eye rolling, fist clenching, sighing, pulling at hair).

3. Motor behavior (e.g., movements of entire body or parts of the body, fidgeting, turning, picking, thrashing).

4. Attitude toward the nurse (e.g., smiles, turns toward or from the nurse, avoids eye contact, makes no response).

5. Response to nursing care (e.g., attempts to keep the nurse longer, is not satisfied, is grateful, tries to prevent or interfere with care).

Speech Activity

1. Presence or absence of verbal communication

2. Rate of speech (e.g., rapid, slow, lack of pauses)

3. Tone (e.g., high pitched, shrill, flat, barely audible, deep)

4. Quality of response (e.g., repetitive statements, monosyllabic answers, avoidance of certain subjects)

5. Unique characteristics (e.g., pressure of speech, loosening of associations, slurring and stuttering, peculiar use of words, irrelevance)

Affective Behavior

1. Mood (e.g., depressed, elated, apathetic, anxious, hostile, spontaneous, negativistic, cheerful, labile, irritable)

2. Methods used to deal with or control emotions (e.g., crying, throwing objects, complaining, swearing, shouting, remaining silent, talking, joking, rationalizing, displacing or projecting feelings, sexually acting out, denying concern, withdrawing, regressing)

3. Manifest needs (e.g., need for security, need to be cared for, need to be submissive)

4. Patient's evaluation or description of mood or feelings. It is extremely important to record the patient's words exactly so that all who care for him will be aware of his feeling state.

Thought Content

1. Describe the patient's spontaneous thought.

2. Observe the patient for:
   A. Hallucinations (imaginary sense perceptions), such as hearing voices or seeing bugs.

B. Delusions (false, fixed beliefs that cannot be changed by logic) such as, "You are putting poison into that IV."
C. Ideas of reference (interpretation of incidents incorrectly as having direct reference to self), such as a patient who hears staff members talking about someone who is dying assuming that they are referring to him.
D. Suicide ideation, such as when a patient states, "I'm not going to take this any longer; I'd rather be dead."
E. Phobias, obsessions, grandiose ideas.
F. Psychotic ideation.

Intellectual Functioning

1. Orientation to person, place, time
2. Memory for recent and remote past, as well as for immediate recall of what was just discussed
3. Insight concerning current situation
4. Judgment (tested by asking a question such as, "What would you do if you found an addressed, stamped letter on the sidewalk?")
5. Abstract thinking (tested by asking patient to interpret proverbs)
6. General information (tested by asking the patient to name the presidents or the states)

A mental status evaluation done on admission to a critical care setting serves as a baseline to which future mental status evaluations can be compared.

Other tools to help nurses assess their patients' feelings and reactions are the Holland-Sgroi Anxiety-Depression Scale for Medically Ill Patients [25], the Hackett-Cassem Denial Scale [26] and the tool Murray has developed to assess the psychological status of the patient in a surgical intensive care unit [54].

Mattsson [51] offers a theory by which one can better understand the patient's psychological response to trauma. Mattsson theorizes that the general psychological response to severe physical injury has six phases: (1) the emergency reaction, (2) the psychological shock, (3) the contrashock, (4) the psychological resistance, (5) the psychological convalescence, and (6) the psychological outcome. Each phase has its unique characteristics, and the nurse who becomes familiar with them can plan appropriate nursing measures to diminish anxiety and enhance psychological support.

Factors Affecting Feeling Responses and Coping Mechanisms

What determines a critically ill patient's feeling responses to illness and the coping mechanisms he will use? In the following paragraphs, four major categories of determinants are discussed: (1) the "personhood" of the patient, (2) the nature of the illness, (3) the environment in which the patient finds himself, and (4) the timing of the illness. In the discussion of each of these categories, areas for consideration in nursing assessment and intervention are included.

"Personhood" of the Patient

The term personhood refers to the sum total of what makes the patient a unique human being: his strengths, weaknesses, life-style, goals, aspirations, character traits, previous experiences, as well as his demographic characteristics.

Assessment of the patient's physiological responses to illness is crucial when a patient arrives in the critical care setting. Yet, while the assessment is being carried out and appropriate life-saving and maintenance measures are introduced, the nurse can also begin to determine the following:

1. Who is this patient? What are his age, sex, religion, ethnic background, life-style, marital and family status, education, employment? What are his activities, interests, plans, goals?
2. What are the patient's strengths and weaknesses? What are some of his personality traits [41]? To what in him will the nurse appeal to elicit his cooperation and increase his comfort—his "guts," intellect, sense of order, desire to comply? What are his areas of vulnerability?
3. What are his previous experiences with hospitalization?
4. How has he coped with illness or other stressors in the past? How effective were his coping mechanisms? How is he coping now, and how effective are his coping mechanisms right now?
5. How does he express his concerns? Does he ask questions about his illness and its outcome?
6. What is his predominant mood? What are his feelings? What are his needs?
7. How does illness seem to affect his place in the family?

If the patient is unable to supply this information, family members may be a source of help. The information is collected not to change the patient's personality or strip him of his defenses. Rather, the nurse can use the information to help him become an active participant in his care, to support those coping mechanisms that help him deal with his illness, and to provide other supportive measures when his alone are not adequate or helpful. This assessment also says to the patient that someone cares about him and his reactions to illness. The patient may experience some relief from tension just through talking about and sharing his experience.

The nurse uses the data she and other members of the health care team have gained from their observations and assessments to begin a patient care plan that is supportive of the patient, as the following two examples show:

1. The following comments are appropriate for the patient who prides himself on his intestinal fortitude ("guts"): "You've told me it took guts to get out alive from Vietnam despite great odds. It takes guts to tolerate a place like this. Not everyone can. Let's help you use your guts here."
2. If the patient finds it important to be in control of the situation, the nurse can look for what aspects of his care he can control.

Case Study

A 49-year-old psychiatrist was admitted for double valve replacement. His history included problems with emboli causing transient aphasia. He was knowledgable in all aspects of his care, including the possibility of complications. The nurses became increasingly uncomfortable caring for the patient. His comprehension and free discussion of his illness, his interrogation of them about everything being done, and his strong desire to manage his care seemed to contribute to their discomfort.

The patient's primary nurse initiated a discussion of the patient at the nurses' weekly meeting with the psychiatric nurse clinician. In the discussion, the nurses grew more aware of the patient's anxiety and fear of permanent aphasia occurring during or after surgery. As the patient's anxiety increased, so did his need to control. One outcome of the discussion was the suggestion that the patient be asked to help write his own patient care plan.

The patient's primary nurse explained to him that care plans were sent with each patient to the operating room and the intensive care unit. Those plans included information about the patient's responses to illness and suggestions for helping the patient deal with stressful situations. Because the patient knew himself better than anyone else did, he was the best one to give them the information.

The patient welcomed the opportunity, and he wrote a logical, concise care plan that, among other things, mentioned his need to be in charge. He stated that it would be difficult for him to feel helpless and dependent on others to meet all his needs and make all decisions concerning him. However, he determined that if he were allowed to have control over one thing, he could tolerate the staff's being in charge of all other things. That one thing was to hold his small transistor radio while he was in the unit and to have the freedom to turn it on and off or change stations at will.

The nurses in the intensive care unit were told in advance about his request and they were highly supportive of the patient during their preoperative visits to him as well as in the postoperative period. They gave him his radio as soon as he entered the unit, and they tried hard to foster his feelings of control and competence. The patient had an uneventful recovery and, on his discharge, he thanked the staff for having allowed him to help direct his care.

In planning nursing care that supports the personhood of the patient, the nurse should:

1. Observe social amenities. It has been said that patients receive more courtesy and respect in an airline terminal than in a hospital. Although some patients may enjoy being called by their first names or nicknames, others may be offended by the practice. Ribbons in the hair of a 70-year-old woman may look cute to the staff but be a source of embarrassment to the patient. Determining the patient's preferences in those and similar instances is essential.
2. Foster independence. While dependency is initially useful because it helps the patient to tolerate being cared for, it contributes to depression and interferes with rehabilitation. The nurse should look for ways, however small, for the patient to help himself.
3. Emphasize the patient's active role in his health care, such as coughing, deep breathing, notifying her when he is in pain.
4. Allow the patient to participate in decision making in keeping with his needs and the state of his health. Yet the nurse should be alert to the danger of expecting or forcing a patient to make decisions that he is not able to make.
5. Recognize the importance of the patient's personal hygiene and his personal belongings to his self-image. The inability to care for oneself as one is accustomed to fosters feelings of powerlessness. Stripped of his clothes, hairstyle, makeup, jewelry, teeth, or money, the patient may feel naked and exposed to others. The nurse's scrupulous attention to those aspects of personal hygiene that the patient cannot care for, coupled with her flexibil-

ity in individualizing and personalizing care, do much to foster self-esteem.
6. Use resource people who could be helpful to the patient—the chaplain, social worker, volunteer, psychiatric nurse, and psychiatrist.

Nature of the Illness

This is the second major category of factors contributing to a patient's response to illness and the coping mechanisms he uses. It can be subdivided into two sections: (1) the nature of the illness as perceived by the patient and (2) the nature of the illness as it is in reality.

THE ILLNESS AS PERCEIVED BY THE PATIENT

The patient's perception of his illness includes the knowledge, understanding, fantasies, and misconceptions that he has of his illness. The nurse is interested in his perception of not only the physical functioning of the organs involved and the effects of illness on his physical well-being but also the emotional or psychological "functioning" of the organs involved and how they contribute to his total body image. For example, the woman with a pelvic exenteration is probably concerned not only with what organs have been removed and the resulting functioning of specific body systems but also with her image as a woman in whatever roles she functions.

The patient with a heart involvement perceives the heart as more than a pump, as do people with healthy hearts. Literature, folklore, poetry, and songs abound with images of the heart as the seat of love and affection. Male patients often associate the heart with virility or masculinity. They view an insult to the heart, such as a myocardial infarction, as an attack on their maleness, and they are concerned about their functioning as men.

The following suggestions may help the nurse to determine the patient's perception of his illness and to lessen the anxiety associated with his perceptions.

1. Find out what the patient thinks is wrong with him. Ask him. Be sure to include his statements in his medical record; they are a good barometer of his adjustment to illness when noted throughout his hospitalization.
2. Encourage the patient to elaborate on or clarify whatever words he has used.

Patient: I've had a heart attack.
Nurse: What do these words mean to you?
Patient: Why, they mean that my heart was attacked by germs.

(or another response)

Patient: A heart attack means you die.
Nurse: Heart attack means death?
Patient: Sure, all my friends who had heart attacks died.

3. Assess what immediate feelings, fears, or threats may be present. The nurse might ask something like, "What does it feel like to hear the word tumor?" or, "What's it like to be so sick?" or, "Patients normally have many feelings concerning their illness. What are some of your feelings?" or, "What are some of your thoughts?" or, "What do you find yourself thinking about?" or, "What are some of the worries on your mind?"

Patient: I feel sad.
Nurse: What does this feel like? (or, Can you describe this feeling? or, Tell me what it's like to feel sad.)
Patient: Like being half a man.
Nurse: Half a man? What do you mean?
Patient: What the hell good am I? They might just as well dig a hole in the ground, put me in a box, and cover me up.

4. Listen for the patient's ideas about what caused his illness. Does the patient feel he is being punished for past sins or misdeeds? Does the patient feel that his behavior directly led to illness (e.g., driving too fast or taking drugs), or does he blame others? What feelings does he express? If the patient expresses guilt, the nurse should allow the patient to talk without telling him he ought not to feel the way he does.
5. Determine the patient's perception of the progress of his recovery. Does he feel he is progressing satisfactorily? Too slowly? Not at all? Does he envision complications or problems in recovery? Does he feel that death is the inevitable outcome? What disabilities, losses of function, or disfigurement does he anticipate?
6. Clarify what long-range concerns the patient may have as a result of his illness. That clarification is appropriate when the nurse feels that a patient's immediate progress may be hampered by his con-

cern over the future (e.g., whether he will have a job or be able to resume sexual activities). She might inquire, "What do you think your life will be like as a result of this illness?" Some of the concerns he mentions may be dealt with at the time. Others must wait until the convalescent period for resolution. Nevertheless, she does the patient a great service (1) by listening, (2) by helping him focus on and clarify his concerns, (3) by agreeing that, indeed, they are a source of worry, and (4) by assuring him that they will be placed on record and that personnel will help him deal with them later in his hospitalization.

7. Listen for what the patient does not say as well as to what he does say. If the patient never mentions his illness, diagnosis, medications, or procedures, the nurse might broach those subjects. She might comment, "We've talked about so many things this morning, but one thing we haven't talked about is your illness. What is it like for you to be a patient?" If the nurse meets resistance, she does not push the patient to talk. Rather, she might say something like, "Patients often have questions or concerns about being sick and all the things we are doing for them. Asking questions and talking about any concerns seems to help them. If you would like to talk with us at any time, be sure to let us know."

8. Provide updated information. Health care personnel constantly receive data about the patient in the form of vital signs, ECG readings, laboratory tests, and x rays that are used to update their picture of the patient's health. Yet the patient is rarely given information that he can use to reinterpret his condition. That lack of updated information can interfere with the patient's acceptance of progressive ambulation, increased responsibility for self-care, and transfer. It is extremely important for the patient to be as involved in his care as he can be.

9. Realize that a patient's perceptions of his illness may be affected by folklore, literature, experiences with others with the same illness, and the responses of his family, employer, community, and hospital personnel. It does little good to tell the patient that he will be well enough to return to work if his company prohibits anyone with his diagnosis from returning to his job. For example, a young taxicab driver was prevented by company policy from driving a cab after he had had a myocardial infarction.

10. Assess what gains or benefits the patient perceives he gets by being ill, such as more attention or permission to be dependent. Does he tell the nurse that as long as he has a certain illness or symptom he cannot be transferred from the unit, assume new activities, or be discharged from the hospital?

11. Provide accurate information as the patient is ready for it. Once the nurse has clarified the patient's perceptions and understanding of his illness and determined his need for learning, she plans and implements a teaching program to meet his needs. Pictures, brochures, anatomical models, samples of equipment (e.g., valves and catheters), on-the-spot drawings, and other visual aids have been mentioned by patients as having been extremely helpful to them. Some kind of ongoing record of the specific topics that were discussed with the patient contributes to the continuity of his teaching program.

THE ILLNESS AS IT IS IN REALITY

In addition to the patient's perceptions of his illness, the reality aspects of the illness affect the patient's responses to and methods of coping with his illness. The following points must be considered:

1. Did his illness or trauma occur suddenly, or did it occur over a period of time? Did he lose consciousness during that period?

2. What is the effect of the illness on his body systems here and now? What are his vital signs, electrolyte levels, blood gas levels, metabolic status, fluid balance?

3. Does he have cerebral hypoxia?

4. Is he in pain, sedated, recovering from anesthesia, withdrawing from drugs or alcohol?

5. What medications is he receiving? Is he receiving atropine? Is the lidocaine infusion dripping too fast? Is he receiving steroid therapy? If so, what kind and for how long? Does he have a drug reaction?

6. Is he septic?

7. Is he in casts, traction, or splints? Is he covered with dressings, bandages? Is he immobile? Are his body movements restricted? Is he isolated from others?

8. Does he have his body assaulted with tubes, intravenous infusions, wires, leads, catheters? Is he dependent on tubes and machines to assist and/or carry out body functions?

9. Does he require suctioning, chest physiotherapy, injections? Is he dependent on the nurses for feeding, bathing, turning, positioning, and other aspects of care?
10. Are any body parts missing or deformed? Do any odors emanate from his body?
11. What is his normal sleep pattern, and to what degree are treatments and procedures interfering with it? Does he have nightmares?
12. Is he on reverse isolation precautions so that anyone coming into his presence requires a gown and mask?
13. Does he have a malignancy? Is he terminally ill?
14. Does he require painful and repeated procedures, such as the changing of burn dressings?

To lessen the patient's anxiety generated by the illness and its treatment, the nurse should:

1. Continually evaluate what the patient's feelings and concerns are about what the staff are doing and what is happening to him. A routine intravenous infusion may not seem so routine to the patient whose father died while an infusion was being started. The taking of a blood pressure is a simple enough procedure, but the patient may view it as the vehicle by which he is kept awake at night. And since he equates being awake with better chances of surviving his illness, he cooperates by trying to stay awake.
2. Provide brief explanations about treatments and procedures before touching the patient or pulling off his sheets.
3. Maintain the patient's sense of dignity and modesty by closing curtains or doors and exposing only the parts of the body that must be exposed. It is not uncommon in some critical care settings to see catheters inserted, tracheostomies performed, dressings changed, and patients exposed during rounds—all without appropriate screening.
4. Always identify herself (by name and position) and tell what she is going to do to the patient—and continue to do so until the patient calls the nurse by name or shows in some other way that he recognizes her. The nurse's name pin may be absent or the print may be too small for the patient to read. Keep in mind that in many critical care settings, nurses wear clothes that do not identify them as nurses. One patient in a respiratory intensive care unit thought that the nurse in her scrub dress was a cleaning woman trying to begin an

intravenous infusion. He attempted to push her away.
5. Emphasize the temporary nature of those aspects of treatment or the effects of illness that are temporary. Give the patient goals that are realistic for him and point out the progress he has made, however minute.
6. Frequently evaluate the need for specific procedures or treatments. The nurse should ask herself, "Am I doing this for the patient's benefit or am I doing this to allay my feelings of inadequacy or my anxiety?" "Am I doing this to feel in charge or in control?" The nurse's assessment of her actions might result in her either discontinuing procedures that are unnecessary or rearranging the times of the procedures to allow the patient more uninterrupted sleep.
7. Assess frequently the patient's degree of orientation and level of awareness. If a patient is not completely oriented, he requires repeated simple explanations of who he is, where he is, and the time of day. It is also helpful to tell him why he is where he is and to remind him of the progress he has made.
8. If the patient is having nightmares after his accident, burns, or surgery, give him reassurance that they are not unusual, are temporary, and do not mean that he is losing control or becoming mentally ill. Allowing the patient to talk about his nightmares and arranging for someone to remain with him during his sleeping hours diminish the patient's anxiety and help him get the rest he needs.

Environmental Characteristics

The third major category of factors contributing to a patient's response to illness and the methods of coping he uses is the environmental characteristics. The following considerations come under this category:

1. The physical characteristics of the room. How many windows? Beds? Are there cubicles, or are there curtains between patients? Are the bright lights on constantly, or are they lowered at night? Does the patient have any control over the lighting at his bedside? Where is the nurses' station in reference to the patient? How close is the patient to doors, hallways, utility areas?

2. Equipment. Kind? Amount? Size? Sounds? How close is the equipment to the patient?

3. The other patients in the room. How many? What sex? How close are they to the patient? How sick are they? What sounds do they, their relatives, or their equipment make?

4. What objects meaningful to the patient are present? Does the patient have any personal possessions, such as pictures, clothes, Bible, or other books?

5. Are there any signs of affection from others, such as cards, letters, flowers, or fruit?

6. What kinds of conversations occur within the patient's hearing?

7. What people come in contact with the patient (e.g., the personnel who care for the patient, his family, or other visitors)?

8. How much activity can the patient see and hear (e.g., noise [74], confusion, many people moving about, emergencies)?

The environment of a critical care unit can be highly traumatic for the patient [43]. Yet, with appropriate nursing intervention, the environment can become less stressful for some patients and highly positive and supportive for others. The nurse should:

1. Assess the patient's response to his environment. Look at the room from the patient's vantage point (Fig. 13-1A, B). Is there anything in his line of vision that is not in an ordinary hospital room? If there is, assume that the patient at least wonders about it and at most is frightened by it. Mention it in conversation if the patient does not. For example, ask the patient, "What is it like to be a patient here?" or, "Is there anything you see or hear that you wonder about?" or, "Do you have any questions you'd care to ask me?" The nurse can preface her questions with, "This is a strange and unfamiliar place. Usually patients have many questions and feelings about being here. What are some of yours?" The words she uses are not so important as the feelings she conveys; namely, that she cares about the patient's comfort and is open to hearing about his concerns and worries.

2. Explain the equipment—its purpose, sounds (e.g., hissing), side effects (e.g., alarms), sights (e.g., wavy lines)—in terms the patient understands. In some instances, the nurse may demonstrate the functioning of the equipment first, or the patient

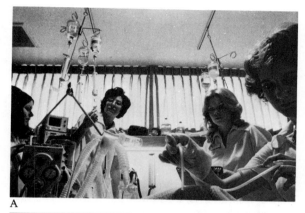

A

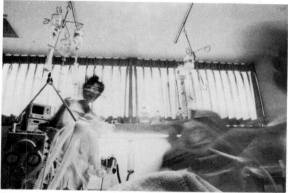

B

Figure 13-1

Look at the room from the patient's vantage point (A) and remember that movement may blur what the patient sees and perceives (B). (Courtesy Brian Anderson.)

may be taken to see the equipment being used by another patient. The nurse's aim is to help the patient tolerate the equipment rather than be made anxious by it. In fact, with the nurse's help, the patient may focus more on the positive aspects of the equipment and have his anxiety lessened as he sees how the equipment helps the nurse care for him. If at all possible, equipment should be positioned in such a way that it does not block the patient's line of vision.

3. Control sounds. In one recovery room, nurses routinely put empty intravenous bottles into a large metal trash can. They had become accustomed to the resultant din, but the patients found it extremely disturbing. Some noises (like the one

just described) can be eliminated as soon as the nurses become aware of their deleterious effects on the patients, but some sounds cannot be lessened. It is essential that the nurse explain those sounds in simple terms to the patients. A special attempt should be made to control noise during the night.

Conversations with a patient should be as concrete as possible to avoid distortion or confusion. It is important to remember that a patient's hearing may extend beyond his immediate bedside area. One patient in a coronary care unit who was recovering without incident from a myocardial infarction heard a nurse outside his room say, "That old thing won't last much longer." He assumed that the nurse was talking about him. In reality, she was discussing a piece of equipment.

4. Control lighting so that patients can experience a day-night cycle as close to normal as possible.

5. Control sights. Patients are often in close proximity to staff members, and they can observe their facial expressions and gestures. They may also be exposed to frightening or anxiety-provoking activities. One patient in a surgical intensive care unit recovering from open-heart surgery witnessed resuscitation attempts on a patient across the room. His impression of all the people on and around the bed was that a sexual orgy was taking place. Another patient who witnessed a tracheostomy being performed on the patient in the bed next to him assumed that the patient was being murdered. His suspicions seemed to him confirmed when he later saw that the bed was empty.

If a patient witnesses a cardiac arrest, resuscitation efforts, and death, it is important to allow him to discuss what he has heard, seen, and felt. Some patients may express sorrow over the loss, anger over the inconvenience or noise, relief that it was the "other guy," reassurance at the speed and competence of staff. They may feel, but not directly express, anxiety that the same fate awaits them. The anxiety may be manifested in elevated blood pressure or pulse, more frequent requests for pain medication, or increased use of the call buzzer, especially in the 24-hour period following the incident [12]. As the patient talks about the incident, the nurse should listen for indications that he is repressing those aspects of similarity between himself and the deceased and focusing instead on the differences ("He was

much older than me" or, "He didn't follow the doctor's orders" or, "His heart attack was worse than mine"). If the patient is unable to do that, the nurse must point out the differences so that he can identify with the living and not with the one who died.

6. If the patient has no window in his cubicle or room, he has no visual contact with the outside world. He cannot see the sun, rain, or snow; he cannot tell whether it is day or night. He cannot see familiar, comforting objects, such as trees, birds, or clouds. Even with a window he may need a radio, newspaper, television, telephone, calendar, clock, family, and the nurse to help him maintain contact with the world outside the critical care unit.

7. Realize that a patient may be made anxious by his close proximity to a patient of the opposite sex. Also, the patient may feel uncomfortable expelling flatus, talking about bowel movements and other body functions, or giving out other information he considers personal.

8. Make the environment as personal as possible. Try to include some objects that are meaningful to the patient. For example, if a dog is the most important object to a patient, perhaps someone can bring the patient a picture of the dog. Perhaps the dog can be brought to a window or, in some circumstances, even in to the patient.

9. Give the patient some control of his environment, if possible; for example, let him turn a radio off or lights down to support his feelings of competence and effectiveness. Shortly before Christmas, a young man was hospitalized in an intensive care unit with multiple injuries he sustained in a motorcycle accident. Christmas carols were played constantly on a piped-in music system, and the patient was too ill to request that the music be turned off occasionally. Ten years later, his only recollection of that painful and life-threatening experience was that of hearing Christmas music played continuously. He no longer enjoys Christmas carols.

10. Recognize the importance of a patient's space or territory. Patients who are not acutely ill have an opportunity, when they are admitted, to walk around the new surroundings and familiarize themselves with its sights, sounds, and activities. They can unpack their own suitcases, arrange their belongings, and thus, in a sense, delineate their own space or territory. Patients in a critical

care unit cannot. The nurses take over as soon as the patient comes in, and the nurses decide what belongings go where and what ones are sent home. The patients have no opportunity to explore, define, or identify what is their territory. That can heighten their feelings of helplessness and powerlessness. To diminish those feelings, the nurse can help the patient delineate his territory. She can give the patient a brief verbal orientation to the nursing unit and a description of the space that "belongs" to him. Also, she can ask his advice about the placement of his personal objects.

11. Realize that in a critical care unit several kinds of sensory alterations can occur. The term *sensory deprivation* refers to the elimination, reduction, or stereotyping of sensation from vision, hearing, or touch [9]. The term *sensory monotony* refers to continuous sensory input along with the elimination or reduction of other sensations (e.g., the constant sound of the cardiac monitor which virtually blocks the input of other sounds). The term *sensory overload* refers to a condition of highly intense stimulation that is not patterned, such as a patient might experience in the recovery room.

The patient who is experiencing sensory alteration may show cognitive signs (e.g., decreased ability to solve problems and reason), perceptual signs (e.g., loss of accuracy in tactual, spatial, and time orientation, deficiencies in visual and motor coordination, and change in size, shape, and color perception), and affective signs (e.g., boredom, restlessness, fatigue, drowsiness, feelings of being dazed, confused, or disoriented). Thus the patient may fall out of bed because his perception of the boundaries of the bed have been altered. He may turn left when the nurse says right because left-right discrimination is readily lost in fatigue and early sensory deprivation. The patient may be unable to decide what to eat, may not absorb teaching, or may not remember directions or other kinds of information.

The nurse should repeatedly assess what effects the sights, sounds, and smells the patient receives have on him. In addition, the nurse should determine what effect the illness and its treatment have on the patient's ability to receive and sort out sensory input. She should find the answers to the following questions: Does the patient usually wear dentures, glasses, or a hearing aid? Does the patient have dressings or patches over his eyes or ears? Is the patient restrained from moving or touching anything? Is he as physically active as his medical condition allows? Can the patient understand the language spoken to him, the expressions used? Does the patient's position in bed prevent him from seeing the activities and people around him? Does he have adequate uninterrupted rest periods? Is the patient taking medications? Does he have a fever or some other medical problem that interferes with his perception and integration of stimuli? Knowing the answers to those questions can help the nurse to plan care that diminishes the effects of sensory alteration.

12. Realize that the presence of people important to the patient is probably the single most important factor in making the environment a secure, caring one. The category includes the people in the patient's life who are dear to him as well as the members of the health care team who care for him. It is important that the nurse have control over visiting hours so that she can exercise her judgment in determining who can visit the patient and for how long, basing her decisions on the patient's needs and the effect visitors have on him [11, 49] rather than on a rigid hospital rule. Nurses have long known that some patients become more relaxed, less fretful, and less restless when someone they love is near. Yet, nurses often do little to encourage others to remain with the patient.

Although it is becoming more widely accepted that parents visit ill children, hospital personnel are still not comfortable allowing children to visit their ill parents. The values and attitudes of hospital personnel in regard to children's visiting a critical care unit may keep them from assessing and meeting the needs of the hospitalized patient and the children. Short, frequent visits may be highly beneficial for both. If children cannot be brought into the unit, possibly the patient can be taken outside the unit in his bed to visit with his children. Also, children can be encouraged to send in drawings and notes, and the patient can be helped to respond to them in some fashion. The exchange of cassette tapes and telephone calls can help maintain family ties.

Nurses play a vital role in not only monitoring the environment and its effects on the patient but also sharing themselves. Through the use of touch [52], presence, listening [56], talking, observing, as well as through giving care, carrying out procedures and treatments, monitoring vital signs, they can share their personhood, their caring, their expertise, their vigilance [19], their acceptance, their concern, and their health. Conversely, for a variety of reasons, including her own responses to working in a critical care unit, the nurse can contribute to a patient's anxiety and diminish his feeling of self-worth. The nurse can have a deleterious effect on the patient by:

A. Offering him superficial reassurance (e.g., "Don't worry. Everything will be all right").
B. Showing a lack of sensitivity to his feelings; for example, by saying "There's really nothing to cry about."
C. Making such statements to the patient as, "I've never seen this reaction before" or, "I don't like the looks of that."
D. Belittling or contradicting other personnel.
E. Checking equipment too frequently.
F. Ignoring the patient when she comes to his bedside to do a procedure or to check equipment.
G. Not responding promptly when summoned by the patient.
H. Telling the patient how busy she is and how many other patients she has to care for.
I. Belittling the patient's concerns.
J. Changing the subject when the patient asks questions that make the nurse feel uncomfortable (e.g., questions about his diagnosis).
K. Rushing in and out of the patient's room.
L. Asking the patient a question and then either not listening to his answer or being annoyed because he takes time to answer it.
M. Disregarding common courtesy.
N. Removing equipment from a patient on which he had become dependent without appropriate psychological weaning and support.
O. Ignoring or minimizing the learning needs of the patient.
P. Overprotecting the patient for a period of time and then suddenly expecting him to do much for himself.
Q. Promising to visit a patient after his transfer and not following through.
R. Shouting or calling out to other staff members across the room.

Even those actions that are viewed by personnel as benign or routine (e.g., taking a pulse, walking into the patient's room, and giving the patient a pill) can arouse both physiological and psychological responses [49, 72].

13. Prepare the patient for transfer from the critical care environment. Because of the patient's dependence on personnel, equipment, and the caring, secure environment, transfer from the critical care unit may be threatening and symptom-provoking for him. The incidence of dysrhythmias, reinfarctions, and extensions of infarction is higher around the time that patients are transferred from coronary care units [42, 53].

To prevent transfer from being fraught with anxiety, the nurse should prepare the patient for transfer as early as possible after his admission and encourage him to share his feelings and reactions to the transfer. Many patients speak about feelings of sadness and loss at leaving the unit and feelings of anxiety over what the new unit will be like, whether their needs will be met, whether the staff will know how to care for them and for emergencies that might arise, and whether the necessary equipment and medications will be present. The nurse can be helpful by not only accepting those feelings but also pointing out the gains the patient will make after the transfer; for example, he will be able to do more for himself. She should emphasize that while the staff members on the receiving unit have the skills, equipment, and medications necessary to handle any emergency that could occur, no emergencies are expected. If possible, the patient should not be weaned from equipment (such as a monitor or respirator) at the same time as he is being transferred.

If possible, the transfer should occur during the day, with familiar people accompanying the patient. The patient should be introduced to someone on the receiving unit, and he should be told that information about his care has been given to the proper people both in writing and verbally. Later, members of the critical care unit staff with whom the patient has established rapport and developed a relationship might visit him.

Timing of the Illness

The timing of the illness, the fourth major category of factors that affect a person's response to illness and the methods of coping with illness, has until recently received relatively little attention. Under that category are discussed the role of stress and the "anniversary reaction."

ROLE OF STRESS

It has long been accepted that loss is a response to illness but only recently has it been accepted that illness and death can be responses to loss and other agents producing stress [24, 31, 57, 59, 60, 65, 71]. Stress is the nonspecific response of the body to any demand made upon it. Each agent calls forth specific and nonspecific responses from the body. The specific response would be the localized response of the body to the agent; e.g., the skin's response to heat. No matter what the specific responses are, all agents have something in common: they increase demand for readjustment. It is immaterial whether that agent or stressor (that which produces stress; i.e., any stimulus that upsets physiological homeostasis) is pleasant or unpleasant, desirable or undesirable. What is important is the intensity of the demand for readjustment or adaptation. The more stressful an event or happening is perceived to be (i.e., the more intense is the demand on the organism to adapt), the greater is the body's physiological response to the stressor. The energy necessary to acquire and maintain adaptation, apart from caloric requirements, is called "adaptation energy [65]."

Selye [65] has coined the term General Adaptation Syndrome (GAS) to describe a three-phased generalized physiological response to stressors. Throughout this response, the autonomic nervous system and endocrine glands attempt to help the body fight off the stressor and regain its former equilibrium.

Researchers in recent years have attempted to develop tools to measure stress and its effects on people's health. Holmes and Rahe [38] compiled a list of life events that they observed occurred around the time of disease onset. Each of those events appeared to place an adjustment demand (stress) upon the person involved. Holmes and Rahe developed a device called a Social Readjustment Rating Scale which measures, in "life change units," the amount of readjustment required by each event on the list. Rahe and others [59] found that people with high total readjustment scores were more likely than those with low scores to become ill within six months.

In 1974 Rahe reported on recent life change data gathered from 279 survivors of documented myocardial infarction and from 226 cases of abrupt coronary deaths in Helsinki [60]. In all but one group of subjects there were marked rises in the magnitude of life changes during the six months immediately before infarction or death compared to the same time interval one year earlier. For sudden death victims, elevation was particularly evident.

Holmes and Rahe suggest that when enough change occurs in one year to total a score of 300, a danger point has been reached. In a study of subjects who had scores of more than 300, 80 percent had heart attacks or other serious illnesses or became seriously depressed [68].

The fact that whatever is perceived as stressful by the individual evokes a physiological as well as a psychological response has enormous implications for the nurse in the critical care setting. The patient who comes to the hospital in the process of dealing with stressors (e.g., the patient who is newly unemployed, recently divorced, or grieving over a parent's death) may need help. The burden of coping with additional stressors in the hospital setting—illness, isolation, fatigue, and other factors mentioned earlier—and the autonomic stimulation evoked by them may be more than the patient can tolerate. Without appropriate intervention, he may succumb to his illness or its complications.

Whatever nurses can do to (1) identify recent life events (e.g., by using the Social Readjustment-Rating Scale), (2) assess the degree of the patient's unresolved conflicts about them, (3) identify what is stressful to the patient in his present situation, and (4) intervene with appropriate measures to lessen the effects of the stressor [36, 53, 54, 69, 71] will enhance the patient's psychological comfort as well as foster his physical well-being.

Some techniques now being used to lessen the impact of stressors may in the future be more widely used in critical care areas. Those are the techniques of biofeedback, meditation, and relaxation, used individually or in combination. Benson's relaxation response counteracts the physiological effects of stressors; that is, it lowers the heart rate and metabolism and decreases the breathing rate [6]. Lown and others discussed the effective use of meditation in a 39-year-old patient who twice experienced ventricular fibrillation and exhibited numerous ventricular premature beats [48]. Biofeedback, a technique using instrumentation to give a person immediate and continuing information of specific bodily function of which he is unaware, has been used to teach patients greater awareness of mind-body correlates and conscious control of certain body functions [8, 61, 64]. Lowering of blood pressure and pulse, reduction of tension headaches and lower back pain, and improved muscle function have been cited as results of those techniques (see Chap. 1).

"ANNIVERSARY REACTION"

Another factor to consider in the category of timing is that of the "anniversary reaction." It is essential for the nurse to determine if anyone else in the patient's family contracted or died of a similar illness on the same date, at the same time, or at the same age. For example, a 50-year-old patient with a myocardial infarction whose father, uncle, and brother died from infarction at the same age may feel that his death is inevitable. If there is evidence of an anniversary reaction, the patient may need help in grieving over the loss of the relative, in expressing anxiety over his own diagnosis, and in pinpointing how his case is different from that of the deceased relatives.

The four categories—personhood of the patient, nature of the illness, environmental characteristics, and timing of the illness—have been discussed separately, but in fact, they are not separate. They interact and together affect how a patient responds to illness.

Nursing Interventions in Specific Situations

Besides the general nursing measures discussed in conjunction with the factors that determine what feeling responses and coping mechanisms are used, there are certain nursing interventions applicable to specific situations that help patients cope with their feelings. The situations to be discussed in this chapter involve (1) the patient who uses denial, (2) the patient who is acutely anxious, (3) the patient who is depressed, (4) the patient who is sexually aggressive, (4) the patient who is suspicious, (5) the patient who is delirious, (6) the patient who is unable to communicate verbally, (7) the patient who is dying, and (8) the patient who is suicidal.

The Patient Who Uses Denial

Denial is a protective mechanism used by a large majority of patients. It can take several forms [63]:

1. Verbal denial (e.g., "I don't have cancer.")
2. Minimizing severity (e.g., "Yes, I had a heart attack yesterday, but it's all gone now.")

3. Displacing symptoms on another organ system (e.g., "It wasn't my heart; it was indigestion.")
4. Behavior contrary to medical advice (e.g., "Sure I still smoke. Cigarettes aren't going to bother *my* lungs.")

Some of the manifestations of denial are excessive cheerfulness, joking, use of terms like "invincible" to describe oneself, use of clichés in reference to death, conversation focused on issues other than illness, use of dismissive gestures when referring to distressing events [15].

If a patient is verbally denying the seriousness of his illness but allows treatments and care to be carried out, his denial may be serving a highly useful purpose [27, 29]. However, his denial may be viewed as maladaptive when a patient's behavior interferes markedly with his care, as would pulling off monitor leads, refusing medication, or getting out of bed. In those instances, arguing with a patient using denial tends to make both the nurse and the patient angry and reinforces the patient's denial. Teaching is likewise generally ineffective: if a patient does not believe he has a particular illness, why should he learn about that illness?

The nurse can attempt to clarify what the patient is defending himself against without challenging the denial directly. She can do that by asking the patient to talk about the illness without having to agree he has the illness. For example, she should ask, "What does the word colostomy mean to you?" rather than, "What does *your* colostomy mean to you?" The nurse should acknowledge what the patient tells her and let him know that others have responded in a similar fashion. She can also ask for his cooperation rather than intellectual assent. For example, she can say, "You tell me you don't believe you had a heart attack. Most people feel the same as you do; they don't believe it either. In fact, at this point we're not expecting you to believe it. We're just asking you to go along with us and keep these leads on."

Rather than chiding the patient for his behavior, the nurse can encourage him to talk about the difficulties he is experiencing. Then she can use the "single solution" approach to see if there is some way to make the experience less threatening.

Case Study

A 54-year-old man was admitted to a four-bed coronary care unit with the diagnosis of massive myocardial infarction. The day after his admission, he pulled off the leads and began walking in the hall. When told by the staff he could not do this, he threatened to sign out of the hospital.

Nurse: You've removed the monitor leads several times today and gotten out of bed. What makes it so hard to keep them on and stay in bed?

Patient: I'm an ex-con. Being strapped with those things and the siderails up reminds me of solitary confinement. I can't stand it; I'm getting out of the hospital.

Nurse: I hear you say you can't stay here with your activities so restricted. If there were one thing I could change that would make the situation tolerable enough for you to stay, what would it be? (Fig. 13-2).

In such a way, the nurse communicates to the patient her concern for him, her recognition of his need to control, and her willingness to compromise. Modifications of what nursing personnel consider the "ideal" are not always easy for them to make; yet those modifications may permit the patient to remain in the hospital and receive the care he desperately needs.

The Patient Who Is Acutely Anxious

The acutely anxious patient may not be able to use denial at all to allay his anxiety. Or he may have used denial to a point, but as he has developed more awareness of his situation, denial no longer relieves his anxiety. The patient may exhibit one or more of the following: rapid, high-pitched voice; incessant talking; fidgeting, twisting, restless movements; rapid pulse, increased respirations, elevated blood pressure; increased perspiration; difficulty sleeping; worried, tense expression; wide, staring eyes [26, 54]. The patient may say outright, "I'm scared" or, "What's going to happen to me?" or, "Am I going to die?" Another patient, not directly stating his anxiety, may call for the nurse frequently and cling to her verbally or physically once she is at his bedside. In either instance, the nurse should help the patient talk about his feelings. She should reassure him that his feelings are normal and not a sign of cowardice.

Nurse: You tell me you are feeling anxious. What does this feel like?

Patient: I don't know; I just don't feel right.

Nurse: Tell me what you do feel.

Patient: Well [pause], I feel restless, nervous. I want to get this over with.

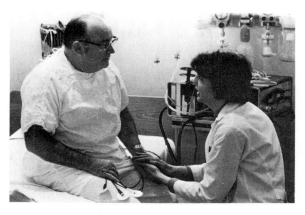

Figure 13-2
"I hear you say you can't stand being so restricted. If there was one thing I could change that would help, what would it be?" (Courtesy Brian Anderson.)

Nurse: Get what over with?

Patient: They tell me I have to go back for another operation to change these dressings.

Nurse: What about that?

Patient: I don't know. [Pause] I wonder if it will hurt. I know it will. Will I have anesthesia? I want to be asleep. I don't want any more pain.

The more the patient can identify the factors that contribute to his feeling of anxiety, the more the nurse has to work with. Each factor should be examined individually with the patient. Some problems can be solved with simple explanations. Others may require the help of resource people. Some problems cannot be fully solved, but at least the nurse and the patient have become aware of what they are and can face them openly.

The presence of a significant other—a family member or someone else the patient trusts—may diminish anxiety and help induce rest. Likewise, consistently having the same nurses, with whom he can develop a relationship, is highly supportive. Planned, frequent visits by the nurse give the patient something to count on and diminish his need to call for attention repeatedly. Once the nurse has developed a relationship with the patient, she can transfer the confidence and trust the patient has in her to one of her colleagues. When the patient's primary nurse plans to be off duty, she ought to tell him that she is leaving and who will be caring for him in her absence, introduce him to that nurse, and review with her in the patient's presence any procedures or routines with which the patient feels comfortable. Doing so enhances the trust the patient will have in the second nurse.

The acutely anxious patient needs reassurance about the routine aspects of treatments and the progress he is making, as well as preparation for what is to come. Anticipating the patient's reactions to surgery or procedures (e.g., pain or nausea), along with reassuring him that medication to lessen the impact of those reactions will be available, also diminishes anxiety. However, explanations, directions, or information should be brief and simple and may have to be repeated at frequent intervals. Some patients also seem calmed by the knowledge that they are being treated in a specialized unit by highly competent personnel who know exactly how to care for them. The effect of the verbal assurance is strongly enhanced if the nurse goes about her work calmly and expertly, appears to be in control of what is happening, and is flexible within a structured framework.

In addition to those measures, the patient may need medication for sleep or the reduction of anxiety. Some patients need reassurance that such medication is an important adjunct to their treatment. The anxious patient, however, should not be expected to be responsible for determining the need for and requesting this medication; that is the nurse's responsibility.

The Patient Who Is Depressed

Depression is a response to a narcissistic injury, a blow to the image of oneself as whole, intact, and independent. As the patient becomes more aware of the reality of his situation, he may become withdrawn, listless, apathetic, and pessimistic; show retarded speech and motor activity; cry; have a decrease in appetite; express feelings of hopelessness; and look sad [26]. He may ruminate about what life will be like as a result of his illness.

It is helpful to anticipate those feelings and reassure the patient that they are normal. The nurse can encourage the patient to share his feelings with her. If he continues to ruminate about his illness to the exclusion of all other topics, the nurse may need to change the subject and focus on some other time in the patient's life when he felt happier. She should allow the patient to cry if he feels comfortable doing so, but she should realize that for some, crying may enhance

their feeling that they have lost control. A matter-of-fact acceptance rather than an overly sympathetic approach seems most supportive.

Nurses do not join the patient in feeling that the situation is hopeless, nor are they overly optimistic. They can refer to the future in their conversations and promote future-oriented thinking. Taking an activity history and beginning a program of planned activity early in the patient's hospitalization will lessen the incidence of depression and foster the patient's sense of well-being [16].

It is helpful to look for ways to increase the patient's self-esteem. The nurse can point out small gains as signs of progress. She can encourage the patient to focus not so much on the total illness, which may be quite discouraging, but on some aspects of it. The patient needs input from the nurse, however, in order to do that. For example, a nurse might say, "From now on, we plan to take your blood pressure every hour instead of every 15 minutes" or, "You will be off this respirator five extra minutes because you are doing so well." The nurse can accentuate the positive—point out all that the patient can do, rather than all that he is unable to do.

Recognize that the depressed patient does not appreciate an exuberant approach; it serves only to heighten his feeling of sadness. Sometimes superficial attempts to be cheerful are seen as just that—superficial. It would be more helpful to say, "I notice that you look sad and have been crying. [Pause] Tell me about it." Again, the words the nurse uses are not so important as the message of concern and caring she transmits to the patient. Sometimes, words are not necessary. Just being with the patient, touching him, and sharing herself with him is a source of great comfort.

The patient may begin to express anger as a means of diminishing his feeling of helplessness. The anger is not a personal attack on the nurse. Rather than respond to the patient defensively, the nurse can encourage the patient to focus on what he is really upset about.

Patient: The food is always cold, the nurses sure don't know much about giving shots, and then there's that parking lot! Why they charge my wife $3.50 every time she comes in!

Nurse: Seems like many things are really upsetting you today. Wonder if you are also upset about being sick and being here in the unit?

Patient: No, it's not that. It's the parking lot. I hate it with a purple passion.

The patient's use of denial signaled that he was not ready to confront the issue of his illness and all that it meant. The nurse listened as the patient expressed more anger. Two days later, during a similar conversation, she again raised the point of his illness and how it affected his feelings. At that time he was able to talk about his feelings of sadness and anxiety.

The Patient Who Is Sexually Aggressive

Sexual acting-out can occur verbally—the patient tells off-color jokes, cites details of past sexual accomplishments, or invites the nurse to talk about her personal life or engage in sexual activities with him. It can also occur behaviorally—pinching, poking, fondling, or kissing the nurse, exposing himself, or masturbating in the nurse's presence.

Sexual acting-out may be the result of anxiety over an altered self-image [63, 73]. The patient no longer sees himself as a functioning, whole man, and he wonders how others view him. He acts out his concern through his comments and behavior. Nurses often become anxious, angry, frightened, or embarrassed by that and respond in such a way that the patient feels he is a naughty boy, a dirty old man, or an inadequate male incapable of arousing a woman. He may then try harder through words and actions to communicate that he is indeed competent.

The nurse's aim is to help the patient express his anxiety verbally and stop his inappropriate behavior. In whatever words she feels comfortable with, she attempts to communicate the following to him:

1. She has noticed the behavior.
2. The behavior is not appropriate at this time in this place.
3. She senses he is concerned about his image as a man and his future sexual functioning.
4. Many patients have that concern; it is a normal concern and one that he may discuss if he wishes.
5. She is willing to listen, to help him clarify his concerns, and to help him get the information he needs.

In some instances a patient is not aware of his verbal preoccupation with sexual topics. Pointing out the content, not as an accusation but as a means of communicating how the patient seems to others, is sometimes helpful [32]. The patient may also respond to the nurse's statement that she feels uncomfortable with the behavior. If the nurse should walk in to a patient's room while he is masturbating, she can excuse herself and say, "I'll close the door (pull the curtain) to give you some privacy" or, "Excuse me; I'll be back in later," and close the door as she leaves.

The Patient Who Is Suspicious or Paranoid

The more suspicious a patient is before his admission to the critical care setting, the more apt he is to become paranoid during acute stress. A suspicious preoperative patient should be prepared for that possibility.

Example
In the ICU you will see many people and won't know most of them. You might sometimes wonder if they know you and know what to do for you. You may even get the idea that they are trying to hurt you. If you do, remember what I'm telling you now—that patients often have those ideas after surgery, but they are temporary and will soon go away. In reality, the staff will know who you are, will know exactly what to do for you, and will do only what will help you get better sooner.

It is important for the patient to meet preoperatively with the critical care unit staff who will be on duty when the patient arrives in the unit. The nurse should encourage the patient to ask questions and give him simple, honest, *consistent* answers. Writing on his record what information he was given may ensure consistent responses from everyone.

In the critical care setting, the nurse may know from his care plan that a patient is suspicious, or she may observe symptoms of such: eyes darting about as if to observe everything, reluctant to eat or sleep, questioning everything the nurse is doing, and not seeming to believe the answers she gives. To allay some of the patient's anxiety, the nurse should always call him by name, give her name and purpose before touching him, and offer simple explanations of things the patient appears to be concerned about.

Example
You may wonder why this solution is colored yellow. (Look for some sign of affirmation from the patient and then go on.) It's the color of _____, a medication I put into the
                        (name)
solution to _____.
                  (purpose)

The nurse should help the patient have as much control as possible. She should encourage him to ask questions by asking, "Is there something you wonder about?" or, "Do you have any questions?" The more anxious the patient becomes, the more suspicious he may be. If the nurse can learn the source of his anxiety and can deal with it, the patient may become less suspicious.

If the patient becomes paranoid, he may hear voices telling him to escape. He may try to pull out his intravenous infusion and tubes and get out of bed. He may scream for the police and attempt to push people away when they come near him. Despite the difficulties encountered in approaching the paranoid patient, it is important to maintain some kind of contact or rapport with him.

Example

Right now you tell me it's hard to believe anyone. You feel we're trying to poison you. Even though you're in _____ hospital because _____, we know it's
    (name)   (diagnosis)
hard for you to believe us. What makes it so hard?

or

What do you think is happening to you? Is there something you're really concerned about?

or

I know you're really uncomfortable now. I'd like you to feel a little less so. What can I do to help you?

or

Right now you seem terribly frightened and are trying to get away. You'd like to be back home with your family, away from here, from sickness, and from all the things we've been doing to you. Being here can be very upsetting. What about being here is upsetting to you?

The last example includes many suppositions that have to be confirmed by the patient. This confirmation might be done by pausing between statements and observing the patient's facial expressions and behavior for signs of agreement. Providing that confirmation is done, this particular style of attempting to reach the patient may be extremely useful in facilitating communication.

A family member whom the patient trusts may need to stay with the patient during his period of paranoid thinking. Only then might the patient eat, take medication, sleep, and tolerate care.

The Patient Who Is Delirious

Delirium is a reversible psychotic state related to a variety of factors, including the nature and severity of the illness, degree of cerebral hypoxia, metabolic disturbances, medications, procedures, treatments, environment, sadness, pain, and anxiety [2, 46, 47, 55, 58, 62]. Symptoms may include restlessness, agitation, mild confusion, memory loss, disorientation, fluctuating states of consciousness, and perceptual distortions. The delirium seems to occur more in surgical intensive care units than in medical intensive care units.

Many of the nursing measures discussed earlier appear useful in minimizing the possibility that delirium will occur; namely, measures to provide adequate sleep, to monitor and minimize the harmful effects of the environment, to determine a patient's emotional responses to illness, to prevent sensory alterations, and to isolate and deal with factors that contribute to anxiety. Establishing rapport with a patient preoperatively, teaching him about his coming experience, and preparing him for the possibility that bad dreams will occur after surgery may also lessen the chances that delirium will occur.

If delirium does develop, the nurse must assess what physiological factors might have contributed to its onset (e.g., a very high temperature, a too rapid infusion of lidocaine or atropine, a low PaO_2), as well as assess the impact of environmental and psychological factors. The patient who is delirious may find it helpful to talk about what he is experiencing and feeling. Family members may be extremely helpful to the staff and supportive to the patient. Their presence may calm the patient and diminish his need for restraints. While the patient needs protection from hurting himself, restraints may only increase his agitation.

Once the delirium has passed, the patient may wish to talk about his experience. He needs reassurance that he had nightmares that sometimes occur in acute illness but are not a sign of mental illness.

The Patient Who Is Unable to Communicate Verbally

The patient who cannot communicate verbally faces the task of coping not only with his illness but also with the loss of verbal expression, a tool that he has had since birth. Even patients who have been prepared for intubation find it a frightening and anxiety-provoking experience.

Some of the commonly experienced fears are the fear of never being able to speak again, of being dependent on the respirator forever, of not breathing adequately when taken off the respirator, of death, and of equipment malfunction. Some patients may also feel depressed over the long-term nature of their illness, their apparent lack of progress, and their dependence on equipment and personnel.

Because the patient cannot communicate verbally, he writes, signals a response to questions (e.g., he blinks his eyes or squeezes the nurse's hand), uses body language (e.g., he cries or changes his body position or facial expression), signals a response by using cards with letters, words, or pictures, or takes specific actions (e.g., he pulls at equipment). The nurse, using her sensitivity and empathy, can help the patient define and express his feelings even more. While carrying on a monologue, she observes the patient's reactions and uses them to determine the trend of the conversation. To do this she needs to stand or sit close to the head of the bed so that she and the patient can see each other's face. The nurse's hand on the patient can be reassuring as well as sensitive to movements the patient may make in response to her. The following is an example of the words the nurse might use:

Example

I'd like to spend a few minutes talking with you about what it's like for you to be a patient here. [Pause] Most people tell us it's not easy to be a patient. [Pause] They have many questions, concerns, or worries about being ill. [Pause] Talking about those concerns and getting answers to questions seem to help them feel more comfortable. [Pause] I wonder what some of your thoughts might be or what some of your questions are. [Pause] Let's work together at looking at these.

After such a beginning, the nurse can become more specific. The more she uses such an approach and the broader her understanding of the common areas of concern becomes, the easier and more helpful the approach becomes. Whatever assumptions the nurse makes should be confirmed by the patient. The nurse should accept whatever feelings are expressed, assure the patient that they are normal, and plan for appropriate supportive measures. She should realize that when a patient's anxiety is lessened, he is freer to concentrate and relax during potentially stressful procedures, such as being taken off the respirator.

The Patient Who Is Dying

Much has been written about the needs of the dying patient, the stages he may pass through in the process of dying, and his predominant feelings during those stages [14, 44]. The information is extremely helpful in viewing the entire dying process and in planning appropriate nursing intervention and support for the patient and his family.

Most patients hospitalized in a critical care setting have considered at one point or another the possibility that they are dying. Those who survive their illness find that the thoughts of death lessen and finally disappear as they progress toward health. But the others, the dying patients, face the awesome task of traveling the last part of their journey through life.

The warm, empathetic critical care nurse recognizes that she can play a significant part in guiding and supporting the patient while he completes that journey. She realizes that only with good communication can there be real caring; without it, the patient will be isolated, alone, and without the solace and comfort of others. How can she improve her communication with the dying patient? She must be willing to be in close contact with the patient, to touch him, to meet his physical needs. She must not turn away from repugnant wounds or malodorous drainage. She must be aware of the patient's need for fresh air, mouth care, frequent turning and positioning, light, and the like.

She must also be willing to listen to what the patient says, regardless of the discomfort she herself experiences. If the patient gives verbal or nonverbal clues that the subject of dying is on his mind and he wants to discuss it, she gives him the opportunity to do so.

Patient: Am I going to die?
Nurse: You ask me about dying. What are your thoughts about it?

or

You ask about dying. Is this something that's been on your mind? Let's talk about it.

For some patients, an appropriate answer to the question "Am I going to die?" might be

I don't know but I wonder what you feel.

or

That's a question I don't know the answer to but what do you think?

As in other issues, the words the nurse uses are not so important as the message she communicates; namely, that she has heard the words the patient has used, she is willing to hear more, and she wonders what thinking and feeling, wondering or worrying on the part of the patient prompted the question he raised or the statement he uttered. Whatever the patient answers, the nurse invites him to elaborate and explain further (but allows him to refuse the invitation at any point in the discussion). She does not jump in and answer questions immediately or superficially before being certain what the questions really are. She considers the factors of honesty, appropriateness, and maintaining hope for the future and trust in the present. If she hears that the patient has misinterpreted some information, she may be able to clarify or correct his interpretations. The nurse also encourages the patient to raise questions and discuss his concerns with his physician.

As the patient talks more about his approaching death, he may share with the nurse his concerns, needs, or fears. Careful listening to the patient helps the nurse find areas for intervention and support.

Patient: I'm dying, you know.
Nurse: [Gets closer to patient] What's it like to feel you're dying?
Patient: Oh, it's not so bad, I guess, once you get over the shock of it. I mean, there's nothing I can do to stop it; that's the worst of it. It's like looking up and seeing this avalanche of rocks and dirt coming down toward you and knowing you can't get out of the way, no matter what. [Note the denial, then the expression of loss of control, helplessness, and fear of a catastrophic ending]
Nurse: That seems pretty frightening.
Patient: It is. [Begins to sob]
Nurse: [Reaches out to patient and puts her hand on his arm. Remains silent while patient cries]

After that exchange the nurse might look for ways, however small, to increase the patient's feelings of control over his care. She also institutes measures to help the patient either view death as less catastrophic or feel not so alone while going through the catastrophe. Those measures include (1) telling the patient she will be there to go through the experience with him, (2) asking the patient if there is anything she can do to make death seem less frightening and then incorporating his suggestions into his care plan, (3) en-

suring effective pain control, (4) administering medication for anxiety or sleep as indicated, (5) allowing the patient either to talk about whatever seemed important to him or to keep silent, (6) helping the patient have his needs for closeness, security, affection met by his family, friends, or members of the health care team, and (7) accepting the patient's expressions of feelings.

In the course of listening to a dying patient, the nurse may be struck by the patient's enumeration of and preoccupation with the failures, poor decisions and missed opportunities in his life. Although she does not deny nor attempt to argue the patient's statements away, the nurse helps the patient focus on what he has accomplished, created, or contributed, such as his children, his garden of fresh vegetables, his getting to work on time, his tolerance of the tragedy of illness, his jokes for the fellows at work, his bowling score. Death may be easier to accept if one feels that in some small way he has made his mark in this world and that others will remember him with fondness and pride.

The following is a list of other nursing measures that are appropriate to the care of the dying patient:

1. Providing the patient and his family with as much privacy as possible
2. Providing the patient with the opportunity to complete his "unfinished business"
3. Meeting the patient's requests to see a member of his family, a lawyer, a clergyman, or his physician
4. Evaluating which procedures and treatments can be discontinued to make the patient more comfortable
5. Making provisions for someone to stay with the patient all the time if he wishes it

The nurse cannot take away a patient's death. But through sharing her presence, her caring, her being, she can help the patient live in such a way that he dies feeling loved and cared for. And when death comes, she can contribute to its peacefulness and dignity.

The Patient Who Has Attempted Suicide

The patient who is admitted to a critical care unit after having made a suicide attempt presents a special challenge to nursing personnel [37]. Nurses may experience conflicting feelings while caring for such a patient: loathing and contempt, compassion and concern, annoyance and anger, anxiety and fear. Although some may feel committed to doing all that they can to save the patient, others may question why so much time, energy, and effort are spent to save someone who wanted to die. Feelings may be heightened (1) if the patient tried to commit suicide before, especially if the same nurses cared for him, (2) if the suicide attempt seems manipulative, (3) if the patient had no "good" reason (in the staff's judgment) to attempt suicide, or (4) if the patient expresses hostility toward those who "saved" him. If the patient acknowledges his foolishness, expresses remorse, vows not to attempt suicide again, accepts psychiatric intervention, or has "good" reason for his attempt, staff members tend to respond more positively to him.

Feelings may also be increased as the nurse observes the reactions of the family members and interacts with them.

Example

A 31-year-old married mother of two girls was admitted to the respiratory intensive care unit following an overdose of glutethimide. As she regained consciousness, she attempted to pull off the respirator and pull out her intravenous infusion. Given a pad of paper and pencil, she scribbled on the pad, "Let me die." Her husband remained in the waiting room, alternately wringing his hands in despair and asking angrily, "Why did she do this to me? What's wrong with her?" The patient's mother shouted to the husband through her tears, "It's all your fault. You drove her to it!" Two small girls were huddled together on the waiting room couch crying quietly for their mother. Their father and grandmother appeared unaware of their presence.

It is important for the nurse to acknowledge her feelings and responses to caring for the patient who has attempted suicide so that the patient's nursing care is not hindered. It is not necessary for her to accept or agree with the patient's desire to die in order to accept the patient as someone who needs her care. In addition to the general nursing measures stated earlier in this chapter, the nurse should:

1. Use psychiatric resource personnel as soon as possible after admission to interview the patient, assess his mental status and suicide risk, offer suggestions for management and treatment, and provide ongoing support or therapy.
2. Allow the patient to talk about his suicide attempt with her but not force him to do so.

3. Evaluate the patient's mental status periodically and report any changes promptly.
4. Participate in assessing the patient's current suicide risk. The patient may require constant observation and protection from further injury to self.
5. Observe the patient's reactions to telephone calls, mail, and visitors, as well as the visitors' responses to the patient. The nurse may need to shield the patient from the wrath of his family.
6. Be aware of the patient's mood and the content of his conversation. Is the patient talking about attempting suicide again? Is the patient crying, euphoric, ashamed, angry, calm?
7. Use resources to help the family members deal with their feelings about the patient, as well as to gain vital information about the circumstances surrounding the event.
8. Chart any observations about the patient's behavior or appearance, as well as comments made by the patient.

Family Responses

Just as the patient experiences a variety of feelings in response to his illness so do his relatives: anger, sadness, guilt, frustration, fear, anxiety, and hope. They cope with those feelings in many ways, including being overprotective of the patient, crying, holding a "living wake" at the bedside, complaining about care, blaming the patient, constantly seeking reassurance, expressing anger, and using denial. Nurses are appropriately concerned about how relatives express their need, how those needs are met, and how they affect the patient [10, 11, 21, 30, 34, 39, 49, 67].

As soon as possible, the nurse should orient the family to the unit. She should give them a tour, introduce them to the staff, and acquaint them with protocol. They should be told whom to go to with questions and what the patient's care will be like. They should be encouraged to write down questions as they occur to them at home to facilitate their asking what they want to know when they come in to visit. Relatives can be given written information about the unit to read at a less anxious moment. If possible, provide a visitor's lounge with a rest area and hot plate, where visitors can relax, rest, wait, cry, eat, and talk informally with members of other families experiencing crises too. Volunteer personnel assigned to the visitors' lounge may be useful in supporting family members, answering simple questions, and explaining hospital routine.

The patient's relatives or significant others should be interviewed by the patient's nurse to complete gaps in her information about the patient, as well as to assess the relative's response to illness and need for support. A question like, "Your husband is stable today. How have you been holding up through all of this?" gives the wife an opportunity to share her reactions to the patient's illness. The nurse may learn that the wife (or some other relative) feels guilty about having contributed to the patient's trauma or illness, such as driving the car in which the patient was injured or carelessly disposing of cigarettes that started the fire in which the patient was burned. Relatives may express anger that the patient became ill or that the patient is not cooperating enough in getting better. Some people may have ambivalent feelings toward the patient and feel frightened or guilty about their wish to see the patient not recover. In addition to meeting the initial needs expressed by the relative, the nurse can introduce family members to one or more resource people available for support: a social worker, psychiatric nurse clinician, psychiatrist, dietitian, chaplain, or volunteer.

Many relatives are reluctant to approach a critically ill patient. Initially the nurse can take them to the bedside and encourage them to touch and talk with the patient. She should, if possible, move any equipment that is in the way of their doing this. If there is something specific they should do (e.g., wear gowns) or should not do (e.g., feed the patient), the nurse must explain the rule to the relatives. Evaluation of the relatives' attitudes toward the patient tells the nurse much about their responses to the patient and gives her information for planning appropriate intervention. Do the patient's relatives want to be involved or uninvolved? Do they want to know or not know about the diagnosis and prognosis? How do they communicate their fears to the patient? How supportive are they of the patient: Do they have a need to keep the patient ill? Are they pushing the patient to be independent too soon or keeping the patient dependent too long?

Often, relatives want to be supportive of the patient but they need help. They need preparation in regard to questions patients may ask, such as questions about dying, or in regard to behavior the patient may exhibit, such as attempting to get out of bed. Those who show a willingness to become involved in the patient's care can be given tasks (e.g., helping bathe

the patient, reading to the patient, or bringing him some special food from home). The nurse can determine from her observations and from talking with the family which relative is most supportive to the patient. He may be willing to be "on call" if the patient requires a visit, especially during the night. He ought to be informed promptly of changes in the patient's condition so that he can communicate the news to other family members.

Relatives might also help the patient maintain an interest in life. Perhaps they can contact employers, friends, or organizations who might wish to remember the patient with cards or notes. Feeling remembered is especially important for the patient who has been ill over a long period of time.

Some units allow the relative closest to the patient to call at any time. Relatives find the privilege highly supportive, and staff members say the relatives rarely abuse it. Other units have a calling hour in which one phone call per family is allowed. Still others have the policy by which every morning the nurse caring for the patient calls the family and gives them a report on the patient. Regardless of the method, there should be some provision for relatives to talk with the nurses to ask questions about the patient, relay messages, and alleviate their anxiety without having to come to the hospital.

The group setting can be an effective means of providing support to family members. I was involved in establishing a program for relatives of patients in a surgical intensive care unit. When a patient was admitted to the unit, relatives were given a card stating that group discussions for relatives were held twice a week and giving the day, time, and place. When the family members arrived, the nurse leader asked them to introduce themselves. They were told that the purpose of the meeting was to give them an opportunity to share their reactions and feelings to the experience of having a relative in the unit. Information about the condition of specific patients was not given in the meeting, but issues of general concern were discussed and questions were answered. Those meetings were both informative for the staff and supportive to the family members. The relatives who attended the discussions appeared later to be more comfortable at the patient's bedside, developed rapport with and trust in the staff, and felt their needs for information and support were well met. Others have used the technique of group intervention for relatives of patients who had myocardial infarction [34, 39] and relatives of burned patients [10].

Regardless of the method of support (telephone, individual contact, or group contact), the staff's caring about relatives and their reactions diminishes their feelings of neglect or of jealousy about the care and attention the patient is receiving.

Relatives of dying patients may have additional needs and heightened emotional reactions [21, 30]. Some may need help in dealing with their feelings so that they can be available and supportive to their loved one. Most need to hear that it is all right to talk about the patient's illness and coming death with the patient and to show emotion; for example, by crying or hugging the patient. They also need to hear that laughter and joking—a sense of humor—have their place in relating to the patient. Those who say they do not want the patient to know he is dying may need to hear that the patient already "knows" his diagnosis even though he has not been "told." Some relatives need to talk about what they think might occur if indeed the patient were "told" [14]. The anticipated "falling apart" might happen to the relative rather than to the patient. Some relatives who have good rapport with the nurse may ask her opinion about having an autopsy. Referring to the procedure as an "examination after death" rather than as an autopsy may make it more acceptable to family members.

When the patient dies, the relatives need to hear from the physician what occurred and why. While many people are never prepared for the death of a loved one, the relatives of the patient who dies suddenly have had no time at all to prepare for their loss, and they may be in severe shock. They require privacy, support, and an opportunity to talk about and react to their loss. An unaccompanied relative should not leave the hospital alone but should wait with someone from the staff until other arrangements have been made.

After relatives have dealt with their initial feelings in response to the death of a loved one, they may wish to learn and talk more about the circumstances surrounding the patient's death. That need for information and closure may not occur for several days or even weeks. One hospital has attempted to meet relatives' needs for support not only while the patient is hospitalized but also after he has died. During the patient's hospital stay, a chaplain of the relatives' religion visits frequently with family members and establishes a relationship with them. After the patient dies, the chaplain participates in whatever rituals are observed or burial services held. He also makes periodic telephone calls to the relatives. Once a month a religious memorial service is held at the hospital in which all the patients who died that month are remembered. Relatives of those patients, as well as staff members who participated in their care, are invited to attend. At that time many relatives finish their "unfinished business." They approach staff members who cared for their loved one and ask, "How was it?" or, "What did he say?" or, "Did he ask for me?" or, "Did he suffer?" Staff members, too, find the occasion a time to say good-bye in another way to the patient and his family.

The Nurse's Responses

Highly motivated, highly dedicated, highly skilled—those adjectives only partially describe the nurses working in critical care settings. Critical care nursing requires technical competence, knowledge of physiological and psychological responses to injury or illness, ability to make perceptive observations and critical judgments, and, above all, compassion for and commitment to the patient for whom one is caring. At its best, critical care nursing can be rewarding, challenging, satisfying, and fulfilling. At its worst, it can be depressing, demoralizing, frustrating, heart rending.

A wide range of feelings are evoked in the critical care setting—joy, fulfillment, satisfaction, sadness, anger, guilt, fear, and anxiety. Those feelings can be uncomfortable, threatening, and even frightening to the nurse who experiences them, as well as to the nurse who perceives them in her colleagues. Nurses deal with these feelings in a variety of ways. Many of the ways are maladaptive in that they do not diminish the nurse's anxiety, increase her self-esteem, enhance patient care, or foster job satisfaction. The following are examples of maladaptive ways the nurse may handle her feelings:

1. Forming too close bonds with staff with whom she works (cliques) and isolating herself from all others
2. Withdrawing from or avoiding the patient
3. Having no energy after work
4. Having nightmares about work
5. Displacing her feelings on others
6. Denying or repressing her feelings
7. Criticizing the involvement or performance of others

8. Fostering overdependent behavior by the patient
9. "Acting-out" her feelings by calling in ill, coming to work late, drinking excessively, taking drugs, smoking excessively, not completing her assigned responsibilities
10. Focusing on technical aspects of care
11. Exercising excessive control, such as by enforcing rigid visiting hours
12. Expressing an overwhelming urge to run and hide
13. Manifesting hyperkinetic behavior
14. Regressing
15. Rationalizing actions or behavior

Nurses in critical care settings have consistently identified the following as sources of stress in their work that generate many uncomfortable feelings [7, 17, 18, 23, 28, 35, 40, 66]: the patient and his care, nurse-nurse relationships (including relationships with peers, head nurse, supervisor, and nurses on other units), nurse-doctor relationships, families, and the nursing environment itself. In addition, there are some sources of stress peculiar to the individual unit, such as the wearing of gowns and masks in a burn unit, too few ancillary or clerical staff members, and lack of supportive resources.

In each critical care unit, nurses need to continually assess their responses to work as a whole, as well as to particular aspects that are stressful. Sometimes that assessment is done in an informal way, such as over coffee or after the change-of-shift report. Other nursing staffs have regularly scheduled weekly meetings with a resource person or facilitator, as well as informal "as needed" meetings to (1) identify, acknowledge, and share their feelings, (2) clarify and review the reality aspects of the situation, and (3) receive feedback and support. Nurses often feel relieved, replenished, and supported by those meetings and are able to integrate what they have learned and experienced into their care of patients. Often, continuing sources of stress are identified, and as a group the nurses plan how to eliminate or lessen them. Likewise, nurses can collectively identify the satisfying aspects of their work and look for ways to enhance or increase them.

The nurse who can accept her feelings and express them appropriately, who can cope effectively with the stressors she experiences not only feels happier and more satisfied but also can be more open and giving to patients, families, and colleagues.

Summary

Patients' responses to acute illness, the assessment of those responses, and the factors affecting those responses have been discussed. Suggestions have been offered for nursing intervention in general and specific situations. The responses of families and nurses have been discussed briefly.

The critical care nurse has among her objectives the reduction of the patient's anxiety and the promotion of his comfort. Her intervention, therefore, includes learning and fostering that which is essential, desirable, or supportive to the patient. She also learns about and attempts to minimize anything that is demeaning, frightening, anxiety provoking, or nonsupportive to the patient. The nurse does not carry that burden alone; there are numerous resources within the community and hospital setting that can help the nursing staff identify and meet the emotional needs of patients. Yet, the nurse in the critical care setting plays a unique and meaningful role in assessing reactions, identifying needs, and initiating the action to meet those needs. Thus she contributes not only to the patient's immediate comfort but also in some instances to his long-range adjustment to illness [27].

References

1. Abram, H. Psychological aspects of intensive care units. *Med. Ann. D.C.* 43:59, 1974.
2. Adams, M., Hanson, R., Norkool, D., et al. Psychological responses in critical care units. *Am. J. Nurs.* 78:1504, 1978.
3. Adler, M. L. Kidney transplantation and coping mechanisms. *Psychosomatics* 13:337, 1972.
4. Andreasen, N. J. C., Noyes, R., Hartford, C. C., et al. Management of emotional problems in seriously burned adults. *N. Engl. J. Med.* 286:65, 1972.
5. Benoliel, J. Q., and VanDeVelde, S. As the patient views the intensive-care unit and the coronary-care unit. *Heart Lung* 4:260, 1975.
6. Benson, H. *The Relaxation Response.* New York: Morrow, 1975.
7. Bilodeau, C. B. The nurse and her reactions to critical-care nursing. *Heart Lung* 2:358, 1973.
8. Blanchard, E. B., and Young, L. D. Clinical applications of biofeedback training: A review of evidence. *Arch. Gen. Psychiatry* 30:573, 1974.
9. Bolin, R. H. Sensory deprivation: An overview. *Nurs. Forum* 13:240, 1974.
10. Brodland, G. A., and Andreasen, N. J. C. Adjustment Problems of the Family of the Burn Patient. In R. H.

Moos (ed.), *Coping with Physical Illness*. New York: Plenum, 1977.

11. Brown, A. J. Effect of family visits on the blood pressure and heart rate of patients in the coronary-care unit. *Heart Lung* 5:291, 1976.

12. Bruhn, J. G., Thurman, A. E., Jr., Chandler, B. C., et al. Patient's reactions to death in a coronary care unit. *J. Psychosom. Res.* 14:65, 1970.

13. Carson, D. I. Personality Development, Conflict, and Mechanisms of Defense. In G. Usdin and J. M. Lewis, *Psychiatry and General Medical Practice*. New York: McGraw-Hill, 1979.

14. Cassem, N. H. What you can do for dying patients. *Med. Dimensions* 2:29, 1973.

15. Cassem, N. H., and Hackett, T. P. Psychiatric consultation in a coronary care unit. *Ann. Intern. Med.* 75:9, 1971.

16. Cassem, N. H., and Hackett, T. P. Psychological rehabilitation of myocardial infarction patients in the acute phase. *Heart Lung* 2:382, 1973.

17. Cassem, N. H., and Hackett, T. P. Sources of tension for the CCU nurse. *Am. J. Nurs.* 72:1426, 1972.

18. Cassem, N. H., and Hackett, T. P. Stress on the nurse and therapist in the intensive-care unit and coronary-care unit. *Heart Lung* 4:252, 1975.

19. Cassem, N. H., Hackett, T. P., Bascom, C., et al. Reactions of coronary patients to the CCU nurse. *Am. J. Nurs.* 70:319, 1970.

20. Davidson, S. P. Nursing management of emotional reactions of severely burned patients during the acute phase. *Heart Lung* 2:370, 1973.

21. Dracup, K., and Breau, C. Helping the spouses of critically ill patients. *Am. J. Nurs.* 78:51, 1978.

22. Dudley, D. L., Wermuth, C., and Hayne, W. Psychosocial aspects of care in the chronic obstructive pulmonary disease patient. *Heart Lung* 2:389, 1973.

23. Eisendrath, S. J., and Dunkel, J. Psychological issues in intensive care unit staff. *Heart Lung* 8:751, 1979.

24. Engel, G. L. Sudden and rapid death during psychological stress: Folklore or folk wisdom? *Ann. Intern. Med.* 74:771, 1971.

25. Froese, A., Hackett, T. P., Cassem, N. H., et al. Trajectories of anxiety and depression in denying and nondenying acute myocardial infarction patients during hospitalization. *J. Psychosom. Res.* 18:413, 1974.

26. Froese, A., Vasquez, E., Cassem, N. H., et al. Validation of anxiety, depression and denial scales in a coronary care unit. *J. Psychosom. Res.* 18:137, 1974.

27. Garrity, T. F., and Klein, R. F. Emotional response and clinical severity as early determinants of six-month mortality after myocardial infarction. *Heart Lung* 4:730, 1975.

28. Gentry, W. D., Foster, S. B., and Froehling, S. Psychologic response to situational stress in intensive and nonintensive nursing. *Heart Lung* 1:793, 1972.

29. Gentry, W. D., and Haney, T. Emotional and behavioral reaction to acute myocardial infarction. *Heart Lung* 4:738, 1975.

30. Goldberg, E. B. Family tasks and reactions in the crisis of death. *Social Casework* 54:398, 1973.

31. Greene, W. A., Goldstein, S., and Moss, A. J. Psychosocial aspects of sudden death: A preliminary report. *Arch. Intern. Med.* 129:725, 1972.

32. Hackett, T. P. Management of the disruptive patient in the intensive care setting. *Cardiovasc. Nurs.* 11:45, 1975.

33. Hackett, T. P., and Cassem, N. H. Development of a quantitative rating scale to assess denial. *J. Psychosom. Res.* 18:93, 1974.

34. Harding, A. L., and Morefield, M. A. Group intervention for wives of myocardial infarction patients. *Nurs. Clin. North Am.* 11:339, 1976.

35. Hay, D., and Oken, D. The psychological stresses of intensive care unit nursing. *Psychosom. Med.* 34:109, 1972.

36. Hoffman, M., Donckers, S., and Hauser, M. The effect of nursing intervention on stress factors perceived by patients in a coronary care unit. *Heart Lung* 7:804, 1978.

37. Holland, J., and Plumb, M. Management of the serious suicide attempt: A special ICU nursing problem. *Heart Lung* 2:376, 1973.

38. Holmes, T. H., and Rahe, R. H. The social readjustment rating scale. *J. Psychosom Res.* 11:213, 1967.

39. Holub, N., Eklund, P., and Keenan, P. Family conferences as an adjunct to total coronary care. *Heart Lung* 4:767, 1975.

40. Huckabay, L., and Jagla, B. Nurses' stress factors in the intensive care unit. *J. Nurs. Adm.* 9:21, 1979.

41. Kahana, R. J., and Bibring, G. E. Personality Types in Medical Management. In N. E. Zinberg (ed.), *Psychiatry and Medical Practice in a General Hospital*. New York: International Universities Press, 1964.

42. Klein, R. F., Kliner, V. A., Zipes, D. P., et al. Transfer from a coronary care unit: Some adverse responses. *Arch. Intern. Med.* 122:104, 1968.

43. Kornfeld, D. S. The Hospital Environment: Its Impact on the Patient. In R. H. Moos (ed.), *Coping with Physical Illness*. New York: Plenum, 1977.

44. Kübler-Ross, E. *On Death and Dying*. New York: Macmillan, 1969.

45. Langsley, D. G. The Mental Status Examination. In G. Usdin and J. M. Lewis, *Psychiatry and General Medical Practice*. New York: McGraw-Hill, 1979.

46. Lasater, K. L., and Grisanti, D. J. Postcardiotomy psychosis: Indications and interventions. *Heart Lung* 4:724, 1975.

47. Layne, O. L., Jr., and Yudofsky, S. C. Postoperative psychosis in cardiotomy patients. The role of organic and psychiatric factors. *N. Engl. J. Med.* 284:518, 1971.

48. Lown, B., Temte, J. V., Reich, P., et al. Recurring ventricular fibrillation in the absence of coronary heart disease. *N. Engl. J. Med.* 294:623, 1976.

49. Lynch, J. J., Thomas, S. A., Paskewitz, D. A., et al. Human contact and cardiac arrhythmia in a coronary care unit. *Psychosom. Med.* 39:188, 1977.

50. Maron, L., Bryan-Brown, C. W., and Shoemaker, W. C. Toward a unified approach to psychological factors in the ICU. *Crit. Care Med.* 1:81, 1973.

51. Mattsson, E. I. Psychological aspects of severe physical injury and its treatment. *J. Trauma* 15:217, 1975.

52. McCorkle, R. Effects of touch on seriously ill patients. *Nurs. Res.* 23:125, 1974.

53. Minckley, B. B., Burrows, D., Ehrat, K., et al. Myocardial infarct stress-of-transfer inventory: Development of a research tool. *Nurs. Res.* 28:4, 1979.

54. Murray, R. L. E. Assessment of psychologic status in the surgical ICU patient. *Nurs. Clin. North Am.* 10:69, 1975.

55. Nadelson, T. The psychiatrist in the surgical intensive care unit. 1. Postoperative delirium. *Arch. Surg.* 111:113, 1976.

56. Obier, K., and Haywood, L. J. Enhancing therapeutic communication with acutely ill patients. *Heart Lung* 2:49, 1973.

57. Pranulis, M. F. Loss: A factor affecting the welfare of the coronary patient. *Nurs. Clin. North Am.* 7:445, 1972.

58. Rabiner, C. J., Wellner, A. E., and Fishman, J. Psychiatric complications following coronary bypass surgery. *J. Nerv. Ment. Dis.* 160:342, 1975.

59. Rahe, R. H., McKean, J. D., and Arthur, R. J. A longitudinal study of life change and illness patterns. *J. Psychosom. Res.* 10:355, 1967.

60. Rahe, R. H., Romo, M., Bennett, L., et al. Recent life changes, myocardial infarction, and abrupt coronary death. *Arch. Intern. Med.* 133:221, 1974.

61. Ryan, B. J. Biofeedback training: The voluntary control of mind over body and mind. *Nurs. Forum* 14:48, 1975.

62. Sadler, P. D. Nursing assessment of postcardiotomy delirium. *Heart Lung* 8:745, 1979.

63. Scalzi, C. C. Nursing management of behavioral responses following an acute myocardial infarction. *Heart Lung* 2:62, 1973.

64. Segal, J. Biofeedback as a medical treatment. *J. Am. Med. Assoc.* 232:179, 1975.

65. Selye, H. *Stress of life* (2nd ed.). New York: McGraw-Hill, 1976.

66. Simon, N. M., and Whitely, S. Psychiatric consultation with MICU nurses: The consultation conference as a working group. *Heart Lung* 6:497, 1977.

67. Skelton, M., and Dominian, J. Psychological stress in wives of patients with myocardial infarction. *Br. Med. J.* 2:101, 1973.

68. Slay, C. L. Myocardial infarction and stress. *Nurs. Clin. North Am.* 11:329, 1976.

69. Solack, S. D. Assessment of psychogenic stresses in the coronary patient. *Cardiovasc. Nurs.* 15:16, 1979.

70. Spicer, M. R. What about the patient? Patient-centered management in an intensive care area. *Nurs. Clin. North Am.* 7:313, 1972.

71. Stephenson, C. A. Stress in critically ill patients. *Am. J. Nurs.* 77:1806, 1977.

72. Thomas, S. A., Lynch, J. J., and Mills, M. E. Psychosocial influences on heart rhythm in the coronary-care unit. *Heart Lung* 5:746, 1975.

73. Van Bree, N. S. Sexuality, nursing practice, and the person with cardiac disease. *Nurs. Forum* 14:397, 1975.

74. Woods, N. F., and Falk, S. A. Noise stimuli in the acute care area. *Nurs. Res.* 23:144, 1974.

V. The Critically Ill Adult with Pulmonary Problems

How do body-mind-spirit concepts affect our ideas about death?

We have seen how these considerations lead to the concept of nurse-patient unity and integration. Because of this unity, what affects the patient in some way affects the nurse. Patient experiences are *always* nurse experiences.

But what of death?

Answers to this question, if not ineffable, will be personal. One personal resolution of this problem was voiced by Whitman:

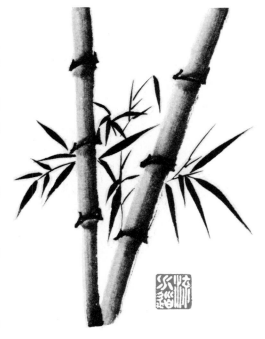

What do you think has become of the young and old
    men?
And what do you think has become of the women and
    children?

They are alive and well somewhere,
The smallest sprout shows there is really no death,
And if ever there was it led forward life, and does not
    wait at the end to arrest it,
And ceas'd the moment life appear'd.

All goes onward and outward, nothing collapses,
And to die is different from what any one supposed, and
    luckier.

Walt Whitman
"Song of Myself"

Acute Respiratory Failure

Martha L. Tyler

14

Acute respiratory failure (ARF) is defined as a rapidly occurring inability of the lungs to maintain adequate oxygenation of the blood with or without impairment of carbon dioxide (CO_2) elimination. The nurse should note that hypercarbia is not necessary to the definition of acute respiratory failure. ARF is present when there is hypoxemia *with or without* hypercarbia. Keeping that definition of ARF clearly in mind results in an ordering of priorities of management and therapy that best protects the patient from permanent damage, disability, or death due to tissue hypoxia in vital organs. The definition is also important because many nurses do not consider the possibility of ARF unless there is gross alteration in ventilation. Closer observation of patients with acute hypoxemia would reveal that many patients actually have an increased minute ventilation due to hypoxic stimulation of respiratory chemoreceptors.

The arterial blood gas levels that have been used to objectively define ARF are an arterial oxygen tension (PaO_2) of 50 mm Hg or less with or without an elevation of the arterial CO_2 tension ($PaCO_2$) to 50 mm Hg or more [18, 28, 29].

When the major blood gas derangement is an increase in $PaCO_2$ the descriptive term *acute ventilatory failure* is used. Acute ventilatory failure will, of course, result in acute respiratory failure if the level of ventilation is so decreased that hypoxemia occurs. *Pulmonary failure* is sometimes used to indicate respiratory failure due specifically to lung disorders. *Pulmonary insufficiency* is another term that is also used as a synonym for acute respiratory failure. Pulmonary insufficiency is properly defined, however, as altered function of the lung that produces clinical symptoms, such as dyspnea [31].

Objectives

Acute respiratory failure occurs as a sequel to a wide variety of diseases and trauma as well as to primary disturbances in the respiratory system. If respiratory failure is to be prevented, controlled, and treated, the critical care nurse must be constantly alert to the possibility of acute respiratory failure in all patients. With a patient in respiratory failure, the nurse will be able to identify precipitating factors, evaluate signs and symptoms, and anticipate complications.

Achieving the Objectives

To achieve the objectives the nurse should be able to:

1. Define acute respiratory failure.
2. List and explain the physiologic basis of the signs and symptoms of acute respiratory failure.
3. Describe four major pathophysiological mechanisms of hypoxemia.
4. Describe two pathophysiological mechanisms of hypercarbia.
5. Compare and contrast the effects of oxygen therapy in four mechanisms of hypoxemia.
6. Describe methods of facilitating secretion clearance.
7. Describe a safe suctioning technique.
8. Assess the success or failure of therapy by interpretation of arterial blood gas values.

How to Proceed

To develop an approach to acute respiratory failure the nurse should:

1. Analyze a case study for the manifestations of ARF.
   A. What is the cause of ARF in the patient?
   B. What are the clinical signs and symptoms?
   C. What is the most likely pathophysiological cause of the patient's hypoxemia?

2. Make an assessment of the patient's status and draw up a nursing problem list.
3. Outline short-term and long-term goals in regard to the problems identified.
4. Review the anatomy and physiology of the respiratory system, with emphasis on how malfunction or disruption of any component of the system—lung parenchyma, airways, chest wall, central nervous system, respiratory muscles (diaphragm and intercostal), and chemoreceptors—affects gas exchange.

Case Study

Ms. C., a 59-year-old woman, was admitted to the hospital with a diagnosis of deteriorating chronic obstructive pulmonary disease. She had been seen in the hospital's chest clinic the day before her admission. Her complaints included increased weakness, fatigue, loss of appetite, and decreased activity tolerance due to shortness of breath. She also felt that her secretion clearance was not as effective as usual despite the use of inhaled bronchodilators and steam.

Two weeks before her admission she had attended the clinic, where a recent, sudden weight gain (from 88 to 95 pounds in two weeks) and ankle edema (3+) were noted. While her neck veins were not distended, chest film showed some evidence of pulmonary artery dilatation. Pulmonary heart disease (cor pulmonale) was suspected, and the patient was given digoxin (0.25 mg/day), along with furosemide (40 mg) and potassium chloride (2 teaspoons) daily. On the day before her admission, Ms. C. basically felt no better despite the institution of those medications. Her weight, however, was down to her usual 87 pounds. It was decided that she should be admitted to the hospital the following day for (1) reevaluation of her current medication regimen, (2) the possible institution of continuous (home) oxygen therapy, (3) a more thorough work-up of her peripheral edema and increased shortness of breath (SOB), and (4) evaluation of her decrease in appetite.

Past Medical History

Ms. C. has a long history of chronic cough with sputum production and progressively worsening shortness of breath. For four years she has been followed in the chest clinic for those symptoms. The results of her pulmonary function test are shown in Table 14-1.

Ms. C.'s cough has been productive of approximately one cup of grayish mucoid sputum per day; the cough is worse in the morning, but it continues throughout the day. Periodically, she wakes at night with paroxysms of coughing and sputum production. She has a total of 80 to 90 "pack years" of smoking, and continues to smoke about one pack per day. Until recently she had been able to keep up with her daily housework and only had dyspnea after walking three level blocks. Now, even minimal exertion, such as walking a few hundred feet, makes her so short of breath that she must

Table 14-1
Ms. C.'s Pulmonary Function Test Values

Test	% Predicted	% Predicted After Bronchodilator
Vital capacity (VC)	52	68
Residual volume (RV)	216	
Total lung capacity (TLC)	111	
Forced expiratory flow 25–75% (FEF25–75%)	8	23
Forced expiratory volume in 1 second (FEV₁)	24	28
FEV₁/VC ratio	35 (normal > 76%)	
Nitrogen elimination rate	9 (normal < 2.5%)	
Blood gases		
pH 7.48		
PaCO₂ 42 mm Hg		
HCO₃⁻ 28 mEq/L		
PaO₂ 51 mm Hg		
SaO₂ 86%		
Base excess + 2.8 mEq/L		

sit down. Her usual medications and therapies have been theophylline (150 mg) and bronchodilator inhalation every four hours, and steam inhalation twice daily after the bronchodilator therapy (to loosen secretions). Last year a course of steroids was tried but Ms. C. showed no significant improvement. Antibiotics have been used as necessary for purulent sputum.

Ms. C. broke her hip several years ago. She has had no operations other than one for hip pinning, she reports no allergies, and the results of the review of systems were unremarkable. She has been treated in the dermatology clinic for five years for psoriasis, mainly of the scalp; the condition is controlled with fluocinolone acetonide.

Family and Social History
Ms. C's mother is alive and well at 85; her father died at age 30 of unknown cause; one sister died from toxemia during childbirth; two brothers are alive, one has arthritis. She was married (once), but she has been separated from her husband for 12 years. She has no children. Ms. C. has not worked in the past six years. Her financial support comes from Medicaid and Supplemental Security Income programs. In the past she worked as a beauty operator and a mail order clerk. She sees her mother and one of her brothers daily; the brother lives directly across the street from her and helps her with shopping and heavy household tasks.

Clinical Presentation
Ms. C. was ambulatory when she was admitted to a general medical nursing unit. She was in "no acute distress." The arterial blood gas values, determined on her admission, were a pH of 7.48, a PaCO₂ of 41 mm Hg, a bicarbonate (HCO₃⁻) level of 30 mEq/L, and a PaO₂ of 27 mm Hg on room air. Apparently, those blood gas values were not believed, because a half hour later a second blood gas analysis was made, again on room air, with the following results: pH, 7.48, PaCO₂, 45 mm Hg, HCO₃⁻, 33 mEq/L, and PaO₂, 36 mm Hg. On confirmation of the extent of her hypoxemia, Ms. C was transferred to the medical intensive care unit (MICU). After the institution of oxygen therapy at 2 liters per minute, by nasal cannula, the pH was 7.48, PaCO₂, 39 mm Hg, HCO₃⁻, 28 mEq/L, and PaO₂, 47 mm Hg.

Physical Examination
Physical examination revealed a temperature of 36.5°C and blood pressure (120/70) and a pulse (88) without postural change. The head, eyes, ears, and throat were remarkable only for bluish membranes. Ms. C. wears glasses. She has clubbing of the fingers and toes and 1 to 2+ ankle edema. Her weight was 87 pounds. Her lungs had markedly decreased breath sounds; there were no rales, wheezes or rhonchi. The diaphragm was low and did not move on percussion. There was increased tympany on percussion over the lung fields. A cardiovascular examination showed no venous distention and no murmurs.

Laboratory Data
The pertinent laboratory data were:

Hematocrit	63%	Sodium	116
White blood count	9800	Potassium	4.4
Blood urea nitrogen	8	Chloride	70
Glucose	151	CO₂	36

The chest film showed hyperinflation compatible with chronic obstructive pulmonary disease (COPD). There were no acute infiltrates. The ECG showed a normal sinus rhythm at a rate of 80 beats per minute. The axis was positive at 102°; P-pulmonale and loss of R-wave forces in leads V_2 through V_6 were present.

Hospital Course
Ms. C. was transferred to the MICU because of extreme hypoxemia, for monitoring, and for institution of a vigorous bronchial hygiene routine. The routine consisted of the inhalation of a bronchodilator from a gas-powered, small volume nebulizer, followed by the inhalation of warm moist air from a heated nebulizer. Those procedures were followed by postural drainage and chest percussion to facilitate secretion removal. The treatments were done every three hours throughout the day and night in the hope of (1) improving oxygenation by bringing the patient to optimal ventilation-

perfusion status and (2) preventing the need for assisted ventilation. Oxygen therapy was increased to 3 liters per minute, resulting in a pH of 7.48, a $PaCO_2$ of 54 mm Hg, a HCO_3^- of 39 mEq/L, and a PaO_2 of 76 mm Hg. A subsequent and final adjustment of flow rate to 2.5 liters per minute resulted in a pH of 7.47, a $PaCO_2$ of 52 mm Hg, a HCO_3^- of 37 mEq/L, and a PaO_2 of 56 mm Hg. A sputum Gram stain showed numerous polymorphonuclear leukocytes with many gram-negative diplococci. Ms. C. was given penicillin (250 mg four times a day). A phlebotomy was done (300 ml whole blood), lowering her hematocrit to 53%. The furosemide and digoxin had been discontinued on her admission. With the bronchial hygiene regimen she was able to bring up large amounts of sputum, and her general condition improved markedly. After three days, she was moved from the MICU to a general medical nursing unit. Her bronchial hygiene treatments were reduced to four times a day because of a decrease in sputum production. But her oxygenation did not improve despite what appeared to be optimal therapy. Therefore it was decided that she would require continuous oxygen therapy to control and/or prevent further episodes of right heart failure and to possibly permit her to be more active.

During her hospitalization, Ms. C. was examined by the physical medicine and rehabilitation service and was started on a graduated exercise tolerance program that she was to continue as an outpatient. She was told how to do postural drainage at home and arrangements were made for oxygen to be delivered to her house. The visiting nurse service was contacted to supervise her medications, help in the use of continuous home oxygen therapy, and instruct a family member in chest percussion therapy to be done while the patient was in postural drainage positions. One week after her admission, Ms. C. was discharged ambulatory with oxygen and, once again, information about the benefits of stopping smoking.

Reflections

Gas exchange is basic to life. Therefore the critical care nurse must be completely familiar with the components of normal respiratory function. There is absolutely no way a critical care nurse can be ignorant of the pathophysiological processes that lead to disturbed respiratory function and be a "good nurse." When the lungs fail, the whole body fails. The patient knows this as well as do the medical and nursing personnel caring for him. One needs only to have been held under water once by a too aggressive friend to know the panic that occurs when one's ventilation is disrupted. The nurse can simulate the discomfort of the patient who has pulmonary emphysema or asthma by inhaling a large breath and exhaling only part of the breath, keeping the chest fixed at a partially inflated position. The technique simulates air trapping. The nurse should then breathe from the new end-expiratory position. To do so is uncomfortable and anxiety producing. In fact, it can cause feelings of panic. Respiratory patients are often described as "crabby" and "difficult." Is it any wonder?

The care of patients with acute respiratory failure is often carried out amid high anxiety. Often, the nurse is not capable of relieving the patient's distressing symptoms. That gives her feelings of guilt and failure. Added to the nurse's anxiety is the patient's fear of death. A thorough understanding of (1) the nature of the patient's problems and his expectations in regard to their resolution, (2) the goals of the medical therapy as related to the problem, and (3) a *reasonable* assessment of the possible outcome will help make the nurse feel less anxious in caring for the patient with acute respiratory failure. When the nurse is not anxious, her energies can be more fully directed to making the patient comfortable. Understanding the normal physiology of the lungs and the pathophysiology of ARF allows the nurse to care for the patient in a way that best supports the physiological and psychological processes that are needed for adequate gas exchange.

Physiology

A brief review of respiratory physiology is presented in the following paragraphs. It is designed to organize the nurse's knowledge and to enable her to recall pertinent facts promptly. For a more comprehensive discussion of the many factors that interact in normal respiratory function, the reader is directed to Chapter 9 and to the references at the end of this chapter [5, 6, 8, 9, 24, 26, 32, 41].

Functions of the Lung

The major purpose of the respiratory system is to provide O_2 for the combustive process of metabolism and to remove CO_2, the waste product of metabolism, from the body. The secondary functions of the respiratory system are acid-base balance, speech, the expression of emotion (laughing, crying, sighing), and, in a relatively minor way, to maintain body water and heat balance.

Ventilation

To provide O_2 and remove CO_2, air must be moved in and out of the lungs. The movement of air is properly termed ventilation, and the term respiration refers to the exchange of gases [31]. Ventilation can occur without effective gas exchange taking place. That is the case in severe ventilation-perfusion inequality or intrapulmonary shunt. It is also true that only a minimal amount of gas exchange (respiration) can occur without ventilation. In such a situation (ventilatory arrest) gas exchange can occur only at the rate allowed by passive diffusion of the gas molecules. Life can be sustained for only four to six minutes under those circumstances. Therefore ventilation and respiration are practically synonymous in the clinical setting although they are defined differently and theoretically are separate concepts.

Movement of air in and out of the lung requires coordinated action of the diaphragm and intercostal muscles against a relatively fixed chamber, the rib cage. In addition, the pathway for air flow—the upper and lower (large and small) airways—must be patent. The alveolar-capillary membrane is the site of gas exchange. It must be of adequate size and normal structure for normal diffusion of O_2 and CO_2 into and out of the blood.

Control of Respiration

The muscular pump of respiration is controlled by the central nervous system (CNS), which, in turn, responds to the metabolic needs of the body. Voluntary control of ventilation is also possible and can override metabolically set respiratory rates, resulting, at times, in grossly abnormal blood gases. The CNS receives its input from central and peripheral chemoreceptors that respond to (1) $PaCO_2$ and (2) PaO_2 and pH, respectively. The ventilatory response to those humoral stimulants is determined by their combined effect. For example, a decrease in PaO_2 increases ventilation, which, in turn, decreases $PaCO_2$ and raises the pH, thus limiting the overall response to hypoxia. Under usual circumstances, CO_2 is the primary determinant of minute ventilation, and the PaO_2 and pH are secondary determinants.

Perfusion

Another major factor in normal respiration is perfusion of the lung by blood with normal hemoglobin in adequate amounts. Not only must blood flow through the lungs, there must also be a reasonable match between ventilation and perfusion. There are different gradients for perfusion and ventilation in the lung due to the different effects of gravity on lung tissue and blood. That phenomenon results in wasted ventilation at the top of the lung and excess perfusion at the bottom [41]. Nevertheless, overall there is a fairly good match of ventilation and perfusion, resulting in normal gas exchange.

Measurement of Lung Function

The definitive physiological indicator of pulmonary function is the arterial blood gas values. It is vital that the critical care nurse know the range of normal values for PaO_2, $PaCO_2$, and pH and be able to interpret blood gas test results. Priority must always be given to the PaO_2 value because hypoxemia is the major cause of the morbidity and mortality associated with respiratory dysfunction. Next, in order of importance, is the pH. A high $PaCO_2$ level is a problem only if it is causing, or is associated with, severe acidemia.

Other tests of pulmonary function are measurements of (1) lung volumes, (2) flow rates, and (3) the distribution and diffusion of gases within and through the lungs. The patient's test results are compared to "normal" values established for people of the same sex, age, and height. The pattern and degree of deviation from normal and the improvement (if any) following bronchodilator therapy are indications of the pathology that underlies any changes observed [8].

Pathophysiology

Mechanisms of Hypoxemia and Hypercarbia

From the definition of acute respiratory failure it is evident that any cause of hypoxemia or hypercarbia is potentially a cause of acute respiratory failure. There are four major mechanisms causing hypoxemia: (1) hypoventilation, (2) diffusion (or gas transfer) impairment, (3) ventilation-perfusion ($\dot{V}A/\dot{Q}$) inequality, and (4) right-to-left shunt. The two mechanisms that produce hypercarbia are (1) hypoventilation and (2) $\dot{V}A/\dot{Q}$ inequality [41]. In clinical practice, hypoventilation is the major cause of hypercarbia; however, $\dot{V}A/\dot{Q}$ inequality does add to the CO_2 retention seen in the later stages of diseases associated with low $\dot{V}A/\dot{Q}$ ratios.

In addition to the four primary causes of a low PaO_2, a fifth cause of hypoxemia is possible. At high altitudes the inspired O_2 tension (PIO_2) is reduced owing to the lower barometric pressure. The reduction results in a low alveolar O_2 tension (PAO_2), which in turn lowers the PaO_2 and can ultimately result in hypoxemia. PIO_2 is also reduced when the person breathes mixtures with a low oxygen concentration. That circumstance occurs infrequently and is usually the result of an error in valving systems during the administration of anesthestic gases.

The four major causes of hypoxemia are briefly reviewed in the following paragraphs. (For additional information, the reader is referred to Chap. 36.)

HYPOVENTILATION

Hypoventilation means that the amount of new or fresh gas reaching the alveoli is reduced. The reduction causes both hypoxemia and hypercarbia. The degree of hypercarbia is an index to the degree of hypoventilation, and it is readily assessed by arterial blood gas analysis. The $PaCO_2$ reflects the balance between CO_2 production by the body cells and its elimination by the lung. Therefore an increase in $PaCO_2$ (hypercarbia) indicates alveolar hypoventilation. Conversely, a decrease in $PaCO_2$ (hypocarbia) occurs during alveolar hyperventilation.

Hypoxemia caused by hypoventilation alone is usually not severe [42]. The reason for that is evident from the alveolar gas equation. The following example shows that when the $PaCO_2$ rises 20 mm Hg from a normal 40 mm Hg, the PAO_2 falls to only 72 mm Hg.

$$PAO_2 = PIO_2 - \frac{PaCO_2}{R}$$

$$= 147 - \frac{60}{0.8}$$

$$= 147 - 75$$

$$= 72 \text{ mm Hg}$$

The PaO_2 is lower, of course (see the discussion of the alveolar-arterial gradient in Chap. 36), but it would not be in the range of ARF (less than 50 mm Hg) unless, in addition to hypoventilation, one of the other causes of hypoxemia is present. Compared to the effect the un-

compensated respiratory acidosis $(PaCO_2$ of 60 mm Hg) will have on the pH, it can be seen that the major concern in a patient with acute hypoventilation is likely to be a severe acid-base imbalance rather than severe hypoxemia.

Hypoventilation often occurs as a result of dysfunction or disease outside the respiratory system. The lung tissue itself may be normal. When hypoventilation is the cause of hypoxemia, it is easily corrected by the administration of small amounts of O_2 or correction of the ventilatory defect. Patients with pure hypoventilation who require support with a mechanical ventilator can often be ventilated with room air. However, when hypoventilation is combined with another cause of hypoxemia, such as $\dot{V}A/\dot{Q}$ inequality or shunt, the hypoxemia will be much greater than would be anticipated with hypoventilation alone. In mixed causes of hypoxemia, the response to O_2 therapy depends primarily on whether the additional problem is one of shunt or $\dot{V}A/\dot{Q}$ inequality.

Examples of frequent causes of hypoventilation are brain and spinal cord injuries, respiratory center depression caused by narcotics, barbiturates, and tranquilizers, and neuromuscular diseases such as Guillain-Barré syndrome (see Chap. 28), myasthenia gravis, or muscular dystrophy. In addition, some patients with increased work of breathing let their $PaCO_2$ drift up (hypoventilate) rather than do the work necessary to keep their $PaCO_2$ normal. Still other patients appear to have a primary lack of sensitivity to increased $PaCO_2$ and/or hypoxemia as stimuli to ventilation. Consequently they fail to maintain normal arterial blood gas levels. Another less frequently recognized cause of hypoventilation and ARF is extreme obesity. The mechanism(s) of hypoventilation in the obese patient is not known for certain, but the increased work of breathing is probably contributory.

DIFFUSION (GAS TRANSFER) IMPAIRMENT

Diffusion is a passive process due to the pressure gradient for the gases from the alveolus to the pulmonary capillary in the case of O_2 and from the capillary to the alveolus in the case of CO_2. Loss of lung surface area or thickening of the alveolar-capillary surface are the two processes associated with gas transfer impairment. That is so because diffusion is directly proportional to the surface area available and inversely proportional to the distance the gases have to travel.

Also, in the liquid phase, diffusion is proportional to the solubility of the gas divided by the square root of its molecular weight.

Diffusion impairment means that equilibration between the pulmonary capillary blood and the alveolar gas has not occurred. Under resting conditions it takes only about one third (0.25 second) of the total time the blood is in the capillary (0.75 second) to equilibrate; therefore, there is time for equilibration in reserve [41]. Even during severe exercise, when contact time is reduced to about 0.33 second, gas equilibration is still assured. Thus, diffusion abnormalities, although undoubtedly a factor in many diseases in which loss of surface area or thickening of alveolar-capillary membrane is present, are almost never a physiological cause of hypoxemia at rest [4, 9, 42]. People with such diseases as diffuse interstitial fibrosis, collagen diseases, such as scleroderma and lupus erythematosus, or severe emphysema (with loss of alveolar-capillary tissue) may have a decreased diffusion capacity during exercise. But those diseases are also associated with $\dot{V}A/\dot{Q}$ inequalities. Therefore, it is difficult to say how much hypoxemia should be attributed to $\dot{V}A/\dot{Q}$ inequality and how much to diffusion limitation.

Hypoxemia caused by diffusion impairment can be corrected by small increases in the inspired O_2 concentration and can always be completely corrected with 100% O_2. That is so because the increase in PaO_2 increases the pressure gradient for diffusion, which overcomes the increased resistance to diffusion due to thickened alveolar membrane. Loss of diffusing surface, on the other hand, greatly increases the amount of ventilation necessary to maintain O_2 content, but it does not cause hypoxemia until the patient is unable to do the necessary work of breathing. Overall, diffusion impairment usually has little clinical significance in the critical care unit.

VENTILATION-PERFUSION INEQUALITY

When ventilation and blood flow to lung units are mismatched, both oxygenation and carbon dioxide elimination are affected. Although there are many possible combinations of $\dot{V}A/\dot{Q}$ ratios, the ratio that produces hypoxemia is when ventilation is less than perfusion in many areas of the lung. In the opposite case, when perfusion is less than ventilation, much of the effort expended in the ventilatory portion of gas exchange is wasted. The ventilation is described as wasted or deadspace. Unless very severe, an increased

$\dot{V}A/\dot{Q}$ ratio does not cause hypoxemia or hypercarbia. It does, however, cause a significant increase in the amount of ventilation necessary to maintain the $PaCO_2$ within normal range.

"Good" regions of the lung, where ventilation and perfusion are evenly matched, cannot compensate for "bad" regions, where ventilation is poor but blood flow continues (low $\dot{V}A/\dot{Q}$ units). That concept is easy to understand when it is recalled that oxygen is carried in the blood mainly in combination with hemoglobin. Blood from areas of perfect $\dot{V}A/\dot{Q}$ can never have an arterial oxygen saturation (SaO_2) of more than 100% and therefore cannot make up for blood coming from areas of low $\dot{V}A/\dot{Q}$, where little or no increase in PaO_2 (and therefore no increase in SaO_2) over the venous level takes place. For example, if blood that is only 75% saturated (that corresponds to a PaO_2 of 40 mm Hg–venous blood) mixes with the blood that is 100% saturated, the overall saturation for the blood returning to the left side of the heart has to be less than 100%. The actual saturation level depends on what portion of the total cardiac output was passing low $\dot{V}A/\dot{Q}$ units. For example, in the example just given if 75% of the cardiac output goes to low $\dot{V}A/\dot{Q}$ units and 25% to normal units, the result would be a saturation of approximately 80% (PaO_2 of 45 mm Hg).

The role of low $\dot{V}A/\dot{Q}$ units in the production of hypoxemia is well recognized. It is less well known, however, that those same units cause hypercarbia. Since poorly ventilated units are unable to contribute to the elimination of the CO_2 from blood passing those units, blood leaving those units still have near venous CO_2 levels. Why is it then, that at least in early stages of some diseases (e.g., chronic obstructive pulmonary disease), hypoxemia is often seen without an elevation in the $PaCO_2$? It is because when CO_2 retention due to $\dot{V}A/\dot{Q}$ inequality develops there is an immediate response to the elevated $PaCO_2$, and alveolar ventilation promptly increases. The increase in alveolar ventilation results in a decrease of $PaCO_2$, usually to normal. The increase in ventilation also affects the PaO_2, which is raised slightly, but it cannot return to normal because, as explained, even overventilated lung units cannot raise the saturation of the blood above 100% [41].

Some patients with $\dot{V}A/\dot{Q}$ abnormalities do not make the extra effort required to increase their ventilation when $\dot{V}A/\dot{Q}$ inequality causes the $PaCO_2$ to increase. Or, perhaps for a time the patients do increase the ventilation, but later, with further increases in work of breathing, they abandon the effort, with the result that CO_2 retention develops. Why some patients let their $PaCO_2$ and hypoxemia increase rather than expend the energy required to increase their alveolar ventilation is not known. Central neurogenic and peripheral chemoreceptor respiratory drives are different from patient to patient. Patients are sometimes categorized as "pink puffers" or "blue bloaters." It is theorized that pink puffers have strong respiratory drives and consequently keep their PaO_2 and $PaCO_2$ at near normal levels despite large increases in work of breathing and ventilation. Blue bloaters are thought to allow their $PaCO_2$ to rise and their PaO_2 to fall owing to a lower-than-normal respiratory drive (central hypoventilation). Blue bloaters become hypoxemic sooner and with equal or less derangement in pulmonary function than do pink puffers because blue bloaters are relatively insensitive to changes in blood gas levels.

Oxygen therapy results in almost complete elimination of hypoxemia in $\dot{V}A/\dot{Q}$ inequality. To determine the full effect of the therapy, one must allow time for the poorly ventilated areas of the lung to equilibrate to the new alveolar gas levels before the arterial blood gas levels are determined. That is the basis for the traditional 15 minute "wait" before drawing blood for arterial blood gas tests after the institution of, or a change in, O_2 therapy. When the patient is given 100% O_2, the widened alveolar-arterial gradient seen in $\dot{V}A/\dot{Q}$ inequality will be eliminated.

SHUNT

In broad terms, "shunt" refers to any blood that reaches the arterial side of the heart without passing through ventilated regions of the lungs. Shunts can be extrapulmonary, but those of interest here are intrapulmonary shunts. Anatomic shunts exist in the lung, but the most common cause of clinically important pulmonary shunting are areas of the lung that are totally unventilated but continue to be perfused. Two clinical examples are areas of consolidated pneumonia and/or atelectasis. Shunts can be thought of as the worst possible $\dot{V}A/\dot{Q}$ inequality that one can imagine, but because the response of shunts to O_2 is so characteristic, it is useful to consider shunt separately from $\dot{V}A/\dot{Q}$ inequality. One hundred percent O_2 breathing does not (cannot) obliterate the widened alveolar-arterial gradient seen in shunt. Shunt is the only situation in which O_2 is ineffective in reducing the gradient. Even a lung with many low $\dot{V}A/\dot{Q}$ areas will eventually reach a normal alveolar-arterial O_2 gra-

dient if enough time is given for O_2 to wash into the poorly ventilated areas of the lungs. In contrast, even when the ventilating gas has an FIO_2 of 1.0, oxygen cannot be taken into blood that passes *totally* unventilated areas of the lung.

SUMMARY

The four causes of hypoxemia—hypoventilation, diffusion impairment, $\dot{V}A/\dot{Q}$ inequality and shunt—constitute the major pathophysiological aspects of acute respiratory failure. The four causes of hypoxemia do not always occur separately. For instance, the patient with chronic obstructive pulmonary disease who has pneumonia with consolidation will have lung areas that are totally unventilated (shunt) due to the pneumonia, as well as areas of $\dot{V}A/\dot{Q}$ inequality due to his underlying COPD.

Oxygen Transport

While hypoxemia and hypoventilation are major factors in acute respiratory failure, the critical care nurse must not forget that O_2 transport to the tissues also requires an adequate supply of hemoglobin that has normal O_2-carrying characteristics as well as an adequate cardiac output for distribution of oxygenated blood to the tissues. An example is anemia, which is a particularly serious problem in the patient who has a low PaO_2 due to lung disease. In such a patient, both his O_2 carrying capacity and his ability to load O_2 are impaired. If he also has a low cardiac output (circulatory failure) tissue O_2 delivery is even more impaired. Such a patient requires skillful management in a critical care unit.

Diagnosis

The diagnosis of acute respiratory failure is simple. Arterial blood gas levels give immediate objective information about the ability of the lungs to provide O_2 and remove CO_2 from the arterial blood. The degree and possible mechanisms of ARF are immediately apparent from the direction and amount the PaO_2 and/or the $PaCO_2$ deviates from normal. If the $PaCo_2$ is elevated, hypoventilation is at least a partial cause of the hypoxemia. Calculation of the alveolar gas equation permits a quick estimate to be made of the contribution of hypoventilation to any hypoxemia present. If hypoventilation is not the sole cause of hypoxemia, the alveolar-arterial oxygen gradient will be widened more than would be expected due to CO_2 retention alone. Widened alveolar-arterial gradients can be caused by either shunt or low $\dot{V}A/\dot{Q}$ ratios. The next step is to note the response of the PaO_2 to O_2 therapy. That allows one to separate shunt from $\dot{V}A/\dot{Q}$ abnormalities as the cause of hypoxemia. One hundred percent O_2 breathing is not needed to get a clinical indication of the presence of shunt. If the PaO_2 remains below 100 mm Hg when the inspired O_2 fraction is 0.3–0.4, shunted blood is contributing significantly to the hypoxemia [1, 2].

Clinical Signs and Symptoms of ARF

More important than the mechanics of making the diagnosis is the ability to recognize the clinical signs and symptoms of ARF. ARF cannot be diagnosed unless its presence is suspected. The clinical signs and symptoms of ARF fall into three categories: pulmonary, cardiovascular, and neurological.

PULMONARY SIGNS AND SYMPTOMS

Pulmonary symptoms can be misleadingly mild or even absent. Dyspnea, usually assumed to be a classic symptom of ARF or hypoxemia, is often absent despite marked hypoxemia. Remember the blue bloater just described. The blue bloater seldom complains of dyspnea or "looks" short of breath because he may have a blunted respiratory drive. The reverse can also be true—marked dyspnea (with close to normal blood gas levels) is often observed in the pink puffer. Dyspnea is a subjective symptom that appears to correlate more frequently with disturbances in the stretch receptors of the lung and/or with a person's feeling that the work of breathing is inappropriate to the situation than with blood gas disturbances [4]. To illustrate, people expect to be "short of breath" after having run hard to catch a bus, and they seldom consider the feeling a particularly noxious one. However, patients who have increased work of breathing even while at rest (e.g., during an asthmatic attack) interpret the symptom as undesirable and uncomfortable even though their minute ventilation during the attack may be less than that required to run for the bus.

Cough and sputum production may increase, or they may decrease. A sudden decrease in sputum production in the patient who has chronic bronchitis is often a more serious indication of impending ARF than is a sudden increase in cough and sputum production. Decreased sputum expectoration may indicate that secretion retention is occurring, which in turn will cause hypoxemia due to an increase in $\dot{V}A/\dot{Q}$ inequality. The retained secretions fill the airways and decrease air flow, creating areas of low $\dot{V}A/\dot{Q}$ throughout the lung.

CARDIOVASCULAR SIGNS AND SYMPTOMS

The presence or absence of cardiovascular signs of acute respiratory failure is determined by the amount of tissue hypoxia present. When arterial oxygenation falls, the usual response is to increase cardiac output in an attempt to bring more oxygen to the myocardium and other vital tissues. Therefore, tachycardia is often a sign of hypoxemia. Dysrhythmias may develop if hypoxemia is severe and cardiovascular compensation is inadequate to prevent myocardial hypoxia. Both supraventricular and ventricular arrhythmias occur as frequently in ARF complicating COPD as they do in myocardial infarction [20, 36]. Changes in the transmembrane action potential in cardiac conducting tissue can result from hypoxemia, increased $PaCO_2$ and changes in pH (not associated with changes in $PaCO_2$). In this setting dysrhythmias can be caused by a change in automaticity of the conducting tissue or the development of a reentry circuit, or both [19].

Coldness of the extremities is another cardiovascular sign of hypoxemia. Peripheral vasoconstriction is a homeostatic mechanism by which blood is shunted from the extremities to vital organs. In contrast (but equally homeostatic), cerebral arteries dilate as hypoxemia and hypercarbia increase, often resulting in the symptom of headache. If acidemia occurs in addition to hypoxemia, peripheral, renal and coronary artery dilatation result. Diaphoresis is seen in this setting [28].

Cyanosis is an unreliable sign of hypoxemia. Many patients in ARF are severely hypoxemic without evidence of cyanosis. Cyanosis does not appear until at least five grams of hemoglobin per 100 ml blood are reduced (deoxygenated). That means that even with severe hypoxemia the anemic patient may not appear cyanotic, whereas the patient with polycythemia may appear cyanotic when his PaO_2 is normal. Added to those physiological variables is the subjective nature of the observation. Central cyanosis is a more reliable sign of low PaO_2, but it also may be a result of low cardiac output independent of a low PaO_2. The principle should be to investigate (by analyzing an arterial blood gas sample) any patient with generalized cyanosis while remembering that the *absence* of cyanosis does not guarantee normoxemia.

NEUROLOGICAL SIGNS AND SYMPTOMS

Central nervous system signs of ARF include restlessness, agitation, confusion, somnolence, and coma. Headache is also frequent, as noted. Sometimes families report subtle personality changes in the patient as the first sign of decreasing cerebral oxygenation. Far too often those nonspecific signs of cerebral dysfunction are misinterpreted. Judging from nursing and medical actions often taken when patients are described as restless, agitated, and confused, one would assume that the most reasonable physiological cause of those symptoms was a low blood tranquilizer level rather than a low blood oxygen level. Any patient exhibiting changes in mentation should be carefully assessed. ARF and all the many other causes of neurological dysfunction should be ruled out before tranquilizers are given.

The Clinical Setting of ARF

The ability to diagnose ARF is related to the diagnostician's index of suspicion about certain clinical settings. A review of the many clinical problems and diseases known to be associated with ARF (Table 14-2) should alert the critical care nurse to the fact that almost every patient in the unit is a candidate for acute respiratory failure.

Treatment

Emergency Care

The priorities set for the treatment of acute respiratory failure are based on the severity and duration of hypoxemia and/or hypercarbia. If the PaO_2 is less than 20 mm Hg, death due to cardiorespiratory arrest will usually occur within minutes. Oxygen must be administered immediately. Do not be concerned about low-flow versus high-flow oxygen in any patient, even the patient with COPD. Cerebral and myocardial hypoxia causes death in minutes. If hypoventilation is also present or becomes a problem during therapy, ventilation must be assisted. Resuscitation

Table 14-2

Clinical Problems Associated with Acute Respiratory Failure

Central nervous system (CNS) depression
  Drug overdose—self-administered or iatrogenic
    Barbiturates, narcotics, tranquilizers
    Uncontrolled high-flow oxygen therapy
  CNS infection
  Cerebral vascular accidents
  Head injury
Chest wall and diaphragm dysfunction
  Trauma
    Flail chest, diaphragmatic rupture, phrenic nerve transection
  Defect in neuromuscular transmission
    Disease states
      Myasthenia gravis, muscular dystrophy, Guillain-Barré syndrome, poliomyelitis, spinal cord injury, amyotrophic lateral sclerosis, multiple sclerosis, botulism, tetanus
    Drug effects or side effects
      Aminoglycosides, curarelike drugs
  Thoracic surgery
  Subdiaphragmatic abscess
Restrictive defect
  Pulmonary: generalized
    Interstitial fibrosis
    Infiltrative lung disease
    Diffuse atelectasis (ARDS)
    Pulmonary edema (cardiogenic or noncardiogenic, ARDS)
  Pulmonary: localized
    Pleural space alteration (pneumothorax, hemothorax, effusion, empyema)
    Pulmonary embolism
    Pneumonia
    Local atelectasis (focal, segmental, lobar)
  Extrapulmonary
    Kyphoscoliosis
    Ascites
    Intestinal distention (ileus)
    Obesity
    Pain
Obstructive defect
  Upper airway
    Severe maxillofacial injury
    Neoplasia
    Laryngeal edema
    Prolapsed tongue
    Foreign objects
  Lower airway
    Foreign objects
    Tracheal stenosis or collapse
    Bronchoconstriction
    Retained secretions, mucus plugging
    Bronchial wall edema
    Airway collapse
    Neoplasia

without oxygen is, of course, less satisfactory than resuscitation using a well-fitting bag-mask resuscitator with an O_2 reservoir, but time should not be wasted getting one [30, 33]. Mouth-to-mouth resuscitation should be begun immediately. On the other hand, if O_2 is available and attempts at mouth-to-mouth breathing are unsuccessful (or endotracheal intubation attempts are prolonged), the highest possible concentration of oxygen should be delivered to the patient's nose and mouth. Diffusion of gases is possible even if ventilation is not taking place, provided that the upper airway is not occluded by foreign objects, edema, or a prolapsed tongue.

If hypoxemia is severe, there is almost always an increase in $PaCO_2$ due to hypoventilation caused by hypoxia of the respiratory centers or $\dot{V}A/\dot{Q}$ inequality. Acute CO_2 retention causes profound acidemia. In addition, lactic acid is produced during anaerobic metabolism, which always occurs when hypoxemia is severe and prolonged. The result is a combined metabolic and respiratory acidosis. Correction of the ventilation and O_2 defects will reverse the acid-base abnormalities. When correction of hypercarbia and hypoxemia is delayed, bicarbonate can be administered to control acidemia. One can "buy time" in hypercarbia but not in hypoxemia—the hypoxemia must be corrected with supplemental O_2 or improved ventilation.

Principles of Management

Once life-threatening alterations in blood gas tensions have been controlled or if the presenting situation is less critical, the general rules for the management of ARF are: (1) maintain or provide an open airway, (2) maintain an adequate PaO_2 at the lowest possible fraction of inspired oxygen, (3) maintain acid-base status within clinically acceptable range, usually a pH of 7.35–7.45, (4) support cardiac output as necessary, (5) assure adequate hemoglobin, and (6) give appropriate therapy to the underlying disease process [5, 7, 10, 18, 28, 32, 33, 37].

Blood gas levels are not only diagnostic in acute respiratory failure but are also the basis of monitoring the efficacy of treatment and resolution of the underlying disease process. The cause of hypoxemia in ARF is often bronchospasm, inflammatory edema of the airway, or retained secretions. Those conditions are usually at least partially reversible and require relatively simple methods of treatment. With therapy

there is often an improvement in oxygenation; however, the *primary* treatment for hypoxemia is the administration of oxygen.

Oxygen Therapy

The basic rule for O_2 administration is to use the lowest amount of O_2 enrichment (FIO_2 or liter flow) that produces an acceptable SaO_2. Adhering to that rule prevents pulmonary O_2 toxicity, a time- and dose-related phenomenon. Oxygen toxicity should never occur as a result of O_2 therapy in the treatment of hypoxemia due to hypoventilation or $\dot{V}A/\dot{Q}$ inequality since in those situations hypoxemia can be corrected with low FIO_2. The patients most at risk of pulmonary oxygen toxicity are those with large intrapulmonary shunts (severe pneumonia, ARDS) who are much less responsive to O_2 administration [1, 6, 42].

A patient's response to a particular FIO_2 can be used to roughly determine the amount of shunt present or, conversely, if the percentage of shunt is known, to predict the FIO_2 required to obtain, if possible, an adequate PaO_2 [2, 26].

For example, when the PaO_2 is less than 100 mm Hg on an FIO_2 of 0.3–0.4—around 6 Lpm (liters per minute) by nasal cannula, a significant part of the hypoxemia is due to shunt. Also, if an increase in FIO_2 to 1.0 produces no change in PaO_2, the shunt is 50% (or greater) [2]. Despite the threat of O_2 toxicity, sometimes very high inspired O_2 tensions are required and *must be used* to preserve life until the underlying process is resolved.

Unfortunately, maneuvers such as continuous positive airway pressure (CPAP) or positive end expiratory pressure (PEEP) that are helpful in reducing FIO_2 in ARDS (see Chap. 17) are seldom helpful in COPD because of the differences in the underlying disease process. However, it is unusual for the COPD patient to require a high FIO_2, although it may be required when the patient has a severe pneumonia. Resolution of the pneumonia usually occurs quickly enough that oxygen toxicity is not a concern even though a high FIO_2 must be used for a while.

Nearly complete O_2 saturation (90–94%) is desirable but that goal is not possible in some patients. The patient with preexisting CO_2 retention who "can't" or "doesn't" respond to increased CO_2 levels is often, but not always, the patient who retains CO_2 when given O_2 [4, 10, 17, 18, 28, 29]. Such a patient relies on hypoxemic stimuli to drive ventilation instead of

CO_2. In most people, the hypoxic stimulus to ventilation is not very strong until the PaO_2 falls below 50 to 60 mm Hg [9, 24, 26, 41]. When high concentrations of O_2 are administered to patients depending on a low PaO_2 to stimulate ventilation, the PaO_2 may be raised past their threshold of hypoxic stimulation. Blunting of the hypoxemic drive occurs, alveolar ventilation falls, and CO_2 retention increases. The problem is avoided in almost all COPD patients with CO_2 retention by the administration of low doses of O_2. A safe starting point is two Lpm by nasal cannula or 24% to 28% O_2 by Venturi mask. The PaO_2 need only be raised to 60 mm Hg since that level will provide a saturation of about 90% to 92%.

Careful monitoring of blood gases during the institution of O_2 therapy in the COPD patient with chronic CO_2 retention is mandatory, but often the benefits gained from the relief of hypoxemia (e.g., increased mental ability and therefore increased cooperation with treatment) offset the increases in $PaCO_2$ (unless this causes significant acidemia).

Oxygen therapy must *never* be discontinued abruptly if unacceptable acidemia due to CO_2 retention does occur. That is so because the elevation in the arterial CO_2 level causes an elevation in the alveolar CO_2 level. When O_2 enrichment of the alveolar gas is stopped, the PAO_2 and, consequently, the PaO_2, falls to a new low because of the higher $PACO_2$. Overall the patient's hypoxemia will be worse than it was before O_2 therapy was started. Ventilation should increase when the PaO_2 falls, but before the increased ventilation can blow off the CO_2, there is a potentially very dangerous period when hypoxemia is worse.

The following, a theoretical example taken from Ms. C.'s case study, illustrates the mechanism just described.

Oxygen	PaO_2 (mm Hg)	$PaCO_2$ (mm Hg)
Room air	27	41
Nasal cannula: 3 Lpm	76	54
Room air	14*	54

* Calculated from the alveolar gas equation with R = 1.

When oxygen was given at 3 Lpm, the $PaCO_2$ rose 13 mm Hg (from 41 to 54 mm Hg). Although an increase in ventilation can be expected when O_2 therapy is discontinued, the $PACO_2$ does not change

rapidly because of the large body stores of CO_2. Consequently, the alveolar PO_2 must fall by at least the amount of the increase in $PACO_2$ [42]. Therefore, unless there had been a reduction in Ms. C.'s original alveolar-arterial gradient of approximately 70 mm Hg (from 97 to 27 mm Hg), the PaO_2 must be at least 13 mm Hg lower than the original value of 27 mm Hg, resulting in a PaO_2 of 14 mm Hg.

OXYGEN DELIVERY METHODS

Oxygen delivered by nasal cannula results in a varied FiO_2, depending on the flow rate used and the patient's rate, depth, and pattern of inspiration. Rapid, gasping inspirations result in a lower inspired FiO_2, at the same O_2 flow rate, than that achieved during a "quieter," less tachypneic, respiratory pattern. That is so because more room air will dilute the inspired O_2 in the first situation than it will in the second [1, 7, 10]. Despite the variations in FiO_2 obtained with the cannula, it is usually possible to achieve satisfactory levels of oxygenation in the majority of hypoxemic patients. In addition, it is easier for the patient to cough out secretions, eat, and communicate when a cannula is used rather than a mask [16, 22, 29]. Mouth breathing is not a contraindication for using a nasal cannula to deliver low-flow O_2. Studies have shown that the inspired PO_2 is at least as high in "mouth breathers" as in those breathing through the nose (if not higher) [22, 32]. Nasal O_2 catheters are capable of delivering approximately the same FiO_2 as are cannulas. But because of associated discomfort and the possibility of misplacement into the esophagus and resultant gastric distention, catheters should be avoided. A possible candidate for their use is the restless patient who frequently dislodges his cannula [1].

In cases in which a cannula does not provide adequate oxygenation, the use of O_2 masks or even intubation is required. Those modes of delivery are usually necessary when shunt is the underlying mechanism of hypoxemia. Examples of disease processes causing shunt are pneumonia and ARDS (see Chap. 17). When a mask is used, the O_2 flow must be high enough to wash exhaled CO_2 from the mask; usually flows greater than 6 Lpm are necessary. The adequacy of the washout can, of course, be monitored by following the arterial $PaCO_2$. A mask with a reservoir bag (rebreathing or nonrebreathing) provides higher concentrations of O_2 than does the simple mask because it has 100% O_2 "stored" in the reservoir. For efficient use of such a mask, the O_2 flow into the mask must be high enough to prevent the reservoir bag from collapsing on inhalation [5, 6, 32]. When a patient requires extremely high percentages of O_2, no external system is stable enough to guarantee consistent O_2 therapy, and intubation becomes necessary, even though assisted ventilation may not be contemplated. Heated, moisturized, and O_2-enriched gas can then be delivered *directly* to the lungs from a nebulizer. Most nebulizers are equipped with a diluter that, without modification, provides 40, 70, or 100% O_2 via a large-bore tubing and a T-piece adapter attached to the endotracheal or tracheostomy tube. It should be remembered that at high concentrations of O_2 (70 to 100%), little air is entrained through the diluter. Thus the patient's inspiratory flow rates may exceed the flow capabilities of the nebulizer. In a tachypneic patient, the inspiratory flow rate may sometimes be in the range of 50 or 60 liters per second, and so even running the nebulizer at flush will not prevent dilution of the inspired gas with room air drawn in from the open (exhalation) side of the T-connector. The dilution can be controlled by adding tubing on the exhalation side of the T-piece. The extra tubing is filled with gas from the constant flow of the nebulizer and acts as an O_2 reservoir [38]. It does not act as dead space because the constant flow of gas through the tubing from the nebulizer also flushes exhaled CO_2 out of the tubing and prevents the patient from rebreathing the CO_2.

Adjunctive Therapies

Elimination of retained secretions often results in improved oxygenation. However, some methods used to clear airway secretions are themselves associated with falls in PaO_2. It has been known for several years that transtracheal suctioning can cause serious hypoxemia [12]. It is less well known, however, that nasotracheal (NT) suctioning causes similar falls in oxygenation. Those falls have been observed to occur despite a preoxygenation regimen (100% oxygen via bag–mask resuscitator) that prevents hypoxemia when used in conjunction with endotracheal (ET) suctioning [27]. NT suctioning probably interrupts ventilation longer than does ET suctioning because of difficulty in passing the catheter through the larynx, coughing and gagging, and the patient's tendency to hold his breath when his airway is being manipulated. To eliminate or lessen some of those problems

a nasopharyngeal airway is useful in guiding the catheter more consistently to the glottis and in protecting the nasal mucous membranes from repeated trauma [40]. The airway is lubricated with anesthetic jelly before it is inserted; it can be left in place for several days. In addition to the use of the nasopharyngeal airway and preoxygenation, the patient's usual O_2 therapy should not be discontinued; in fact, it should be temporarily increased during suctioning so that any air he gets contains a high percentage of O_2.

One of the common fallacies in the management of secretion problems in ARF is that once a patient is intubated there need be no more concern about secretion retention because suctioning is "easy" and "effective" when an artificial airway is in place. *A good cough is always better than suctioning.* Suction catheters reach only the central airways, frequently only the right side. Also, cough is less effective when the patient is intubated because it is impossible to generate the high intrathoracic pressures needed to produce the high expiratory flow rates required to blast mucus out of the lung. For those reasons, intubation for secretion control should always be a last resort unless a patient is completely obtunded and/or has no gag reflex and must have his airway protected.

Postural Drainage

When intubation is required, drainage of secretions from peripheral airways is facilitated by changes in position that elevate the usually gravity-dependent portions of the lung; e.g., the posterior basal segments of both lower lobes of the supine patient. Probably the best drainage of those segments occurs when the patient lies prone with his hips raised or with his bed in the Trendelenburg position; however, it has been noted that the horizontal prone position also results in improved oxygenation [11]. Changes in amount and location of air in the lung at end expiration (FRC) are thought to be mechanisms associated with the increased PaO_2 seen in the prone position, as well as with the increased flow of secretions from those areas.

Frequent position changes to prevent pressure sores have long been a part of nursing management. That frequent position changes are effective also in secretion management and gas exchange in the lung is less well known. However, "routine" position changes or "routine" postural drainage may also be associated with falls in oxygenation. Falls in PaO_2 were seen in almost all the subjects receiving routine postural drainage in two studies done in seriously ill patients [15, 21, 39]. One explanation for the fall in PaO_2 is that when a patient with a unilateral lung infiltrate (e.g., the patient with single lobe pneumonia) is turned so that the affected lung is dependent, an increase in venous admixture and a consequent fall in the PaO_2 can be predicted [43]. That is so because blood flow is increased in the dependent lung owing to gravity, and therefore more blood passes the area of the infiltrate, where there is poor or no ventilation, resulting in an increase in venous admixture. This physiologically predictable result was seen in one of the studies just cited [21, 39]; however, since some of the subjects with evenly distributed infiltrates also had falls in PaO_2, other mechanisms of hypoxemia must also have been operative. Since drainage is definitely not facilitated when a lung with a unilateral infiltrate is dependent, use of this position should be minimized. Simply increasing the FIO_2 may not overcome the problem since the fall in PaO_2 is due mainly to increased intrapulmonary shunt, which, by definition, is unresponsive to O_2 therapy. Patients who have signs of hypoxemia or who are significantly distressed during postural drainage or when they are in a particular position should have their blood gases analyzed while in that position.

Commentary on Case Study

The general principles of nursing and medical management of ARF were discussed in the sections on treatment. Some of those principles are illustrated in the following discussion of the case study presented earlier in the chapter. Therapy for ARF is always adapted to the particular cause of the failure so this case highlights those aspects of ARF therapy pertinent to patients with underlying COPD.

Pulmonary Function Tests

Ms. C.'s pulmonary function tests were typical of severe COPD, with striking decreases in FEV_1, FEV_1/VC, an FEF25–75%. The apparent restriction noted in the vital capacity (51% of predicted) is not true restrictive lung disease since the total lung capacity is 111% of predicted. Although restrictive and obstructive diseases can occur together, more often the small vital capacity seen in COPD is a function of the marked increase in the residual volume (in

this case 216% of predicted) due to air trapping. Further evidence of air trapping is seen in the nitrogen elimination rate, which is prolonged. Slow washout of nitrogen from the lung indicates that there are areas of lung with very poor communication with the outside [8]. These areas of low $\dot{V}A/\dot{Q}$ are also responsible for the patient's hypoxemia.

The FEV_1 is also greatly reduced. Patients with this degree of air flow obstruction have a very limited ability to increase their ventilatory rate to meet increased metabolic demands. They cannot be hurried through procedures; simple activities of daily living, such as bathing, require more time than usual because the patient must pace himself [37].

Arterial Blood Gases

Without any knowledge of Ms. C.'s history, one would conclude from the evaluation of her blood gas levels, both on admission and those reported earlier in conjunction with her pulmonary function tests, that Ms. C. had mild alkalemia due to metabolic alkalosis. Diuretics taken without sufficient chloride replacement result in metabolic alkalosis and a compensatory elevation of the $PaCO_2$. However, Ms. C. also has severe air-flow obstruction (FEV_1 24% of predicted), so it is possible that the HCO_3^- level is elevated in compensation for a *usually* more elevated $PaCO_2$. Hyperventilation often occurs because of discomfort to the patient while blood is being drawn for tests. Ms. C.'s $PaCO_2$ may have been suddenly lowered to 42 mm Hg, resulting in a temporary increase in pH to the limits of the normal range on the alkalemic side. Because Ms. C.'s admission electrolyte tests showed a low chloride value, a combination of those two mechanisms seems to be the cause of her alkalemia.

Electrolyte Imbalance

The low serum sodium and chloride values are apparently secondary to diuretic therapy and an inappropriate antidiuretic hormone level. Hyponatremia was resolved by fluid restriction during part of Ms. C.'s hospital stay. Potassium chloride supplement had been ordered when digoxin and diuretics were started two weeks before admission (but may not have been taken). In addition, there can be an obligatory loss of Cl^- ion when HCO_3^- is retained to maintain ionic balance.

Metabolic alkalosis from any cause is a particular problem in COPD because the normal compensatory mechanism for metabolic alkalosis is CO_2 retention. When CO_2 retention is already present in COPD, the additive effects of the two processes can cause particularly severe decreases in PaO_2 due to the increased $PaCO_2$. Ms. C. could not possibly afford to breathe less and retain CO_2 to balance her metabolic alkalosis. Any further decrease in ventilation would have increased her already life-threatening hypoxemia (PaO_2 of 27 mm Hg).

Signs and Symptoms of ARF in COPD

The nonspecific symptoms of decompensation seen in Ms. C.—increased shortness of breath, difficulty with raising sputum, decreased effectiveness of cough, generalized malaise and anorexia—are typical of the patient with chronic obstructive disease [17, 29]. It is often difficult to know when to hospitalize a patient with longstanding COPD because it is difficult to assess what aspects of the disorder will be amenable to therapy. Also, prolonged and gradual deterioration of oxygenation blunts the usual symptoms of hypoxemia. Some patients develop an amazing tolerance for "anaerobia." Ms. C., however, had indications of right ventricular failure, which is potentially reversible, in addition to the nonspecific complaints just mentioned. She was admitted to the hospital so that her condition could be stabilized and she could be treated with O_2 if necessary. Her admission blood gas levels were remarkable in that she had a strikingly low PaO_2 (27 mm Hg). According to an admission note, 45 minutes before blood for the test was drawn, the patient said that it was hard for her to breathe and that she had been unable to eat solid food of any kind. Despite her condition, Ms. C. was ambulatory. That amazing adaptation to tissue hypoxia is possible only in slowly developing hypoxemia. Oxygen administration was finally started after the severe hypoxemia was confirmed. Ms. C. had clubbing, an unusual finding in COPD even with long-standing hypoxemia. When clubbing is present, it is usually associated with cancer or bronchiectasis. The latter is more likely in Ms. C.'s case.

Polycythemia

Polycythemia is one of the adaptations to hypoxemia. It occurs as a result of hypoxic stimulation of the erythropoietin system, which in turn stimulates red cell production by the bone marrow. Ms. C. had a hematocrit of 63%. That was one reason she was able to "tolerate" the extremely low PaO_2. An increase in the amount of hemoglobin enables more O_2 to be carried per unit volume of blood. However, the increased "thickness" of the blood also causes increased resistance to blood flow, a particularly negative side effect in patients who also have increased pulmonary vascular resistance due to hypoxic vasoconstriction of the pulmonary capillary bed [23]. The two mechanisms produce an additive effect in terms of cardiac work, particularly for the right ventricle. For those reasons, Ms. C. had a phlebotomy, which in conjunction with hydration, lowered her hematocrit to 53%. A similar reduction in hematocrit would also have occurred, although more gradually, after the institution of O_2 therapy alone, because the stimulus for excessive production of red cells would have been removed.

Cardiovascular Compensation and Decompensation

Remarkably, Ms. C.'s extremely low PaO_2 was not accompanied by an increase in her cardiac rate. An increase in cardiac output, usually by increasing rate, is one of the mechanisms that prevent tissue hypoxia in the face of extreme arterial hypoxemia. Failure of the heart rate to increase is unusual with such a degree of hypoxemia; however, in Ms. C.'s case pulmonary hypertension and right ventricular failure may have resulted in a "fixed" cardiac output [4, 14, 29].

Pulmonary Heart Disease

Pulmonary heart disease (cor pulmonale) is a frequent complication of hypoxemic COPD [3, 13, 14]. The primary therapy for right heart failure is relief of pulmonary artery hypertension. Increased pulmonary vascular resistance due to alveolar hypoxia is the major mechanism of pulmonary hypertension [23]. In this setting, pulmonary hypertension is usually responsive to increases in PaO_2. If therapy such as inhalation of a bronchodilator and postural drainage improves ventilation enough to normalize the alveolar gases, cor pulmonale is reversible. If therapy is not successful, supplemental O_2 must be given to raise the PaO_2 to control hypoxic vasoconstriction [25, 35]. It is of interest that Ms. C. had no signs or symptoms of left heart failure. The two sides of the heart can fail independently [3, 14]. Ms. C.'s digoxin therapy was discontinued on her admission to the hospital; the efficacy of digoxin therapy when right heart failure is the only cardiac problem has been questioned [4, 13, 14]. In addition, digoxin is well known for its toxicity when the myocardium is hypoxic.

Anorexia and Weight Loss

Anorexia and weight loss are frequent complaints in severe chronic obstructive pulmonary disease [17, 37]. The symptoms are apparently due to poor digestion associated with hypoxemia of the digestive tract. Recent true tissue weight loss was actually difficult to document in Ms. C.'s case because her weight fluctuated frequently owing to right heart failure and diuretic therapy. Her anorexia and general well-being improved after O_2 therapy was instituted.

Inability to Perform Activities of Daily Living

The scaling and flaking associated with psoriasis, particularly of her scalp, was of great concern to Ms. C. In the two weeks before her admission, shortness of breath and decreased exercise tolerance made it impossible for her to wash her hair often enough to control the psoriasis. One of the ways Ms. C. judged her well-being was by her ability to control her psoriasis. Because she was unable to control it, she felt particularly disabled at the time of her admission. That is probably one reason she agreed to hospitalization —Ms. C. was usually stoic about her respiratory symptoms.

Respiratory Care

Ms. C. was given intensive bronchial hygiene therapy designed to improve ventilation and oxygenation by enhancing secretion clearance. The regimen included inhalation of a bronchodilator from a gas-driven, small-volume nebulizer, followed by inhalation of warm humidified air from a heated nebulizer, followed by chest physical therapy (percussion and coughing) in various postural drainage positions. Positions suitable for general drainage of the right and left posterior lung bases were used since no localized infiltrate was seen on the chest film.

It has been customary to administer bronchodilator

therapy with an intermittent positive pressure breathing (IPPB) device; however, there is no evidence that that method of delivery produces greater bronchodilatation than having the patient inhale the medication during a voluntary deep breath [34]. In addition, Ms. C. has significant air trapping (residual volume = 216% of predicted). Her problem is getting the air *out* of the lungs. She does not need assisted inhalation. But that does not mean, of course, that no patient needs IPPB assistance. The modes of therapy are selected on the basis of the pathophysiology to be treated.

Oxygenation

Oxygen therapy at 2 Lpm resulted in a PaO_2 of 47 mm Hg. Later the O_2 flow rate was adjusted to 2.5 Lpm, resulting in a PaO_2 of 56 mm Hg. At that level of oxygenation there was also an increase in CO_2 retention (15 mm Hg) to 54 mm Hg. However, it was not associated with a fall in pH. Ms. C. also had a metabolic alkalosis that may have fortuitously acted as a buffer for the CO_2 retention. The point to be stressed, however, is that CO_2 retention should be tolerated unless there is a significant fall in pH (usually pH < 7.3), since the benefits of improved oxygenation outweigh the disadvantages of mild acidemia. During Ms. C.'s hospitalization, it was decided that even with optimum therapy her hypoxemia would not be resolved and that she met the criteria for continuous home O_2 therapy. Those criteria are: (1) the patient's right ventricular failure is controlled by O_2 therapy, (2) the patient's exercise tolerance is increased by O_2 therapy, and (3) the patient's polycythemia is controlled by O_2 therapy.

Antibiotic Therapy

Pencillin (250 mg four times a day by mouth) was used to treat the gram-negative diplococci seen on Gram stain. The most common organisms seen on culture in COPD are *Diplococcus pneumoniae* and *Hemophilus*. But in this setting, patients are often treated without waiting for culture results. In addition, as the *Hemophilus* strains are frequently not type B, penicillin is a satisfactory choice although the use of broad-spectrum antibiotics, such as tetracycline and ampicillin, is more common.

Discharge Planning

The visiting nurse service was contacted for supervision of Ms. C.'s medications, including the patient's use of O_2 in the home and her secretion clearance. The visiting nurse also instructed the patient's brother in percussion and postural drainage.

Ms. C.'s therapy on discharge was a bronchial hygiene program consisting of the use of (1) an inhaled bronchodilator, (2) inhaled steam for moisturizing the airways, followed by (3) postural drainage (with percussion when possible). Theophylline was given (one tablet four times a day) and O_2 therapy was continued at 2 Lpm for as much of 24 hours as was practical. To facilitate continuous O_2 therapy, the patient was given 50 feet of extension tubing to enable her to walk freely around her house.

Adjusting to chronic O_2 therapy is difficult for most patients. Wearing nasal cannula, or "prongs," is a sign of their disease that cannot be disguised. And storing five or six O_2 tanks in the home is often a problem. Ms. C.'s hospitalization was successful not only because she got "better" but also because she accepted her need for continuous O_2 therapy. Also, Ms. C. and her family understood the proper use of O_2 *as a medication.*

General Comments

Ms. C.'s case clearly shows that acute respiratory failure need not always be associated with ventilatory failure. In fact Ms. C.'s $PaCO_2$ was always below 50 mm Hg until the institution of O_2 therapy. Mild rises in $PaCO_2$ during controlled O_2 therapy are usually well tolerated by patients with COPD; however, acute ventilatory failure with significant acidemia can occur if O_2 is administered in an uncontrolled fashion and/or if blood gases are not monitored carefully.

Did Ms. C. need to be admitted to a critical care unit? Careful monitoring is required when a patient has acute hypoxemia. Dysrhythmias are as likely to occur in patients with ARF as in patients with acute myocardial infarction [19, 20]. Also, the frequency and intensity of the treatments needed for sputum clearance are sufficient indications that such a patient should be treated in a critical care unit until her condition is stable [5, 6, 29]. On a general nursing floor, it is seldom possible to provide patients with intensive assistance in chest physiotherapy and postural drainage, bronchodilator therapy, and inhaled moisture therapy at frequent intervals.

Nursing Orders

OBJECTIVE NO. 1
Maintain patent upper and lower airways.

1. Encourage and help the patient to cough and clear mucus.
2. Use suctioning as needed to stimulate cough and clear the upper and lower (central) airway secretions.
3. Position the comatose patient in a way that helps prevent aspiration.
4. Change the position of the ventilated patient every hour to promote the clearance of secretions from the peripheral airways.
5. Monitor the patient's breath sounds regularly to assess: (a) his need for suctioning (indicated by rhonchi), (b) any development of or change in wheezing, (c) the sudden absence of breath sounds (for example, pneumothorax), and (d) any development of or change in rales* (for example, pulmonary edema).

OBJECTIVE NO. 2
Maintain adequate oxygenation.

1. Observe the patient constantly for changes in mental, cardiac, or pulmonary status that indicate hypoxemia: confusion, restlessness, disorientation, headache, unconsciousness, tachycardia, peripheral vasoconstriction, diaphoresis, central cyanosis, hypotension, increased dyspnea.
2. Monitor O_2 therapy equipment to make sure that the ordered liter flow or concentration is maintained.
3. Observe the patient regularly for the correct placement of O_2 cannula, catheter, mask, or T-piece connection.
4. Observe the ventilator pressure dial to assure the maintenance of PEEP.
5. Assume responsibility for recording blood gas values, *including* the corresponding FIO_2 or liter flow, PEEP level, patient position (right/left lateral, sitting, supine, prone).

*Also termed crackles [31].

6. Check the patient's hemoglobin and/or hematocrit level.

OBJECTIVE NO. 3
Maintain adequate ventilation.

1. Note and record regularly the character of respirations (labored, shallow, pursed lips).
2. Record the objective measures of ventilation: $PaCO_2$, rate, minute ventilation.
3. Support the patient in the position that best facilitates his respiration.
4. Turn and reposition the patient frequently to promote ventilation of the dependent areas of the lung.
5. Prevent unnecessary increases in work of breathing by limiting or requiring the patient to be active only to his tolerance level and by keeping him stable emotionally (e.g., by explaining procedures to him and reassuring him as needed).

OBJECTIVE NO. 4
Maintain mechanical ventilation when required.

1. Check all ventilator settings for accuracy and the *alarm system* every hour.
2. Assure *constant* observation of patients who are apneic without ventilatory support (patients with head injury or paralysis due to trauma, disease, or curarelike drugs).
3. Monitor and record changes in the patient's response to mechanical ventilation.

OBJECTIVE NO. 5
Maintain normal cardiovascular function.

1. Gather objective data regarding the patient's cardiovascular status from central venous pressure and central and peripheral arterial lines; make sure the tracings are accurate and the catheters are patent before recording data.
2. Monitor the patient's cardiovascular functioning by regular assessment in regard to cyanosis, edema, neck vein distention, respiratory rales (crackles), urinary output, pulse amplitude, and blood pressure.

3. Observe the cardiac monitor for any dysrhythmias, particularly during suctioning and postural drainage; make a rhythm strip when dysrhythmias occur.

OBJECTIVE NO. 6
Maintain adequate drug therapy.

1. Administer drugs at scheduled intervals.
2. Make sure that the patient receives the entire dose ordered when drugs are given by IPPB or nebulizer.
3. Monitor and record the patient's response to therapy (e.g., decreased wheezes, improved breath sounds or improved FEV_1) when monitoring bronchodilator therapy.

OBJECTIVE NO. 7
Maintain adequate hydration.

1. Observe the patient's skin, mucous membranes and sputum viscosity for changes indicative of dehydration.
2. Record total system intake and output (oral, parenteral, urinary, upper and lower gastrointestinal tract).
3. Weigh the patient and record his weight daily.
4. Monitor the equipment used to hydrate the respiratory tree (humidifiers and nebulizers) to make sure they are working properly.

OBJECTIVE NO. 8
Maintain adequate nutrition.

1. Monitor the patient's weight for true tissue weight loss.
2. Provide the dyspneic patient with small, frequent, high-calorie, high-protein feedings.
3. Institute supplemental (gastric or parenteral) feedings *early*.
4. If the patient has trouble swallowing after prolonged intubation, arrange for a speech therapist to help him reestablish the proper swallowing sequence.

OBJECTIVE NO. 9
Prevent loss of physical function.

1. Use proper positioning for the bedfast patient, using foot boards when necessary.
2. Make sure that the patient receives (or does) full range of motion exercises as indicated.
3. Help the patient to become ambulatory as soon as possible; ventilatory support can be maintained with a self-inflating bag (oxygen enriched) for short walks.
4. Lift the patient to a chair if he cannot walk.

OBJECTIVE NO. 10
Maintain psychological function.

1. Provide sensory stimulation for the comatose patient.
2. Limit sensory stimulation for the dyspneic patient.
3. Support the coping mechanisms the patient has developed.
4. Reduce stress and anxiety by talking often with the patient about procedures, dates, times, place, and names of staff.
5. Provide uninterrupted periods for visits from his family.

References

1. Beall, C. E., Braun, H. A., and Cheney, F. W., Jr. *Physiologic Bases for Respiratory Care.* Missoula, Mont.: Mountain Press, 1974.
2. Benatar, S. R., Hewlett, A. M., and Nunn, J. F. The use of iso-shunt lines for control of oxygen therapy. *Br. J. Anaesthesiol.* 45:711, 1973.
3. Bhargava, R. K. *Cor Pulmonale (Pulmonary Heart Disease).* Mt. Kisco, N.Y.: Futura, 1973.
4. Burrows, B., Knudson, R. J., and Kettel, L. J. *Respiratory Insufficiency.* Chicago: Year Book, 1975.
5. Burton, G. G., Gee, G. N., and Hodgkin, J. E. (eds.). *Respiratory Care: A Guide to Clinical Practice.* Philadelphia: Lippincott, 1977.
6. Bushnell, S. S. *Respiratory Intensive Care Nursing.* Boston: Little, Brown, 1973.
7. Campbell, E. J. M. The management of acute respiratory failure in chronic bronchitis and emphysema. *Am. Rev. Respir. Dis.* 96:626, 1967.
8. Cherniack, R. M. *Pulmonary Function Testing.* Philadelphia: Saunders, 1977.
9. Cherniack, R. M., Cherniak, L., and Naimark, A. *Respiration in Health and Disease* (2nd ed.). Philadelphia: Saunders, 1972.
10. Cherniack, R. M., and Hakimpour, K. The rational use of oxygen in respiratory insufficiency. *J.A.M.A.* 199:146, 1967.
11. Douglas, W. W., Rehder, K., Beynen, F. M., et al. Improved oxygenation in patients with acute respiratory failure: The prone position. *Am. Rev. Respir. Dis.* 115:559, 1977.
12. Fell, T., and Cheney, F. W. Prevention of hypoxemia during endotracheal suction. *Ann. Surg.* 174:24, 1971.
13. Ferrer, M. I. Cor pulmonale (pulmonary heart disease): Present-day status. *Am. Heart J.* 98:657, 1975.
14. Fishman, A. P. Chronic cor pulmonale. *Am. Rev. Respir. Dis.* 114:775, 1976.
15. Gormezano, J., and Branthwaite, M. A. Effects of physiotherapy during intermittent positive pressure ventilation. *Anesthesiology* 27:258, 1972.
16. Green, I. D. Choice of method for administration of oxygen. *Br. Med. J.* 3:593, 1967.
17. Hodgkin, J. E., Balchum, O. J., Kass, I., et al. Chronic obstructive airway disease: Current concepts in diagnosis and comprehensive care. *J.A.M.A.* 232:1243, 1975.
18. Hudson, L. D. The acute management of the chronic airway obstruction patient. *Heart Lung* 3:93, 1974.
19. Hudson, L. D. Significance of arrhythmias in acute respiratory failure. *Geriatrics* 31:61, 1976.
20. Hudson, L. D., Kurt, T. L., Petty, T. L., et al. Arrhythmias associated with acute respiratory failure in patients with chronic airway obstruction. *Chest* 63:661, 1973.
21. Huseby, J. S., Hudson, L. D., Stark, K., et al. Oxygenation during chest physiotherapy. *Chest* 70:430, 1976.
22. Kory, R. C., Bergmann, J. C., Sweet, R. D., et al. Comparative evaluation of oxygen therapy techniques. *J.A.M.A.* 179:767, 1962.
23. Lloyd, T. C., Jr. Effect of alveolar hypoxia on pulmonary vascular resistance. *J. Appl. Physiol.* 19:1086, 1964.
24. Murray, J. F. *The Normal Lung.* Philadelphia: Saunders, 1976.
25. Neff, T. A., and Petty, T. L. Long-term continuous oxygen therapy in chronic airway obstruction. *Ann. Intern. Med.* 72:621, 1970.
26. Nunn, J. F. *Applied Respiratory Physiology* (2nd ed.). London: Butterworth, 1977.
27. Peterson, G. M., Pierson, D. J., and Hunter, T. Arterial oxygen saturation during naso-tracheal suctioning. *Respir. Care* 23:68, 1978.
28. Petty, T. L. Answers to questions on acute respiratory failure. *Hosp. Med.* 70:36, 1970.
29. Petty, T. L. *Intensive and Rehabilitative Respiratory Care* (2nd ed.). Philadelphia: Lea & Febiger, 1974.
30. Pribble, A. H., and Tyler, M. L. Emergency! On-the-spot cardiopulmonary resuscitation. *Nurs. '75* 5:45, 1975.

31. Pulmonary terms and symbols. A report of the ACCP-ATS joint committee on pulmonary nomenclature. *Chest* 67:583, 1975.

32. Shapiro, B. A., Harrison, R. A., and Trout, C. A. *Clinical Application of Respiratory Care.* Chicago: Year Book, 1975.

33. Shibel, E. M., and Moser, K. M. (eds.). *Respiratory Emergencies.* St. Louis: Mosby, 1977.

34. Smelzer, T. H., and Barnett, T. B. Bronchodilator aerosol: A comparison of administration methods. *J.A.M.A.* 223:884, 1973.

35. Stewart, B. N., Hood, C. I., and Block, A. J. Long-term results of continuous oxygen therapy at sea-level. *Chest* 68:486, 1975.

36. Thomas, A. J., and Valabhji, P. Arrhythmia and tachycardia in pulmonary heart disease. *Br. Heart J.* 31:491, 1969.

37. Traver, G. A. Nursing the Patient Having a Problem in the Removal of Carbon Dioxide and/or in Maintaining the Supply of Oxygen. In I. L. Beland and J. Y. Passos, *Clinical Nursing: Pathophysiological and Psychosocial Approaches* (3rd ed.). New York: Macmillan, 1975.

38. Tyler, M. L. Artificial airways: Suctioning, tubes and cuffs, weaning and extubation. *Nurs. '73* 3:21, 1973.

39. Tyler, M. L. Arterial Blood Gases, Arterial Oxygen Saturation, Heart Rate and Blood Pressure During Chest Physiotherapy. Master's thesis, University of Washington, 1977.

40. Wanner, A., Zighelboim, A., and Sackner, M. A. Nasopharyngeal airway: A facilitated access to the trachea. *Ann. Intern. Med.* 75:593, 1971.

41. West, B. *Respiratory Physiology—the Essentials.* Baltimore: Williams & Wilkins, 1974.

42. West, B. *Pulmonary Pathophysiology—the Essentials.* Baltimore: Williams & Wilkins, 1977.

43. Zack, M. B., Pontoppidan, H., and Kasemi, H. The effect of lateral positions on gas exchange in pulmonary disease: A prospective evaluation. *Am. Rev. Respir. Dis.* 110:49, 1974.

Chest Trauma

Cornelia Vanderstaay Kenner
Kathleen MacKay White

Chest injuries are frequently lethal injuries. Approximately 75 percent of people who die as a result of a motor vehicle accident have sustained significant chest trauma [38]. Thoracic injury alone is the cause of death in 25 percent of those people and a major contributing factor in another 50 percent [6, 23]. Other causes of chest injury that require hospitalization are falls, missiles, crush injuries, recreational accidents, and violence [26]. Nursing care administered to patients with chest injuries must be comprehensive and specific in every detail.

Objectives

In her encounter with a person with chest trauma the nurse should be able to:

1. Obtain pertinent historical information.
2. Systematically assess the patient's physical condition, using inspection, palpation, percussion, and auscultation.
3. Record pertinent data.
4. Anticipate the physician's management.
5. Outline the nursing management.
6. Anticipate, prevent, and detect complications.

15

Achieving the Objectives

To achieve the objectives, the nurse should be able to:

1. Elicit and interpret historical data pertinent to the mechanism and severity of the injury.
2. Perform the essential components of the physical examination.
3. Assess the problems in regard to priority.
4. Quickly form a plan of action.
5. Implement the plan.
6. Evaluate the results and continue to assess.

How to Proceed

To develop an approach to chest trauma, the nurse should:

1. Review information about the anatomy and physiology of the respiratory system and the information in Chapters 9, 17, and 36; study the overview of chest injuries given in the next sections.
2. Practice rapid techniques of history taking and physical examination.
3. Improve her skills by caring for postoperative patients.
4. Assess patients in the emergency room with a preceptor.
5. Assess patients just before the preceptor's assessment so that the nurse's findings can be validated.
6. In the emergency room and in the intensive care unit, plan nursing care for patients with various types of injuries. Validate her care using the information presented in this chapter.
7. Practice in the following order the management techniques to be acquired: (a) in a simulation situation, (b) if possible, in an animal laboratory, (c) in a nonemergency situation, and (d) in an emergency situation.

Case Study

To make the problems of chest trauma more realistic and relevant, a case example of a patient who has a severe chest injury is presented in the following paragraphs. The data presented include information about the patient's history, the events that occurred before he reached the emergency room, the physical findings demonstrated, the abnormalities found, and how his treatment was carried out. Following the case study, interpretive comments are made about the patient's entire admission experience, why some things were done, why others were not, and what considerations underlay planning and executing the plan for his initial care.

Mr. R. T., a 35-year-old retail store manager, was brought to the emergency room because of injuries he sustained in a high-speed car accident. Witnesses claimed that Mr. T. lost control of his car, which was traveling at 50 to 60 mph, and crashed it into a telephone pole. At the scene of the accident, Mr. T. was found pinned against the steering wheel, but he was awake and responsive. The paramedics who were present at the scene of the accident said that Mr. T. was in obvious respiratory distress and that he complained of chest pain and shortness of breath. Examination of his chest revealed a right chest deformity. His right chest was immediately splinted with three-inch tape placed over a small towel. The patient's vital signs at the scene of the accident were BP 98/60, P 110, R 32 and labored. The patient's skin was pale, cool, and clammy. An intravenous infusion of 1000 ml of Ringer's lactate solution was begun by the paramedics; the patient had received 700 ml by the time of his admission to the hospital.

In the emergency room, Mr. T. was found to be in acute respiratory distress, with BP 82/40, P 150, R 26 with obvious right-sided paradoxical motion of a portion of his chest (flail chest). His respiratory pattern was also characterized by severe intercostal and sternal retraction. No air exchange could be felt at his mouth or nares. His breath sounds were absent. Airway maneuvers and suctioning failed to open his airway. Therefore, a #8 French endotracheal tube was inserted, and Mr. T. was ventilated with 100% oxygen for 20 breaths. Because of the severe flail chest, he was placed on a pressure-cycled respirator.

Assessment of Mr. T.'s condition after intubation revealed improvement in his cardiopulmonary status. A stat upright portable chest x ray showed multiple rib fractures, including a clavicular fracture on the right. The mediastinum appeared widened.

Mr. T.'s condition stabilized, with BP 102/80, P 100, R 12, central venous pressure (CVP) 4 cm H_2O. A Foley catheter was connected to straight drainage; it drained clear, yellow urine. A nasogastric tube was placed and connected to low suction; it drained a small amount of blood and then normal gastric contents. A complete physical examination was then carried out. It revealed no abnormalities other than minimal abdominal tenderness and hypoactive bowel sounds. No masses were palpable, and there was no rebound tenderness or distention. Peritoneal taps were negative bilaterally, and peritoneal lavage was also negative. The rest of the physical examination was essentially negative.

After Mr. T.'s condition had sufficiently stabilized, he was taken to the operating room, where an aortogram was done. The aortogram revealed an intact aorta with no intimal tears or lacerations. Mr. T. was then taken to the trauma critical care unit and placed on a volume ventilator with a tidal volume of 1000 ml and an FIO_2 of 40%.

Clinical Presentation of Case Study

On Mr. T.'s arrival in the critical care unit, the primary care nurse made her initial assessment of him and recorded her findings on the assessment sheet (see the accompanying assessment sheet) used in the unit. The following notes, a synopsis of Mr. T.'s pulmonary management based on his hospital record, document the care he received and his progress during his hospital stay.

3/1 4:30 P.M. Arterial blood gases (ABG) on FIO_2 of 40%: PO_2 146, pH 7.37, PCO_2 34, HCO_3^- 19.6, delta base −5. CVP < 3 cm H_2O. For increasing restlessness and pain, diazepam (5 mg IV) and meperidine (75 mg, one-half IV and one-half IM).

5:00 P.M. ABG on FIO_2 of 100%: PO_2 264, pH 7.32, PCO_2 42, HCO_3^- 21, delta base −4. Vital signs: BP 110/74, P 96, R 10. For hyperventilation and restlessness, morphine sulfate (5 mg IV).

6:00 P.M. BP 112/72, P 94, R 10, urine 50 ml/hr. Restlessness continues. Laboratory reports serum potassium of 3.1 mEq/L. 30 mEq/L potassium added to peripheral IV per physician order.

8:00 P.M. BP 76/42, P 146, R 40, CVP < 3 cm H_2O. Physician notified, Ringer's lactate solution opened wide, and patient's legs elevated. X-ray technician and blood bank notified. Patient progressively more agitated and tachypneic. Chest examination by the primary care nurse revealed dull percussion note and absent breath sounds right lower base. Equipment for chest tube placement assembled.

8:05 P.M. Doctor here. Right posterior chest catheter inserted, with the immediate return of 800 ml gross blood. Right anterior tube placed. Two units whole blood started. Twelve-lead ECG showed sinus tachycardia.

8:15 P.M. Stat portable chest film. Blood sent for CBC.

8:20 P.M. ABG on FIO_2 of 40%: PO_2 103, pH 7.34, PCO_2 37, HCO_3^- 19, delta base −6. Vital signs: BP 92/60, P 104, R 26. Chest tubes connection to Emerson pump with −20 cm of suction.

10:00 P.M. Vital signs: BP 108/70, P 96, R 12, CVP 15 cm H_2O. Hgb 8 gm/100 ml and Hct 22.7%. Urine 25 ml/hr. Alert. Two units whole blood completed. Ringer's lactate solution slowed and foot elevation discontinued. Patient asked to see his wife. Seemed more relaxed in her presence.

10:45 P.M. Lasix 25 mg IV push.

11:15 P.M. Vital signs: BP 110/70, P 90. Alert. Urine output increased.

3/2 12:30 A.M. Alert. Urine output 60 ml/hr. ABG on FIO_2 of 40%: PO_2 80, positive end-expiratory pressure (PEEP) of 4 cm H_2O started. Vital signs stable. Anterior chest tube oscillating, posterior tube shows minimal increase in drainage (25–30 ml). Both tubes stripped. Turned. Gastric pH maintained at 7. TED stockings applied.

2:00 A.M. PO_2 81 on FIO_2 of 50%. Morphine sulfate 4 mg given IV for hyperventilation and restlessness.

3:30 A.M. PO_2 122 on FIO_2 of 50%. Alert. Urine output 50 ml/hr. Vital signs stable. Demerol (50 mg IM) for pain.

5:00 A.M. Alert. Urine output decreased to 34 ml/hr.

6:00 A.M. Alert. Urine output 60 ml/hr. Vital signs stable. Posterior chest tube drainage total 875 ml (anterior 75 ml). Both tubes connected to Emerson pump. Diazepam (10 mg IM) given.

7:30 A.M. Forced vital capacity 1400 ml. PEEP decreased to 2 cm H_2O.

8:00 A.M. Alert. Urine 40 ml/hr. BP 150/80, P 90, R 10, T 100°F. Visited by family; seemed less tense during visit.

NOON Arterial line separated. Estimated blood loss 200 to 250 ml. No change in vital signs.

1:00 P.M. Swan-Ganz catheter inserted via subclavian vein; pulmonary artery pressures (PAP) 22/10 mm Hg and pulmonary capillary wedge pressure (PCWP) 10 mm Hg.

2:00 P.M. Restless and complaining of pain; meperidine (50 mg IM). Pulmonary artery catheter permanently wedged with a reading of 13 mm Hg. Doctor notified.

2:15 P.M. Doctor here. Pulmonary artery catheter repositioned. Cardiac output 7 Lpm.

2:45 P.M. Lasix (20 mg IM) and one unit packed cells per order.

4:00 P.M. BP 82/40, P 52. Minimal response to command. Pupils equal and react to light. Bilateral breath sounds present. Doctor notified.

4:05 P.M. Doctor here. BP 80/40, P 56. Atropine (0.25 mg) IV per order. Rate of fluid administration increased. Suctioned.

4:30 P.M. PCWP 9 mm Hg. Twelve-lead ECG shows normal sinus rhythm, no evidence of ischemia. P 84.

5:00 P.M. BP 120/80, P 96. Alert. Urine 60 ml/hr,

Critical Care Nursing Admission Assessment
Major Systems Approach

PATIENT'S NAME: _Mr. R.T._ DATE: _3/1_ TIME: _2 p.m._

DIAGNOSIS: _Flail Chest_ T: _99_ A.P.: _104_ R.P.: _104_ R.: _12_

B.P.: _100/70_ E.C.G. RHYTHM: _NSR_ ECTOPY: _____ WT: _—_ HT: _—_

ADMITTED VIA: _stretcher_ INFORMANT: _wife_ LAST MEAL: _9 am_

I. CHIEF COMPLAINT: _High-speed motor vehicle accident_

II. PATIENT PROFILE:

1. Age _35_ 2. Sex _male_

3. Marital Status (M) W D S

4. Race _W_ 5. Religion _Catholic_

6. Occupation _retail store manager_

7. Availability of Family _wife at home or hospital, parents live 40 mi. away_

8. Dietary _deferred_

9. Sleeping _deferred_

10. Activities of Daily Living _deferred_

III. HISTORY OF PRESENT ILLNESS: _multiple rib fractures and right clavicular fracture. In E.R., respiratory distress improved after endotracheal intubation and mechanical ventilation_

IV. PAST MEDICAL HISTORY:

1. Pediatric & Adult Illnesses _usual childhood illnesses_

2. Cardiac _____

3. Hypertension _____

4. Respiratory _____

5. Diabetes Mellitus _____ _negative_

6. Renal _____

7. Jaundice _____

8. Infections _____

9. Other _____

10. Hospitalizations & Surgeries _Fx. ® arm age 10 healed s complications_

11. Current Medication _and immunizations_ _no current medications, tetanus booster 3 yrs. ago_

12. Allergies _Sulfa_

13. Habits _½ pack/day cigarettes· 10 yrs occasional beer_

V. FAMILY HISTORY: _M + F., A + W_

VI. PSYCHOSOCIAL:

1. Behavior During Assessment _Responsive Cooperative Seemingly distressed since unable to talk_

2. Specific Problems _None noted at this time Closely knit family able to work together_

VII. PHYSICAL EXAMINATION:

1. General _No obvious distress O₂ volume ventilator per ET tube_

2. Respiratory System _____

Airway _ET tube_

Inspection _Flail chest, vol. ventilator c̄ 1000 ml. TV, sigh 1400 ml. F₁O₂ 40%_

Rate _12_

Rhythm _Normal, even amplitude_

Chest Wall _Paradoxic motion apparent only on inspiration at ® Ant. 2-6 ICS MCL + axillary line_

Palpation _Crepitus palpable ® axilla + supraclavicular fossa_

Percussion _dull RLL Generalized tenderness_

Auscultation
Voice Sounds _____ *deferred* _____
Breath Sounds _____
   Normal ___ Increased ___ Decreased *R base*
   Adventitious Sounds *rhonchi and rales* RLL
_____
_____

3. Cardiovascular System
   A.P. *104* R.P. *104*
   B.P. Supine   R _____   L *monitor 100/70*
   P.M.I. _____ *5th ICS*   *MCL*
   Heart Sounds _____ *Normal S₁ S₂* _____

   Thrills _____
   Peripheral Pulses _____ *all 3⁺*

4. Neurological System
   Level of Consciousness *Alert*

   Respiratory Pattern *Even*

   Cranial Nerves *Grossly intact*

   Eyes _____
   (1) Pupils   OD   OS
       Size   *4 mm*   *4 mm*
       Shape   *round*   *round*
       Light   *react*   *react*
       Consensual   *react*   *react*
       Accommodation *react*   *react*
   (2) Ocular Movements *Intact*

   Motor *moves all extremities*

   Sensory *Reactive*
   Coordination *intact*

   Reflexes *2⁺*

5. Gastrointestinal System
   Nose & Mouth *Levine tube*

   Stomach *no bleeding*

   Abdomen *tender, esp. RUQ; no distention or palpable tenderness*
   Bowel Sounds *hypoactive*
   Liver *not palpable*
   Spleen *deferred*

6. Renal & Genitourinary Systems
   I. _____ O. *100 ml.*
   Urinary Bladder & Urethra *deferred*

   Kidneys *deferred*

7. Musculoskeletal System
   Spine *no tenderness*
   Extremities *skin color and capillary refill good; warm extremities*
   Sacral Edema *none*
   Masses *none*

8. Hematologic System
   Petechiae ⎫
   Ecchymosis ⎬ *negative*
   Gingiva ⎭

9. Endocrine System
   Breath ⎫ *negative*
   Skin ⎭

VIII. LABORATORY:
   1. Hematology
      HGB *12.7 gm%* HCT *36.1*
      W.B.C. *10,500*
   2. Chemistry
      Na *138* K *3.4*
      CO₂ *24* CL *101*
      Blood Sugar *240* Amylase *<320*
      BUN *13* Cr *.6*
   3. Urinalysis *cath, pH 3.0, sp. gr. 1.010, no sugar or acetone, no RBC's*
   4. Electrocardiogram
      Rate *104* Rhythm *NSR*
      P-R *0.16* QRS *0.08* ST *0.12*
      Interpretation *normal sinus rhythm*
   5. Chest x-ray *multiple R lateral rib fractures, Fx R distal clavicle, sub-emphysema mediastinum appears slightly widened*

IX. PROBLEM LIST:
   450 1. *Incomplete date base*

ACTIVE	INACTIVE
2. *Flail chest 2° blunt chest trauma*	*Fx arm, age 10*
3. *Hx deceleration c̄ widened mediastinum on x-ray*	
4. *Airway obstruction 2/, Endotracheal tube → resp. dysfunction*	
5. *Anxiety over hospitalization*	
6. *Impaired mobility*	
7. *Pain*	

Kathy White R.N.
NURSE'S SIGNATURE

pale yellow. Maintained on FIO_2 of 40% with 2 cm H_2O PEEP. Blood from pulmonary artery catheter for mixed venous blood gas (MVBG) studies could not be drawn.

5:30 P.M.   ABG on FIO_2 of 40%: PO_2 101, pH 7.49, PCO_2 35, HCO_3^- 26.5, delta base +3.

6:30 P.M.   BP 110/70, P 110. Alert. Digoxin (0.25 mg IV) per order.

7:30 P.M.   BP 110/72, P 92.

9:00 P.M.   ABG on FIO_2 of 40%: PO_2 110, pH 7.47, PCO_2 32, delta base 0. Hgb 11.3 gm/100 ml, Hct 32.6%.

10:00 P.M.   BP 150/90, P 88. Alert. Urine 60 ml/hr. Electrolytes: sodium 139 mEq/L, potassium 3.4 mEq/L, CO_2 29.5 mEq/L. PEEP discontinued. Repositioned at hourly intervals. Linen changed and patient made comfortable for sleep. Meperidine (25 mg IM) for pain. Pulmonary protocol maintained.

11:00 P.M.   ABG on FIO_2 of 40% one hour after PEEP discontinued: PO_2 99, pH 7.49, PCO_2 34, HCO_3^- 26.8, delta base +2.

11:30 P.M.   MVBG: PO_2 35, pH 7.43, PCO_2 39.8, HCO_3^- 26.

3/3   4:00 A.M.   BP 130/70, P 84. Alert. PAP 28/12, PCWP 10. Back care and position change. Demerol (25 mg IM) for discomfort.

8:00 A.M.   BP 150/80, P 84, R 12, T 101, PAP 20/10, PCWP 10. Alert. Urine 30 ml/hr, Lasix (20 mg IV) per order. Bilateral rhonchi significantly decreased after suctioning. Being digitalized.

9:00 A.M.   Urine 300 ml/hr.

10:00 A.M.   Urine 460 ml/hr. Less restless. Bed bath and mouth care given, after which patient smiled and rested for a period.

11:45 A.M.   ABG on FIO_2 of 40%: PO_2 100, pH 7.52, PCO_2 32. MVBG on FIO_2 of 40%: PO_2 34, pH 7.5, PCO_2 37. Wife visited; patient seemed much more relaxed during visit. Primary care nurse remained at the bedside during visit to answer questions and help with communication.

12:15 P.M.   ABG on FIO_2 of 100%: PO_2 391, pH 7.54, PCO_2 31. MVBG on FIO_2 of 100%: PO_2 43, pH 7.49, PCO_2 35.5. Hgb 9.9 gm/100 ml, Hct 28.6%.

12:30 P.M.   Typed and crossmatched for four units packed cells.

1:15 P.M.   Two units packed cells ordered. Chest bottles changed.

4:00 P.M.   BP 120/70, P 86, PAP 15/3, PCWP 3. Alert. Urine 50 ml/hr. Packed cells started.

6:00 P.M.   PAP 17/5, PCWP 5.

8:00 P.M.   BP 150/90, P 108, R 12, T 101°F, PAP 17/8, PCWP 3. Alert. ABG on FIO_2 of 40%: PO_2 99, pH 7.49, PCO_2 34.6, delta base +3. Second unit packed cells nearly completed.

10:00 P.M.   BP 164/76, P 96, R 12, T 101.6°F, PAP 17/3, PCWP 3. Alert. Urine 50 ml/hr. Hgb 11.5 gm/100 ml, Hct 33.1%. Posterior chest tube drainage 75 ml. Linen changed and patient made comfortable for sleep.

3/4   Mr. T.'s vital signs remained stable throughout the day. He was alert and his urinary output was within satisfactory limits. Cardiopulmonary parameters included PAP measurements ranging from 16/8 to 20/5, PCWP measurements ranging from 3 to 8, and cardiac output measurements averaging 6.8 Lpm. Oscillation in his anterior chest tube ceased. Mr. T. was able to use a Magic Slate to communicate, and he seemed to understand all explanations. In general, he was more relaxed and able to sleep for long periods of time.

3/5   Mr. T.'s vital signs remained stable, and his anterior chest tube was removed. PCWP readings were not obtainable due to catheter malfunction. He moved about actively in bed, remembered to do his bed exercises, and was out of bed twice during the day. He enjoyed longer visits with his family, who were a great support to him. The primary care nurse remained in close proximity during family visits to answer questions, offer information, and help in communication.

3/6   The Swan-Ganz catheter was removed, and Mr. T. sat in a chair for three 15-minute periods.

3/7   At 2 A.M. an air leak was noted in Mr. T.'s endotracheal tube, and at 8 A.M. a tracheotomy was performed with a #8 Portex. Later the Emerson pump was discontinued.

3/10   Mr. T.'s posterior chest tube was removed, and he was transferred to the intermediate care unit. His pulmonary condition was stable, but he was still observed closely by the health team. His family members had learned a great deal about his care from the critical care nurses, and they were able to assist in most aspects of his care. Having his wife help pleased Mr. T., and he rapidly assumed more and more responsibility for his own care.

3/17   Mr. T. was weaned from the respirator according to established protocol without any problems. He was quite active, assumed total responsibility for himself, and participated in the patient education program.

3/22   After the completion of discharge teaching, Mr. T. left the hospital with his family.

Interpretation of the Case Study

To clarify the pathophysiological aspects of chest trauma, the following paragraphs explain the significant physical findings in Mr. T.'s case. The findings and problems in Mr. T.'s case are typical of patients who are taken to the emergency room of a hospital after a high-speed motor vehicle accident. Obviously, how and when the problems are managed depends on how soon they are detected, on their severity, and on what priorities are set by those responsible for patient care. The process of detecting the signs and symptoms of specific injury, interpreting the findings, setting priorities, and then instituting appropriate care extends from the moment the ambulance arrives at the scene of the accident, to the emergency room, and through the patient's hospital stay. Furthermore, the information gained at each stage helps to narrow each problem to the point at which the management designed is as specific and appropriate as possible.

The process of assessing and managing Mr. T.'s injury was begun by the ambulance team. From the information gathered at the scene, the team learned that the accident occurred at high speed. That clue to the possible mechanisms of injury warned the health care team to consider the severe internal injuries that can result from the tearing, torsional forces of rapid deceleration. The aorta is especially vulnerable to that type of injuring mechanism. Next the team learned that the patient had been thrown against the steering wheel, information that quickly alerted them to the possibility of blunt chest injury with rib fracture and/or lung damage. The patient's complaint of shortness of breath and chest pain narrowed the injury to chest involvement. Inspection of the chest revealed the presence of flail chest. Splinting the flail segment with 3-inch tape over a small towel was the best available first-aid method of stabilizing the segment. The paradoxical motion of the flail segment was controlled to some degree, and the patient's ability to expand his chest on inspiration and recoil on expiration was somewhat improved. That improvement helped to reduce the work of breathing and to maintain minimal respiratory function with adequate gas exchange while the patient was being transported to the hospital.

En route, Mr. T.'s falling blood pressure, a sign that another problem was developing, was detected by the ambulance crew. Considering the force of the blow that caused the patient's severe chest injury, the possibility of shock due to internal bleeding from intrathoracic or intraabdominal injury had to be considered. Since the blood pressure remained lower than 90 mm Hg despite the administration of 700 ml of Ringer's lactate solution, the hypotension most likely had hypovolemic causes.

Little or no response to the rapid infusion of 500 ml of Ringer's lactate solution indicates that 5 to 10% of the blood volume has been lost—unless, of course, the problem is decreasing cardiac output secondary to mediastinal shift seen in tension pneumothorax, which also would not respond to Ringer's lactate solution.

Had Mr. T.'s condition remained the same in the emergency room as it had been before transport, with his airway, breathing, and cardiac function maintained, attention would have been directed toward (1) quickly assessing his injuries, (2) treating the shock and uncovering and correcting its cause, and (3) ensuring adequate stabilization of the flail so that sufficient gas exchange continued. That would have been followed by a complete and orderly examination to detect the less serious or occult injuries that might have been overlooked in the initial assessment. But that course of management, however, had to be set aside temporarily when a more serious problem, airway obstruction, demanded a rearrangement of priorities. Management of that problem proceeded from the simple to the complex; that is, when simple airway maneuvers failed to establish an airway, the more complex maneuver of endotracheal intubation became necessary. Had intubation also failed, cricothyreotomy would have been appropriate, since at that point failure to correct the obstruction could have led to Mr. T.'s death.

But the intubation not only corrected the airway obstruction but combined with the use of positive pressure, provided the most efficient means of stabilizing the flail. Positive intrathoracic pressure prevented the sinking in of the flail on inspiration, the work of breathing was greatly reduced, and gas exchange improved.

Once Mr. T.'s condition had been stabilized, a thorough physical examination was carried out. It is important to conduct a systematic examination after the crises have been resolved so that minor or occult injuries that may have gone unseen or unattended can be found and evaluated.

Because Mr. T. had undergone rapid deceleration, and was found to have a first rib fracture and a widened mediastinum, the possibility of aortic injury had to be considered. Therefore additional radiographic studies were necessary to determine if aortic injury was present. Mr. T. was taken to the operating room, not the x-ray department, for an arteriogram, because operative repair of an aortic tear must be done immediately. Having the patient in the operating room prevents unnecessary delay and prevents the aorta from rupturing in the x-ray department, where immediate surgical intervention is not available. Also, the arteriographic study itself might cause a torn aorta to rupture, and it should not be undertaken without operative interventions being immediately possible. After Mr. T.'s arrival in the trauma unit, he showed agitation, tachypnea, and tachycardia, which signaled that his hypoxia had become worse. The person with a thoracic injury is usually in shock primarily because of hemorrhage and/or pericardial tamponade and only secondarily because of respiratory distress or pain. Mr. T.'s continued shock, absent breath sounds, and dullness to percussion of the right lower lobe pointed to hemothorax. Again, the history of injury strongly warned of intrathoracic vessel tear and bleeding. The ineffectiveness of the positive pressure suggests a space-occupying lesion of the chest—hemothorax. Positive pressure would also have been ineffective with tension pneumothorax, but that condition was ruled out on physical examination, when hyperresonance was not found. An immediate chest x ray confirmed the suspicion of hemothorax, and a blood gas analysis documented the hypoxia and hypercapnia already suspected. Continued hypoventilation, followed by acute respiratory failure and death, would occur inevitably if the space-occupying blood was not removed.

Once the chest tubes were inserted (the posterior tube was placed first since evacuation of the pleural blood took priority over the evacuation of air by the anterior tube), Mr. T.'s condition quickly stabilized. Administration of two units of whole blood helped reduce the volume loss and increase the circulating red blood cells so that the oxygen-carrying capacity of the blood was adequate for tissue demands. The chest tubes were connected to underwater seal drainage. Emerson suction with -20 cm H_2O, though rarely necessary, was ordered for Mr. T. to help evacuate the intrapleural air. That degree of negative pressure safely evacuates intrapleural air without damage to the delicate pulmonary structures near the end of the chest tube. Pressures greater than -20 cm H_2O can create such great transpulmonary pressure gradients that pulmonary edema results as capillary fluid is literally suctioned into the alveolar spaces [7].

Although Mr. T.'s initial chest drainage was 800 ml, the rate of continued blood loss after chest tube insertion is the usual factor that determines whether open thoracotomy is necessary. Since Mr. T.'s bleeding slowed soon after the insertion of the tube, it was assumed that the bleeding was venous and capillary in origin and that hemostasis could be maintained by the chest tube's expansion of the injured lung. But had the rate of bleeding exceeded 500 ml per hour or had the first episode of bleeding been more than 1500 ml, exploratory thoracotomy would have been indicated for repair of the larger intercostal and internal mammary arteries.

Pulmonary artery and radial artery catheters were inserted so that cardiopulmonary function could be closely monitored. Pulmonary complications are particularly likely to occur in trauma patients who have been in shock, have had direct pulmonary injury, have had transfusions, or have been hypoxic (see Chaps. 17 and 36). In severe cases or in cases detected and treated too late, refractory hypoxemia, hypercapnia, acidosis, pulmonary failure, and death may result.

Reflections

At the monthly nursing grand rounds, Mr. T.'s hospital course was discussed. The main topic of the conference was to have been care of a patient with tube thoracostomy, but, as usually happens, the meeting centered on the problem of greatest concern to most of those present. A discussion of the role of the nurse in life-threatening situations was prompted by the mention of two salient events that occurred during Mr. T.'s course of treatment: (1) his respiratory failure, which required endotracheal intubation, and (2) his sudden deterioration, which required chest tube placement.

The discussion was heated. Many different points of view were expressed. "A nurse is a nurse is a nurse, a physician is a physician is a physician, and the roles of the two do not overlap" was a repeated theme. Several nurses brought up some "gray" areas of practice (e.g., what is the nurse to do when a physician is not present?). Still others discussed the moral and ethical questions posed by the nurse's not acting in an emergency to the fullest extent of her knowledge and ability. Discussion of the Good Samaritan laws in various states led to a discussion of the public's concern about the failure of medical personnel to stop and render aid at the scene of an accident, a problem that has prompted the enactment of legislation.

In summarizing and concluding the meeting, the nurses said that they considered the session so rewarding that they would have a committee write up the feelings and ideas expressed in the form of a journal article. They agreed about the nurse's role in life-threatening situations; namely, that when a person in crisis is brought to an emergency room or a critical care unit, the nurse must be able to assess the patient's injuries systematically and to work with the physician in managing the problems. In the physician's absence, the nurse must make the decisions. Those conclusions were based on the assumption that the nurse would be expert in assessing and managing critical situations, precise in assessment, and reasonably well versed in the pathology suggested by the physical signs. That expertise, combined with (1) an understanding that has been reached with administrative personnel and (2) nursing protocols and legal observances appropriate to the state, should precede the nurse's performance of critical care procedures. For too long nurses have committed sins of omission because they felt commission was not within the realm of nursing. Today that attitude must be reexamined. If the nurse is to assume responsibility for patients' lives in the absence of a physician, she must be knowledgeable, expert, and accountable for her actions.

Mechanics of Breathing

For a further understanding of the different problems associated with chest trauma and how the priorities of treatment are determined, certain basic concepts must be clarified and it must be remembered that any alteration in a person's respiratory cycle can significantly disturb his oxygenation.

The thoracic cavity is divided into three compartments: (1) the pleural space, which is occupied by the lungs, (2) the mediastinum, which is occupied by the trachea, esophagus, and large blood vessels, and (3) the pericardial space, which is occupied by the heart. The parietal pleura separates each compartment from the other and partitions off the three compartments by lining the entire thoracic cavity (i.e., the internal surface of the chest wall), part of the superior surface of the diaphragm, and the mediastinum. The lungs are covered by the visceral pleura and are thus separated from the rest of the thoracic structures. In fact, the lungs are attached to the body only at their hila.

To understand the mechanics of many types of

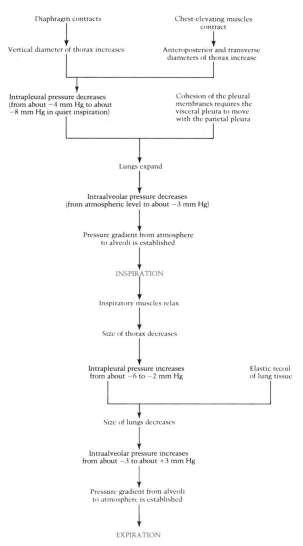

Figure 15-1
Inspiration-expiration.

chest injuries, it is important to understand the normal mechanics of respiration (Fig. 15-1). The outer surface of the lungs, the visceral pleura, is a smooth, moist membrane that lies in complete contact with the smooth, moist membrane lining the inner thoracic wall, the parietal pleura. Those two layers slide over one another during inspiration and expiration. Between those two layers of pleura is a "potential space"; that is, the presence of any type of fluid or air will create a space between the thoracic wall and the lung. The membranes, however, constantly absorb any fluid or gas that enters the potential space. In other words, the visceral and parietal pleural membranes are in an apposition that is maintained by the surface tension of a thin layer of fluid separating them. Furthermore, a partial vacuum exists between the two membranes, partly as a result of the constant reabsorption of fluid or air but largely as a result of two opposing forces: the natural elastic recoil of the lungs and the outward expansion of the chest wall. Together those forces establish a constant vacuum in the potential pleural space that not only keeps the lung from collapsing but also is the mechanism by which negative pressures (pressures less than that of the atmosphere) are produced within the thorax. Intrapleural pressure is always less than (negative to) atmospheric pressure. Also, one should understand that although the mechanics of respiration are most clearly described using the concept of intrapleural pressures, the description is academic under normal conditions since no real space exists within which to measure pressures.

Air moves into and out of the lungs for the same reason blood flows through vessels—a pressure gradient exists. Air moves from an area of greater pressure to an area of lesser pressure. At the end of expiration, the intrapleural pressure is −4 mm Hg (because of a naturally occurring vacuum). The pressure within the lungs (intraalveolar or intrapulmonic pressure), having been exposed to the atmosphere via bronchi and the trachea, is 0 mm Hg. At that point, no pressure gradient exists between the airways and the atmosphere. However, a pressure gradient is produced by increasing the size of the thorax. As volume increases, pressure decreases (Boyle's law).

Thoracic size and volume are increased by (1) the downward movement of the diaphragm and (2) the elevation of the ribs, which increases the anteroposterior diameter of the chest cavity. Although normal inspiration is caused principally by contraction of the diaphragm, 70 percent of the expansion and contraction of the lungs is caused by the anteroposterior movement of the chest cage and only 30 percent by movement of the diaphragm. In normal breathing, the diaphragm contracts and descends several centimeters so that approximately 500 ml of air enters the lungs. If the body needs more air (as it does during excitement), additional muscles are needed for inspiration, and the external intercostals contract and move the ribs outward.

Once the size of the thorax is increased, the pressure in the potential pleural space (the intrapleural or intrathoracic pressure) falls from its end-expiratory pressure of −4 mm Hg to the more negative pressure of −8 mm Hg, and the pressure in the intraalveolar space is lowered from atmospheric pressure to −3 mm Hg. At that point, the pressure gradient between the airways and the atmosphere produces air movement into the airways.

In expiration, the muscles of inspiration (the diaphragm and the external intercostals) relax and spring back to the resting position. If for some reason (e.g., airway obstruction) one has to use muscles to help in expiration, he cannot use the diaphragm since it is a muscle of inspiration. Instead, the abdominal and internal intercostal muscles contract and help in expiration. As the expiratory muscles contract, the intraalveolar pressure and the intrapleural pressure increase. The intraalveolar pressure is now +3 mm Hg (i.e., higher than atmospheric pressure) and so air moves out of the lungs. The following pressure cycles are repeated with each respiration.

Intraalveolar Pressures for Normal Quiet Breathing (Are All Variable, Depending on the Force of Inspiration and Expiration)

Inspiration	−3 mm Hg
Expiration	+3 mm Hg
Pressure at the end of expiration before inspiration begins	0 mm Hg

Intrapleural Pressures

During inspiration	−8 mm Hg
During expiration	−2 mm Hg
At the end of expiration	−4 mm Hg
At the end of inspiration	−6 mm Hg

Blunt Trauma and Penetrating Trauma

When caring for the patient with chest trauma, consideration should be given to the type of injury sustained by the patient. The patient may be suffering from blunt (nonpenetrating) trauma to the chest, or he may have received a penetrating injury. Blunt trauma is defined as closed injury without communication to the outside (unless a fractured rib has penetrated the chest wall). Direct impact causes the greatest injury to the chest wall. Injuries to the structures within the chest may result from the forces of acceleration-deceleration, shearing, and compression-decompression. Direct impact with severe force may grossly deform the chest, pressing the sternum almost against the spinal column [54]. Sudden compression increases the pressure intravascularly and may result in vascular damage and bleeding. Since the glottis is usually closed during injury, the chest acts as a closed system and pressure is transmitted anywhere in the system. Thus injuries following blunt trauma may occur anywhere in the chest, and the injuries can be severe even though there are few external signs. Compression injuries commonly occur to the chest wall, pleura, trachea, bronchi, lung (pneumothorax and/or hemothorax), heart, great vessels, esophagus, and/or diaphragm [5]. The forces of acceleration-deceleration cause the greatest injury to the vascular system. Rapid deceleration from a high speed, as in a highway accident, can cause major vessels to undergo extreme stretching and bowing. Stretching forces that exceed the elasticity of those vessels can produce shearing damage of the vessel walls, which then tend to tear, dissect, rupture, or form an aneurysmal deformity. Also, shearing damage occurs in vessels that decelerate at a rate different from that of the structures they perfuse. Hence organs may be torn from the source of their blood supply.

Penetrating chest injuries usually are less of an assessment problem than are blunt injuries. The presence of entrance and exit wounds helps greatly in determining the site of injury. A line plotted between an entrance wound and an exit wound would allow one to determine what structures lie in the path and hence what types of pathology are likely to occur.

When penetrating injuries are encountered, consideration must be given to the injuring instrument.

1. Gunshot wounds have special injuring mechanisms in that the ballistics of certain missiles produce injury beyond just the missile's tract (see Chap. 34).
2. Missiles do not always travel in a straight line, and so they can injure more than just the structures lying beneath the entrance wound.
3. Missiles do not always exit, and thus it is not always possible to plot the path between entrance and exit and to estimate the extent of injury.
4. Missiles are not sterile, and they expose the chest wound to considerable contamination.
5. All apparent gunshot wounds of the chest are not always *just* gunshot wounds of the chest. Due to the extreme mobility and upward excursions of the diaphragm, a missile to the fifth intercostal

space can cut a path through not only the chest but also the dome of the diaphragm and structures that lie beneath it—the spleen and the liver. What may initially appear to be chest trauma may actually be complicated thoracoabdominal trauma [28].

In regard to knife-blade–type injuries, the following considerations must be kept in mind.

1. If the patient is admitted to the hospital with the instrument (e.g., knife, arrow, or screwdriver) in place, it must not be removed. In most cases, the blade, despite the lacerating injury produced, serves as a "mechanical" tamponade for the lacerated vessels. Removing the instrument may release the temporary hemostasis and precipitate instant hemorrhage. In such a situation, the blade must be *immobilized*, and nothing, not even a sheet, must be allowed to exert its weight on the blade. Even the slightest movement could disturb the tamponade and result in internal bleeding and death before operative intervention could be undertaken.
2. Stab wounds can have amazing depth, and they may contain pieces of broken blade or other foreign material.
3. It is important to obtain information about the size of the knife and about the angle at which it was thrust. Estimating the angle of entry can help determine what structures are likely to be involved in the trauma.

Rib Fracture

Flail Chest

When multiple adjacent rib fractures and/or costosternal separations result in the "floating" of a segment of the rib cage, a flail chest is said to exist (Fig. 15-2). The segment, having lost continuity with the rest of the chest wall, moves paradoxically [13]. On inspiration, when the chest wall is expanding in an attempt to establish the negative intrathoracic pressures necessary for air to enter the lungs, the free (floating) segment sinks inward [38]. That phenomenon negates some of the chest expansion brought about by the anteroposterior and diaphragmatic movement and begins to abolish the pressure gradients essential for inspiration. Consequently, movement of air is diminished. The same is true on expiration. As the patient tries to reduce the size of

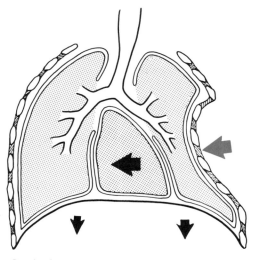

Inspiration

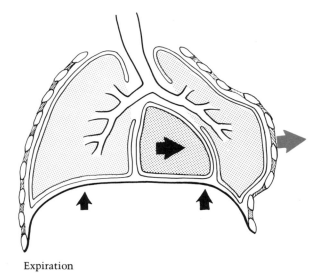

Expiration

Figure 15-2
Flail chest.

gress to respiratory failure with reduced gas exchange, hypoxemia, and hypercapnia [25, 40].

It was once thought that one of the problems associated with flail chest was that a large segment of air moved back and forth between the lungs, resulting in increased dead space ventilation. Now the movement of air back and forth (sometimes called *pendelluft*) is considered not as significant as was once thought.

A flail chest may result in the movement of other structures within the chest. There may be a shift of the mediastinal structures toward the uninjured lung, with reduction in the amount of gas going to the normal lung [39, 42]. That reduction may further impair gas exchange. Furthermore, the shifting of the mediastinal structures may cause the great vessels to kink and obstruct, thus decreasing the venous return to the heart, thereby decreasing the cardiac output and producing a shock of cardiac origin [35].

A sternal flail, in which fractured ribs or costochondral separations around the sternum result in the sternum itself becoming a free-floating segment, is also potentially a detriment to the patient's cardiac function [4, 11]. If the condition is severe enough, the sternum may compress the mediastinum and the heart at the time of initial injury, resulting in myocardial contusion or pericarditis. Heart failure due to myocardial injury, pericarditis, blood in the pericardial space, or mechanical compression of the heart as the sternal segment flails may result.

ASSESSMENT OF LATERAL FLAIL CHEST

The patient is examined for obvious deformity of the chest wall with associated paradoxical movement. The examiner should be aware that, owing to splinting, initially the paradox may not be apparent. Damage to the chest wall musculature may cause spasm and initially conceal the severity of the underlying injury. However, as the patient becomes exhausted from the work of breathing, the paradoxical movement becomes apparent. Respiratory difficulty increases, and the patient tries to increase his rate and depth of breathing (as carbon dioxide increases and oxygen decreases). Later cyanosis, noisy breathing, and a moribund appearance complete the clinical picture [31].

The patient should also be examined for the presence of other clues. He may be tachypneic and have painful respirations. He may be apprehensive, anxious, and/or dyspneic. He may have diastolic hypertension. If the person was previously normotensive,

the thoracic cavity and create the pressure gradient necessary for expiration, the flail segment bulges outward. The pressure gradient necessary for expiration is then partially lost and complete exhalation cannot occur. The larger the free-floating segment, the less efficient inspiration and expiration become, causing increased work of breathing that may pro-

diastolic hypertension suggests carbon dioxide retention. Particularly in younger persons, progressive skin changes from red to white may be seen. First the skin is flushed from carbon dioxide retention and vasodilatation, next it is pale from diastolic hypertension, and then it has a bluish hue from cyanosis. The patient may have decreased air flow on expiration, suggesting ventilatory inadequacy. His ventilation can be grossly evaluated by having him expire forcefully against the examiner's hand. He must be observed for any signs that indicate the degree of respiratory embarrassment. The signs of hypoxia are irritability, restlessness, confusion, cyanosis, and tachycardia. The signs of hypercapnia are headache, dizziness, lethargy, stupor, confusion, and disorientation.

Using palpation, the examiner may find point tenderness, crepitus indicative of rib fracture, changing site of the apex beat, and tracheal deviation. Using percussion, the examiner may find pronounced tenderness, hyperresonance due to pneumothorax, and decreased resonance due to an associated hemothorax. Using auscultation, the examiner may hear noisy respirations.

ASSESSMENT OF STERNAL FLAIL CHEST

To detect a flail chest produced by the sternum's acting as a free-floating segment, the patient should be examined for paradoxical movement of the sternum during respirations and the following signs of cardiac involvement: (1) weak and slow pulse, (2) falling blood pressure, (3) rising central venous pressure, and (4) dysrhythmias. The examiner should palpate the area around the sternum for rib fracture and the trachea for normal positioning (no deviation is present with a sternal flail). Also, the patient may show signs of accompanying traumatic asphyxia, in which the anterior crush of the chest not only produces sternal flail but also forces blood to surge suddenly out of the thorax into the head and neck. The visible signs are edema of the face, lips, tongue, and conjunctivae and gross cyanosis of the face and neck [41].

MANAGEMENT OF FLAIL CHEST

The objective of whatever type of emergency treatment is used is maintenance of adequate pulmonary oxygenation and ventilation. Reduction of the mobility of the flail segment and of the detrimental effects of its paradoxical movement is followed by drainage of the pleural space and maintenance of respiratory excursion [19].

As an immediate first-aid measure, the palm of the hand may be used to exert firm but gentle pressure against the flail segment and thus to stabilize it. Occasionally, a pressure dressing or an adhesive strapping may be ordered by the physician as a temporary method of stabilization. The dressing is applied over a thick, firmly rolled pad of cotton or folded towels to conform to the size and shape of the mobile area. Since the method is restrictive, it may cause impairment of the normal volume of ventilation, interfere with the cough mechanism, and thus predispose the person to atelectasis and pneumonia. To avoid those complications and despite the discomfort and pain, the nurse must continuously encourage the patient to cough, deep breathe, and turn.

The method of choice in the management of flail chest by improving respiratory exchange and decreasing shunting is internal stabilization with endotracheal intubation and positive pressure breathing [2]. Most important, adequate ventilation averts the complications of hypoxemia since the rate and depth of respiration may be controlled. Abnormalities in ventilation and perfusion are produced by the underlying pulmonary parenchymal contusion and splinting of the chest wall. Splinting inhibits coughing and allows tracheobronchial secretions to accumulate and atelectasis to develop. Also, since with positive pressure applied within the lung on inspiration it is not necessary to create negative pressure on inspiration, the paradoxical motion of the flail segment is thus prevented. Stabilization of a flail chest requires several weeks; the positive pressure "splints" the flail segment during that time [13].

If when a patient with a severe flail chest and respiratory distress enters the hospital, a physician is not available and the nurse is not skilled in endotracheal intubation, a temporary means of stabilization employing traction may be instituted. The effectiveness of external splinting is questionable, but in such a situation it is the only alternative. Traction can be applied with the use of towel clips. First either side of the ribs is anesthetized with 0.5 ml of a 1% lidocaine solution, and the towel clips are applied through the skin to the ribs. A cord is tied to the clips and attached to an intravenous pole with enough traction (5–15 lb) to reduce retraction of the flail on inspiration. With a sternal flail, mechanical compression of the mediastinal structures may be treated by elevation of the flailing sternal segment. A uterine tenaculum may be used to grasp the mobile sternum and lift it off the pericardium. Later, the towel clips or tenaculum may be replaced with Kirschner wire placed behind the ribs or sternum. Certain potential problems exist with external splinting: (1) difficulty in identifying the appropriate ribs, (2) inadequate control of the paradox, (3) infection, (4) necrosis, (5) hemothorax, (6) pneumothorax, and (7) subsequent bony deformity.

At some time during the period of artificial ventilation, the endotracheal tube may be replaced by a tracheostomy tube, which offers the advantage of convenience for suctioning [10]. When the airway is artificially maintained, therapy is directed toward normalizing cardiopulmonary parameters, such as the arterial oxygen level, the alveolar arterial gradient, and the shunt fraction, and toward maintaining adequate pulmonary hygiene [42].

A refinement of positive pressure therapy that uses intermittent mandatory ventilation (IMV) often accompanied by positive end-expiratory pressure (PEEP) may be used. According to some authors that refinement has shortened the time needed for mechanical respiratory support [16, 47]. The technique is based on the premise that the fundamental problem in flail chest is pulmonary, not orthopedic. The patient suffers from a form of acute respiratory failure, with pulmonary contusion producing congestion, edema, decreased surfactant production, pain, decreased compliance, and increased work of breathing. With IMV, the patient breathes spontaneously between ventilatory cycles and thus determines his own arterial carbon dioxide levels. He is prevented from developing a significant degree of subatmospheric intrapleural pressure, which might dislodge the fibrosing rib cage, and because he has less pain, he has less need of sedation or respiratory paralysis. With PEEP, the patient's lung is maintained at a greater degree of inflation during expiration, thus increasing the functional residual capacity [52]. Small airway and alveolar collapse is prevented, and the resulting larger lung volume improves arterial oxygenation [36]. The hazards of oxygen administered in high concentrations are avoided. In managing patients with that form of therapy, the end-expiratory pressure is titrated to produce the smallest intrapulmonary shunt [51].

Uncomplicated Rib Fracture

Fractured ribs are frequently overlooked as a sign of potential chest trauma. The medical advice to the patient with a fractured rib often is, "Strap it, take aspi-

rin for the pain, don't cough too much, the pain will go away in about two weeks." However, even though most people with uncomplicated fractured ribs have relatively minor injuries and can be treated as outpatients, the nurse must remember that serious associated injuries do occur with rib fracture. One study showed that among people with severe rib fractures, as many as 20 percent have an associated hemothorax, 25 percent have a pneumothorax, and 30 percent have both [23]. Those numbers mean that only 25 percent of people with severe rib fractures have an uncomplicated rib fracture. Naclerio [33] says that, "This high frequency of underlying complications should be recalled whenever one treats a broken rib as a matter of little consequence." In other words, when the chest x-ray report indicates a rib fracture, the nurse should remember that more serious problems may be present and she should observe the patient for underlying internal chest trauma.

The key factors during the assessment process that lead to the diagnosis of fractured rib are the history, pain with point tenderness, and confirmation by chest x ray. Management for the patient with uncomplicated rib fracture with no associated injury basically is pain relief and the prevention of complications.

Several techniques for pain relief may be chosen by the physician: chest strapping, intercostal nerve block, local infiltration, and/or paravertebral block. A review of the literature [27, 32, 45] shows that chest strapping is not recommended, except in selected cases of very minor injury. Increased splinting may be fostered by strapping, and the risk associated with shallow respirations is thus compounded. Also, local skin irritation may result from the tape. The intercostal nerve block is considered effective and is generally recommended. The usual procedure is that the physician injects an anesthetic proximal to and including the intercostal spaces below and above the injured rib. Usually the injections are given every 4 to 6 hours for 8 to 24 hours. Occasionally, plastic cannulas are inserted and used for intermittent injections. The major potential complication is pneumothorax.

The nurse greatly helps the patient by explaining to him the very real danger of the complications of inadequate pulmonary ventilation as well as their signs and symptoms. It is important for the nurse to remember that with any technique the physician uses, ventilation may be restricted, predisposing the patient to atelectasis and pneumonia. The patient should be instructed about deep breathing exercises, coughing with support, and prompt return for medical care if fever or a productive cough develops. Analgesics should be used carefully and supplemented with relaxation therapy or other measures to make the patient as comfortable as possible while keeping him alert and actively participating in his care. The patient must remain mobile, turn and move about frequently, breathe deeply, and cough.

Pneumothorax

Pneumothorax may accompany blunt trauma or penetrating trauma [7]. In pneumothorax, an injury to either pleural membrane through the chest wall or through a punctured lung will allow air from the atmosphere to enter the pleural space [46]. The normal negative intrapleural pressure having been lost, there is nothing to counteract the elastic recoil of the lung. Consequently, the lung collapses. Both circulatory and respiratory functions are affected, to a degree dependent on the volume of air accumulated. Small amounts of air may cause no symptoms and few if any physical signs. Massive accumulations, however, can lead to rapid respiratory and circulatory failure if they are not reduced. The pathophysiology of the two most serious forms of pneumothorax, open pneumothorax and tension pneumothorax, usually accounts for the grave condition of patients with pneumothorax.

Open Pneumothorax

An open pneumothorax is the result of air entering the pleural space through a large chest wall defect, usually one caused by a penetrating injury from a stab wound, a gunshot wound, or an explosion (Fig. 15-3). On inspiration, a characteristic swishing or sucking noise can be heard as air rushes from an area of greater pressure (the atmosphere) to an area of lesser pressure (the pleural space). Negative intrapleural pressure is then lost, resulting in collapse of the lung, shift of the mediastinal structures toward the unaffected side, and impairment of the lung's ventilation. On expiration, as pressure on the unaffected side increases, the mediastinal structures shift to the area of lesser pressure (i.e., the side of the collapsed lung). As it does in flail chest, the mediastinal flutter results in kinking of the great vessels, with reduced venous return and cardiac output [50]. The problem with reduced venous return is compounded because negative pressure

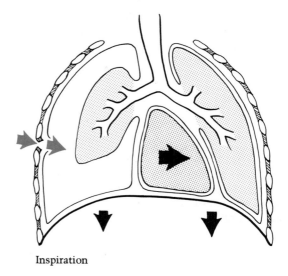

Inspiration

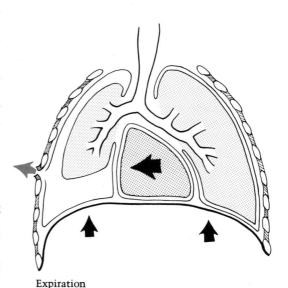

Expiration

Figure 15-3
Open pneumothorax.

is no longer present to draw blood into the thorax. The degree of seriousness of open pneumothorax depends on the size of the opening; air enters the wound in preference to the trachea when the wound is larger than the upper airway.

ASSESSMENT AND MANAGEMENT

In assessing the patient for the presence and seriousness of open pneumothorax, he should be examined for chest wall defect, cyanosis, dyspnea, and hyperpnea. Using palpation, the examiner should note any deviation of the trachea from side to side as the mediastinum shifts from side to side. Using percussion, the examiner should listen for hyperresonance on the affected side. Using auscultation, the examiner should listen for a sucking sound audible to the unaided ear for decreased or absent breath sounds detectable with the stethoscope.

Since open pneumothorax can be quickly lethal, management of the patient entails immediate closure of the wound by any means available [12]. Petrolatum gauze is best, but if nothing else is available, the palm of the hand can be used to prevent further pneumothorax and mediastinal shift. An additional 100 to 200 ml of air can be evacuated from the pleural space if the occlusive dressing is applied after the patient coughs or exhales forcibly [8]. The edges of the wound should not be approximated with tape or suture at this time since subcutaneous air may invade the area. Care must be taken not to convert the open pneumothorax into a more lethal condition, tension pneumothorax. An emergency dressing of petrolatum gauze will close the open wound so that tension pneumothorax will not develop. The dressing is applied to cover the wound and extend 6 to 8 in. beyond the wound edges. It is then covered with gauze and three-inch adhesive tape [44]. A new dressing must be applied when the old dressing becomes sodden with blood, is stiff, and stands away from the chest.

After the emergency care, decompression and drainage of the pleural space are achieved by the use of chest tubes. Since the wounds are inevitably contaminated, attention to the details of asepsis is needed to prevent further infection.

Tension Pneumothorax

A tension pneumothorax results when the volume of air accumulating in the pleural space continues to in-

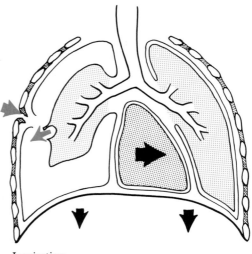

Inspiration

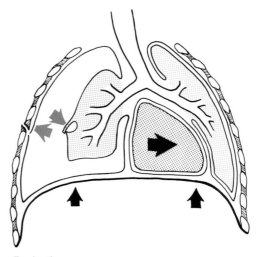

Expiration

Figure 15-4
Tension pneumothorax.

crease in size with each breath, adding more and more air to a pleural space that has no outlet (Fig. 15-4). Air enters the pleural space during inspiration and cannot escape during expiration through the wound in the trachea, bronchus, lung, or chest wall. For several reasons, the effects of a tension pneumothorax are more severe and pronounced than in any other type of pleural involvement. As the size of the pneumothorax increases, pressure begins to build, forcing the mediastinal structures toward the unaffected side. Each breath adds to the expanding volume and exerts more pressure on the mediastinum. If the situation is allowed to continue, a progressive mediastinal shift occurs that impairs the function of the uninjured lung. Venous return is reduced by the rising positive intrathoracic pressure to a much greater extent than in even an open pneumothorax. Since there is no escape for the accumulating air and no mediastinal flutter, the progressive shift to the uninjured side continues unabated.

ASSESSMENT AND MANAGEMENT

In assessing the patient in order to determine the presence of tension pneumothorax, the patient should be examined for (1) severe agitation and apprehension accompanied by cyanosis and air hunger (signs of hypoxia), (2) an intact chest wall but a history of crushing, blunt, or blast injury to the chest, (3) a thorax that appears larger on one side than the other, (4) asymmetrical chest excursion (the affected side lags behind the unaffected side during inspiration), (5) deviation of the trachea toward the unaffected side, and (6) circulatory embarrassment, with falling blood pressure, weak rapid pulse, cold, clammy skin, distended neck veins, and rising central venous pressure. Using palpation, the examiner should note any deviation of the trachea toward the unaffected side, shifting of the apex beat away from the affected side, and subcutaneous emphysema. Using percussion, the examiner should note any resonance (which could reach extreme hyperresonance) on the affected side. Using auscultation, the examiner should listen for diminished or absent breath sounds on the affected side with absent voice sounds and vocal fremitus.

Management of the patient with tension pneumothorax requires providing a route for the escape of air from the pleural space. Introduction of a chest tube or needle aspiration is the technique generally used to remove the air.

An emergency maneuver that offers temporary relief involves the insertion of a 16-gauge intravenous catheter or a large needle attached to a large syringe with a stopcock into the second intercostal space in the midclavicular line on the affected side. Intercostal vessels and nerves may be avoided by entering at midpoint in the intercostal space. When the tension inside the chest is encountered, the high intrapleural pressure will suddenly push the plunger out of the syringe. In using the intravenous catheter, the inner needle stylet is removed from the catheter so that the

air will have a larger pathway through which to escape and the slowly reexpanding lung will not be further traumatized by a needle present at the chest wall. The soft plastic catheter will not harm the reexpanding lung.

Pleural decompression can be maintained by attaching a flutter valve to the end of the catheter so that air will continue to escape on expiration but not enter the thorax on inspiration, as would happen with an open pneumothorax. Pleural decompression can be improvised by taping a perforated finger cot to the hub of the intravenous catheter. The finger cot, which is pliable, will allow air to escape through the perforation on expiration, and it will collapse and seal on inspiration. Commercially prepared flutter valves are available under the tradenames Heimlich valve and McSwain dart.

Hemothorax

Hemothorax, the accumulation of blood in the pleural space, involves not only the cardiorespiratory impairments of chest trauma, but also the problems of shock from blood loss. As much as 2 liters of blood, enough to induce profound levels of hemorrhagic shock, may accumulate in the chest cavity. Furthermore, the amount and severity of the "internal chest bleed" cannot be seen but only estimated by the signs produced [11]. Detection is a key part of the management of that type of chest involvement.

Hemothorax may occur in both blunt and penetrating trauma. Although more common in penetrating trauma, it must also be considered in severe blunt and/or decelerating accidents, both of which may rupture intrathoracic vessels by pressure and torsional mechanisms. Rapid deceleration is particularly notorious for producing aortic tears, which bleed into the chest slightly at first, dissect through the intimal layers of the aorta, and eventually end in a ruptured aneurysm. The association of hemothorax with traumatic pneumothorax suggests laceration of the pulmonary parenchyma. Additional sources of bleeding may be lacerated intercostal muscles and vessels, torn pleural adhesions, and injury to the heart or great vessels and at the site of fractured ribs [20, 30].

There are four usual sources of bleeding in hemothorax:

1. The pulmonary parenchyma and vessels. Since the pulmonary artery pressure is one-third that of systemic pressure, bleeding from the pulmonary artery branches infrequently continues.

2. The intercostal and internal mammary arteries. Bleeding from those sites is usually longer and greater than bleeding from the lung. However, the bleeding may be massive and continuous, requiring thoracotomy and ligation due to the high flow in the internal mammary artery (the flow is similar to that in the radial artery). In particular, the bleeding is greater when the artery is only partially lacerated because on complete transection, retraction and spasm will usually cause thrombosis.

3. The mediastinum—heart, aorta, and great vessels. Bleeding from those sites is not difficult to detect; the patient will be moribund, in profound shock, and unresponsive to even the most vigorous resuscitative measures. The bleeding may be occult initially and clinically apparent only later, when the traumatic aneurysm ruptures into the pleura.

4. The spleen or liver. Because of their vascularity, those subdiaphragmatic organs are potential sources of bleeding.

Hemothorax impairs cardiorespiratory function much as does any other space-occupying lesion of the thorax. As the size of the accumulation increases, greater and greater pressures are exerted on the lung of the involved side, leading to compression atelectasis. Eventually, the mediastinal structures are encroached on by the growing mass and progressively shift away from it, toward the unaffected side, thus impairing the function of the good lung. Again, the mediastinal shift produces kinking of the great vessels, which with the obstructing pressure of the blood mass, reduces venous return and cardiac output. Hence shock of both cardiac and hemorrhagic origin occurs in hemothorax. The rate at which the shock occurs, as well as its severity, depends on the source and rate of the bleeding.

Assessment and Management

If the accumulation of blood is less than 350 ml, the patient is usually asymptomatic. Also, accumulations of less than 300 ml are commonly not seen on chest x ray. If the accumulation of blood is greater than 350 ml but less than 1500 ml, the patient probably is short of breath and has distant breath sounds, dullness on the affected side, and decreased arterial oxygen tension. A chest x ray taken with the patient in the upright position shows a shadow curving upward and laterally on the involved side. An accumulation of more than 1500 ml of blood produces: (1) deviation of the trachea toward the unaffected side, (2) dullness, absence of breath sounds, limited excursions on the affected side, and an even further decreased arterial oxygen tension, (3) profound shock, from both blood loss and compression, (4) tightness and severe pain in the chest, shortness of breath, faintness, and pain radiating to the neck, shoulder, and upper abdomen, and (5) cyanosis and cardiopulmonary compromise.

Management depends in part on the size of the hemothorax. If less than 350 ml has accumulated, no treatment is indicated; the clot will be defibrinated by normal respiratory excursions and absorbed in 10 to 14 days [37]. Serial chest x rays are needed to rule out continuing bleeding if a chest tube is not placed. With accumulations of up to 1500 ml, thoracentesis and/or tube thoracostomy is indicated, and with accumulations of more than 1500 ml, immediate chest tube drainage, possibly followed by emergency surgery, may be indicated.

As an emergency measure, when the accumulation of blood in the chest begins to produce both circulatory and respiratory impairment, needle aspiration may be performed. The procedure is similar to that used in tension pneumothorax, except that the site is different. One of two sites may be used: (1) the fifth or sixth intercostal space or (2) the seventh or eighth intercostal space between the anterior and posterior axillary lines. Insertion of the needle into a lower intercostal space may injure a high-lying diaphragm and an underlying organ, such as the liver or spleen. Thoracentesis may be repeated or even continued intermittently through the use of stopcock maneuvering as long as the bleeding continues and until tube thoracostomy can be performed.

Chest tube drainage should be instituted as soon as possible since it is the only really effective method of maintaining and monitoring the drainage. Serial chest x rays are essential in monitoring the effectiveness of treatment and the success in evacuating the blood from the pleural space. Once the dangerous level of intrathoracic blood is reduced, attention must be directed to restoring the blood volume. Thoracic blood loss of less than 1000 ml requires replacement with Ringer's lactate solution in an amount two to three times the volume of blood loss.

Tracheal and Bronchial Injuries

Tracheal rupture and bronchial rupture are rare problems caused more often by a crushing than by a penetrating injury. They usually occur as a result of the victim's hitting the steering wheel in a motor vehicle accident. Patients with tracheal rupture are frequently dead before they arrive at the hospital. The tears may vary from small lacerations to complete rupture of the cervical and intrathoracic trachea and even avulsion of the bronchi. Rupture is more likely to result from a blow to the anterior chest when the glottis is closed.

Assessment and Management

Phenomena to be assessed include a persistent air leak uncontrolled by the use of chest tubes, massive amounts of subcutaneous air, massive hemoptysis, refractory hypoxemia (usually associated with pneumothorax), and stridor. Mediastinal emphysema or a pneumothorax may be the only sign of a ruptured airway. Prompt endoscopic examination by the physician with a fiberoptic bronchoscope is imperative.

Fractures of the first and second ribs should alert the examiner to the possibility of a bronchial rupture. Physical signs are demonstration of the fracture by x ray, respiratory distress, hemoptysis, cyanosis, and massive air leak, which may be followed by a pneumothorax. On x ray, retropharyngeal air may be seen. If there is no improvement after chest tube placement, the patient should undergo endoscopic examination to establish the diagnosis. Surgery to repair the rupture may be necessary.

Cardiovascular Injuries

Penetrating Injuries

Penetrating injuries of the heart are the gravest of injuries, and most victims die instantly at the scene of the accident or crime. For the few who live long enough to reach the hospital, the mortality is 50 percent. Death is the result of major cardiac injury, involving large atrial, ventricular, or aortic disruption followed by sudden and massive hemorrhage.

Treatment often requires seemingly drastic, desperate measures, including thoracotomy and open cardiac massage by the physician. The nurse must keep the necessary equipment readily available and workable, ventilate the patient during the resuscitation, administer large amounts of whole blood, and support the family emotionally in the event the patient dies.

PERICARDIAL TAMPONADE

In less severe cardiac injuries, such as ones inflicted by a small knife, immediate death from massive blood loss may be averted by the development of a pericardial tamponade. The pericardial sac is a tough, fibrous, inelastic membrane surrounding the heart. With small knife wounds and (rarely) with small-caliber, low-velocity gunshot wounds, the wound in the pericardial sac may seal, trapping the blood that escapes from the myocardial wound. Blood trapped by the pericardial sac can exert enough pressure to arrest, or "tamponade," the hemorrhage. The pericardial tamponade, which can last from several minutes to several hours, provides the patient with a temporary, lifesaving reprieve from massive blood loss from the cardiac wound, often allowing time to reach emergency care and to take an orderly approach to the management of the injury. The inelasticity of the pericardial sac, however, does not allow much trapped blood to accumulate without the development of excessively high intrapericardial pressure. Eventually, the tamponading effect of a small amount of trapped blood gives way to the restrictive effects of a pericardium full of a large amount of trapped blood. Compression of the atria and ventricles prevents adequate cardiac filling. As the mounting pericardial pressure begins to exceed the pressure within the thin-walled venae cavae and pulmonary veins, it impedes the venous return to the heart. Increasing intrapericardial pressure begins to impede coronary artery blood flow. Eventually the stroke volume and cardiac output fall, and the patient develops profound cardiogenic shock. If the situation is not remedied, pressure continues to build within the pericardial sac until the fibrous membrane tears. At that point, the patient is in the same condition as the victim who dies of massive blood loss at the scene of the accident.

Assessment and Management

Assessing pericardial tamponade is a challenge. Initially the tamponade produces only the most subtle of changes in the patient's condition, changes that can easily go unnoticed. A typical example is the patient with cardiac injury who presents with an obvious penetrating injury in the vicinity of the heart but no apparent signs of cardiac compromise. The patient may be alert, his vital signs may be within normal limits, and the wound may even be dismissed as superficial. If the need for continued close monitoring is not appreciated, the potentially lethal nature of the patient's injury may go undetected. To prevent that from happening, early detection is needed.

A cardiac injury with possible accompanying tamponade should be suspected in any patient with a wound in the cardiac area. The patient should be examined for:

1. Distended neck veins.
2. Deep shock that seems out of proportion to the severity of the wound and the amount of apparent blood loss.
3. Falling arterial pressure.
4. Narrowing pulse pressure.
5. Rising central venous pressure.
6. Pulsus paradoxus—more beats palpated on expiration than on inspiration, loss of the palpated pulse on inspiration, or a fall in systemic arterial blood pressure greater than 10 mm Hg during inspiration. During inspiration, the limited output from the right heart may pool in the lungs and thus reduce the amount of blood delivered to the left heart. The descent of the diaphragm on inspiration pulls on the pericardium to further decrease its volume and further constrict the venae cavae. Expiration, however, pumps blood out of the lungs to augment left ventricular filling and cardiac output.
7. Tachycardia with distant heart sounds.
8. Reduced cardiac pulsation shown by fluoroscopic examination and cardiac enlargement shown by physical examination and chest x ray.

The four key signs of pericardial tamponade are easily detected by the nurse. They are (1) falling arterial pressure, (2) rising central venous pressure, (3) distant heart sounds (Beck's triad), and (4) distended neck veins. Unfortunately, all four signs do not usually appear in every patient with pericardial tamponade. Severe imminent compromise can be detected by use of the "rule of 20s": (1) central venous pressure increased by more than 20 cm H_2O, (2) pulse increased by 20 beats per minute, (3) systolic blood pressure decreased by 20 mm Hg, and (4) pulsus paradoxus greater than 20 mm Hg.

When the amount of blood in the pericardial space is so great that myocardial compression is apparent, immediate aspiration of the pericardial sac is mandatory to prevent death. If aspiration is not performed immediately, the patient will die either as the tamponade's mechanical compression restricts cardiac filling, resulting in shock, or from the exsanguination that follows the eventual rupture of the sac and release of the tamponade. With pericardiocentesis, however, the removal of as little as 15 to 20 ml

of blood may be enough to relieve the pressure and revive even a moribund patient. The procedure is as follows:

1. Unless the patient's condition requires that he be in the supine position, the patient is placed in a semi-Fowler's position (so that accumulated blood will be dependent), and he is monitored continuously with a 12-lead ECG.
2. An area to the left of the fifth or sixth intercostal space at the sternal margin or a few centimeters below the left intercostal margin and to the left of the midline is antiseptically prepared.
3. A large-bore, short-beveled spinal needle attached to a 50-ml syringe with a three-way stopcock is directed superiorly and posteriorly at a 30-degree angle to the chest wall. The chest lead is attached to the needle by an alligator clamp. If the needle touches the epicardium, ST segment elevation occurs. If the needle is in the pericardial space, the ECG reading, including the ST segment, is normal. The needle is inserted by the physician upward through the diaphragm and then gently into the pericardial sac. The blood is checked for clotting. If it clots, the tap is probably intraventricular.

Emergency open thoracotomy with a midsternal incision is used by some physicians. The protocol varies from physician to physician, but most physicians do the pericardiocentesis procedure once or twice, and if bleeding continues, they turn quickly to the surgical approach [9].

Blunt Injuries

Blunt chest trauma results in myocardial injury much more often than is clinically recognized [15, 22]. If one considers the anatomy of the heart and the surrounding structures, it becomes obvious that the heart's position behind the sternum is a vulnerable one. The heart may be severely damaged from an external force without any visible injury to the chest wall. Myocardial damage may be slight or severe. The injury may be forgotten in the initial assessment, particularly if there are associated injuries. Interestingly, myocardial injuries seem to be well tolerated by most patients.

The myocardium, pericardium, endocardial structures, and coronary artery may be contused, lacerated, and/or ruptured, resulting in (1) myocardial contusions, (2) rupture of the cardiac wall, (3) tears of the valves and chordae tendineae, (4) rupture of the interventricular septum, (5) coronary artery injury, (6) rupture of the pericardium and formation of a left ventricular aneurysm, and (7) rupture of the aorta and/or great vessels. Injury results from a direct blow, a transmitted blow, compression, deceleration, and/or blast effects.

ASSESSMENT AND MANAGEMENT

In assessing the degree of myocardial damage, the injury is usually described as mild, serious, or critical. With a mild injury, the patient shows such findings as pericardial friction rub, benign, dysrhythmias, and ST-T wave abnormalities on the ECG. With a serious injury, the likely findings are pericardial or angina-type pain, persistent sinus tachycardia, systolic or diastolic murmurs consistent with valvular regurgitation, atrial or ventricular dysrhythmias on serial ECGs, bundle branch block, enlarged heart on serial chest x rays, abnormal uptake with radionuclide imaging with a tracer substance, and (rarely) myocardial infarction (for example, one demonstrated by transient, abnormal Q waves with an intraventricular conduction defect). With a critical injury, the findings include low cardiac output, severe ventricular dysrhythmias, progressive tamponade, congestive heart failure, ventricular aneurysm, and mural thrombi with systemic or pulmonary embolism.

Management depends largely on the actual injury. A surgical or medical approach is chosen according to the ramifications of the injury and the clinical prognosis [22]. Anticoagulant therapy is often instituted if the danger of mural thrombi is present or if musculoskeletal injuries and prolonged immobilization are associated. In selected patients, the injury may not be diagnosed for weeks or years after the trauma, and so repeated follow-up examinations are mandatory.

AORTIC INJURY

Blunt trauma subjects the thoracic aorta and the great vessels to a variety of forces. Sudden acceleration or deceleration may create shearing forces between different parts of the aorta, between the heart and the aorta, and between the aorta and the great vessels. Compression of the aorta or the great vessels over the vertebral column may cause an aneurysm or rupture.

Aortic trauma must be suspected in all patients

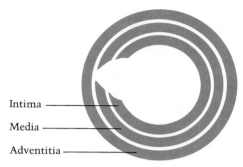

Intima

Media

Adventitia

Figure 15-5
Aortic laceration.

surviving a motor vehicle accident that occurred at speeds greater than 45 mph [17]. Aortic injury occurs with sudden deceleration, typically a head-on collision and when the victim is wearing a seat belt. Because of the sudden deceleration, the descending aorta literally bows forward in a whiplash movement and undergoes severe bending and shearing stress [21]. That segment of aorta is relatively mobile and unrestrained by attachments to nearby structures. The two points at which the stresses most commonly produce damage are (1) where the aorta is fixed, just distal to the subclavian artery, where the ductus arteriosus once was, and (2) at the root of the aorta, where it bifurcates into the femoral arteries. The sudden whiplash stress results in extensive stretching and tearing of the aortic wall, which is sheared. Blood then escapes through the tears, producing a traumatic aneurysm.

When the patient arrives at the hospital, the outer layer of the aneurysm may be all that is keeping the aorta intact (Fig. 15-5). Blood escaping through the tears into the vessel wall may exert great pressure on that outer layer as the aneurysm expands, leaving the patient vulnerable to spontaneous rupture and death from severe intrathoracic hemorrhage.

Assessment and Management
In the assessment and monitoring of all patients with chest trauma, a high index of suspicion must be maintained in regard to the possibility of aortic damage. Prompt investigation and surgical repair by the physician will avert a potential catastrophe. The important signs and symptoms to look for are mediastinal widening, a systolic murmur, hypertension localized to the upper extremities, hoarseness from

pressure on the laryngeal nerve, an enlarged neck, severe back pain, feelings of apprehension, the patient's involvement in a motor vehicle accident at a speed greater than 45 mph, a patient in adolescence or young adulthood (possibly because the physical stamina of people in that age range is such that they are able to survive the initial injury), and positive findings on arteriography.

One-third of all patients with an aorta rupture had little or no evidence of chest trauma on first examination. Serial monitoring is mandatory. The most ominous sign is a widened mediastinum shown by chest x ray, a finding that is reason enough for further diagnostic study involving arteriography to identify and locate the site of the lesion. (Anteroposterior chest x rays occasionally give the impression that the mediastinum is slightly widened when it is normal.) Also, since there is a high incidence of subclavian artery and bronchial injuries, as well as aortic injuries, associated with clavicle and first rib fractures many authorities recommend arteriography for a patient, even when the mediastinum appears normal. Once the diagnosis of aortic injury is made, the patient is moved to the operating room for immediate surgical repair.

Patient Care Delivery

If patients are to be cared for properly, their presenting signs and symptoms must be assessed and their problems managed. The question arises, what should the nurse do to help the patient on his arrival in the emergency room? The nurse must know how to assess the patient and how to set the priorities of care.

Certain historical information should be gathered to help estimate the location and extent of injury. As much information as possible should be obtained by radio from the paramedics in the ambulance or the helicopter before the patient arrives at the hospital [48]. Once the patient is in the emergency room, emphasis is on the examination, but the staff continues to try to gather as much information as possible about the injury. Firemen, policemen, eyewitnesses, other less severely injured victims, and family members are possible sources of information. The information they supply is often invaluable in the patient assessment.

Certain questions should be asked. If the injury was a penetrating one, what was the weapon? Was it a knife? A gun? What was the length of the knife or the caliber of the gun? What was the angle from which the assailant attacked the patient? If the injury followed blunt chest trauma, did it involve rapid deceleration? Was the patient sitting in the driver's seat or in the front passenger's seat, where the energy from the impact against the steering wheel or dashboard was absorbed by the body? All the details of the accident and any treatment given after it are important.

The examination begins even while the patient is being brought into the emergency room. His level of consciousness, any obvious blood loss, his color, and the appearance of any distress should be noted. A systematic examination should follow, with relevant questions being asked and answered as the examination proceeds. His respiratory and cardiac status should be evaluated. Is his airway patent? If not, emergency room personnel should perform the airway maneuvers, airway insertion, endotracheal intubation, or cricothyreotomy as indicated. Is he exchanging air? If not, artificial ventilation should be instituted. Is his trachea in the midline? If not, does he have a mediastinal shift from a pneumothorax or hemothorax and should chest tube(s) be inserted? Is his carotid pulse palpable? It is important to remember that the ABCDs of resuscitation have first priority [43]. Are his neck veins distended? If so, he should be further evaluated for cardiac tamponade and prepared by pericardiocentesis. Does he have a penetrating chest injury? If so, where are the entry and exit wounds? Does he have a blunt chest injury? Does he have a flail segment? What are his respiratory rate and depth? Does he retract or does he use his accessory muscles? Does he have stridor? Does his chest expand equally on both sides, or is one side larger than the other? Does he show paradoxical motion? Does he have hemoptysis? Does his chest expand equally on palpation? Does the examiner feel rib movement, crepitation, or a deformity? Does the patient complain of a painful or tender area? Where is the point of maximal impulse? Are there areas of hyperresonance or dullness on percussion? What are the pattern and equality of breath sounds on auscultation? Are the sounds diminished or absent? Are adventitious sounds present?

Additional information about the patient is essential to his assessment and management. His response to the treatment for shock must be determined. It is important to remember that MAST trousers (see Chap. 34) are contraindicated in chest injuries. Laboratory reports of the arterial blood gas determinations must be evaluated. The chest x ray must be examined.

As soon as possible, the data base should be completed by the addition of a complete history of the injury, pertinent points in the patient's past medical history, and the findings from a thorough physical examination. Throughout the emergency phase, the health team should continue to monitor and reassess the patient to determine his condition and his response to resuscitation.

The data obtained from the assessment must be put into action. If the nurse does not know what the assessment data mean, she should give them to someone who can interpret them. Her ability to describe is of the utmost importance. If the physician is not present, the nurse can transmit to him a description of the patient that may give the physician a basis for decision making. The tools of assessment are essential to the nurse.

Tube Thoracostomy

In the critical care unit, all supportive measures to prevent the complications of injury must be given the patient. Unless the nursing measures are comprehensive and detailed, the patient may suffer from the side effects of immobility, pulmonary dysfunction, psychological alterations, sepsis, and altered metabolism. Those complications are discussed in other chapters of the text. The nursing care specific to the patient with chest tubes is discussed in the following paragraphs.

Patients in critical care units frequently have problems that require the placement of chest tubes [49]. There are some variations in the type of drainage system, but the basic principles remain the same. Chest tubes are primarily used to return the lung to functioning at normal pressure and dynamics. Various types of injury allow air and/or fluid to enter the pleural space so that the normal negative pressure (−8 mm Hg intrapleural pressure and −3 mm Hg intraalveolar pressure during inspiration) is lost and proper lung inflation cannot occur. Chest tubes are used to evacuate the pleural space so that the pressure may be reestablished. The fluid and/or air removed may be monitored and changes noted. Coughing and the removal of secretions are mandatory for the adequate reexpansion of the lung [3].

The drainage system that is connected to the chest tube must include the safety feature of an underwater seal. The water functions as the flutter valve, permitting air and/or fluid to escape from the chest on expiration and preventing its reentrance into the pleural space on inspiration. Also, the device permits persistent air leaks, as well as continuing hemorrhage, to be evaluated. Other problems are prevented: compression of the trachea, mediastinal shift, and infection.

A person who has been injured naturally positions himself to decrease pain and restrict movement of the affected part. When the injury is a lung injury, the inadequate lung expansion due to the restricted movement results in stasis, with the accumulation of secretions and the occlusion of lung passages. Atelectasis progresses rapidly and the entire lung can be involved. Atelectatic areas are perfused but not ventilated, and right-to-left shunting results in hypoxia and hypercarbia [9]. Those problems must be prevented.

CHEST TUBE DRAINAGE SYSTEM

The chest tube drainage system has several components [24, 29]. Essentially a chest tube (catheter) drains the pleural space and is attached to a valve arrangement. The valve arrangement can be (1) a one-way valve, (2) a waterseal drainage system, or (3) a waterseal drainage system with suction.

The one-way valve is a simple unidirectional system, such as the Heimlich flutter valve, in which a Penrose-type material is used in the tube so that the tube collapses on inspiration and opens on expiration. Thus air and fluid drain from the chest. The thin, wide rubber tube is open at the end of the valve proximal to the chest tube and compressed at the end distal to the chest tube so that the flat sides remain in contact with each other. The apparatus is encased in clear plastic, making it possible to see what is draining through the valve.

The most common drainage system is a water-sealed valve arrangement (Fig. 15-6). The chest tube drains the pleural space and is connected to another tube or glass rod, which remains under water (usually saline solution is used). The water acts as a seal. Since the tube remains under water and the intrapleural pressure is negative, water rises in the tube. Thus the underwater seal valve must remain at a level sufficiently below the chest to prevent the column of water from reentering the pleural space. The pressure in the valve is determined by the depth the tube extends under the water (the fluid level should not be more than 3 to 4 cm above the end of the water column). Any intrapleural pressure that is greater than the valve pressure forces air and/or fluid

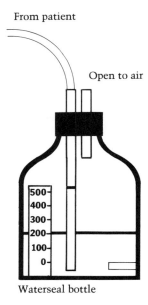

Figure 15-6
Simple water-sealed drainage system.

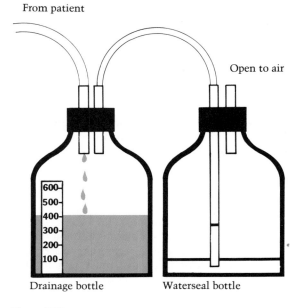

Figure 15-7
Water-sealed drainage system with added drainage bottle.

through the system. Thus the waterseal is important because it seals the chest so that the air cannot leak back. The waterseal drainage system is sufficient if the fluid or air that has collected is well localized and in a walled space. Any accumulation that exerts more than 3 to 4 cm H_2O will be drained. The patient is instructed to cough forcefully and frequently to help evacuate the trapped air. How successful the patient is in coughing out the air can be monitored by watching the column of water in the underwater tube: the column will fluctuate with the respirations, and bubbles will escape from the tube on forced expiration or cough.

The chest bottle is also important because it allows for gravity drainage of fluid and allows air to escape from the pleural space. The drainage bottle is closed except for two openings in the rubber stopper. The long tube for the waterseal goes through one opening, and a short glass rod (air vent) for the egress of air and stabilization of the pressure in the system goes through the other opening. The drainage bottle and all tubing are kept sterile. The system is maintained as a leakproof system in case suction must be added. If the drainage is of sufficient quantity so that the bottle is more than about two-thirds full, the bottle must be changed. The amount of fluid is measured and the difference between that and the amount of saline solution originally placed in the bottle is calculated and recorded.

The tubing must always hang straight from the patient's bed to the drainage bottle since any fluid in the dependent tubing will alter pressures and obstruct flow. The intrapleural pressures will have to be higher to force air and/or fluid from the chest.

In an alternate—but still simple—drainage system, a second bottle or reservoir is used (Fig. 15-7). The bottle acts as a drainage bottle and is placed between the patient and the waterseal bottle. The same principle is used with the disposable plastic drainage apparatus shown in Figure 15-8, in which the first chamber is for drainage and the second chamber is for the waterseal (the open air vent at the top of the well makes it a simple drainage system). In both types, the waterseal valve apparatus is maintained in a fixed system, and the volume of drainage can be accurately measured. Drainage accumulates in the first bottle, displacing air into the second bottle's underwater tube. When intrapleural pressure is higher than atmospheric pressure, air escapes through the second bottle's waterseal into the atmosphere.

Oscillation (also called fluctuation or tidaling) in

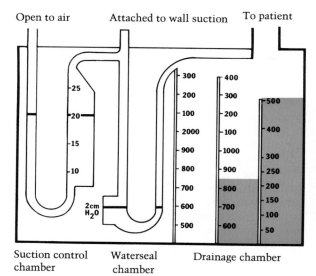

Open to air   Attached to wall suction   To patient

Suction control chamber   Waterseal chamber   Drainage chamber

Figure 15-8
Disposable chest-drainage unit.

Figure 15-9
Water-sealed drainage with added suction.

the glass connector tube ending under the water must also be monitored. The level in the water column fluctuates in accordance with lung compliance and acts as a manometer for intrapleural pressure. During inspiration, the intrapleural pressure is at its peak, and fluid in the water column rises (2-6 cm). Inspiratory effort can be evaluated by the oscillation. During expiration, intrapleural pressure is less negative, and the level in the connector tube falls. Different pulmonary mechanisms alter the amount of oscillation. For example, the deep inspiration before coughing will cause the level to rise to a higher level. Fluctuation is reversed with the patient on a ventilator; that is, on inspiration, fluid in the water column falls, and on expiration, the fluid rises.

Even after chest tubes have ceased to function, they are left in place another 24 hours. The amount of time is increased to 48 hours and serial x rays are reevaluated if the leak is persistent and the possibility of recurrence remains.

In the third type of system, controlled suction is added in order to apply negative pressure to the chest (Fig. 15-9). Suction is necessary if the flow of air and fluid must be increased (as it must be when there is a large air leak or a large amount of fluid that reaccumulates) or when the negative intrathoracic pressure must be reestablished. For example, the egress of air is thus increased in order to evacuate the continued pneumothorax if the tear in the lung is large.

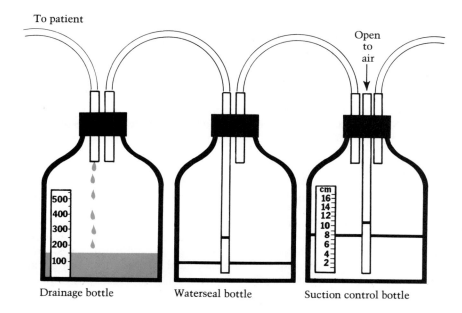

To patient

Open to air

Drainage bottle   Waterseal bottle   Suction control bottle

Suction is connected to the air vent in the water-seal bottle and is maintained between -15 and -30 cm H_2O pressure since higher degrees of subatmospheric pressure may result in large transpulmonary pressure gradients with the precipitation of acute pulmonary edema. With added suction, two chest bottles are most frequently used. Negative pressure applied to the thorax may be adjusted from 1 to 15 cm H_2O by varying the level of fluid within the two waterseal bottles and by varying the inflow of atmospheric air allowed in the waterseal bottle adjacent to the source of suction. With the disposable plastic chest drainage apparatus, the third chamber is used for suction. However, many surgeons consider the commercial appliances inadequate when suction must be added. In all suction systems, the suction is temporarily discontinued to assess tube patency since oscillation is sometimes difficult to observe with added suction.

INSERTION SITES

Various sites are used for chest tube insertion. The more common site for the anterior tube is the second intercostal space in the midclavicular line, and the more common site for the posterior tube is the seventh to eighth intercostal space between the anterior and the posterior axillary lines. Tubes are usually used in both sites for a hemopneumothorax. However, it must be noted that an increasing number of surgeons place chest tubes in the fourth to fifth intercostal space in the midaxillary line in a posterosuperior direction since that site has been seen to be clinically effective to treat pneumothorax following trauma.

The second intercostal space in the midclavicular line is chosen for many reasons. Since air rises, when that site is used, quick, complete reexpansion commonly occurs. Few injuries are associated with insertion since there are no major anatomical hazards. The mammary artery is close to the sternal border, and the subclavian artery and vein are near the first intercostal space. If the patient is lying in the supine or semi-Fowler's position, the area is easily accessible. Last, but certainly not least, the tube is out of the way during many procedures (for example, cardiopulmonary resuscitation).

The posterior tube is placed in a dependent position for drainage. Although the tube is posterior, a site is chosen so that the patient in the supine position will not compress the tube or be uncomfortable. The lowest position possible is chosen; the seventh or eighth intercostal space is commonly used since the diaphragm bulges into the thoracic cavity at the eighth or ninth intercostal space. In cases in which the tube is lower, it is usually placed as a drain rather than as a chest tube.

Chest tubes are inserted in patients with pneumothorax to reestablish normal chest functioning, to relieve the dyspnea, and to correct imbalances of the arterial blood gases. Repeated needle aspiration, an alternate method, is rarely used because of the ease of inserting a chest tube and because a tube allows for continuous evacuation. When the potential for tension pneumothorax exists, chest tubes are mandatory.

Chest tubes are also used for patients with hemothorax; they allow for continuous evacuation so that the lung is expanded more quickly and completely. The amount the patient is bleeding can be seen and monitored. The blood in the chest cavity remains liquid if it is not mixed with air. However, when it is mixed with air—the more likely case—a clot forms that is difficult to remove with a chest tube. If a large amount of clotted blood forms, the lung will not reexpand. The thrombus progresses and forms a fibrothorax, which then physically restricts expansion. Usually a #34 or #36 tube (large-bore, to allow the passage of blood clots) is placed posteriorly to drain the dependent regions of the thorax, where the blood accumulates. The chest tube is connected to underwater seal drainage, which serves as a collection system for the blood drained from the thorax while it keeps atmospheric air from entering the thoracotomy wound and thus compounding the hemothorax with a pneumothorax. The tube—or tubes, since two may be inserted beside each other in case severe bleeding occurs or one tube clots—must be managed scrupulously—to maintain patency, encourage evacuation of the blood from the thorax, and determine the amount and extent of the bleeding.

COMPLICATIONS

Many problems can arise with chest tubes. The nurse must think through whatever problem situations arise. If by some accident, the chest tube is pulled out, the problem is simple and rarely life threatening (unless the danger of tension pneumothorax is present). The patient is asked to cough, and the area is covered with petrolatum gauze and a dry sterile dressing. The physician is notified, and a stat portable chest x ray is ordered from the x-ray department.

If the chest tube is accidentally disconnected from the chest tube drainage, the solution is to reconnect the two in the patient who has a continuing air leak. It is best not to clamp the chest tube but to reconnect it to avoid a tension pneumothorax. If reconnection is not possible, it is better to let the chest tube act as an open pneumothorax.

When the patient with a tension pneumothorax is to be transferred from the emergency department or if the bottles break, the chest tubes should not be clamped. If the tubes are clamped, by the time the patient has arrived on the next service, a tension pneumothorax may not only have redeveloped but be worse if positive pressure ventilation is used. On the other hand, if the chest tube has stopped functioning prior to disconnection, there is no danger in clamping the tube next to the chest wall. Also, when a continuing air leak is not present and the chest tube is pulled loose from the bottle or the connector or bottle breaks, the chest tube may be clamped close to the chest while the bottle is changed or the connector quickly replaced.

Problems can also exist with the drainage bottle. One simple problem is that the chest tube is connected to the air vent rather than to the glass connector tube. In such a case, air in the pleural space could not leave and room air would enter the pleural space. A persistent air leak may be present in the apparatus rather than in the patient. Usually the leak is caused by a loose connection. Replacement of the tubing may be necessary. If it is, the chest tube is clamped at the patient's chest wall, and the system is evaluated inch by inch. If the bubbling continuous leak is in the tubing, it can be pinpointed by putting a clamp distal to each connection. Each portion is closely observed since the leak is often difficult to find. On the other hand, the problem may be obvious but simply overlooked. If no leak is found in the tubing, the leak is in the patient or at the insertion site.

Nursing Orders

Problem/Diagnosis

The patient has a respiratory dysfunction secondary to hemopneumothorax due to motor vehicle accident.

OBJECTIVE NO. 1

The patient should demonstrate the return of adequate pulmonary function.

To achieve the objective, the nurse should:

1. Assess the patient before assessing the equipment.
2. Monitor the patient's pulmonary status as evidenced by the assessment. She should:
   a. Measure the patient's temperature and respiration every two to four hours.
   b. Perform a respiratory examination, including percussion notes and breath sounds.
   c. Measure the central venous pressure and pulmonary artery pressures.
   d. Calculate compliance if the patient is mechanically ventilated.
   e. Draw an arterial blood sample and send it to the laboratory for the determination of PO_2, pH, PCO_2, HCO_3^-, and delta base [55].
   f. Order a chest x ray daily as directed by the physician.
   g. Send specimens to the laboratory for a white blood cell count with a differential count and a sputum smear or culture.
3. Turn the patient every hour he is awake. The nurse should plan a schedule with him so that he assumes all positions and so that he is as comfortable as possible. For example, she should turn him every one to two hours from a left semiprone position to a right semiprone position (and vice versa). She should turn him slowly, using pillows to position him. She should put him in the semi-Fowler's position once or twice a day for 30 minutes.
4. Maintain the patient's pulmonary hygiene. The nurse should:
   a. Have the patient deep breathe every hour. She should remain with him and remind him to inhale slowly and evenly, hold his breath for three seconds, and exhale normally. The procedure should be repeated five times.
   b. Have him cough at least five times every hour. Have him take several deep breaths and then cough. Splint his chest with hands or pillow. Check any tubes and connections.
   c. Move him out of bed to chair as soon as possible and begin ambulation as ordered.
   d. Perform nasopharyngeal suctioning if he is unable to clear his own secretions. Be sure he understands the procedure and knows that he should not hold his breath. Use a nasopharyngeal airway that has been lubricated with a local anesthetic. Administer oxy-

gen before suctioning and maintain oxygen therapy if possible during suctioning. Suction carefully. Remember that a good cough is more effective than suctioning.

e. Perform chest physiotherapy and postural drainage every four to six hours, as indicated by the findings from auscultation and chest x rays.

5. Maintain the patient's airway when an endotracheal tube is placed.

a. Monitor the patient frequently to make sure there is no obstruction, which is evidenced by lack of air movement, restlessness, absence of chest excursions, absent breath sounds, tachycardia, noisy breathing, and cyanosis.

b. Monitor the placement of endotracheal tube by auscultating the patient's chest for bilateral breath sounds. Remember that the endotracheal tube is much more likely to move down the right mainstem bronchus and obstruct the left side than it is to come out of the patient.

c. Use a low-pressure high-volume cuff. Inflate the cuff, using the minimal air-leak technique.

d. Determine the patient's need for suctioning by monitoring his breath sounds for rhonchi, a change in or sudden absence of sounds, the development of rales, and arterial blood gas imbalances. Do not withhold suctioning when patient is on PEEP. The levels will be reestablished in three to five minutes after suctioning [14].

e. Explain the suctioning procedure to the patient.

f. Give the patient oxygen by lung hyperinflation, using a higher concentration of inspired oxygen. Promote lung hyperinflation by deep breaths or the use of manual breathing bag or if the patient is being ventilated mechanically, increase oxygen to 100% and sigh. Assess the patient and the suctioning procedure variables that affect hypoxemia related to endotracheal suctioning: the suction pressure, catheter-to-endotracheal tube ratio, catheter lumen-to-suction orifice ratio, length of suctioning, hyperinflation before and after suctioning, administration of oxygen during suctioning, arterial oxygen tension, vital signs, ECG, magnitude of the pulmonary shunt, and patient's susceptibility to suction-induced small airway closure [1, 34].

g. If the patient is hypoxic, give him oxygen with FIO_2 of 100% for three minutes before suctioning. Endotracheal suctioning is more likely to reduce arterial oxygen levels and produce complications in a hypoxemic patient than in a patient with normal or elevated oxygen levels. If the patient is ventilated mechanically, give him oxygen before, during, and after suctioning [34]. Do not interrupt the ventilations of patients who are not responsive to increased FIO_2 or who have large pulmonary shunts. Use hyperinflation carefully, assessing first the level of respiratory secretions and the acid base status (since an increase in pH may increase myocardial and central nervous system irritability).

h. Suction through the aperture of the swivel adapter if the patient is being ventilated mechanically (another way to maintain oxygen levels while suctioning is to administer oxygen through a second catheter lumen) [5].

i. Turn the patient's head from left to right to facilitate the removal of secretions from both mainstem bronchi. (Although that nursing procedure has been commonly accepted, preliminary research evidence now questions its effectiveness.)

j. Use a suction catheter long enough to stimulate coughing and to obtain secretions (use of a multiple side hole catheter probably does less damage than a whistletip catheter; the catheter diameter should not be more than one-half the diameter of the lumen of the tube through which it is passed).

k. Instill 5 to 30 ml sterile saline solution before suctioning if needed to loosen thick secretions.

l. Limit the time of suctioning to 10 to 15 seconds. The nurse performing the procedure should hold her breath while suctioning.

m. Be gentle. Important variables in trauma resulting from repeated suctioning are frequency, manner of insertion, duration of prolonged suction, and pressure magnitude (less than 150 mm Hg is recommended for an adult).

n. Use a rotating motion while removing the catheter and apply suctioning intermittently. Remove the catheter if the patient becomes cyanotic or dyspneic or has dysrhythmias.

o. Deep breathe or sigh the patient several times

following suctioning and oxygenate him with FIO_2 of 100% for three minutes.

p. Auscultate the patient after suctioning to determine what changes have taken place and whether repeated suctioning is needed.

q. Maintain the sterility of the system.

r. Change the bite block daily. Make sure no significant pressure is applied to the patient's mouth or nose.

s. Change the tapes that secure the endotracheal tube daily.

t. Give mouth care every four hours. Use a mouthwash and swabs. Lubricate the patient's nares with a water-soluble lubricant to prevent dryness and irritation.

6. Maintain mechanical ventilation. The nurse should:

a. Assess the pulmonary parameters.

b. Measure the FIO_2 and other settings every hour to see that the dials have not been inadvertently changed.

c. Ensure the sterility of the system.

d. Ensure constant humidification.

e. Auscultate the patient for breath sounds hourly.

f. Facilitate communication with the patient by observing the patient's mouthing of words. Have a paper and pencil or Magic Slate available.

g. Observe the patient for signs of decreased venous return to the heart: falling blood pressure, weak pulse, rising central venous pressure or distended neck veins, and fall in the oxygen level in a mixed venous sample.

h. Refer to Chapter 17, which has a detailed description of patient care.

i. To assist with respiratory control, administer diazepam or morphine sulfate as ordered.

j. If controlled respiratory manuevers are ordered, prepare to administer pancuronium bromide (initial dose 0.04–0.1 mg/kg body weight; maintenance dose 0.01 mg/kg body weight). Determine the need for additional medication by monitoring the patient's muscle activity and the pressure gauge on his ventilator to determine whether the patient is assisting ventilation. Continue to administer analgesics, which have no adverse side effects. Since the muscles that control eyelid movement are paralyzed, take precautionary measures to avoid dryness of the eyes.

7. Apply and maintain the chest-tube drainage system for hemothorax.

a. Strip, or milk, the tubes every five minutes until the flow significantly decreases (an accepted nursing procedure, but one whose validity has not been established by research).

b. Measure the amount of drainage at 5-minute intervals until the flow of blood begins to slow, and then measure it at 15-minute intervals.

c. Encourage the patient to lie with his affected side down so that the chest tube, which is now dependent, can collect the intrathoracic blood more efficiently.

8. Monitor the patient for shortness of breath, subcutaneous emphysema, and cyanosis.

9. Evaluate the entire chest-tube drainage system for proper assembly every four hours. Starting at the patient's chest, the nurse should make certain that:

a. The airtight dressing is in place.

b. The tubing is free of kinks, loops, and obstructions.

c. The air outlet is open.

d. The chest tube is connected to the long glass column, the end of which is submerged 2 to 4 cm. (If it is submerged deeper, the resistance to drainage of air or fluid is increased.)

e. The waterseal is intact.

f. The end of the glass column does not touch the bottom of the bottle.

g. All connections are secured by adhesive tape.

h. To prevent tube kinking, a tongue blade is taped to the drainage tubing where it enters the drainage bottle.

i. The bottles are in protective cradles.

j. The bottles are kept at a level lower than the chest.

10. Check the chest-tube drainage system every hour to see that:

a. The oscillations in the glass column occur with respiration (up on inspiration, down on expiration, except during positive pressure ventilation, when the opposite is true). If the work of breathing is increased, the oscillations will be seen at a greater level.

b. Bubbles occur on expiration or cough only (with positive pressure, on inspiration). The nurse should report to the physician any continuous bubbling because it usually means that there is a leak in the system.

c. The level, consistency, color, and rate of drainage have not changed significantly.

d. The blood loss is not greater than 100 ml/hr. If it is, the physician should be notified.

11. Maintain the proper functioning of the chest tubes. The nurse should:

a. Strip the tubes every hour. Gently compress the tube in the direction of the drainage apparatus (away from the patient to remove fluid, air, or blood clots). Clasp the tube and slide the hand over the tube in a direction away from the chest and toward the drainage. Use alcohol sponges or a water-soluble lubricant to facilitate sliding. Be gentle—the procedure can be painful.

b. Reconnect any tube that is disconnected and do not clamp it.

c. If a bottle breaks, (a) not clamp the anterior tube; rather, submerge the end of the tube in a convenient container of sterile water or saline solution and then prepare a new bottle (if the tube had already stopped functioning, it may be clamped), and (b) clamp the posterior tube and prepare a new bottle.

d. Not clamp the tube if the patient is to be moved to another unit.

e. Monitor the patient closely if the physician orders the tubes clamped.

f. Position the patient on the affected side for hemothorax and in the semi-Fowler's position for pneumothorax.

g. Keep the tubes hanging straight from the bed to the bottles; the tubes should not be left in a dependent position.

h. Observe the following procedure for chest tube removal: Have petrolatum gauze and a sterile dressing ready for the physician. The tube should be removed with a steady, quick motion during expiration or following a deep inspiration and the dressing should then be applied. Follow-up chest x rays are mandatory.

12. Apply added suction as ordered. The nurse should:

a. With a disposable plastic controlled suction apparatus, fill the control tube to the prescribed distance and keep the upper end of the control tube open to air.

b. With two waterseal bottles, adjust the fluid levels and the amount of atmospheric air entering the bottle nearest the suction source to obtain the desired pressure.

c. Open the tubing from the motor to the air if the motor goes off.

d. Refill the control bottle as the fluid evaporates.

e. Check for constant bubbling, a sign of proper functioning.

f. Know that with hemopneumothorax, two systems are often used. The system with the greater negative pressure is used for the hemothorax, and the system with the lesser pressure is used for the pneumothorax.

OBJECTIVE NO. 2

The patient should demonstrate the return of adequate cardiovascular functioning.

To achieve the objective, the nurse should:

1. Provide volume replacement as ordered, using whole blood, packed cells, Ringer's lactate solution, and/or colloid solution.

2. Monitor cardiovascular functioning by measuring blood pressure, pulse, pulmonary capillary wedge pressure, pulmonary artery pressures, central venous pressure, sensorium, urinary output, cardiac output, capillary refill, ECG results, and hemoglobin and hematocrit levels.

3. Monitor and replace electrolytes as ordered.

4. Administer diuretics as ordered.

OBJECTIVE NO. 3

The patient should maintain psychological equilibrium.

To attain the objective, the nurse should:

1. Explain to the patient in simple terms what has happened and what is happening to him.

2. Provide the patient with some means of communication.

3. Offer the patient support and reassurance.

4. Involve the patient's family and encourage their support.

5. Plan care to permit the patient periods of uninterrupted sleep.

6. Refer to Chapter 36, which has a detailed description of patient care.

7. Remember that even the simplest nursing act is never a neutral event; it should be performed with skill and understanding (Fig. 15-10).

8. If the patient is paralyzed for respiratory control,

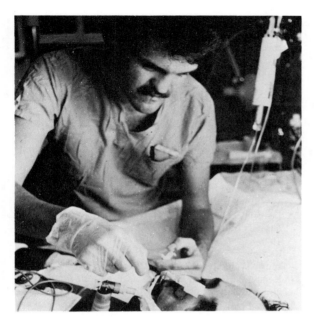

Figure 15-10
Even the simplest nursing act should be performed with skill and understanding since it is never a neutral event.

remember that his vision is blurred, that he can still hear and feel, and that he is totally powerless.

OBJECTIVE NO. 4

The patient should not have an inordinate amount of pain.

To attain the objective, the nurse should:

1. Give the patient a chance to tell her about any pain and what makes it better and what makes it worse.
2. Splint the patient's chest with her hands or with pillows to make coughing and deep breathing easier.
3. Strip the chest tubes carefully.
4. If possible, relieve any other sources of discomfort, including worry.
5. Use the established techniques for making the patient comfortable: changing his bed linens, giving him backrubs, and changing his position.
6. If possible, involve the family in the patient's care.
7. Use deep breathing and other relaxation techniques.

8. Use pain medication as ordered in conjunction with the other measures that have been effective for the individual patient. Remember that the patient paralyzed for respiratory control still has pain and requires analgesics.

OBJECTIVE NO. 5

The patient should maintain his fluid and electrolyte balance.

To attain the objective, the nurse should:

1. Explain to the patient why and how intravenous therapy is to be given.
2. Weigh the patient every day.
3. Monitor the patient's fluid intake and output.
4. Administer intravenous fluids as ordered.
5. Maintain the patient's intake by mouth (when he is able to take nourishment by mouth). Refer to Chapter 36, which discusses nutritional requirements.
6. Monitor the patient's electrolyte status (see Chap. 34).
7. Monitor the patient's nasogastric drainage and urinary output, determining the amount of both and the loss of electrolytes.
8. Check the infusion site every four hours for phlebitis, evidenced by swelling, redness, pain, and heat. If infiltration is suspected, the bag should be lowered below the patient's arm level and blood should be watched for at the distal end of the intravenous catheter.
9. Check the tubing for kinks, obstructions, and improper connections.
10. Maintain the rate of flow constantly as ordered.
11. Add any intravenous medication that is ordered to the volutrol. Dilute the medication and allow it to be infused before filling the volutrol. Observe the patient for any untoward reactions (e.g., dyspnea, an allergic reaction, or a rash).

OBJECTIVE NO. 6

The patient should maintain functional range of motion.

To achieve the objective, the nurse should:

1. Use active, active-assisted, and passive range-of-motion exercises for each joint three to four times each day.
2. Maintain appropriate body alignment when doing positioning techniques. Think carefully of each

body part and whether or not it has been positioned for ultimate functioning.

3. Use a footboard or a commercial device, such as Bunny Boots or Space Boots, to maintain the lower extremity positioning.

4. Use a trochanter roll, which often can prevent hip and leg abduction.

5. Remember that contracture complications are much more easily prevented than treated.

References

1. Adlkofer, R., and Powaser, M. The effect of endotracheal suctioning on arterial blood gases in patients after cardiac surgery. *Heart Lung* 7:1011, 1978.

2. Avery, E. E., Morch, E. T., and Benson, D. W. Critically crushed chests: New method of treatment with continuous mechanical hyperventilation to produce alkalotic apnea and internal pneumatic stabilization. *J. Thorac. Cardiovasc. Surg.* 32:291, 1956.

3. Barchelder, T. L., and Morris, K. A. Critical factors in determining adequate pleural drainage in both the operated and non-operated chest. *Ann. Surg.* 28:302, 1962.

4. Bartlett, J. G., and Gorbach, S. L. The triple threat of aspiration pneumonia. *Chest* 68:560, 1975.

5. Belling, D., Kelley, R., and Simon, R. Use of the swivel adaptor aperture during suctioning to prevent hypoxemia in the mechanically ventilated patient. *Heart Lung* 7:320, 1978.

6. Blair, E., Topuzlu, C., and Deane, R. S. Chest Trauma. In J. P. Hardy (ed.), *Critical Surgical Illness.* Philadelphia: Saunders, 1971.

7. Blanco, G. Pneumothorax. *Hosp. Med.* 2:40, 1975.

8. Borrie, J. *Management of Emergencies in Thoracic Surgery.* New York: Appleton-Century-Crofts, 1972.

9. Breaux, E. P., Dupont, J. B., Albert, H. M., et al. Cardiac tamponade following pentrating mediastinal injuries: Improved survival with early pericardiocentesis. *J. Trauma* 19:461, 1979.

10. Bryan-Brown, C. W. Tissue blood flow and oxygen transport in critically ill patients. *Crit. Care Med.* 3:103, 1975.

11. Clarke, R., and Fisher, M. R. Assessment of blood loss following injury. *Br. J. Clin. Pract.* 10:746, 1956.

12. Committee on Trauma of the American College of Surgeons. *Early Care of the Injured Patient.* Philadelphia: Saunders, 1976, p. 32.

13. Cullen, P., Modell, J. H., Kirby, R. R., et al. Treatment of flail chest. *Arch. Surg.* 110:1099, 1975.

14. De Campo, T., and Civetta, J. The effect of short-term discontinuation of high level PEEP in patients with acute respiratory failure. *Crit. Care Med.* 7:47, 1979.

15. Doty, D. B., Anderson, A. E., Rose, E. F., et al. Cardiac trauma: Clinical and experimental correlations of myocardial contusion. *Ann. Surg.* 180:452, 1974.

16. Downs, M. D., and Klein, E. F. Intermittent mandatory ventilation: A new approach to weaning patients from mechanical ventilators. *Chest* 64:331, 1973.

17. Eisenman, B., and Rainer, W. G. Clinical management of posttraumatic rupture of the thoracic aorta. *J. Thorac. Cardiovasc. Surg.* 35:347, 1958.

18. Gabel, J., and Drake, R. Pulmonary capillary pressure and permeability. *Crit. Care Med.* 7:92, 1979.

19. Geiger, J. P. Diagnosis of chest injuries. *Hosp. Med.* 7:109, 1971.

20. Grant, H., and Murray, R. *Emergency Care.* Washington, D.C.: Brady, 1971.

21. Haeck, W. T. Motor Vehicle Trauma. In C. Jelenko (ed.), *Emergency Medical Services—an Overview.* Washington, D.C.: Brady, 1976.

22. Jackson, D. H., and Murphy, G. W. Nonpenetrating cardiac trauma. *Mod. Con. Cardiovasc. Dis.* 45:123, 1976.

23. Kemmerer, W. T. Patterns of thoracic injuries in fatal traffic accidents. *J. Trauma* 1:595, 1961.

24. Kersten, L. Chest-tube drainage system—indications and principles of operation. *Heart Lung* 3:97, 1974.

25. Kish, M. P. The battered lung syndrome. *Emergency Med.* 7:183, 1975.

26. Kulowski, J. *Crash Injuries.* Springfield, Ill.: Thomas, 1960.

27. Love, J. W. Chest injuries. *J.A.M.A.* 232:385, 1975.

28. Martin, J. D. *Trauma to the Thorax and Abdomen.* Springfield, Ill.: Thomas, 1969.

29. Morgan, C. V., and Thomas, W. O. The care and feeding of chest tubes. *Am. J. Nurs.* 72:305, 1972.

30. Moseley, R. V., Vernick, J. J., and Dotz, D. B. Response to blunt chest injury: A new experimental model. *J. Trauma* 10:673, 1970.

31. Moser, K. Oxygen and carbon dioxide transfer. *Respir. Care* 20:480, 1975.

32. Murray, J. *The Normal Lung.* Philadelphia: Saunders, 1976.

33. Naclerio, E. A. Chest trauma. *Clin. Symp.* 22:75, 1970.

34. Naigow, D., and Powaser, M. The effect of different endotracheal suction procedures on arterial blood gases in a controlled experimental model. *Heart Lung* 6:808, 1977.

35. Pomerantz, M., Delgado, F., and Eiseman, B. Unsuspected depressed cardiac output following blunt thoracic or abdominal trauma. *Surgery* 70:865, 1971.

36. Powers, S. R. The use of PEEP for respiratory support. *Surg. Clin. North Am.* 54:1125, 1974.

37. Powley, P., Garfield, J., and Thexton, R. *Trauma Surgery.* Baltimore: Williams & Wilkins, 1973.

38. Ramsay, B. Surgical Emergencies of the Chest. In J. C. Sharpe (ed.), *Surgical Management of Medical Emergencies.* New York: McGraw-Hill, 1969.

39. Sankaran, S., and Wilson, R. F. Factors affecting prognosis in patients with flail chest. *J. Thorac. Cardiovasc. Surg.* 60:402, 1970.

40. Schaal, M. A., Fischer, R. P., and Perry, J. F. The unchanged mortality of flail chest injuries. *J. Trauma* 19:494, 1979.

41. Scott, M., Arens, J., and Ochsner, J. Fractured sternum with flail chest and post-traumatic pulmonary insufficiency. *Ann. Surg.* 15:386, 1973.

42. Shackford, S. R., Smith, D. E., Zarins, C. K., et al. Flail chest. *Am. J. Surg.* 132:759, 1976.

43. Shapter, R. K. Cardiopulmonary resuscitation: Basic life support. *Clin. Symp.* 26:11, 1974.

44. Shefts, L. M. *The Initial Management of Thoracic and Thoraco-Abdominal Trauma.* Springfield, Ill.: Thomas, 1956.

45. Shires, G. R. *Care of the Trauma Patient.* New York: McGraw-Hill, 1978.

46. Steier, M., Ching, N., and Roberts, E. B. Pneumothorax complicating continuous ventilatory support. *J. Thorac. Cardiovasc. Surg.* 67:17, 1974.

47. Sugerman, H. J., Rogers, R. M., and Miller, L. D. Positive end-expiratory pressure (PEEP); indications and physiologic considerations. *Chest* 62:865, 1972.

48. Thompson, H. K., Jackson, P. M., Mattox, K. L., et al. Impact of ambulance life support on outcome of cardiovascular emergencies. *Heart Lung* 8:486, 1979.

49. Von Hippel, A. *Chest Tubes and Chest Bottles.* Springfield, Ill.: Thomas, 1970.

50. Webb, W. R. Thoracic trauma. *Surg. Clin. North Am.* 54:1179, 1974.

51. Weled, B. J., Winfrey, D., and Downs, J. B. Measuring exhaled volume with continuous positive airway pressure and intermittent mandatory ventilation. *Chest* 76:166, 1979.

52. Wilson, R. F. Lung injury—direct or indirect? *Emergency Med.* 5:109, 1973.

53. Wilson, R. F., Murray, C., and Antonenko, D. R. Nonpenetrating thoracic injuries. *Surg. Clin. North Am.* 57:17, 1977.

54. Wilson, R., Arbulu, A., Bassett, J., and Walt, A. Acute mediastinal widening following blunt trauma. *Arch. Surg.* 104:551, 1972.

55. Woodson, R. Physiological significance of oxygen dissociation curve shifts. *Crit. Care Med.* 7:368, 1979.

Acute Pulmonary Embolism

Barbara Montgomery Dossey

Pulmonary embolism is one of the most important and problematical diseases in medicine, both because of its frequency and because of the difficulties in diagnosis and treatment. Pulmonary embolism is one of the most common causes of death in hospitalized patients, and yet it is correctly diagnosed in less than 50 percent of the victims at the time of its occurrence. The primary objective of therapy when pulmonary embolism occurs is to prevent recurrence. Therefore, anticoagulant drugs, notably heparin and the warfarin compounds, are most effective in the majority of cases. In spite of anticoagulants and other forms of therapy, embolic phenomena recur. Prophylactic and therapeutic measures are extremely effective if used early and adequately. Such a troublesome problem as embolism requires the utmost alertness and the most careful management that physician and nurse can provide.

Objective

Given a patient with suspected pulmonary embolism, the nurse should be able to evaluate the signs and symptoms, identify the precipitating factors, and anticipate the complications of acute pulmonary embolism.

16

Achieving the Objective

To achieve the objective the nurse should be able to:

1. Perform a systematic assessment of the patient.
2. Recognize the urgent symptoms of acute pulmonary embolism.
3. Construct a problem list for the patient with acute pulmonary embolism.
4. List the precipitating factors of acute pulmonary embolism.
5. Identify the factors that constitute a high risk for acute pulmonary embolism.
6. Write appropriate nursing orders for a patient with acute pulmonary embolism.
7. Teach the patient self-care during his convalescence.

How to Proceed

To develop an approach to the patient with acute pulmonary embolism the nurse should:

1. Identify the characteristics of acute pulmonary embolism that are present in the patient in the case study that follows.
   a. List the clinical manifestations (signs and symptoms).
   b. Identify the causative and precipitating factors.
   c. Explain the pathophysiology.
2. Write a problem list immediately after reading the patient's case history.
3. Develop a system of patient assessment and apply it to the patient.
4. Anticipate the problems that the patient will face.
5. Outline the major objectives of patient care and management.

Case Study

Ms. J. C., age 25, was hospitalized for elective cholecystectomy. Her chief complaint was increasingly frequent episodes of right upper quadrant abdominal pain over the preceding year, with the recent onset of nausea and vomiting. The pain was associated most often with the evening meal.

In the patient's profile and social history, Ms. C. was described as a 5'8", 220-lb Caucasian, a married housewife, and a mother of six-month-old female identical twins. Ms. C.'s husband, age 27, was an unemployed automobile mechanic. Ms. C. was a Roman Catholic. Her hobbies were baking and sewing. Her alcoholic intake consisted of an occasional beer.

She smoked half a pack of cigarettes a day. She was not nursing her infants.

Ms. C.'s current medical history included diabetes mellitus (since age 19) and significant varicose veins in her lower extremities (three years' duration). She had no history of pulmonary disease. She had never had complications of diabetes mellitus. Her medications included NPH insulin (25 units daily), Valium (5 mg as needed), and, occasionally, aspirin for tension headaches. She had no known drug allergies. She was using oral contraceptives.

Ms. C.'s medical history listed an appendectomy at age 12. Her family history noted that her mother had adult onset diabetes mellitus that was controlled with diet. She had two sisters and one brother and they were alive and well.

The physical examination disclosed no abnormalities of the pulmonary, cardiovascular, renal, or nervous system. The abdominal examination revealed tenderness of the right upper quadrant.

The initial diagnostic studies included tests of renal and hepatic function, a complete blood count, a platelet count, a prothrombin time determination, and x-ray examinations of the chest and abdomen. All the tests were normal. An oral cholecystogram confirmed the diagnosis of cholelithiasis.

On the morning after Ms. C.'s admission, a cholecystectomy with operative cholangiography (revealing no choledocholithiasis) was performed. Multiple stones and chronic inflammatory changes were found in the gallbladder. After the operation, which was uncomplicated, thigh-length stockings were put on Ms. C., and she was given 5000 units of heparin subcutaneously every eight hours because she was felt to be at high risk for pulmonary embolism. Because Ms. C. had pain from her incision, she refused to get out of bed or cough and deep breathe on her own. Only when a nurse or physician insisted did she perform those activities—and then only minimally.

Superficial thrombophlebitis on the inner aspect of the left thigh appeared on the second postoperative day. Ms. C. complained of anterior chest pain, which was attributed to her recent surgery. She had a fever of 100°F. She did not complain of calf tenderness.

Late on the third postoperative day, Ms. C. complained of shortness of breath of sudden onset. Her blood pressure was 130/90, pulse 120, and respiration 30 per minute. Coarse rales were heard at both lung bases, and a pleural friction rub was present in the right anterolateral chest. Arterial blood gas analysis revealed a PO_2 of 74 mm Hg (normal is 80 to 100 mm Hg), a PCO_2 of 34 mm Hg (normal is 35 to 45 mm Hg), and a pH of 7.48 (normal is 7.35 to 7.45). A chest x ray revealed a density in the right lateral lung base that was not present preoperatively and elevation of the right hemidiaphragm. The heart's size was normal; the left lung appeared normal. A lung scan revealed perfusion defects at the right base and in the right upper lobe. The diagnosis of pulmonary embolism was made, and the patient was transferred to the critical care unit (see assessment sheet).

The patient remained in the critical care unit for four days, and she had an uncomplicated recovery thereafter. She received a total of 14 days of intravenous heparin therapy, and when she was discharged she was taking the oral anticoagulant warfarin. Her physician prescribed a weight-reduction diet.

Reflections

Ms. C. had a difficult medical problem that was eventually resolved. In multidisciplinary conferences, the nurses caring for Ms. C. decided that they must be aware of many factors in caring for the patient with pulmonary embolism, especially the patient at high risk for pulmonary embolism. They discussed the nurse's responsibility in making a nursing diagnosis and writing nursing orders for patients experiencing embolism. Specific factors for the nurse to remember are given in the section of the case study that discusses assessment and management.

Particularly instructive to the nurses was the fact that they lost their incentive to make Ms. C. perform specified activities such as coughing, deep breathing, and walking. Ms. C. refused to perform such activities because she was in pain. One nurse said that she became extremely angry at Ms. C. because Ms. C. would not cough, deep breathe, or do leg exercises after she had been made aware of the need for those activities. The nurse said also that she felt guilty because she was aware that she was cool to Ms. C. and that she avoided her when she could. She also said that she felt that "Ms. C. probably caused her present situation [the pulmonary embolism]." She felt that although many of the factors that predisposed Ms. C. to the development of the embolism were beyond Ms. C.'s control, Ms. C. had control over some other predisposing factors—her obesity, the varicose veins that resulted from obesity, and her refusal to cough, deep breathe, and walk after the cholecystectomy.

At the end of a long conference, the nurses agreed that anger and guilt on the part of nurses is an aspect of illness, especially when the patient does not follow the instructions for his own care. The nurses also agreed that the nurse should not judge the patient she is angry at; rather, she should try to understand why she is angry at the patient. The person who is now the patient must be treated. The nurse's feelings of guilt are heightened when she blames a patient. Blaming a patient also distorts the normal empathetic reactions of the nurse to the patient.

Pathophysiology

Pulmonary embolism occurs when there is an obstruction in the pulmonary vascular bed. The acute events of pulmonary embolism are subject to rapid change as resolution of the embolism proceeds. The clinical picture varies according to the size and location of the embolus. The nurse must continue to develop her assessment skills because subtle changes are often the first sign of pulmonary embolism.

Precipitating Factors

A variety of factors predispose one to intravascular thrombosis [9–14, 20, 22, 29, 32, 33]:

1. The postoperative state
2. Obesity
3. Diabetes mellitus
4. Venous stasis secondary to immobility
5. Infection
6. The postpartum state
7. A high concentration of estrogen
8. Occult carcinoma
9. Oral contraceptives
10. Trauma to vessel walls
11. Varicose veins
12. Other circulatory disorders, such as shock and congestive heart failure

Acute Embolization

Once a thrombus has developed, it may loosen and break from its attachment. A flowing clot is known as an embolus. An embolus travels from the systemic venous circulation through the right heart and into the pulmonary arterial system. There it eventually reaches a branch too small for it to pass through, and it becomes impacted, obstructing the flow of blood in that vessel.

Pulmonary Consequences

Pulmonary embolism produces alveolar dead space since it results in a lung zone that is ventilated but not perfused. Alveolar dead space refers to a portion of tidal volume that ventilates alveoli that have a reduced or nonexistent flow of blood. In the physiolog-

Critical Care Nursing Admission Assessment
Head to Toe Approach

Date	Time	
		Pt. Name: *Ms. J.C.* Age: *25* Allergies: *NKA*
3-4-78	1³⁰ PM	Admitted Bed No: *7* Via: *Bed from surgical floor* Ad. Dx.: *Cholecystitis; Pulmonary Embolism*
		T.: *100⁷(o)* A.P.: *120* R.P.: *120* R.: *30* B.P. Supine R: *130/90* L: *130/90* Sitting: *134/90*
3ʳᵈ day post-op		Wt. (unit scale): *220 lbs* Ht.: *5'8"* ECG Rhythm: *Sinus Tach* Ectopy: *none*
		Informant: *pt.; floor nurse; chart (done on admission 2-29)* Last meal: *clear liquid breakfast 8³⁰ AM*
	1.	Chief complaint: *SOB; chest pain c̄ inspirations*
	2.	Hx. of present illness: *cholecystectomy 3 days ago; superficial thrombosis; phlebitis 2 days ago; sudden SOB + chest pain*
	3.	Past medical Hx. (include all surgeries, hosp., diseases, injuries, blood trans.): *Appendectomy -1965; Diabetes Mellitus diagnosed - 1971; Varicose veins last 3 yrs.; Pregnancy - healthy identical twins 1977*
	4.	Family Hx.: *Mother - diabetes mellitus - diet controlled; Father alive + well; 2 sisters and 1 brother alive and well*
	5.	Current drugs: *NPH Insulin 25u daily; Valium 5 mg PRN, oral contraceptive; Heparin 5,000 u. SQ q 8h; Demerol 75 mg q 4h PRN*
	6.	Alcohol and tobacco habits: *½ pkg. cigarettes/day; an occasional beer*
	7.	Dietary and fluid needs: *clear liquids post surgery*
	8.	Sleep and rest patterns: *poor last month due to twins being sick*
	9.	Bowel and bladder habits: *daily B.M. requires no laxative*
	10.	Hygienic needs: *dental care poor; skin dry*
	11.	Psychosocial needs: *disruption of home life; need to verbalize feeling*
	12.	Occupation and education: *housewife and mother; graduated from H.S.*
	13.	Exercise habits: *none*
	14.	Spiritual needs: *attends Catholic church; pt. wants to see her priest tonight*
	15.	Personal interests: *sewing and baking*
	16.	Family member interaction and availability: *Demanding of husband, anxious about twins; pt.'s mother and husband visit 2x daily*
	17.	Attitude towards illness and hospitalization: *pt. very anxious - asks same questions many times: "Why am I in this unit?", or "I'm not that sick."*

Physical Examination

Date	Time	
	18.	Gen. appearance: *obese white female* color: *pale* skin: *no lesions warm and dry*
	19.	Neurological:
		a) level of consciousness: *L.O.C.: oriented and anxious*
		b) cerebellar: *posture: deferred gait: deferred*
		c) motor function: upper: *normal* lower: *normal*
		d) sensory function: upper: *normal* lower: *normal*
		e) reflexes: *deferred*
	20.	Head and face: *no abnormalities*
	21.	Eyes: *PERRLA; does not wear glasses*
	22.	Ears: *no drainage; membrane intact*
	23.	Nose: *no drainage*
	24.	Mouth/throat: *dry (mouth breathing); poor mouth care*
	25.	Neck: *no neck vein distention; no scars*
	26.	Chest: *increased respirations; decreased excursion due to chest pain*
	27.	Breast: *negative* *c̄ inspirations*
	28.	Respiratory: *course rales at both lung bases; pleural friction rub rt. anterior lat chest*
	29.	Cardiac: *heart sounds normal; tachycardia present; PMI left 5th ICS at MCL*
	30.	Abdomen: *abdominal dressing c̄ tube in place; dressing dry, drainage slight*
	31.	Genitourinary: *voided 400 cc on adm. to unit; SAD neg./neg.* *bowel sounds present Levine tube pulled*
	32.	Extremities (all pulses): *bilateral equal pulses; superficial thrombophlebitis this AM*
	33.	Back: *no deformities or scars* *inner aspect left thigh; no calf tenderness*
	34.	Problems requiring possible referral service: *husband unemployed; pt. expressed financial concerns to floor nurse yesterday; assess c̄ pt. and pt. needs*
	35.	Teaching needs: *weight reduction diet, diabetic diet, foot care, insulin, anticoagulants post-pulmonary embolism, self-care post pulmonary embolism*
	36.	Other:

		PROBLEM LIST: **ACTIVE**	**INACTIVE**
3-4		1. Cholecystitis *cholecystectomy →*	8. Appendectomy *1965 →*
		2. Diabetes Mellitus	9. Pregnancy *1977 →*
		3. Varicose Veins	
		4. Pulmonary Embolism	
		5. Obesity	
		6. Anxiety	
		7. Lack of knowledge of diet, meds, diabetes	

Barbara Dossey, RN, CCRN
NURSE'S SIGNATURE

ical sense, such ventilation is "wasted" because the lung zone involved fails to participate in gas exchange. Overall ventilation in the uninvolved lung zones must be increased to maintain normal gas exchange. For that reason, dyspnea and tachypnea are common in patients with pulmonary embolism.

PNEUMOCONSTRICTION

Pneumoconstriction in the embolized lung zone is the second pulmonary event. Alveolar hypocapnia is responsible for constriction of the distal airways. Normally the major source of alveolar carbon dioxide is pulmonary arterial blood. An embolus interrupts the pulmonary arterial blood flow, and constriction of the distal airways occurs. Pneumoconstriction shifts ventilation away from the poorly perfused lung zone so that less ventilation is wasted.

Loss of Alveolar Surfactant

Pulmonary embolism also causes a loss of alveolar surfactant. Surfactant, the lipoprotein material that stabilizes and prevents the collapse of alveoli, is produced by type II alveolar cells. When the supply of nutrients to those cells is cut off by the embolus, the production of surfactant ceases. When surfactant decreases, alveoli collapse, and atelectasis results.

Hemodynamic Consequences

The patient's previous physical condition and the number and size of emboli determine the severity of the acute pulmonary hemodynamic events. Embolism causes a decrease in the cross-sectional area of the pulmonary vascular bed that results in an increase in pulmonary vascular resistance. Pulmonary arterial pressure and right ventricular work will increase if enough of the pulmonary arterial circulation is occluded. The most extreme and serious consequences of embolism therefore are acute right ventricular failure, reduced left ventricular filling, and systemic hypotension.

Pulmonary Infarction

A rare but often serious complication of pulmonary embolism is pulmonary infarction. Pulmonary infarc-

tion and pulmonary embolism are not synonymous. Approximately 80 to 90 percent of occlusive emboli fail to cause infarction since the involved lung continues to receive adequate blood perfusion from the bronchial arterial system [2]. There are two circulations in the lung: the pulmonary and the bronchial. The pulmonary circulation promotes gas exchange, and the bronchial circulation supplies the pulmonary structure down to, but not including, the alveoli. Pulmonary infarction appears to result from embolism to middle-sized vessels when pulmonary congestion due to systemic hypotension or to left ventricular failure interferes with bronchial collateral circulation [2].

Diagnosis of Pulmonary Embolism

The characteristic history of pleuritic pain and dyspnea in the presence of one or more predisposing factors should always make one suspect pulmonary embolism. The most typical physical finding is a pleural friction rub. Rales, tachypnea, and tachycardia are common. Hemoptysis is less common (Fig. 16-1). X-ray manifestations are nonspecific, and they frequently include atelectasis and pleural effusion. When an embolus lodges in a segmental artery, the parenchyma distal to the segment may become infarcted. Typically, the segment extends to the pleura, causing a peripheral concave infiltrate (Hampton's hump), which strongly suggests pulmonary infarction [7]. The ECG is usually normal, but it may show signs of right ventricular strain if the embolism is massive [27, 31]. Atrial dysrhythmias are also seen frequently. Arterial blood gas analyses frequently show hypoxemia, but oxygen tension is normal in a minority of cases [2].

The most useful diagnostic procedure is the lung scan (Fig. 16-2) [3, 19, 26, 30, 33]. It involves external measurement of the intrapulmonary distribution of injected radioactive particles (e.g., iodine 125 attached to aggregates of albumin). Obstruction of pulmonary blood flow by an embolus denies the radioisotope access to a segment of the lung and appears on the scan as a "perfusion defect" (Fig. 16-3). Unfortunately, such a defect may also appear in a variety of other pulmonary disorders, such as pneumonia, pulmonary edema, chronic bronchitis, and emphysema. But in the absence of those other conditions, the lung scan

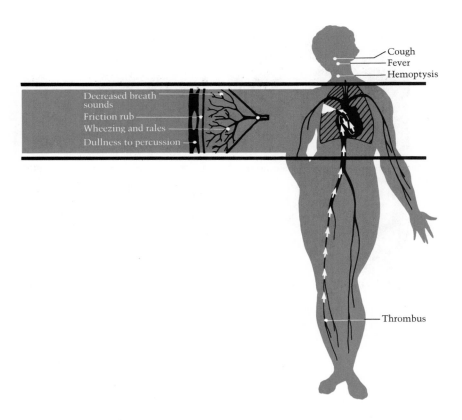

Figure 16-1
Clinical features.

may be a reliable diagnostic tool for pulmonary embolism.

If the scan fails to provide a definitive answer and if the patient's condition is unstable, most physicians resort to pulmonary angiography (Fig. 16-4). That test requires right-sided cardiac catheterization with injection of radiographic contrast material into the pulmonary circulation. Obstruction or diversion of the stream of contrast medium shows the presence of emboli in pulmonary vessels [7, 8].

Massive Pulmonary Embolism

Diagnostic tests such as pulmonary angiography can differentiate between non-life-threatening and life-threatening embolism. Life-threatening massive pulmonary embolism is said to occur when there is a sudden mechanical obstruction of 50 percent or more of the pulmonary arterial bed [2]. The clinical picture of massive pulmonary embolism includes cyanosis, tachypnea with confusion or anxiety, and sudden hypotension. Pulmonary angiography usually provides a definitive diagnosis. Treatment may include thrombolysis or surgical intervention to interrupt the passage of emboli through the inferior vena cava, such as the placement of a Mobin-Uddin umbrella filter. If the patient meets certain criteria, embolectomy may be necessary.

The lung scan and pulmonary angiography are complementary, not competitive, procedures for arriving at a sometimes difficult diagnosis. The less invasive procedures are done first, and the physician proceeds to more complicated diagnostic procedures, depending on the clinical evidence shown by each patient suspected of having pulmonary embolism.

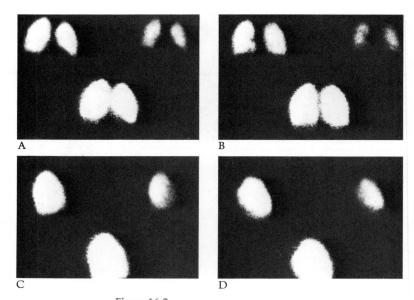

Figure 16-2
A normal lung scan. A. Anterior view. B. Posterior view. C. Right lateral view. D. Left lateral view. Each view contains three exposures, representing different degrees of intensity. The lungs are smooth and regular in outline, without evidence of "perfusion defects."

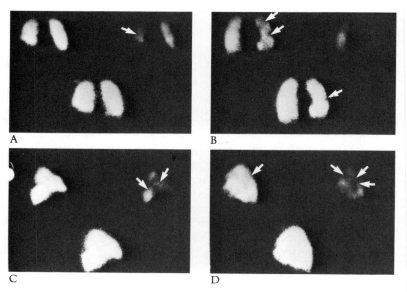

Figure 16-3
An abnormal lung scan. The views are the same as those in 16-2. There are a number of dark areas, or "perfusion defects," mostly in the middle and lower regions of the right lung *(arrows)*. Those defects represent pulmonary emboli.

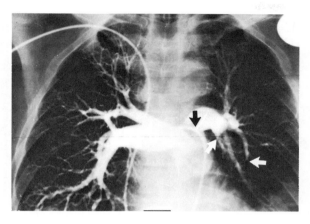

Figure 16-4
A pulmonary angiogram. The catheter enters from the right arm, and the contrast medium is being injected into the pulmonary artery, filling its right and left branches to give a treelike appearance. The main trunk of the left pulmonary artery appears shorter and more irregular than normal ("cut-off"), and it has several areas that are poorly opacified ("filling defects") *(arrows)*. Those abnormalities represent pulmonary emboli.

Treatment

Recognition and Prevention of Deep Venous Thrombosis

The support of vital functions and the prevention of further emboli are the primary goals of the treatment of pulmonary embolism. Physical assessment is the easiest and most effective way for nurses to screen patients who are at risk for pulmonary embolism.

Since 90 percent of the patients who have pulmonary embolism have thrombi originating in the deep veins of the legs [2], the nurse must be aware of the appropriate preventive nursing measures, described in the following paragraphs. She should not rely on the patient's having symptoms of thrombophlebitis, since 50 to 60 percent of patients with deep vein thrombosis have no signs or symptoms [33].

Bed rest is necessary to prevent further embolism. However, that treatment is paradoxical since immobilization has its own hazards. Elastic stockings are used to promote effective venous return. To avoid venous stasis, the patient should be told not to cross his legs in bed. Also, his legs can be elevated since gravity helps venous return. To avoid congestion in

the inguinal area, the legs should be elevated no more than 10 to 15 degrees. Leg exercises using active flexion and extension of muscles and frequent turning are the best activities for patients at bed rest. The patient must receive instruction on proper exercise. Isometric exercises should be avoided because they increase left ventricular end-diastolic pressure and cardiac oxygen consumption. The nurse should encourage the patient to do breathing exercises on his own. The patient should understand that doing so increases venous return and prevents atelectasis.

The patient's legs should be inspected routinely for tenderness, redness, swelling, or pain, especially in the calf and popliteal areas. Deep vein tenderness can be detected by having the patient dorsiflex his foot. If that maneuver causes pain in the patient's calf, Homan's sign has been elicited, information that should be given to the physician as soon as it is uncovered. Deep vein thrombosis is extremely difficult to diagnose; it often cannot be detected with safe noninvasive procedures, such as (1) the ^{125}I–labeled fibrinogen test, which is frequently used to detect deep vein thrombosis in the calf and lower thigh; (2) the Doppler ultrasound technique used to detect deep vein thrombosis in the popliteal and iliofemoral veins; and (3) phlebography, used for radiographic visualization of the deep venous system [12, 21].

When pulmonary embolism is suspected, oxygen may be given to the patient by mask or cannula, depending on the clinical picture. Narcotics, such as meperidine and morphine, may be used to relieve the patient's apprehension and pain. The nurse must keep in mind the hypotensive effects of narcotics. Codeine sulfate may be given for minimal pain.

Fluids are given intravenously to treat shock. For patients with severe circulatory collapse, vasopressors may be needed.

Since the drug therapy of patients with pulmonary embolism is based on the dynamics of the coagulation system, clotting, lysis, and routine tests for hemostatic function are discussed briefly before the medical and surgical treatment of pulmonary embolism is discussed.

Clotting and Lysis

Clotting and lysis are well-balanced mechanisms in humans, and when either mechanism is unbalanced, the patient may demonstrate hemorrhage or thrombosis.

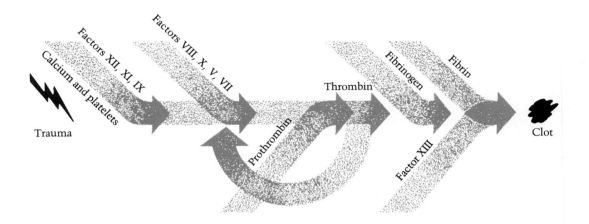

THE CLOTTING MECHANISM

The clotting mechanism can be initiated by an extrinsic mechanism or by an intrinsic mechanism (Fig. 16-5). After trauma, a normal clotting sequence occurs that results in clot formation. When a blood vessel is damaged, the extrinsic mechanism goes into effect. The intrinsic mechanism goes into effect when blood has been traumatized directly—for example, when it has been removed from the body by venipuncture.

The clotting of blood involves 13 well-defined factors. An inactive proenzyme is converted into an active factor, which initiates the next step. Calcium is required at many points. Three major stages occur in coagulation: (1) procoagulants (from platelets, plasma proteins, and tissue factors) combine in the presence of calcium to form thromboplastin, (2) thromboplastin activates prothrombin to form thrombin, and (3) thrombin enzymatically converts fibrinogen to insoluble fibrin. That fibrin clot is stabilized by a factor, and it can be broken down by fibrinolysins [10].

The basic concepts of clotting that the reader must know are [10] (see Fig. 16-5, which depicts this process):

1. Inactive factor XII is the first factor to be activated. Factor XIIa is the active enzyme of factor XII.
2. Next, factor XIIa acts on inactive factor XI. Factor XIa is the active enzyme of factor XI. The process continues in the same manner.
3. Factor X requires factor VIII for activation.
4. Prothrombin requires factor V for activation.
5. Platelet cofactor −3 (a fatty lipid substance from platelets) must be present to activate factors VIII and V.

Figure 16-5
Clotting factors.

6. The activation of factor X through the effects of thrombin on factor VIII perpetuates the cycle.
7. Thrombin converts fibrinogen to soluble fibrin, which is stabilized by factor XIII.

THE FIBRINOLYTIC SYSTEM

The fibrinolytic system functions through the conversion of enzymes that are capable of dissolving fibrin clots. Plasminogen is one such proenzyme normally found in whole blood that may be converted to plasmin, a major lytic (dissolving) enzyme that can dissolve fibrin.

Because of the normal turbulence of blood flow, the endothelial surface of blood vessels constantly undergoes wear and tear. Whenever an area is denuded, platelets adhere to the damaged area. Platelets, produced by megakaryocytes in the bone marrow, are important factors in hemostasis. Platelets not only plug the injured vessel site, they also release vasoactive substances that cause local vasoconstriction. They also contribute several factors to promote coagulation. Eddy currents that are set up by the adhered platelets may activate the intrinsic clotting mechanism, causing further clot formation. If it were not for the fibrinolytic system, total vessel occlusion might occur; however, the fibrinolytic system keeps a normal balance between clotting and lysis.

The tests for hemostatic function that are discussed in the following paragraphs are the Lee-White clotting time, the activated partial thromboplastin time (APTT), and the prothrombin time. (There are other tests of blood coagulation, but they are not discussed.)

LEE-WHITE CLOTTING TIME

The Lee-White clotting time test is used in a clinical setting to regulate heparin dosage. It is a relatively insensitive test, and it can give values that are within a normal range in patients with mild-to-moderate clotting deficiencies. The normal clotting time is 8 to 12 minutes. Heparin is given intravenously in the treatment of pulmonary embolism to maintain the Lee-White clotting time at 2 to 2.5 times the control level an hour before the next scheduled dosage [23]. The test is done by placing 2 ml of venous blood into three separate test tubes. As soon as the blood is drawn, the time is recorded with the use of a stopwatch. Five minutes after the drawing of blood, the first tube is tilted to check for a clot. The same tube is then tilted at one-minute intervals until it can be inverted without loss of blood from the tube. Then the second tube is tilted at one-minute intervals until a firm clot is present. The same procedure is followed for the third tube. The clotting time is the time a firm clot forms in the third tube.

ACTIVATED PARTIAL THROMBOPLASTIN TIME

The activated partial thromboplastin time (APTT), a laboratory test, is more reliable at low levels of anticoagulation than is the Lee-White clotting time.

PROTHROMBIN TIME

The prothrombin time (PT) is probably the most common routine test of blood coagulation. It is used to monitor anticoagulation therapy with warfarin (Coumadin). This drug suppresses the vitamin K— dependent factors produced by the liver. Warfarin is given until the prothrombin time rises to a therapeutic range of 2 to 2.5 times control, which is the range that seems necessary to prevent most venous thrombotic complications [23].

In determining a prothrombin time, a sample of venous blood is drawn from the patient and a sample of plasma is placed in an anticoagulated tube. Next, calcium and tissue thromboplastin are added. Usually a clot forms in 11 to 14 seconds. Thromboplastin activity varies with each test, so a control must be done on normal plasma with each test. The values that are recorded give the number of seconds for clot forma-

tion in the test blood and the number of seconds for clot formation in the normal blood.

Drug Therapy

Drug therapy for patients with pulmonary embolism is based on the dynamics of the coagulation system. After embolism and damage to the pulmonary vessel wall, secondary sites of thrombus formation occur in the lung. Thrombi may continue to form either at the site of origin in the legs or in the lungs. The pulmonary arterial endothelium damaged by the embolus releases fibrinolysins, which lyse the primary clot. However, there may be a continuous formation of a secondary thrombus in response to the primary embolus. The major components of the secondary thrombus are platelets and fibrin. High levels of fibrinogen contribute to the fibrin formation.

Heparin is used to arrest an active thrombotic state [5, 6]. Heparin is given intravenously either by continuous drip or by intermittent intravenous doses, preferably through a heparin lock every four hours. Heparin should not be administered through intramuscular or subcutaneous routes in patients with acute pulmonary embolism due to unpredictable absorption with variations in systemic blood pressure and tissue perfusion. After a loading dose of 5000 to 10,000 units, sufficient heparin should be administered to prolong the clotting time to 2 to 2.5 times the control level an hour before the next dose. Generally, 5000 to 6000 units of heparin is required on a four-hour schedule, and 7500 to 10,000 units is required on a six-hour schedule. Heparin acts quickly to block the chain of clotting reactions at several points. It prevents the action of thrombin in converting fibrinogen to fibrin, and it impairs the activation of several other clotting factors [5]. Anticoagulant therapy should usually continue for at least 10 to 14 days after acute pulmonary embolism. Protamine is used to antagonize heparin; it should always be available for emergency use when a patient is given heparin. It is a low-molecular-weight protein that contains large amounts of arginine, an amino acid. It combines with heparin to form a stable compound that has no anticoagulant properties.

The goal of oral anticoagulant therapy is to prevent the recurrence of an active thrombotic process. That goal is achieved by using coumarin derivatives, of which warfarin is the one most commonly used after the acute phase of pulmonary embolism and during the recovery phase after discharge from the hospital [6, 23]. Warfarin interferes with the biochemical reactions that cause the liver to synthesize several clotting factors (prothrombin and factors VII, IX, and X). It acts as a competitive inhibitor of vitamin K, which is essential for the production of those factors. Increasingly large doses of warfarin are given until the prothrombin time rises to a therapeutic range (2 to 2.5 times the control time). The antagonist of warfarin is vitamin K, which rapidly neutralizes the effects of warfarin. It should be available for patients who are taking oral anticoagulants.

Oral administration of warfarin may begin toward the end of heparin therapy or simultaneously at the beginning of heparin therapy. Oral anticoagulant drugs reduce the levels of clotting factors in plasma. Approximately three to five days are required to reduce sufficiently the circulating levels of factors IX and X, the key factors for the antithrombotic effect [5]. Therefore heparin is continued for that length of time after the initiation of oral anticoagulants. The dosage of heparin is tapered and discontinued.

Several factors determine how long a patient should take oral anticoagulants. The physician considers (1) the events that occurred with the embolism, (2) whether the patient has a predisposition to further thromboembolism, (3) how well the patient tolerates anticoagulants, and (4) how reliable the patient is about taking his medications. The exact length of anticoagulation therapy is debatable, but most patients remain on oral anticoagulants for a three- to six-month period. The patient should be checked regularly for signs of bleeding. Bleeding secondary to the deficiency or inhibition of clotting factor generally presents as deep dissecting hematomas. Therefore the circumference of the extremities should be determined. Other common signs of bleeding are large, often solitary, ecchymoses, gingival oozing, and delayed bleeding from puncture wounds. Discharged patients taking oral anticoagulants should know the signs of over-anticoagulation, such as easy bruising, minor cuts that stop bleeding normally (in the platelet phase of bleeding) but begin bleeding later, black stools, blood in the urine or stool, coughed-up blood, swelling and pain in the joints, and severe headaches. They should be told not to take medications other than those prescribed by the physician since many drugs interfere with the action of the coumarin anticoagulants. They should be told to avoid foods that are high in vitamin K. If the patient

taking an anticoagulant requires dental surgery or other minor surgery, he should tell his dentist or physician about his anticoagulant therapy.

When the patient is taking coumarin, particular attention should be given to the other medications he takes. Many medications can increase or decrease the effect of coumarin anticoagulants in several ways: (1) by altering the bioavailability of vitamin K, (2) by displacing coumarin from its binding sites on serum albumin, and (3) by altering the concentration of prothrombin complex.

The most common medications that increase the effect of coumarin anticoagulants are salicylates, indomethacin, phenylbutazone, diphenylhydantoin, quinidine, clofibrate, chloral hydrate, thyroxine, bowel-sterilizing antibiotics, chloramphenicol, sulfonamides, and anabolic steroids. Drugs that decrease the effect of coumarin anticoagulants include most antacids, barbiturates, adrenocorticosteroids, estrogen, oral contraceptives, mercurial and thiazide diuretics, and cholestyramine.

Certain phenomena are contraindications to anticoagulant therapy. Among them are an actively bleeding or a symptomatic gastrointestinal or genitourinary lesion that may bleed, acute cerebrovascular accident, severe systemic hypertension, recent surgical procedures in which bleeding may constitute a risk, renal or hepatic insufficiency, and platelet or coagulation factor abnormalities. When any of those phenomena are present, the physician must consider having an inferior vena caval interruption done to prevent recurrent pulmonary embolism.

During pregnancy, anticoagulant therapy presents special problems. Since heparin does not cross the placental barrier, it is the safest drug for the patient and the fetus; however, its use outside the hospital setting is not practical. Coumarin derivatives cross the placental barrier, and not much is known about the extent and duration of resulting fetal clotting derangements. Oral anticoagulants should be avoided (1) during the first trimester of pregnancy because of their possible teratogenic effects and (2) during the last three weeks of pregnancy because of the increased risk of perinatal hemorrhage.

THROMBOLYTIC DRUGS

Another form of therapy is thrombolysis using urokinase and streptokinase. Those drugs cause rapid lysis of large thrombi. They act by enhancing the activation of fibrinolytic mechanisms. They are currently being used primarily in patients with severe hemodynamic impairment [1].

In patients who have untreated pulmonary embolism, the plasminogen activator that is released from the endothelium of the pulmonary artery lyses emboli. That phenomenon occurs automatically, without the use of exogenous fibrinolytic drugs. The level of lysis depends on the level of fibrinolysis inhibitor. Patients with myeloma, congestive heart failure, or carcinoma of the liver have a high level of fibrinolysis inhibitor. Their platelets have a large quantity of fibrinolytic inhibitor. In patients with pulmonary embolism, serial pulmonary arteriographs often demonstrate rapid clot lysis due to the high fibrinolytic activity of the pulmonary arterial endothelium.

Urokinase appears to be safer than streptokinase [6, 28]. Urokinase dosage is relatively easy to regulate and is monitored by the euglobin lysis time. Since urokinase is extracted from human urine, it is not antigenic. It is expensive to produce. Streptokinase is antigenic, because it is a secretory protein of hemolytic streptococci. The dosage depends on the patient's history of streptococcal infection. Since anaphylactic reactions have been reported, some physicians routinely give hydrocortisone (100 mg) with streptokinase.

Streptokinase and urokinase show great promise in the management of massive pulmonary embolism and extensive deep vein thrombosis. In spite of these new drugs, pulmonary embolectomy remains the procedure for those patients with extremely poor prognosis. Improvements in the current therapy regimes is still necessary [1].

ANTIPLATELET SUBSTANCES

Antiplatelet substances may play a significant role in the prevention of deep venous thrombosis [3, 4, 11, 23]. Platelets play a role in secondary thrombus formation; histological examination of pulmonary emboli reveals that platelets are a substantial component of clots. Aspirin prevents platelet aggregation by the acetylation of certain chemicals on the platelet membrane. That effect of aspirin lasts about eight days, or as long as platelets are viable. Dextran seems to reduce platelet adhesiveness, especially in areas of damaged endothelium. Dipyridamole (Persantine), a mild vasodilator, may reduce platelet aggregation that

is induced by adenosine diphosphate (ADP). At present, the role of antiplatelet drugs is unclear.

SURGICAL PROCEDURES

Vena Caval Interruption
Surgical procedures are used only for patients who cannot be helped with heparin therapy or who are not candidates for anticoagulant therapy.

The inferior vena cava is interrupted to prevent the transmission of additional clots from the lower extremities to the lungs. Vena caval interruption is usually done when the results of anticoagulant therapy are unsatisfactory [23]. Indications for vena caval interruption are different in different medical centers, but the most common indications are recurrent embolism during adequate heparin treatment, bleeding or other contraindications to anticoagulation, massive pulmonary embolism, or septic embolism. A number of techniques have been used; the most popular one is simple ligation, which results in complete occlusion of the flow of blood (Fig. 16-6). Other approaches use fenestrating sutures or partially occluding clips, which are designed to allow at least partial maintenance of venous return [17].

The Umbrella Filter

A unique device has been developed for use with local anesthesia in patients who cannot tolerate major surgery. A so-called umbrella filter can be inserted percutaneously or transvenously by cutdown (usually in the jugular vein) and advanced to the inferior vena

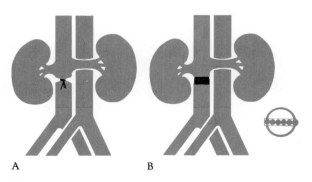

A   B

Figure 16-6

A. Ligation. B. Partially occluding clip.

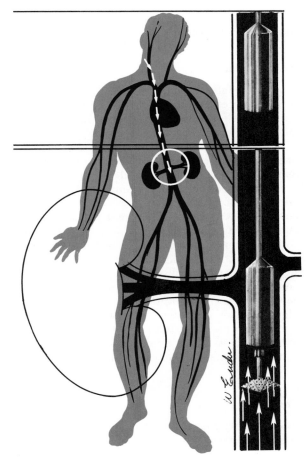

Figure 16-7
An umbrella filter.

cava, below the level of the renal veins. The filter, which is folded about the catheter tip, is then opened like an umbrella to obstruct the flow of emboli [16, 17, 23] (Fig. 16-7).

None of those procedures for vena caval interruption is completely effective in preventing the recurrence of embolism.

PULMONARY EMBOLECTOMY

Pulmonary embolectomy is a dramatic procedure. In the appropriate clinical situation, it may be lifesaving [1]. When the decision is made to do a pulmonary embolectomy, certain criteria must be met since the procedure has been shown in different studies to carry a mortality of 40 to 100 percent [24].

Embolectomy is reserved for a select group of patients who show evidence of severe hemodynamic compromise due to embolism that does not respond to other measures. Those patients must show clear evidence of massive pulmonary embolism to the main pulmonary artery or its major branches involving more than 60 percent of the pulmonary vasculature [16, 24]. When therapy and/or circulatory assist procedures do not bring dramatic improvement, emergency cardiopulmonary bypass and pulmonary embolectomy must be considered [1, 24].

Prognosis in Acute Pulmonary Embolism

When long-term anticoagulation therapy or interruption of the inferior vena cava following an acute pulmonary embolism is done in the patients just described, recurrent symptomatic pulmonary embolism is rare. The long-term prognosis is excellent, and it is adversely affected only by associated diseases.

Before he is discharged from the hospital, the patient must be educated about several aspects of his condition—and the nurse must make sure that the patient understands the information he is given. The patient must be educated about the need (1) to do the proper leg exercises, (2) to take his medications exactly as they are prescribed, (3) to recognize the signs of excessive anticoagulation, (4) to know the antidote to oral anticoagulants and to take it as needed, (5) to adhere to his diet, (6) to seek his physician's approval of any new medications, and (7) to tell his dentist or any other physician who suggests doing a surgical procedure that he is taking an anticoagulant. The patient must also understand the need to keep his follow-up appointment with his physician and to have laboratory work done when it is ordered.

Assessment and Management of the Patient with Pulmonary Embolism

OBJECTIVE NO. 1

The patient should not have a recurrence or further complications of pulmonary embolism.

To achieve the objective, the nurse should:

1. Assess the patient for the signs and symptoms of hypoxia: (a) restlessness, (b) headache, (c) ap-

prehension, (d) euphoria, (e) hallucinations, (f) delirium, (g) unconsciousness, and (h) color (pallor, cyanosis).

2. Assess the lung functioning of the patient suspected of having pulmonary arterial embolism.
    a. Inspection. Does the patient show splinting, supraclavicular, suprasternal, or intercostal retractions, tachypnea, or dyspnea?
    b. Palpation. Does the patient show decreased chest excursion unilaterally, nonsymmetrical diaphragmatic excursion, rubs (thrills), an accentuated PMI, or a decrease in vocal fremitus?
    c. Auscultation. Does the patient have abnormal breath sounds (whispered pectoriloquy, bronchial or bronchovesicular sounds), abnormal voice sounds, or a friction rub (an accented pulmonic second sound)?

3. Assess the right heart functioning of the patient who is suspected of having pulmonary arterial embolism.
    a. Inspection. Does the patient have peripheral edema or distended neck veins?
    b. Palpation. Does the patient have an enlarged liver?
    c. Auscultation. Does the patient have abnormal heart sounds, such as accented pulmonic sounds, pulmonic murmurs, gallop rhythms, or tachycardia?

4. Give oxygen in an emergency situation and as ordered.

5. Give pain medication as ordered—meperidine or morphine. (The nurse should be aware of the hypotensive effects of these drugs.)

6. Be alert to any cardiac dysrhythmias and treat appropriately any that are found.

7. Be alert to signs of shock. If shock occurs, fluids and/or vasopressors should be given as ordered.

8. Give intravenous fluids as ordered.

9. Maintain the patency of any intravenous line.

10. Be aware of the patient's intake, output, and daily weight.

11. Arrange for arterial blood gas analyses when ordered. Record the FIO_2 and the duration of administration of oxygen when blood gas analyses are made.

12. Obtain daily chest x rays as ordered.

13. Order diagnostic tests for pulmonary evaluation as ordered. Explain the tests to the patient and have the patient sign the necessary consent forms.

14. Initiate anticoagulant medication as ordered.

15. Obtain the Lee-White clotting time one hour before the previous dose of heparin as ordered and record the results. Notify the physician if the clotting time is not within the desired range. If the patient is also taking warfarin, obtain the prothrombin time as ordered.

16. Check the patient regularly for signs of bleeding. Bleeding secondary to clotting-factor deficiency or inhibition generally is manifested as a deep dissecting hematoma (the circumference of the extremities should be measured) or large, often solitary, ecchymoses, gingival oozing, and delayed bleeding from puncture wounds.

17. Keep anticoagulant antagonists available (protamine is the antagonist for heparin, and vitamin K is the antagonist for warfarin).

18. Give stool softeners to prevent constipation and straining.

19. Prevent pressure at the popliteal space or against the calf of the leg. Do not raise the bed at knee level, which places the patient's lower extremities in a dependent position.

20. Tell the patient not to cross his legs in bed and not to sit in a chair with his legs dependent. When he sits, he should elevate his legs slightly.

21. Put on the patient fitted elastic stockings that extend above his knee and thus support the walls of the leg veins [25].

22. Encourage the patient to do active and passive leg exercises at least twice a shift. Do frequent movement and position changes (at least twice an hour) for the patient with limited mobility.

23. Encourage the patient to walk in accordance with his level of activity.

24. Offer reassurance and support to the patient, especially when he is in pain. Such help will encourage him to take a positive attitude toward recovery from pulmonary embolism.

25. Alleviate the anxiety of the patient in the acute phase of his illness by, for example, reassuring him and teaching him as the occasions arise.

26. Prepare the patient for pulmonary embolectomy or vena caval interruption when indicated.

OBJECTIVE NO. 2

The nurse should be able to assess the patient's grasp of information before his discharge from the hospital.

To achieve the objective, the nurse should discuss the following subjects with the patient.

1. The patient's need to take his medications as ordered and to have his laboratory work done as ordered.
2. The signs of excessive anticoagulation.
   a. Easy bruising
   b. Minor cuts that stop bleeding normally (in the platelet phase of bleeding) but begin bleeding later
   c. Severe nosebleed
   d. Black stools
   e. Blood in the urine or stool
   f. Coughing up blood
   g. Joint swelling and pain
   h. Severe headaches
3. The advisability of using an electric razor for shaving (it is easier to cut oneself when shaving with a blade).
4. The need to contact the physician before he takes any new medications (many medications interfere with the action of the coumarin anticoagulants).
5. The use of vitamin K as an antidote to oral anticoagulants.
6. The need to avoid foods that are high in vitamin K (e.g., cauliflower, dark-green vegetables, bananas, and tomatoes).
7. If any surgical procedure is necessary, the need to tell his dentist or other physician that he is taking anticoagulants.
8. The need to learn and do leg exercises (active flexion and extension of leg muscles) to enhance venous circulation, especially while at work and during long automobile and airplane trips.
9. The need for correct posture and activities.
10. The need for the patient to follow through with continued medical guidance and to keep his medical appointments.
11. The need for the patient to carry a card or to wear a bracelet that states he is taking an anticoagulant.

Summary

The frequency with which pulmonary embolism occurs in hospitalized patients demands that everyone caring for hospitalized patients be thoroughly familiar with the causative and the high-risk factors in pulmonary embolism. The signs and symptoms of pulmonary embolism are usually nonspecific. Routine laboratory studies, chest x rays, arterial blood gas analyses, and ECGs are helpful but not diagnostic. The lung scan and pulmonary angiograms are the best diagnostic techniques. Treatment is aimed at preventing further embolism by anticoagulation. The nursing and medical professions are concerned with the prevention of deep venous thrombosis and early recognition of it when pulmonary embolism is suspected.

Study Problems

1. Outline an assessment protocol for follow-up of a patient who has had an initial episode of pulmonary embolism.
2. Fibrin and platelets are the major components of the secondary thrombus.
   a. True
   b. False
3. List two anticoagulants that inhibit secondary thrombus formation.
4. (Choose one answer.) Once thrombi have begun to form, they:
   a. Are resorbed within 48 hours in 50 percent of patients.
   b. Will continue to form at the site of origin and in the lungs following embolism.
   c. Cause secondary complications in about 40 percent of patients.
   d. Grow slowly at primary and secondary sites in patients undergoing heparinization.
   e. Are resorbed within 24 hours in patients undergoing heparinization.
5. What sign is present when deep vein tenderness is elicited when the patient dorsiflexes his foot?
6. List two procedures for detecting pulmonary embolism.
7. What is the clinical picture of massive pulmonary embolism?

Answers

1. a. Check the patient's vital signs every 15 minutes.
   b. Observe the patient's sputum for hemoptysis.
   c. Monitor the patient's ECG.
   d. Give oxygen and watch for the patient's response.

e. Elevate the head of the bed to relieve the discomfort due to dyspnea.

f. Observe the patient's level of consciousness; look for signs of increased restlessness or anxiousness.

g. Determine whether the elastic stockings are properly fitted on the patient's lower extremities.

2. True.
3. Heparin, warfarin.
4. b.
5. Positive Homan's sign.
6. Lung scan, pulmonary angiogram.
7. Cyanosis, tachypnea with confusion or anxiety, and sudden hypotension.

References

1. Cudkowicz, L., and Sherry, S. Current status of thrombolytic therapy. *Heart Lung* 1:97, 1978.

2. Dexter, L. Pulmonary Embolism and Acute Cor Pulmonale. In J. W. Hurst and R. B. Logue (eds.), *The Heart* (4th ed.). New York: McGraw-Hill, 1978. Pp. 1472–1481.

3. Fitzmaurice, J., and Sasahara, A. Current concepts of pulmonary embolism: Implications for nursing practice. *Heart Lung* 3:209, 1974.

4. Genton, E. Therapeutic aspects of pulmonary embolism. *Heart Lung* 3:233, 1974.

5. Genton, E., and Hirsh, J. Observation in Anticoagulant and Thrombolytic Therapy in Pulmonary Embolism. In A. Sasahara (ed.), *Pulmonary Emboli.* New York: Grune & Stratton, 1975.

6. Gracey, D., Kwaan, H., and Cugell, D. The Treatment of Pulmonary Embolism. Clinical Conference in Pulmonary Disease. Chicago: Northwestern University, McGraw Medical Center, 1972.

7. Grollman, J. Radiological diagnosis of pulmonary thromboembolism. *Heart Lung* 3:219, 1974.

8. Grollman, J. H., Jr., Gyepes, M. T., and Helmer, E. Transfemoral selective bilateral pulmonary arteriography with a pulmonary-artery-seeking catheter. *Radiology* 96:202, 1970.

9. Gruber, U. F. Dextran and the prevention of postoperative thromboembolic complications. *Surg. Clin. North Am.* 55:679, 1975.

10. Guyton, A. *Textbook of Medical Physiology* (5th ed.). Philadelphia: Saunders, 1976.

11. Harris, W. H., Salzman, E. W., Athanasoulis, C., et al. Comparison of warfarin, low-molecular-weight dextran, aspirin, and subcutaneous heparin in prevention of venous thromboembolism following total hip replacement. *J. Bone Joint Surg.* [*Am.*] 56A:1552, 1974.

12. Hirsh, J., and Gallus, A. S. ^{125}I-labeled fibrinogen scanning. Use in the diagnosis of venous thrombosis. *J.A.M.A.* 233:970, 1975.

13. Joffe, S. N. The incidence of postoperative deep vein thrombosis. *Thromb. Res.* 7:141, 1975.

14. Maeder, E. C., Jr., Facog, A. B., and Mecklenburg, F. Obesity: A maternal high-risk factor. *Obstet. Gynecol.* 45:669, 1975.

15. McIntyre, K. M., and Sasahara, A. A. The hemodynamic response to pulmonary embolism in patients free of prior cardiopulmonary disease. *Am. J. Cardiol.* 28:288, 1971.

16. Mobin-Uddin, K., Bolooki, H., and Jude, J. R. Intravenous caval interruption for pulmonary embolism in cardiac disease. *Circulation* 41:152, 1970.

17. Mobin-Uddin, K., Trinkle, J. K., and Bryant, L. R. Present status of the inferior vena cava umbrella filter. *Surgery* 70:914, 1971.

18. Moore, K., and Maschak, B. How patient education can reduce the risks of anticoagulation. *Nurs. '77* 9:24, 1977.

19. Moser, K. M. *Diagnostic Measures in Pulmonary Embolism. Basics of Respiratory Diseases.* American Thoracic Society 3:1, 1975.

20. Paraskos, J. A., Adelstein, S. J., Smith, R., et al. Late prognosis of acute pulmonary embolism. *N. Engl. J. Med.* 289:55, 1973.

21. Pollak, E. W., Webber, M. M., Victery, W., et al. Radioisotope detection of venous thrombosis. Venous scan versus fibrinogen uptake test. *Arch. Surg.* 110:613, 1975.

22. Rao, G., Zikria, E. A., Miller, W. H., et al. Incidence and prevention of pulmonary embolism after coronary artery surgery. *Vasc. Surg.* 9:37, 1975.

23. Sasahara, A. Therapy for pulmonary embolism. *J.A.M.A.* 299:1795, 1974.

24. Sautler, R. D., Meyers, W. O., Ray, J. F., et al. Pulmonary Embolectomy: Review and Current Status. In A. Sasahara (ed.), *Pulmonary Emboli.* New York: Grune & Stratton, 1975.

25. Smith, T. C., Glassford, E. J., and Wood, G. D. Effects of two elastic hospital stockings on fluid accumulation and tissue perfusion in calf and thigh. *Curr. Ther. Res.* 17:206, 1975.

26. Stein, M., Stevens, P., and Soffer, A. Recognition and management of pulmonary embolism. *Heart Lung* 1:650, 1972.

27. Stein, P. D., Dalen, J. E., McIntyre, K. M., et al. The Electrocardiogram in Acute Pulmonary Embolism. In A. Sasahara (ed.), *Pulmonary Emboli.* New York: Grune & Stratton, 1975.

28. The urokinase-pulmonary embolism trial: A national cooperative study. *Circulation* 4:1, 1973.

29. Vorherr, H. Contraception after abortion and post partum. An evaluation of risks and benefits of oral contraceptives with emphasis on the relation of female sex

hormones to thromboembolism and genital and breast cancer. *Am. J. Obstet. Gynecol.* 117:1002, 1973.

30. Wagner, H. N., and Strauss, H. W.   Radioactive Tracers in the Differential Diagnosis of Pulmonary Embolism. In A. Sasahara (ed.), *Pulmonary Emboli.* New York: Grune & Stratton, 1975.

31. Wenger, N. K., Stein, P. D., and Willis, P. W.   Massive acute pulmonary embolism. The deceivingly nonspecific manifestations. *J.A.M.A.* 220:843, 1972.

32. Williams, J. W., Britt, L. G., and Sherman, R. T.   Pulmonary embolism associated with surgically proved deep venous thrombosis. *Am. J. Surg.* 129:500, 1975.

33. Wright, I.   Pulmonary embolism: A most underdiagnosed and untreated disorder. *J. Am. Geriatr. Soc.* 22:433, 1974.

Bibliography

Dickie, K. J., deGroot, W. J., Cooley, R. N., et al. Hemodynamic effects of bolus infusion of urokinase in pulmonary thromboembolism. *Am. Rev. Respir. Dis.* 109:1, 1974.

Micheli, L. J.   Thromboembolic complications of cast immobilization for injuries of the lower extremities. *Clin. Orthop.* 108:191, 1975.

Adult Respiratory Distress Syndrome

Yvonne Lawton Wagner

Definition

Adult respiratory distress syndrome (ARDS) is a form of noncardiogenic pulmonary edema resulting in a failure of oxygenation. The causative mechanisms for ARDS are discussed in this chapter after the presentation of the case study. ARDS occurs in the critically ill, in the severely injured, and in major surgical patients following a profound clinical insult [5]. ARDS is frequently associated with low perfusion of blood to a single organ, to several organs, or to the total body system (shock). The patient's primary or admitting illness frequently is not respiratory in nature, but because of a distressful clinical episode, the patient develops a progressive, relentless respiratory complication that is often fatal [22].

Objective

The nurse will be able to discuss the anatomy, pathophysiology, clinical manifestations, therapeutic regimen, nursing responsibilities, and prognosis of the patient having ARDS.

Achieving the Objective

To achieve the objective, the nurse should be able to develop:

17

1. A meaningful definition of ARDS.
2. An awareness of the incidence of ARDS.
3. A knowledge of the prognosis of ARDS, with an appreciation of its severe morbidity and high mortality.
4. A clinical impression of whether early institution of vigorous prophylactic measures for patients in the high-risk group lowers the morbidity or mortality.
5. Criteria by which to identify patients in the high-risk group.
6. The assessment skills necessary for early recognition of ARDS.
7. The analytical ability to interpret case studies.
8. A concept of the interrelationships between gross and microscopic structural changes, physiological changes, clinical manifestations, and therapeutic regimens.
9. The ability to participate in the aggressive management of patients who are candidates for ARDS or who have already developed it. That ability must cover:
   a. The administration of prophylactic pulmonary hygiene.
   b. The performance of pulmonary function tests.
   c. The interpretation of pulmonary function tests, blood gas analyses, and other laboratory studies pertinent to respiratory functioning.
   d. The skillful use of complex monitoring equipment and ventilatory support equipment.
   e. The participation in clinical research.

How to Proceed with Academic Objectives

To achieve those goals the nurse must make rigorous efforts in the academic area and in the clinical setting. She must:

1. Read extensively the materials listed in the bibliography.
2. Learn the definition of medical terms.
3. Study the tables, figures, symbols, and abbreviations.
4. Evaluate the case study, using the bases of the nursing process:
   a. Assessment: (1) data collection, including patient history, physical examination, laboratory results, and diagnostic tests, and (2) organization and presentation of data in a precise and concise format.
   b. Analysis of data (collation): (1) verification of the data, (2) close critical comparison of the data, (3) integration of the data, and (4) synthesis of the data and the nurse's own knowledge.
   c. Statement of the patient's resolved, existing, and potential problems.
   d. Formulation of nursing diagnoses, nursing care plans, and nursing orders.
   e. Rationale for nursing actions based on an understanding of pathophysiology and psychopathology.
   f. Nursing intervention with the application of highly sophisticated skills at the maximum level of competency.
   g. Continuous reevaluation of the patient and of his responsiveness to nursing and interdisciplinary professional management.
5. Use simulators and demonstration equipment in a supervised laboratory setting to improve technical skills. The nurse should:
   a. Listen to recordings of normal and abnormal breath sounds.
   b. Study anatomical models of the thorax and the respiratory system.
   c. Work with various ventilators, oxygen analyzers, and spirometers, performing various tests of lung function until she becomes competent.
   d. Perform animal dissections to study the anatomy of the chest.
   e. Engage in animal experiments using ventilatory support, positive end-expiratory pressure (PEEP), pulmonary function tests, and blood gas analyses.

How to Proceed with Clinical Objectives

To develop an approach to adult respiratory distress syndrome the nurse should:

1. Improve her physical assessment skills by working with a proctor in the clinical environment.
2. Practice independently, placing emphasis on the physical examination of the chest and on the interpretation of laboratory data and pulmonary function tests.
3. Review patient charts, nursing care plans, and the medical management of patients with ARDS.
4. Assess the chronology of the pathophysiological changes and make alterations in therapeutic regimens as the patient's condition varies.

5. Carry out—first under supervision and then independently—the following methods of caring for patients with ARDS.
   a. Physical assessment
   b. Aggressive pulmonary hygiene
   c. Endotracheal and tracheostomy care
   d. Ventilatory support and oxygen therapy
   e. Assessment of the effects of PEEP on cardiovascular responses, including blood pressure, heart rate, cardiac output, ECG data, central venous pressure, pulmonary artery pressure, and pulmonary wedge pressure
   f. Interpretation of blood gas analyses
   g. Weaning techniques
   h. Monitoring of the patient's fluid status. The nurse should monitor plasma volume, hematocrit, hemoglobin, fluid intake and output, blood pressure, central venous pressure, pulmonary artery pressure, pulmonary wedge pressure, and daily weight

Case Study

Mr. R. F., a 46-year-old man, underwent both an emergency laparotomy and surgery for fixation of a crushed femur. He had received multiple injuries in an automobile accident, and he suffered from hypovolemic hemorrhagic shock.

Surgical Management

Abdominal Exploration

The exploratory laparotomy revealed that the right lobe of the patient's liver was shattered and that the lower pole of his spleen was lacerated. A resection of the right lobe of the liver and a splenectomy were performed. Intestinal perforation and pancreatic injury were not evident on inspection. The serum amylase level was 240 Somogyi units, indicating that there was no pancreatic involvement. During surgery, the patient's blood pressure oscillated about 70/40 mm Hg, except on two brief occasions when his blood pressure was not recordable.

Wound Exploration

The thigh wound was incised and debrided widely to remove necrotic tissue. Noncontractile muscle tissue was considered nonviable and was also excised. Foreign material and blood clots were removed to avoid a nidus for infection. Drainage tubes were placed in the wound; the wound was packed and allowed to granulate (second intention healing).

Orthopedic Surgical Procedure

Strict aseptic technique was used during the insertion of a Steinmann's pin into the proximal portion of the right tibia. Balanced surgical traction using a Thomas' knee splint with a Pearson attachment and 25 pounds of weight were to be used postoperatively to stabilize the fractured femur.

The operation took five hours. Blood loss from injury and during surgery was estimated at 3000 ml. Fluid replacement during surgery consisted of 6 units of appropriately typed and crossmatched acid citrate dextrose blood, 10 ml of a 10% calcium gluconate solution intravenously for each 3 units of blood to replace calcium chelated with citrate, and 3 liters of Ringer's lactate solution. Unfortunately, freshly banked blood (less than 24 hours storage time) was not available. A stat postoperative chest x ray showed correct placement of a central venous pressure line in the superior vena cava and no pulmonary infiltration in the lung fields.

Postoperative Course and Management

Phase I of ARDS

Injury, Resuscitation, and Respiratory Alkalosis (First 24 Hours After the Insult)
After the patient's recovery from anesthesia, his respirations were spontaneous but guarded because of pain from the abdominal trauma and from the high laparotomy incision. The respiratory rate was 28 breaths per minute, but the patient did not complain of dyspnea and the increased rate did not seem to fatigue him. His breath sounds were normal. There were no rales or adventitious sounds. The patient was encouraged to inspire deeply and to cough. Intravenous morphine was given slowly and titrated according to the patient's level of pain in order to enable the patient to breathe deeply. No adverse respiratory depression or cardiac slowing resulted from the judicious use of morphine. His chest x rays were negative.

During the first 12 postoperative hours, the patient's cardiovascular parameters stabilized; his blood pressure was 110/70 mm Hg, pulse 90 per minute, hematocrit 32%, hemoglobin 10 gm per 100 ml, cardiac output 8 liters per minute by dye dilution technique, and central venous pressure 9 to 13 cm H_2O. His urine output averaged 50 to 60 ml per hour; there was no evidence of red blood cells in the urine. The ratio of blood urea to urine urea was 1:20, which is normal.

Strong peripheral pulses were felt in all his extremities. No bleeding was evident at the thigh wound or abdominal site. The level of fibrinogen after the liver lobectomy and multiple transfusions was not significantly depressed (the fibrinogen level was 195 mg/100 ml; normal is 200–450 mg/100 ml).

Neurologically, the patient appeared alert and oriented in regard to time, person, place, and circumstance. His cranial nerves and peripheral nerves seemed intact.

Although the patient's severe hemorrhagic shock had been complicated by (1) the administration of large quantities of balanced crystalloid fluids, (2) massive transfusions with "old" banked blood, (3) long-term general anesthesia, (4) the additional trauma of surgical intervention, and (5) the imposed dorsal recumbency of balanced surgical traction, clinically the patient seemed to be doing well.

During the next 12 to 24 hours, the patient had persistent unexplained tachypnea not associated with pain or anxiety, and a slight hypocarbia ($PaCO_2$ 32 mm Hg) with mild respiratory alkalosis (pH 7.47).

Phase II of ARDS

Circulatory Stabilization and Beginning of Respiratory Difficulty (Second Postoperative Day)

The clinical improvement and relative stability that the patient showed during the first postoperative day were short lived. The patient began to complain of progressive dyspnea and fatigue. The patient's respiratory difficulty was manifested by (1) increasing tachypnea and hyperventilation, (2) use of accessory muscles of respiration with supraclavicular and suprasternal retractions, (3) fine rales audible in the dependent portions of both lungs, and (4) x-ray suggestions of patchy irregular infiltrations.

Serial blood gas analyses showed a falling $PaCO_2$ (30 mm Hg), a rising pH (7.50), and a PaO_2 that had fallen to a borderline hypoxic value of 60 mm Hg on room air. The patient seemed restless and agitated.

His serum potassium level was decreased (K^+ 2.9 mEq/L) owing to the renal exchange of hydrogen ions and potassium ions to compensate for the respiratory alkalosis. Potassium was administered intravenously.

Phase III of ARDS

Progressive Pulmonary Insufficiency (Third to Fourth Postoperative Day)

By the third to fourth postoperative day, the patient's unrelenting respiratory difficulty was manifested by (1) tachypnea (35/min), (2) progressive dyspnea, (3) moderate cyanosis of the tongue, (4) decreased tidal volume (3 ml/kg), (5) a minute volume of 8 liters, (6) an alveolar-arterial oxygen gradient of 520 mm Hg when 100% oxygen was inhaled for 10 minutes, (7) a progressive hypoxia that was unresponsive to increasing fractions of inspired oxygen, and (8) a deteriorating sensorium. In spite of the patient's extreme hyperventilation, paradoxically his $PaCO_2$ level began to rise ($PaCO_2$ 49 mm Hg), his CO_2 content was 29, his base deficit was -1.0, his PaO_2 continued to fall (to 40 mm Hg), and his pH decreased to 7.36.

Fine-to-medium rales were audible bilaterally and progressed to musical rhonchi that were accentuated on expiration. A serial pulmonary x ray revealed extensive progressive infiltrations with widespread areas of consolidation.

Serial thermal dilution cardiac outputs and measurements of pulmonary wedge pressures with a Swan-Ganz catheter did not indicate that the patient was suffering from congestive heart failure.

On the basis of the patient's clinical deterioration and the criteria for ventilatory support, a cuffed nasotracheal tube was inserted and the patient was placed on a positive pressure volume ventilator adjusted to deliver a tidal volume (TV) of 1050 ml (15 ml/kg) at a rate of 18 per minute with a sigh volume of 1500 ml delivered at six-minute intervals and FIO_2 of 40%. Initially, the peak airway inspiratory pressure (PAIP) required to administer that selected TV was 25 cm of H_2O pressure, but it rose to 45 cm H_2O. Intravenous morphine sulfate was titrated to gain control during assisted ventilation.

A tracheostomy was performed in the operating room to facilitate aspiration of secretions that were increasing in quantity and viscosity. The Portex tube with a soft cuff was used to minimize tracheal damage secondary to pressure-induced ischemia.

Gram-stain microscopic smears made from the tracheal aspirate indicated the presence of *Klebsiella pneumoniae* sensitive to gentamicin and cephalothin. Antibiotic therapy was adjusted because of alterations in liver function following lobectomy. Kidney function was considered adequate, as indicated by normal blood urea nitrogen and creatinine levels, blood urea to urine urea ratio, and a urinary output of 60–100 ml/hr. The initial penicillin therapy was continued.

The patient's hematocrit was 33% and his hemoglobin was 11 gm/100 ml. One unit of packed red blood cells was given to enhance his oxygen-carrying capacity.

Phase IV of ARDS

Terminal Hypoxia and Hypercarbia with Asystole (Fifth Postoperative Day)

The patient's PaO_2 was 35 mm Hg with an FIO_2 of 40%. Adequate PaO_2 was unobtainable even after the FIO_2 was increased to 60%. An increasing lactic acidosis indicated by a rising lactate to pyruvate ratio occurred secondary to tissue hypoxia and was superimposed on the patient's respiratory acidosis ($PaCO_2$ 55 mm Hg, PaO_2 40 mm Hg, pH 7.12).

The PAIP required to delivery the same TV had slowly risen to 60 cm H_2O. The patient was placed on 10 cm H_2O PEEP, and his blood pressure fell. His PEEP was reduced to 7.5 cm H_2O, his blood pressure returned to baseline, and his serial blood gas analysis showed a slight improvement in the PaO_2.

The chest x rays showed excessive pulmonary infiltration and consolidation. The opacity of the chest film was termed a "white out" by the radiologist.

The patient's sputum samples were mucopurulent, with rusty, blood-stained streaks.

On the fifth day, the patient died from a combined metabolic and respiratory acidosis leading to bradycardia and asystole.

On autopsy, gross examination revealed wet, dark, consolidated, and heavy lungs with scattered patches of necrosis and abscess formation. Histopathological examination showed focal hemorrhage into the alveoli, hypertrophy of the alveolar lining cells, alveolar edema, cellular infiltration, and perivascular hemorrhage.

Reflections

Death is an intense, complex affair, and the nurse as a survivor of the patient's death suffers the reactions of all survivors—feelings of loss and experiencing the stages of grief. Death is especially hard for the nurse to cope with when it is the death of a "salvageable" patient, a patient who was thought to have a number of years to live and who had potential and responsibilities. The loss of such a patient in spite of the nurse's heroic efforts, superb skills, and dedication is a demoralizing experience; it is fraught with feelings of grief, guilt, and inadequacy. Death is a mockery of the nurse's advanced knowledge, sophisticated skills, and elite classification as a critical care specialist. The critical care nurse is driven to acquire even more sophisticated skills, but frequently suppresses the need to think about a personal concept of death. Some nurses fail to develop a meaningful philosophy of life and death. Often the nurse reacts to the death of a patient with shock, embarrassment, inappropriate comments, or even laughter. The nurse is overwhelmed by the death of a salvageable patient.

Death of the nonsalvageable patient may be easier to bear provided the nurse accepted the imminent eventuality of death and perceived the patient as having died with dignity. The death of a patient may even be a positive experience for the nurse if the patient dies without pain, surrounded by loved ones, with dignity, and reconciled to the inevitability of death. Perhaps the negative feelings that arise when a nonsalvageable patient dies are related to the degree that life support efforts are applied when the patient is near death and to the time when a decision is made to let the illness take its fatal course.

The death of each patient is unique, and it evokes a unique response from each nurse. Nurses cannot be impervious to the deaths of their patients without diminishing the significance of life.

The Etiology of ARDS

There seems to be no single exogenous or endogenous precipitating factor acting on pulmonary tissue that induces the alterations that occur in lung ultrastructure and function during ARDS [6]. However, there does appear to be a common pathological response that occurs in lung tissue after a profound stressful event. The lung reacts to an insult in a limited manner, regardless of the cause of the stressor [6, 104]. Efforts should be made to prevent stressors from occurring and to prevent the progression of lung alterations before the point of irreversibility is reached.

Blaisdell and Schlobohm [6] have drawn up a list of conditions associated with ARDS (Table 17-1), as well as a list of synonyms for the syndrome (Table 17-2). McClelland [55] and Horovitz [43] have added the following to the associated conditions: peritonitis, severe head injury, oxygen intoxication, and inappropriate assisted ventilation techniques. Causative mechanisms are thought to be intracellular enzymes and vasoactive amines released into the circulation during a stressful episode (Table 17-3) [6, 108, 122]. Those intrinsic factors may be released at a distal site and transported to the lung, or they may be generated in the lung, or they may arise from both sites.

Factors acting in concert within the lung tissue cause (1) vascular endothelial wall damage, (2) pulmonary vasoconstriction, and (3) bronchoconstriction. The lung ultimately reacts as a leaky alveolar capillary membrane, causing transudation of plasma into alveolar air spaces. That leads to hypoxemia due to diffusion abnormalities, shunts, and ventilation-perfusion abnormalities. Those changes may be listed as alterations in:

1. The pulmonary capillary permeability, with transudation of plasma into the interstitial space and ultimately into the intraalveolar space (pulmonary capillary permeability defect and alveolar epithelial defect).
2. The diffusion capacity of gases to move through edematous alveoli and across the alveolar capillary membrane unit (alveolar capillary gas exchange defect).
3. The blood flow and distribution through the pulmonary region and microcirculation with increases in pulmonary vascular resistance (pulmonary perfusion defects).
4. The ventilatory flow and distribution of gases through regional and alveolar spaces (ventilation defects).
5. The ventilation-perfusion ratio (ventilation-perfusion imbalance; shunts).

A more precise definition of the specific causative

Table 17-1
Conditions Associated with Adult Respiratory Distress Syndrome

Amniotic fluid embolism	Malaria
Arterial embolism	Multiple transfusions
Bowel infarction	Peripheral vascular disease
Burns	Ruptured aneurysm
Carcinomatosis	Shock
Cardiopulmonary bypass surgery	Transfusion reactions
Clostridial sepsis	Transplantation
Drug abuse	Trauma
Eclampsia	Peritonitis
Multiple fractures	Severe head injury
Gram-negative sepsis	Oxygen intoxication
Heatstroke	Excessive tidal volume and pressure during assisted ventilation
High-altitude pulmonary edema	
Major surgery	

Source: Blaisdell and Schlobohm [6], McClelland and Fry [55], and Horovitz and Luterman [43].

Table 17-2
Synonyms of Adult Respiratory Distress Syndrome

Adult respiratory insufficiency (ARI) syndrome	Progressive pulmonary consolidation
Bronchopulmonary dysplasia	Progressive respiratory distress
Centroneurogenic pulmonary edema [64]	Pulmonary edema
Congestive atelectasis	Pulmonary hyaline membrane disease
Da Nang lung	Pulmonary microembolism
Fat embolism	Pump lung
Hemorrhagic atelectasis	Respirator lung
Hemorrhagic lung syndrome	Shock lung
Hypoxic hyperventilation	Stiff lung syndrome
Oxygen intoxication	Transplant lung
Postperfusion lung	Traumatic wet lung
Posttransfusion lung	Wet lung
Posttraumatic pulmonary insufficiency	White lung syndrome

Source: Blaisdell and Schlobohm [6].

factors and their mechanisms awaits further investigation. It is possible to arbitrarily categorize the postulated causative factors into two groups (Table 17-4) [22].

To best manage the critically ill patient, the actual and potential causative factors of ARDS must be dealt with and/or prevented when possible. Paradoxically, some of the adaptive mechanisms that the body uses to overcome the initial critical stress and some of the medical maneuvers used to treat critical insults may lead to ARDS in 24 to 72 hours.

Attention should be directed to the harmful effect of excessive fluid administration in producing pulmonary edema. The role of fluid overload in the production of ARDS is not completely understood. Recent experimental animal studies have shown that pulmonary edema induced solely by fluid overload can be cleared without development of the progressive anatomical and functional changes characteristic of ARDS [6]. Acting with other causative factors or acting on an already damaged lung, excessive fluid may be catastrophic.

Table 17-3

Intrinsic Factors Responsible for Adult Respiratory Distress Syndrome

Frequently shock plus
  Endotoxin
  Fatty embolism
  Collagenase
  Elastase
  Anaerobic acids (e.g., lactic acid)
  Lysosomal enzymes (e.g., killikriens and phospholipase A)
  Catecholamines
  Histamine 5-hydroxytryptamine
  Aggregated leukocytes
  Platelet aggregations
  Platelet vascular permeability factor
  Necrotic tissue debris
  Microembolism
  Serotonin
  Complement
  Prostaglandins

Source: Blaisdell and Schlobohm [6], Thompson [108], and Wilson [122].

Although the exact causative mechanism(s) is not known, measures to prevent the occurrence or to halt the progression of ARDS must be undertaken by the medical team in order to reduce the morbidity of the syndrome in the high-risk group of patients. Because of the many potential causes of ARDS, it follows that the syndrome is not uncommon. Until recently, the incidence of ARDS was rising rapidly. The increasing incidence was probably a reflection of the more accurate recognition of the syndrome and a concomitant increase in the number of patients surviving the initial severe stress.

Morbidity and Mortality

The morbidity and mortality of ARDS are related to the time of onset of the syndrome. When ARDS becomes evident *early* after an episode of shock, massive trauma, and/or fluid overload, the mortality is approximately 11 percent. When ARDS develops *late* and is related to sepsis, the mortality rises to 85 percent [115]. The site of the bacterial seeding of the bloodstream is extrapulmonary 90 percent of the time [85]. In surgical units, ARDS is the cause of death in many patients.

Historical Perspective

After World War II, the "limiting organ" system that appeared after injury, major surgery, or during a severe illness was the cardiovascular system. With the use of fluid replacement therapy to stabilize the cardiovascular system, the kidneys emerged as the limiting organ. Therapeutic emphasis was placed on supporting renal circulation and enhancing renal function. During the war in Vietnam, patients who survived cardiovascular and renal failure developed pulmonary complications, and the lung emerged as the limiting organ [3]. At present, with identification of the high-risk group for ARDS, early prophylaxis, early recognition of pulmonary compromise and aggressive therapeutic management (both circulatory and respiratory), the incidence of ARDS is being kept to a minimum [5]. The next problem that will emerge in the care of the critically ill patient will be multiple-systems failure and/or sequential-systems failure secondary to metabolic derangements and/or low tissue perfusion [3].

Today there is an acute awareness of potential pulmonary problems in patients at high risk. According to Horovitz and Luterman, high-risk patients include those with a history of (1) systemic and pulmonary sepsis, (2) massive soft-tissue injury with or without long-bone fracture, (3) direct pulmonary injury, (4) massive transfusion of whole blood, (5) aspiration of gastric contents, and (6) multiple-systems trauma, including trauma of the chest and head [43]. Those problems may have a wide spectrum of clinical manifestations, from mild respiratory dysfunction to the progressive and highly lethal ARDS. Both of those extremes occur less frequently than does an intermediate type of abnormality. Nevertheless, vigilance must be maintained and aggressive management instigated in the high-risk group to avert the development of ARDS with its high mortality. The hallmarks of ARDS are (1) hyperventilation, (2) atelectasis, interstitial edema, and intraalveolar edema, (3) progressive hypoxia that is relatively unresponsive to elevations of inspired oxygen concentrations, (4) decreased pulmonary compliance, and (5) a relative decrease in the functional residual capacity of the lung.

Characteristically, in the early stages of ARDS chest x rays are normal. However, with progression of the syndrome, the x rays show spotty and then diffuse pulmonary infiltrates that in the terminal stages may progress to widespread areas of consolidation.

Table 17-4
Classes of Causative Factors in Adult Respiratory Distress Syndrome

Group 1. Causative factors not readily prevented by medical means
  Injured peripheral tissue with release of factors that traumatize the lung
    Skeletal fractures with release of fatty emboli from bone marrow
    Massive soft tissue injury with release of necrotic and catabolic products (crush injuries and thermal trauma)
    Infected tissue with release of bacterial by-products (e.g., endotoxins, exotoxins, and septic emboli)
    Low perfusion state (shock) with release of anaerobic acids, lysosomal enzymes, and bradykinins secondary to cellular
      hypoxia
    Disseminated intravascular coagulation with release of microembolic clots and with alterations in the fibrinolytic sys-
      tem
    Cerebral injury or hypoxia with reflex centroneurogenic effects on the lung
  Injured lung tissue from direct trauma to the lung
    Inhaled chemical irritants
    Recognized or unrecognized aspiration of acid gastric contents
    Lung contusion secondary to a physical force acting on the chest wall or diaphragm
  Sepsis. Once sepsis occurs, the mortality in ARDS is high despite rigorous therapeutic efforts
Group 2. Causative factors that are relatively easily modified by medical means
  Side effects of massive transfusions
    Cellular debris
    Stored blood with red blood cells depleted in 2,3-diphosphoglycerate
    Use of citrated blood with chelated calcium
    Transfusion reactions (incompatibility or contamination)
  Oxygen intoxication secondary to prolonged use of oxygen at high concentrations ($FIO_2 > 50$ mm Hg)
  Inadequate or excessive fluid administration with wrong quantity, rate, or type of fluid replacement
  Microatelectasis secondary to
    Monotonous ventilatory support
    Prolonged recumbency
    Sedation
    General anesthesia
    Inadequate pulmonary hygiene
  Prevention of local infections
    Adequate debridement of injured soft tissues
    Proper wound care
    Correct pulmonary hygiene and careful management of endotracheal or tracheostomy tubes
    Sterile techniques in regard to the use of urinary catheter and intravenous cannula
  Prevention of dissemination of local infections
    Culture and sensitivity monitoring
    Specific antibiotic therapy
    Maintenance of nutrition for optimal wound healing

Moore has made a classic division of ARDS into four major clinical stages (Table 17-5) [62]. The first phase of ARDS is very difficult to detect because the signs and symptoms are so few. A medical history that includes a known precipitating factor of ARDS should alert the medical team. It is imperative that early diagnosis be made so that an appropriate medical regimen can be employed that will prevent the progression of ARDS to more serious, even fatal, stages. It is mandatory that the patient at risk:

1. Be recognized early.
2. Be assessed carefully and continuously.
3. Be given excellent pulmonary physiotherapy.
4. Be given baseline pulmonary function tests so that

subsequent testing will reveal any deterioration in pulmonary function.

The case study presented earlier in the chapter shows the dynamic progressive clinical changes that occur in the various stages of ARDS.

The Pathophysiology of ARDS

To comprehend the significance of the progressive clinical changes occurring during the various phases of ARDS and to apply the appropriate diagnostic test and optimal therapeutic management for a particular phase, it is necessary to correlate the molecular, cellular, functional, and gross pathological changes as

Table 17-5
Progressive Stages of Adult Respiratory Distress Syndrome

Normal	Phase I	Phase II	Phase III	Phase IV
	Clinical picture History of critical insult	Clinical picture Circulatory stability	Clinical picture Progressive respiratory insufficiency	Clinical picture Terminal hypoxia (modus exodus)
	High-risk category	Evidence of respiratory distress	Signs and symptoms of CNS hypoxia	↓ BP ↓ HR or asystole
	No dyspnea	Complaints of dyspnea	Severe dyspnea	
	No cyanosis		Moderate central cyanosis	
	Normal breath sounds	Basilar fine rales	Moderate rales ↑ in pulmonary secretions ↑ in tenaciousness of secretions	Diffuse rhonchi Rusty sputum
	Unexplained hyperventilation	Fatigue secondary to hyperventilation		
	Normal chest film	Chest film Normal to patchy infiltrates	Chest film Diffuse infiltrates	Chest film White out, consolidation
	Normal CO	Slight increase in CO	Increase in CO	Decrease in CO
pHa units 7.42	Slight ↑ in pHa (7.49)	pHa 7.50 respiratory alkalosis	Falling pHa (7.36)	pHa 7.12 (severe acidosis)
PaCO₂ 35–40 mm Hg	Slight ↓ in PaCO₂ (34 mm Hg)	PaCO₂ 30 mm Hg	PaCO₂ 45 mm Hg	↑ in PaCO₂ (55 mm Hg)
PaO₂ room air 90–100 mm Hg	Compensated PaO₂ room air (90 mm Hg)	PaO₂ room air 60 mm Hg	PaO₂ 40 mm Hg (on room air) unresponsive to ↑ % of administered O₂	↓ in PaO₂ (25 mm Hg) on room air
CO₂ content 24–27 mEq/L	Normal CO₂ content (26 mEq/L)	CO₂ content 23.5 mEq/L	CO₂ content 25 mEq/L	CO₂ content 18.5 mEq/L
No base excess (0)	↑ in base excess + 3	Base excess + 1	Base deficit − 1	Base deficit − 13
PaO₂ on 100% O₂ for 10 min 400–600 mm Hg	PaO₂ on 100% O₂ × 10 min (500 mm Hg)	PaO₂ on 100% O₂ × 10 min (250 mm Hg)	PaO₂ 100% O₂ for 10 min (80 mm Hg) (↑ in P[A-a]O₂)	PaO₂ on 100% O₂ for 10 min (45 mm Hg) (great ↑ in P[A-a]O₂)
Physiological shunt < 5% CO	Physiological shunt ≥ 5% CO	≥ 10% CO	≥ 18% CO	Shunt ≥ 35% CO
RR 16	Slight ↑	Exaggerated tachypnea	Tachypnea or bradypnea	↓ in RR
TV 7 cc/kg	Slight ↑	Moderate ↑ in TV	Slight ↑ or ↓ in TV	↓ in TV
MV 5 Lpm	Slight ↑	Moderate ↑ in MV	Slight ↑ or ↓ in MV	
Compliance normal	? ⎫	or ↓ in compliance	Moderate ↓ in compliance	Great ↓ in compliance
	⎬ Studies are needed			
FRC normal	? ⎭	or ↓ in FRC	Moderate ↓ in FRC	↓ in FRC

Key: BP = blood pressure; CNS = central nervous system; CO = cardiac output; FRC = functional residual capacity; HR = heart rate; Lpm = liters per minute; MV = minute volume; P(A-a)O₂ = alveolar-arterial oxygen difference; RR = respiratory rate; TV = tidal volume; ↑ = increase; ↓ = decrease.

they present themselves concurrently or sequentially. In the following pages, consideration is given to six pathophysiological processes that exist to some degree and at some point in ARDS:

1. The pulmonary capillary endothelial defects and alveolar epithelial defects
2. The alveolar-capillary gas exchange defect
3. The ventilation defect
4. The pulmonary perfusion defect
5. The ventilation-perfusion imbalance
6. Immunological defects

Pulmonary Capillary Endothelial Defects and Alveolar Epithelial Defects

In the severely injured or critically ill patient with ARDS, initially there occurs an episode of low tissue perfusion and cellular hypoxia that may go unrecognized. Consequently, peripheral tissues are deprived of essential nutrients. Intracellular metabolic derangements result secondary to an inadequate supply of oxygen and essential substrates. It is speculated that chemical factors (e.g., lysosomal enzymes, vasoactive amines, activated complement, metabolic acids, collagenase, or histamine) are released from the compromised peripheral tissue into the systemic circulation [6]. Those blood-borne factors are carried to the pulmonary microvasculature and cause a response in the lung tissue that is characterized by an increase in the permeability of the pulmonary capillary endothelium [104].

PULMONARY CAPILLARY ENDOTHELIAL DEFECTS

The pulmonary capillary wall damage resulting from the systemically derived factors may be aggravated by direct insults that occur within the lung per se (Table 17-6).

During shock episodes, the complement system becomes activated [67]. There are two principal mechanisms by which complement activation affects lung capillary permeability: (1) directly, complement activation impairs the biological membrane of the cell and (2) indirectly, the activated complement causes the mast cells (cells that are found in abundance in the lungs) to release histamine, which acts on the pulmonary capillary endothelial cells.

With rheological changes (e.g., low blood flow) in lung tissue, a stagnation of platelets and leukocytes in the pulmonary microvasculature results. Platelets release a platelet permeability factor and leukocytes release histamine, bradykinin, collagenase, and elastase. Those substances tend to increase capillary permeability.

Other insults that cause damage directly to the lung [26] are: (1) overt or silent aspiration of acidic gastric contents, (2) reflex centroneurogenic effects secondary to cerebral hypoxia [64–66], (3) inhalation of chemical irritants [45], and (4) high concentrations of oxygen administered for prolonged periods of time [69, 112].

The stressed lung may have a lowered tolerance for oxygen administered at concentrations greater than 60 percent for prolonged periods. The stressed lung may also be more sensitive to oxygen administered under hyperbaric conditions [88]. Unfortunately, it is sometimes necessary to utilize a fraction of inspired oxygen (FIO_2) greater than 60 percent in the patient

Table 17-6
Factors Within the Lung That Increase Pulmonary Capillary Permeability

Pulmonary low flow with pulmonary hypoxia → pulmonary lactic acidemia → vasoconstriction in pulmonary vascular bed → increased pulmonary vascular resistance
Complement activation
Platelet aggregates in the lung that release a platelet permeability factor

Key: → = leads to.

with ARDS in an effort to achieve adequate arterial oxygenation.

Peripheral and local insults to the lung act together to damage the pulmonary capillary endothelial cells by altering either cellular membrane structure or cellular membrane function or both. According to Snyder [98], the mechanism and nature of the endothelial insult have not been clearly defined.

Structural derangements in cell membrane integrity may result from changes in the lipid and protein composition of the cell wall [94] or from changes in the interactions between those lipids and proteins [111]. Teplitz [104] has demonstrated through transmission electron micrographs a widened gap "between" the endothelial cells of the pulmonary capillary that could permit excessive water movement into the interstices, resulting in interstitial pulmonary edema.

Functional alterations in cell membranes may be manifested by deficits in transport systems. A deficit is exemplified when the energy required for the membrane's sodium-potassium pump to maintain normal intracellular volume is considered. That active transport system utilizes adenosine triphosphate (ATP) for its supply of energy. The primary site of ATP production is in the mitochondria. In shock the mitochondria become abnormal in appearance [3, 9, 83], and subsequently inadequate amounts of ATP are produced. Consequently, the sodium-potassium pump has an inadequate amount of energy to maintain normal cell volume. The cell swells as its permeability increases. The deprivation of ATP is eloquently described by Baue as "an energy crisis in the cell" [3]. Simionescu and his associates [92, 93] have performed laboratory experiments evaluating the two hypotheses advanced to explain water transport across muscle capillaries. One hypothesis favors water transport through intercellular junctions, and the other hypothesis favors water transport through pinocytosis and plasma vesicles. Research is needed to ascertain the type of water transport that is present in the normal and in the pathological lung capillary walls. Once the pulmonary capillary wall has become more permeable due to either a widening of the "pores" between the endothelial cells or an increase in pinocytosis and vesicle transport across cells, plasma, which is rich in large protein molecules, cells, and cellular debris, leaks from the intravascular compartment across the capillary wall and into the interstitium (the condition is known variously as wet lung, pulmonary edema, or interstitial edema).

The exudate contains albumin, fibrinogen, elastase, and collagenase. Elastase and collagenase are proteolytic enzymes that cause disruption of the elastic and collagen fibers that are found in the interstitium. The plasma protein exudate and the products of the breakdown of interstitial fibers increase the tissue oncotic pressure of the lungs. The increase in tissue pressure tends to pull water from the blood into the interstitium, aggravating the interstitial edema.

In his hypothesis of the capillary, Starling listed four factors that regulate the movement of fluids across the capillary. All four of those factors are involved in ARDS (Fig. 17-1):

1. The hydrostatic pressure of the blood increases in the lungs secondary to an increase in pulmonary vascular resistance.
2. The plasma oncotic pressure decreases secondary to the exudation of albumin and other plasma proteins from the vascular bed (albumin has a smaller molecular size and passes through small pores more readily than does fibrinogen).
3. The tissue oncotic pressure increases secondary to the accumulation of excessive proteinaceous material in the interstitial fluid.
4. The capillary endothelial membrane permeability increases secondary to the loss of membrane stability and alterations in transport function.

ALVEOLAR EPITHELIAL DEFECTS

As the disease progresses, changes occur not only in the capillary endothelial cells but also in the epithelial cells lining the alveoli. Figures 17-2 to 17-4 show comparisons between normal lung architecture, an early phase of ARDS in which interstitial edema predominates, and a later phase of ARDS, in which in-

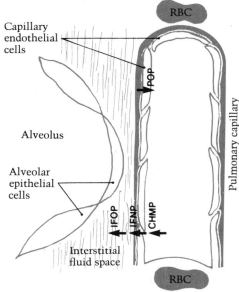

Figure 17-1
Starling's hypothesis of fluid exchange at the pulmonary capillary.

IFOP = Interstitial fluid oncotic pressure
IFNP = Interstitial fluid negative pressure
CHMP = Capillary hydrostatic mean pressure
POP   = Plasma oncotic pressure
RBC   = Red blood cell

The arrows indicate the direction of fluid movement at the pulmonary capillary venous blood and arterial blood ends.

traalveolar edema and a hyaline membrane are the dominant features.

The early architectural derangements of ARDS (Fig. 17-3) are swollen capillary endothelial cells, widened interendothelial junctions, diapedesis of cells, disrupted basement membranes, disorganized collagen in the interstitium, and swollen interstitial fluid spaces. If irreversible damage has not occurred, the interstitial edema can be removed by the lymphatic transport of the lungs. Serial chest x rays appear essentially normal when early interstitial edema is present. As the paravascular and interstitial spaces become moderately edematous, the chest x ray shows diffuse opacity indicative of profuse pulmonary infiltration.

Late architectural deterioration (Fig. 17-4) includes changes in the two types of epithelial cells that line the alveoli. Those changes correlate with the clinical symptoms of phase III and phase IV of ARDS. Alveo-

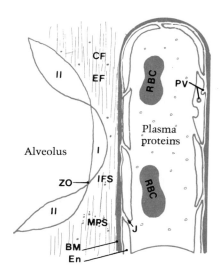

Figure 17-2
Normal architecture of the alveolus and capillary.

I   = Type I alveolar epithelial cell (gas exchange pneumocyte)
II   = Type II alveolar epithelial cell (surfactant producing pneumocyte)
ZO   = Zona occludens (tight junction between epithelial cells)
IFS   = Interstitial fluid space (narrow)
CF   = Organized arrangement of collagen fibers
EF   = Elastic fibers
BM   = Basement membrane (narrow)
En   = Capillary endothelium
J   = Interendothelial junction, or gap
MPS   = Mucopolysaccharide ground substance
PV   = Pinocytotic vesicles

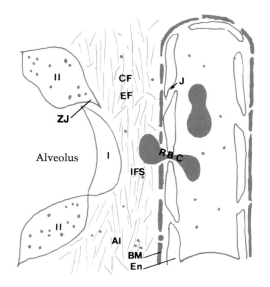

Figure 17-3
Abnormal architecture of the alveolus and capillary in early adult respiratory distress syndrome (phase 1 and phase 2) with interstitial edema.

I   = Swollen type I alveolar epithelial cell
II   = Granular type II alveolar epithelial cell
ZJ   = Widening of the interalveolar epithelial tight junction
IFS   = Marked edema of the interstitial fluid space
CF, EF = Disorganization of collagen fibers and elastic fibers
Al   = Increase in the quantity of albumin in the IFS
J   = Interendothelial junction, or gap
BM   = Disruption of the basement membrane
En   = Swollen capillary endothelial cells
RBC   = Diapedesis of red blood cells through the widened interendothelial junctions

lar type I epithelial cells (gas-exchange pneumocytes) are swollen. Alveolar type II epithelial cells (surfactant-producing cells) show more granulation. The tight junctions between alveolar lining cells appear tortuous. The intraalveolar spaces are filled with proteinaceous material, making alveolar ventilation difficult and compromising gas exchange. Red blood cells are found in the alveoli and account for the rusty sputum. Hyaline membranes form along the alveolar surface and represent denatured inspissated and coagulated protein (the condition is known as adult pulmonary hyaline membrane disease). Teplitz [100] suggests that fibrinogen exudate in the alveolar edema polymerizes to form intraalveolar fibrin that cannot be resorbed in the fluid state but must be enzymatically lysed or phagocytized. It has been postulated that proteinaceous alveolar edema serves as a culture medium for bacterial proliferation. Many patients die from a fulminating bronchopneumonia secondary to a bacterial infection. Those who survive long enough (weeks to months) may have as a terminal lesion a pulmonary fibrosis [5].

As intraalveolar edema and fibrosis occur, serial chest x rays show progressive opacity until the x-ray film appears white (the condition is known as white out or white lung syndrome). Gross examination of the lung at necropsy, however, shows a heavy, wet, boggy lung, deep red in color, with areas of consolida-

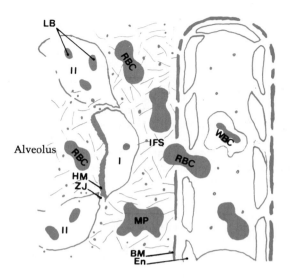

Figure 17-4
Abnormal architecture of the alveolus and capillary in late adult respiratory distress syndrome (phase 3 and phase 4) with intraalveolar edema. The alveolar space is filled with protein, red blood cells, and edema fluid.

HM = Deposition of hyaline membrane
I   = Swollen type I alveolar epithelial cell
ZJ = Tortuous, widened interalveolar epithelial junction
II = Granular type-II alveolar epithelial cells increased in number, granulation, lamellar bodies, and disrupted membranes
IFS = Marked edema of the interstitial fluid space
BM = Disruption of the basement membrane
MP = Macrophages
LB = Lamellar bodies
WBC = White blood cells

tion and focal abscesses (the condition is known as wet lung, hemorrhagic lung, or progressive pulmonary consolidation).

FUNCTIONAL DISORDERS

Physiologically, the leakage of fluid resulting in interstitial edema leads to progressive compression of the small bronchiolar airways and causes some compression of the alveoli. Teplitz [104] thinks that atelectasis has no relationship to progressive ARDS whereas Lucas and his associates [52] consider extensive alveolar atelectasis and resultant progressive hypoxemia the hallmarks of ARDS. Patients with ARDS who are placed on PEEP have an increase in

PaO_2. That reponse to PEEP indicates that atelectasis plays a role in the pathogenesis of ARDS.

Advancing interstitial-intraalveolar edema results in a less compliant lung (stiff lung). Compliance is defined as the relationship of the change in volume to the change in pressure required to produce the volume change. In ARDS, as the lung compliance decreases, a greater inspiratory effort is required during spontaneous breathing to expand the stiff lung. That results in increased work on inspiration. If the patient is being mechanically ventilated, higher positive pressures are necessary during the inspiratory phase to deliver the same volume of gas. For that reason, some physicians prefer using a positive-pressure volume-controlled ventilator for mechanical assistance in ARDS. The lung's decrease in compliance can be monitored by (1) observing a gradual rise over a number of hours in the inspiratory negative force a patient must generate to initiate an unassisted inspiration or (2) by observing a slow rise in the peak airway inspiratory pressure (PAIP) when a patient is ventilated with a volume-controlled respirator. It is possible to calculate both the dynamic and the static compliance of the lung. Dynamic compliance is obtained by dividing the tidal volume (TV) by the PAIP:

$$\text{Dynamic compliance} = \frac{\text{tidal volume}}{\text{PAIP}}$$

Normal = 45–55 ml/cm H_2O

Since inspiratory airway pressure evolves during an inflow of air with turbulence, perhaps a more sensitive measurement would be that of compliance calculated when no air flow is occurring. That measurement is referred to as static compliance, and it is calculated by dividing the tidal volume by the pressure existing at the end of inspiration (plateau inspiratory pressure):

$$\text{Static compliance} = \frac{\text{tidal volume}}{\text{plateau inspiratory pressure}}$$

Normal = 65–75 ml/cm H_2O

Plateau pressure is observed when the exhalation tube of a ventilator is pinched for a moment at the end of inspiration. The plateau pressure will always be somewhat lower than the PAIP.

DISORDERS IN TYPE II EPITHELIAL CELLS

Another factor contributing to decreasing compliance and progressing alveolar collapse is a reduction in the

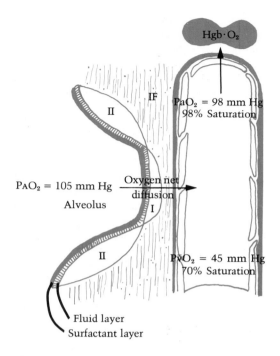

Figure 17-5
The alveolar capillary membrane (gas exchange unit).

PaO$_2$ = Alveolar oxygen tension
P$\bar{v}$O$_2$ = Mixed venous oxygen tension (dissolved oxygen)
PaO$_2$ = Arterial oxygen tension (dissolved oxygen)
Hgb·O$_2$ = Oxygen chemically combined with hemoglobin

The arrows indicate the direction of net diffusion of oxygen down the pressure gradient.

production of surfactant by the type II alveolar epithelial cells (type II pneumocytes) [40]. Surfactant is a surface-acting lipoprotein that lines the alveoli and separates the air-water interface (Fig. 17-5), thereby decreasing the surface tension of water. A high surface tension tends to collapse the alveoli. Surfactant stabilizes the alveoli and decreases their tendency to collapse. The production and release of surfactant from type II alveolar cells is stimulated by active ventilation, adequate tidal volumes, and intermittent hyperventilation (sighing). Continuous hyperventilation, continuous excessive tidal volumes, and ventilation with excessively high concentrations of oxygen decrease surfactant synthesis [55]. Failure to mechanically deep sigh a patient periodically during prolonged anesthesia or imposed re-

cumbency or continuous support of a patient on monotonous positive-pressure volume may lead to diminished surfactant production and consequent alveolar collapse. It has been suggested (but not adequately documented) that surfactant production decreases in shock. That decrease could be secondary to low perfusion of lung tissue with a resultant circulatory insufficiency to type II alveolar cells. According to Moser [63], surfactant production requires the continuous delivery of nutrient materials to type II alveolar cells. Control studies are needed to determine the role of surfactant production, release, and degradation in the pathology of ARDS.

STRUCTURAL DISORDERS IN TYPE II EPITHELIAL CELLS

Changes occur not only in the function of type II alveolar cells but also in their structural integrity following ischemia and resuscitation [40]. The type II pneumocytes are found (1) to be increased in number, (2) to contain large lamellar bodies (in which surfactant is produced) and lipid inclusion bodies, and (3) to have disrupted cell membranes (see Figs. 17-3, 17-4). Surfactant is inactivated by the presence of fibrin in the alveolar space [68].

Knowledge of the pathophysiological changes that follow an increase in pulmonary capillary permeability and alveolar epithelial defects is necessary for an understanding of the progression of ARDS and of the clinical manifestations of this progression. The clinical manifestations vary in accordance with the various pathological processes that are occurring [5]. The various phases of ARDS are defined on the basis of the clinical picture produced by the underlying pathophysiological mechanism(s). Further investigation is needed to identify the specific pathophysiological mechanisms.

Alveolar-Capillary Gas Exchange Defects

Respiration must be discussed in regard to: (1) internal (intracellular) respiration, which refers to the cellular utilization of oxygen for metabolic processes, and (2) extracellular respiration, which can be thought of as a multicomponent system by which air is acquired from the ambient environment, diffused into the blood, combined with hemoglobin, transported to the peripheral systemic tissues, and released at the capillary level for cellular uptake. That complex extracellular system also removes carbon dioxide from the peripheral tissues, transports the gas back to the lungs, and excretes it into the atmosphere. A dynamically balanced relationship must exist between the mechanisms that supply oxygen to (and remove carbon dioxide from) the cells and the utilization of oxygen by the cells in aerobic metabolism.

The functions of the extracellular respiratory multicomponent system are:

1. Dead space ventilation.
2. Alveolar ventilation.
3. Alveolar-capillary gas diffusion.
4. Physical dissolving of oxygen and carbon dioxide in plasma.
5. Chemical combining of oxygen with hemoglobin in the red blood cells.
6. Distribution of oxyhemoglobin to the microcirculation.
7. Release of oxygen from oxyhemoglobin at the capillary level.
8. Removal, transport, and excretion of carbon dioxide.

Various components of the system will be discussed in the following paragraphs in order to point out their importance in the pathophysiology of ARDS.

DEAD SPACE VENTILATION

Dead space ventilation (V_D) refers to the movement of air into and out of the large and small airways, starting with air inflow at the nasal orifices and ending at the terminal bronchioles. Since there is no gas exchange between air and blood as air traverses those conduits, V_D makes no contribution to the supply of oxygen to the blood or the removal of carbon dioxide from the blood. In a normal adult, the V_D is approximately 1.5 to 2 cc/kg ($\approx$150 cc). In patients with ARDS, the airway conduits do not change in volume, and therefore the anatomical dead space is unaltered. Those patients may, however, have difficulty in moving air through the dead space airway conduits. People who have ARDS produce an excessive amount of pulmonary secretions and may have a decreased ability to mobilize and remove those secretions. Without optimal pulmonary hygiene and adequate humidification, those people may develop inspissated mucous plugs in the larger airways. In the smaller airways, which have no supporting cartilaginous rings, the formation of interstitial edema tends to compress the diameter of the bronchioles. As a consequence, airway resistance increases and the patient is required to expend more energy in the movement of air (increased work on exhalation). A premature closing of small airways on expiration causes trapping of air in the alveoli and can be monitored by "closing volumes" in a cooperative patient [12, 85].

ALVEOLAR VENTILATION AND PHYSIOLOGICAL DEAD SPACE

Air filling the normal alveolus comes in contact with the alveolar-capillary membrane unit, where gases are exchanged between the alveolus and the blood in the pulmonary capillary. The volume of gas reaching the alveolus might be referred to as a useful ventilation. During normal quiet inspiration, only enough air is inhaled to fill the anatomical dead space (150 cc) and a portion of the total potential alveolar volume (350 cc). The sum of those two volumes is referred to as the tidal volume (TV), and it is approximately 6 to 8 cc/kg (500 cc) in an adult. Normally the ratio between the anatomical dead space (V_D = 150 cc) and the tidal volume (TV = 500 cc) is:

$$\frac{V_D}{TV} = \frac{150 \text{ cc}}{500 \text{ cc}} = 0.3 \text{ or } 30\% \text{ (normally} \leq 30\%)$$

In ARDS there are changes in blood flow through the pulmonary capillaries secondary to increased pulmonary vascular resistance or to microembolism to the microvasculature. Consequently, an inadequate amount of blood reaches the alveolar–capillary membrane unit in some alveoli. Those underperfused alveoli may have normal ventilation of their air space but optimal gas exchange does not take place. Those ventilated but poorly perfused alveoli are nonfunctional in regard to oxygenation of the blood. Ventilation to underperfused alveoli may be referred to as "wasted ventilation" [88]. The sum of the anatomical dead space (150 cc) and the alveolar wasted ventilation (e.g., 100 cc) is termed the physiological V_D. If a comparison is made between the physiological V_D and the TV in ARDS, the ratio will be elevated due to an increase in V_D and a decrease in TV:

$$\frac{\text{Physiological } V_D}{TV} = \frac{150 + 100}{400 \text{ cc}} = 0.63 \text{ or } 63\%$$

The V_D/TV ratio is one of the criteria used to assess the ventilatory capability of a patient with ARDS. An increase in the physiological dead space must be compensated for when determining the volume needed for assisted ventilation. A normal unassisted TV is 6 to 8 cc/kg, but a ventilator TV should be set at about 15 cc/kg (depending on the patient's response).

ALVEOLAR-CAPILLARY GAS DIFFUSION

The diffusion of gases between the alveolus and the pulmonary capillary occurs across the alveolar-capillary membrane (Fig. 17-5). Gases diffuse passively down their pressure gradients, requiring no expenditure of energy. The following factors facilitate the diffusion of oxygen across the alveolar-capillary membrane [16]:

1. The tension of oxygen in the alveolus (PaO_2 = 105 mm Hg) is greater than the tension in the blood returning to the lungs (PvO_2 = 45 mm Hg).
2. The distance across which diffusion occurs is small due to the thinness of the alveolar-capillary membrane unit.
3. The extensive surface area of the alveolar-epithelial type I cells and the capillary endothelial cells.
4. The large blood flow through the pulmonary capillary bed ($\geq$95% of the cardiac output).

In ARDS, several parameters change that could alter the rate of gas exchange. Due to intraalveolar edema, hyaline membranes, and a swollen alveolar-capillary membrane unit, gases must diffuse across a greater distance. This results in a decrease of diffusing capacity that contributes somewhat to the severe hypoxemia seen in the later phases of ARDS, but it is not considered to be the major cause of hypoxemia [25, 27, 57]. The alveolar surface area across which diffusion occurs is reduced secondary to the degeneration of the alveolar cells, the disruption of intraalveolar septa [40], and the presence of atelectatic alveoli and fluid-filled alveoli [121].

McLaughlin and his associates [57] state that "the major factor producing arterial desaturation is a ventilation-perfusion abnormality (shunt-like effect)" due to blood flow through multiple underventilated areas. Several studies [36, 61, 63] support the theory that hypoxemia in ARDS is due to alterations in the ventilation-perfusion imbalance and shunting. Rarely is hypoxemia due to changes in gas diffusion capacity.

OXYGEN IN PHYSICAL SOLUTION

Plasma has a very low solubility coefficient for oxygen, and therefore only a small percentage (<2%) of the total oxygen transported by the blood is carried in

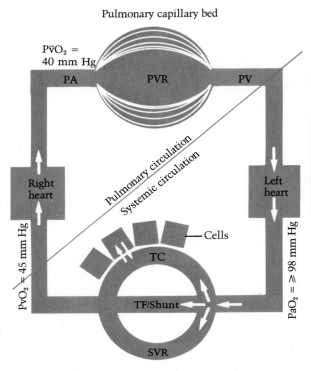

Figure 17-6
The circulatory system.

PA   = Pulmonary artery
PV   = Pulmonary veins
PVR = Pulmonary vascular resistance
SVR = Systemic vascular resistance
TF   = Thoroughfare channel, site of extrapulmonary arteriovenous shunting
TC   = True capillary
$P\bar{v}O_2$ = Mixed venous oxygen tension
PvO_2 = Venous blood oxygen tension
PaO_2 = Arterial blood oxygen tension

The single arrows show the direction of blood flow.
The double arrows indicate the nutrient and waste exchange between cells and blood perfusing the true capillaries.

physical solution. That dissolved oxygen remains in a gaseous state and therefore exerts a partial pressure (PO_2). Normally, the partial pressure of oxygen in the arterial blood (PaO_2) is $\geq$ 95 mm Hg pressure. This level decreases with age. At the peripheral capillary level, oxygen is extracted from the blood for consumption by the cells, and consequently the partial pressure of oxygen in the venous blood is about 45 mm Hg tension (PvO_2) (Fig. 17-6). Oxygen consumption can be evaluated by the arteriovenous oxygen content difference ($C(a\text{-}v)O_2$).

During the progression of ARDS there seems to be no alteration in the solubility coefficient of plasma for oxygen. The capacity of oxygen to dissolve in plasma remains constant, but the quantity of oxygen actually dissolved is reduced because less oxygen is moved across the alveolar-capillary membrane unit and into the pulmonary capillary blood. Although the quantity of oxygen transported as a dissolved gas is small ($< 2\%$ of total) the significance of the dissolved gas cannot be overlooked. Oxygen must be physically dissolved in plasma to diffuse through the plasma, through the red blood cell membrane, and through the red cell cytoplasm to reach the hemoglobin molecule. The driving force by which oxygen reaches the hemoglobin-binding sites is the oxygen tension (PO_2).

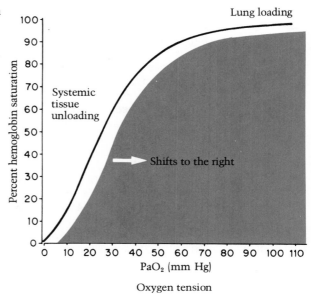

Figure 17-7

The oxyhemoglobin desaturation curve. The hemoglobin saturation is approximately 95% at a PaO_2 of 90 mm Hg. The slope of the curve is steep at a PaO_2 of less than 60 mm Hg. Shifts of the curve to the right release more oxygen at the systemic (peripheral) tissue level.

OXYHEMOGLOBIN

The largest quantity of oxygen (98%) is carried chemically combined with hemoglobin as oxyhemoglobin ($HgbO_2$). The total oxygen-carrying capacity (oxygen content) of the blood is equal to the sum of the amount carried in physical solution plus the amount carried in chemical combination.

$$\text{Arterial } O_2 \text{ capacity WB} = (PaO_2)(0.003) + (Hgb)(1.39) \times (\% \text{ saturation})$$

where

O_2 capacity WB = total oxygen-carrying capacity of 100 ml of arterial whole blood
  0.003 = solubility constant for O_2 in plasma
  Hgb = gm hemoglobin/100 ml WB
  1.39 = cc oxygen affinity/gm hemoglobin

Any change in the hemoglobin level, the percentage of saturation, or the quantity of dissolved oxygen causes a decrease in the total oxygen content. The portion of oxygen bound to hemoglobin is, however, the primary determinant of the total oxygen-carrying capacity. Patients with ARDS have decreased PaO_2 levels and decreased hemoglobin saturation. As the oxyhemoglobin desaturation curve in Figure 17-7 shows, at a PaO_2 of 60 mm Hg or less, the percentage of hemoglobin saturated with oxygen is critically reduced. That leads to a decrease in the total oxygen content. At a PaO_2 above 60 mm Hg, if the hemoglobin level is normal, total oxygen content will usually be adequate.

OXYHEMOGLOBIN DISTRIBUTION

Blood that is rich in oxyhemoglobin must be adequately distributed to the microvasculature of all tissues. In the systemic circulation, at the peripheral cellular level blood must flow through the true capillaries in order for substances to be exchanged between the blood and the peripheral cells. Blood perfusing through the thoroughfare channels [28] passes from the arterial side of the systemic circulation to the venous side without being exposed to nutrient and gas exchange at the peripheral tissue level. Such systemic arteriovenous "shunting" is called an extrapulmonary shunt. For adequate distribution of blood through the true capillary beds to occur, there must be cardiovascular proficiency and stability. Constant assessment must be made of the circulating volume, the cardiac efficiency, the peripheral perfusion, and the cellular oxygen consumption and utilization. During the early phases of ARDS, cardiac output is usually increased. In phase IV of ARDS, severe hypoxemia leads to myocardial compromise, decrease in cardiac output, and the subsequent failure of adequate cellular oxygenation. That failure results in anaerobic cellular metabolism with an increased production of lactic acid and a metabolic lactic acidemia. Declining perfusion of multiple organs with resulting hypoxia is manifested by a decreasing level of consciousness, convulsions, a diminished urinary output, and cardiac irregularities. Low flow of blood deficient in oxygen to the coronary arteries may result in ventricular fibrillation and sudden death or in bradycardia that progresses to asystole.

Both hemodynamic and ventilatory studies are necessary for a complete profile of patients with pulmonary physiological disturbances [109]. Tissue oxygen demands vary from organ to organ; they also vary in resting, active, and diseased states. A determination of the difference between the total arterial oxygen content and the total venous oxygen content can generally be used to evaluate the processes of oxygen delivery, unloading, and utilization by cells. Venous sampling from a central venous line does not accurately measure the mixed venous oxygen tension ($P\bar{v}O_2$) or the mixed venous oxygen content ($C\bar{v}O_2$). Samples of mixed venous blood should be drawn from a catheter placed in the pulmonary artery. An increase or a decrease in mixed venous oxygen values will not pinpoint what alteration(s) has occurred at the peripheral capillary exchange site. The alterations that are reflected by both elevated and lowered $P\bar{v}O_2$s are summarized in Table 17-7.

RELEASE OF OXYGEN AT THE SYSTEMIC CELLULAR LEVEL

The combining of oxygen with hemoglobin at the pulmonary alveolar-capillary level is of no value unless the oxygen can be dissociated from the hemoglobin at the systemic capillary cellular level. The percentage of oxygen loading onto hemoglobin at the lung is called the percentage of hemoglobin saturation. It is depicted in Figure 17-7 by the upper, flat portion of the oxyhemoglobin dissociation curve. The unloading of oxygen from oxyhemoglobin at the systemic level is represented by the steep portion of the curve.

There are certain physical and chemical changes that facilitate oxygen uptake by hemoglobin in the lungs. The reverse of these changes facilitates oxygen release from hemoglobin at the periphery. Factors that increase oxygen release to the cells (a shift of the curve to the right) are listed in Table 17-8.

As Figure 17-8 shows, the pressure of oxygen in the

Table 17-7
Alterations in Pulmonary Artery Oxygen Tension

Alterations that produce increases in mixed venous oxygen tension ($P\bar{v}O_2 > 40$ mm Hg)
  Decreased utilization of oxygen by peripheral tissues
  "Inappropriately" increased cardiac output
  Arteriovenous shunting at the peripheral tissue level
  Decreased ability of oxyhemoglobin to unload oxygen to the peripheral cells (leftward shift of the oxyhemoglobin dissociation curve)
  An excessively high PaO_2 (i.e., increased PaO_2 secondary to oxygen administration)
Alterations that produce decreases in mixed venous oxygen tension ($P\bar{v}O_2 < 40$ mm Hg)
  Increased utilization of oxygen by peripheral tissues
  Decreased cardiac output
  Increased ability of oxyhemoglobin to unload oxygen (shift of the oxygen dissociation curve to the right)
  An excessively low PaO_2 (i.e., a low PaO_2 secondary to abnormal pulmonary shunting)

Source: Snyder [98].

Table 17-8
Factors That Increase Oxygen Release at the Systemic Cellular Level

Physical factors
  Large capillary-to-cell-oxygen diffusion gradient
  Increase in body temperature
  Increase in PCO_2
Chemical factors
  Increase in hydrogen ion (increase in acidity)
  Increase in 2,3-diphosphoglycerate in red blood cells
  Increase in adenosine triphosphate

arteriolar sections of the capillary (PaO_2 98 mm Hg) and the pressure of oxygen in the venular section of the capillary (PvO_2 45 mm Hg) are greater than the oxygen tension in the interstitial fluid ($PIFO_2$ 10–20 mm Hg) and the intracellular water ($PICWO_2$ 5 mm Hg). Since gases diffuse down a pressure gradient, oxygen diffuses toward the cell. Any increase in temperature gives more kinetic energy to a molecule. An elevation of body temperature consequently enhances the rates of oxyhemoglobin dissociation and of oxygen diffusion.

Chemically, oxygen has to compete with other molecules for combination on hemoglobin-binding sites. Hydrogen ions combine with hemoglobin to form reduced acid hemoglobin ($H \cdot Hgb$). An increase in the number of hydrogen ions tends to increase the release of oxygen. It has been observed that an eleva-

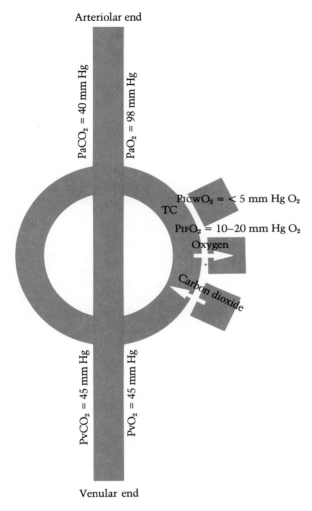

Arteriolar end

$PaCO_2 = 40$ mm Hg

$PaO_2 = 98$ mm Hg

$PIcwO_2 = < 5$ mm Hg O_2
TC

$PIFO_2 = 10-20$ mm Hg O_2

Oxygen

Carbon dioxide

$PvCO_2 = 45$ mm Hg

$PvO_2 = 45$ mm Hg

Venular end

Figure 17-8
Gas diffusion gradients in the peripheral capillary bed.

PaO_2 = Arterial oxygen tension
$PIFO_2$ = Interstitial fluid oxygen tension
$PIcwO_2$ = Intracellular water oxygen tension
TC = True capillary

The arrows indicate the direction of passive gas diffusion down pressure gradients.

tion in PCO_2 also enhances oxygen release, perhaps through the formation of carbonic acid [36].

A patient with ARDS has several problems in regard to oxygen release. During phase I and phase II of ARDS, a respiratory alkalosis and a decreased PCO_2 impede oxygen unloading. If the patient's condition progresses to phase III or phase IV, the PaO_2 is significantly lowered to abolish the steepness of the pressure gradient of oxygen from the blood to the interstitial fluid and the cell. A metabolic acidosis exists secondary to hypoxia, and therapy consists of increasing the FIO_2. Correcting the acidosis by administering bicarbonate may interfere with oxygen release. A patient in the terminal phase of ARDS has a decreased body temperature and a depletion of cellular adenosine triphosphate (ATP). If such a patient requires blood transfusions, fresh blood with high levels of 2,3-diphosphoglycerate should be administered. The appropriate medical regimen incorporates the application of factors that improve oxygen uptake in the lung and oxygen release in the systemic tissue. Management practices that improve oxygen loading include the administration of oxygen to saturate hemoglobin and the application of positive end-expiratory pressure (PEEP) to expand the functional residual capacity (FRC).

REMOVAL OF CARBON DIOXIDE

Systemic cells that are supplied with sufficient quantities of oxygen engage in aerobic metabolism (oxidative phosphorylation) within the mitochondria. Carbon dioxide, water, and energy in the form of ATP are the by-products of aerobic catabolism. The final function of the multicomponent extracellular respiratory system is to rid the body of excess carbon dioxide. Carbon dioxide diffuses from its site of production (the cell) down a pressure gradient to the blood.

Carbon dioxide is transported by the blood in physical solution and in chemical combination. Although the solubility of carbon dioxide in plasma is greater than the solubility of oxygen in plasma, the amount of carbon dioxide transported as a dissolved gas (PCO_2) is only about 6 to 8 percent of the total carbon dioxide content of the blood. The remaining 92 percent of carbon dioxide is transported in chemical combination. Harper [36] and Ganong [28] describe those chemical fractions as: (1) a small amount in the form of carbonic acid (H_2CO_3), (2) a moderate amount combined with proteins as carbamino compounds (e.g., $HgbCO_2$), and (3) a large amount carried as sodium or potassium bicarbonate (NaHCO$_3$, KHCO$_3$).

In the early phases of ARDS, tachypnea causes an excessive loss of carbon dioxide, the pH becomes elevated, and respiratory alkalosis ensues. The alkalosis may be exaggerated in the postsurgical patient who has received an intraoperative alkaline load. According to Moore and his associates [62], a metabolic alkaline component may exist due to the massive transfusion of citrated blood with oxidation of the citrate. In the oxidative metabolism of sodium citrate, sodium bicarbonate is produced. The sodium bicarbonate load is difficult for the surgically stressed patient to excrete because of his reduced glomerular filtration rate and transient hyperaldosteronism. As a result of the patient's inability to excrete bicarbonate, a paradoxical aciduria may occur. Those who monitor the patient's urine pH should be aware that the urine pH may be acidic when the blood pH is alkaline.

The elevated serum pH in early ARDS might reflect a mixed respiratory-metabolic alkalosis. The increased pH (increased hydrogen ion level) shifts the oxyhemoglobin curve to the left, impeding the release of oxygen to the peripheral cells. Paradoxically, then, in phases I and II of ARDS, the patient's PO$_2$ might appear adequate but his oxygen unloading might be inadequate. At present, for patients in phases I and II of ARDS, some physicians recommend the administration of oxygen in low concentrations plus 3% carbon dioxide to correct the hypocarbia [110]. That mode of therapy is controversial, however, and until the exact cause of the tachypnea is known, any therapy to correct hypocarbia is probably not warranted. Further research is needed to determine the causes of tachypnea, the underlying pathological states, the preventive measures, and the containing measures for the early stages of ARDS.

In the later stages of ARDS (phases III and IV), the PaCO$_2$ is abnormally high (a condition called hypercarbia or hypercapnia). That is so primarily because of hypoventilation, and because adequate carbon dioxide exchange does not occur at the alveolar-capillary membrane unit. A respiratory acidosis results. During phases III and IV of ARDS, a metabolic acidosis also develops secondary to hypoxia and intracellular anaerobic metabolism with lactic acid formation (lactic acidemia). Excessive hypercarbia heralds the terminal stage of ARDS and the patients die with a mixed respiratory-metabolic acidosis [110].

Ventilation Defects in ARDS

The simplest way to obtain an overview of the multiple defects occurring in the ventilation of patients who have ARDS is to group the defects by anatomical sites and by pulmonary function tests.

AIRWAY ALTERATIONS

Three major problems arise in the upper airways. First, there is a decrease in the escalator effect of the cilia lining the respiratory tree. That decrease in the ability of the cilia to lift and clear secretions may be secondary to low perfusion. After shock, the ciliated cells may be depleted of the energy that they require for normal functioning. Ciliary transport may also be directly disturbed by hypoventilation and hypoxia [124]. Second, in the later phases of ARDS, an increase in the quantity and viscosity of pulmonary secretions occurs that impedes the removal of mucus. In addition, any superimposed infections in the respiratory tract intensify the production of pulmonary secretions.

In the smaller airways, the primary ventilatory problem is an increase in airway resistance, with premature closure of the small airways. The increase in airway resistance results from humoral factors causing constriction of the bronchial smooth muscles and from mechanical compression of the airway conduits by interstitial edema. Increased airway resistance leads to a turbulence in airflow and a harshness of breath sounds, and it makes artificial ventilation of the patient more difficult. Extended research is needed to evaluate alterations in closing volumes, closing capacities of the lungs, flow volume loops, and functional residual capacity (FRC).

ALVEOLAR ALTERATIONS

At the alveolar level, a number of pathological changes interfere with effective alveolar ventilation:

1. Some alveoli are ventilated but nonperfused, resulting in an increase in physiological dead space.
2. Some alveoli are compressed secondary to interstitial edema (atelectasis) and therefore are nonventilated.
3. Some alveoli are collapsed due to inadequate amounts of surfactant (atelectasis), again resulting in nonventilation.
4. Some alveoli are filled with transudate, red blood

cells, and cellular debris (intraalveolar edema and hemorrhage), which form a diffusion barrier.

5. Some alveoli are lined by exudates that form a hyaline membrane and impede gas exchange (diffusion barrier, increased physiological dead space).
6. Some alveoli have disrupted type I and type II pneumocytes, with loss of structure and function.
7. Some alveoli have lost septae and consequently have decreased surface areas for gas exchange.

MIXED VENTILATORY PATTERNS

Those airway and alveolar alterations produce uneven and ineffective alveolar ventilation. Mixed patterns of ventilation result. Overventilated, underventilated, and nonventilated alveoli are distributed throughout each lung field. If hyperventilated alveoli dominate the mixed pattern, (a) blood gas analysis shows a normal PO_2, hypocapnea, and respiratory alkalosis and (b) pulmonary function tests show increased TVs, increased minute volumes (MVs), and increased FRC. If hypoventilated alveoli predominate, the blood gases indicate hypoxemia, hypercarbia, and acidosis, while the TV, MV, and FRC are decreased.

By performing serial blood gas analyses and serial pulmonary function tests, a quantitative description of the progressive alterations in ARDS can be obtained [27]. Ventilatory volume and lung capacity tests are designed to study the mass movement of gas. *Capacity* refers to the sum of two or more volumes. *Flow* refers to the rates of movement of air into and out of the lungs. *Force* refers to the pressures generated during inspiration and expiration. Further investigation of pulmonary functions in patients at high risk for ARDS and in patients in the early phases of ARDS is needed. Patients in phases III and IV are not usually able to participate in complex or strenuous tests.

MECHANICS OF BREATHING

Pulmonary function tests are used to evaluate the mechanics of breathing. Changes that have been observed in breathing mechanics during ARDS are as follows:

1. An early increase in the rate of respiration (tachypnea), which converts in phases II and III to a decrease in the rate of respiration
2. An early increase in work of breathing
3. An early increase in total lung capacity but a late decrease in total lung capacity

4. An early increase in vital capacity but later a decrease in vital capacity
5. A decrease in lung compliance
6. An increase in airway resistance
7. An increase in PAIP
8. An increase in TV in phases I and II of ARDS and a decrease in TV in phases III and IV of ARDS
9. An increase in MV in phases I and II of ARDS and a decrease in MV in phases III and IV of ARDS
10. A late decrease in absolute FRC (studies of relative FRC are needed)
11. An increase in the V_D/V_T ratio

Research using more sophisticated pulmonary function tests for diagnosing and managing patients with early ARDS is needed. Investigations should use

1. Nitrogen washout techniques to evaluate FRC.
2. Flow rates to evaluate peak flow and flow at 25, 50, and 75 percent of vital capacity.
3. Dynamic and static compliance calculations.
4. Closing volumes and closing capacities.
5. Flow-volume loops to check small airway function.

Serial ventilatory function tests do not indicate the pattern of air flow in the lung to any given region. They indicate only a change in the mass movement of air. In ARDS, alterations in ventilation are not localized to any particular region of the lung; they are widely spread. Scintiphotographs (ventilation scans) using the inhalation of a radioactive gas (xenon 133) show a diffuse maldistribution of ventilation in patients suffering from smoke inhalation [73]. Serial scintiphotographs of patients with ARDS may be of value in diagnosis in determining the effectiveness of therapy. The point must be stressed that routine chest x rays are not reliable indicators of the early phase of ARDS. Clinical deterioration is usually one or two days ahead of routine radiographic findings [123].

Serial x rays, however, show progressive changes in the later phases of ARDS. The x-ray appearances vary as the underlying disease process varies. At first, the chest x rays appear normal, then random interstitial edema appears, and as the disease progresses, widely dispersed patchy alveolar infiltrates appear. The location of the alveolar process varies from film to film, depending on the patient's response to fluid administration and positioning. When bacteria colonize in the

Table 17-9
Physiological Profile of Patient with Adult Respiratory Distress Syndrome

Clinical Appearance	Ventilatory Status	Gas-Exchange Capacity	Hemodynamic Status	Metabolic Status	Immunological Status
Work of breathing	Lung volumes	PaO_2	CO	Lactate level	WBC
Labored breathing	Lung capacities	$PaCO_2$	CI	Pyruvate level	
Rate of breathing	Flow-volume loops	$P\bar{v}O_2$	PAP	L/P ratio	Schick/Dick test
Rhythm of breathing	Flow rates	$P(A-a)O_2$	CVP PAWP	pH	Protein determination
Pattern of breathing	Scintiphotographs	Shunts Berggren test ^{133}Xe test	RBC	Acid or base excess or deficit	Gram stains
Complaints of dyspnea	X rays		Hgb	O_2 consumption $P(A-a)O_2$	Cultures and sensitivity tests
Color of skin	Bronchoscopy		Hct		History of immunosuppressant therapy
Temperature of skin			Plasma volume		History of recurrent infections
			Blood volume		Debilitating disease

Key: CI = cardiac index; CO = cardiac output; CVP = central venous pressure; Hct = hematocrit; Hgb = hemoglobin; L/P = lactate/pyruvate; $P(A-a)O_2$ = alveolar-arterial oxygen difference; PAP = pulmonary artery pressure; PAWP = pulmonary artery wedge pressure; $P\bar{v}O_2$ = mixed venous oxygen tension; RBC = red blood cells; WBC = white blood cells.

respiratory tract, the x ray may show pneumonia characterized by segmental or lobar infiltrates or even by pulmonary abscesses, depending on the causative organism.

Gravitational effects have a profound influence on the distribution of both air and blood in the lungs. By raising the head of the bed 15 degrees, the FRC can be increased. Thus "positional effects" must be kept in mind when pulmonary function tests are performed and when caring for the patient. For comparative studies, the patient should be in the same position each time a battery of tests is given. Unfortunately, the seriously ill or confused patient may not be able to successfully complete many of the tests. Efforts must be made to design techniques for determining ventilation mechanics that will (1) yield the desired information with minimal stress to the patient, (2) be moderately easy for the investigator, (3) allow maximal diagnostic efficiency, and (4) be economically feasible for widespread use.

PHYSIOLOGICAL PROFILE

If the clinical personnel are to cope with the many problems arising in ARDS, they must develop a series of physiological profiles, beginning with the initial assessment of the at-risk patient and then proceeding sequentially through each phase of ARDS. The profiles note any physiological changes that precede or follow any changes in types of treatment. The physiological profile (Table 17-9) should include an evaluation of the patient in regard to his:

1. General clinical appearance.
2. Ventilation status.
3. Hemodynamic status, including his pulmonary hemodynamic status.
4. Metabolic status [40].
5. Immunological status [16].

BASIS OF HYPERVENTILATION

The patient in phase I of ARDS characteristically demonstrates tachypnea and hyperventilation. Several explanations of the cause of hyperventilation have been offered. One hypothesis is that an underlying hypoxia exists secondary to atelectasis and pulmonary physiological shunting. The compensatory hyperventilation corrects the hypoxia so that no unusual decrease in PaO_2 is evident when infrequent blood gas analyses are made.

Another hypothesis is based on the fact that the carotid and aortic bodies normally have a very large flow of blood (2000 ml/min/100 gm tissue). Those chemoreceptors increase their rate of oxygen utilization during low-flow states. The concomitant decrease in oxygen delivered to the chemoreceptors, along with their increase in oxygen demand, results in the chemoreceptors' detecting an oxygen deficiency [37, 62]. An imbalance between blood flow and oxygen demand causes excitation of the chemoreceptors and respiratory stimulation occurs via afferent fibers to the central nervous system. The hyperventilation leads to respiratory alkalosis.

Several points should be made about the patient's clinical appearance during the alkalosis of phases I and II of ARDS. Since it is more difficult to release oxygen to cells when the pH is elevated, less oxygen is available for central nervous system function. Consequently, the patient may appear restless or even irrational. The undissociated oxyhemoglobin passes through the systemic arterial tree, traverses the peripheral capillaries without releasing much oxygen, and appears on the venous side of the circulation $C(a-v)O_2$. Since oxyhemoglobin is a red pigment, the patient's skin is pink. Alkalosis causes vasodilatation, and therefore the patient's skin is warm. Again it is paradoxical that in the early stages of ARDS a patient may have a warm, pink skin, a PaO_2 that is within normal limits, an acid urine, and yet be in respiratory distress with alkalosis.

As the ventilation problems in ARDS are considered, the perfusion problems to the lungs must also be considered. There are dynamic interrelationships between alterations in alveolar ventilation and pulmonary perfusion.

Pulmonary Perfusion Defects

PULMONARY CAPILLARY VASOCONSTRICTION WITH INCREASED PULMONARY VASCULAR RESISTANCE

Several alterations are thought to occur in the microvasculature of the lungs at the onset of ARDS. Various intrinsic factors involved in the precipitation of ARDS (see Table 17-3) may act on the pulmonary capillary bed, causing vasoconstriction. Heightened vascular resistance in the pulmonary capillary results in edema and hemorrhage, and may lead to atelectasis—the complex noted in ARDS [66]. This increase in pulmonary vascular resistance (PVR) is manifested by a sudden rise in pulmonary artery pressure.

Moss and Stein [66] demonstrated in one group of dogs that cerebral hypoxia of two hours' duration will produce pulmonary impairment bilaterally and an increase in PVR. In a second group of dogs, Moss and Stein denervated the left lungs while leaving the nerve supply to the right lungs unaltered. After inducing cerebral hypoxia in the second group of dogs, they found the denervated left lungs unimpaired and the right innervated lungs impaired. Those findings were offered as evidence that ARDS may have a centroneurogenic origin. Moss and Stein postulated the following sequence of pathophysiological alterations: " 'Shock' causes cerebral (probably hypothalamic) cellular oxygen deprivation and dysfunction; there is autonomically mediated increased resistance of the pulmonary venules ('postcapillary sphincters'); this leads to capillary hypertension, congestion, hemorrhage, edema, surfactant inactivation, and atelectasis." Theodore and Robin [106] reviewed a number of studies that propose a neurogenic mechanism for pulmonary edema. They suggest that a relationship exists between pulmonary edema secondary to head injury and pulmonary edema secondary to heroin overdose, high altitude, and cerebral hypoxia. They also suggest that after a central nervous system insult, there is a massive sympathetic discharge that produces an intense but transient vasoconstriction in the systemic circulation.

Kim and Shoemaker [48] demonstrated that during hemorrhagic shock in dogs (a) the duration of the elevated pulmonary vascular resistance and (b) the degree of acidosis in the early stages of shock were good predictors of total postshock pulmonary complications. In their study, Kim and Shoemaker concluded that severe metabolic acidosis during the hemorrhagic shock episode was the major factor causing a prolonged increase in PVR.

If a prolonged increase in PVR occurs in a patient with preexisting cardiac compromise, failure of the right heart may occur. If a right ventricular failure occurs, the central venous pressure (CVP) rises. Obviously, between pulmonary artery pressure (PAP) and CVP, the earlier, more sensitive indicator of changes in vascular resistance is the PAP. To monitor PVR, a Swan-Ganz catheter must be placed in the pulmonary artery.

OBSTRUCTION OF THE PULMONARY MICROCIRCULATION

Macroemboli and microemboli can be transported from the systemic circulation to the pulmonary circulation, causing obstruction in the pulmonary capillary beds. Blaisdell [5] has indicated that debris from injured tissues, platelet aggregations, and fibrin clots may cause microembolism in the lungs. Trauma may also upset normal coagulation states and in turn contribute to embolism. Trauma may impair the fat transport systems and cause premature conversion of fatty acids to neutral fats with resultant pulmonary vascular embolism.

Emboli in the pulmonary microcirculation could have several sequelae:

1. Platelet aggregates might release a platelet permeability factor.
2. Fibrin clots might undergo lysis, releasing fibrin split degradation products.
3. Septic emboli might seed bacteria, causing hematogenous pneumonia.
4. Fat emboli [14] might break down, producing a lipid irritation of the pulmonary parenchyma leading to an exudative pneumonia.
5. Any emboli might cause a redistribution of blood flow to unobstructed vessels [121]. Consequently, some pulmonary capillary beds would be underperfused, some would be normally perfused, and some would be overly perfused. When underperfused alveoli have normal ventilation, the ventilation-perfusion imbalance called physiological dead space (wasted ventilation) occurs.

PULMONARY CAPILLARY COMPRESSION

Pulmonary capillary compression can occur secondary to the pressure exerted by interstitial fluid edema, positive pressure ventilatory assistance, or the application of PEEP. Evaluation of cardiac output and of left ventricular end-diastolic filling pressure (pulmonary artery wedge pressure) should be made in the ARDS patient during the syndrome's severe phases (III and IV).

PULMONARY REGIONAL BLOOD FLOW

Normally, pulmonary blood flow is greater to the lower lobes of the lung, as is ventilation. Posture has a significant effect on pulmonary regional blood flow

[16]. With elevation of the head of the patient's bed, blood flow to the lower dependent zone increases. During hypotension, the pulmonary vascular resistance increases 16 times above normal in the upper segments of the lungs but only 2 times above normal in the lower segments [91]. With elevation of the head of the patient's bed, blood flow to the lower segments will be increased in the areas of the lung where pulmonary vascular resistance elevation is minimized. That may delay the formation of pulmonary edema. By maximizing ventilation (FRC) to the lower dependent segments of the lung and by maximizing blood flow to the lower segments where PVR is minimally increased, a better balance between ventilation and perfusion is struck.

COMPENSATORY CHANGES IN THE BLOOD FLOW TO THE ALVEOLI

With the early appearance of atelectatic nonventilated alveoli, there occurs a compensatory redistribution of pulmonary arterial blood flow. Blood is directed away from the collapsed alveoli and to the ventilated alveoli. As alveolar collapse progresses, it offsets the homeostatic mechanism that balances ventilation and blood flow. Consequently, in phases III and IV of ARDS, blood perfuses nonventilated alveoli. The perfusion is "wasted" since no gas exchange can occur (a condition called shunting).

Ventilation-Perfusion Imbalances

SHUNTING; PHYSIOLOGICAL DEAD SPACE

The term ventilation-perfusion imbalance may refer to shunting or to an increase in physiological dead space. In shunting, wasted perfusion occurs through nonventilated alveoli. Physiological dead space is present when the alveoli receive an adequate expansion with air but an inadequate blood flow. Each of those derangements exists in ARDS, but the defect causing the most severe problem is shunting (blood flow without ventilation).

Normally, the amount of ventilation delivered to the lungs during a one-minute interval is matched by approximately the same amount of blood perfusing the lung in one minute. Since the heart and lung are in series (see Fig. 17-6), the quantity of blood flowing through the heart (CO) in one minute represents the quantity of blood flowing through the pulmonary capillary bed in the same minute (Q), with the exception of a small percentage (3–5%) that is anatomically shunted through bronchial veins and thebesian vessels. By comparing alveolar ventilatory minute volume in liters per minute (Lpm) to CO in Lpm, a ventilation-perfusion ratio can be calculated.

Example of a $\dot{V}/\dot{Q}$ ratio in a 70-kg man:

1. CO or $\dot{Q}$ = stroke volume × heart rate
    = 70 ml × 72
    = 5.04 Lpm
2. $\dot{V}_A$ = (tidal volume − dead space) × respiratory rate
    = (500 cc − 150 cc) × 16
    = 5.6 Lpm
3. $\dot{V}/\dot{Q}$ ratio = $\dfrac{5.6\ \text{Lpm}}{5.04\ \text{Lpm}}$
    = 1.1

NORMAL VENTILATION-PERFUSION RATIO

An ideal ventilation-perfusion ratio is illustrated in Figure 17-9, in which alveoli A and B are each shown to be receiving normal ventilatory volumes and normal blood flow while normal gas exchange is occurring. The results are a normal PaO_2 and a normal percentage of oxyhemoglobin saturation, provided that there is no impairment to diffusion across the alveolar capillary membrane.

Shunting
In ARDS, large numbers of widely distributed alveoli are underventilated secondary to atelectasis or intraalveolar edema. The total alveolar ventilation is decreased and at the same time cardiac output is increased in a compensatory effort to supply oxygen to the cells. Consequently, a ventilation-perfusion imbalance occurs, with "wasted perfusion," as illustrated in Figure 17-10 (shunting). The gas exchange of the blood that perfuses alveolus B is inadequate; therefore, its PO_2 remains low and its reduced hemoglobin remains high. Low PO_2 and high reduced hemoglobin are characteristics of venous blood. When the venous blood of alveolus B and the arterial blood of alveolus A mix, the process is called venous admixture.

The consequences of abnormal pulmonary shunting may be summarized as an increase in venous admixture leading to a decrease in systemic arterial oxygen content and a decrease in oxygen transport, resulting in tissue hypoxia. The severity of the pa-

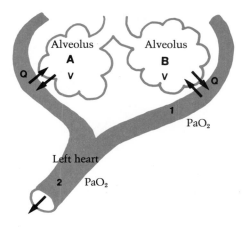

Figure 17-9
The normal ventilation-perfusion relationship.

V   = Normal ventilation in alveolus A and alveolus B
Q   = Normal blood perfusion
$PaO_2(1)$ = Normal oxygen tension in the pulmonary veins
$PaO_2(2)$ = Normal oxygen tension in the systemic arterial blood

The single arrow shows direction of blood flow. The double arrows indicate normal gas exchange at the alveolar capillary membrane units.

tient's condition depends on the degree of the shunting and the consequent degree of hypoxemia.

Lucas [52] indicates that there is a strong correlation between the degree of shunting and the patient's morbidity. Lucas called physiological shunting greater than 40 percent excessive shunting. He called shunts greater than 50 percent of the cardiac output lethal shunts. He found that some patients whose acid-base studies were normal and who had shunts greater than 40 percent died. Therefore, the degree of shunt is a better prognosticator of the patient's condition than are serial blood gas analyses alone. The degree of shunt also is used to evaluate the need for mechanical ventilation. Shunting is considered to be the major factor producing hypoxemia in ARDS.

At present, tests performed to measure the amount of pulmonary shunting do not separate out the normal anatomical pulmonary shunt of 3 to 5 percent from pathophysiological pulmonary shunts. Any shunt greater than 25 percent that occurs despite respiratory therapy strongly suggests acute ARDS and has a dire prognosis.

Several techniques to measure shunting have been

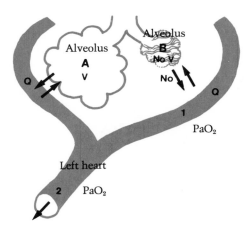

Figure 17-10

The abnormal ventilation-perfusion relationship of shunting.

Alveolus A = A normally ventilated alveolus
Alveolus B = A fluid-filled atelectatic alveolus
No V = No ventilation
No ↕ = No gas exchange
Q = Normal perfusion
PaO₂(1) = Decreased oxygen tension in the pulmonary veins
PaO₂(2) = Decreased oxygen tension in the systemic arterial blood

used. West [119] described a method for determining the degree of disturbance of ventilation-perfusion ratios in critically ill patients in the intensive care setting. West's method is based on the infusion of a mixture of inert gases into the venous circulation with subsequent analysis of gas concentrations in the air exhaled and in the arterial blood. His studies indicate that 100% oxygen breathing as a means of determining shunting may result in an overestimate of the shunt and could possibly be detrimental to the patient who has existing lung damage.

Horovitz and his associates [42] compared the technique of determining pulmonary shunts by the Berggren oxygen inhalation method and the xenon 133 inert gas method. In the ^{133}Xe method, the xenon gas was injected intravenously and then arterial samples were drawn and assayed for xenon content. Xenon should be almost totally cleared from the blood by the first transit of blood through the lung. Any appearance of xenon in the arterial blood indicates that as perfusion occurred, some blood was passed through nonventilated alveoli and xenon was

not removed by means of gas exchange in the lung. The higher the arterial blood content of ^{133}Xe, the greater the degree of shunt.

The 100% oxygen inhalation method of Berggren is the accepted standard means of determining shunt. "In both clinical and research use the Berggren method is universally adopted" [42] to determine shunts. Horovitz indicates that there are clinical problems with both the 100% oxygen method and the ^{133}Xe method.

DISADVANTAGES OF THE 100% OXYGEN METHOD

1. The administration of an inspired oxygen concentration of 99.6% is essential in the oxygen challenge test. This can be achieved by placing an endotracheal tube or a tracheostomy tube in the patient or by using a special mouthpiece in the cooperative patient.
2. Samples must be drawn from the pulmonary artery to obtain a true venous blood gas analysis. The procedure involves the placement of a pulmonary artery catheter.
3. The effects of breathing 100% oxygen may result in an increase in any existing shunt.
4. The administration of high concentrations of oxygen may abolish the hypoxic drive in patients with chronic obstructive pulmonary disease and result in respiratory arrest.
5. Nitrogen washout (denitrogenation) that occurs secondary to 100% oxygen administration may cause alveolar collapse.
6. Studies in experimental animals have shown that 100% oxygen administration for only 30 minutes causes anatomical changes in the lung.

DISADVANTAGES OF THE ^{133}Xe METHOD

Disadvantages of the xenon method are:

1. A slight fixed error is introduced by the fact that less than 100 percent of the injected ^{133}Xe is removed in one passage through the lung. (The error is less than 2–3%.)
2. ^{133}Xe and oxygen have solubility differences. Therefore, the two elements may measure somewhat different shunt fractions under some circumstances.
3. The ^{133}Xe method requires more elaborate measuring equipment.

SHUNT DETERMINATIONS

Horovitz recommends the ^{133}Xe method for clinical and research use because it is not complicated, there is good correlation between the xenon and oxygen methods for variable large shunts, and the xenon method avoids the use of high inspired oxygen concentrations.

The oxygen challenge test of Berggren for measuring pulmonary shunt flow is based on the fact that all causes of arterial hypoxemia, except shunting, are almost wholly reversible with the administration of 100% oxygen. Consequently, if a patient is permitted to breathe 100% oxygen for 10 to 15 minutes to the point of denitrogenation and the expected improvement in his arterial PaO_2 does not occur, the difference between the expected improvement and the actual measurement of PaO_2 indicates the degree of shunt. The shunt fraction (Qs/Qt) is determined as follows [42, 105]:

$$Qs/Qt = \frac{Cc'O_2 - CaO_2}{Cc'O_2 - C\bar{v}O_2}$$

where
Qs = quantity of blood shunted
Qt = total CO
CaO_2 = O_2 content of the systemic arterial blood
$C\bar{v}O_2$ = O_2 content of mixed venous blood from the pulmonary artery sampling
$Cc'O_2$ = O_2 content of the pulmonary capillary blood. It cannot be measured directly; an estimate is made from the (PaO_2)

The content of arterial oxygen (CaO_2) is calculated from equation 1 by using the PaO_2, the solubility constant for oxygen in plasma (0.003), the hemoglobin concentration (Hgb) in gm/100 ml, the oxygen-carrying capacity per gram of hemoglobin and the percentage of oxygen saturation of the hemoglobin.

$$CaO_2 = (PaO_2 \times 0.003) + (Hgb \times 1.39 \times \% Hgb \text{ saturation}) \quad (1)$$

The content of mixed venous blood is calculated from equation 2, where the mixed venous oxygen pressure ($P\bar{v}O_2$) is used in the computation.

$$C\bar{v}O_2 = (P\bar{v}O_2 \times 0.003) + (Hgb \times 1.39 \times \% Hgb \text{ saturation}) \quad (2)$$

Since the pulmonary capillary oxygen pressure ($Pc'O_2$) cannot be sampled and used to calculate the content of oxygen in the capillary blood ($Cc'O_2$), an assumption is made. It is assumed that the alveolar oxygen pressure (PAO_2) is the same as the pulmonary capillary oxygen pressure, and equation 3 is used to calculate the content of oxygen in the pulmonary capillary.

$$Cc'O_2 = (PAO_2 \times 0.003) + (Hgb \times 1.39 \times \% Hgb \text{ saturation}) \quad (3)$$

A direct measurement of PAO_2 is difficult to obtain, and therefore the PAO_2 is calculated from equation 4.

$$PAO_2 = Pb - PACO_2 - PAH_2O - PAN_2 \quad (4)$$

where
Pb = barometric pressure
PAH_2O = the pressure of water vapor in the alveoli at body temperature (normal = 47 mm Hg)
PAN = the alveolar nitrogen tension

In equation 4, the term for PAN_2 may be dropped, because with 100% oxygen breathing for 10 to 15 minutes all nitrogen is washed out of the lungs. The $PACO_2$ is not measured directly but is assumed to be the same as the $PaCO_2$; therefore, $PaCO_2$ may be substituted in the equation and a simplified equation (5) may be used to calculate PAO_2.

$$PAO_2 = Pb - PaCO_2 - 47 \text{ mm Hg} \quad (5)$$

ESTIMATED SHUNT

For simplicity and expedience, a reasonably good estimate of the degree of shunt may be made by comparing the difference between the PAO_2 and the PaO_2 when an oxygen challenge has been administered. The result is referred to as the alveolar-arterial oxygen difference $P(A-a)O_2$. In the normal patient, there is a 5 to 6 percent shunt for each 100 mm Hg oxygen pressure difference between PAO_2 and PaO_2. For example, a normal person breathing 100% oxygen for 15 minutes has a measured PaO_2 of approximately 550 or more mm Hg, a measured $PaCO_2$ of 40 mm Hg, and a calculated PAO_2 of approximately 653 mm Hg:

$$PAO_2 = Pb - PaCO_2 - PAH_2O$$
$$= 740 - 40 - 47$$
$$= 653 \text{ mm Hg}$$

$$P(A-a)O_2 = PAO_2 - PaO_2$$
$$= 653 - 550$$
$$= 103 \text{ mm Hg}$$

Since there is a 5 to 6 percent shunt for each 100 mm Hg difference in pressure, it can be surmised that the person in question (who is normal) has a shunt of about 5 to 6 percent.

The following is an estimate of a shunt in a patient with ARDS who has been given a 15-minute oxygen challenge test:

$PaO_2 = 320$ mm Hg after O_2 challenge

$Pb = 740$ mm Hg

$PACO_2$ is assumed to equal $PaCO_2 = 45$ mm Hg

$PAH_2O = 47$ mm Hg

$$PAO_2 = Pb - PACO_2 - PAH_2O$$
$$= 740 - 45 - 47$$
$$= 648 \text{ mm Hg}$$

$$P(A\text{-}a)O_2 = PAO_2 - PaO_2$$
$$= 648 - 320$$
$$= 328 \text{ mm Hg}$$

Estimated shunt = 5% per 100 mm Hg oxygen difference × 328 mm Hg
= 16.4%

FUNCTIONAL RESIDUAL CAPACITY

In patients with ARDS, an increase in venous admixture (shunting) is closely related to a decrease in functional residual capacity (FRC). A linear relationship exists so that as the FRC decreases, the percentage of venous admixture increases. Medical management is directed toward improving FRC through the use of positive end-expiratory pressure (PEEP). When shunt volumes approach 30 to 40 percent of the cardiac output, survival is unlikely. Patients who can maintain a reasonably high cardiac output have somewhat better survival rates. Therapeutic efforts must be made to increase FRC, maintain adequate cardiac output, decrease the degree of shunting, improve arterial oxygen content, and allow time for sealing of the capillary membrane permeability defect.

Immunological Defects

Following a severe stress (shock), the ability of the reticuloendothelial system to clear bacteria and particulate matter from the circulation is impaired. Thal

[105] indicates that the severity of the reticuloendothelial dysfunction appears to be directly related to the duration and degree of shock; one factor common to all forms of posttraumatic pulmonary insufficiency is sepsis. Careful studies of patients with ARDS will reveal obvious sepsis and in over half it will be extrapulmonary in nature [1]. Sepsis poses a challenge to the medical team involved in patient care. It is very important that measures be taken to prevent sepsis in the high-risk group. The medical team must guard against extrapulmonary and pulmonary infections. "Subclinical infections in patients rendered immunologically incompetent by trauma, surgery, or shock may have devastating effects on pulmonary function" [1]. Not only is the systemic immune response incompetent but the pulmonary immune response is deficient.

The lung plays an essential role in the body's defenses against a hostile environment [80]. The respiratory system is exposed to injurious substances from the internal environment (endogenous insults) and from the external environment (exogenous insults). The normal lung is remarkable in its ability to maintain function despite continued bombardment from the environment.

NONSPECIFIC DEFENSE MECHANISMS

The lung's immune response is dual, being nonspecific and specific. Nonspecific defenses of the lung include: (1) the cilia, which remove inhaled substances, including bacteria, (2) the nasal secretions, which contain lysosomes that kill bacteria nonspecifically, and (3) the alveolar macrophages, which act as scavengers and engulf inhaled particles. Patients with ARDS have decreased ciliary motility. Patients requiring an endotracheal or tracheostomy tube have air flow that by-passes nasal filtering and the bactericidal activity of nasal secretions. Further evaluation needs to be made of the ability of polymorphonuclear phagocytes, mononuclear phagocytes, and alveolar macrophages to ingest and digest particulate matter and bacteria. Research studies should try to determine whether leukocytes from at-risk patients have normal phagocytic activity and whether they have normal bactericidal activity after ingestion.

SPECIFIC DEFENSE MECHANISMS

Specific immunity of the body involves both cellular and humoral factors. The mechanisms of immunity used by the body vary, depending on the nature of the invasive microorganism [19, 80]. Specific immunity to most bacterial infections depends largely on antibody formation. Antibodies are protein molecules, now known collectively as immunoglobulins. Five major immunoglobulins have been found in man: IgG, IgA, IgM, IgE, and IgD. The IgA antibodies are found in immune reactions that occur in the serum (serum IgA) and in reactions that occur at secondary surfaces (secretory IgA). The secretory IgA antibody is found in secretions bathing the mucous membranes of the respiratory and gastrointestinal tracts. The role of secretory IgA in immunity is being investigated intensively. Secretory IgA has been shown to prevent colonization of the mucous membrane by viruses. Serum IgA prevents the hematogenous dissemination of viruses. Richardson [80] postulates that local immunization of the respiratory tract with intranasal instillation of vaccine is theoretically possible but not yet a reality. Investigation of the immune response of patients with ARDS should incorporate the principles of both systemic and pulmonary immunology, as well as of specific and nonspecific responses.

At present, little is known about the immune response of patients who have sustained major injury, surgery, or shock. It is, however, a well-established fact that the mortality of patients in acute respiratory failure rises sharply when gram-negative pneumonia supervenes [95, 101] or systemic sepsis occurs. Prophylactic measures to prevent infection in the at-risk patient are obligatory.

Nursing Management

Patient Problem List

To establish a patient problem list, the nurse must (1) review the patient's history, (2) perform an examination of the patient, and (3) interpret the laboratory data (Table 17-9). On the basis of the patient's history, the nurse should determine what the patient's problems have been and are, and anticipate what they might be in the future. Before the patient's transfer to a unit, the medical team should prepare equipment and personnel to meet the patient's immediate needs. The team must manage existing problems, try to prevent potential problems, recognize developing problems, and intercede with the correct medical and nursing actions. The team's responsibilities necessitate an immediate assessment of the patient on his arrival in the unit and continuous reevaluation of the patient. Medical management is adjusted continu-

ously on the basis of the patient's evolving needs. An illustration of the complexity of a patient problem list follows. This problem list is based on the information provided in the case study.

A PROBLEM LIST FOR THE PATIENT DESCRIBED IN THE CASE STUDY

Existing Problems
1. Respiratory compromise

2. Cardiovascular instability (hemorrhagic episode)
3. Multiple transfusions

4. Large fluid administration and electrolyte imbalance

5. Transient change in urinary output

Potential Problems
1. Respiratory depression secondary to anesthesia
   Obstruction of respiratory tract
   Postanesthetia atelectasis
   Splinting secondary to abdominal surgery
   Pulmonary edema secondary to long-term bed rest
   ARDS in at-risk category
   Pneumonia (endogenous or exogenous)
   Complications of respiratory therapy
2. Recurrence of bleeding
   Shock
3. Bleeding diathesis
   Transfusion reactions
   Hepatitis
   Pulmonary microembolism
4. Fluid overload
   Pulmonary edema
   Congestive heart failure
   Alkalosis
   Serum potassium increase secondary to tissue injury
   Calcium loss secondary to blood and immobility
5. High output renal failure
   Myoglobinuria

Hemoglobinuria
Acute tubular necrosis
Oliguria/anuria

6. Abdominal trauma and surgery	6. Recurrence of bleeding Paralytic ileus Wound dehiscence or infection Peritonitis/sepsis Abdominal splinting
7. Multiple soft-tissue injury	7. Wound infection Release of septic emboli Tissue necrosis Release of tissue breakdown products
8. Fractured femur	8. Failure of correct alignment Delay of ambulation Release of fatty emboli Osteomyelitis
9. Imposed recumbency secondary to surgical traction	9. Pulmonary emboli Decubitus ulceration Loss of calcium secondary to immobility and no weight bearing Loss of muscle mass Psychological problems Atelectasis
10. Depressed immune response after the traumatic insult	10. Wound sepsis Peritonitis/osteomyelitis Systemic sepsis Septic shock leading to death
11. Hypermetabolic state (endocrine and metabolic response to injury)	11. Progressive energy expenditure Increased oxygen consumption Increased respiratory demands Exhaustion leading to total systems failure
12. Depressed gastrointestinal motility	12. Acute gastric distention with resultant hypotension

Aspiration of gastric contents
Paralytic ileus

13. Nutritional status	13. Negative nitrogen balance Weight loss following injury Anorexia
14. Wound healing	14. Delay in healing due to: Negative nitrogen balance Necrotic tissue Infection Depressed food intake
15. Pain/analgesics	15. Depression of respiration Development of dependency
16. Drug responses	16. Development of resistant strains of organisms to antibiotics Allergic reactions Development of sensitivity Harmful side effects (e.g., nephrotoxicity, hepatotoxicity, and ototoxicity)
17. Psychological impact of illness	17. Anxiety Fear Long-term recovery or deterioration or death Family anxiety and separation Financial burden Institutional dehumanization Altered body image Interference with self-actualization

Nursing Management Objectives for Patients with ARDS or at Risk for ARDS

Management of the patient necessitates early recognition of the patient at risk, establishment of a patient problem list, formation of nursing goals and

Table 17-10
Phenomena to Measure in Patients in the At-Risk Groups

Patients at Moderate Risk	Patients at High Risk
Routine vital signs: TPR, BP	All tests from at-risk group are positive
Ventilatory functioning	Ventilatory functioning
TV	VC
IF	FEV
Compliance	FRC
Chest x ray	V_D/V_T
Alveolar-capillary gas exchange	Alveolar-capillary gas exchange
Arterial blood gases	$HgbO_2$ saturation; PaO_2
F_IO_2	$P(A-a)O_2$
$P(A-a)O_2$ by "flow concept"	Pulmonary venoarterial shunt
$\dfrac{PaO_2}{F_IO_2} = 3$ (satisfactory)	Pulmonary vascular resistance
$\dfrac{PaO_2}{F_IO_2} = <3$ "suspect" a problem and do a 100% O_2 challenge test	
$P(A-a)O_2$ in 100% O_2 challenge test for "suspect" patient	
Perfusion and tissue oxygenation	Perfusion and tissue oxygenation
Pulse, skin temperature, BP	$P\bar{v}O_2$
Urine	$C(a-v)O_2$
CVP	P50
Sensorium	CO
	PADP
	PAWP
	O_2 delivery and utilization computation

Source: Snyder [98].
Key: BP = blood pressure; $C(a-v)O_2$ = arteriolar-venous oxygen content difference; CVP = central venous pressure; FEV = forced expiratory volume; F_IO_2 = fraction of inspired oxygen; FRC = functional residual capacity; IF = inspiratory force; $P(A-a)O_2$ = alveolar-arterial oxygen difference; PADP = pulmonary artery diastolic pressure; PAWP = pulmonary artery wedge pressure; P50 = oxygen tension at which 50% of the hemoglobin is saturated; $P\bar{v}O_2$ = mixed venous oxygen tension; TPR = temperature, pulse, respirations; TV = tidal volume; VC = vital capacity; V_D/V_T = dead space ventilation ratio.

finally a plan of action to meet the goals. Identification of patients who are at risk for ARDS is made on the basis of:

1. The patient's history.
2. Table 17-10.
3. The nurse's physical assessment.
4. The nurse's performance of or assistance in pulmonary function testing.
5. Data collection and comparison of values with those in Table 17-5.

The patient's problems serve as a basis for the establishment of nursing goals. Nursing goals for the patient in the case study would include:

1. Achievement of efficient ventilation.
2. Maintenance of cardiovascular stability.
3. Acquisition of normal renal function.
4. Prevention of wound complications.

5. Prevention of systemic sepsis.
6. Evaluation and control of pain and anxiety.
7. Maximizing of patient's (and patient's family's) coping mechanisms.
8. Maintenance of normal gastrointestinal functioning.
9. Early institution of optimal nutrition.
10. Facilitation of maximal wound healing.
11. Restoration of normal mobility.
12. Return of patient to optimal life-style.

Nursing actions that should be taken immediately in the at-risk group to prevent pulmonary complications include:

1. Institution of vigorous pulmonary hygiene; prevention, recognition, and control of infections and hematogenous seeding of infections; prevention of pulmonary microemboli; and guarding against additional clinical stresses.

2. Continuous surveillance as needed of the signs and symptoms that indicate the development of phase I of ARDS (see Table 17-5).
3. Continual recording on a progress flow sheet of changes in the patient's status is essential.

Upon recognition of signs and symptoms of early ARDS, instigation of appropriate nursing intervention would include:

1. Alerting of the physician to any improvement or deterioration in the patient's status.
2. Adjustment of nursing management to respond to changes in the patient's status.
3. Continuing vigorous pulmonary hygiene.
4. Assisting with serial blood gas analyses, serial chest x rays, and serial pulmonary function tests (Table 17-10).
5. Determination from laboratory data of the adequacy of the blood's oxygen transport capacity and immediate reporting of deficits in hemoglobin and hematocrit levels.
6. Appropriate use of oxygen therapy.
7. Institution of intermittent positive pressure breathing (IPPB) or oxygen therapy as ordered by the physician.
8. Administration of bronchodilators.
9. Control of gastric dilatation.
10. Maintenance of optimum hydration.
11. Lowering of oxygen consumption.
12. Applying PEEP.
13. Use of endotracheal suctioning when indicated.

Upon recognition of signs and symptoms of phase III of ARDS the appropriate nursing response would be:

1. Evaluation of the patient based on the criteria for ventilatory support.
2. Institution of proper endotracheal care.
3. Being alert to indications for elective tracheostomy.
4. Applying detailed tracheostomy care.
5. Correctly managing the patient on assisted ventilation with a positive-pressure volume-controlled ventilator.
6. Application of PEEP, following the physician's orders and monitoring the patient's cardiopulmonary response to PEEP.
7. With a Swan-Ganz catheter, continuous monitoring of the patient's pulmonary artery pressure (PAP), pulmonary artery wedge pressure

(PAWP), central venous pressure (CVP), and thermal dilution cardiac output.
8. Performance (or assistance with performance) of pulmonary function tests on the ventilated patient (TV, MV, effective compliance, and peak airway pressure).
9. Administration of medications to "control" the patient on the ventilator (as needed).
10. Reassurance of the patient who is being ventilated; support to his family.
11. Assistance in weaning the patient from ventilatory support and continuous evaluation of his response to weaning.

When the signs and symptoms of phase IV of ARDS are evident, a difficult decision must be made as to whether complex technical procedures will be initiated. This decision should be a collaborative decision. Nursing intervention would be to either assist the physician with "exceptional life-saving measures" (pulmonary lavage and extracorporal membrane oxygenators) or assist the family with coping with the patient's terminal illness and approaching death.

Nursing and Medical Management Procedures of the Patient with ARDS or at Risk for ARDS

IDENTIFICATION OF PATIENTS IN THE AT-RISK GROUP

Once it has been ascertained from the patient's clinical history that he falls into the category of at risk for ARDS, it becomes necessary to measure certain parameters to acquire detailed information regarding ventilation, oxygenation, and perfusion. These data make it possible to determine whether the patient has a slight or high probability of developing ARDS. The information serves as the data base for future comparisons. Table 17-10 indicates the parameters that should be measured in the patient at moderate risk and in the patient at high risk. By using the results from those measured parameters and comparing them to the stages of ARDS as depicted in Table 17-5, one can determine what phase of ARDS the patient is in. The therapeutic regimen varies, depending on the phase of the patient's disease.

IMMEDIATE INTERVENTION TO PREVENT PULMONARY COMPLICATIONS IN THE AT-RISK PATIENT

Early and Vigorous Pulmonary Hygiene
Vigorous pulmonary hygiene is aimed at preventing small airway closure and the retention of secretions

in the tracheobronchial tree. The absorptive microatelectasis that follows small airway closure can be minimized either by applying positive pressure inflation or by voluntary maximal inspiration [2]. Periodically, the patient should be encouraged to deep breathe, to change his position frequently, to assume an upright position, and, when possible, to ambulate. Optimal fluid balance should be achieved to prevent pulmonary edema, which causes sequential compression microatelectasis.

Macroatelectasis secondary to tracheobronchial secretion retention can be reduced by encouraging the patient to forcibly expire (cough) or by inducing coughing through stimulation of the trachea with a catheter. During coughing, an abdominal or thoracic incisional site must be supported. Chest percussion and vibration, postural drainage, humidification of inspired air, and administration of bronchodilators enhance the expectoration of secretions. It may become necessary to use endotracheal suctioning or bronchoscopic aspiration to remove tenacious mucus.

Vigorous pulmonary hygiene can definitely prevent minor pulmonary problems and reduce the severity of major pulmonary problems. It may prevent the progression of pulmonary dysfunction to florid ARDS. Objective evidence is needed to determine whether vigorous pulmonary hygiene decreases the incidence of ARDS.

The Prevention, Recognition, and Control of Infections and Hematogenous Pulmonary Problems
A host-oriented approach is necessary to prevent and control infections [17, 84]. Each patient must be evaluated in regard to his capacity to ward off infection. In accumulating the patient's data base, his host resistance factors must be ascertained. The patient's history should include: (1) the status of immunizations, (2) the documentation of recurrent infections, (3) the presence of underlying disease entities (e.g., diabetes or malignancies), (4) any treatment with immunosuppressants, and (5) the presence of risk factors (e.g., obesity, malnutrition, or edema). Laboratory evaluation of the patient's resistance factors includes: (1) a white blood cell count with differential and morphology, (2) a nitroblue tetrazolium test to check leukocyte metabolism and bactericidal activity and a Schick/Dick test to determine immunoglobulin level and activity (not usually available), (3) a protein determination, (4) Gram stains and cultures of wounds and blood for aerobic and anaerobic bacteria and for fungi, (5) a *Candida* skin test and (6) tests of sensitivity of bacteria to specific antibiotics (see Table 17-9).

Emphasis must be placed on the fact that mortality is exceptionally high in patients with ARDS who develop sepsis. Hospital pathogens are essentially opportunistic [84]; that is, they take advantage of the patient with impaired resistance and the patient whose body has been invaded by surgical procedures, trauma, intravenous cannulas, urinary catheters, or ventilatory procedures. Nonpathogenic organisms may become pathogenic when the patient undergoes antibiotic therapy that is directed against competitive organisms. Bacterial patterns in hospitals change rapidly, and therefore it is necessary to have continuous surveillance of hospital microflora to control nosocomial infections.

To prevent infection, emphasis must be placed on (1) handwashing to decrease the transmission of infection by hospital personnel and (2) the correct management of special risk factors (e.g., intravenous and urinary catheters, wounds, and inhalation equipment) [53, 82, 84, 120].

Attention should be called to the fact that even though ARDS patients are at increased risk for superimposed bacterial infection, antimicrobials are generally not administered until evidence suggesting a bacterial pneumonia or sepsis is present. Pneumonia is suggested by an x ray that shows progressive pulmonary infiltration, fever, leukocytosis, and purulent tracheal secretions [34]. Sputum and blood samples are obtained for culture and sensitivity tests before antibiotic therapy is initiated. Sepsis is suggested by nonspecific neurological symptoms, nonspecific gastrointestinal symptoms, hyperventilation, thrombocytopenia, leukocytosis or leukopenia, glucosuria, tachycardia, hyperthermia or hypothermia, and severe refractory hypotension [53, 54].

In a few exceptional cases prophylactic antibiotics are administered before there is any evidence of infection. Those cases are listed by Shires [89] as:

1. Gross soiling of tissues, especially soiling with intestinal contents
2. The presence of foreign objects that cannot be retrieved (e.g., clothing and rock)
3. Massive crush injuries or contusions
4. Gangrene of an extremity
5. Suitable media for clostridial multiplication (hematomas)
6. Obstructed hollow viscus

The Prevention of Pulmonary Microemboli
The number of pulmonary microemboli can be minimized by the debridement of necrotic tissues, by

the prevention of septic embolism, and by the use of micropore filters for intravenous and blood administration [22]. Careful attention should be paid to the mixing of drugs and intravenous solutions to avoid incompatibility and microprecipitation. There is some controversy about the extent of reduction of pulmonary damage by micropore filtering of blood in humans. The evidence available at present indicates that micropore filters should be used with multiple transfusions [55].

Efforts should be made not to disturb long-bone fractures and fractures of the pelvis because fatty emboli might be released from bone marrow [72]. The patient should be observed for the fat embolism syndrome, which is characterized by pulmonary, neurological, and systemic symptoms [55].

Guarding Against Additional Clinical Stresses

A patient who is in the at-risk group because of the severity of his illness, surgery, or trauma does not tolerate any additional clinical insults well. Such a patient must be carefully observed for hemorrhage, infection, and shock. Efforts should be made to prevent him from becoming fatigued. Since shivering, anxiety, and pain increase oxygen demands, patients should be kept warm, be reassured, and be given appropriate analgesics. Any increased work of breathing should be reported to the physician.

RECOGNITION OF THE SIGNS AND SYMPTOMS OF PHASE I AND PHASE II OF ARDS AND THE APPROPRIATE NURSING INTERVENTION

Since the only obvious sign of phase I of ARDS is unexplained tachypnea, it is necessary to perform serial assessments according to the criteria for ventilatory assistance listed in Table 17-11. If the physician determines that the patient is in phase I or phase II of ARDS, the therapeutic regimen should include:

1. Continuation of pulmonary hygiene procedures
2. Utilization of oxygen therapy
3. Maintenance of a hemoglobin concentration greater than 10 gm/100 ml (Wilson [123] suggests a 12.5% to 14% hemoglobin concentration)
4. Institution of IPPB
5. Administration of bronchodilators to decrease airway resistance
6. Insertion of a nasogastric tube to decrease abdominal distention
7. Regulation of fluid therapy to avoid volume deficits or excesses

8. Judicious administration of diuretics and/or albumin (a controversial therapy)
9. Attenuation of oxygen consumption by controlling pain, temperature, and anxiety and by preventing shivering
10. Insertion of an endotracheal tube for application of positive end-expiratory breathing and endotracheal suctioning
11. Administration of steroids [123] in a few situations (steroid therapy is controversial)
12. Administration of digitalis only in patients in whom congestive heart failure is clearly indicated

Optimal Pulmonary Inflation

Emphasis is placed on maneuvers to inflate the alveoli optimally and to maintain a normal FRC [2] and a normal total lung capacity. Bartlett and his associates [2] state that properly applied positive pressure inflation of the lungs by a flow-generating, pressure-controlled ventilator or by manual assistance with an anesthesia bag can maximally inflate the lungs. Bartlett and his associates state also that a study showing the effectiveness of properly applied positive pressure breathing has not been reported. McConnell and his associates [56] compare the effects of applying IPPB and encouraging voluntary inhalation. The most important conclusion of the McConnell study was that the greatest increase in alveolar and bronchial expansion is achieved by voluntary maximal inhalation maneuvers aided by incentive spirometry, which is less costly and more convenient [55] than using IPPB machines.

Oxygen Therapy

Oxygen therapy alleviates the symptoms of hypoxia (in phase II of ARDS) and is frequently needed for the support of vital functions, but oxygen has no known effect on repair of basic pathological defects. The following is a guideline for oxygen therapy in phases I and II of ARDS:

1. Oxygen therapy should be used, along with a therapeutic approach to the basic pathophysiology.
2. Efforts should be made to keep the FIO_2 less than 50% to avoid oxygen toxicity. Pontoppidan and his associates give a detailed discussion of the controversy regarding oxygen toxicity [75, 76, 77].
3. A PaO_2 greater than 60 mm Hg is generally adequate if hemoglobin levels are adequate. Hemoglobin is approximately 89% saturated at a PaO_2 of 60 mm Hg unless the curve has shifted [28].

Table 17-11
Criteria for Ventilatory Assistance

| | | Deterioration in Patients in the High-Risk Group[a] | | | |
	Normal	Intubation	Ventilatory Assistance	PEEP[b]	Wean
Mechanics of ventilation					
RR/min	12–16/min	>30/min	>35		<30
TV (ml/kg)	6–8 ml/kg	<5 ml/kg	<3.5		>5
VC (ml/kg)	50–60 ml/kg	<10 ml/kg	<10–15		>10–15
MIF cm H_2O	> − 25 cm H_2O	< − 20	< −25		> −20 cm H_2O or
MV resting Lpm	<10 Lpm				<10 Lpm
Oxygenation					
PaO_2 (mm Hg) 21%	80–90	Face mask <70 mm Hg on 40%	<50	Ventilator<65	>60
PaO_2 (mm Hg) 100%	550–630		<200		
P(A-a)O_2 21%	5–20	20–50	>50		
P(A-a)O_2 100%	20–60	>60	>350	>400	<350
Qs/Qt 5% CO	3–8%	>15%	>40%	<20%	<15%
FRC					>50% of that predicted
pHa	7.35–7.40	<7.25			
Ventilatory capability					
$PaCO_2$ (mm Hg)	30–40	>50	>55		<40 or equal to preoperative level
VD/VT ratio	0.3–0.4	>0.6	>0.6		<0.6
Chest x ray	Clear		Diffuse infiltrates		

Source: Blaisdell and Schlobohm [6], Stemmer, Oliver, Corey, et al. [100], and Wilson [123].
Key: CO = cardiac output; FRC = functional residual capacity; Lpm = liters per minute; MIF = maximum inspiratory force; MV = minute volume; P(A-a)O_2 = alveolar-arterial oxygen difference; PEEP = positive end-expiratory pressure; pHa = pH of the arterial blood; Qs/Qt = shunt fraction; RR/min = respirations per minute; TV = tidal volume; VC = vital capacity; VD/VT = dead space volume/tidal volume ratio.
[a] Any deterioration in patients in the high-risk group should be evaluated.
[b] Studies are needed for early PEEP.

When serial blood gases are being monitored for a patient receiving oxygen therapy, the percentage of oxygen that is being delivered and the duration of oxygen administration should be recorded on the laboratory slips and in the patient's laboratory report.

Fluid Management

The efficacy of some of the therapeutic measures just described is controversial; and some of the measures are not without hazards (e.g., oxygen, diuretics, albumin, steroids, digitalis, and PEEP). Fluid regulation and diuretic and albumin administration should be aimed at decreasing edema gradually without compromising intravascular volume and incurring the dangers of systemic dehydration [114]. Snyder [48] considers crystalloid therapy superior to colloid therapy in the high-risk group, but he still suggests that an accurate definition of what constitutes optimal fluid administration is needed.

Care should be taken when using diuretics that rapidly deplete effective circulating volume (e.g., furosemide). Such diuretics should be titrated in broken doses while the patient's response [123] is closely monitored. The fluid response is adequate when the cardiac output is adequate, the urinary output is greater than 30 ml per hour, central venous pressures and pulmonary artery wedge pressure are within normal range, there is evidence of good peripheral perfusion [22], and the patient is alert [33]. Daily monitoring of the patient's weight indicates any rapid fluid loss or retention. Careful attention must be given to serum electrolytes. Hypokalemia and hypochloremia may be aggravated by diuretic therapy.

Ethacrynic acid causes a prompt diuresis within 10 to 15 minutes after intravenous administration, but there are several problems associated with its use [96]. Ethacrynic acid causes severe ototoxicity in patients who have poor renal function. The drug may increase capillary permeability for albumin, or it may stimulate pinocytotic transfer of albumin so that albumin is lost more rapidly from the vascular bed. When plasma albumin is decreased, the plasma oncotic pressure may be diminished. That allows an increase in the rate of the movement of water into the interstitial space and accentuates the pulmonary interstitial edema. A diuresis of 1000 ml of urine following the administration of ethacrynic acid may represent only a 50 to 100 ml loss of lung water.

Following severe stress, several physiological alterations occur that affect the plasma level of albumin: (1) there is a catabolic loss of protein, including albumin, and (2) there is an increase of capillary permeability with extravasation of small molecular-size proteins, especially albumin. Colloid therapy should not be started until the "capillary leak" has sealed. After "capillary seal," salt-poor albumin may be given, based on the rationale that albumin represents about 50 percent of the total plasma protein and is responsible for about 65 percent of the plasma oncotic pressure. The duration of the capillary endothelial leak has not been accurately determined and therefore the use of albumin is indicated only infrequently in patients with ARDS. Pontoppidan and his associates state that no one has shown that albumin mobilizes water from the lungs [77]. Further studies are necessary to determine whether albumin significantly mobilizes lung water in selected patients.

Steroid Therapy
There are conflicting reports from both experimental studies in animals and control clinical studies regarding the beneficial effects of adrenal corticosteroids in the treatment of pulmonary edema [34]. Because of the conflicting reports, Pierce suggests that a double-blind randomized control study is needed to determine the correct role of corticosteroids.

Murray [68] suggests that steroids be reserved for those patients in whom chemical injury to the lung is evident (e.g., aspiration of gastric contents or fat embolism). Despite the lack of conclusive evidence, steroid therapy for the treatment of aspiration is used by some management teams [55].

Digitalis Therapy
ARDS is not an indication for digitalization. Digitalis and/or other cardiotonic drugs are reserved for use in patients who have a history of left heart failure [123] or patients who have acute myocardial dysfunction. It is wise not to use digitalis in the early management of the ARDS patient unless there is evidence of left ventricular failure [34].

RECOGNITION OF THE SIGNS AND
SYMPTOMS OF PHASE III OF ARDS;
APPROPRIATE NURSING INTERVENTION

As a patient moves into phase III of ARDS, it becomes mandatory to place him on ventilatory assistance. That should be done early in phase III. A delay in placing the patient on the respirator makes correction of the respiratory failure extremely difficult.

Criteria for Intubation and Ventilatory Support
By using Table 17-11, which lists the criteria for ventilatory assistance, and by continuing to evaluate the patient's clinical status, the physician can determine when continuous mechanical ventilation should be used. When any deterioration occurs in patients in the high-risk group, they should be assessed to determine their need for continuous positive pressure ventilatory support (CPPV). Not a single test, but rather trends in the clinical and laboratory data determine the need. When increasing fractions of inspired oxygen (FIO_2) are required to maintain an adequate PaO_2, when shunt fractions exceed 40% of the cardiac output, when the difference between the PAO_2 and PaO_2 during the 100% oxygen challenge test exceeds 350 mm Hg, when the $PaCO_2$ continues to rise and the PaO_2 continues to fall, ventilatory assistance is obligatory.

Artificial Airways
A patient requiring ventilatory support for prolonged intervals must have an artificial airway [34]. For the initial artificial airway, a cuffed endotracheal tube that is constantly monitored is the device of choice [33]. The criteria for intubation are present somewhat earlier than the criteria for assisted ventilation (Table 17-11). With an artificial airway in place, it is possible to administer warmed humidified oxygen through a T tube while the patient spontaneously breathes, to irrigate the trachea with normal saline solution and readily suction tracheobronchial secretions, to place the patient on PEEP, to nebulize the tracheal tree with bronchodilators, to intermittently hyperventilate the patient mechanically, and, when necessary, to place the patient on a positive pressure volume ventilator. Intubation is required when excessive tracheobronchial secretions are unresponsive to pulmonary hygiene and when the upper respiratory tract is compromised.

Endotracheal tubes may be inserted through the nose or through the mouth. Tubes with low-pressure inflatable cuffs should be used. High-pressure cuffs cause tracheal ischemia, leading to tracheal necrosis, tracheal fistula, and tracheal stenosis following extubation.

Nasal endotracheal tubes are better tolerated by the conscious unsedated patient than are oral endotracheal tubes. Patients tend to bite oral tubes, salivate excessively, and retch. Nasal endotracheal tubes permit the patient to close his mouth and to continue oral intake. They are more easily anchored in place and are less likely to slip in and out. The disadvantages of the nasotracheal tube are: (1) the tube size is limited by the diameter of the nostril and the presence of the turbinates, (2) the tube is longer and narrower, causing greater resistance to air flow, (3) the tube is difficult to keep patent and is more likely to kink due to acute angulation, and (4) the tube may obstruct drainage from the cranial sinuses [34, 75], cause nasal necrosis, or cause minor epistaxis. Some physicians think that the nasotracheal tube is more difficult to insert than is the oral endotracheal tube.

Tracheostomy tubes are sometimes required as the artificial airway when prolonged intubation is required, but they are generally not used as the initial or emergency airway. "While tracheostomy has a widespread use, it is rarely used in an *emergency situation*" [86]. Instead, early control of the airway is acquired with the endotracheal tube. When tracheostomy is performed, the endotracheal tube is left in place until the tracheostomy is completed and the tracheostomy cannula is inserted [99]. That technique allows the anesthesiologist to have continuous control of the airway. Endotracheal tubes are usually left in place four to five days. Sometimes they may be left in place longer. If it then becomes clear that a tracheostomy is needed, it is performed under optimal (elective) operative conditions [33]. Before, during, and after surgery, blood gas monitoring allows early detection of ventilatory insufficiency before severe hypoxia, hypercapnia, and acidosis result [100].

Grillo [33] and Selecky [86] have described concisely the indications and the operative techniques for tracheostomy and the postoperative management and the complications of tracheostomy.

The Complications of Tracheostomy

The intraoperative and postoperative complications of tracheostomy include acute hemorrhage from the operative site, pneumothorax, air embolism, aspiration, subcutaneous and mediastinal emphysema, left recurrent laryngeal nerve damage, obstruction of the tracheostomy tube, failure of the tracheostomy cuff, placement in the right mainstem bronchus, dislodgment of the tube, wound infection, swallowing dysfunction, tracheoesophageal fistula, erosion into the innominate artery with sudden exsanguination, and delayed tracheal stenosis [33, 125].

Efforts should be made during surgery to select the correct tube size and angulation, to control bleeding, to position the tube correctly between the second and third tracheal rings, and to secure the tube.

Suctioning should be performed immediately after placement of the cannula to remove blood and secretions, but suctioning should not be traumatic (and thus aggravate bleeding) nor excessive (and thus bring on hypoxia). Ample numbers of disposable catheters should be on hand postoperatively to facilitate removal of blood from the tracheostomy tube.

A rare but often fatal complication of tracheostomy is innominate artery erosion (it occurs in less than 1% of tracheostomies). The peak incidence of innominate artery erosion falls between the first and second weeks. Jones and his associates [46] suggest that patients having more than 10 ml of blood from the tracheostomy stoma or cannula 48 hours or more after tracheostomy must be assumed to have innominate artery erosion until it is proved otherwise. Patients who have abnormal neck positions, low-placed tracheostomy stomas (below the third tracheal cartilage), or very high-placed tubes (at or above the first tracheal ring), high-pressure tracheostomy tube cuffs, an asthenic body habitus, gram-negative tracheal cultures, minor bleeding after 48 hours, and/or pulsation of the tracheal cannula should be watched carefully [13, 46]. Sites of erosion are the cannula tip, the balloon, and the stoma. If delayed bleeding occurs, cuff inflation should be the first procedure used to control bleeding. According to Utley and his associates [113], if cuff inflation fails, blunt digital dissection with the index finger along the fascial plane anterior to the trachea but pressing on the trachea and inferiorly along the trachea to the carina traps the innominate artery between the finger and the posterior surface of the sternum. By pressing the finger firmly against the sternum, bleeding can be controlled. Intravenous infusions should be pushed to reverse hemorrhagic hypovolemia; the patient should be taken immediately to surgery while digital compression is maintained. On occasion this emergency measure must be performed by the nurse. If it is not done, massive exsanguination and death ensue.

Early dislodgment can often be avoided if the surgeon selects a tube of the proper size and shape and secures the flange with sutures as well as ties about the neck. The sutures may be left in place for four or five days until a tract is well formed. Before a tract is well formed, it is often difficult to replace a cannula following accidental (or with tube obstruction, intentional) dislodgment.

Several maneuvers that can be done by physicians during surgery facilitate replacement of the tube if it is dislodged. The skin margin can be sutured to the edge of the trachea, a window can be made in the trachea, or traction sutures can be placed in the edges of the trachea. Those maneuvers help to locate the tracheostomy stoma and tract. If the tracheostomy outer cannula or plastic tracheostomy tube is dislodged before a tract has been well formed (i.e., 4–5 days postoperatively), reinsertion should be attempted with adequate lighting and retraction [13]. Retraction may be accomplished using the traction sutures, a tracheal hook, and a Trousseau dilator. After the reinsertion, the patient must be evaluated in regard to ventilation. Unfortunately, tubes have sometimes been "reinserted" into the soft tissues of the neck and mediastinum.

Immediately after the placement or replacement of the tracheostomy tube and suctioning of the trachea, the position of the tube should be determined. Intubation of the right mainstem bronchus is one of the more serious complications of tracheal intubation [125]. Observation of the patient for bilateral symmetrical chest excursions and auscultation for bilateral breath sounds should be performed. A chest x ray is needed immediately after intubation or reintubation to check the position of the tube. Serial chest x rays reveal any malplacement, pneumothorax, atelectasis, or bleeding [33].

Nursing Care of the Tracheostomized Patient

Posttracheostomy care consists of constant monitoring by nurses who are attuned to the needs of the tracheostomized patient. Such a patient has lost his ability to communicate verbally, to cough effectively enough to clear the airway, and to swallow readily. The alert patient should be given a signal light, bell, or paper and pencil [13]. The patient's airway must be kept clear of secretions by appropriate cleaning and suctioning techniques, and maneuvers must be employed to avoid aspiration.

Management of the tracheostomized patient can be discussed under five categories: (1) airway care, (2) wound care, (3) cuff care, (4) care of swallowing dysfunction and prevention of aspiration, and (5) psychological care.

Airway Care. Two primary causes of obstruction of the artificial airway are plugging by blood clots or inspissated mucus and occlusion by a herniated tracheostomy tube cuff. Regardless of the cause, immediate action to move the obstruction is necessary. Frequent postoperative suctioning is needed until bleeding ceases. Adequate humidification using a T tube and humidifier when a patient breathes spontaneously or using a cascade when a mechanical ventilator is used decreases the incidence of inspissated mucous plugs. When metal double-cannula tubes are used, periodic cleaning of the inner tube and prompt replacement of it are required. During the first 72 postoperative hours [86], the outer cannula is not disturbed, but thereafter infrequent changes of the outer cannula are necessary (i.e., once a week). Cleansing only the inner tube does not prevent all crust obstruction since mucous plugs can form at the tip of the outer cannula. A plug in that position can act as a one-way valve, permitting a suction catheter to pass inward but not allowing air to flow outward. Prompt change of the entire tube is necessary [33]. Too early removal of a tracheostomy tube allows the stoma to collapse, impeding tube replacement. A change of the tube may be accomplished by inserting a suction catheter into the initial tracheostomy tube, carefully slipping out the tracheostomy tube without dislodging the catheter, then sliding the new tracheostomy tube into place over the "guiding" suction catheter. A bronchoscope should be kept at hand for the first four postoperative days in case the physician needs to reexplore the wound. Correct replacement of the tube is confirmed by x ray.

The most effective ways of preventing mucous obstructions are correct humidification, optimal suctioning, effective coughing, and adequate systemic hydration. Inspired gas is warmed to body temperature and saturated with water vapor. A thermometer should be placed in the inspiratory line near the patient to monitor the temperature of the inspired gas. The gas temperature at the point of entry should be near the normal body temperature (i.e., 37°C), but it must not exceed 39°C [34]. The heated humidifier used to deliver water vapor must be changed or decontaminated at least once each 24 hours. If it is not, it becomes a reservoir for gram-negative bacilli [34]. Ideally, sterile tubing should be replaced every 8 hours, sterile water changed every 8 hours, condensed water removed from tubing as often as necessary, and the humidifier sterilized every 24 hours [86].

Coughing is provoked by passing a suction catheter into the trachea or by instilling approximately 2 to 5 ml of bacterostatic sterile normal saline solution into the tracheostomy tube. If cultures of tracheal secretions are needed, the bacteriostatic saline solution should be replaced by plain sterile saline solution for tracheal irrigation several hours before sampling. For a forceful cough to occur, intrapulmonary pressure must build up against a closed glottis. An endotracheal or a tracheostomy tube prevents that build-up of pressure. The nurse may simulate the sudden opening of the glottis by having the patient inspire deeply, quickly placing a sterile gloved finger over the tube orifice as the patient strains to expire, then quickly removing the finger.

Equipment for suctioning should include a tracheal suction gauge, clear-plastic connection tubing, a plastic disposable collection container, disposable clear-plastic sterile suction catheters with thumbholes, sterile gloves, a bottle of sterile bacteriostatic saline solution, sterile syringes for the instillation of saline solution, a sterile basin with sterile distilled water, an anesthetic ventilation bag (or respirator), and an oxygen supply. The catheter size should be no greater than one-half the diameter of the tracheostomy tube, and a few catheters with bent tips should be available to facilitate suctioning of the left mainstem bronchus. The left mainstem bronchus diverges from the carina at a more acute angle and is narrower than the right bronchus. Consequently, it is difficult to insert a straight-tipped catheter into the left bronchus. It is commonly supposed that turning the patient's head to the right will enhance left bronchus suctioning, but studies that support that theory have not been performed.

Before beginning the suctioning, the nurse should explain the suctioning procedure to the patient, procure all the materials needed for suctioning, and make sure the equipment is functional. The areas to be suctioned are the trachea and bronchi below the tube, the tube itself, the trachea above the cuff, and the posterior pharynx and mouth. Suctioning of those areas may be approached in several ways, but it must be remembered that the oropharynx is naturally contaminated and the trachea must be kept free of contamination. Suctioning may be done as often as every 15 minutes, but it should be done no less than once every hour routinely. The duration of suctioning should be as brief as possible; it should not exceed 15 seconds for each catheter insertion. Prolonging the aspiration induces hypoxia that may lead to dysrhythmia and/or cardiac arrest. Hypoxic patients should receive a few deep inspirations with 100% oxygen before each catheter insertion. Patients with chronic obstructive pulmonary disease who maintain a low PaO_2 should not be ventilated with 100% oxygen, because such ventilation may remove their hypoxic drive and lead to respiratory arrest.

The procedure for suctioning involves:

1. Auscultating the chest for adventitious sounds before suctioning.
2. Washing the hands properly.
3. Drawing up 10 to 15 ml of normal saline solution or 5% $NaHCO_3$ solution.
4. Adjusting the suction control gauge to the tracheal suction range for adults (120–150 mm Hg).
5. Making sure there are no leaks in the suction apparatus by placing the suction connection tubing into a basin of tap water and flushing the tubing.
6. Opening the sterile catheter package, exposing the connector end.
7. Connecting the catheter to the suction tubing. (The catheter should not be removed from the package until it is time to use it.)
8. Adjusting the oxygen flow to the disposable ventilation bag. The bag should be changed every 24 hours.
9. Putting on sterile gloves.
10. Removing the connection to the T tube or to the ventilator or removing the disk from the swivel adapter so as to have access to the tracheostomy tube. The connector or disk should be placed on a sterile field.
11. Ventilating the hypoxic patient with 100% oxygen with several deep breaths. The respirator or the ventilation bag may be used to deep sigh the patient. (Caution: The FIO_2 should be changed from 100% to the prescribed FIO_2 following deep sighing. High concentrations of oxygen for prolonged periods damage the ultrastructure of the lung [11].)
12. Inserting the sterile catheter with the thumbhole open to the desired depth.
13. Applying suction (with the thumbhole closed) only on withdrawal. The suctioning should be intermittent, and it should be applied as the catheter is withdrawn with a twirling motion.

14. Limiting the suctioning and withdrawal time to 15 seconds.
15. Ventilating the patient between each catheter insertion.
16. Instilling 5 ml of normal saline solution or 5% sodium bicarbonate solution to liquefy thick secretions, ventilating quickly, and aspirating immediately. (Caution: The instillation should not be done through a needle, because the needle could fall into the tracheostomy tube.)
17. Observing the ECG monitor during suctioning for any dysrhythmias secondary to hypoxia. The patient should be hyperoxygenated if dysrhythmia occurs.
18. Suctioning the posterior pharynx.
19. Deflating the cuff and hyperventilating the patient while suctioning the pharynx. The air forces mucus up into the pharynx to the site of suctioning.
20. Hooking the tracheostomy tube to the T tube or the respirator tube again. (The entire system should be checked.)
21. Assessing the patient for bilateral chest excursions, rate of respiration, and heart rate and rhythm and auscultating the chest to see if the suctioning has decreased rales or rhonchi.
22. Disposing of the catheter and flushing the suction tubing with distilled water.
23. Turning off unneeded equipment.

Wound Care. The tracheostomy must be treated as a surgical wound; that is, strict attention must be paid to the sterility of the equipment, the humidifier, the tracheal dressings, and the suctioning technique [74, 86, 112]. Local wound care involves:

1. Keeping the area free from secretions and exudate.
2. Cleaning the area from the operative site outward with a 3% hydrogen peroxide solution as needed.
3. Applying as needed (or at least once a day) a sterile tracheostomy dressing (the edges must not be frayed).
4. Adequately fixing the tube with tape. The decision must be made whether to use a bow tie or a knot. Bow ties tend to come loose easily, possibly causing decannulation; however, if knots are used, the nurse must have bandage scissors at hand in order to snip the ties should an obstruction occur that necessitates the removal of the cannula.
5. Using a swivel adapter to connect the tube to ventilator hoses in order to minimize mechanical damage to the tracheal wall.

6. Applying topical water-based antimicrobials to minimize wound colonization.
7. Recognizing whether any clinical indicators are present as those of wound colonization or those of pulmonary infection. The diagnosis of infection is based on purulent tracheal secretions, the presence of or changes in pulmonary infiltrates, and evidence of sepsis, such as fever or leukocytosis. The management of pulmonary infection includes the administration of specific systemic antibiotics.

Cuff Care. The adult patient who has had a tracheostomy must have a functioning tracheostomy cuff to achieve optimal mechanical ventilation. A number of problems can be associated with tracheostomy cuffs:

1. Unbonded or noncemented cuffs on metal tubes can slip over the tip of the cannula, causing acute obstruction.
2. Cuffs can suddenly rupture or slowly leak, making adequate ventilation impossible.
3. A cuff can herniate over the tip, serving as a one-way valve and thus causing air trapping.
4. High-pressure cuffs or overinflated low-pressure cuffs can exert excessive pressure against the tracheal wall, impeding perfusion to the tracheal wall and resulting in ischemic necrosis.
5. Cuffs may fail to inflate if crusts have formed about them during deflation.
6. Cuff pressure transmitted across the tracheoesophageal wall may result in swallowing dysfunctions or tracheobronchial fistulae.
7. Cuff pressure and friction may cause erosion of the tracheal ring or cause cicatrization after the removal of the cannula, with subsequent circumferential stenosis [38].

The following factors may affect the degree of damage to the trachea resulting from pressure at the site of the cuff: (1) the intracuff pressure, (2) the number of days the cuff is in place, (3) the peak inspiratory pressure (which determines how firmly a cuff must be seated to prevent excess airway leakage), (4) the materials, size, and shape of the cuff, (5) the patient's degree of debilitation and healing potential, (6) the presence of tracheal sepsis, (7) the blood perfusion to the trachea (i.e., the level of systemic and local hypotension), (8) the use of ethylene oxide for gas sterilization of nondisposable cuffs or tubes [38], and (9) the prolonged use of nasogastric tubes. Ideally, a soft cuff bonded to an endotracheal or a tracheostomy tube should have a large sealing area, inflate evenly so that it molds to the tracheal contour, center the tube within the lumen, and have large volumes but low tracheal-wall sealing pressure, even with over-inflation (i.e., less transmural pressure than the tracheal arterial pressure) [8, 38]. Soft cuffs should be inflated gently to a sealing volume and then deflated to the point of a minimum leak. The sealing volume and minimal leak volume can be ascertained by auscultating with a stethoscope over the trachea or hearing or feeling an air leak out of the mouth during inflation of the lungs with a ventilator.

If cuff slippage or herniation causes airway obstruction, the cuff should be immediately deflated and the tracheostomy tube removed and replaced. "Cuff herniation should be suspected immediately if a patient receiving assisted ventilation begins acutely to lose tidal volume and fails to cycle the ventilator properly" [55].

Thomas [107] notes that in the last few years tracheoesophageal fistula (TEF) resulting from cuffed tracheal tubes has been widely recognized. TEF may appear early at about seven days of cuff use (on the average it appears on the thirtieth day). A nasogastric tube in the esophagus promotes impingement and erosion of the esophageal and treacheal wall by the tracheal cuff. Clinical signs that suggest TEF (but are not definitive for it) result from: (1) the abnormal flow of materials from the esophagus into the trachea or (2) the abnormal flow of air from the trachea into the esophagus by way of the TEF. Violent coughing following swallowing; food, gastric juice, or bile in or about the tracheostomy; and swallowed methylene blue or contrast media in the tracheal aspirant suggest a fistula. Those materials could have been aspirated through the vocal cords and therefore do not verify the presence of TEF. Similarly, the presence of air in the stomach does not verify TEF, although gastric distention seen on a routine chest x ray may be the first sign of TEF. Air movement through a TEF may cause bubbling in the hypopharynx or in the stomach synchronous with the ventilator's inspiratory phase. However, an inadequately sealed cuff allows bubbling in the throat and may lead to gastric distention. Although those clinical signs are suggestive of TEF, a definitive diagnosis must be based on one of the following: (1) direct visualization with a tracheoscope through the TEF and into the esophagus where the nasogastric tube is seen, (2) direct visualization with an esophagoscope through the TEF where the tracheostomy tube is seen, (3) a cineradiographic study that clearly shows the TEF, or (4) verification by operation or by autopsy.

The nurse should suspect a TEF when she observes the following signs:

1. Food, gastric juice, or bile in the tracheal aspirate
2. Copious secretions in the trachea
3. An increase in coughing, especially after swallowing
4. Gastric distention
5. Gurgling of air in the stomach or mouth during positive pressure inspiration
6. The appearance of methylene blue in the tracheal secretions after swallowing

Nursing action should include adequately suctioning the patient, placing the patient on a nothing-by-mouth regimen, contacting the physician, and obtaining the necessary equipment for placing a longer tracheal tube between the carina and the fistula. Since air will continue to reach the stomach because of aerophagia or the TEF, a properly functioning nasogastric or gastrotomy tube is essential. The nurse may prepare the patient for the definitive diagnostic procedures. Should a TEF be found by direct visualization, early operative repair is indicated as soon as the patient's overall condition permits [107].

Swallowing Dysfunction. Since many severely ill patients with ARDS are metabolically depleted (as evidenced by weight loss, anemia, hypoalbuminemia, and negative nitrogen loss), hyperalimentation by oral, gastrointestinal, or intravenous methods may be mandatory. The presence of an inflated tracheal cuff may interfere with oral feedings because of posterior pressure on the esophagus. Not all patients can tolerate cuff deflation, and oral ingestion when the cuff is inflated is difficult. By flexing their necks, some patients are able to swallow liquids and/or very soft foods when high-compliance cuffs are inflated. Before the patient is given fluids or foods by mouth, his swallowing ability should be evaluated by the methylene blue test, first with the cuff up and then with it down. After the removal of an endotracheal or tracheostomy tube, many patients have swallowing dysfunction, and aspiration should be carefully guarded against (e.g., by having the patient in an upright position for feeding and in a semisitting position after eating, by having the patient first take liquids and then small bites of soft food, and by observing the patient for gastric distention).

Psychological Care. The anxiety level of the conscious patient who has a tracheostomy is intensified because of his inability to communicate verbally. Such a patient needs to be reassured by the nurse's continual presence at his bedside and should be told of a system by which he can communicate with the nurse (by tongue clicking or by tapping). The patient's anxiety level, sensory overloads and deprivations, and problems of communication, as well as the dehumanization of the intensive care patient, are discussed in Chapters 34 and 36.

Ventilatory Equipment

Classification. According to Hill and Dolan [39], there is an almost bewildering number of different makes of automatic lung ventilators. Cox and Chapman [15] give a comprehensive account of modern ventilator design. A classification of ventilators may be made by grouping them into (1) pressure generators, (2) flow generators, and (3) combinations of both types. When pressure generators are used, pressure is applied to the airway for a specified length of time or until a preset pressure has been attained. The pressure-limited, patient-sensitive machines are useful in simple ventilatory failure when the lung is dry, without alveolar or interstitial edema [59], and trauma, pain, and splinting of the chest are not present.

The flow-generator ventilator is designed to drive a steady flow of gas into the lungs for a definite time or until a preset volume has been delivered. For safety, there is a preset limiting pressure that causes an automatic release of excessive pressure if exceeded. In patients with ARDS, the lungs become progressively stiffer, requiring higher and higher force to deliver the gas. The preset pressure of a pressure generator might be reached before an adequate amount of gas has been delivered to the patient's airway. As compliance decreases and lung stiffness increases, the pressure limit is exceeded at lower and lower tidal volumes. Consequently, volume-generated machines are primarily useful in ARDS [4, 10]. The preset volume is delivered at whatever pressure is required up to the safety pressure setting. One serious hazard of the volume-cycled ventilator is pneumothorax resulting from the high pressures required to deliver the preset volume. In ARDS, larger-than-normal tidal volumes are preferable since they increase alveolar ventilation and decrease shunt (10–15 cc/kg).

Hill and Dolan [39] state that once means have been provided to drive gas into the lungs, a need arises to cycle the ventilator; that is, to change over from the inspiratory to the expiratory phase. There are four kinds of cycling: pressure cycling, volume cycling, time cycling, and patient-assist cycling. Ventilators may provide an optional triggering mechanism that responds to a patient's attempts at spontaneous respiration. The mechanism (1) senses the negative inspiratory effort (e.g., −5 cm H_2O) initiated by the patient and (2) then delivers the gas to the preset pressure, volume, and/or time limits. When a patient is spontaneously triggering the ventilator, the "machine-rate-of-breathing" should be set slightly lower than the "patient-rate-of-breathing" so that if the patient tires or his respirations become depressed, the machine assumes control of breathing. In the patient-assist mode, the patient determines the rate of respiration, but the machine-setting determines the tidal volume to be delivered.

Newer mechanical ventilators are able to deliver deep intermittent sigh volumes (e.g., volumes 1.5 times the tidal volume every six minutes for 1 to 3 breaths) and PEEP. If a machine does not mechanically sigh a patient, the nurse must use an anesthetic bag and deep breathe the patient for two or three breaths every 30 minutes.

The purpose of PEEP is to expand collapsed small airways and atelectatic alveoli, thus improving alveolar ventilation without interfering with intrathoracic pressure relations or impeding pulmonary blood flow. If a drop in arterial systolic pressure of more than 10 mm Hg occurs, with the initiation of PEEP, the PEEP level should be decreased and the patient should be evaluated for hypovolemia and the need for additional intravenous fluid administration. An increase of capillary wedge pressure following an increase in PEEP of 5 cm H_2O suggests that the PEEP pressure has impeded blood flow to the left ventricle.

In hypervolemia, the following points should be remembered:

1. Prolonged continuous positive pressure ventilatory support and/or PEEP have been shown (by Sladen and his associates [97]) to increase the secretion of antidiuretic hormone (ADH) about threefold, thus aggravating any fluid overload.
2. Daily recording of weights is necessary for mechanically ventilated patients to assess the syndrome of positive water balance.

PEEP is generally administered at pressures not exceeding 7 to 10 cm H_2O. PEEP up to 20 cm H_2O may occasionally be required in some ARDS patients with very low compliance and severe respiratory insufficiency. PEEP pressures that exceed pulmonary artery wedge pressure impede pulmonary capillary blood flow. The use of PEEP, especially high levels of PEEP in lungs with low compliance, may cause an increase in the incidence of subcutaneous and mediastinal emphysema and tension pneumothorax. PEEP should therefore be maintained at the lowest level possible for optimal pulmonary function on a nontoxic concentration of oxygen. According to Powers [78, 79], PEEP is most effective (and least dangerous) when airway obstruction is minimal. The patient's airway should be cleared frequently by maximal pulmonary hygiene and endotracheal suction before and during PEEP administration. An optimal level of PEEP is characterized by:

1. A decrease in the percentage of shunt.
2. An increase in the FRC.
3. No significant increase in pulmonary capillary wedge pressure, as monitored by a Swan-Ganz catheter.
4. Maintenance of blood pressure.
5. An increase in the PaO_2.
6. An increase in lung compliance.
7. An improvement in serial cardiac outputs.

Attention should be focused on the response of cardiac output to PEEP. A decrease in cardiac output following the initiation of PEEP or an increase in the amount of pulmonary artery wedge pressure (PAWP) may be the result of deterioration in pulmonary capillary perfusion secondary to excessive PEEP. Conversely, a decrease in cardiac output may indicate an improved state of arterial oxygenation, abolition of cellular hypoxia, and a decreased demand on the heart.

Complications of Ventilatory Assistance. The prognosis of patients with ARDS has improved with the increased use of assisted ventilation; however, as the use of assisted ventilation has increased so has the incidence of its complications. Zwillich and his associates [125] have grouped (Table 17-12) and studied prospectively 18 complications of mechanical ventilation. Their study indicates that three of the complications—intubation of the right mainstem bronchus, tracheal tube malfunction, and alveolar hypoventilation—are associated with decreased survival.

Before the nurse can care competently for a patient

Table 17-12
Complications Observed Prospectively in Assisted Ventilation

Complications attributable to intubation or extubation
Prolonged intubation attempt
Intubation of the right mainstem bronchus
Premature extubation by physician
Extubation by patient
Complications associated with endotracheal and tracheostomy tubes
Cuffed tube malfunction (e.g., herniation of cuff, cuff leak, or tube obstruction)
Nasal necrosis and tracheal erosion
Complications attributable to operation of the ventilator
Machine failure
Alarm failure
Alarm "turned off"
Inadequate nebulization or humidification
Overheating of inspired air leading to mild hyperthermia
Fluid overloading compounded by humidified inspired air
Medical complications occurring during assisted ventilation
Alveolar hypoventilation leading to hypoxia, hypercarbia, and respiratory acidosis
Alveolar hyperventilation leading to hypocapnia and respiratory alkalosis
Massive gastric distention
Pneumothorax
Macroatelectasis secondary to obstruction of the left mainstem bronchus
Microatelectasis following hypoventilation
Nosocomial pulmonary infections
Depressed cardiac output and hypotension
Positive water balance

Source: Modified from Zwillich, Pierson, Creagh, et al. [125].

on a ventilator, she must (1) be aware of the potential complications; (2) be able to assess thoroughly the patient's ventilatory status, oxygen transport capacity, and peripheral oxygenation; (3) be skilled at managing the endotracheal or tracheostomy tube; and (4) be able to operate efficiently and troubleshoot the ventilator. The nurse must give priority to assessing the patient for problems (e.g., obstructed airway, extubation, pneumothorax, intubation of the right mainstem bronchus, aspiration, respiratory muscle discoordination, and TEF) before assessing the ventilatory equipment. She must take immediate action to correct the patient's problem and restore adequate alveolar ventilation by "bagging" the patient if necessary.

Constant observation of the patient's mental status, degree of dyspnea, work of breathing, bilateral chest excursions, depth and rate of respirations, air trapping, chest retractions, position of the tracheostomy tube, resonance of the chest, breath sounds, adventitious sounds, pressure parameters (arterial blood pressure, central venous pressure, pulmonary artery pressure, and pulmonary artery wedge pressure), heart rate and rhythm, gastric distention, serial blood gases, and shunt fractions is mandatory.

The nurse must observe the patient's thoracic excursions and determine whether the patient's breathing efforts are "in phase" with the ventilator. Adjustment in rate, tidal volume, or flow may stop the patient from "fighting" the respirator. If those maneuvers (made by the physician) fail, it is necessary to control the patient's respiratory discoordination by titrating intravenous doses of morphine sulfate or Pavulon. Pavulon causes less depression of blood pressure than does morphine sulfate, and it has a short duration of action. Patients with deep respiratory suppression secondary to morphine sulfate and those paralyzed by Pavulon must be continuously monitored by a skilled nurse.

The development of a pneumothorax in a positive pressure-ventilated patient requires immediate surgical intervention with decompression. Steier [99] stresses that a diagnosis should be made on the clinical basis of a sudden and dramatic onset, subcutaneous emphysema occurring initially in the supraclavicular fossa and cervical regions, tachycardia as high as 150 beats per minute, diminished breath sounds, hyperresonance, and systolic blood pressure falling suddenly to 90 mm Hg or lower. Any delay in diagnosis and intervention substantially increase mortality. Waiting for x-ray verification of a tension component in pneumothorax, as evidenced by a mediastinal shift, increases the possibility of death.

Factors that contribute to the incidence of pneumothorax during continuous ventilatory support are [99]:

1. The use of volume-cycled ventilators.
2. Preexisting chronic obstructive lung disease.
3. Application of excessive tidal volumes (i.e., greater than 15 cc/kg).
4. The presence of increased end-inspiratory pressure (i.e., greater than 38 cm H_2O).
5. The application of PEEP, especially with PEEP in excess of 15 cm H_2O.
6. Percutaneous subclavian venipuncture during positive pressure ventilation.
7. Coughing and breathing out of phase with the respirator.

To assess the mechanical functioning of the ventilator adequately the nurse must know [123]:

1. The fraction of inspired oxygen being delivered.
2. The prescribed rate, tidal volume, and minute volume. The rate is usually around 10 to 14 per minute and the tidal volume about 10 to 15 cc/kg. A spirometer should be used to measure the tidal and minute volumes. The tidal volume delivered must include the mechanical dead space of the machine and tubing, the patient's airway dead space, and the desired volume for alveolar ventilation.
3. The peak inflation pressure. Pressures above 35 to 40 cm H_2O to deliver the tidal volume should be avoided when possible. If a sudden rise in peak airway pressure occurs, the nurse should suspect airway obstruction and begin suction. If failure to remove the obstruction occurs, cuff herniation should be suspected.
4. The desired sigh volume, interval, and airway pressure limit. The hyperventilation volume is usually 1.5 times the tidal volume, 6 to 12 times per hour; the airway pressure should not exceed 50 to 60 cm H_2O.
5. The inspiratory air temperature should not exceed 39°C at the point of entry into the patient.
6. Whether the patient is on controlled ventilation or assisted ventilation. In the patient-assist mode, the patient's spontaneous inspiratory efforts trigger the ventilator's cycling.
7. What medications have been ordered to control discoordinate breathing efforts (fighting the respirator). Intravenous morphine may be used to titrate the patient to a control level, or a muscle-paralyzing drug may be used (e.g., Pavulon).
8. Whether "dead space" tubing has been added to correct hypocapnia (or removed to abolish high $PaCO_2$ levels).
9. What level of PEEP is being used (if any) and what the patient's response is to PEEP.
10. Whether drug nebulization therapy is to be administered and how to determine whether the humidification is adequate.
11. How to empty the water condensate in the ventilatory hoses without contaminating the humidifier or "drowning" the patient.
12. The technique for using an oxygen analyzer in the inhalation line to determine whether the patient is receiving the concentration of oxygen or-

dered by the physician. Machine dials for FIO_2 are not always accurate.

13. How to calculate static compliance.
14. That blood gas analysis must be performed within 15 to 30 minutes after any change in ventilator parameters (e.g., changes in tidal volume, minute volume, rate, FIO_2, or PEEP) and repeated again 30 minutes later.
15. How to ventilate the patient manually with or without oxygen if the ventilator fails.
16. Not to turn off the alarm mechanism on the ventilator but instead to use the reset button with a one-minute or less delay.
17. Where the emergency electrical source is.
18. Whom to contact in the event of a patient emergency or a mechanical failure.
19. That daily weight taking and chest x rays are needed.
20. How to record data and how to interpret data from the intensive care unit respiratory flow sheet.
21. How to prevent infection of the respiratory system from contaminated inhalation equipment.

Decontamination of Ventilatory Equipment. There is an obvious need to protect the patient's airway from contamination with nosocomial organisms. Aseptic techniques for handling the patient's tracheostomy tube, for performing tracheal suctioning, and for obtaining cultures of tracheal secretions were discussed previously. Of equal importance is the control of infection by proper decontamination of the ventilator, humidifier, and hoses (especially on the inhalation side of the system). The use of disposable plastic connection hoses, nebulizer swivel adapters, and tracheostomy tubes is becoming increasingly common. Some humidifiers can be autoclaved; some are made of a disposable plastic. Ventilator hoses and humidifiers should be changed every 24 hours. Only sterile water should be placed in the humidifier, and the condensed water in the hoses should never be emptied into the humidifier.

There is a risk that the inside as well as the outside of a ventilator may be contaminated by microorganisms in the air. Hill and Dolan [39] state that "the patient circuit can be treated depending on its construction by autoclaving, low-temperature steam, pasteurization, ethylene oxide gas, formaldehyde vapor or chemical antimicrobials." Various filters have been placed in the air intake or oxygen intake lines of the ventilator. Mitchell and Gamble [60] recommend the use of siliconized bacterial filters between the ventilator and the patient. Copper filters are also used to decrease the bacterial count [20]. A 2% aqueous activated Cidex solution can be used to clean the exterior of the ventilator.

Weaning the Patient from Ventilatory Assistance. Immediately after placing a patient on mechanical ventilation, the physician must begin to evaluate when the patient can be removed from the ventilator. The three major complications of weaning are carbon dioxide retention, hypoxemia, and cardiovascular instability.

The criteria for weaning a patient from the ventilator are the reverse of those for instituting ventilatory support (Table 17-11) [24, 81]. However, as Klein [49] states, "There are few, if any, simple determinations that signify when mechanical ventilatory support should be terminated. Once gas tension levels in arterial blood indicate reasonable cardiopulmonary function, there are few tests that accurately predict success or failure of weaning and discontinuance in ventilatory support." Weaning should not be attempted in a patient who has (1) too little strength to inspire (the inspiratory force should be greater than -25 cm H_2O), (2) a vital capacity of less than 15 cc/kg, (3) hypovolemia, (4) life-threatening dysrhythmias, (5) a low cardiac index, (6) an increased oxygen consumption, (7) uncorrected acidosis or alkalosis, or (8) a VD/VT ratio of 60% or greater. When a patient with chronic obstructive pulmonary disease is weaned from the ventilator, his arterial PaO_2 and $PaCO_2$ should be as close as possible to what his baseline levels were before he developed ARDS.

Weaning is done in a stepwise manner, with the baseline and serial objective parameters monitored. For example, a patient on controlled support should be evaluated for his ability to breathe spontaneously in a patient-assist mode. Once he is on "spontaneously triggered" breathing, the patient should be assessed for weaning from PEEP. Weaning from PEEP usually precedes weaning from the ventilator. If the patient's alveolar-arterial oxygen gradient is shown to be less than 350 mm Hg on a 100% oxygen challenge test, PEEP may be decreased in steps of 3 to 5 cm H_2O every four to six hours. Blood gas and shunt fraction analyses must be performed within 10 to 20 minutes after each decrease in PEEP. If the patient becomes hypoxic or if his shunt fraction increases, PEEP must be started again. If a shunt increase occurs, it usually appears within 30 minutes of the PEEP decrease or discontinuation. However, occasionally a shunt increase is not seen for 18 hours [24]. For that reason, the patient is monitored for 24 to 36 hours after his removal from PEEP before he is weaned from mechanical ventilation.

Most patients are weaned from mechanical ventilation by means of a T-piece adaptor, with a heated nebulizer connected to the inspirator oxygen source and to the patient's tracheostomy tube [24]. The patient with a chronic obstructive pulmonary disease must be closely observed during the administration of oxygen while he breathes unassisted.

A baseline assessment is made to determine whether the patient meets the criteria for weaning. The nurse or inhalation therapist explains the procedure to the patient. The patient should be assured that the nurse will remain at his bedside. The FiO_2 to be administered with the T piece should be the same as or slightly higher than the FiO_2 being delivered with the ventilator. The patient should be placed in a sitting position, suctioned adequately, and then placed on the T piece. His vital signs and cardiac dynamics are monitored every 5 to 10 minutes during a trial period of 15 minutes. If the patient experiences no distress during the 15 minutes, blood gas analyses samples should be made and the patient should be placed back on the ventilator until the results of the blood gas analyses have been obtained. If the arterial blood gas values are satisfactory, a 30-minute trial can be made. If the patient manifests any distress (e.g., tachycardia, hypertension, hypotension, pallor, agitation, a new dysrhythmia, or a respiratory rate that is highly abnormal), a sample of arterial blood should be drawn immediately for blood gas analysis, and the patient should be returned to continuous positive pressure ventilation.

An assessment of the gas flow rate should be made while the patient is on the T adapter [34]. There should be a continuous visible flow of humidified gas out of the exhalation port on the T piece. If the mist stream disappears during inspiration, the flow rate of gas is too low and the patient is inhaling room air as well as humidified oxygen. Increasing the flow rate corrects that problem. Since the nebulizer setting (e.g., 40%, 70%, or 100%) controls the FiO_2, an increase in the flow rate does not alter the percentage of oxygen being delivered by the inspiratory hose. However, if the flow rate is inadequate, the FiO_2 reaching the patient is decreased by the amount of room air inhaled through the exhalation port. According to Feeley [24] and Wagner [116], patients should not be given 100% oxygen during weaning since that leads to an increase in the right-to-left shunt. After two to four hours on the T adapter, the patient with an endotracheal tube may be extubated, provided that he has manifested no respiratory or cardiovascular distress and the results of his blood gas analysis are satisfactory. The patient with a tracheostomy tube should be left on the T adapter for 18 to 24 hours. The patient who has had prolonged respiratory failure and/or high closing volumes may have hypoxia secondary to rapid alveolar collapse once he has been placed on the T adapter. Rather than placing the patient back on the mechanical ventilator, PEEP may be started while the patient is breathing spontaneously and without assistance. The patient with a T adapter may be placed back on the respirator if he tires or if it is time for sleeping.

Weaning from the Artificial Airway. If a patient tolerates spontaneous breathing on the T adapter without undue anxiety or inadequate cardiopulmonary function, extubation may be performed. The physician must evaluate the cause of any undue anxiety prior to extubation.

Before the removal of his endotracheal tube, the patient should be suctioned adequately and placed in a sitting position. The cuff should be deflated and the tube removed quickly. Usually supplemental oxygen delivered through a face tent or Venturi mask is used after extubation to ensure a PaO_2 of 70 mm Hg. After extubation, the patient may be hoarse and have some difficulty swallowing. Food and fluids by mouth are withheld for the first few hours [34], and then bland liquids are given to determine the patient's swallowing ability. Upper airway obstruction secondary to edema of the vocal cords or larynx may occur. The patient should be observed for stridor and dyspnea. It may become necessary to reestablish an artificial airway. Upper airway edema may necessitate an emergency tracheostomy or cricothyreotomy. A mixture of 80% helium and 20% oxygen administered before reintubation may be beneficial since this mixture is less dense than room air and will increase the flow rates through obstructed areas where there is turbulent flow.

A patient with a tracheostomy tube who has tolerated 18 to 24 hours of spontaneous breathing may (1) have his cuffed tracheostomy tube replaced by a noncuffed fenestrated tracheostomy tube or (2) have his tracheostomy tube removed and the stoma covered with a sterile nonocclusive dressing. A fenestrated tube has a window that allows the patient to breathe through his own upper respiratory tract, to talk, and to cough if the external outlet is plugged. There should be no inner cannula in place when the external outlet of a fenestrated tube is plugged.

Weaning from the inspired oxygen concentration may take several days. When supplemental oxygen therapy is discontinued, blood gas analyses should be made 30 minutes and 90 minutes after the discontinuation. If the patient seems hoarse, warm humidified air may be administered through a face tent.

A new type of ventilation that eliminates much of the tedium of weaning patients from their ventilators has been introduced [21, 49]. The technique is called intermittent mandatory ventilation (IMV). It combines the patient's spontaneous breathing of an oxygen-enriched gas with a mechanically delivered volume of oxygen-enriched gas from the ventilator. While the patient is spontaneously breathing at his own rate and at his own tidal volume, the machine intermittently delivers a preset tidal volume. Initially, the machine may be set to frequently deliver a preset volume, perhaps 8 to 10 times per minute. Weaning is accomplished by a gradual decrease in the number of breaths per minute that the mechanical ventilator delivers, and the patient is allowed to take over more of the work of breathing. Spontaneous ventilation by the patient progressively assumes a greater proportion of alveolar minute ventilation as mandatory machine breaths become fewer. Serial monitoring of respiratory and cardiovascular status must be done as with other weaning techniques. When the mandatory machine rate has been lowered to one or two breaths per minute, most patients can be weaned safely by using the T bar, as discussed. No control study has been carried out to determine whether IMV significantly accelerates the weaning process [34]. Feely and Hedley-Whyte [24] state that IMV has the advantage of allowing weaning to be accomplished with one piece of equipment in a controlled manner but the disadvantage of having an inadequate humidification system. Klein [49] explains why dissynchronous breathing (in which the machine begins driving gas into the airway before the patient expires his spontaneous breath) is not dangerous. Klein says that the pressure-safety valve in the ventilator will be released if the preset safety limit for airway pressure is exceeded, and he points out that

the FRC of such a patient is substantially lower than normal; therefore, the sum of the patient's tidal volume and the machine's tidal volume is well below the total lung capacity.

Repeated failure to wean a patient from the ventilator, a distressing event, is usually caused by three basic problems:

1. An increase in the alveolar ventilation requirement in the presence of an increase in V_D/V_T ratio and/or an increase in the $PaCO_2$.
2. A decrease in muscle strength secondary to metabolic wasting, inadequate nutrition, or respiratory discoordination.
3. An increase in the work of breathing following a decrease in lung compliance or an increase in airway resistance due to bronchospasm or mucous obstruction or narrowing of the air conduits with edema.

Daily efforts should be made to strengthen the patient's respiratory muscles and ventilation ability by placing him on a T adapter for a few minutes and then returning him to mechanical ventilation. The period during which he is off the ventilator should be lengthened as the rest periods are shortened. The patient should be kept on the ventilator at night. Maximal nutritional efforts should be made to provide the energy needed for the work of spontaneous breathing.

RECOGNITION OF THE SIGNS AND SYMPTOMS OF PHASE IV OF ARDS; APPROPRIATE NURSING INTERVENTION

It is important that the medical team recognize the patient for whom volume-cycled ventilator management is failing before his status deteriorates to the point of irreversibility (phase IV of ARDS). Moore [62] has described phase IV of ARDS as the terminal hypoxic event. The patient has severe acidosis, depressed cardiovascular parameters, a pulmonary shunt greater than 35 percent, and unresponsive drastic hypoxemia (see Table 17-5).

Membrane Oxygenation
When it is ascertained that ventilatory support and PEEP cannot maintain an adequate PaO_2, the patient should be evaluated for placement on extracorporeal membrane oxygenation (ECMO). When all other techniques have failed, membrane oxygenation is

used as a temporary lifesaving measure [22] to allow time for the lung parenchyma to recover [35].

Murray [68] thinks that the criteria for ECMO are not clear, that more studies of it are needed, and that at present its use should be reserved for the desperately ill. The criteria for patient selection given by Hanson [35] stress evaluating the response of the PaO_2 to various procedures applied to increase ventilation and deciding early on the use of ECMO. According to Hanson, the patient should have had a trial period on a volume-cycled ventilator with the tidal volume and rate set to give the highest possible minute volume without exceeding a PAIP of 60 cm H_2O and with a PEEP of at least 10 to 15 cm H_2O. He recommends a trial administration of diuretics and an FIO_2 of 60%. If despite that therapy the PaO_2 remains below 45 mm Hg and if the patient can tolerate heparinization, he should be placed on ECMO. The management team cannot wait for the neurological and/or myocardial hypoxic signs to become manifest. The membrane oxygenator should be used before brain, cardiac, or lung damage is irreversible. "The ideal patient for membrane oxygenator support is an individual with potentially reversible pulmonary disease in whom deterioration of respiratory function has been documented (PaO_2) during maximum ventilatory support" [35]. The nursing team at the patient's bedside plays a significant role in the monitoring, data collecting, and administration of ventilatory support to the patient. Nursing assessment and data documentation are integral aspects of the decision to use ECMO. ECMO should not be used in patients over 65 years of age or in patients who have:

1. Left heart failure.
2. Chronic kidney or liver failure.
3. Debilitating systemic disease.
4. Contraindications for anticoagulation.
5. Chronic lung disease.

ECMO is difficult to use because of the complexity of resources and personnel involved in its use and because of the detailed attention that must be paid to the management of (1) the fluid balance, (2) anticoagulation, (3) renal function, (4) levels of oxygenation, and (5) the continuation of mechanical ventilation without interruption. The most common fatal complications of ECMO are bleeding and infection. The length of the illness preceding ECMO is directly proportional to the mortality [29].

Continuous systemic and pulmonary pressure monitoring by the nursing staff during fluid management is mandatory. Small changes in the patient's blood volume while he is on ECMO affect his systolic pressure. Changes in his flow rate affect his diastolic pressure. Pulmonary artery pressure monitoring helps to prevent pulmonary circulatory overloading [35].

Blood clotting is a problem in maintaining a patient on prolonged ECMO, but excessive use of heparin leads to excessive bleeding. Heparin should be titrated with an infusion pump, and the clotting time should be evaluated every 20 minutes to obtain a twice-normal value [35]. Packed red cells are given to maintain a hematocrit of 36 to 40%. Patients on ECMO may suffer red blood cell losses from bleeding and from cellular destruction in the membrane oxygenator system. Efforts to improve the oxygen-carrying capacity of the blood by administering stroma-free hemoglobin [31, 71] or a soluble dextran-hemoglobin complex [103] are still in the experimental and clinical trial stages.

Bleeding coagulopathy induced by heparin is aggravated by thrombocytopenia secondary to platelet deposition on the artificial membrane surfaces [51] of the oxygenator. The thrombocytopenia is corrected during bypass by the transfusion of platelets. Following discontinuation of the bypass, the platelet count reverses spontaneously toward normal.

There are two different cannulation techniques: arteriovenous and venovenous. When the femoral artery has been cannulated, the ipsilateral leg must be monitored for adequacy of circulation by assessment of pedal pulses, blood flow, warmth, color, temperature, and evidence of edema.

The efficacy of the pulmonary bypass is ascertained by PaO_2 measurements. The distinction must be made between an improvement in oxygenation secondary to ECMO and an increase in PaO_2 secondary to lung healing. According to Hanson [35], the only valid blood sample showing improvement in lung gas exchange must be taken by a retrograde arterial catheterization into the left ventricle. Since ventricular catheterization is not always feasible, Hanson suggests the use of a right radial sample, which minimizes the mixing of blood being oxygenated by the lungs with that being oxygenated by ECMO.

As the patient's pulmonary artery oxygen tension ($P\bar{v}O_2$) improves with ECMO, the effects of pulmonary hypoxia (vasoconstriction) decrease. Consequently, pulmonary vascular resistance decreases, the pulmonary artery pressure descends toward normal, the interstitial edema attenuates, and the pulmonary pathological shunt lessens.

Serial monitoring of an improving PaO_2 (from a radial or other arterial sample) will permit (1) a decrease in the FIO_2 administered by the volume ventilator, (2) a decrease in PEEP (although PEEP should be maintained throughout and following bypass), and (3) a decrease in tidal volume so that the PAIP is less than 50 cm H_2O. Those measures remove some of the potential problems of vigorous ventilatory therapy and establish ventilation circumstances that are more conducive to lung healing.

Although the patient's blood is being oxygenated by adequate bypass, the patient's ventilation mechanics cannot be ignored. The management team (especially the nurse) must continue vigorous respiratory therapy through appropriate tracheostomy care, tracheal suctioning, postural drainage, frequent turning, hand clapping and vibration, and optimal humidification and nebulization. Periodically, the physician may lavage the lungs, and tracheal samples may be collected for culture and sensitivity tests.

Serial x rays should show a decrease in the diffuse pulmonary infiltration. The weaning process consists of gradually decreasing the amount of blood flow through the membrane oxygenator while monitoring arterial oxygen tensions that indicate lung gas exchange capacity (using left ventricular or right radial artery samples). By his "lung gas exchange," the patient should maintain a "nonmixed blood" PaO_2 of 60 to 80 mm Hg and a $P\bar{v}O_2$ of 35 to 40 mm Hg with the following ventilatory support values: (1) an FIO_2 of 40 to 60%, (2) tidal volume and rate to give a PAIP of less than 50 cm H_2O, and (3) a PEEP maintained at 10 cm H_2O.

In a series of cases treated by Lefrak (51), patients were maintained on the membrane oxygenator from 6 hours to 11 days. Unfortunately, long-term use of ECMO depends on the availability of space in the intensive care unit, pump operators, physicians, and a large number of highly skilled nurses.

ASSISTING THE FAMILY IN COPING WITH THE PATIENT'S DYING

If the patient's condition deteriorates to the point of irreversible lung damage, the nurse's primary focus of "caring" shifts from the unconscious, unresponsive patient to the grieving family. The nurse enters what is perhaps the most difficult phase of working with the dying ARDS patient. The nurse (1) is continuously assessing a multitude of physical parameters, (2) is aware of the patient's impending death, (3) is using complex technical equipment to prolong his life, perhaps while questioning the ethics of doing so, and (4) is also psychologically involved with the patient's family on a self-conscious professional basis.

According to Kübler-Ross [50], the patient's family are participants in the drama of dying, and they undergo stages of adjustment similar to those of the patient. The nurse must avoid the game of mutual pretense, and must assume the professional role of therapist in helping the family go through the stages of denial, anger, guilt, resentment, and depression. By helping the family face the reality of the impending separation, the nurse allows them to experience "preparatory grief," and thus facilitates their acceptance of the patient's "appropriate death."

One of the most felicitous contributions to the field of thanatology is the concept of appropriate death [90]. Weisman [118] has defined an appropriate death as "one in which there is reduction of conflict, compatibility with the ego ideal, continuity of significant relationships, and consummation of prevailing wishes. In short, an appropriate death is one which a person might choose for himself had he an option. It is not merely conclusive; it is consummatory." Dying with dignity is integral to the concept of appropriate death, and the family must be helped to overcome their repudiation of death.

In the contemporary intensive care unit setting, the family is often isolated from the patient and staff, especially as the patient moves closer to death and the demands on the staff increase. The family often feels excluded from matters that affect their loved one. That "abandonment" of the family prevents the staff from closely observing the family for dysfunctioning behavior and affect.

The act of dying has many aspects, and there are many attitudes toward death. The professional nurse must perceive the attitude of each family member, develop an awareness of his affect, and understand his behavior. The medical team must be honest and must talk with the family about the seriousness of the patient's illness. Truth and what sustains one's sense of reality are more supporting and beneficial to the family than are deception and denial. Opening the channels of communication can lessen feelings of inadequacy, guilt, isolation, and hostility in the family and in the professional people who are involved in "caring."

Communication must be tailored to the needs of the family, and it must be a professional exchange, not merely a social conversation. Professional exchange focuses on affect at the latent level, seeking unconscious feelings the family members need to express. Inappropriate communication and disinheriting the family psychologically leads to a falsification of the essence of their dying loved one.

To the family member, the nurse must be not only a highly scientific, technically skillful practitioner struggling to prolong the life of their loved one but also a humanistic person. That combination encompasses more than just respectful ministering to a dying body. The "caring" nurse feels deep compassion for each person who wrestles with grief and the acceptance of death. Progress in technology may complicate the relationship between the nurse and the family. Therefore the human process of expressing compassionate caring takes on even greater significance.

THE CRITICAL CARE NURSE AND THE DYING PATIENT

Nurses in critical care units must have in-depth knowledge, sophisticated skills, an analytical approach to problem solving, decision-making abilities, a rational philosophy of life and death, and the coping mechanisms to function optimally in the stressful setting of the critical care unit.

The nurse who cares for the critically ill patient must show human concern while using technical skills. The numerous tasks of caring for such a patient require knowledge and the application of advances in science and in the technology of medicine. However, one of the essential parts of caring for the critical care patient is a continuing personal interest in him. That means emotional involvement. While the patient's disease is being monitored and coped with, the patient's emotions must not be neglected.

Emphasis in training and in evaluating performance is often placed on a core of critical care knowledge and on observable skills. The high turnover rate of the staff of the critical care unit, the investment of time and money needed to train their replacements, the tension, the feelings of inadequacy, the incidences of disharmony among the staff, and the failure to support the patient and his family emotionally make it mandatory to train nurses in the techniques of coping with stress. The nurse who cares for the critically ill should be able to (1) identify stressors, (2) recognize personal response to stressors, and (3) know strategies of stress management. The nurse should also be able to analyze accurately professional colleagues' responses to stress and to help them cope with stress. The professional's management of intrapersonal stress is related to the chronicity and degree of severity of the stressful experience, the nature and number of compensating positive experiences, the person's coping skills, and the support given the individual by other important professional persons.

The environment in which the critically ill are cared for provides the external stressors of complex equipment, crowding, constant flow of people, and rigid time schedules. The nurse who works in such an environment should be involved in decision making relating to these stressful factors.

The management of the physical stressors is easy compared to the management of intrapersonal and interpersonal stressors. Nurses are inundated with emotional stimuli, physically drained by the many demands made of them, required to be constantly alert, and emotionally involved with the critically ill, the dying, and the stressed or dysfunctioning family. Critical care nurses are often denied the reward of seeing their patients improve significantly because their patients die or are transferred to stepdown units. Since stressors are unavoidable in a critical care unit, nurses must be skilled in the techniques of managing stress by using appropriate adaptive responses.

The holistic philosophy of nursing should give the nurse an awareness of self and strategies that help to achieve self-actualization. Before working in critical care settings, the nurse should have developed a philosophy of life and of death. The nurse should be able to communicate, negotiate, and control negative thoughts; be self-motivating, self-monitoring, and self-reinforcing; be realistic in goal setting; and relate to meaningful persons. The nurse who cares for the critically ill must know something of philosophy, thanatology, interpersonal communications, and psychology.

The humanistic approach to nursing implies that nurses not only are concerned for their patient but also are compassionate toward others, including their colleagues. The humanistic approach requires that the "coping nurse" recognize any maladaptive coping responses of colleagues and help them with their coping strategies. To do that, the nurse must be skilled in:

1. Assessing attitudinal changes.
2. Accepting (and not feeling threatened by) the values of others.

3. Utilizing appropriate professional resources.
4. Developing a system to improve the coping strategies of the staff of the critical care unit.

Negative attitudes and maladaptive responses of critical care personnel are shown by excessive criticism, procrastination, anger, hostility, denial, overprotectiveness, complaints, depression, transference of blame, deficits in or lack of social skills, self-justification, fatigue, blunting of sensitivities, psychological numbness, profound guilt, and inability to resume meaningful activities or make optimal decisions.

The professional nurse must not only recognize maladaptive responses of colleagues (as well as of self) but also must quickly perceive without condemnation the feeling that lies beneath some attitude or statement of a colleague.

There should be readily available professional consultants to help manage stress in critical care units—not only the stress of the patients and their families but also the stress of the staff. The consultants should be clearly identified and their functions delineated. The boundaries of their authority, the areas of their responsibility, their availability, and the channels of communication with them should be made clear. Ministers, psychiatrists, psychiatric nurses, and psychologists should schedule regular times for working in a formal setting with the critical care staff and should be readily available for informal evaluation and intervention.

Since stressors and responses to them are permanent parts of a critical care unit, they must be handled effectively. A system in which the critical care staff learns to cope with stressors must be established. If the system achieves its goal of teaching the staff how to cope with stress well, the staff can give the patients the best possible care. Stress in a critical care unit cannot be removed or ignored, but it can be handled by the critical care staff so that it does not harm the care of the patients.

The process by which the best possible patient care is achieved may consist of (1) determining what are the stressors in the critical care unit, (2) group input and planning in regard to ways of reducing stressors, (3) awareness of and involvement in the responses of the staff to stress, (4) analysis of one's own stress and the freedom to discuss that stress with one's colleagues, (5) finding people who can help one cope with stress, (6) formalizing short-term and long-term goals, (7) establishing evaluation tools and feedback mechanisms to help one adapt to change, and (8)

planning the content of the system that helps one cope with stress.

Some anticipated results of the systems approach just outlined are a reduction in the turnover of the staff of the critical care unit, a decrease in absenteeism, a reduction in the number of accidents and poor judgments, an increase in skill, an improvement in the speed of decision making, and an improvement in the attitude of the personnel.

An improvement in the affect of the personnel is shown by (1) a decrease in the number of complaints, criticism, procrastinations, and hostile reactions and (2) an increase in warm, receptive attitudes, responsible self-direction, positive attitudes despite upsetting routines, a sense of pride about one's work, and a feeling of confidence and "OK-ness" about oneself.

To incorporate the content of the systems approach to stress management, the following should be done:

1. Formal group sessions should be held at which qualified people should discuss the systems content.
2. Informal group sessions should be held that allow open participation and discussion of stressors and responses to stressors under the direction of a qualified counselor.
3. Techniques of constructive peer evaluation should be taught to the critical care personnel.
4. Self-evaluation and awareness of stressors and feelings should be encouraged. People may be encouraged to keep a private record of their own stress cues and responses.
5. Professional counseling and/or support should be readily available to the critical care personnel.
6. Communication between all staff levels should be improved, lines of communication should be defined, and friendly conversations in places other than the critical care unit (e.g., the cafeteria) should be encouraged.
7. Recognition conferences should be held at which the successes of the critical care unit staff (and not their failures) are pointed out and at which other types of positive reinforcement are given to the staff.

The content of the stress management system should be based on the critical care unit staff's identification of their needs and on the professional consultants' evaluation of their existing ways of coping with stress. Since the mortality in the critical care unit is high, cultural attitudes toward death must be explored and anxiety about death must be faced. The idea that death is ugly is pervasive, and it must be dealt with. Man's sense of his own immortality should be explored. Life must be defined in terms of tasks, objective behavior, feelings, and philosophy. When a person learns strategies for coping with stress, he gains an appreciation of his own psychological processes and a heightened awareness of the feelings of others. He acquires an increased capacity to translate his feelings of rage, anxiety, and aggression into constructive action. When stress is managed successfully, life and death can be coped with in an open, dignified way. A person's evolving ability to cope with life crises brings a wholeness to his personal values and maximizes his humanistic ability to care (in every sense of the word) for others.

References

1. American College of Surgeons Committee on Trauma. *Early Care of the Injured Patient* (2nd ed.). Philadelphia: Saunders, 1976.
2. Bartlett, R. H., Gazzaniga, A. B., and Geraghty, F. R. Respiratory maneuvers to prevent postoperative pulmonary complications: A critical review. *J.A.M.A.* 224:1017, 1973.
3. Baue, A. E. Mitochondrial Function in Shock. In *A Cell in Shock: Proceedings of a Symposium on Recent Research Developments and Current Clinical Practice in Shock.* Kalamazoo, Mich.: UpJohn, Scope Publication, 1975.
4. Bendixen, H. H. Rational ventilatory modes for respiratory failure. *Crit. Care Med.* 2:225, 1974.
5. Blaisdell, W. F. Pathophysiology of the respiratory distress syndrome. *Arch. Surg.* 108:44, 1974.
6. Blaisdell, W. F., and Schlobohm, R. M. The respiratory distress syndrome: A review. *Surgery* 74:251, 1973.
7. Brown, P. P., Coalson, J. J., Alkins, R. C., et al. Response of the edematous isolated lung to static positive end-expiratory pressure. *J. Surg. Res.* 16:248, 1974.
8. Carroll, R., Hedden, M., and Safar, P. Intratracheal cuffs: Performance characteristics. *Anesthesiology* 31:275, 1969.
9. Chaudry, I. H., Sayeed, M. M., and Baue, A. E. Effects of adenosine triphosphate-magnesium chloride administration in shock. *Surgery* 75:220, 1974.
10. Chusid, E. L., and Bryan, H. Application of ventilation in acute respiratory failure. *Med. Clin. North Am.* 57:1551, 1973.
11. Coalson, J. J., Beller, J. J., and Greenfield, L. J. Effects of 100% oxygen on pulmonary ultrastructure and mechanics (abstract). *Am. Rev. Respir. Dis.* 101:997, 1970.
12. Comroe, J. H., Jr., and Gowler, W. S. Lung function studies. VI. Detection of uneven alveolar ventilation during a single breath of oxygen. *Am. J. Med.* 10:408, 1951.
13. Conner, G. H., Hughes, D., Mills, M. J., et al. Tracheostomy. *Am. J. Nurs.* 72:68, 1972.
14. Cook, W. A. Shock lung: Etiology, prevention, and treatment. *Heart Lung* 3:933, 1974.
15. Cox, L. A., and Chapman, E. D. W. A comprehensive volume cycled lung ventilator embodying feedback control. *Med. Biol. Eng.* 12:160, 1974.
16. Crofton, J., and Douglas, A. *Respiratory Disease* (2nd ed.). London: Blackwell, 1975.
17. Cushing, R. Pulmonary infections. *Heart Lung* 5:611, 1976.
18. Daly, B. D., Hughes, D. A., and Norman, J. C. Alveolar morphometrics: Effects of positive end-expiratory pressure. *Surgery* 76:624, 1974.
19. Davis, B. D., Dulbecco, R., Eisen, H., et al. *Microbiology.* New York: Harper & Row, 1967.
20. Deanne, R., Mills, E., and Hamel, A. Antibacterial action of copper in respiratory therapy apparatus. *Chest* 58:373, 1970.
21. Dowens, J. B., Klein, E. F., Jr., Desautels, D., et al. Intermittent mandatory ventilation: A new approach to weaning patients from mechanical ventilators. *Chest* 64:331, 1973.
22. Edelist, G. Post-traumatic pulmonary insufficiency following chest trauma: Identification and prophylaxis. *Can. J. Surg.* 18:323, 1975.
23. Ellertson, D. G., McGrough, E. C., Rasmussen, B., et al. Pulmonary artery monitoring in critically ill surgical patients. *Am. J. Surg.* 128:791, 1974.
24. Feely, F. W., and Hedley-White, J. Weaning from controlled ventilation and supplemental oxygen. *N. Engl. J. Med.* 292:903, 1975.
25. Fenn, W. O., and Rahn, A. (eds.). *Handbook of Physiology-Respiration* (vol. 1). Baltimore: Waverly, 1964.
26. Flint, L., Gosdin, G., and Carrico, C. J. Evaluation of ventilatory therapy for acid aspiration. *Surgery* 78:492, 1975.
27. Gaensler, E. A., and Wright, G. W. Evaluation of respiratory impairment. *Arch. Environ. Health* 12:146, 1966.
28. Ganong, W. F. *Review of Medical Physiology* (7th ed.). Los Altos, Calif.: Lanae, 1975.
29. Gille, J. P., and Bagniewski, A. M. Ten years of use of extracorporeal membrane oxygenation (ECMO) in the treatment of acute respiratory insufficiency (ARI). *Trans. Am. Soc. Artif. Intern. Organs* 22:102, 1976.
30. Giordano, J., and Harken, A. Effect of continuous positive pressure ventilation on cardiac output. *Am. Surg.* 41:221, 1975.
31. Greenburg, A. G., Christopher, E., Levine, B., et al. Hemoglobin solution and the oxyhemoglobin dissociation curve. *J. Trauma* 15:943, 1975.

32. Gregory, G. A., Kitterman, J. A., Phibbs, R. H., et al. Treatment of the idiopathic respiratory-distress syndrome with continuous positive airway pressure. *N. Engl. J. Med.* 284:1333, 1971.

33. Grillo, H. C. *Current Problems in Surgery: Surgery of the Trachea.* Chicago: Year Book, 1970.

34. Guenter, C. A., and Welch, M. H. (eds.). *Pulmonary Medicine.* Philadelphia: Lippincott, 1977.

35. Hanson, E. L. Membrane oxygenator support for pulmonary insufficiency. *Surg. Clin. North Am.* 54:1171, 1974.

36. Harper, H. A. *Review of Physiological Chemistry* (13th ed.). Los Altos, Calif.: Lange, 1971.

37. Heironimus, L. W., III, and Bageant, R. A. *Mechanical Artificial Ventilation: A Manual for Students and Practitioners* (3rd ed.). Springfield, Ill.: Thomas, 1977.

38. Hermes, C. G., Cooper, J. D., Geffin, B., et al. A low-pressure cuff for tracheostomy tubes to minimize tracheal injury. A complete clinical trial. *J. Thorac. Cardiovasc. Surg.* 62:898, 1971.

39. Hill, D. W., and Dolan, A. M. *Intensive Care Instrumentation.* New York: Grune & Stratton, 1976.

40. Hillen, P. G., Gaisford, W. D., and Jansen, C. G. Pulmonary changes in treated and untreated hemorrhagic shock: Early functional and ultrastructural alterations after moderate shock. *Am. J. Surg.* 122:639, 1971.

41. Hobelmann, C. F., Smith, D. E., Virgilo, R. W., et al. Hemodynamic alterations with positive end-expiratory pressure: The contribution of the pulmonary vasculature. *J. Trauma* 15:951, 1975.

42. Horovitz, J. H., Carrico, C. J., Maher, J., et al. Pulmonary shunt determinations: A comparison between oxygen inhalation (Berggren) and Xenon-133 methods. *J. Lab. Clin. Med.* 78:785, 1971.

43. Horovitz, J. H., and Luterman, A. Postoperative monitoring following trauma. *Heart Lung* 4:269, 1975.

44. Horton, W. G., and Cheney, F. W. Variability of effect of positive end expiratory pressure. *Arch. Surg.* 110:395, 1975.

45. Hunt, J. L., Agee, R. N., and Pruitt, B. A. Fiberoptic bronchoscopy in acute inhalation injury. *J. Trauma* 15:641, 1975.

46. Jones, J. W., Reynolds, M., Hewitt, R. L., et al. Tracheo-innominate artery erosion. *Ann. Surg.* 184:194, 1976.

47. Kasnitz, P., Druger, G. L., Yorra, F., et al. Mixed venous oxygen tension and hyperlactatemia. *J.A.M.A.* 236:570, 1976.

48. Kim, S. I., and Shoemaker, W. C. Role of the acidosis in the development of increased pulmonary vascular resistance and shock lung in experimental hemorrhagic shock. *Surgery* 73:723, 1973.

49. Klein, E. F. Weaning from mechanical breathing with intermittent mandatory ventilation. *Arch. Surg.* 110:345, 1975.

50. Kübler-Ross, E. *On Death and Dying.* New York: Macmillan, 1969.

51. Lefrak, E. A., Stevens, P. M., Noon, G. P., et al. Current status of prolonged extracorporeal membrane oxygenation for acute respiratory failure. *Chest* 63:773, 1973.

52. Lucas, C. E., Ross, M., and Wilson, R. F. Physiologic shunting in the lungs in shock or trauma. *Surg. Forum* 19:35, 1968.

53. Maki, D. G., Goldman, D. A., and Rhame, F. S. Infection control in intravenous therapy. *Ann. Intern. Med.* 79:867, 1973.

54. Marvin, J., Heck, E., Lobel, E., et al. Usefulness of blood cultures in confirming septic complications in burn patients: Evaluation of a new culture method. *J. Trauma* 15:657, 1975.

55. McClelland, R. N., and Fry, W. J. (eds.). Overview of papers on cardiorespiratory disease. *Sel. Read. Gen. Surg.* 4:1, 1977.

56. McConnel, G. H., Maloney, J. V., and Buckberg, G. D. Postoperative intermittent pressure breathing treatments: Physiological considerations. *J. Thorac. Cardiovasc. Surg.* 68:944, 1973.

57. McLaughlin, J. S., Suddhimonda, C., Mech, K., et al. Pulmonary gas exchange in shock humans. *Ann. Surg.* 169:42, 1969.

58. Mellins, R. B., Chernick, V., Doershuk, C. F., et al. Respiratory care in infants and children. *Am. Rev. Respir. Dis.* 105:461, 1972.

59. Meyer, J. A. Mechanical support of respiration. *Surg. Clin. North Am.* 54:1115, 1974.

60. Mitchell, N. J., and Gamble, D. R. Evaluation of the new "Williams" anaesthetic filter. *Br. Med. J.* 2:653, 1973.

61. Monaco, V., Burdge, R., Newell, J., et al. Pulmonary venous admixture in injured patients. *J. Trauma* 12:15, 1972.

62. Moore, F. D. *Post Traumatic Pulmonary Insufficiency.* Philadelphia: Saunders, 1969.

63. Moser, K. M. Diagnostic measures in pulmonary embolism. *Basics RD* 3:1, 1975.

64. Moss, G. The role of the central nervous system in shock: The centroneurogenic etiology of the respiratory distress syndrome. *Crit. Care Med.* 2:181, 1974.

65. Moss, G., Staunton, C., and Stein, A. A. The centrineurogenic etiology of the acute respiratory distress syndrome. *Am. J. Surg.* 126:37, 1973.

66. Moss, G., and Stein, A. A. The centrineurogenic etiology of the respiratory distress syndrome: Induction by isolated cerebral hypoxemia and prevention by unilateral pulmonary denervation. *Am. J. Surg.* 132:352, 1976.

67. Müller-Eberhard, H. J. The significance of complement activity in shock. *Shock Cell* Feb.:35, 1975.

68. Murray, J. F. Shock lung. *Clin. Notes Respir. Dis.* 13:3, 1971.

69. Nash, G., Bowen, J. A., and Langlin-Ais, P. C. "Respirator lung": A misnomer. *Arch. Pathol. Lab. Med.* 21:234, 1971.

70. Osborn, J. J.   Monitoring respiratory function. *Crit. Care Med.* 2:217, 1974.

71. Palami, C. K., DeWoskin, R., and Moss, G. S.   Scope and limitations of stroma-free hemoglobin solution as an oxygen carrying blood substitute. *Surg. Clin. North Am.* 55:3, 1975.

72. Pazell, J. A., and Pettier, L. F.   Experience with sixty-three patients with fat embolism. *Surg. Gynecol. Obstet.* 135:77, 1972.

73. Petroff, P. A., Hander, E. W., Clayton, W. H., et al.   Pulmonary function studies after smoke inhalation. *Am. J. Surg.* 132:346, 1976.

74. Pierce, A. K., and Sanford, J. P.   Bacterial contamination of aerosols. *Arch. Intern. Med.* 131:156, 1973.

75. Pontoppidan, H., Geffin, B., and Lowenstein, E.   Acute respiratory failure in the adult (2). *N. Engl. J. Med.* 287:743, 1972.

76. Pontoppidan, H., Geffin, B., and Lowenstein, E.   Acute respiratory failure in the adult (3). *N. Engl. J. Med.* 287:799, 1972.

77. Pontoppidan, H., Geffin, B., and Lowenstein, E.   *Acute Respiratory Failure in the Adult.* Boston: Little, Brown, 1973.

78. Powers, S. R.   The use of positive end-expiratory pressure (PEEP) for respiratory support. *Surg. Clin. North Am.* 54:1125, 1974.

79. Powers, S. R., Mannal, R., Neclerio, M., et al.   Physiologic consequences of positive end expiratory pressure (PEEP) ventilation. *Ann. Surg.* 178:265, 1973.

80. Richardson, H. B.   Immunology of the respiratory system. *Basics RD* 2:1, 1974.

81. Sahn, S. A., Lakshminarayan, S., and Thomas, P. L.   Weaning from mechanical ventilation. *J.A.M.A.* 235:2208, 1976.

82. Sanford, J. P.   Infection control in critical care units. *Crit. Care Med.* 2:211, 1974.

83. Sayeed, M. M., and Baue, A. E.   Mitochondrial metabolism of succinate, beta-hydroxybutyrate, and alpha-ketoglutarate in hemorrhagic shock. *Am. J. Physiol.* 220:1275, 1971.

84. Schering Pharmaceutical Corporation. *Schering Infectious Disease Hospital Handbook: Host Immunity and Hospital Infection* (No. 2). Kenilworth, N.J.: Schering Corporation, 1974.

85. Schmidt, C.   Closing volumes: What good are they? *J. Cardiovasc. Pulm. Technol.* Mar./Apr.:19, 1974.

86. Selecky, P. A.   Tracheostomy: A review of present day indications, complications, and care. *Heart Lung* 3:272, 1974.

87. Seriff, N. S., Skan, F., and Lazo, B. J.   Acute respiratory failure: Current concepts of pathophysiology and management. *Med. Clin. North Am.* 57:1539, 1973.

88. Shapiro, B. A., Harrison, R. A., and Trout, C. A.   *Clinical Application of Respiratory Care.* Chicago: Year Book, 1975.

89. Shires, G. T. (ed.).   *Care of the Trauma Patient.* New York: McGraw-Hill, 1966.

90. Shneidman, E. S. (ed.).   *Death: Current Perspectives.* Palo Alto, Calif.: Mayfield, 1976.

91. Shoemaker, W. C.   Pattern of pulmonary hemodynamic and functional changes in shock. *Crit. Care Med.* 2:200, 1974.

92. Simionescu, M., Simionescu, N., and Palade, G. E.   The blood vessel wall, hemorheology, and hemodynamics: Characteristic endothelial junctions in different segments of the vascular system. *Thromb. Res.* 8:247, 1976.

93. Simionescu, N., Simionescu, M., and Palade, G. E.   Structural-functional correlates in the transendothelial exchange of water-soluble macromolecules. *Thromb. Res.* 8:257, 1976.

94. Singer, S. J., and Nicolson, G. L.   The fluid mosaic model of the structure of cell membranes. *Science* 175:720, 1973.

95. Skillman, J. J.   The role of albumin and oncotically active fluids in shock. *Crit. Care Med.* 4:55, 1976.

96. Skillman, J. J., Bipinchandra, M. P., and Lanenbaum, B. J.   Pulmonary arteriovenous admixture: Improvement with albumin and diuretics. *Am. J. Surg.* 119:441, 1970.

97. Sladen, A., Laver, M. B., and Pontoppidan, H.   Pulmonary complications and water retention in prolonged mechanical ventilation. *N. Engl. J. Med.* 279:448, 1968.

98. Snyder, W., III.   Personal communication, 1976.

99. Steier, M., Ching, N., Roberts, E. B., et al.   Pneumothorax complicating continuous ventilatory support. *J. Thorac. Cardiovasc. Surg.* 67:18, 1974.

100. Stemmer, E. A., Oliver, C., Corey, J. P., et al.   Fatal complications of tracheotomy. *Am. J. Surg.* 131:289, 1976.

101. Stevens, R. M., Teres, D., Skillman, J. J., et al.   Pneumonia in an intensive care unit: A thirty month experiment. *Arch. Intern. Med.* 134:106, 1974.

102. Suter, P. M., Fairley, H. B., and Isenberg, M.   Optimum end-expiratory airway pressure in patients with acute pulmonary failure. *N. Engl. J. Med.* 292:284, 1975.

103. Tam, Sui-Cheung, Blumenstein, J., and Tze-Fei Wong, J.   Soluble dextran-hemoglobin complex as a potential blood substitute. *Proc. Natl. Acad. Sci. U.S.A.* 73:2128, 1976.

104. Teplitz, C.   The core pathobiology and integrated medical science of adult acute respiratory insufficiency. *Surg. Clin. North Am.* 56:1091, 1976.

105. Thal, A. P., Brown, E. B. Jr., Hermreck, A. S., et al.   *Shock: A Physiologic Basis for Treatment.* Chicago: Year Book, 1971.

106. Theodore, J., and Robin, E. D.   Speculations on neurogenic pulmonary edema (NPE). *Am. Rev. Respir. Dis.* 113:405, 1976.

107. Thomas, A. N.   The diagnosis and treatment of tracheoesophageal fistula caused by cuffed tracheal tubes. *J. Thorac. Cardiovasc. Surg.* 65:612, 1973.

108. Thompson, W. L.   A perspective. *Shock Cell* Feb.:3, 1975.

109. Tietjen, G. W., Gump, F. E., and Kinney, J. M.   Cardiac output determinations in surgical patients. *Surg. Clin. North Am.* 55:521, 1975.

110. Trimble, C., Smith, D. E., Rosenthal, M. H., et al. Pathophysiologic role of hypocarbia in post-traumatic pulmonary insufficiency. *Am. J. Surg.* 122:633, 1971.

111. Trump, B. F.   The Role of Cellular Membrane Systems in Shock. In *A Cell in Shock: Proceedings of a Symposium on Recent Research Developments and Current Clinical Practice in Shock.* Kalamazoo, Mich.: Upjohn, Scope Publication, 1975.

112. Urgena, R. B.   Oxygen toxicity: Basic and clinical conditions. *J. Iowa Med. Soc.* 62:583, 1972.

113. Utley, J. R., Singer, M. M., Benson, B. R., et al.   Definitive management of innominate artery hemorrhage complicating tracheostomy. *J.A.M.A.* 220:577, 1972.

114. Vaisrub, S.   What's in the cards for ARDS? *J.A.M.A.* 236:960, 1976.

115. Walker, L., and Eisman, B.   The changing pattern of posttraumatic respiratory distress syndrome. *Ann. Surg.* 181:693, 1975.

116. Wagner, P. D., Laravuso, R. B., Uhl, R. R., et al.   Continuous distribution of ventilation-perfusion ratios in normal subjects breathing air and 100% O_2. *J. Clin. Invest.* 54:54, 1974.

117. Weinstein, R. A., Stamm, W. E., Kramer, L., et al. Pressure monitoring devices: Overlooked source of nosocomial infections. *J.A.M.A.* 236:936, 1976.

118. Weisman, A. D.   *On Dying and Denying: A Psychiatric Study of Terminality.* New York: Behavioral Publications, 1972.

119. West, J. B.   Pulmonary gas exchange in the critically ill patient. *Crit. Care Med.* 2:171, 1974.

120. Wilmore, D. W.   The future of intravenous therapy. *Am. J. Nurs.* 71:2334, 1971.

121. Wilson, J. W.   Pulmonary microcirculation cellular pathophysiology in acute respiratory failure. *Crit. Care Med.* 2:186, 1974.

122. Wilson, J. W.   Some Effects of Shock on the Lung's Cellular Components. In *A Cell in Shock: Proceedings of a Symposium on Recent Research Developments and Current Clinical Practice in Shock.* Kalamazoo, Mich.: Upjohn, Scope Publication, 1975.

123. Wilson, R. F.   The diagnosis and treatment of acute respiratory failure in sepsis. *Heart Lung* 5:614, 1976.

124. Ziskind, M. M.   The acute bacterial pneumonias in the adult. *Basis RD* 3:1, 1974.

125. Zwillich, C. W., Pierson, D. J., Creagh, C. E., et al. Complications of assisted ventilation, a prospective study of 354 consecutive episodes. *Am. J. Med.* 57:161, 1974.

VI. The Critically Ill Adult with Cardiovascular Problems

The critical care nurse, in applying body-mind-spirit concepts to patient care, *experiences* these concepts. She and the patient form a unit. Because of this integration and unity, *patient* therapy is *nurse* therapy.

These experiences become a *part of* the critical care nurse. When she leaves the critical care setting they go with her, so that she is never really "off the job." She redefines her previous distinctions between "working" and "not working."

But yield who will to their separation,
My object in living is to unite
My avocation and my vocation
As my two eyes make one in sight.

Robert Frost
"Two Tramps in Mud Time"

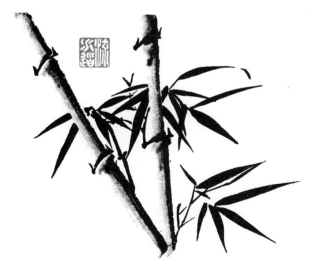

Cardiopulmonary Arrest and Resuscitation

Cathie E. Guzzetta

A cardiopulmonary arrest is perhaps the gravest of all medical and surgical emergencies. It is recognized by the cessation of breathing and circulation, signifying clinical death. Ordinarily, unless definitive action is taken within four to six minutes, biological death will occur, and the patient will suffer irreversible brain injury. Immediate and effective cardiopulmonary resuscitation (CPR) administered to the victim of sudden death often prevents that fatal complication. CPR is divided into basic life support and advanced life support. The standards governing both modes of management have recently undergone major changes and revisions. Because sudden death is a potential problem associated with all critically ill patients, the critical care nurse must keep abreast of the principles, revisions, and performance skills involved in CPR.

This chapter is divided into two sections—(1) basic life support and (2) advanced life support.

Objectives

The critical care nurse must understand thoroughly the standards of basic and advanced life support and should be able to perform perfectly the five major modes of resuscitation: (1) one-person rescue, (2) two-person rescue, (3) obstructed-airway rescue in the

18

unconscious patient, (4) obstructed-airway rescue in the conscious patient, and (5) obstructed-airway rescue in the conscious-to-unconscious patient.

Achieving the Objectives

To achieve the objectives, the nurse should be able to:

1. List the major causes of sudden death.
2. Recognize the signs of unconsciousness.
3. Describe the rationale and principles involved in one-person, two-person, and obstructed-airway resuscitation.
4. On a manikin, perform with 100 percent accuracy the psychomotor skills for one-person, two-person, and obstructed-airway resuscitation.
5. Contrast the advantages and disadvantages of each of the airway and breathing adjuncts.
6. Describe the indications for artificial circulatory adjuncts.
7. Describe the rationale and principles involved in a monitored, witnessed cardiac arrest.
8. On a manikin, perform with 100 percent accuracy the psychomotor skills for a monitored, witnessed cardiac arrest.
9. List the principles involved in defibrillation and synchronized cardioversion.
10. Perform defibrillation and synchronized cardioversion.
11. List the reasons for and the placement of intravenous lifelines.
12. Perform a venipuncture.
13. List the indications, dosage, and precautions for the drugs used during CPR.
14. List the indications, dosage, and precautions for the drugs used after CPR.
15. Write a paragraph explaining why acidosis occurs during cardiac arrest.
16. Using the patient's arterial blood gas measurements, calculate the dosage of sodium bicarbonate that should be given during CPR.
17. List the indications for temporary artificial cardiac pacing.
18. Describe the principles of demand cardiac pacemakers.
19. List the nursing actions that are taken to eliminate the various problems of pacemaker malfunctioning.

How to Proceed

To develop an approach to cardiopulmonary arrest and resuscitation, the nurse should:

1. Read the material that follows.
2. Practice her skills using airway adjuncts.
3. Practice her skills using circulatory adjuncts.
4. Become thoroughly familiar with the defibrillator in her institution.
5. Frequently review the indications, dosage, and precautions for all drugs used in advanced life support.
6. Maintain her competency in evaluating blood gas measurements.
7. Be able to assist with the placement of an artificial cardiac pacemaker.
8. Practice her psychomotor skills on a manikin every three to six months.

Case Study

The emergency medical service received a call for help from a secretary working in a large metropolitan office building in regard to an unconscious person who was trapped on a ledge of the building. When they arrived at the scene of the accident, the paramedics learned that the injured person, Mr. C. S., age 40, had been working on an overloaded transformer bank. He had been on the job for about 30 minutes when the power was inadvertently turned back on. Mr. S. had been thrown to a landing on the fourth floor. Ladders from a fire truck were raised to enable the paramedics and equipment to reach the patient. Basic life support was immediately begun. Radio contact was established with a physician at a local hospital to receive orders to proceed with advanced life support measures. An intravenous lifeline was begun. Based on the patient's body weight of 70 kg, 70 mEq of sodium bicarbonate was given intravenously. The cardiac monitor revealed that the patient had a fine ventricular fibrillation. Epinephrine (5 ml of a 1:10,000 solution) was ordered by the physician and administered intravenously by the paramedics. An esophageal airway was quickly inserted and attached to a manually triggered mechanical ventilator that supplied 100% oxygen. The cardiac rhythm revealed a coarse ventricular fibrillation. The patient was defibrillated with 200 watt-seconds of delivered energy and the fibrillation was converted into a normal sinus rhythm with frequent premature ventricular contractions (PVCs). A 100-mg bolus of lidocaine was given intravenously, followed by the administration of a lidocaine drip (1 gm in 250 ml of a 5% dextrose and water solution to run at 4 mg per minute). The patient had a palpable pulse for 30 seconds, but he reverted to ventricular fibrillation. He was again defibrillated, and his dysrhythmia was converted to a sinus rhythm. His systolic blood pressure was palpated by pulse at 94 mm Hg. He had not resumed spontaneous respirations. Artificial ventilation was continued at 12 times per minute. The patient was lowered to the ground and transported to the hospital, where he was admitted to the intensive care unit. The family was notified of the accident by the primary physician.

On arrival at the intensive care unit, the patient was intubated with an endotracheal tube and the esophageal airway was removed. A nasogastric tube was inserted. He was placed on a volume ventilator and a cardiac monitor. His blood pressure was 94/64, pulse 74, temperature 98°F. His pupils were dilated and fixed. There was no response to stimuli, no muscular movement, and no elicitable reflexes. His EEG showed no cerebral activity. The primary physician requested a neurology consultation to confirm his findings.

When the patient's wife and two sons arrived, the primary physician explained the events surrounding the accident. The primary care nurse explained the patient's general appearance and what to expect when they first saw the patient. The physician and nurse accompanied the family to the patient's bedside and later took them to a conference room to discuss the situation further. The physician told the family that he thought the patient suffered from total brain death and had no chance of recovery. He added that he would observe the patient carefully and would repeat his examination in 24 hours.

After the physician left, the primary care nurse stayed with the family to answer their questions and to support them in their crisis. She realized that the family was in the stage of shock and disbelief. The nurse helped the family explore their feelings about the patient's condition and prognosis. They began to talk about the possibility of the patient's death. The nurse learned that the patient was Catholic. The parish priest was notified. He arrived several hours later and gave the patient the last rites.

Twenty-four hours after the patient's admission the EEG and neurological tests were repeated, with the same results. The neurologist confirmed the findings. The patient was pronounced dead. The priest, primary care nurse, and a psychologist were present when the primary physician told the family of the patient's death. The family said that they wished to donate the patient's corneas, kidneys, and portions of skin from his legs and back. The patient remained oxygenated on the volume ventilator until those organs could be removed. The priest, primary care nurse, and psychologist continued to support the family. Arrangements were made for the psychologist to continue contact with the family to reduce the emotional trauma caused by the patient's death.

Basic Life Support

In 1973, the American Heart Association and the National Academy of Sciences—National Research Council sponsored the National Conference on Standards for Cardiopulmonary Resuscitation (CPR) and Emergency Cardiac Care (ECC). Those standards, which were prepared by authorities from a number of related fields, established a guide for the development and implementation of programs in CPR and ECC. Further revisions and changes were incorporated in an update of the Standards and Guidelines for CPR and ECC in 1980 [1].

A cardiopulmonary arrest is defined as the absence of ventilation and circulation in a person who is not expected to die [28]. In the United States, over 650,000 people die each year of ischemic heart disease [1]. Approximately 350,000 of those deaths occur outside the hospital. It is reasonable to assume that many deaths could be prevented by the prompt application of CPR and ECC whether in or out of the hospital setting [39]. Also, CPR may save the lives of victims of drowning, carbon monoxide poisoning, smoke inhalation, electrocution, drug intoxication, automobile accident, anaphylactic reactions, and suffocation.

A primary objective of the National Conference on Standards for CPR and ECC was the development of a protocol for a total, communitywide system of emergency medical services (EMS) capable of identifying and responding to all types of life-threatening situations [1]. Traditionally, it has been recommended that physicians and nurses receive adequate training in CPR. Until recently, however, basic life support training had not been extended to the general public, particularly groups with specific needs, such as families of cardiac patients, firemen, policemen, lifeguards, rescue workers, military personnel, and workers in industry. Currently, emphasis has been placed on developing a broad national program to train those groups and others in basic life support skills. With CPR programs extending into the community, industry, and schools, all hospital personnel should certainly be well trained and certified in basic life support. It is recommended that psychomotor manikin skills be practiced every three to six months and that all people trained in CPR be recertified annually.

Many states are developing and implementing basic life support courses in their schools. The philosophy of CPR is, "Teach your best friend."

The critical care nurse may wish to ask herself the following questions in regard to CPR:

1. Are my CPR skills up to the national standards?
2. Does my spouse know CPR?

3. Do my parents, children, relatives, neighbors, and friends know CPR?
4. What groups do I come in contact with that could benefit from learning CPR (e.g., a scuba divers' club, a golfers' club, a PTA chapter, a baseball team, a bridge club, a church group, a charity organization, a sailing club, a skiing club, or a scouting club)?
5. Does my community have enough instructors and instructor trainers to teach CPR?
6. Does my community need to establish basic life support units staffed by qualified personnel in such places as civic auditoriums, stadiums, bus, train, and airline terminals, state fair grounds, convention centers, sports arenas, and apartment complexes?
7. Did the last nursing or medical convention I attended have a basic life support station?

Definition of Basic Life Support

Basic life support (BLS) involves recognition and immediate treatment of an airway obstruction or cardiac or respiratory arrest by the application of CPR. CPR consists of establishing an airway, administering breathing, and establishing circulation. The following paragraphs discuss the principles of basic life support, the techniques and procedures of one-person rescue, two-person rescue, and obstructed-airway rescue of the unconscious patient, of the conscious patient, and of the conscious-to-unconscious patient. BLS does not require any equipment. It can be taught to the general public, and it can be used inside or outside the hospital.

Technique of Basic Life Support

DIAGNOSING UNCONSCIOUSNESS

A nurse who comes upon an unconscious person should always assume that the person has suffered a respiratory and/or cardiac arrest until it is proved otherwise. The first step in the management of unconsciousness is assessment of the patient's condition. People who seem to be unconscious might be sleeping, resting, or intoxicated. To determine whether the patient is unconscious, the nurse should

"shake and shout"—shake the patient's shoulders while shouting, "Hey! Are you okay?"

CALLING FOR HELP

If the patient does not respond, the nurse should call for help. In the hospital, help is summoned by turning on the emergency light or call light in the patient's room or simply shouting for assistance. Outside the hospital, even if no one is in sight the nurse should shout for help in the hope that someone will be within hearing distance. Once the nurse has discovered an unconscious patient, she is morally responsible for staying with that patient and beginning CPR.

POSITIONING THE PATIENT

After the nurse has determined that the patient is unconscious and has called for help, she positions the patient so that she can begin CPR. Many unconscious people are discovered lying face down. The nurse, raising the patient's arm above his head, log rolls him to the supine position to prevent aggravation of any fractures or other injuries, and positions herself at the patient's side.

AIRWAY

Establishing an airway in the unconscious patient must be done quickly. It can be accomplished without using any equipment. In an unconscious patient, the head becomes flexed on the cervical vertebral column, the jaw muscles become relaxed, and the tongue falls back against the wall of the pharynx, obstructing the flow of air into the trachea (Fig. 18-1A).

Head Tilt–Chin Lift Maneuver
The head tilt–chin lift maneuver has been found to be more effective than the head tilt–neck lift maneuver in opening the airway. If the patient is trying to inspire, the negative pressure created may cause the tongue to occlude the airway. If the head is tilted back and the neck extended, as it is in the head tilt–neck lift maneuver, the lower jaw may still need to be supported to lift the tongue off the posterior pharyngeal wall to provide a patent airway. Therefore, the head tilt–chin lift is now the preferred method of opening

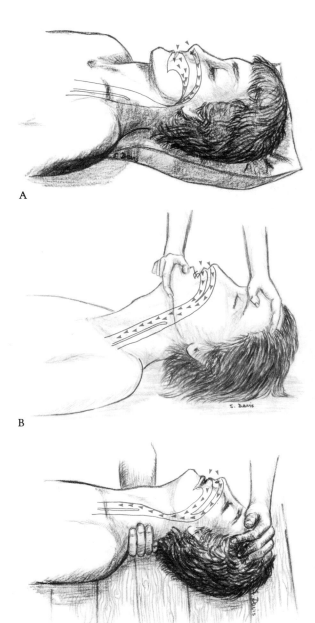

Figure 18-1
A. Airway obstruction. B. Head tilt–chin lift maneuver. C. Head tilt–neck lift maneuver.

the airway. The head tilt–neck lift maneuver is, however, still considered an acceptable alternative [1].

To perform the head tilt–chin lift maneuver, the nurse should place the fingers of one hand under the patient's lower jaw while lifting the patient's chin forward, taking care not to obstruct his airway further by compressing the soft tissue under his jaw. The chin should be lifted so that the teeth are brought almost together. The mouth, however, should not be completely closed. The thumb may be used to slightly depress the patient's lower lip but should never be used for lifting the chin. The other hand should be placed on the patient's forehead to tilt the head backward (Fig. 18-1B). For some patients, the head tilt–chin lift maneuver may be all that is needed to establish spontaneous ventilation.

Head Tilt–Neck Lift Maneuver
The head tilt–neck lift maneuver is accomplished by placing one hand under the patient's neck and the other hand on his forehead while applying pressure to the forehead and lifting the neck and head backward (Fig. 18-1C). The hand lifting the neck should be placed close to the back of the head to reduce cervical spine hyperextension. Using excessive force to hyperextend the head may cause a cervical spinal injury.

Jaw Thrust Maneuver
If the head tilt maneuvers do not open the patient's airway, the jaw thrust (triple-airway maneuver, mandible thrust) should be attempted. The nurse positions herself at the patient's head, placing her fingers behind the angle of the mandible. The head is tilted backward while the mandible is forced forward (Fig. 18-2). A thumb may be used to retract the lower lip if the mouth is completely closed. If artificial ventilation is also necessary, the nurse places her cheek tightly against the patient's nostrils.

If a cervical spinal injury is suspected (the nurse should look for lacerations of the head or face of a patient involved in a motor vehicle accident), caution should be used to avoid moving the patient's neck. In such a case, the jaw-thrust maneuver is used to maintain a fixed neutral position of the patient's neck without hyperextension. The head is carefully supported without tilting it backward or turning it from side to side. If the maneuver is unsuccessful, the head

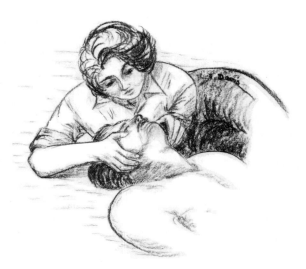

Figure 18-2
Jaw thrust maneuver.

is tilted back very slightly in an attempt to open the airway.

BREATHING (VENTILATION)

Checking for Breathing
After the patient's airway is established, the nurse must proceed with the next step of CPR—administering ventilation. While using the head tilt (or other) method, the nurse should look, feel, and listen for breathing for three to five seconds. The nurse's ear is placed over the patient's mouth while she looks for the rise and fall of the patient's chest, feels for the movement of air against her face, and listens for air exchange (Fig. 18-3A).

Mouth-to-Mouth Ventilation
When the nurse has diagnosed that the patient is not breathing, artificial ventilation is started immediately. The nurse maintains the head tilt–chin lift position, pinching off the patient's nostrils while taking in a deep breath and establishing a tight seal over the patient's mouth (Fig. 18-3B). She then forcefully delivers four quick, full breaths without allowing time for the patient to completely deflate his lungs between breaths.

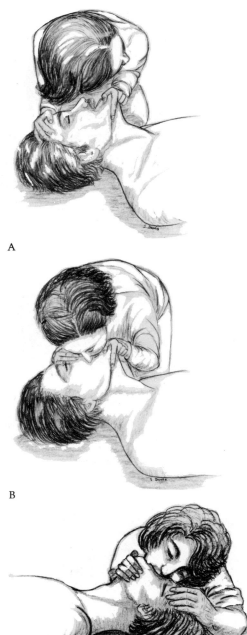

A

B

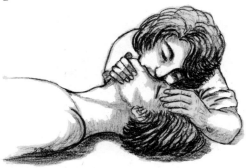

C

Figure 18-3
A. Look-feel-listen for breathing. B. Mouth-to-mouth ventilation. C. Mouth-to-nose ventilation.

If artificial ventilation is effective, the nurse should observe the rise and fall of the patient's chest, hear air escape during exhalation, and feel the patient's airway resistance and compliance during ventilation. For most adults, volumes between 800 and 1200 cc are adequate for ventilation. If the patient has a strong carotid pulse, artificial ventilation should be given once every five seconds, or 12 times per minute, until he resumes spontaneous ventilation. The carotid pulse should be rechecked after each 12 ventilations (or after one minute).

Artificial ventilation is effective because of the large tidal volumes that are given during each breath. The oxygen concentration given to the patient is approximately 16%, an amount sufficient to sustain life. Artificial ventilation should never be delayed in order to obtain or use adjunctive airway equipment (e.g., endotracheal tubes) since that equipment is not needed for effective CPR [1].

Mouth-to-Nose Ventilation
Mouth-to-nose ventilation is used when it is impossible to ventilate through the patient's mouth, when the mouth is seriously injured, or when a tight seal cannot be established around the mouth. The nurse tilts the patient's head back, placing one hand on the forehead while lifting the lower jaw with the other hand in order to seal the lips. Artificial ventilation is performed by sealing the nurse's lips around the patient's nose and blowing until his lungs expand (Fig. 18-3C).

Mouth-to-Stoma Ventilation
Breathing for the laryngectomy patient is accomplished directly—by mouth-to-stoma ventilation. For the patient with a temporary tracheostomy tube, direct mouth-to-tube ventilation is administered after the cuff is inflated. Because of the anatomical locations, neither the head tilt nor the jaw thrust maneuver is needed.

CIRCULATION

Checking for a Pulse
Once the airway has been established and artificial ventilation has been performed in the unconscious patient, the nurse must quickly continue with the next step of CPR—starting artificial circulation. While maintaining the head tilt with one hand on the patient's forehead, the nurse uses her other hand to gently locate the patient's larynx, sliding her fingers laterally into the groove between the trachea and sternocleidomastoid muscle to palpate the carotid pulse (Fig. 18-4). The carotid pulse closer to the nurse should be felt without applying firm pressure. If pulsation is absent for 5 to 10 seconds, artificial circulation must be started.

Activating the Emergency Medical Services System
In the hospital, the procedure used to set the cardiac arrest team in motion depends on the institution's policies. The procedure should include an alert system to summon trained personnel and equipment to the scene of the emergency. If a cardiac arrest occurs outside the hospital, the nurse should ask a bystander to call the local emergency medical services (EMS) system. The EMS should be activated after the breathing and pulse check so that the essential information can be given to the dispatcher.

If the nurse is alone, she should administer CPR for about one to two full minutes. If no help has arrived at the end of that time, the nurse should telephone for help and then resume CPR as quickly as possible. If a telephone is not available, the nurse should continue CPR.

Performing External Cardiac Compression
External cardiac compression produces an artificial, pulsatile blood flow. In a cardiac arrest, it establishes a systolic blood pressure of over 100 mm Hg, but the diastolic pressure is zero. The mean pressure in the carotid arteries, therefore, is approximately 40 mm Hg—or one-fourth to one-third normal.

External cardiac compressions must be done on a hard, flat surface with the patient supine to ensure that the downstroke of the compression is effective. The floor is an ideal place to perform CPR because it provides firm support and allows the patient to be easily positioned. If the arrest occurs while the patient is in bed, a board should be placed beneath him. It should extend from his shoulder to his waist and across the width of the bed. Venous return and artificial circulation may be improved by elevating the patient's lower extremities while keeping the rest of his body horizontal [1].

The nurse positions herself close to the patient's side, locates the tip of the patient's xiphoid process with her middle finger, and places her index finger be-

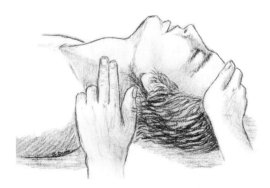

Figure 18-4
Palpation of carotid pulse.

side it (Fig. 18-5A). The heel of the other hand is placed next to her index finger on the lower half of the sternum (Fig. 18-5B). The heel of the second hand is placed directly over the heel of the first so that both hands are parallel and directed straight away from the nurse. Only the heel of the hand should be in contact with the patient's chest (Fig. 18-5C). To keep the fingers from touching the chest wall, some people prefer to interlock the fingers of both hands (Fig. 18-5D). The hands should not be crisscrossed over each other. Crisscrossing can cause unequal downward pressure during compression, resulting in rib fracture. The nurse positions her shoulders directly over the patient's sternum, keeping her arms straight while exerting vertical pressure downward to depress the sternum 1.5 to 2 in. (Fig. 18-5E). The compressions are regular and smooth and without interruptions or bouncing and snapping movements. Fifty percent of the cycle should be done during compression and 50 percent of the cycle should be done during relaxation. The heel of the hand should never lose contact with the chest during the upstroke of the compression although pressure on the sternum should be completely released before the next downstroke.

CHECKING THE EFFECTIVENESS OF CPR

The carotid pulse is palpated during CPR to check both the effectiveness of the external cardiac compressions and the return of a spontaneous cardiac rhythm. It is checked during the first minute of CPR and every four to five minutes thereafter. When there

is a two-person rescue team, the pulse is checked by the person administering the ventilations.

The patient's pupillary reaction may be checked periodically to assess the effectiveness of the CPR. If there is adequate oxygenated blood flow to the brain, the pupils should constrict when they are exposed to light. Persistently dilated, nonreactive pupils, on the other hand, may indicate serious cerebral damage. Widely dilated pupils that react to light usually indicate that cerebral oxygenation is not adequate but that serious brain damage has probably not occurred. It should be remembered, however, that pupillary reaction may not always indicate the patient's condition. Specific drugs, such as narcotics and atropine, diminish the pupillary reaction and so make it difficult to assess. The elderly patient with glaucoma or cataracts may be equally difficult to evaluate. As a result, checking pupillary reaction during CPR is optional [54].

INTERRUPTING CPR

CPR must not be interrupted for more than five seconds, except during endotracheal intubation or when the patient must be carried up or down stairs. In those cases, the interruption may be extended to 30 seconds (see Advanced Life Support). The critical care nurse has the responsibility to keep an accurate count of the seconds that elapse during defibrillation, intubation, placement of subclavian or jugular venous lines, and transport of the patient.

REDUCING GASTRIC DISTENTION

Gastric distention occurs frequently in CPR. It often occurs when excessive pressure is used during ventilation or when the airway is partially or completely obstructed. Gastric distention can be reduced by limiting the ventilatory volume to the point at which the chest wall rises, thereby avoiding excessive esophageal opening pressures. Severe gastric distention is dangerous, because it may induce regurgitation and aspiration and can reduce the ventilatory capacity of the lungs by elevating the diaphragm.

If gastric distention is observed, the nurse should *re*check and *re*position the airway, observe the volume of air needed to raise the chest wall, and avoid excessive airway pressure. Artificial breathing should be continued without attempting to relieve gastric

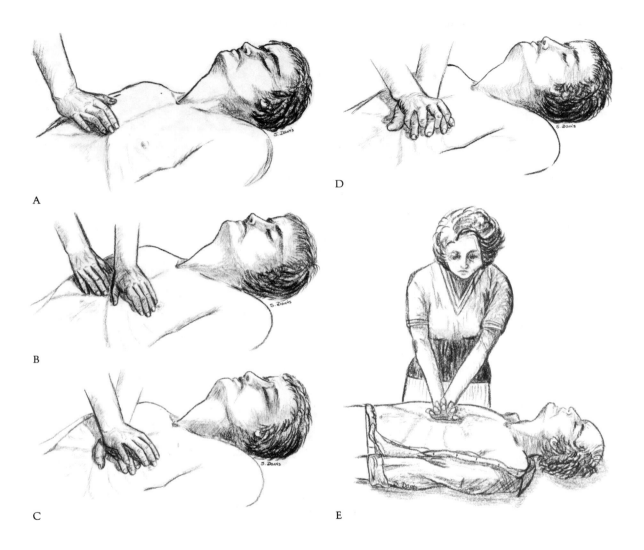

Figure 18-5
A. Xiphoid process. B. Hand placement on the lower half of the sternum. C. Hand position for cardiac compression. D. Interlocking fingers (alternate hand position). E. Body position for cardiac compression.

distention. Manual pressure applied to the patient's upper abdomen usually provokes regurgitation and aspiration. Such a maneuver, although it was once recommended, should not be used [54]. If the patient does regurgitate during CPR, his head should be turned to the side, his mouth should be wiped out, and CPR should be continued.

COMPLICATIONS OF CPR

A common complication of CPR is rib fracture, which generally occurs because of improper hand positioning. Other complications are sternal fracture,

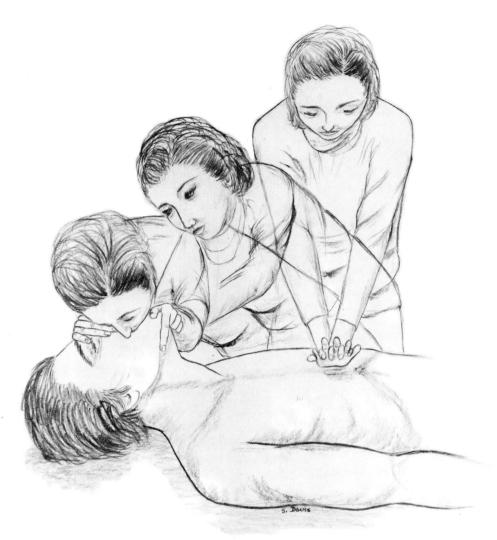

Figure 18-6
One-person rescue.

costochondral separations, pneumothorax, hemothorax, liver lacerations, and fat embolism.

The complications of CPR are reduced by carefully assessing the situation and developing proper techniques. Although complications should be avoided, obviously, no complication is more serious than death.

One-Person Rescue

The person who is found in a state of cardiac arrest is described as having had an unwitnessed arrest. The nurse must perform both external cardiac compression and artificial ventilation at a ratio of 15:2. She positions herself to administer two quick full breaths after each 15 compressions by leaning over from the waist while keeping her knees in place (Fig. 18-6). The two lung inflations are delivered rapidly (within four to five seconds) without allowing full exhalation between breaths.

Each time the nurse resumes compressions, she must relocate the sternal landmarks before placing the heel of her hands on the patient's chest. If the nurse is alone, she must compress the chest at a rate of 80 times per minute in order to achieve an overall compression rate of 60 times per minute because of the interruptions that occur when she gives artificial ventilation. For timing purposes, the compressions should be counted aloud as "1-and, 2-and, 3-and, 4-and, 5-and, 6-and . . . 15-and."

After one full minute, the nurse should check the patient for the return of spontaneous breathing and circulation. After delivering two quick full breaths, she should look, feel, and listen for breathing while maintaining the head tilt–chin lift maneuver. If she observes no spontaneous ventilation, she should keep her hand on the patient's forehead while palpating for the carotid pulse. If no pulse is felt, she should continue CPR. Checking the pupils at this time is optional. If CPR is continued alone, the nurse should check for the return of spontaneous breathing and of the pulse every four to five minutes thereafter. The procedure for one-person rescue is outlined in Table 18-1.

Two-Person Rescue

The most effective way to deliver CPR is by means of a two-person rescue team, which ensures that cardiac compressions and ventilations are given without interruption. When a second rescuer arrives to assist the nurse with two-person CPR, she positions herself opposite the nurse. The second rescuer first palpates the carotid pulse to check the effectiveness of the chest compressions. Then she calls out, "Stop compressions." The nurse stops chest compressions for five seconds while the second rescuer checks the patient for a spontaneous pulse. If no pulse is found, two-person CPR is begun (Fig. 18-7).

The compression rate is 60 times per minute. The ratio is five compressions to one breath. The spoken expression "1-one thousand" represents one second. Thus the nurse performing cardiac compressions (the compressor) counts out loud the sequence "1-one thousand, 2-one thousand, 3-one thousand, 4-one thousand, 5-one thousand," and, without pause, begins the sequence again. While the compressor counts out loud, the nurse performing ventilation (the

Table 18-1
CPR Procedure for One-Person Rescue

1. Shake and shout
2. Call for help
3. Position the patient
4. Establish an airway (do the head tilt–chin lift maneuver)
5. Look, feel, and listen for breathing (3–5 sec)
6. Give four quick, full breaths (3–5 sec)
7. Palpate the carotid pulse (5–10 sec)
8. Activate the EMS system
9. Locate the sternal landmarks
10. Do cardiac compression and ventilation
    a. Depress the sternum 1.5–2 in.
    b. Do compressions at the rate of 80/min (saying, "one and, two and . . . 15 and")
    c. Do 15 compressions to 2 breaths
11. Check for the return of spontaneous respirations and pulse after the first minute and every 4–5 min thereafter. Checking the pupils is optional

ventilator) takes in a deep breath on the count of 3, places her mouth over the patient's mouth on the count of 4, and ventilates the patient on the count of 5. The ventilator delivers the tidal volume during the upstroke of the fifth compression. The compressor should not interrupt the compressions to allow the ventilator to interpose breaths.

The return of ventilation and circulation should then be checked every four to five minutes. The pupils can also be checked at that time. The procedure for a two-person rescue is outlined in Table 18-2.

SWITCH TECHNIQUE

In the two-person rescue sequence, it is possible for the nurses to exchange positions. To prevent unnecessary interruption, the nurses are positioned on opposite sides of the patient. The compressor signals the switch to the ventilator by saying, "Change on 3 next time," using one word for each compression.

When a breath is given after the signal for changing, the compressor stops and checks the pulse for five seconds. The ventilator moves down to the patient's chest, locates the sternal landmarks, and begins compressions. The original compressor moves to the patient's head to perform the next ventilation.

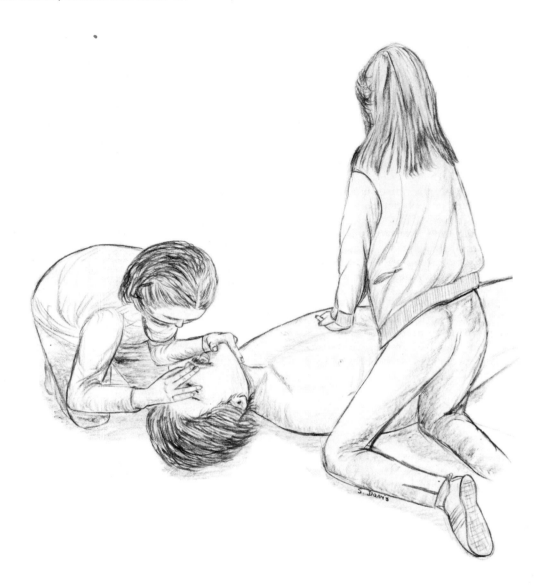

Figure 18-7
Two-person rescue.

Obstructed Airway in the Unconscious Patient

Unconsciousness and cardiopulmonary arrest can result from an upper-airway obstruction. The National Safety Council has estimated that approximately 3000 deaths per year are caused by obstruction of the upper airway by a foreign body [42]. Obstruction of the airway usually occurs when a person chokes while eating. It may be mistaken for a heart attack, giving rise to the name "café coronary" [20]. Intoxication, dentures, and poorly masticated food, particu-larly meat, are some common factors associated with choking.

When a person is found unconscious, the cause of the unconsciousness cannot be determined immediately. Early recognition of airway obstruction is essential to successful management. Any person who is discovered unconscious must be managed as if in a

Table 18-2
CPR Procedure for Two-Person Rescue

1. Shake and shout
2. Call for help
3. Position the patient
4. Establish an airway (do the head tilt–chin lift maneuver)
5. Look, feel, and listen for breathing (3–5 sec)
6. Give four quick, full breaths (3–5 sec)
7. Palpate the carotid pulse (5–10 sec)
8. Activate the EMS system
9. Locate the sternal landmarks
10. Do cardiac compression and ventilation
    a. Depress the sternum 1.5–2 in.
    b. Do compressions at the rate of 60/min (saying, "1-one thousand, 2-one thousand . . .")
    c. Do 5 compressions to 1 breath
11. Ventilator checks for the return of spontaneous respiration and pulse when she arrives and every 4–5 min thereafter. The pupils may be checked at this time. The ventilator should also palpate the carotid pulse frequently during chest compression to evaluate the effectiveness of the compressions

state of cardiopulmonary arrest. The technique for an obstructed airway is used only when the diagnosis of airway obstruction is made. Once the diagnosis is made, the nurse must administer back blows, do manual thrusts, and use the finger-probe-and-sweep technique [20].

The nurse should begin BLS in the unconscious patient—shake and shout, call for help, establish an airway, check for breathing, and deliver four quick full breaths. If the nurse is unable to ventilate the patient, the patient's head is repositioned and rehyperextended, and a second attempt to ventilate is made.

The most common cause of a nurse's inability to ventilate a patient is improper head tilt positioning, which causes the tongue to block the airway. Once the head has been repositioned and ventilation has been unsuccessfully attempted a second time, the diagnosis of upper-airway obstruction is established. The obstruction must be managed and removed before the nurse proceeds with the rest of the resuscitative maneuvers.

BACK BLOWS

The first step in the management of an airway obstruction is to deliver a series of back blows. To do

so, the arm of the patient that is closer to the nurse's body is raised above the head and the patient is rolled onto his side toward the nurse with his chest against the nurse's knees. Using the palm of her hand, the nurse delivers four sharp blows over the patient's spine between the scapulae. The blows are forceful, glancing toward the patient's head, and they are administered in rapid succession (Fig. 18-8A).

THE ABDOMINAL THRUST

Before the nurse returns to CPR, she uses one of two types of manual thrusts. The first type is the abdominal thrust, which is delivered to the upper abdomen. The nurse places the patient in the supine position and turns the patient's head to the side, away from her, while positioning herself with her knees close to the patient's hips. She places the heel of one hand against the patient's abdomen between the xiphoid process and the umbilicus, with her fingers pointing toward the patient's hip or side. Her other hand is crisscrossed on top of the first hand, with her fingertips pointing toward the patient's head (Fig. 18-8B). No part of either hand should touch the sternum or the ribs. The nurse's shoulders should be directly over the patient's abdomen while she administers four quick upward abdominal thrusts.

THE CHEST THRUST

The second manual maneuver (the chest thrust) may be used in place of the abdominal thrust. The nurse places the patient in the supine position and positions herself at the patient's hips. The patient's head is turned to the side. The nurse's hands are placed in the same position as for external cardiac compression (see Fig. 18-5E). The nurse compresses the chest four times quickly [54].

The differences between the effects of the abdominal thrust and of the chest thrust on airway flow, pressure, and volume are not significant [1]. Table 18-3 outlines the indications for and complications of each maneuver.

THE FINGER-PROBE-AND-SWEEP TECHNIQUE

If the back blows and the abdominal or chest thrusts have dislodged a foreign body, it must be removed. With the patient's head turned to the opposite side,

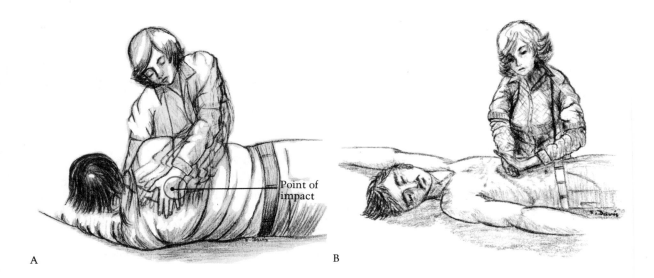

Point of impact

A   B

his mouth may be opened if he is unconscious by the tongue–jaw lift or the crossed-finger technique. Using the tongue–jaw lift technique, the nurse opens the patient's mouth by grasping both the tongue and lower jaw between the thumb and fingers of one hand and lifting (Fig. 18-9A). That maneuver, which draws the tongue away from the back of the pharynx, may be effective in partially relieving the obstruction. If the tongue–jaw lift does not open the patient's

Figure 18-8
A. Back blows (the patient is unconscious). B. Abdominal thrust (the patient is unconscious).

mouth, the crossed-finger technique is used. In that technique, the patient's head is turned in the opposite direction while the nurse's thumb and index fingers are placed between the upper corners of the patient's lips. The thumb is crossed over the index finger to provide maximum leverage to separate the jaws by bracing the thumb on the upper teeth and the index finger on the lower teeth (Fig. 18-9B).

While holding the patient's mouth open with either the tongue–jaw lift or the crossed-finger technique, the nurse runs the index finger of her other hand down the side of the cheek deeply toward the base of the tongue and across the back of the throat using a hooking action and sweeping the debris out through the lower part of the mouth (the finger-probe-and-sweep technique) (Fig. 18-9B).

The sequence of the techniques used to manage an obstructed airway is based on important physiological principles. Repositioning the patient's head and ventilating him a second time rules out improper head tilt positioning and establishes the diagnosis of upper-airway obstruction. The back blows raise the pressure in the respiratory passages to dislodge the foreign body. The manual thrusts produce a sustained

Table 18-3
Guidelines for the Use of the Abdominal and Chest Thrusts

Type of Thrust	Indications	Complications
Abdominal	Elderly patients with brittle ribs	Gastric regurgitation Internal organ injury, laceration, or rupture Rib fracture if any portion of the hand is allowed to touch the patient's lower rib cage
Chest	Obese patients Patients in advanced stage of pregnancy	Rib fracture Internal organ injury, laceration, or rupture

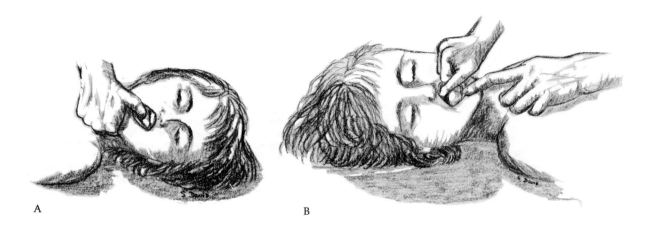

A   B

Figure 18-9
A. Tongue–jaw lift to open mouth. B. Crossed-finger technique to open mouth and finger-probe-and-sweep technique.

pressure flow to force up the foreign body. The foreign body becomes accessible for removal by the finger-probe-and-sweep technique. The combination of those maneuvers is recommended because it is the most effective method for relieving an upper-airway obstruction [1] (Table 18-4). It should be noted that maneuvers used to relieve the obstruction may be ineffective initially. As the patient becomes anoxic, however, the respiratory muscles become relaxed and efforts to relieve the obstruction may become effective.

Obstructed Airway in the Conscious Patient

Since upper-airway obstruction in a conscious patient may constitute a medical emergency, it is discussed here. It is important to distinguish that emergency from heart attack, fainting, stroke, intoxication, drug overdose, or any other condition. For that reason, the general public should be taught to use the distress signal for choking—clutching the neck between the thumb and index finger (Fig. 18-10).

PARTIAL AIRWAY OBSTRUCTION—GOOD
AIR EXCHANGE

Foreign bodies may cause either partial or complete airway obstruction. Almost everyone has at one time

Table 18-4
CPR Procedure for Obstructed Airway in the Unconscious Patient

1. Shake and shout
2. Call for help
3. Position the patient
4. Establish an airway (do the head tilt–chin lift maneuver)
5. Look, feel, and listen for breathing
6. Give four quick, full breaths. If unable to ventilate the patient:
7. Reposition the head (do the head tilt–chin lift maneuver again)
8. Activate the EMS system
9. Give four quick, full breaths. If still unable to ventilate the patient:
10. Roll the patient toward you onto his side and administer four back blows
11. Roll the patient onto his back
12. Turn the patient's head to the opposite side
13. Administer four abdominal (or chest) thrusts
14. Open the patient's mouth with the tongue–jaw lift or the crossed-finger technique. Do the finger-probe-and-sweep technique to clear the airway of any foreign body
15. Establish an airway (do the head tilt–chin lift maneuver)
16. Look, feel, and listen for breathing
17. If the patient is not breathing spontaneously, give four quick, full breaths. If still unable to ventilate the patient, repeat steps 10 to 17
18. Palpate the carotid pulse
19. Locate the sternal landmarks
20. Do cardiac compression and ventilation
21. Check for the return of spontaneous respirations and pulse after the first minute and every 4–5 min thereafter

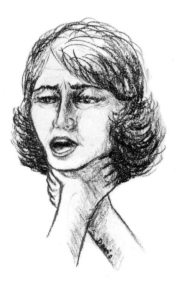

Figure 18-10
Universal distress signal for choking.

Table 18-5
CPR Procedures for Obstructed Airway in the Conscious Patient

Condition	Procedure
Partial airway obstruction with good air exchange	1. Assess the patient. Ask "Can you speak?" 2. Look for good air exchange; forceful, spontaneous cough; good color 3. Management: Do nothing. Do not interfere with the patient's efforts to expel the foreign object. Observe the patient closely for any signs and symptoms of complete obstruction
Partial airway obstruction with poor air exchange; complete airway obstruction	1. Assess the patient. Ask "Can you speak?" 2. Look for poor air exchange; weak, ineffective, or absent cough; stridor; inability to speak; and cyanosis 3. Management: Deliver four, quick, glancing back blows while stabilizing the chest with the other hand. Administer four abdominal (or chest) thrusts 4. Alternate the two maneuvers in step 3 until your efforts are successful or until the patient becomes unconscious. If the patient becomes unconscious, follow the procedure for obstructed airway in Table 18-6

or another suffered from a partial airway obstruction but has had good air exchange. In such a situation, the person has a forceful, spontaneous cough, good color, and is exchanging air well. The treatment of choice is to do nothing [20]. The person should be allowed to use his own protective physiological mechanisms to expel the foreign object.

PARTIAL AIRWAY OBSTRUCTION—POOR AIR EXCHANGE; COMPLETE OBSTRUCTION

The person may, however, progress to a partial airway obstruction with *poor* air exchange. That condition is evidenced by a weak, ineffective cough, stridor, increasing respiratory distress, inability to talk, and cyanosis. The patient may also progress to or initially suffer from a complete airway obstruction, evidenced by an inability to speak, breathe, or cough. The condition must be treated immediately, preferably while the patient is still conscious.

Back Blows

The techniques used for a partial airway obstruction with poor air exchange or a complete airway obstruction in a conscious patient include back blows and manual thrusts (Table 18-5). With the patient standing or sitting, the nurse should first position herself at the side of or slightly behind the patient and deliver four sharp glancing blows to the spine between the scapulae with the heel of her hand. To support and stabilize the patient, the nurse's other hand is placed on the front of his chest (Fig. 18-11A). If possible, the patient's head should be lower than his chest.

The Abdominal Thrust

After delivering the back blows, the nurse delivers either the abdominal or the chest thrust. The nurse performs the abdominal thrust by standing behind the patient and wrapping her arms around the patient's waist. The nurse grabs one fist with her other hand and places the thumb side of her fist against the patient's abdomen, between the xiphoid process and the umbilicus (Fig. 18-11B). Pressing her fist into the patient's abdomen, the nurse gives four quick upward thrusts. The indications for and complications of the abdominal thrust are listed in Table 18-3.

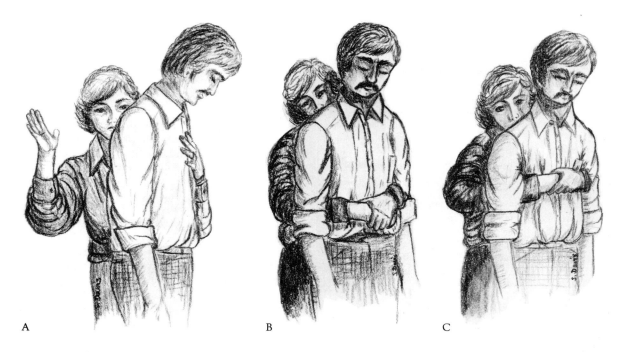

A   B   C

Figure 18-11
A. Back blows (the patient is conscious; the airway is obstructed). B. Abdominal thrust (the patient is conscious; the airway is obstructed). C. Chest thrust (the patient is conscious; the airway is obstructed).

The Chest Thrust
An alternate procedure to the abdominal thrust is the chest thrust (see Table 18-3). With the patient standing or sitting, the nurse wraps her arms under the patient's arms to encircle his chest. The nurse grabs one fist with her other hand, placing the thumb side of the fist against the patient's lower sternum above the xiphoid process, and she delivers four quick backward thrusts (Fig. 18-11C).

**Obstructed Airway in the
Conscious-to-Unconscious Patient**

If the efforts to relieve the airway obstruction are not effective in the conscious patient in a short period of time, he may lose consciousness. If that occurs, the management involves a combination of the techniques used for the conscious and the unconscious pa-

tient with an obstructed airway. The procedure is outlined in Table 18-6.

Terminating CPR

The nurse should initiate CPR for all victims of cardiac arrest according to the standards discussed. Resuscitation efforts should be continued until one of the following events occurs: (1) effective circulation and ventilation have been restored, (2) other qualified people have arrived who can continue the resuscitation efforts, (3) a physician or a physician-directed team assumes basic life support efforts, (4) resuscitation efforts have been transferred to a properly qualified emergency medical service team, or (5) the nurse becomes exhausted and is unable to continue CPR.

Advanced Life Support

Advanced life support (ALS) is provided by highly trained personnel who use special equipment to prevent or reverse cardiopulmonary arrest and to supplement basic life support measures. ALS involves

Table 18-6
CPR Procedure for Obstructed Airway in the Conscious-to-Unconscious Patient

1. Follow steps 1 to 4 listed in the lower part of Table 18-5
2. If the patient becomes unconscious, put him in the supine position
3. Establish an airway (do the head tilt–chin lift maneuver)
4. Give four quick, full breaths. If unable to ventilate the patient:
5. Activate the EMS system
6. Roll the patient toward you onto his side and administer four back blows
7. Roll the patient onto his back
8. Turn the patient's head to the opposite side
9. Administer four abdominal (or chest) thrusts
10. Do the finger-probe-and-sweep technique to clear the airway of any foreign body
11. Establish an airway (do the head tilt–chin lift maneuver)
12. Give four quick, full breaths. If still unable to ventilate the patient, repeat steps 6 to 12
13. Palpate the carotid pulse
14. Locate the sternal landmarks
15. Do cardiac compression and ventilation
16. Check for the return of spontaneous respirations and pulse after the first minute and every 4–5 min thereafter

BLS, stabilization and transport of the patient, adjunctive breathing and circulation equipment and techniques, cardiac monitoring, monitored witnessed cardiac arrest and resuscitation, defibrillation, intravenous infusion, artificial cardiac pacing, drug administration, and correction of acid-base imbalance [1]. ALS also involves identification of a patient who might be considered at high risk for cardiac arrest.

Prearrest Phase of ALS

When CPR is administered to a patient outside the hospital, in the emergency room, or in a general hospital ward, the patient should not be transported to a critical care area until his condition has been stabilized. Stabilization of the unconscious patient involves establishing ventilation, circulation, and an intravenous lifeline. BLS must never be interrupted for more than 30 seconds, even for transporting the patient up or down stairs or for the placement of an endotracheal tube. For the conscious patient suffering from an acute myocardial infarction, stabilization involves monitoring the cardiac rhythm, administering

oxygen, inserting an intravenous lifeline, stabilizing the cardiac rhythm, relieving pain, and maintaining blood pressure.

Adjuncts for Airway and Breathing

Adjuncts for airway and breathing maintenance include oxygen, oropharyngeal, nasopharyngeal, and esophageal airways, endotracheal intubation, bag-valve devices, mechanical ventilation, transtracheal catheters, cricothyreotomy, and endotracheal suctioning. Those devices and techniques are discussed in the following paragraphs.

The first step of CPR—establishing an airway by means of the head tilt–chin lift maneuver—should be attempted before any airway adjuncts are used. For some patients that maneuver is all that is needed to begin spontaneous respirations.

OXYGEN THERAPY

Supplemental oxygen is administered to any patient suspected of suffering from an acute myocardial infarction or from respiratory distress. Oxygen therapy is not dangerous when used over a short period of time, and it is effective in reducing tissue hypoxia resulting from a low cardiac output.

The fraction of inspired oxygen (FIO_2) of room air is 21%. The exhaled air delivered to the patient during artificial ventilation contains approximately 16% oxygen, which produces an alveolar oxygen tension of 80 mm Hg, or torr (see Acid-Base Balance [19]), making it adequate to sustain life. During cardiac arrest, however, several ventilatory problems exist, including ventilation-perfusion abnormalities, intrapulmonary shunting, and a large arteriovenous oxygen content difference produced by a lowered cardiac output during artificial circulation. Consequently, hypoxemia develops, leading to anaerobic metabolism and metabolic acidosis. For that reason, 100% oxygen should always be administered when bag-valve tubes or bag-valve masks are used [1, 19].

OROPHARYNGEAL AIRWAY

The oropharyngeal airway is used to move the patient's tongue away from the posterior wall of his pharynx as a means of maintaining an open airway. The oropharyngeal airway is semicircular, and it is made of plastic, rubber, or metal. It is inserted back-

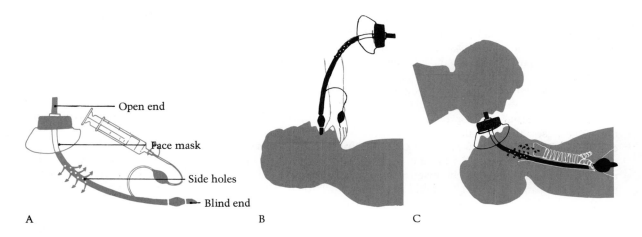

Open end

Face mask

Side holes

Blind end

A   B   C

Figure 18-12

A. Esophageal airway. B. Placement of esophageal airway: the lower jaw is pulled forward and the tube is passed into the esophagus. C. The face mask is seated, and the patient is being ventilated.

ward to enter the patient's mouth and then rotated to its proper position as it reaches the base of the tongue near the posterior pharyngeal wall. A tongue blade may also be used to move the tongue out of the way in order to place the airway. Care is taken to make sure that the patient's lips are not caught between his teeth and the airway. When the oropharyngeal airway is used, the head tilt position must be maintained. Improper placement of the airway traps the patient's tongue against his posterior pharynx and results in airway obstruction. Placement of the airway in an alert patient is not recommended because it generally causes retching and vomiting [56]. Oropharyngeal airways should always be used whenever a bag-valve mask or an automatic breathing device is used.

NASOPHARYNGEAL AIRWAY

A nasopharyngeal airway is used to maintain a patent airway in a semiconscious patient. It is inserted along the floor of the patient's nostril behind his tongue into the posterior pharynx, allowing air to pass into the lower pharynx and larynx. It is inserted gently with a water-soluble lubricant or a local anesthetic to prevent trauma to the mucous membranes. The patency of the tube is checked after insertion. The nasopharyngeal airway also provides a less traumatic passageway for deep tracheal suctioning.

ESOPHAGEAL AIRWAY

The esophageal airway, which resembles an endotracheal tube [1, 19, 52], may be used to maintain a patent airway. The esophageal airway has an open end at the top and a closed, or blind, end at the bottom (with a 30-cc inflatable cuff) (Fig. 18-12A). The lower (blind) end is inserted into the esophagus. The tube is approximately 15 in. long, and it has a universal adapter on its proximal end. Below the adapter, and extending approximately one-third of the way down the tube, is a series of side holes that are located at the level of the pharynx when the tube is inserted. Above the adapter is a removable cushion-seal face mask that accommodates the tube.

The tube is inserted into the patient's mouth and oropharynx without visualization while his lower jaw is pulled forward with the thumb and forefinger (Fig. 18-12B). The tube follows the normal curvature of the pharynx when the head is flexed forward, passing into the esophagus. It is advanced until the mask is seated on the patient's face to ensure that the cuff is below the level of the carina (Fig. 18-12C).

During placement of the esophageal airway, there is a slight chance that the tube will be passed into the trachea instead of the esophagus. After the airway has been inserted, therefore, the nurse should ventilate the patient by the mouth-to-tube or bag-valve-to-tube approach so that she can evaluate the location of the tube by observing the chest expansion and by auscultating the lungs. If the trachea has been intubated, the chest will not rise, breath sounds will not be heard, and the esophageal airway should be removed immediately. When the tube is properly placed in the esophagus, the cuff is then inflated with 30 to 35 cc of air, thus sealing off the esophageal opening. The air that is blown into the tube during ventilation escapes through the side holes and passes down the trachea. The inflatable cuff prevents air from entering the stomach.

Inserting the esophageal airway is simple, and it does not require extensive practice. It prevents stomach insufflation and aspiration of gastric contents because the inflatable cuff blocks the esophagus. The airway, however, can cause retching or vomiting in the conscious or semiconscious patient and it should therefore be inserted only in the unresponsive patient [19, 52]. It should not be used in cases of caustic-poison ingestion or esophageal disease or in children under the age of 16 [3].

The esophageal airway is only for short-term use in emergencies. If the patient requires esophageal intubation for longer than two hours, an endotracheal tube should be inserted. The mask is removed from the esophageal airway, and the endotracheal tube is inserted with a laryngoscope while the esophageal tube is left in place with the cuff inflated. To prevent possible aspiration of gastric contents, the endotracheal cuff is then inflated before deflating the esophageal cuff and removing the esophageal airway. Insertion of a nasogastric tube also helps to decompress the stomach before removing the tube. Because regurgitation is a common complication, the esophageal airway should not be removed until the patient is fully awake and responsive when endotracheal intubation is not required. Also, suction should be available, and the patient should be placed on his side when the tube is removed.

ESOPHAGEAL GASTRIC TUBE

The esophageal gastric tube comprises both an esophageal airway and a nasogastric tube. The nasogastric tube is inserted through a separate port on the face mask of the airway, and it is passed through a separate channel of the airway that opens to the stomach. The patient is ventilated through another port on the mask. The esophageal gastric tube permits ventilation of the lungs and decompression of the stomach while the esophagus is occluded to prevent the possibility of vomiting and aspiration.

ENDOTRACHEAL INTUBATION

Adequate oxygenation of the patient's lungs by means of artificial ventilation must always precede any attempts at endotracheal intubation. Because adequate lung ventilation requires high pharyngeal pressures, gastric distention often occurs during mouth-to-mouth ventilation. Gastric distention causes elevation of the diaphragm, which reduces the patient's tidal volume and is associated with regurgitation and aspiration. Consequently, endotracheal intubation should be performed as soon as skilled personnel and equipment arrive. It is indicated when the patient has cardiac or respiratory arrest. It may also be necessary when the patient cannot be ventilated by means of rescue breathing or if the patient is unable to protect his own airway (e.g., when he is in a coma). To avoid the problems of hypoxemia, no more than 30 seconds should be allowed for the procedure.

The endotracheal tube is passed directly into the trachea by means of laryngoscopic visualization of the glottis, larynx, and trachea (Fig. 18-13A). The endotracheal tube contains a standard 15-mm adapter for attachment to a bag-valve or a similar device. The end of the tube has an inflatable cuff that is used to seal off the airway, thereby protecting the lungs from aspiration (Fig. 18-13B). The tube isolates the airway, allowing high concentrations of oxygen to be delivered to the patient while providing a nontraumatic passage for deep tracheal suctioning.

The most common problem associated with placement of the endotracheal tube is accidental esophageal intubation. It is also possible to insert the tube into the right mainstem bronchus, which results in ventilation of only the right lung. For that reason, it is important to auscultate the lungs to determine the presence of bilateral breath sounds and to obtain a chest x ray after the tube has been inserted.

BAG-VALVE DEVICES

Bag-valve devices generally provide lower ventilatory volumes than does mouth-to-mouth ventilation. Specialized training and proficiency are required to use a bag-valve device. The acceptable bag-valve device is self filling, should not contain sponge rubber (to ensure proper cleansing and disinfecting), and should have a nonjam valve that allows a 15-liters-per-minute oxygen inlet flow. Moreover, it should have a transparent plastic face mask with a contoured cuff so that the patient can be observed for regurgitation [1]. As discussed earlier, a 15-mm adapter must be available for connection to the endotracheal tube.

The resuscitation bag delivers an FiO_2 of 21% (the FiO_2 of room air). When supplemental oxygen is at-

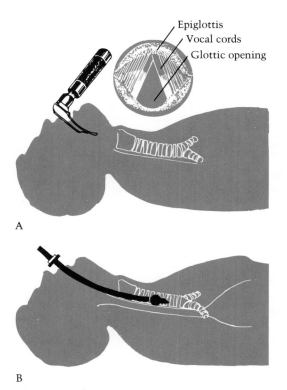

Epiglottis
Vocal cords
Glottic opening

A

B

Figure 18-13
A. Laryngoscopic visualization of glottis, larynx, and trachea. B. Endotracheal tube placement.

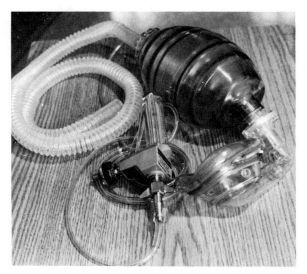

Figure 18-14
Bag-valve device with oxygen reservoir.

tached to the bag at a flow rate of 12 liters per minute, approximately 40% oxygen is delivered [19]. To achieve an FIO_2 of 90% or greater, an oxygen reservoir should be placed over the bag inlet (Fig. 18-14) [19].

When a bag-valve mask is used, an oropharyngeal airway must be inserted. The nurse should position herself at the head of the patient and maintain the head tilt position by using two or three fingers of one hand to force up the patient's mandible. The thumb and index finger are placed on either side of the valve while the nurse exerts pressure on the mask with her hand to achieve a tight seal. The free hand compresses the bag with an even squeezing motion.

The major advantages of the bag-valve mask are that it provides a means of administering an enriched oxygen mixture and that it can be used immediately during an arrest. The primary disadvantage of the device is that the tidal volume delivered to the patient is reduced because of the difficulty in establishing an airtight seal around his mouth. For that reason, it is recommended that the bag-valve mask be used only in conjunction with a cuffed endotracheal tube or a cuffed esophageal airway [1].

MECHANICAL VENTILATORS

Most types of mechanical ventilators should not be used during CPR. Pressure ventilators are not recommended because effective external cardiac compression prematurely stops the inspiratory cycle on the machine, resulting in ineffective ventilatory volumes [19]. Volume ventilators also should not be used because of the difficulty of coordinating chest compressions with ventilation.

Manually triggered or time-cycled devices are acceptable for use during CPR if they are used by skilled personnel. They allow for proper timing between compressions and ventilation, deliver high-flow rates, provide an FIO_2 of 100%, and are generally equipped with an inspiratory pressure safety pop-off valve that opens at pressures of 50 cm H_2O [19]. Those devices deliver high pressures to the patient and usually cause stomach distention unless a cuffed endotracheal tube or an esophageal airway is used.

TRANSTRACHEAL CATHETER AND CRICOTHYREOTOMY

If the airway obstruction cannot be relieved by any of the methods described, the use of a transtracheal catheter or a cricothyreotomy is indicated [19]. Those procedures are used only when ventilatory efforts have failed, and they are performed only by skilled personnel. The transtracheal catheter ventilation procedure is accomplished by inserting a 14-gauge plastic intravenous catheter into the trachea to establish a patent airway. To perform a cricothyreotomy, an incision is made in the cricothyroid membrane through which a tube or a large-bore needle is placed as a means of ventilation.

SUCTIONING

Tracheal suctioning equipment must be available during all resuscitation attempts. It should be powerful enough to provide an air flow of more than 30 liters per minute at the end of the delivery tube and a vacuum of more than 300 mm Hg when the tube is clamped [19]. Tracheal suctioning has been discussed in Chapter 17.

Adjuncts for Artificial Circulation

THE CARDIAC PRESS

BLS must be performed wherever a person who has suffered a cardiac arrest is found. Although no circulatory adjuncts are needed to perform CPR, a manually operated chest compressor (cardiac press) can be used for effective cardiac compression, particularly when transportation of the patient is necessary. Those adjuncts should provide an adjustable sternal depression of 1.5 to 2 in. Artificial ventilation must be given during the upstroke of the fifth chest compression. Manual CPR should not be interrupted for more than five seconds when applying the device. Skilled personnel must be in constant attendance because of the problems associated with its use, such as the tendency of the compressor to shift position or of the plunger to loosen, resulting in inadequate chest compression and general mechanical malfunction [19].

GAS-POWERED CHEST COMPRESSORS

Automatic gas-powered chest compressors are generated by compressed gas and perform both external cardiac compression and artificial ventilation. The use of those devices is indicated during prolonged resuscitation efforts or during transportation of the patient. When they are used, manual CPR must always be initiated first. Critical care personnel must practice extensively the technique for using the device so

that CPR is not interrupted for more than five seconds. The device must be very carefully observed for compression or ventilation malfunction.

MEDICAL ANTISHOCK TROUSERS

The garment known as medical antishock trousers (MAST) has been developed for use in patients with hypovolemic shock [36]. It is a one-piece garment that is placed over the patient's legs and abdomen. When it is inflated, it compresses the patient's legs and viscera, performing as an autoinfusion device and increasing central volume. If the shock is due to hypovolemia, the patient's clinical condition should improve with the use of the trousers. Fluids are infused until an adequate volume is achieved, and the trousers are then slowly deflated.

INTRAAORTIC BALLOON PUMP

The intraaortic balloon pump is another circulatory adjunct. It is indicated for use in patients with left ventricular failure and cardiogenic shock (see Chap. 19).

INTERNAL CARDIAC COMPRESSION

Internal cardiac compression should be attempted only by qualified personnel. It should not be substituted for external cardiac compression. Internal cardiac compression is generally not successful if external cardiac compression, coupled with appropriate ventilatory and pharmacological therapy, has failed. Internal cardiac compression may be indicated, however, in patients with anatomical deformities of the chest, in chest trauma, in cardiac tamponade, or when the patient's chest is already open (i.e., during surgery).

Cardiac Monitoring

Continuous cardiac monitoring should be provided as an essential part of ALS. Critical care personnel must be familiar with monitoring equipment, lead placement, and individual equipment problems. Nurses providing ALS should be able to recognize the following dysrhythmias: sinus bradycardia, sinus tachycardia, premature atrial contractions, atrial tachycardia, atrial flutter, atrial fibrillation, junctional rhythms, first-, second-, and third-degree atrioventricular heart blocks, premature ventricular contractions, ventricular tachycardia, ventricular fibrillation, and cardiac standstill.

Training and testing of all personnel providing ALS should be done periodically to ensure that they are competent in recognizing dysrhythmias and in treating the patient. (Cardiac monitoring and the recognition of dysrhythmias are discussed more fully in Chapter 10.)

Monitored, Witnessed Cardiac Arrest

A monitored, witnessed cardiac arrest is defined as an arrest that occurs when the potential rescuer actually sees the person experiencing a cardiac arrest resulting from a life-threatening dysrhythmia (e.g., ventricular tachycardia, ventricular fibrillation, or asystole) while the patient's cardiac rhythm is being monitored by the ECG. (That definition represents a major change in the standards for cardiopulmonary resuscitation and emergency cardiac care.*) A monitored, witnessed arrest by definition implies that the person who witnesses it is able to recognize the dysrhythmia (as shown by the ECG) and treat the patient. Thus the resuscitation procedure for such an arrest should be taught as part of ALS training to critical care and emergency room personnel. The witnessed cardiac arrest is no longer considered a part of BLS.

The basic difference between the treatment of a monitored, witnessed cardiac arrest and other resuscitative techniques is the use of a precordial thump. The thump generates a small electrical stimulus to the potentially reactive heart. The stimulus may be effective in reversing the dysrhythmia and in restoring a normal heartbeat if it is performed within one minute of the time the patient goes into arrest. Because the myocardium generally becomes anoxic after the first minute of an arrest, a precordial thump would probably not be effective in an unmonitored, unwitnessed cardiac arrest [19]. The precordial thump is not recommended for patients with anoxic asystole or in patients with ventricular tachycardia who have an adequate pulse and blood pressure.

A single precordial thump is administered by delivering a sharp, quick blow over the midsternum. The midsternum is located first by placing the index finger of one hand in the sternal notch and the index finger of the other on the xiphoid process. The

*Memo from the American Heart Association, May 17, 1977.

Table 18-7
CPR Procedure for Monitored, Witnessed Cardiac Arrest

1. Shake and shout
2. Call for help
3. Position the patient
4. Establish an airway (do the head tilt–chin lift maneuver)
5. Look, feel, and listen for breathing while palpating for the carotid pulse
6. If the patient is not breathing and has no pulse, locate the midsternum and administer a precordial thump*
7. Begin CPR
   a. Establish an airway (do the head tilt–chin lift maneuver)
   b. Look, feel, and listen for breathing
   c. Give four quick, full breaths
   d. Palpate the carotid pulse (determine whether the precordial thump reestablished the pulse)
   e. Activate the EMS system
   f. Locate the sternal landmarks
   g. Do cardiac compression and ventilation
   h. Check for the return of spontaneous respirations and pulse after the first minute and every 4–5 min thereafter

*The precordial thump should be delivered within one minute of the start of the cardiac arrest.

thumbs of both hands are then brought together to locate the midsternum (Fig. 18-15A). The fist should be raised only 8 to 12 in. above the patient's chest. The elbow, hand, and arm should be parallel to the patient's sternum (Fig. 18-15B). A sharp thump is then delivered with the fleshy portion of the fist. If the precordial thump is not effective, CPR must be instituted immediately (Table 18-7).

Defibrillation

Electrical defibrillation causes a simultaneous electrical depolarization of myocardial muscle fibers, resulting in a unified contraction of the myocardium. After depolarization, repolarization of each fiber occurs. Theoretically, the process results in a normal electrical impulse from the sinoatrial node that provides the stimulus for a normal, coordinated cardiac rhythm.

INDICATIONS FOR DEFIBRILLATION

Defibrillation is indicated for the treatment of the disordered cardiac rhythm produced by ventricular fibrillation. It must be delivered to the patient as soon

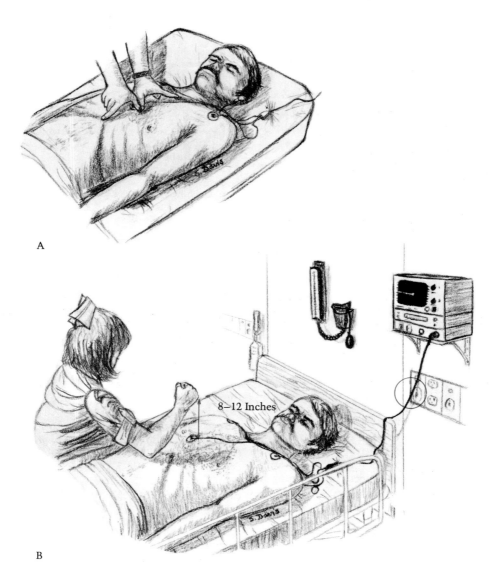

8–12 Inches

A

B

as the diagnosis of ventricular fibrillation has been made (as confirmed by the cardiac monitor in an unconscious and pulseless patient who has been in cardiac arrest less than two minutes) and the equipment becomes available. BLS, however, must never be delayed to obtain the defibrillator. Unmonitored defibrillation is also recommended for the unconscious, pulseless patient (with a presumptive diagnosis of ventricular fibrillation) when a defibrillator is available and a cardiac monitor is not. In such a case, a single shock is delivered by properly trained and authorized personnel.

Figure 18-15
A. Measurement of the midsternum for a precordial thump.
B. Precordial thump in a monitored, witnessed cardiac arrest.

Defibrillation of an anoxic myocardium is generally not successful. If the patient has been in ventricular fibrillation for an undetermined period of time, CPR should be initiated for approximately two minutes to relieve the anoxia before attempting to defibrillate [1]. Defibrillation has not been shown to be useful in asystole, but it may be indicated when it is difficult to determine whether the patient has a fine ventricular fibrillation or a true cardiac standstill.

DIRECT CURRENT DEFIBRILLATORS

The direct current (DC) defibrillator consists of a high-voltage power supply that charges an energy capacitor connected to paddles through a current-limiting inductor. The current that is delivered through the paddles is several thousand volts, and it lasts for only a few milliseconds. Current is expressed as energy. The term energy is also equivalent to the terms joules and watt-seconds. Energy is defined as the product of the charge power and the charge duration, as expressed in the following equation:

Energy = power × duration
(joules)   (watt)   (seconds)

DC defibrillators are light and effective. Since they can be powered by batteries they can be used outside the hospital setting. They may also be preset or synchronized to deliver current to the QRS complex for treatment of dysrhythmias other than ventricular fibrillation (see Elective Cardioversion).

The major disadvantage of DC defibrillators is that the amount of energy they store does not equal the amount of energy they deliver to the patient. Most defibrillator units have a switch to initiate the storage of energy in the capacitor with some type of meter or indicator for measuring that energy. However, the measurement indicates only the amount of stored energy. Some of the newer models are capable of measuring the stored energy and estimating or measuring the delivered energy (the amount of energy received by the patient). The maximum delivered energy that is available in most defibrillators is 300 to 360 watt-seconds. The level of energy required to defibrillate a heart depends on the size of the patient and the size of his heart [40]. For large people, 300 to 360 watt-seconds may not be enough to revert the ventricular fibrillation successfully. Newer models are designed to store up to 900 to 1000 watt-seconds. As those defibrillators become widely available, the medical and nursing staffs must be reeducated so that patients are not shocked with levels of current that are too high for their body mass.

All defibrillators should be tested monthly for proper functioning. The actual energy delivered through a 50-ohm resistance (simulating human body resistance) should be measured for each increment of 50 watt-seconds of stored energy. The results of those measurements should be written on a piece of adhesive tape attached to the side of the defibrillator.

ELECTRICAL RESISTANCE

Electrical resistance must be reduced before the electrical charge is applied to the patient's chest so that the delivered energy will not be wasted. When the skin resistance is high, the amount of electrical energy delivered to the heart will be lost through the production of smoke, heat, and burns. Electrical resistance is reduced by applying saline-soaked 4" × 4" gauze pads to the chest. Saline-soaked pads are not greasy, and so they prevent the hands from slipping if external cardiac compression is continued after defibrillation. Care must be taken to avoid creating a path of saline solution from one paddle to the other on the patient's chest. Such a path provides a low-resistance channel that shunts current away from the heart by producing electrical bridging and skin burns. As a result, defibrillation is generally ineffective because little or no current is delivered to the heart. Alcohol-soaked pads must never be used because they will burst into flames when the electrical current passes through the alcohol.

Electrode paste is also used to reduce skin resistance and is probably more effective than the saline-soaked pads [19]. A large amount of paste is applied to the surfaces of both paddles. Care must be taken to avoid creating a path of paste between the two paddles to prevent electrical bridging. A major disadvantage of electrode paste is that it causes the hands to slip when chest compressions are reinstituted after defibrillation. To ensure proper skin contact, electrode paddles should be periodically examined for pitting and the presence of oxide films.

ELECTRODE PADDLE PLACEMENT

In preparing for emergency defibrillation, one electrode paddle is placed below the right clavicle at the sternoclavicular joint while the other is placed to the left of the cardiac apex (below and to the left of the left nipple) in the anterior axillary line (Fig. 18-16).

After the paddles are in place, 20 to 25 pounds of firm pressure is applied to each paddle. That pressure results in good skin contact and reduces the complications of skin burns. Strong muscular pressure, rather than pressure exerted by body weight (leaning

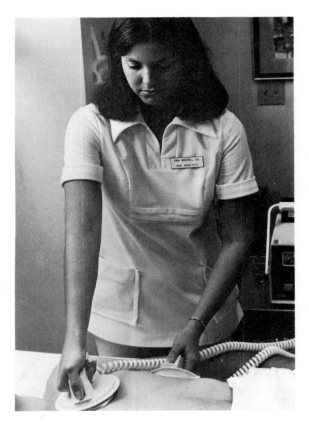

Figure 18-16
Electrode placement for defibrillation (anterior placement of electrode paddles).

on the paddles), should be used to avoid slipping of the paddles and to prevent the nurse from losing her balance [40].

DEFIBRILLATION GUIDELINES

When the patient is in ventricular fibrillation, CPR must be initiated. Personnel and equipment are summoned. The patient's cardiac rhythm is assessed, and the patient is prepared for defibrillation. The entire procedure should not interrupt CPR for more than 10 seconds.

The electrode paste is applied to the paddles, or the saline pads are placed on the chest. Once the paddles are in place, the appropriate energy level is selected and activated. Theoretically, the proper setting is the one that is high enough to defibrillate the heart on the first attempt and low enough to avoid myocardial

damage. It is recommended that 3.5 to 6 watt-seconds/kg be used for patients weighing less than 50 kg. If the patient weighs 50 kg or more, 200 to 300 watt-seconds of delivered energy should be used.

When the capacitor has reached its desired level of energy, the nurse orders the area to be cleared and looks carefully to make sure that no one is in contact with the bed, equipment, or patient. That precaution is taken to avoid accidental shock to the nurse or other personnel. The defibrillator is fired (on most machines, firing requires simultaneously depressing the buttons on both paddles). If the electrical energy is delivered to the patient (and if the machine is working correctly), the muscles of the patient's chest wall will contract. If his muscles do not contract, the nurse should check to make sure that the synchronizer circuit is off, that the defibrillator is plugged in, and, if a battery is used, that it is sufficiently charged (Table 18-8). The patient's pulse and ECG must be assessed immediately after defibrillation.

If the first attempt at defibrillation is unsuccessful, a second attempt should be made using 200 to 300 watt-seconds of delivered energy. If the second attempt is also unsuccessful, CPR should be continued and epinephrine and sodium bicarbonate should be

Table 18-8
CPR Procedure When Defibrillation Is Used*

1. Administer CPR until the equipment and personnel arrive
2. Assess the patient's pulse and ECG
3. Turn on the machine. Check to see that the synchronizer is off
4. Apply electrode paste or saline-soaked 4″ × 4″ gauze pads
5. Position the electrode paddles
6. Set the machine for 200–300 watt-seconds of delivered energy
7. Recheck the ECG
8. Clear the area
9. Apply 20–25 lb pressure to the paddles
10. Activate the firing buttons
11. Assess the patient's pulse and ECG
12. If unsuccessful, repeat steps 4–11. If still unsuccessful after second attempt at defibrillation:
13. Administer CPR. Give epinephrine and sodium bicarbonate as appropriate
14. Repeat steps 4–11 using 360 watt-seconds of delivered energy

*Defibrillation should not interrupt CPR for more than 10 seconds.

administered as appropriate. A third attempt at defibrillation is then made using 360 watt-seconds of delivered energy.

Elective Cardioversion

Cardioversion is used to deliver an electrical current to the myocardium approximately 10 milliseconds after the peak of the R wave. It is used to treat patients with dysrhythmias other than ventricular fibrillation, such as rapid ventricular and supraventricular dysrhythmias associated with a low cardiac output.

With a few minor exceptions, the procedure for cardioversion is similar to that for defibrillation. During elective cardioversion, the anteroposterior placement of the electrode paddles is preferred because it provides more delivered energy to the heart than does the standard position. The anteroposterior placement involves positioning one electrode paddle anteriorly over the precordium and the other electrode paddle behind the heart in a posterior position (Fig. 18-17). Because the posterior paddle is difficult to place, it should not be used in emergencies.

The QRS complex on the monitor must produce a tall R wave before cardioversion. If the R wave is inverted or if the amplitude of the R wave is small, it may not trigger the synchronizing circuit on the defibrillator. The synchronizer switch on the defibrillator is turned on and the energy level set. When the defibrillator is fired, the paddles must be left in place, and the firing buttons must be depressed (sometimes for several seconds) until the synchronizer discharges the stored energy. That is necessary because when the synchronizer is activated, it controls the release of the energy until the RS segment of the QRS complex. That avoids delivering the current during the vulnerable period of the T wave and reduces the probability of causing ventricular fibrillation. Should the patient's rhythm be cardioverted into ventricular fibrillation, however, the defibrillator should be recharged, the synchronizer circuit turned off, and the patient immediately defibrillated.

What energy levels are needed for cardioversion depends on the associated dysrhythmia. The potential for myocardial damage increases as the level of electrical energy increases. Maximal settings should not be used when they are not required. Ventricular tachycardia, for example, can be converted with en-

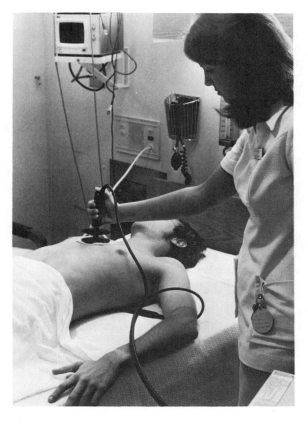

Figure 18-17
Electrode placement for cardioversion (anteroposterior placement of electrode paddles).

ergy levels as low as 20 watt-seconds although in clinical practice 50 to 200 watt-seconds are generally used. When repeated shocks are given, the interval between shocks should be three minutes or longer when possible. Myocardial damage has also been found to be reduced by the use of larger electrode paddles [19].

Intravenous Therapy

Intravenous cannulation is essential to the administration, uptake, and distribution of fluids and drugs. It is also used to obtain blood specimens for laboratory tests and to provide a route for physiological monitoring or artificial cardiac pacing.

It is necessary to establish an intravenous lifeline as

quickly as possible during a cardiac arrest. Because blood is shunted away from muscle and skin during low-flow states, subcutaneous and intramuscular medications should not be given. For the administration of medications, peripheral veins rather than internal jugular or subclavian sites should be used because their use does not cause any interruption of CPR [19]. The use of either a peripheral or central vein, however, is preferred in all cases to intracardiac injection [1, 19]. Because it is not always possible to maintain strict asepsis during an emergency, an unsterile catheter should be removed after a new sterile venipuncture has been started (and the patient's condition has been stabilized).

INTRAVENOUS INFUSION OF DRUGS

All intravenous drugs must be administered cautiously to critically ill patients. Most drugs are diluted in a 5% dextrose in water solution unless contraindicated, or they are given undiluted in a bolus form. Diluted medications should always be infused using a microdrip administration chamber (60 drops = 1 ml) and an infusion pump to ensure absolute control of the administration rate.

Drugs Used During CPR and ECC

Intravenous drugs are administered to most patients who receive CPR. Drugs used in ALS are divided into two groups: (1) drugs used during CPR and ECC and (2) drugs used after CPR [1]. Drugs in group 1 include oxygen, sodium bicarbonate, epinephrine, calcium, atropine, lidocaine, procainamide, bretylium, and morphine (Table 18-9).

OXYGEN THERAPY

Oxygen therapy is considered essential to CPR and ECC. Supplemental oxygen is administered as soon as it is available to any patient suffering a cardiopulmonary arrest or suffering from a cardiac emergency (see Oxygen Therapy under the head Adjuncts for Airway and Breathing).

SODIUM BICARBONATE

Anaerobic metabolism is caused by a lack of oxygen that results in the formation of lactic acid, producing metabolic acidosis during a cardiopulmonary arrest.

Respiratory failure leads to the retention of carbon dioxide (hypercarbia), producing a respiratory acidosis. Acidosis decreases the electrical threshold required to produce ventricular fibrillation. Moreover, it decreases ventricular contractility and cardiac responsiveness to catecholamines.

The treatment of choice for respiratory acidosis is prompt and effective ventilation. The administration of sodium bicarbonate ($NaHCO_3$), on the other hand, is used to combat the metabolic acidosis generated during anaerobic metabolism. Initially, the dosage of 1 mEq/kg $NaHCO_3$ is given. Subsequent doses are determined according to the results of blood gas determinations. When arterial blood gas and pH measurements are not readily available, one-half the initial dose or one-half mEq/kg is administered at 10-minute intervals. If a precordial thump or defibrillation is successful in reviving the patient in less than one to two minutes, the administration of $NaHCO_3$ is not necessary [14].

An intravenous bolus injection of $NaHCO_3$ is the preferred method of administration. Continuous intravenous infusion is not recommended because the dosage is difficult to regulate. Also, a continuous infusion will inactivate the effects of catecholamines or calcium salts if the drugs are administered simultaneously [1, 19].

Excessive $NaHCO_3$ therapy results in metabolic alkalosis, hypernatremia, hyperosmolality, and a reduced oxygen uptake by the tissues [19]. Metabolic alkalosis can be just as lethal as acidosis. Those complications can be avoided by carefully calculating the dosage of $NaHCO_3$, based on body weight, observing the frequency of administration, and assessing blood gas and pH measurements (see Acid-Base Balance).

EPINEPHRINE

Epinephrine (Adrenalin) is an endogenous catecholamine that stimulates both alpha- and beta-adrenergic receptor sites. Its positive inotropic effect increases myocardial contractility. Its positive chronotropic effect increases automaticity and heart rate. Its vasoactive effect elevates perfusion pressure during external cardiac compression, which may enhance coronary blood flow. Systemic vascular resistance and blood pressure are increased [53]. Electrical defibrillation is frequently more successful when epinephrine is administered beforehand to convert a fine ventricular fibrillation into a coarse one. Although epinephrine has been found experimentally to produce ventricular fibrillation, it may be useful in restoring electrical activity during asystole [19].

The dosage of 0.5 to 1 mg (5–10 ml of a 1:10,000 solution) is given intravenously and repeated at five-minute intervals during CPR. (One mg of a 1:1000 solution should be diluted in 9 ml of saline solution.) An intracardiac injection of epinephrine is given only if an intravenous lifeline has not been established. Intracardiac injections have many potential hazards, such as coronary artery laceration, cardiac tamponade, interruption of CPR, pneumothorax, and intramyocardial injection (which may produce intractable ventricular fibrillation). Because of those dangers, the intravenous administration of epinephrine is recommended. Epinephrine can also be directly injected into the endotracheal tube (10 ml of a 1:10,000 solution) where absorption from the lungs is rapid [1, 19]. Epinephrine must not be added directly to a continuous $NaHCO_3$ infusion because catecholamines are inactivated by an alkaline medium.

CALCIUM

Although the exact role of calcium is not understood, it is known to increase myocardial contractility [13]. It is a useful drug in electromechanical dissociation, which is characterized by an orderly electrical cardiac rhythm but an inadequate mechanical ejection or stroke volume. Calcium enhances ventricular excitability and is used to stimulate electrical activity in ventricular standstill [1, 19].

Calcium chloride is administered intravenously in a dose of 5 to 7 mg/kg that is repeated at 10-minute intervals. Calcium chloride contains 1.36 mEq Ca^{++} per 100 mg of salt (100 mg = 1 ml) in a 10% solution. Calcium gluconate provides less ionizable calcium per unit volume and is given in a dose of 10 ml (4.8 mEq Ca^{++}); or calcium gluceptate is given as 5 ml (4.5 mEq Ca^{++}).

The rapid administration of calcium can suppress sinoatrial node activity, resulting in sinus bradycardia or sinus arrest. It must be used carefully in the fully digitalized patient. Because calcium salts precipitate when administered with $NaHCO_3$, those drugs should never be administered simultaneously.

ATROPINE SULFATE

Atropine sulfate is a parasympatholytic drug. Its cardiac action reduces the effects of vagal stimulation, accelerating discharge from the sinoatrial node and thereby increasing the heart rate. Acceleration of a slow heart rate augments cardiac output and reduces the incidence of ventricular fibrillation secondary to ventricular ectopic activity. Atropine is indicated for the treatment of a symptomatic sinus bradycardia when associated with ventricular ectopic activity, or a systolic blood pressure of less than 90 mm Hg [19]. The cardiac vagolytic effects of atropine also improve atrioventricular conduction and may be indicated for patients who have a high-degree atrioventricular block with a slow ventricular response. The recommended dosage of atropine is 0.5 mg given intravenously at five-minute intervals to achieve the desired heart rate. It should be diluted in saline solution and given slowly over a period of several minutes while its effects are observed on the cardiac monitor. The total dosage should not exceed 2 mg [43].

Heart rate is an important determinant of myocardial oxygen consumption. Accelerating the heart rate in a patient suspected of having myocardial infarction or ischemia can produce a rise in myocardial oxygen demand that may be disproportionate to the available myocardial oxygen supply. The area of infarct may thereby extend or the ischemia may increase. Atropine has also been found to produce ventricular tachycardia and fibrillation [19]. It must always be administered with caution.

LIDOCAINE HYDROCHLORIDE

Lidocaine hydrochloride (Xylocaine) is an antidysrhythmic drug that is most useful in the suppression of ventricular dysrhythmias. At therapeutic blood levels, it raises the ventricular fibrillatory threshold (resulting in a need for more current to provoke ventricular fibrillation). It ordinarily has no significant effect on myocardial contractility, systemic arterial pressure, or atrioventricular conduction. It is particularly effective in controlling ventricular ectopic activity, such as frequent (i.e., occurring more often than five times per minute) premature ventricular contractions (PVCs), PVCs on T waves (the R-on-T phenomenon), multifocal PVCs, or runs of two or more PVCs. It is indicated for ventricular tachycardia or ventricular fibrillation, especially when it repeatedly occurs after defibrillation.

Lidocaine is administered as a 50- to 100-mg intravenous bolus (approximately 1 mg/kg) and repeated every three to five minutes to suppress the dys-

Table 18-9
Drugs Used During CPR and ECC

Drug	Actions	Indications	Dosage and Administration	Adverse Effects	Special Considerations
Oxygen	Elevates arterial O_2 Improves tissue oxygenation	Chest pain (cardiac emergency) Cardiac arrest	Administration of 100% O_2. Mask/nasal cannula at 4–6 Lpm. Positive pressure ventilation devices at 8–10 Lpm	No adverse effects with short-term use during CPR. Patients with COPD may need assisted ventilation	
Sodium bicarbonate	Raises serum pH Combats acidosis	Metabolic acidosis	1 mEq/kg IV push followed by blood gas analyses; or 1 mEq/kg IV push followed by 0.5 mEq/kg IV push every 10 min	Metabolic alkalosis Hypernatremia Hyperosmolality Reduced O_2 tissue uptake	Should not be administered as a continuous intravenous infusion Inactivates catecholamines or calcium salts if administered simultaneously
Epinephrine (Adrenalin)	Increases myocardial contractility, automaticity, and heart rate Increases arterial pressure	Asystole Fine ventricular fibrillation	0.5–1 mg (5–10 ml of a 1 : 10,000 solution) given IV and repeated every 5 min 1 mg (10 ml of a 1 : 10,000 solution) given by tracheobronchial injection	Ventricular fibrillation	Should not be given in an alkaline solution Should not be given by intracardiac injection if IV line is already established
Calcium	Increases myocardial contractility Enhances ventricular excitability	Electromechanical dissociation Ventricular standstill	Calcium chloride: 5–7 mg/kg of a 10% solution IV Calcium gluconate: 10 ml IV (4.8 mEq Ca⁺⁺) Calcium gluceptate: 5 ml IV (4.5 mEq Ca⁺⁺) Calcium may be repeated at 10-min intervals as necessary	Sinus bradycardia Sinus arrest	Use cautiously for the fully digitalized patient Calcium salts will precipitate if administered with $NaHCO_3$
Atropine sulfate	Blocks vagal stimulation Increases heart rate Improves atrioventricular node conduction	Symptomatic bradycardia associated with a systolic blood pressure of less than 90 mm Hg or with ventricular ectopic activity High-degree atrioventricular block associated with a slow ventricular response	0.5 mg diluted in a saline solution given slowly at 5-min intervals Total dosage should not exceed 2 mg	Ventricular tachycardia or ventricular fibrillation Increasing heart rate may increase myocardial O_2 consumption, resulting in extension of myocardial infarction or ischemia Small doses may slow heart rate	Continuous cardiac monitoring needed Use cautiously for patients with acute myocardial infarction

Drug	Action	Indications	Dosage	Side effects	Nursing considerations
Lidocaine hydrochloride (Xylocaine)	Suppresses ventricular dysrhythmias Raises ventricular fibrillatory threshold	Ventricular ectopic activity Frequent PVCs (more than 5/min) PVCs on T wave (R-on-T phenomenon) Multifocal PVCs Sequential or paired PVCs Ventricular tachycardia Ventricular fibrillation Acute myocardial infarction (prophylactic use)	50–100 mg IV bolus every 3–5 min; total dosage not to exceed 225 mg Following IV bolus, IV drip of 1–2 gm in 250–500 ml of a 5% dextrose in water solution (4 mg/ml) titrated at rate of 1–4 mg/min	Myocardial and circulatory depression Drowsiness Disorientation Hearing loss Paresthesias Agitation Muscle fasciculations Seizures Heart block	One-half the usual dose is used for patients with impaired hepatic function or documented renal disease Observe patient closely for toxic and therapeutic effects
Procainamide hydrochloride (Pronestyl)	Decrease cardiac excitability Slows cardiac conduction	Ventricular tachycardia Ventricular fibrillation PVCs Supraventricular dysrhythmias	100 mg/5 min IV: dilute 1 gm in 125 ml of a 5% dextrose in water solution (8 mg/ml) administered slowly at 20 mg/min. Total dosage should not exceed 1 gm Maintenance dose is 1–4 mg/min: 500 mg diluted in 250 ml of a 5% dextrose in water solution (2 mg/ml)	Hypotension Widening of QRS complex and PR or QT interval Heart block and asystole	Continuous blood pressure monitoring needed Continuous cardiac monitoring needed Use cautiously for patients with acute myocardial infarction
Bretylium tosylate (Bretylol)	Initially releases norepinephrine; adrenergic blockade follows Increases duration of action potential and prolongs refractory period of normal ventricular muscle and Purkinje fibers Raises ventricular fibrillatory threshold Suppresses ventricular ectopic activity	Ventricular fibrillation resistant to defibrillation and first-line antidysrhythmic drugs (drug administered and patient then defibrillated) Ventricular tachycardia and other ventricular dysrhythmias resistant to first-line antidysrhythmic drugs	For ventricular fibrillation: 5 mg/kg IV undiluted, then 10 mg/kg at 15–30 min intervals. Dosage not to exceed 30 mg/kg For ventricular tachycardia: 500 mg diluted in 50 ml of a 5% dextrose in water solution given at dosage of 5–10 mg/kg IV for 8–10 min Maintenance dose: 1–2 mg/min IV (500 mg diluted in 250 ml of a 5% dextrose in water solution to achieve 2 mg/ml)	Initial effects Transient hypertension Increase in heart rate Increase in PVCs or other dysrhythmias Subsequent effects Hypotension Bradycardia Nausea and vomiting	Continuous blood pressure monitoring needed Continuous cardiac monitoring needed Patient should remain supine Enhances effects of catecholamines Dose diluted for patients with renal impairment Contraindicated for patients with digitalis intoxication or a fixed cardiac output
Morphine sulfate	Is an effective analgesic Pools venous blood Reduces venous return Lowers systemic vascular resistance Reduces left ventricular afterload Reduces myocardial oxygen consumption	Pain associated with acute myocardial infarction Pulmonary edema	2–5 mg diluted in a saline solution and given IV every 5–30 min	Respiratory depression Hypotension	

Key: COPD = chronic obstructive pulmonary disease; Lpm = liters per minute.

rhythmia. The total dosage should not exceed 225 mg. Because the suppressive effects of the lidocaine bolus begin almost immediately but last only for 15 to 20 minutes, a lidocaine drip must always follow a bolus injection. A lidocaine drip, infused at 1 to 4 mg per minute, is prepared by adding 1 gm of lidocaine to 250 ml of a 5% dextrose in water solution or 2 gm to 500 ml (4 mg/ml). The drip reaches therapeutic blood levels 15 to 20 minutes after it is begun. It is decreased gradually—over the next 24 hours if possible.

After a myocardial infarction, lidocaine may be effective prophylactically in reducing the incidence of primary ventricular fibrillation [32]. Thus the drug is useful in both the prevention and treatment of life-threatening ventricular dysrhythmias.

The toxic effects of lidocaine include myocardial and circulatory depression, drowsiness, disorientation, hearing loss, paresthesias, agitation, muscle fasciculations, and focal or grand mal seizures. The treatment for lidocaine intoxication consists of withdrawing the drug and administering diazepam or a central nervous system depressant to control the seizures.

Because lidocaine undergoes hepatic degradation, the dosage must be reduced by one-half when hepatic function is impaired (e.g., in hepatic cirrhosis) and when hepatic blood flow is reduced because of a fall in cardiac output associated with hypovolemic shock, myocardial infarction, or congestive heart failure [19]. Care should be taken when the administration of lidocaine is prolonged for patients with documented renal disease. Occasionally lidocaine has been observed to produce heart blocks or depression of the sinoatrial node when used in large doses [18].

PROCAINAMIDE HYDROCHLORIDE

Procainamide hydrochloride (Pronestyl) is an antidysrhythmic drug that depresses the excitability of cardiac muscle and slows conduction in the atrium, bundle of His, and ventricles [1]. It is generally used for the treatment of ventricular tachycardia, ventricular fibrillation, and PVCs that cannot be suppressed with lidocaine [26], and it is occasionally used for the treatment of supraventricular dysrhythmias that are resistant to quinidine. It generally does not depress myocardial contractility.

One hundred mg is administered every five minutes at a rate of 20 mg per minute until the dysrhythmia is suppressed or until toxic effects are observed. (One thousand mg of the drug should be diluted in 125 ml of a 5% dextrose in water solution to

achieve a concentration of 8 mg/ml.) The total dosage should not exceed 1 gm. The maintenance dosage is 1 to 4 mg per minute. (Five hundred mg procainamide should be added to 250 ml of a 5% dextrose in water solution for a final concentration of 2 mg/ml.) Careful ECG and blood pressure monitoring is necessary to detect acute episodes of hypotension or conduction disturbances (i.e., QRS widening by 50 percent of its original length, lengthening of the PR or QT interval, or heart block). Procainamide must be administered carefully in patients with acute myocardial infarction.

BRETYLIUM TOSYLATE

Bretylium tosylate (Bretylol), an antifibrillatory and antidysrhythmic drug, acts on both adrenergic nerve endings and myocardial muscle. When bretylium is administered, adrenergic activity is altered by two opposing mechanisms. The drug causes an initial release of norepinephrine from adrenergic nerve endings. After the initial release, bretylium blocks the release of norepinephrine from the postganglionic nerve endings. Thus bretylium causes first the release of catecholamines and then peripheral adrenergic blockade [11]. Bretylium also directly affects the myocardium by increasing the duration of the action potential and by prolonging the refractory period of normal ventricular muscle and Purkinje fibers.

The most important action of bretylium is its raising of the ventricular fibrillatory threshold. The principal indication for bretylium is ventricular fibrillation when that dysrhythmia has failed to respond both to repeated defibrillation attempts and to first-line antidysrhythmic drugs, such as lidocaine or procainamide. In that setting, bretylium may be extremely beneficial in terminating ventricular fibrillation by emergency defibrillation after the drug is given.

For recurrent ventricular fibrillation, undiluted bretylium is rapidly administered intravenously in the dosage of 5 mg/kg followed by defibrillation. If ventricular fibrillation continues, 10 mg/kg may be given and repeated at 15- to 30-minute intervals until the maximum dosage of 30 mg/kg has been given. For recurrent ventricular tachycardia or other ventricular dysrhythmias, 500 mg is diluted in a minimum of 50 ml of a 5% dextrose in water solution. The diluted solution is administered intravenously at a dosage of 5 to 10 mg/kg for eight to ten minutes. If the dysrhythmia recurs, a second dose may be given in one to two hours. The maintenance dosage of bretylium may be given by a constant intravenous infusion at 1 to 2 mg per minute. (Five hundred mg of bretylium should be diluted in 250 ml of a 5% dextrose in water solution to achieve a concentration of 2 mg/ml.)

The antifibrillatory action of bretylium is observed within minutes after intravenous injection; the antidysrhythmic effects may not be seen for several hours. The bretylium-induced release of norepinephrine may produce an initial rise in blood pressure, or it may cause transient hypertension shortly after the drug is given. The release of norepinephrine may also produce a positive inotropic effect on the heart, and it may increase heart rate, PVCs, or other dysrhythmias. Careful monitoring of the cardiac rhythm and the blood pressure is essential.

The subsequent adrenergic blocking action of bretylium usually results in hypotension although the mean arterial pressure does not usually fall by more than 20 mm Hg when the patient is in the recumbent position. The drug should not be given to a patient with a fixed cardiac output (i.e., a patient with severe pulmonary hypertension or severe aortic stenosis) since the reduction in peripheral vascular resistance (caused by the adrenergic blockade) without a compensatory increase in cardiac output can produce severe hypotension. If excessive hypotension is observed after administration of the drug, treatment with intravenous fluids and vasopressor drugs may be necessary. When dopamine, levarterenol, or another catecholamine is given, the catecholamine dosage must be decreased because bretylium enhances the effects of catecholamines.

Bretylium may aggravate digitalis intoxication; it should not be used when life-threatening dysrhythmias occur in a fully digitalized patient [37]. Since bretylium is excreted through the kidneys, it must be diluted when it is given to a patient with renal impairment. Nausea and vomiting occur when the drug is administered over a period of less than about eight minutes. Bretylium may be given intramuscularly, but not more than 5 ml should be given in one site. Also, the injection sites must be rotated, because repeated injection into the same area can cause necrosis of the tissue, vascular degeneration, and inflammatory changes.

MORPHINE SULFATE

Morphine sulfate is used to control the pain associated with acute myocardial infarction because its analgesic effect has been proved to surpass that of the other drugs available. Morphine sulfate is useful in the treatment of pulmonary edema because of its ability to increase venous capacitance, thereby peripherally pooling venous blood (pharmacological phlebotomy) and reducing venous return. Morphine also lowers systemic vascular resistance, reducing left ventricular afterload and myocardial oxygen consumption [19].

Morphine is titrated at frequent intervals in doses of 2 to 5 mg given intravenously every 5 to 30 minutes to achieve the desired therapeutic effects. It should be diluted in saline solution so that small increments can be administered safely and easily. Large bolus doses of morphine are dangerous; they may produce respiratory depression or hypotension.

Drugs Used After CPR

Besides the drugs used during CPR and ECC, a second group of medications is used to stabilize the patient after a cardiac arrest or to treat acute myocardial infarction. The drugs in group 2 are dopamine, levarterenol, metaraminol, dobutamine, and isoproterenol (which are sympathomimetic amines) and propranolol, sodium nitroprusside, nitroglycerin, digitalis, the corticosteroids, and the diuretics [1] (Table 18-10).

Most of the drugs in group 2 increase or decrease peripheral vascular resistance and/or change the inotropic or chronotropic status of the heart. In patients with severely impaired cardiac output, many of the drugs alter blood pressure and blood flow; they may be particularly useful in treating a patient with acute myocardial infarction, left or right ventricular failure, shock, or cardiac arrest.

To understand the actions of the sympathomimetic drugs, the nurse needs a working knowledge of the cardiovascular adrenergic receptor system. That system is discussed briefly in the following paragraphs.

CARDIOVASCULAR ADRENERGIC RECEPTOR SYSTEM

Sympathomimetic amines act on the adrenergic receptors found in the heart and blood vessels [2]. The adrenergic receptors are divided into two categories—the alpha-adrenergic receptors and the beta-adrenergic receptors. There are also some adrenergic receptors that respond only to dopamine; they are termed dopaminergic receptors.

When alpha-adrenergic receptors are stimulated (e.g., with norepinephrine), a peripheral arterial vaso-

Table 18-10
Useful Drugs After CPR

Drug	Actions	Indications	Dosage and Administration	Adverse Effects	Special Considerations
Dopamine hydrochloride (Intropin)	1–2 μg/kg/min: stimulates dopaminergic receptors to dilate renal and mesenteric arteries 2–10 μg/kg/min: stimulates beta-adrenergic receptors to increase myocardial contractility, cardiac output, and renal blood flow with no effect on heart rate or blood pressure More than 10 μg/kg/min: stimulates alpha-adrenergic receptors to increase peripheral vasoconstriction and thus elevate blood pressure More than 20 μg/kg/min: additional stimulation of alpha-adrenergic receptors causing vasoconstriction to reverse vasodilatation of renal and mesenteric arteries	Cardiogenic shock Hypotension	Initial dose 2–5 μg/kg/min: dilute 200 mg in 250 ml of a 5% dextrose in water solution (800 μg/ml) or 200 mg in 500 ml of a 5% dextrose in water solution (400 μg/ml) Dosage based on hemodynamic response	Tachydysrhythmias Ectopy Nausea and vomiting Angina pectoris Hypertension Hypotension with low doses Produces ischemic necrosis of superficial tissue with infiltration of peripheral catheter	Hypovolemia should be corrected before drug used Monitoring of intraarterial pressure, cardiac rhythm, pulmonary capillary wedge pressure, cardiac output, and urinary output needed Must be diluted for patients taking monoamine oxidase inhibitors Contraindicated for patients with pheochromocytomas, uncorrected tachydysrhythmias, or ventricular fibrillation Becomes inactivated in an alkaline solution Must be administered through a central line Phentolamine (Regitine), an alpha-adrenergic receptor–blocking drug, should be injected locally for peripheral infiltration Must be discontinued slowly
Levarterenol or norepinephrine (Levophed)	Causes peripheral vasoconstriction and thus elevates blood pressure Increases myocardial contractility	Peripheral vascular collapse producing hypotension Cardiogenic shock	2 ampules (16 mg) in 1 L of a 5% dextrose in water solution or 1 ampule (8 mg) in 500 ml of a 5% dextrose in water solution to produce a concentration of 16 μg/ml titrated IV to maintain a systolic pressure above 90 mm Hg	Hypertension Renal and mesenteric vasoconstriction Ventricular irritability Hypotension with abrupt withdrawal of therapy Ischemic necrosis of superficial tissue with infiltration of peripheral catheter	Hypovolemia should be corrected before drug used Continuous intraarterial pressure monitoring needed Continuous cardiac monitoring needed Must be administered through a central line Must be diluted for patients taking monoamine oxidase inhibitors

					Use with caution for patients with myocardial ischemia or infarction Phentolamine (Regitine), an alpha-adrenergic receptor–blocking drug, should be injected locally for peripheral infiltration Must be discontinued slowly
Metaraminol bitartrate (Aramine)	Releases endogenous catecholamines Increases blood pressure and cardiac output	Peripheral vascular collapse producing hypotension Cardiogenic shock	4 ampules containing 400 mg in 1 L of a 5% dextrose in water solution (400 µg/ml) or 400 mg in 500 ml of a 5% dextrose in water solution (800 µg/ml) titrated IV to maintain blood pressure	Hypertension Ventricular irritability	Hypovolemia should be corrected before drug used Continuous intraarterial pressure monitoring needed Continuous cardiac monitoring needed Effects of drug reduced in patients with chronic heart failure or in those taking guanethidine or reserpine Should be used cautiously for patients taking monoamine oxidase inhibitors Effects of drug not observed for 10 min after administration Must be discontinued slowly
Dobutamine hydrochloride (Dobutrex)	Increases myocardial contractility and cardiac output Reduces ventricular diastolic pressure Enhances sinoatrial node automaticity and atrioventricular node and intraventricular conduction	Heart failure without severe hypotension	2.5–10 µg/kg/min: dilute 250 mg in 500 ml of a 5% dextrose in water solution (500 µg/ml) Dosage based on hemodynamic response	Dysrhythmias Ventricular ectopic activity Tachycardia Hypertension	Hypovolemia should be corrected before drug used Monitoring of blood pressure, cardiac rhythm, pulmonary capillary wedge pressure, cardiac output, and urine output needed Becomes inactivated in an alkaline solution Use with caution for patients with atrial fibrillation Not effective for patients with a fixed cardiac output or for patients taking beta-adrenergic receptor–blocking drugs

Table 18-10 (Continued)

Drug	Actions	Indications	Dosage and Administration	Adverse Effects	Special Considerations
Isoproterenol hydrochloride (Isuprel)	Increases myocardial contractility, heart rate, and O_2 consumption Increases cardiac output Increases systolic pressure Increases venous return Increases myocardial irritability	Symptomatic bradycardias due to heart block or bradycardias resistant to atropine	1 mg in 500 ml of a 5% dextrose in water solution (2 μg/ml) or 1 mg in 250 ml of a 5% dextrose in water solution (4 μg/ml) titrated at 2–20 μg/min to achieve the desired heart rate	Ventricular dysrhythmias Tachydysrhythmias Extension of myocardial infarction or ischemia	Continuous cardiac monitoring needed Should not be used for patients with tachydysrhythmias Use with caution for patients with hypokalemia, acute myocardial infarction or ischemia, or digitalis intoxication
Propranolol hydrochloride (Inderal)	Blocks beta-adrenergic receptor sites Reduces automaticity to cause sinoatrial node slowing Reduces conduction velocity and increases refractory period of atrioventricular node Depresses myocardial excitability Reduces myocardial contractility and cardiac output Reduces myocardial O_2 consumption Lowers blood pressure	Ventricular dysrhythmias refractory to other antidysrhythmic drugs Tachydysrhythmias due to digitalis intoxication or associated with Wolff-Parkinson-White syndrome	1 mg diluted in 10 ml of a 5% dextrose in water solution given IV at 5-min intervals not to exceed a total of 3–5 mg	Hypotension Bradydysrhythmias Asystole Cardiac decompensation	Continuous cardiac monitoring needed Continuous blood pressure monitoring needed Contraindicated for patients with COPD, asthma, atrioventricular block, sinus bradycardia, congestive heart failure, or cardiogenic shock
Sodium nitroprusside (Nipride)	Dilates venous capacitance (reduces preload) Reduces arterial resistance and outflow impedance (reduces afterload) Increases cardiac output Reduces left ventricular filling pressure Reduces myocardial O_2 consumption	Left ventricular failure, refractory congestive heart failure, hypertensive crisis, pulmonary edema	15–400 μg/min; average dosage 50 μg/min; dilute 50 mg in 2–3 ml of a 5% dextrose in water solution. Add solution to 250 ml of a 5% dextrose in water solution (200 μg/ml) or 500 ml of a 5% dextrose in water solution (100 μg/ml) Dosage based on hemodynamic response	Hypotension Nausea and vomiting Diaphoresis Apprehension Restlessness Muscle twitching	Hypovolemia and anemia should be corrected before drug used Monitoring of intraarterial blood pressure, cardiac rhythm, pulmonary capillary wedge pressure, cardiac output, and urinary output needed Wrap bottle in aluminum foil or paper bag Replace solution every 4 hr Do not add other medications to solution Use with caution for patients with hepatic insufficiency Observe patient for thiocyanate intoxication with prolonged infusion

Nitroglycerin (glyceryl trinitrate)	Dilates venous capacitance (reduces preload) Reduces outflow impedance and arterial resistance (reduces afterload) Reduces myocardial oxygen consumption	Angina pectoris Left ventricular failure Pulmonary edema	One tablet sublingually Repeat at 3–5 min intervals	Headache Hypotension Faintness Syncope	Continuous cardiac and blood pressure monitoring needed for critically ill patient
Digitalis (Digoxin, Lanoxin)	Increases myocardial contractility and cardiac output Slows atrioventricular conduction to reduce ventricular rate	Congestive heart failure Atrial fibrillation Atrial flutter Supraventricular tachydysrhythmias	IV loading dose: 1 mg, followed by 0.25 mg orally (or IV) in 4–6 hours for 2–3 doses Oral loading dose: 2–2.5 mg in 48 hours Maintenance dose: 0.125–0.25 mg/day	Noncardiac effects Nausea Vomiting Anorexia Diarrhea Yellow or blurred vision Mental confusion Cardiac effects Frequent premature beats Significant regular or irregular increase or decrease in heart rate Any form of atrioventricular heart block Almost any type of dysrhythmia	Electrolyte monitoring needed For intoxicated patients Continuous cardiac monitoring needed Potassium chloride (if patient hypokalemic) Antidysrhythmic drugs needed Artificial cardiac pacing needed Cardioversion needed (low energy levels) Dosage reduced for patients with hypothyroidism, severe respiratory disease, and hepatic or renal insufficiency
Corticosteroids	Stabilizes lysosomal membranes Prevents release of histamine and bradykinin Prevents lactate accumulation	Cardiogenic shock Adult respiratory distress syndrome Cerebral edema following cardiac arrest	Methylprednisolone (Solu-Medrol): 60–100 mg IV for cerebral edema following cardiac arrest Dexamethasone (Decadron): 12–20 mg IV for cerebral edema following cardiac arrest Repeat dose every 6 hours	Adverse effects with short-term use are rare Adverse effects with long-term use include Peptic ulcer Aggravation of diabetes mellitus Hypernatremia Hypervolemia Hypokalemia Hypotension Masking of infection	
Furosemide (Lasix) Ethacrynic acid (Edecrin)	Inhibits reabsorption of sodium, chloride, and potassium	Cerebral edema following cardiac arrest Acute pulmonary edema	Furosemide: 0.5–1.9 mg/kg IV for 1–2 min (in 10–20 ml saline solution) Ethacrynic acid: 40–50 mg IV for 1–2 min (in 10–20 ml saline solution)	Hypokalemia (causing dysrhythmias) Circulatory collapse due to dehydration and blood volume depletion Alkalosis	Monitoring of serum potassium level needed; patient must be watched for signs and symptoms of hypokalemia Potassium replacement therapy given as needed Monitoring of urinary output and blood pressure needed

Key: CODP = chronic obstructive pulmonary disease.

constriction occurs. There are two types of beta-adrenergic receptors—cardiac beta (β_1) receptors and peripheral beta (β_2) receptors. Stimulation of β_1 receptors (e.g., with isoproterenol) causes an increase in myocardial contractility, heart rate, and atrioventricular node conduction. Stimulation of β_2 receptors (e.g., with isoproterenol) causes vasodilatation of systemic arteries and bronchodilatation in the lungs, effects that are opposite to those of alpha-adrenergic receptor stimulation. The coronary arteries possess both alpha- and beta-adrenergic receptors. The dopaminergic receptors that are stimulated by low doses of dopamine have a vasodilating effect on the renal, mesenteric, coronary, and intracerebral beds that results in increased blood flow [31].

The net effect of any of the sympathomimetic amines depends on their dominant receptor activity and, in some cases, on the dosage of the drug administered.

DOPAMINE HYDROCHLORIDE

Dopamine hydrochloride (Intropin), a precursor of norepinephrine, stimulates both alpha- and beta-adrenergic receptors. The primary indication for the use of dopamine is cardiogenic shock. Its actions, which are unlike those of epinephrine or norepinephrine, depend on the dosage and on the patient's response [29]. In low doses (1–2 μg/kg/min), dopamine has the unique property of stimulating dopaminergic receptors, causing vasodilatation of the renal beds. At doses of 2 to 10 μg/kg/min, dopamine has a beta-adrenergic receptor–stimulating effect, increasing cardiac contractility, cardiac output, and renal blood flow without affecting heart rate or blood pressure. When given at even higher doses (more than 10 μg/kg/min), it has an alpha-adrenergic receptor–stimulating effect that increases blood pressure as a result of peripheral vasoconstriction. Doses above 20 μg/kg/min reduce renal and mesenteric blood flow and may cause the urinary output to drop [19].

Dopamine is given intravenously by diluting 200 mg in 500 ml of a 5% dextrose in water solution to produce a concentration of 400 μg/ml (or 200 mg in 250 ml of a 5% dextrose in water solution to produce a concentration of 800 μg/ml). The initial dose of dopamine is 2 to 5 μg/kg/min. Doses of up to 50 μg/kg/min have been used occasionally. The hemodynamic response is best determined while titrating the drug by monitoring the patient's blood pressure, heart rate, cardiac rhythm, pulmonary capillary wedge pressure, cardiac output, and urinary output. When an optimal hemodynamic response has been achieved, the drug must be discontinued slowly.

The adverse effects of dopamine include tachydysrhythmias, ectopy, nausea, vomiting, and angina pectoris. Severe vasoconstriction may result from extremely high doses. Blood pressure is occasionally reduced because of the vasodilating effect of small doses. Hypovolemia must be fully corrected before treatment with dopamine. Dopamine is metabolized by the enzyme monoamine oxidase. If the enzyme is inhibited, the effects of dopamine are enhanced and prolonged. Thus a patient taking monoamine oxidase (MAO) inhibitors should receive one-tenth the usual dose of dopamine. Dopamine is contraindicated in a patient with a pheochromocytoma because the release of catecholamines may cause acute hypertension. It is also contraindicated in a patient with an uncorrected tachydysrhythmia or ventricular fibrillation. It is inactivated in an alkaline solution and thus should not be diluted with $NaHCO_3$ or other alkaline solutions.

Dopamine should be infused through a central line to prevent its extravasation into tissue near the infusion site. Extravasation may cause necrosis and sloughing of adjacent tissue. If extravasation of the drug occurs in a peripheral venous line, phentolamine (Regitine), an alpha-adrenergic receptor–blocking drug must be used immediately (5–10 mg of phentolamine diluted in 10–15 ml of a normal saline solution). Phentolamine is injected locally around the infiltrated area with a small-bore needle to reduce the amount of skin necrosis produced by the severe vasoconstrictive effects of dopamine.

LEVARTERENOL BITARTRATE

Levarterenol bitartrate (norepinephrine, Levophed) is an endogenous catecholamine whose actions resemble those of epinephrine. The major action of levarterenol is related to its alpha-adrenergic receptor stimulating effect, which causes peripheral vasoconstriction and elevation of blood pressure. Its beta-adrenergic receptor stimulating effect has a powerful inotropic action on the cardiac muscle. Levarterenol produces dilatation of the coronary arteries and raises perfusion pressure to augment coronary blood flow.

Because the major action of levarterenol is on blood vessels while it affects the heart only indirectly, restoring the blood pressure generally produces a rise in cardiac output. Levarterenol is indicated for the patient in cardiogenic shock or with peripheral vascular collapse that has produced hypotension without severe peripheral vasoconstriction. Levarterenol produces an elevation in blood pressure slightly more rapidly than do the other catecholamines, including dopamine.

Levarterenol is given as a continuous intravenous solution. Two ampules (8 ml) containing a total of 16 mg of levarterenol bitartrate (8-mg levarterenol base) are diluted in a liter of a 5% dextrose in water solution (or one ampule [4 ml] containing 8 mg of levarterenol bitartrate [4 mg levarterenol base] is diluted in 500 ml of a 5% dextrose in water solution) to provide a concentration of 16 μg/ml. The drug is titrated intravenously after a cardiac arrest to establish and maintain a blood pressure usually above 90 mm Hg.

Because of the need for accurate arterial blood pressure measurement, an intraarterial line should be inserted for continuous monitoring of the blood pressure [15]. The blood pressure is measured every two to five minutes, and the levarterenol infusion is titrated accordingly. If the blood pressure is elevated to unnecessarily high levels, cardiac output and heart rate may drop. Cardiac monitoring is indicated to detect rhythm disturbances. Hypovolemia must be corrected before administration of levarterenol. Myocardial oxygen consumption may be increased because of the inotropic effects of the drug. Renal and mesenteric vasoconstriction are major adverse effects of levarterenol.

Levarterenol must be used carefully in the patient with acute myocardial infarction or in a patient receiving MAO inhibitors. Levarterenol may be used for several days, but the dosage must be tapered before the drug is discontinued. Severe hypotension may result if the drug is stopped abruptly. Because of its vasoconstrictive effects, levarterenol can cause ischemic necrosis and sloughing of superficial tissue if the catheter is allowed to infiltrate. For that reason, a central line must be used to administer the drug. If extravasation of the drug occurs in a peripheral venous line, phentolamine must be injected immediately (see Dopamine Hydrochloride).

METARAMINOL BITARTRATE

Metaraminol bitartrate (Aramine) is a strong sympathomimetic drug that is useful in the treatment of peripheral vascular collapse that has produced hypotension without impressive peripheral vasocon-

striction [3]. It stimulates both alpha-adrenergic and beta-adrenergic receptors. Its major pressor action is produced by the indirect release of endogenous catecholamines. It elevates blood pressure and cardiac output.

Metaraminol is administered by a continuous intravenous infusion of 400 mg in a liter of a 5% dextrose in water solution to produce a concentration of 400 μg/ml, and it is titrated according to the response in blood pressure. The effects of metaraminol are reduced when endogenous catecholamine stores are depleted, as in patients with chronic heart failure or those receiving guanethidine or reserpine. It must be used carefully in patients on MAO inhibitors. The patient must be monitored closely to avoid unnecessary elevation of blood pressure. Patients are placed on a cardiac monitor so that they can be observed for the development of ventricular irritability. Metaraminol should not be used in cases of hypotension associated with volume depletion.

DOBUTAMINE HYDROCHLORIDE

Dobutamine hydrochloride (Dobutrex) is a synthetic catecholamine that chemically resembles isoproterenol. Dobutamine acts directly on the beta-adrenergic receptors in the myocardium but has only a slight effect on the beta-adrenergic receptors in the peripheral vasculature. When stimulating myocardial beta-adrenergic receptors, dobutamine exerts a more prominent inotropic than chronotropic effect. As a result, it primarily increases myocardial contractility and cardiac output while it reduces ventricular diastolic pressure [49]. Dobutamine enhances atrioventricular and intraventricular conduction and, to a lesser extent, it increases sinoatrial node automaticity. Only minor increases in heart rate occur when the drug is given in normal doses. The arterial pressure is not significantly affected; it tends to decrease slightly with high doses and to increase slightly with low doses. Dobutamine does not specifically affect the dopaminergic vasodilating receptors in the kidney although urinary output has been found to increase during administration of the drug to patients in heart failure [49].

Dobutamine is indicated for patients with heart failure that is not accompanied by severe hypotension and for patients with acute myocardial infarction complicated by heart failure [27, 49].

Like other catecholamines, dobutamine increases myocardial oxygen consumption because it increases myocardial contractility. In a patient with heart failure, however, dobutamine reduces left ventricular filling pressures, decreases heart size and left ventricular wall tension, and improves coronary blood flow, which results in reduced oxygen needs. The net effect is a reduction in myocardial oxygen demand [49]. The combination of nitroprusside and dobutamine results in a higher cardiac output and a lower pulmonary capillary wedge pressure than either drug used alone [41]. Dobutamine increases myocardial contractility and nitroprusside reduces peripheral vascular resistance to enhance ventricular function.

Dobutamine is administered intravenously by diluting 250 mg in 500 ml of a 5% dextrose in water solution to yield 500 μg/ml. The usual dose is titrated from 2.5 to 10 μg/kg/min. The hemodynamic response is evaluated by monitoring blood pressure, cardiac rhythm, urine output, pulmonary capillary wedge pressure, and cardiac output. In doses of greater than 20 μg/kg/min, dobutamine may produce tachycardia and dysrhythmias.

Hypovolemia must be corrected before the drug is given. Dobutamine may precipitate or increase ventricular ectopic activity. It must be used carefully in patients with atrial fibrillation because dobutamine improves atrioventricular conduction and may increase the ventricular response. Hypertension has been observed in some patients receiving the drug. When beta-adrenergic receptor blocking drugs are used in combination with dobutamine, dobutamine may be ineffective and may cause an alpha-adrenergic receptor–stimulating response and thus peripheral vascular constriction. Dobutamine is not effective for a patient with a fixed cardiac output. It is inactivated in an alkaline solution, and it should not be infused simultaneously with $NaHCO_3$.

ISOPROTERENOL HYDROCHLORIDE

Isoproterenol hydrochloride (Isuprel) is a potent sympathomimetic amine whose principal action is related to its beta-adrenergic receptor stimulation. Its chronotropic effects are more powerful than those of dobutamine. It increases sinoatrial node automaticity and atrioventricular node and intraventricular conduction. It augments cardiac output by increasing heart rate and myocardial contractility. It also increases venous return while it decreases peripheral vascular resistance. Diastolic pressure may fall, but

systolic pressure is usually increased because of the rise in cardiac output [19].

Isoproterenol is indicated for patients who have symptomatic bradycardias due to heart blocks, and it is useful for patients who have sinus bradycardias that are resistant to atropine [19]. Under those conditions, the drug is generally used only until artificial cardiac pacing can be achieved.

Isoproterenol is administered in a continuous infusion of 1 mg in 500 ml of a 5% dextrose in water solution (2 μg/ml) or 1 mg in 250 ml of a 5% dextrose in water solution (4 μg/ml). It is titrated at 2 to 20 μg/min to achieve the desired heart rate. Continuous cardiac monitoring is indicated to observe the rhythm response and to detect ventricular irritability.

Because its potent inotropic and chronotropic properties increase myocardial oxygen demand, isoproterenol can increase the degree of myocardial ischemia and necrosis. It can produce lethal ventricular dysrhythmias, and it is contraindicated in patients with existing tachydysrhythmias. It is used with extreme caution in patients with hypokalemia.

PROPRANOLOL HYDROCHLORIDE

Propranolol hydrochloride (Inderal) is a beta-adrenergic receptor blocking drug that works by competing with catecholamines for beta receptor sites [21]. Because it blocks the action of circulating catecholamines, it reduces pacemaker automaticity, and it produces a sinus slowing. Electrocardiographically, propranolol slows the ventricular rate, depresses ectopic foci, and may increase the amplitude of the T wave.

The drug also has a quinidinelike effect on atrial and ventricular muscles. It slows conduction velocity, increases the refractory period of the atrioventricular node, and depresses excitability. It has been found to be most useful in the treatment of atrial dysrhythmias and tachydysrhythmias associated with Wolff-Parkinson-White (WPW) syndrome or digitalis intoxication [19]. The drug is less successful in the treatment of ventricular dysrhythmias, but it is indicated when control has not been achieved with lidocaine or other drugs. Propranolol reduces myocardial contractility and myocardial oxygen consumption. It reduces blood pressure by decreasing cardiac output, lowering peripheral vascular resistance, and reducing plasma volume.

Propranolol is administered intravenously by

slowly giving 1 mg diluted in 10 ml of a 5% dextrose in water solution. The rate of infusion should not exceed 1 mg/5 min, and the total dosage should not be greater than 3 to 5 mg. The cardiac rhythm must be continuously monitored and the patient should be assessed for sudden episodes of hypotension, bradydysrhythmias, or asystole.

Because of its beta-adrenergic receptor-blocking effects, propranolol is contraindicated in patients with chronic obstructive lung disease, bronchial asthma, atrioventricular block, or sinus bradycardia. It can precipitate cardiac decompensation and should be avoided in patients with depressed myocardial function, which frequently occurs following cardiac arrest.

SODIUM NITROPRUSSIDE

Sodium nitroprusside (Nipride) is a potent vasodilator that relaxes both arterial and venous vessels. It dilates venous capacitance and thus produces venous pooling (reducing preload) and it reduces systemic arterial resistance and outflow impedance (reducing afterload).

Left ventricular function is directly affected by both preload and afterload [16]. The cardiac output response to nitroprusside depends on whether the drug affects primarily preload or outflow impedance. In the patient with a normal cardiac function, the effect of nitroprusside is primarily on preload. Because the ventricle is operating on the upslope of the Frank-Starling curve, venous pooling reduces venous return. Ventricular filling is reduced, resulting in a drop in cardiac output. The effect of reducing outflow impedance is minimal, however, because when the left ventricle is normal, decreasing arterial resistance does not increase left ventricular ejection nor does it augment ventricular stroke volume. Blood pressure is reduced in response to the vasodilatation. A reflex tachycardia occurs, increasing the cardiac output to minimize the drop in arterial pressure.

In patients with low output states due to depressed cardiac function, nitroprusside affects primarily outflow impedance. In the presence of severe ventricular disease, systolic emptying of the left ventricle is incomplete, and stroke volume is reduced because of increased outflow impedance. Nitroprusside reduces outflow impedance and systemic arterial resistance. When outflow impedance is reduced, a larger stroke volume can be ejected. Left ventricular emptying is enhanced, reducing left ventricular dia-

stolic pressure, wall tension, pulmonary pressure, and pulmonary congestion [30]. Stroke volume is increased, minimizing the reduction in blood pressure that might occur due to the vasodilating effects of nitroprusside. As a result, reflex tachycardia is not observed. Moreover, myocardial oxygen consumption is reduced because left ventricular end-diastolic pressure is reduced without increasing myocardial contractility or heart rate [44]. In contrast, the effect of nitroprusside on preload in the impaired left ventricle is minor. Decreasing preload by venous pooling has little or no effect on cardiac output because the patient is operating on the flat portion (plateau) of the Frank-Starling curve (i.e., increasing or decreasing filling to the left ventricle has no effect on stroke volume [16]). Nitroprusside is indicated primarily for patients with left ventricular failure, refractory heart failure, hypertensive crisis, and pulmonary edema [17]. To administer sodium nitroprusside, the contents of a 50-mg vial are dissolved in 2 to 3 ml of a 5% dextrose in water solution. No other diluent should be used. The dissolved mixture, which is amber in color, should be added to 500 ml of a 5% dextrose in water solution, yielding a concentration of 100 μg/ml (or 250 ml of a 5% dextrose in water solution, yielding a concentration of 200 μg/ml). The dosage ranges from 15 μg to 400 μg/min, with an average dosage of 50 μg/min.

Because nitroprusside is light sensitive, the bottle containing it must be wrapped with aluminum foil or covered with a paper bag. The solution should be replaced every 4 hours. No other medication should be added to the solution. The drug is titrated to obtain an optimal hemodynamic response. Cardiac rhythm, intraarterial blood pressure, pulmonary capillary wedge pressure, cardiac output, and urinary output should be monitored [59]. The goal of therapy is reducing the pulmonary capillary wedge pressure by 40 to 50 percent without allowing the arterial blood pressure to fall below 90 to 100 mm Hg. The drug begins to act in minutes. Because the duration of action is very brief, there is no need to wean the patient from the drug after his condition has become stable.

The principal adverse effect of nitroprusside is hypotension. Hypotension can be relieved by stopping the infusion and elevating the legs. Other adverse reactions are nausea, vomiting, diaphoresis, apprehension, restlessness, and muscle twitching. Anemia and hypovolemia should be corrected before infusion of the drug. Nitroprusside is metabolized to cyanide and then to thiocyanate. Excessive, prolonged nitroprusside infusion can cause thiocyanate intoxication, as evidenced by blurred vision, tinnitus, and delirium. Because cyanide is converted to thiocyanate by the hepatic enzyme rhodanese, nitroprusside must be used with caution in patients with hepatic insufficiency.

NITROGLYCERIN

A number of nitrates have been used to relax vascular smooth muscle. Nitroglycerin (glyceryl trinitrate [TNG]) has a more profound effect on the venous beds than on the arterial beds, causing venous pooling by increasing peripheral venous capacitance. Also, it causes a dilating effect on arteries, reducing systemic vascular resistance, particularly in patients with left ventricular failure. The more abnormal the function of the left ventricle, the greater the reduction in outflow impedance, resulting in a reduction in left ventricular end-diastolic volumes and an improvement of stroke volume and cardiac output [4]. The work of the myocardium is therefore reduced, causing a decreased myocardial oxygen demand. Reducing myocardial oxygen demand may explain why nitroglycerin is effective in the relief of angina pectoris [6]. An alternate explanation may be that nitroglycerin directly dilates coronary arteries and increases blood flow and thus favorably assists the balance between myocardial oxygen supply and demand.

Nitroglycerin is indicated for patients with angina pectoris, left ventricular failure, and pulmonary edema [17]. The intravenous use of nitroglycerin is still under investigation. One tablet is taken sublingually, and the dose is repeated at three- to five-minute intervals. If nitroglycerin is used for patients with heart failure in the setting of acute myocardial infarction, ECG and blood pressure monitoring are essential. Headache is a common side effect of the drug. Hypotension, faintness, or syncope may also occur.

DIGITALIS

Digitalis (Digoxin, Lanoxin), a cardiac glycoside, exerts a positive inotropic effect on the heart. It increases myocardial contractility, thereby increasing cardiac output. It also exerts a negative chronotropic effect, slowing atrioventricular node conduction to reduce the ventricular rate.

Digitalis is indicated for patients with congestive heart failure, and it is used to slow the heart rate of patients with atrial fibrillation, atrial flutter, and supraventricular tachydysrhythmias.

The intravenous loading dose of 1 mg is given slowly; it is followed by 0.25 mg orally (or intravenously) in four to six hours for two or three additional doses. The average oral loading dose is 2 mg to 2.5 mg in 48 hours. The maintenance dose is 0.125 to 0.25 mg per day.

The noncardiac toxic manifestations of digitalis are nausea, vomiting, anorexia, diarrhea, yellow or blurred vision, and mental confusion. Today those symptoms occur less frequently because the drug is now prepared in a purer form. The cardiac manifestations of digitalis intoxication are more common, and the nurse must be able to recognize them. The cardiac manifestations are frequent premature beats, a significant regular or irregular increase or decrease in heart rate, any kind of atrioventricular heart block, or almost any kind of dysrhythmia. When digitalis intoxication is suspected, the drug should be discontinued and the patient should be assessed carefully. Cardiac monitoring is essential. Further treatment of digitalis intoxication may include the administration of potassium chloride (especially if the patient is hypokalemic), diphenylhydantoin, lidocaine, procainamide, propranolol, artificial cardiac pacing, and cardioversion [22, 33, 38]. Administration of potassium to a patient who does not have a potassium deficit and who is in heart block due to digitalis excess may increase the degree of block. Patients who have atrial tachycardias or heart block caused by digitalis are not good candidates for cardioversion. If cardioversion is necessary in digitalis-intoxicated patients, low energy levels must be used.

Hypomagnesemia and hypercalcemia may also sensitize the heart to digitalis. Monitoring of the electrolyte and serum digitalis levels is important. The dosage of digitalis must be reduced in patients with hypothyroidism, severe respiratory disease, and liver or kidney disease.

THE CORTICOSTEROIDS

The use of corticosteroids for the treatment of shock and other medical problems is controversial. The glucocorticoids are believed to stabilize the lysosomal membranes, prevent the release of histamine and bradykinin, and prevent lactate accumulation [19]. Corticosteroids appear to be useful in patients with cardiogenic shock or adult respiratory distress syndrome associated with cardiac arrest. Methylprednisolone sodium succinate (Solu-Medrol) may be helpful following a cardiac arrest when cerebral edema is suspected.

Methylprednisolone is administered intravenously in doses of up to 5 to 30 mg/kg for cardiogenic shock or shock lung. For cerebral edema, methylprednisolone is given in doses of 60 to 100 mg, or dexamethasone sodium phosphate (Decadron) is given in doses of 12 to 20 mg, intravenously every six hours. The adverse effects of the drug include peptic ulcers, aggravation of diabetes mellitus, sodium and water retention, potassium and calcium excretion, hypotension, and masking of infection. Those problems, however, are relatively uncommon during short-term corticosteroid therapy.

FUROSEMIDE AND ETHACRYNIC ACID

Furosemide (Lasix) and ethacrynic acid (Edecrin) are potent diuretics that inhibit the reabsorption of sodium chloride, potassium, and ammonium ions in the proximal and distal tubules and loop of Henle. Their diuretic action begins within 5 minutes of administration, peaks at 30 minutes, and exerts its effects for two hours. The drugs are used in the management of pulmonary edema and cerebral edema following cardiac arrest [19].

To treat pulmonary or cerebral edema, intravenous furosemide is diluted and administered slowly in doses of 0.5 to 1.9 mg/kg for one to two minutes. Ethacrynic acid is given intravenously in doses of 40 to 50 mg.

Furosemide and ethacrynic acid are associated with circulatory collapse secondary to dehydration and blood volume depletion. Hypokalemia, a common complication, can cause lethal dysrhythmias. Potassium levels must be carefully monitored, especially in patients receiving digitalis or in those suffering from acute myocardial infarction.

Temporary Cardiac Pacing in Emergency Cardiac Care

Temporary cardiac pacing may be an important mode of therapy in a cardiac emergency. The indications for its use in an emergency are related to the development of life-threatening dysrhythmias. Drug therapy used to treat those acute problems, particularly complete atrioventricular block, is less reliable and successful than is artificial cardiac pacing. Cardiac pacing involves delivering an artificial stimulus to the heart to cause electrical depolarization and myocardial contraction.

HISTORY

For centuries, scientists and physicians have been interested in electrical stimulation of the myocardium. Most of the work done was directed toward cardiac arrest. Early experimentation was generally not accepted and was often ridiculed. In 1932, however, Hyman made the first device for myocardial stimulation [35]. He designed a magnogenerator, used as a power supply, to generate pacing pulses that were fed into the heart with a needle. The spring-wound motor was activated by a hand crank used to spin the generator. The apparatus was limited to short-term use because the machine had to be rewound every six minutes. Hyman conceived the device as a substitute for the nonfunctioning sinus pacemaker, and he coined the term artificial pacemaker. Twenty years later, Zoll [60] successfully treated two patients in ventricular standstill by using an artificial external pacemaker to restore and maintain cardiac activity (see Methods).

In the years that followed, improvements were made in the generator devices and pacemaker electrodes. In 1959, Furman and Robertson [25] reported that external cardiac pacing had been achieved by the use of a transvenous endocardial electrode inserted in the jugular vein and placed in the right atrium. One year later, the problem of an external pulse generator was solved by Chardack [10], who reported the first successful long-term use of a self-contained pacemaker inserted through a thoracotomy.

INDICATIONS

The primary indications for temporary cardiac pacing are atrioventricular block, certain atrioventricular conduction defects, and symptomatic bradydysrhythmias or tachydysrhythmias [3, 12]. Those rhythm disturbances may precede, follow, or occur during a cardiac arrest. As a result, temporary pacemakers are used prophylactically as well as therapeutically.

The most common indication for the insertion of a temporary pacemaker is complete atrioventricular block [57]. Complete block develops in 0.5% to 3.4% of patients suffering from acute myocardial infarction [50]. The mortality ranges from 40 to 100 percent in patients without artificial cardiac pacing [23].

Heart block results from congenital defects, or it can be surgically induced as a result of edema or inflammation around the atrioventricular node or bundle of His. It may also be caused by aortic or mitral valvular disease, and it can be linked to myocardial ischemia. Drugs such as digitalis, potassium, quinidine, and procainamide are known to produce atrioventricular block. Infections such as scarlet fever, influenza, measles, pneumonia, and tuberculosis have also been found to be causative factors. In the majority of cases, complete atrioventricular block is due to a sclerodegenerative disease that causes fibrosis of the peripheral bundle branches and their divisions [57].

Bilateral bundle branch block (BBBB) is commonly observed to occur before the development of complete heart block. A common BBBB is right bundle branch block (RBBB) in association with left anterior hemiblock (LAH). That bifascicular block maintains intraventricular conduction by means of the remaining left posterior fascicle of the left bundle. The posterior fascicle, however, can become blocked intermittently, producing a Mobitz type II second-degree atrioventricular block or spontaneous complete atrioventricular block. (Other types of BBBB are described in Chapter 10.) Depending on the situation, temporary cardiac pacing may be needed in the management of any of those conduction disturbances.

Bradydysrhythmias, which frequently are severe enough to produce a drastic reduction in cardiac output secondary to depressed cardiac rates, may require cardiac pacing. Reduced cardiac output can result in dizziness, syncope, ventricular irritability, and cerebral or tissue hypoxia. The bradydysrhythmias associated with sick sinus syndrome (Chap. 10) frequently produce rates below 60 beats per minute. Those dysrhythmias respond poorly to treatment with atropine or isoproterenol. In some cases of sinus arrest, sinus block, or sinus bradycardia, the dysrhythmia is transient and can be demonstrated only intermittently by continuous cardiac monitoring. Sinus bradycardias are commonly seen in patients with acute myocardial infarction, particularly an infarction involving the inferior or posterior wall [57].

Temporary cardiac pacing is occasionally indicated to overdrive, or suppress, atrial or ventricular tachydysrhythmias. Overdrive pacing is used to stimulate the myocardium at a rate above the patient's own intrinsic cardiac rhythm and thus suppress impulse formation [24]. Atrial overdrive pacing may be used to convert atrial flutter, supraventricular tachycardia, and tachycardias associated with Wolff-Parkinson-White syndrome to normal sinus rhythm.

Ventricular overdrive pacing may be useful in treating patients with refractory ventricular dysrhythmias. It is used, for example, to suppress an irritable ventricular focus, such as one that produces ventricular tachycardia or frequent PVCs. The overdrive pacing rate, however, does not need to be faster than the ectopic rate, and it may need to be only slightly faster than the normal sinus pacemaker.

METHODS

Temporary cardiac pacing is accomplished by one of four methods: (1) external pacing, (2) transthoracic pacing, (3) epicardial pacing, or (4) transvenous endocardial pacing.

External Cardiac Pacing

External cardiac pacing was developed in 1952 [60] to manage temporary and permanent heart blocks that arose as complications of open heart surgery. External pacing is accomplished by placing skin electrodes on the patient's precordium and repeatedly shocking him. The method is rarely used today because of the high voltage required to stimulate the myocardium successfully. The technique is also very painful for the conscious patient because it produces skin burns and skeletal muscle contractions.

Transthoracic Cardiac Pacing

Transthoracic cardiac pacing is a rapid procedure that is generally used only in emergencies [24]. A large-bore needle is inserted in the third to fourth intercostal space at the left sternal border to provide an entry into the right ventricle. A pacing wire is inserted through the needle and embedded in the ventricle. The needle is removed and the pacing wire is connected to a pulse generator (a temporary pacemaker). The procedure may be associated with severe complications, such as cardiac tamponade, coronary artery laceration, and pneumothorax.

Epicardial Pacing

Many cardiovascular surgeons insert epicardial pacing wires during open heart surgery prophylactically—to prevent dysrhythmias or conduction disturbances [58]. The wires are sewed loosely to the epicardium and can easily be connected to a pacemaker if postoperative dysrhythmias occur. The wires are easily removed by pulling them through the skin.

Transvenous Endocardial Pacing

Transvenous endocardial pacing is the method of cardiac pacing most commonly used [24]. The pacing wire is passed into the brachial, femoral, subclavian, or jugular vein by a percutaneous stick or by cutdown. The catheter wire is advanced through the vein, into the right atrium, and generally on through the tricuspid valve and embedded in the trabeculae of the right ventricle.

The transvenous endocardial pacing electrode is inserted with the guidance of fluoroscopic monitoring or ECG. Fluoroscopy is not recommended in the emergency situation because it usually involves moving the patient from the critical care area to an x-ray department or cardiac catheterization laboratory [48]. If portable fluoroscopy is not available, electrode placement under ECG control (blind pacemaker insertion) is a relatively rapid procedure that can be carried out at the patient's bedside [47, 48].

The first step in the blind insertion of a pacemaker involves attaching the patient to the limb leads of the ECG. An intravenous line must be in place, and a defibrillator and emergency cardiac drugs should be at the patient's bedside. A balloon-tipped catheter is inserted aseptically into the patient's vein. (The balloon on the catheter must be checked before it is inserted.) When the balloon is inflated, it causes the catheter to float with the venous blood into the right ventricle. After the catheter is inserted, the external end of the catheter is attached to lead V on the ECG with a wire that has two insulated alligator clamps. One clamp is attached to lead V. The other clamp is attached to the electrode on the external catheter that corresponds to the tip electrode (the distal end of the catheter inside the heart); it serves as the exploring electrode within the heart. The lead V selector switch on the ECG is turned on to provide an intracardiac ECG.

As the tip electrode approaches the right atrium, large negative P waves and small QRS complexes are recorded on the ECG. At that point, the balloon on the catheter is inflated to the recommended volume (usually 1.5 cc). As the tip electrode approaches the low right atrium, the P waves become positive and smaller than the QRS complexes. The catheter is passed through the tricuspid valve, and the balloon is deflated. When the catheter is in the right ventricle, a large rS deflection is observed on the ECG, with ST segment elevation as the tip electrode touches the endocardium, indicating good endocardial placement of the catheter [7]. The patient is disconnected from lead V, and the external catheter is connected to the pacemaker.

After the pacemaker settings have been chosen (see Pacemaker Settings), the catheter is sutured in place and the insertion site is covered with an antibiotic ointment and a sterile dressing. A posteroanterior chest x ray is taken to check for the presence of a pneumothorax or other possible complications of the catheter insertion. A lateral chest x ray is also taken to check the positioning of the catheter. If the catheter tip is in the right ventricular apex, it points anteriorly on the lateral chest x ray. But if the catheter is in the coronary sinus or has perforated the right ventricle, it points posteriorly, and it must be repositioned [7].

Right ventricular pacing is also assessed electrocardiographically by observing a wide QRS complex and left axis deviation with deep S waves in leads 2, 3, and aVF and a left bundle branch block pattern in the right precordial leads [57]. Although ventricular pacing is the type of pacing most commonly used, atrial or atrial and ventricular pacing may occasionally be indicated. (The references at the end of the chapter supply additional details [12, 24, 55, 57, 58].)

CLASSIFICATION OF PACEMAKERS

The following paragraphs discuss two major classifications of pacemakers—fixed-rate (continuous asynchronous) pacemakers and demand pacemakers.

Fixed-Rate Pacemakers

The fixed-rate pacemakers deliver continuous, nonsynchronized impulses to the myocardium. The pacemaker rate is preset and is not affected by the intrinsic rhythm of the heart. The pacemaker has a preset timing circuit that measures off the intervals between impulses. At the end of each interval, the pacemaker releases an impulse (Fig. 18-18). A pacer artifact (spike), representing the release of a pacemaker impulse, is seen on the ECG. Pacemaker electrodes are usually placed within the right ventricle. The pacer artifact is observed just before the QRS complex. The ventricle is depolarized (stimulated) by the pacemaker impulse (spike), causing the QRS complex to appear on the ECG and the ventricles to

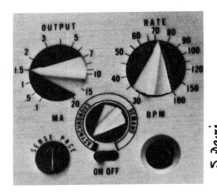

A   Fixed-rate pacer

B   Pacer

Pacer impulse

C   Stimulation level

D

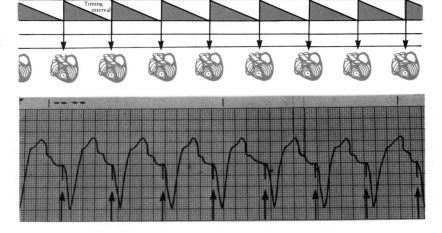

E   ECG

contract. Figure 18-18 illustrates a series of pacemaker impulses resulting in the artificially induced depolarization of the heart.

For example, if the heart is in complete atrioventricular block with a ventricular rate of 30 beats per minute, a fixed-rate pacemaker initiates all ventricular impulses and provides regular ventricular contractions. Therefore, if the fixed-rate pacemaker is set at 78, it will stimulate the heart 78 times per minute. The disadvantage of the fixed-rate pacemaker, however, is that it is insensitive to the inherent electrical activity of the heart. It continues to release impulses even if the heart block disappears and spontaneous conduction is resumed. If the patient's inherent sinus rhythm returns at 90 beats per minute, for example, the fixed-rate pacemaker will continue to fire 78 times per minute. The ventricles, therefore, are receiving impulses from both the natural and the artificial pacemakers. The phenomenon, known as a

Figure 18-18
A. Fixed-rate pacemaker: the rate is 72 beats per minute; the output is 1.5 MA. B. The pacemaker has a circuit that measures off the timing interval to release 72 impulses per minute. C, D. The pacemaker impulse is released at a high enough stimulation (capture) level (C) that the ventricle is depolarized (D). E. The pacemaker impulse is represented on the ECG as a spike (artifact) followed by a wide QRS complex.

competitive rhythm (Fig. 18-19), is the major drawback of the fixed-rate pacemakers (see Pacemaker Malfunction).

The problems associated with a competitive rhythm are related to the vulnerable period that occurs during the T wave, the period when the myocardium is partially but not completely recovered. If the pacemaker spike strikes during that period, ventricular fibrillation may develop [55] (see Pace-

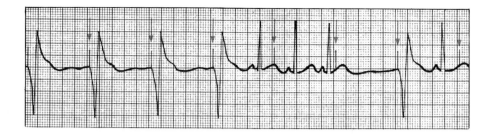

Figure 18-19
Failure to sense: competitive rhythm. The cardiac pacemaker does not sense inherent heart activity, and it inappropriately releases pacemaker impulses (arrows).

maker Malfunction). Fortunately, there is a wide safety margin between the amount of energy needed to pace the heart and the amount of energy needed to produce ventricular fibrillation. The presence of myocardial ischemia, anoxia, infarction, electrolyte disturbances, or metabolic disturbances can reduce the ventricular fibrillatory threshold and narrow the margin of safety [12, 57]. As a result, less energy is needed to produce ventricular fibrillation. Because of those problems, fixed-rate pacemakers have limited clinical use.

Demand Pacemakers
Demand pacemakers are most commonly used [10, 55]. They are not a problem in regard to competitive rhythm because the demand pacemaker is inhibited when the patient's inherent heart rate is faster than the rate at which the pacemaker releases impulses. Pacemaker impulses are delivered to the heart only when the patient's rate falls below a preselected interval (or rate). The demand pacemaker, therefore, fires only when needed.

The circuitry of the demand pacemaker measures off a preset timing interval and then releases a pacemaker impulse. If a spontaneous QRS complex occurs, the circuitry is reset. In the presence of a natural adequate heart rate, information is signaled back to the pacemaker input circuit to interrupt the timing cycle, causing it to reset and inhibit the release of a stimulus (Fig. 18-20). For example, if the demand pacemaker is set at 70 and the patient is in complete atrioventricular block with a ventricular response of 36 beats per minute, the pacemaker releases impulses at the preset interval of 70 times per minute. If the patient's normal sinus rhythm returns at a rate of 80 beats per minute, however, the demand pacemaker senses the spontaneous heart activity (QRS complex) and is recycled and inhibited by each naturally occurring beat. If the patient goes back into complete atrioventricular block, the pacemaker measures the preset timing interval and again releases pacemaker impulses to the heart. The major advantage of demand pacemakers, therefore, is that they sense spontaneous ventricular activity and do not compete with naturally occurring rhythms.

POWER SUPPLY
Most artificial temporary cardiac pacemakers are powered by mercury oxide batteries that have a life span of two to four months. (Keeping the batteries in a cool place, such as a refrigerator, helps them stay charged.) Each time a temporary pacemaker is inserted, new batteries should be installed and tested for proper functioning. The time and date that the battery was inserted should be written on a piece of adhesive tape attached to the back of the pacemaker. The batteries should be replaced at the first sign of failure. It is probably advisable, however, to change them prophylactically every two or three days when the pacemaker is in continuous use (see Electrical Hazards).

TYPES OF ELECTRODES
Artificial pacing is accomplished by means of a unipolar or a bipolar electrode. The impulse generated from the pacemaker must flow between two poles or electrodes to create an electrical circuit.

Unipolar Electrode
In the unipolar electrode, one wire is in the catheter that is positioned in the heart. It is known as the intracardiac electrode, and it senses and stimulates electrical heart activity. It is connected to the nega-

Demand pacer

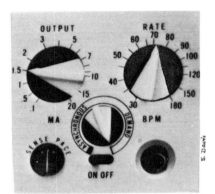

Pacer

Pacer impulse

Stimulation level

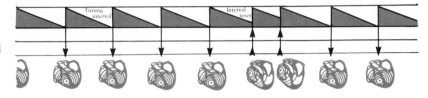

ECG

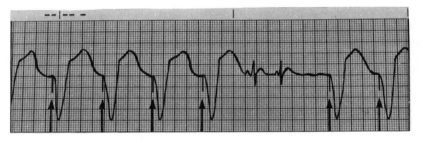

tive terminal on the pacemaker. The other electrode needed to complete the circuit is known as the indifferent, or ground, electrode. It consists of a small metal needle that is inserted subcutaneously and sutured (or taped) to the chest wall. A wire with alligator clamps is then attached on one end to the metal needle and on the other end to the positive terminal on the pacemaker. The advantage of the unipolar electrode is that it needs a lower threshold of stimulation [57]. The ground electrode must be used with caution; it should be insulated and protected from electrical interference.

Bipolar Electrode

The bipolar electrode contains both the sensing (or stimulating) electrode and the ground electrode. It is useful because it provides better contact with endocardial tissue. Depending on which wire is connected to the positive terminal of the pacemaker,

Figure 18-20

A demand pacemaker. The rate is 72 beats per minute; the output is 1.5 MA. The first four beats illustrate the release of pacemaker impulses at 72 beats per minute. The fifth and sixth beats reveal the temporary return of SA node functioning. The timing interval is reset on the demand pacemaker when it senses the return of the inherent rhythm and thus the pacemaker impulse is inhibited. The seventh and eighth beats occur when the heart rate falls below the preselected interval (72 beats per minute) and the pacemaker impulse is released to stimulate the ventricle.

either the distal tip or the proximal tip of the electrode can serve as the sensing (or stimulating) electrode. If one of the bipolar wires malfunctions, it can be converted to a unipolar electrode by the addition of a skin electrode. To convert a bipolar electrode to a unipolar electrode, the distal electrode is connected to the negative terminal, the proximal electrode is disconnected, and the positive pole is grounded to the patient's subcutaneous tissue, as described for the unipolar electrode. Converting the electrode from a bipolar to a unipolar mode is particularly helpful when a pacemaker fails to sense the patient's intrinsic QRS complex because the complex is generating an inadequate intracardiac voltage. Unipolar electrodes act like antennas because of the large interelectrode distance, and they can therefore pick up a greater voltage for a given QRS signal as compared to the bipolar electrode [57].

PACEMAKER SETTINGS

Before artificial pacing is begun, consideration must be given to the (1) mode of pacing, (2) rate of pacing, and (3) stimulation threshold level. Most artificial pacemakers are able to provide either a fixed-rate or a demand mode of pacing. The demand mode, which is more commonly used, has been discussed (see Demand Pacemakers).

Selecting the appropriate pacemaker rate depends on the patient's need for pacing. The lowest rate that controls the dysrhythmia and produces a maximum cardiac output at rest is chosen. Rates above those that are hemodynamically necessary, however, cause a rise in myocardial oxygen consumption and, perhaps, a drop in cardiac output.

The stimulation threshold level (also known as the capture level) is the minimum amount of energy necessary to stimulate the heart. The energy output control, measured in milliamperes (MA), is slowly raised until a QRS complex is seen to occur after every pacer artifact. That point is called the stimulation threshold (the capture level). It is the amount of current needed to produce a 1:1 capture (one QRS complex for every pacer artifact) (Fig. 18-21). The capture level indicates whether the electrode is properly positioned in the endocardium. If less than 1.5 MA is needed to capture the heart, the electrode is properly positioned [10, 24]. The threshold level rarely stays constant after insertion; it often changes in time. Factors that increase the capture level include eating, sleeping, anesthetics, mineralocorticoids, and fibrosis around the tip of the catheter [55]. When one or more of those factors are present, the heart demands a greater amount of energy (a higher MA) for stimulation. (The threshold is lowered by such factors as exercise, a low blood sugar level, glucocorticoids, and sympathomimetics, resulting in the need for less current—or a lower MA—to capture.) Because the threshold level is unpredictable and because resis-

tance generally rises several days after the catheter has been inserted, to ensure consistent pacing the energy level (maintenance level) is set two to three times above the stimulation threshold needed for capture. The energy level should not be set too high, however, because the fibrillation threshold ranges from 10 to 30 times that of the capture level.

SECURING THE PACEMAKER

To prevent catheter dislodgment, most pacemaker electrodes are sutured to the skin. If the catheter is placed in the arm, to prevent displacement of the wire, the arm should be rendered immobile by using armboards, Kling or Ace bandages, and pillows. The reasons for limiting the movement of the arm are explained to the patient. Analgesics can help to relieve the pain and stiffness associated with immobility. After removal of the pacemaker, range-of-motion exercises are begun.

Securing the pacemaker unit to the patient avoids accidental breakage and permits the patient to turn in his bed. Pacemaker or colostomy belts or Kling or Ace bandages are wrapped around the patient's arm or chest or leg and are tied to the pacemaker.

CARE OF THE INSERTION SITE

The area around the insertion site is checked daily for signs and symptoms of infection or inflammation. The dressing is changed daily. The nurse, using sterile gloves, cleanses the area with iodine and applies antibiotic ointment and a sterile dressing. The date and time of the dressing change are recorded on the dressing. That information and information about the general appearance of the insertion site are recorded in the nursing notes. Extreme caution is used to prevent catheter dislodgment during the dressing change, especially if the catheter is placed in the arm.

TEACHING THE PATIENT

When inserting a temporary pacemaker in an emergency, generally there is not enough time to adequately teach the patient about the procedure. Although explanations may need to be brief, reassurance must not be forgotten. In the elective situation or when the patient's condition has been stabilized, he should be told why he needed the pacemaker and taught how it works. A picture can be used to explain

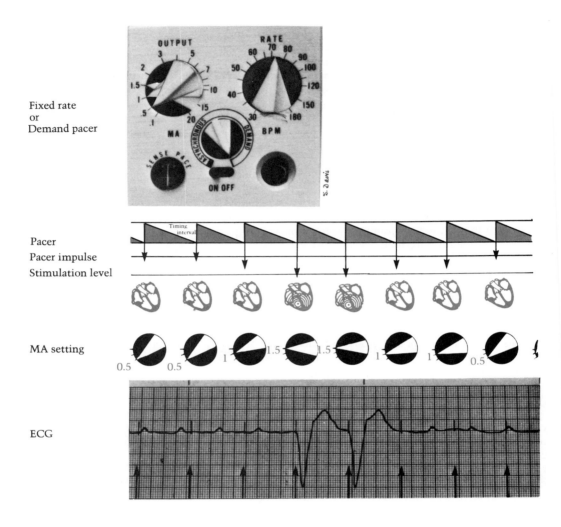

Fixed rate
or
Demand pacer

Pacer
Pacer impulse
Stimulation level

MA setting

ECG

Figure 18-21
Stimulation (capture) level. The first and second pacemaker impulses are released at an energy output of 0.5 MA, and the third impulse is released at 1 MA. The energy output is insufficient to stimulate (capture) the ventricle. The ECG reveals a pacer artifact followed by no QRS complex (*arrows*). The fourth and fifth impulses are released at an energy output of 1.5 MA. That level of energy is sufficient to stimulate the ventricle, and it is known as the stimulation, or threshold, level. The ECG shows a pacer artifact followed by a QRS complex. The output is again turned down to 1 MA and 0.5 MA in the sixth, seventh, and eighth impulses. Once again the ventricle is no longer stimulated, and the ECG reveals loss of capture.

the location of the catheter in the heart. The patient should know that the procedure will take about an hour and that he will be awake. He should be told that he will be connected to a continuous cardiac monitor, have an intravenous line in place, and have his face covered if the site of insertion is the subclavian or the jugular vein. The discomforts associated with the procedure, such as stiffness and pain at the insertion site, should be discussed. The patient should be assured that he will receive analgesics to relieve any discomfort associated with the procedure. If possible, the nurse should explain briefly what the patient can expect in regard to care and management in the postoperative period.

TROUBLESHOOTING TEMPORARY PACEMAKERS

The critical care nurse is often the person responsible for troubleshooting artificial pacemakers. When a problem arises with a temporary pacemaker, the nurse must first assess the patient. A rapid evaluation of the patient's color, pulse, blood pressure, and respiration is essential. Signs and symptoms of confusion, restlessness, or unresponsiveness are looked for. Also, the nurse should observe the patient for rhythmic hiccoughing or diaphragmatic twitching, which indicate electrode perforation of the right ventricle.

The next step in troubleshooting temporary artificial pacemakers involves knowledge of prophylaxis. The nurse must thoroughly understand the principles of cardiac pacing. She must be familiar with the equipment, electrodes, and pulse generators used in her institution. She must know why a pacemaker was inserted in her patient, and she should know her responsibilities. The rate, energy output, mode of pacing, time, date, and site of insertion are written in pencil on the front of the patient's care plan. The settings may change frequently, and the records must be updated as needed.

Troubleshooting must be systematic. First, the nurse should determine whether the pacemaker is turned on. Most temporary pacemakers have a sense/pace dial. If the pacemaker is turned on and the batteries are working, the needle on that dial indicates whether the pacemaker is sensing or pacing the cardiac rhythm. The rate of pacing, the mode of pacing, and the energy output are checked for proper settings. Most pacemaker units have a plastic cover to prevent the patient or the hospital personnel from inadvertently changing the settings. Nevertheless, the settings should be checked. The connection between the pacemaker terminals and electrodes is checked. And finally, the insertion site is checked to be sure that the pacing wire has not been accidentally pulled out.

PACEMAKER MALFUNCTION

A pacemaker malfunction is generally one of three types: (1) failure to pace, (2) failure to sense, and (3) failure to pace *and* sense. Problems associated with failure to pace are seen on the ECG either when there is no pacing artifact observed or when there is a pacer artifact followed by no QRS complex.

Figure 18-22A illustrates a failure to pace because the pacer artifact is absent. The pacemaker is not sending energy through the electrode to stimulate the heart. The problem may be a result of pulse generator malfunction or electrode fracture. Correction of the problem involves assessing the patient, checking the on-off switch and other pacemaker settings, checking the connection between the pacemaker terminals and electrode, and changing the batteries or the pacemaker unit. The pacing catheter can be evaluated by disconnecting the catheter from the pacemaker and connecting first one and then the other electrode terminal of the catheter to lead V on the ECG. The wires in the catheter are intact if the ECG can be recorded through both electrodes. If a wire is fractured, a straight line is recorded on the ECG.

Figure 18-22B illustrates failure to pace; the pacer artifact is not followed by a QRS complex. That problem may be a result of battery failure, catheter dislodgment, electrode perforation of the ventricle, electrode fracture, or an increase in the threshold needed for capture. Occasionally, the amplitude of the pacer artifact is large enough to be interpreted by the cardiac monitor as a QRS complex. Because the cardiac monitor "sees" the pacer spike as a stimulated ventricular complex, the rate meter will continue to function normally and fail to trigger the cardiac monitor alarm system. In that potentially lethal situation, the pacemaker unit continues to release pacemaker impulses (spikes) that fail to stimulate the ventricle. The patient may, however, be in complete ventricular standstill without alarming the monitor. Such a phenomenon demonstrates the importance of carefully observing both the patient and the equipment used to treat him. Correction of the problem involves assessment of the patient and, if necessary, CPR. The nurse can also increase the energy output by one or two MA, reposition the patient on his left or right side, sit the patient up, have the patient lean forward, reverse the electrodes on the terminal, change the batteries or pacemaker units, or convert the bipolar electrode to a unipolar one.

Another serious but less frequently encountered pacemaker malfunction is that of the runaway pacemaker, which fires faster than the preset rate (Fig. 18-22C). Each of the pacer artifacts may capture the myocardium, resulting in a life-threatening rapid heart rate. In most such instances, the electronic circuitry of the pulse generator is malfunctioning, and the pacemaker unit should be exchanged for a new one.

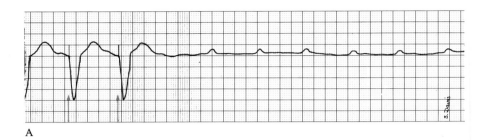

A

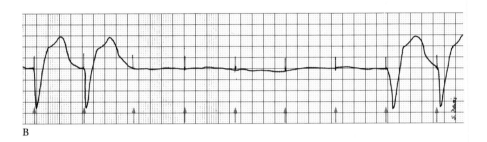

B

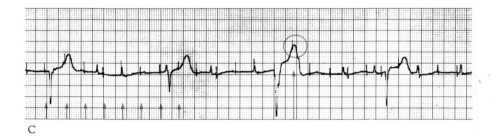

C

Failure of the pacemaker to sense is evidenced electrocardiographically by an intrinsic QRS complex followed by an inappropriately timed pacer artifact. The phenomenon, known as competitive rhythm (see Fig. 18-19), was discussed earlier (see Fixed-Rate Pacemakers). If the patient is being paced at a fixed rate, the pacemaker is changed to the demand mode. Because the electrode may be malpositioned, repositioning the patient may be useful. Other methods of intervention might be turning the pacemaker off, changing the batteries or the pacemaker unit, or converting the bipolar electrode to a unipolar one.

Figure 18-23 shows a pacer artifact hitting the vulnerable period of the T wave in a patient with an

Figure 18-22
A. Failure to pace. No pacer artifact is observed on the ECG after the second beat. B. Failure to pace. The pacer artifact is not capturing the ventricle. The ECG reveals several pacer spikes followed by no QRS complex. C. A runaway pacemaker. The pacemaker impulses are firing faster than the preset rate. Fortunately, each artifact is not followed by ventricular capture. The large arrow indicates a pacer artifact hitting on the T wave.

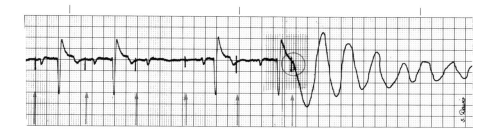

Figure 18-23
Failure to sense: competitive rhythm with a pacer artifact hitting on the T wave to produce ventricular fibrillation.

ischemic myocardium, producing ventricular fibrillation (see Fixed-Rate Pacemakers). The pacemaker is turned off and basic life support is initiated until a defibrillator is available (see Cardiac Arrest and Cardiac Pacing).

ELECTRICAL HAZARDS

The person who does not have an artificial pacemaker is generally protected by the high resistance of the skin and other body tissues against small amounts of electrical current arising from improperly grounded, line-powered equipment. Electrical current seeks the path of least resistance. An electrode that is placed directly in the heart bypasses the protective resistance of the skin and provides a low-resistance pathway to electrical current. Ventricular fibrillation can be produced by low-voltage current if the current is applied directly to the heart [51].

The use of two-pronged plug equipment, extensions, adapters, or cheater cords near the patient with an artificial pacemaker is strictly forbidden because such devices are potential sources of "hot" current [5]. Hot current seeks a ground by using the path of least resistance (the patient). Most patients who have temporary artificial pacemakers are also connected to a well-grounded cardiac monitor. If an ungrounded piece of equipment (one with a two-prong plug), such as an electric radio, is placed at a patient's bedside, it is a potential source of hot current. As the patient turns to change the radio station, the stray current passes through the patient's body to seek the ground of the cardiac monitor. Because of the low resistance provided by the electrode that is placed directly into

the patient's heart, the stray current may cause ventricular fibrillation. That danger can arise if the nurse (or anyone else) simultaneously touches the radio and the patient, causing the current to pass through her and into the patient. Nurses must be careful to avoid contact with the patient while they are operating such electrical equipment. The problem is avoided by ensuring that all electrical equipment is grounded properly and checked periodically. All grounded equipment should be plugged into the same electrical outlet.

The exterior end of the pacer catheter must be carefully insulated to prevent contact with stray current. Most of the newer models have well-insulated pacemaker terminals. Many of the older pacemakers, however, have exposed electrode tips sticking through the terminal poles of the unit. If the tips are exposed, they must be insulated by placing the temporary pacemaker and electrode connections in a dry surgical rubber glove so that they do not come in contact with liquids or other conductive substances. When the nurse handles the electrode terminals, she should wear rubber gloves. If alligator clamps are used, the connections between the electrode terminals and the clamps must be insulated.

Batteries should not be replaced while the pacemaker is in use on the patient. Contact with the battery terminals may be as dangerous to the patient as contact with the electrode terminals. The catheter should be disconnected from the pacemaker (contact with the electrode terminals should be avoided) and the battery replaced. If the patient cannot be disconnected from the pacemaker, rubber gloves should be worn to change the batteries; extreme caution should be used to avoid touching the pacemaker battery terminals. Also, prophylactic pacing wires, which are placed in a patient after open heart surgery, should be insulated with a dry rubber glove. Patients with temporary pacemakers should not use electric razors, electrical bed controls, or other electrical equipment.

ENVIRONMENTAL INTERFERENCE

Demand pacemakers are able to respond to environmental electrical signals, causing the inhibition of their demand function [57]. Many newer pacemakers have developed better shielding and filtering devices, but the danger of external interference still exists. Environmental interference may suppress demand pacemaker functioning, leaving the patient unprotected. Pacemakers may be disrupted by microwave ovens or by radar, diathermy, or electrocautery equipment [7, 8, 55, 57]. Because patients with temporary pacemakers are generally restricted to the critical care area, such disruptions are rare. They occur more frequently in the patient with a permanent pacemaker. Should a problem arise, however, the treatment is to move the patient away from the environmental interference. The demand pacemaker will then resume normal functioning.

COMPLICATIONS OF TEMPORARY PACEMAKERS

The problems of failure to sense, failure to pace, local infection, catheter dislodgment, electrode fracture, electrical hazards, battery failure, and myocardial perforation have been discussed. The nurse must also assess her patient for signs and symptoms of other complications of cardiac pacing. They include pneumothorax, hemothorax, dysrhythmias, septicemia, pulmonary embolism, and venous thrombosis.

CARDIAC ARREST AND CARDIAC PACING

If the patient has a cardiac arrest after the insertion of a temporary pacemaker, CPR must be initiated. Also, the pacemaker unit should be checked to be sure that it is turned on. The energy output level should be raised one or two MA. The rate should be set above 60. The functioning of the pacemaker is assessed by observing the ECG and the sense/pace dial while simultaneously palpating the carotid pulse. A new pacemaker may be needed. If the patient is in ventricular fibrillation, the pacemaker is turned off and disconnected from the patient before defibrillation is attempted—to prevent pacemaker damage and to be sure that the electrical current is not diverted from the cardiac pathway. After defibrillation, the rhythm is checked again and, if necessary, the pacemaker is reconnected and turned on.

Permanent Pacemakers

Some patients requiring temporary pacing suffer from continuous or intermittent rhythm disturbances. Those patients are observed to determine whether they need permanent pacemakers. Permanent pacemakers are indicated for patients with complete, intermittent, or incomplete atrioventricular block with Stokes-Adams syncope or congestive failure, sinus bradycardia, sinus arrest or symptomatic sinoatrial block, permanent postoperative surgical heart block, or uncontrollable tachydysrhythmias.

A permanent pacemaker is inserted with the patient under local anesthesia. An incision is made over the right or left external jugular or subclavian vein. The pacing catheter is passed into the heart and wedged firmly between the right ventricular trabeculae. A subcutaneous incision is made in the upper chest to implant the pacemaker. A tunnel is formed under the skin between the two incisions. The distal end of the pacing catheter is pulled under the skin from the insertion site to the subcutaneous incision. The catheter is attached to the pacemaker and is placed in the subcutaneous pocket and sewed closed.

The general principles for the preoperative preparation of the temporary pacemaker patient apply also to the permanent pacemaker patient. Postoperatively, the nurse must assess pacemaker functioning by checking the patient's apical and radial pulses, blood pressure, and cardiac rhythm. She must help the patient to become independent in regard to his care and to realize his ability to return home to an active and productive life. Following his postoperative instruction, the patient should be able to demonstrate to the nurse how to take his pulse. He should be able to identify the activities that he should restrict. He should be able to discuss the environmental and electrical hazards—how to prevent them and what to do if they occur. The patient should describe his diet, medications, the signs and symptoms of incisional infection, and what to do if his pacemaker malfunctions.

Acid-Base Balance

A thorough understanding of acid-base disturbances is another important part of advanced life support. Arterial blood gas measurements and pH are widely accepted physiological parameters used to assess acid-base balance and cardiopulmonary functioning. In this section, the acid-base balance is discussed in terms of respiratory and metabolic abnormalities and applied to cardiac arrest [19].

pH

Blood is either alkaline or acid as a result of a decrease or increase in free hydrogen ions (H^+). pH, the expression of the acid-base balance, is defined as the reciprocal logarithm of the hydrogen ion concentration expressed as the power of 10. In the following paragraphs, several principles (golden rules) are presented to help the learner understand acid-base disturbances.

Golden Rule 1

H^+ can be thought of as an acid.

1. As the H^+ concentration increases, the blood becomes more acidic.
2. As the H^+ concentration decreases, the blood becomes more alkaline.

Golden Rule 2

The normal serum pH is 7.4 ($\pm$ 0.04) (the range is 7.36 to 7.44).

1. A pH below 7.36 is acidic (H^+ increase).
2. A pH above 7.44 is alkaline (H^+ decrease).

The acid-base balance is maintained by the special buffer systems found in the blood, lungs, and kidneys. An important blood buffer system is the bicarbonate–carbonic acid system, which prevents excessive changes in the hydrogen ion concentration. The system consists of 1 part carbonic acid (H_2CO_3) to 20 parts bicarbonate (HCO_3^-) in the extracellular fluid, and it may be expressed in a modified Henderson-Hasselbalch equation:

$$pH \propto \frac{base}{acid} = \frac{HCO_3^-}{H_2CO_3} = \frac{20}{1}$$
$$\uparrow \qquad \downarrow$$
$$PaCO_2 \times 0.03$$

CARBON DIOXIDE

When the ratio of HCO_3^- to H_2CO_3 is altered, the acid-base balance (pH) will change. H_2CO_3 is formed at the cellular level by the production of carbon dioxide (CO_2) following the uptake of oxygen by the cell. H_2CO_3 then dissociates in the blood to form CO_2 + H_2O ($H_2CO_3 \rightarrow CO_2 + H_2O$). CO_2 is conceptually understood as the acid in the denominator of the Henderson-Hasselbalch equation. As CO_2 builds up, the blood becomes more acidic. The concentration of CO_2 is regulated primarily by the lungs.

Golden Rule 3

CO_2 can be thought of as an acid.

1. As the CO_2 increases, the blood becomes more acidic and the pH decreases.
2. As the CO_2 decreases, the blood becomes more alkaline and the pH increases.

PaCO2

The $PaCO_2$ is defined as the partial pressure exerted by the amount of CO_2 dissolved in the arterial blood. The tension that is produced by CO_2 is measured in torr units (1 torr = 1 mm Hg). The $PaCO_2$ is related directly to the rate and depth of respiration. It is a direct index of the effectiveness of ventilation. The normal value of the $PaCO_2$ is 40 ($\pm$4) torr (the range is 36–44 torr).

Golden Rule 4

When the primary disturbance affects alterations in the $PaCO_2$, a *respiratory* derangement is present.

HCO3−

Changes in the level of HCO_3^-, the numerator of the equation, also affect the acid-base balance. HCO_3^- is used to protect the blood against changes in pH because of its ability to take up and release H^+. The concentration of HCO_3^- is regulated mainly by the kidneys. The normal concentration of HCO_3^- in the blood is 22 to 28 mg.

Golden Rule 5

HCO_3^- can be thought of as a base (alkaline).

1. As the HCO_3^- increases, the blood becomes more alkaline and the pH increases.

Table 18-11
Respiratory Acidosis and Alkalosis

Respiratory Acidosis	Respiratory Alkalosis
Causes	Causes
Hypoventilation	Hyperventilation
COPD	Pulmonary embolism
Sedation	Severe pain
Clinical manifestations	Anxiety
Dyspnea	Brain stem disease
Headache	Chronic overventilation on controlled ventilator
Mental confusion	Clinical manifestations
Pallor	Dizziness
Sweating	Tingling, numbness
Apprehension, restlessness	Restlessness, agitation
ABG measurements (example)	Tetany
pH 7.24	ABG measurements (example)
$PaCO_2$ 60	pH 7.48
HCO_3^- 24	$PaCO_2$ 30
Treatment	HCO_3^- 22
Determine and treat cause	Treatment
Maintain adequate respiratory minute volume	Identify and treat cause
Increase tidal volume and/or increase respiratory	Sedation
rate	Reduce respiratory minute volume
Suctioning	Decrease tidal volume and/or decrease respiratory
	rate
	Reassure and support patient

Key: ABG = arterial blood gas; COPD = chronic obstructive pulmonary disease.

2. As the HCO_3^- decreases, the blood becomes more acidic and the pH decreases.

Golden Rule 6

When the primary disturbance affects alterations in HCO_3^-, a *metabolic* derangement is present.

Acid-Base Abnormalities

Acid-base abnormalities may be produced by a respiratory derangement (expressed by a low or a high $PaCO_2$) or produced by a metabolic derangement (expressed by a low or a high HCO_3^-). Depending on the specific problem, the patient has acidosis (expressed by a low pH) or alkalosis (expressed by a high pH). Those abnormalities are discussed individually in the following paragraphs.

RESPIRATORY ACIDOSIS

Respiratory acidosis is defined as an abnormal physiological process in which there is a primary reduction

in the rate of alveolar ventilation relative to the rate of CO_2 production. Respiratory acidosis is caused by factors that produce hypoventilation. A pure respiratory acidosis is identified from arterial blood gas analyses in which the pH is shown to be low (acidosis) and the $PaCO_2$ (respiratory) is shown to be high (Table 18-11).

RESPIRATORY ALKALOSIS

Respiratory alkalosis is an abnormal physiological process in which there is a primary increase in the rate of alveolar ventilation relative to the rate of CO_2 production. It is caused by factors that produce hyperventilation. An arterial blood gas puncture, for example, is a common cause of hyperventilation [46]. A pure respiratory alkalosis is identified when the pH is shown to be high (alkalosis) and the $PaCO_2$ (respiratory) to be low (Table 18-11).

METABOLIC ACIDOSIS

Metabolic acidosis is an abnormal physiological process characterized by the primary loss of HCO_3^- from the extracellular fluid. It is identified from blood gas

Table 18-12
Metabolic Acidosis and Alkalosis

Metabolic Acidosis	Metabolic Alkalosis
Causes	Causes
Cardiac arrest	Vomiting
Diabetic ketoacidosis	Gastric suctioning
Poisoning (acetylsalicylic acid, methyl alcohol, ethylene glycol, paraldehyde)	Sodium bicarbonate overload
Renal failure	Diuretics
Diarrhea (loss of HCO_3^-)	Adrenal disease
	Corticosteroids
Clinical manifestations	Clinical manifestations
Lethargy	Dullness
Nausea, vomiting	Weakness
Dysrhythmias	Dysrhythmias
Coma	Tetany
	Hypokalemia
ABG measurements (example)	ABG measurements (example)
pH 7.30	pH 7.50
$PaCO_2$ 40	$PaCO_2$ 40
HCO_3^- 15	HCO_3^- 40
Treatment	Treatment
Identify and treat cause	Identify and treat cause
Sodium bicarbonate	Correct dehydration
	Correct hypokalemia
	Acetazolamide (Diamox)
	Ammonium chloride
	Arginine monohydrochloride

Key: ABG = arterial blood gas.

analyses when the pH is shown to be low (acidosis) and the HCO_3^- level (metabolic) to be reduced (Table 18-12).

METABOLIC ALKALOSIS

Pure metabolic alkalosis is an abnormal physiological process characterized by a primary gain in HCO_3^- in the extracellular fluid. Blood gas analyses reveal an elevated pH (alkalosis) and an increased HCO_3^- level (metabolic) (Table 18-12).

COMPENSATION VERSUS CORRECTION OF ACID-BASE ABNORMALITIES

When acid-base abnormalities occur, one of two basic mechanisms may be used to return the pH to normal: (1) compensation or (2) correction.

In compensation, the pH is returned to normal by altering the system not primarily affected by the disturbance. If a primary respiratory disturbance is present, there is a change only in the $PaCO_2$. There is no immediate change in the overall base or bicarbonate system (the secondary system). Changes in $PaCO_2$ occur quite rapidly since changes in respiration cause CO_2 to be excreted or retained. In time, however, the kidneys attempt to compensate for the primary respiratory disturbance. In respiratory acidosis, for example, the kidneys help to compensate for the abnormally low pH by retaining HCO_3^- to return the base-acid ratio to 20:1. It should be noted that when the primary disturbance is respiratory, the secondary (compensatory) changes in the kidneys take place only gradually to help return the pH to normal. The serum HCO_3^- level, therefore, is often useful in determining how acute the situation is [46]. Changes in HCO_3^-, on the other hand, are primarily the result of the renal excretion of H^+ and retention of HCO_3^-. In contrast, if the primary disturbance is metabolic (as, for example, in metabolic acidosis), the lungs (the secondary system) immediately attempt to blow off excess acid as a compensatory mechanism to return the pH to physiological neutrality.

The second mechanism to return the pH to normal is correction, in which the system primarily affected by the disturbance is altered. In the setting of respiratory acidosis, effective ventilation and suctioning may improve the $PaCO_2$ and return the pH to normal.

In metabolic acidosis, a bolus of sodium bicarbonate is generally effective in combating the acidosis and correcting the abnormal pH. The general clinical approach used to deal with acid-base abnormalities is usually aimed at correcting the abnormality as quickly as possible rather than at helping the body to compensate (which may take a long and unpredictable period of time).

The critical care nurse has probably observed that acid-base abnormalities frequently are complicated. Assessing a pure respiratory or a pure metabolic disturbance is generally a simple procedure. More commonly, however, the nurse observes both a primary metabolic and a primary respiratory disturbance (as, for example, in cardiac arrest), or she may observe acid-base abnormalities that are affected by the primary disturbance with compensated or uncompensated changes in the secondary system, as discussed.

In evaluating complicated arterial blood gas measurements, the nurse must use a systematic approach. Blood gas analysis, like the physical examination and the analysis of a cardiac rhythm strip, demands patience and organization. One must first evaluate the patient's total clinical picture, his clinical signs and symptoms, the findings from his physical examination, and his presumptive diagnosis. Keeping those facts in mind, the nurse should evaluate the arterial blood gas measurements, using the golden rules just given and the rules that follow [19]. The method presented here is a relatively easy one to master, and the critical care nurse will quickly discover that blood gas analysis is not a mystery but rather it is exciting and fun and an important tool for determining patient care.

Systematic Approach to Arterial Blood Gas Analysis

ASSESSMENT OF THE RESPIRATORY COMPONENT

Respiratory acidosis is commonly encountered during the first minutes of a cardiopulmonary arrest. In respiratory acidosis, the $PaCO_2$ increases (an increase in H_2CO_3), and the pH is lowered. The following important principle can be used to assess the situation.

Golden Rule 7

As the $PaCO_2$ changes by 10 torr (from the basic unit of 40 torr), it is associated with a change in pH of 0.08 unit (from 7.40) in the opposite direction [19].

Example A: $PaCO_2$ 40 torr; pH 7.40: Normal

Example B: $PaCO_2$ 50 torr; pH 7.32: Respiratory acidosis (50 − 40 torr is an increase in 10 torr units in $PaCO_2$ associated with a decrease in pH of 0.08 unit, or 7.40 − 0.08 = 7.32)

Example C: $PaCO_2$ 55 torr; pH 7.28: Respiratory acidosis (55 torr − 40 torr is an increase in 15 torr units in the $PaCO_2$ associated with a decrease in pH of 0.12 unit, or 7.40 − 0.12 = 7.28)

The same situation applies to respiratory alkalosis that is caused by artificially hyperventilating the patient during or after the cardiac arrest.

Example D: $PaCO_2$ 30; pH 7.48: Respiratory alkalosis (a decrease in $PaCO_2$ of 10 torr increases the pH by 0.08 unit)

Example E: $PaCO_2$ 25; pH 7.52: Respiratory alkalosis (a decrease in $PaCO_2$ of 15 torr increases the pH by 0.12 unit)

Example F: $PaCO_2$ 20; pH 7.56: Respiratory alkalosis (a decrease of _____ torr increases the pH by _____ unit)

When assessing the respiratory component of the acid-base balance, one must proceed through the following steps: (1) determination of the $PaCO_2$, (2) calculation of the change in $PaCO_2$ from 40 torr, (3) calculation of what the pH should be (calculated pH) based on a pH of 7.40, and (4) determination of the measured pH (the actual blood gas measurement).

Example G: Step 1. $PaCO_2$ = 50 torr
Step 2.   Change = 10-torr increase in $PaCO_2$ ($PaCO_2$ 50 torr − 40 torr = 10 torr)
Step 3.   Calculated pH = 7.32 (pH 7.40 − 0.08 = pH 7.32)
Step 4.   Measured blood gas pH = 7.32
Diagnosis: Pure respiratory acidosis

Example H: Step 1. $PaCO_2$ = 50 torr
Step 2.   Change = 10-torr increase in $PaCO_2$
Step 3.   Calculated pH = 7.32
Step 4.   Measured blood gas pH = 7.25
Diagnosis: The calculated pH and the measured pH are not the same (there is a 0.07 difference). The blood gas measurements indicate a respiratory acidosis plus a metabolic disturbance

ASSESSMENT OF THE METABOLIC COMPONENT

After the respiratory component is assessed, the metabolic component is evaluated. The following principle is used to estimate the metabolic involvement.

Golden Rule 8

As the pH changes (from the basic unit of 7.40) by 0.15 unit, it is associated with a change in base of 10 mEq/L [19].

When the base (bicarbonate) decreases, a base deficit exists (acidosis). An increase in base (bicarbonate) is defined as a base excess (alkalosis). The normal base deficit or excess is 0 ± 2.

During a cardiopulmonary arrest, anaerobic metabolism results in the build-up of strong acids and a drop in pH. As strong metabolic acids build up, they combine with a base, such as sodium bicarbonate, to form a weak acid and a neutral salt. To assess the metabolic component of the acid-base balance, one must add the following steps to those just discussed: (5) subtraction of the calculated pH from the measured pH, (6) calculation of the amount of base change associated with step 5. One can apply those principles to the following examples:

Example I: Step 1. $PaCO_2$ = 50 torr
Step 2. Change = 10-torr increase in $PaCO_2$ ($PaCO_2$ 50 torr − 40 torr = 10 torr)
Step 3. Calculated pH = 7.32 (pH 7.40 − 0.08 = 7.32)
Step 4. Measured blood gas pH = 7.17 (lower than it should be)

Golden Rule 8 ⎡ Step 5. Change between calculated pH and measured pH = 0.15 unit (pH 7.32 − pH 7.17 = 0.15)
⎣ Step 6. Base change = 10 mEq/L deficit
Diagnosis: Respiratory acidosis with a metabolic acidosis

Example J: Step 1. $PaCO_2$ = 50 torr
Step 2. Change = 10-torr increase in $PaCO_2$
Step 3. Calculated pH = 7.32
Step 4. Measured pH = 7.25 (lower than it should be)
Step 5. Change in pH = 0.07 unit
Step 6. Base change = 5 mEq/L deficit
Diagnosis: Respiratory acidosis with a metabolic acidosis

Example K: Step 1. $PaCO_2$ = 30 torr
Step 2. Change = 10-torr decrease in $PaCO_2$
Step 3. Calculated pH = 7.48
Step 4. Measured pH = 7.33 (lower than it should be)
Step 5. Change in pH = 0.15 unit
Step 6. Base change = 10 mEq/L deficit
Diagnosis: Respiratory alkalosis and metabolic acidosis

(Question 20 at end of the chapter gives further examples.)

TREATMENT

When the management of acid-base disturbances during a cardiac arrest is being evaluated, the problems of both respiratory and metabolic acidosis are commonly encountered. The treatment of respiratory acidosis involves administering a respiratory minute volume that attains effective alveolar ventilation. The treatment of metabolic acidosis includes neutralizing strong metabolic acids by administering intravenous sodium bicarbonate. Calculation of the dosage of sodium bicarbonate without the use of blood gas measurements has been discussed (see Sodium Bicarbonate). Ideally, however, the dosage should be calculated on the basis of arterial blood gas measurements and by the following equation [19]:

$$NaHCO_3 \text{ dose (mEq)} = \frac{\text{base deficit (mEq/L)} \times \text{body weight (kg)}}{4}$$

Example L: Cardiac arrest in a 70-kg man
Step 1. $PaCO_2$ = 55 torr
Step 2. Change = 15-torr increase in $PaCO_2$
Step 3. Calculated pH = 7.28
Step 4. Measured pH = 7.13
Step 5. Change in pH = 0.15 unit
Step 6. Base change = 10 mEq/L deficit
Diagnosis: Respiratory acidosis with a metabolic acidosis
Treatment: Artificial ventilation to maintain effective minute volume to combat the respiratory acidosis and administration of sodium bicarbonate to combat the metabolic acidosis

To calculate the sodium bicarbonate dosage for the 70-kg patient with cardiac arrest described in example L:

$$NaHCO_3 \text{ dose (mEq)} = \frac{10 \text{ mEq/L} \times 70 \text{ kg}}{4}$$

$$= \frac{700}{4}$$

$$NaHCO_3 \text{ dose (mEq)} = 175$$

The entire dose of sodium bicarbonate is given during a cardiac arrest because of the rapid and acute fall in pH. However, because it is possible to produce serum alkalosis, hyperosmolality, dysrhythmias, and cerebral disturbances by the rapid administration of sodium bicarbonate, the sudden and total correction of acidosis is not indicated in the patient who does not have cardiac arrest. Such a patient is treated with a bolus of sodium bicarbonate to effect a 50 percent correction of the metabolic disturbance, and the rest of the bicarbonate is given over several hours with the aid of further arterial blood gas analyses.

For the patient in metabolic acidosis who does not have cardiac arrest [19]:

$$\text{NaHCO}_3 \text{ dose (mEq)} = \frac{10 \text{ mEq/L} \times 70 \text{ kg}}{4}$$

$$= 175$$

with a 50 percent correction: 88 mEq of NaHCO_3 given in bolus form and 87 mEq given over the next few hours

The Legal Aspects of CPR

Because CPR is rarely rendered with the patient's consent, various legal problems can arise. Currently, 29 states have a "Good Samaritan law," 8 states have relevant legislation pending, and 13 states do not have laws to protect qualified people who give CPR. The Good Samaritan law states that if a person renders CPR in good faith and according to the accepted standards and does not charge a fee or accept a remuneration, he cannot be held liable for any complications or injuries that result from his rendering BLS.

National certification programs in CPR have been established by the American Heart Association and the American Red Cross. The critical care nurse should acquaint herself with the certification programs in her community and with the law (or lack of a law) in her state regarding "immunity" for people who render CPR [39].

Summary

The critical care nurse plays a vital role in the administration of basic and advanced life support. The recent changes in CPR and ECC have made it incumbent on the nurse to update her knowledge and techniques so that she can deliver skilled and compassionate emergency care.

Study Problems

1. The correct compression-ventilation ratio in one-person CPR rescue is:
   a. 5:1.
   b. 15:1.
   c. 15:2.
   d. 5:2.
2. The correct compression-ventilation ratio in two-person CPR rescue is:
   a. 5:1.
   b. 15:1.
   c. 15:2.
   d. 5:2.
3. The treatment of an unconscious patient with an obstructed airway includes:
   a. Back blows.
   b. Abdominal or chest thrusts.
   c. The finger-probe-and-sweep.
   d. All the above.
4. CPR should never be interrupted for more than five seconds, except during endotracheal intubation or while the patient is being carried up or down a flight of stairs. In these situations, CPR may be interrupted for not more than:
   a. 10 seconds.
   b. 15 seconds.
   c. 30 seconds.
   d. 60 seconds.
5. The most common complication of CPR is:
   a. Sternal fracture.
   b. Pneumothorax.
   c. Rib fractures.
   d. Fat embolism.
6. The precordial thump should not be used:
   a. For a patient who is not on a cardiac monitor.
   b. For a person with an unwitnessed cardiac arrest.
   c. For a patient with anoxic asystole.
   d. For any of the above.
7. Esophageal airways should not be used:
   a. For a person with an unwitnessed arrest.
   b. For a person with a witnessed arrest.
   c. For a conscious patient.
   d. For any of the above.
8. Which of the following breathing adjuncts are acceptable for use during CPR?
   a. Volume ventilators.
   b. Pressure ventilators.

   c. Manually triggered ventilators.

   d. All the above.

9. Defibrillation of the fibrillating heart can result in:

   a. Depolarization of the myocardium.

   b. Repolarization of the myocardium.

   c. The return of a normal electrical impulse formation from the sinoatrial node.

   d. All the above.

10. The initial dose of sodium bicarbonate that should be given during a cardiac arrest is:

   a. 0.5 mEq/kg.

   b. 1 mEq/kg.

   c. 5 mEq/kg.

   d. 44.6 mEq.

11. Epinephrine is given:

   a. To convert a fine ventricular fibrillation to a coarse ventricular fibrillation.

   b. During asystole.

   c. By intravenous injection.

   d. All the above.

12. Atropine sulfate can:

   a. Increase myocardial oxygen consumption.

   b. Extend an area of myocardial ischemia or infarct.

   c. Produce ventricular fibrillation.

   d. All the above.

13. Lidocaine:

   a. Decreases myocardial contractility.

   b. Lowers systemic arterial pressure.

   c. Raises the ventricular fibrillatory threshold.

   d. All the above.

14. Calcium chloride:

   a. Increases myocardial contractility.

   b. Decreases myocardial excitability.

   c. Reduces stroke volume.

   d. All the above.

15. Levarterenol:

   a. Is primarily an alpha-adrenergic receptor stimulating drug.

   b. Elevates the blood pressure by causing peripheral vasoconstriction.

   c. May cause tissue necrosis if extravasation of the drug occurs in a peripheral vein.

   d. All the above.

16. The most common indication for insertion of a temporary cardiac pacemaker is:

   a. Tachydysrhythmia.

   b. Bradydysrhythmia.

   c. Heart block.

   d. Asystole.

17. The stimulation threshold of the myocardium is:

   a. The capture level.

   b. The minimum electrical energy necessary to stimulate the heart.

   c. An indication of electrode placement.

   d. All the above.

18. Electrical safety of the patient with an artificial temporary pacemaker includes:

   a. Ensuring that all electrical equipment is properly grounded.

   b. Insulating pacemaker terminals.

   c. Allowing the patient to use only the electrical bed control.

   d. Only a and b of the above.

19. If a patient has a cardiac arrest after the insertion of a pacemaker:

   a. CPR must be initiated.

   b. The pacemaker is evaluated for proper functioning.

   c. The pacemaker should be disconnected from the patient, if possible before defibrillation is attempted.

   d. All the above.

20. The blood gas measurements shown in the following table are those of patients who were suffering a cardiac arrest. Figure the calculated pH, pH difference, base excess or deficit, diagnosis, and treatment.

Weight	PaO_2	$PaCO_2$	Measured pH	Calculated pH	pH Difference	Base ±	Diagnosis	Treatment
70 kg	96 torr	52 torr	7.30					
70 kg	95 torr	40 torr	7.25					
60 kg	75 torr	50 torr	7.26					
50 kg	97 torr	32 torr	7.25					
70 kg	70 torr	55 torr	7.17					

Answers

1. c.
2. a.
3. d.
4. c.
5. c.
6. d.
7. c.
8. c.
9. d.
10. b.
11. d.
12. d.
13. c.
14. a.
15. d.
16. c.
17. d.
18. d.
19. d.
20.

Weight	PaO_2	$PaCO_2$	Measured pH	Calculated pH	pH Difference	Base ±	Diagnosis	Treatment
70 kg	96 torr	52 torr	7.30	7.30	.00	0	Respiratory acidosis	↑ TV
70 kg	95 torr	40 torr	7.25	7.40	.15	−10	Metabolic acidosis	$NaHCO_3$ 175 mEq
60 kg	75 torr	50 torr	7.26	7.32	.06	−4	Respiratory and metabolic acidosis	↑ TV, $NaHCO_3$ 60 mEq
50 kg	97 torr	32 torr	7.25	7.46	.21	−14	Respiratory alkalosis, and metabolic acidosis	↓ TV, $NaHCO_3$ 175 mEq
70 kg	70 torr	55 torr	7.17	7.28	.11	−8	Respiratory and metabolic acidosis	↑ TV, $NaHCO_3$ 140 mEq

Key: TV = tidal volume.

References

1. American Medical Association. Standards and guidelines for cardiopulmonary resuscitation (CPR) and emergency cardiac care (ECC). *J.A.M.A.* 244:453, 1980.
2. Ahlquist, R. P. A study of adrenotropic receptors. *Am. J. Physiol.* 153:586, 1948.
3. Alcock, M., and Wilson, S. Code 66: From anxious "amateurs" to smooth-working code team. *Nurs. '75* 5:17, 1975.
4. Aronow, W. S. Clinical use of nitrates: Nitrates in congestive heart failure. *Mod. Con. Cardiovasc. Dis.* 7:37, 1979.
5. Batstow, R. E. Nursing care of patients with pacemakers. *Cardiovasc. Nurs.* 8:7, 1972.
6. Bernstein, L., Fresinger, G. C., Lichtlen, P. R., et al. The effects of nitroglycerin on the systemic and coronary circulation in man and dogs: Myocardial blood flow measured with xenon. *Circulation* 33:107, 1966.
7. Bing, O. H. L., McDowell, J. W., Hartman, J., et al. Pacemaker placement by electrocardiographic monitoring. *N. Engl. J. Med.* 287:651, 1972.
8. Carleton, R. Environmental influence on implantable cardiac pacemakers. *J.A.M.A.* 190:160, 1964.
9. Chardack, W. M. Cardiac Pacemakers and Heart Block. In J. H. Gibbon (ed.), *Surgery of the Chest* (2nd ed.). Philadelphia: Saunders, 1969.
10. Chardack, W. M., Gage, A. A., and Greatbatch, W. A transistorized, self-contained, implantable pacemaker for the long-term correction of complete heart block. *Surgery* 48:643, 1960.
11. Chatterjee, K., Mandell, W. J., Vyden, J. K., et al. Cardiovascular effects of bretylium tosylate in acute myocardial infarction. *J.A.M.A.* 233:757, 1973.
12. Chawla, N. P. S., Rea, W., and Shapiro, W. The use of an implanted demand pacemaker in bradyarrhythmias. *Arch. Intern. Med.* 124:593, 1969.
13. Chidsey, C. A. Calcium metabolism in the normal and failing heart. *Hosp. Prac.* 8:65, 1972.
14. Cohen, M. Preparing drugs for cardiopulmonary resuscitation. *Hosp. Pharm.* 7:180, 1972.
15. Cohn, J. N. Blood pressure measurements in shock. *J.A.M.A.* 199:148, 1967.
16. Cohn, J. N., and Franciosa, J. A. Vasodilator therapy of cardiac failure: Part 1. *N. Engl. J. Med.* 297:27, 1977.
17. Cohn, J. N., and Franciosa, J. A. Vasodilator therapy of cardiac failure: Part 2. *N. Engl. J. Med.* 297:254, 1977.
18. Collinsworth, K. A., Kalmann, S. M., and Harrison, D. C. The clinical pharmacology of lidocaine as an antiarrhythmic drug. *Circulation* 50:1217, 1974.
19. Committee on Emergency Cardiac Care. *Advanced Cardiac Life Support.* Dallas: American Heart Association, 1975.
20. Committee on Emergency Cardiac Care. *Obstructed Airway Management.* Dallas: American Heart Association, 1976.
21. Conolly, M. E., Kersting, F., and Dollery, C. The clinical pharmacology of beta-adrenoceptor-blocking drugs. *Prog. Cardiovasc. Dis.* 19:203, 1976.
22. Corwin, N. D., Klein, M. J., and Friedberg, C. K. Countershock conversion of digitalis-associated paroxysmal atrial tachycardia with block. *Am. Heart J.* 66:804, 1963.
23. Courter, S. R., Moffat, J., and Fowler, N. O. Advanced atrioventricular block in acute myocardial infarction. *Circulation* 27:1034, 1963.
24. Escher, D. J. W., and Furman, S. Emergency treatment of cardiac arrhythmias: Emphasis on use of electrical pacing. *J.A.M.A.* 214:2028, 1970.
25. Furman, S., and Robertson, G. Stimulation of the ventricular endocardial surface in control of complete heart block. *Ann. Surg.* 159:841, 1959.
26. Giardina, E. G. V., Heissenbuttel, R. H., and Bitter, J. T. Intermittent intravenous procainamide to treat ventricular arrhythmias. *Ann. Intern. Med.* 78:183, 1973.
27. Gillespie, T. A., Ambos, H. D., Sobel, B. E., et al. Effect of dobutamine in patients with acute myocardial infarction. *Am. J. Cardiol.* 39:588, 1977.
28. Goldberg, A. H. Cardiopulmonary arrest. *N. Engl. J. Med.* 290:381, 1974.
29. Goldberg, L. I. Dopamine: Clinical uses of an endogenous catecholamine. *N. Engl. J. Med.* 291:707, 1974.
30. Guiha, N. H., Cohn, J. N., Mikulic, E., et al. Treatment of refractory heart failure with infusion of nitroprusside. *N. Engl. J. Med.* 291:587, 1974.
31. Haddy, F. J. Physiology and pharmacology of the coronary circulation and myocardium, particularly in relation to coronary artery disease. *Am. J. Med.* 47:274, 1969.
32. Harrison, D. C. Should lidocaine be administered routinely to all patients after acute myocardial infarction? *Circulation* 58:582, 1978.
33. Hilmi, K. I., and Regan, T. J. Relative effectiveness of anti-arrhythmic drugs in treatment of digitalis-induced ventricular tachycardia. *Am. Heart J.* 76:365, 1968.
34. Horsley, J. E. *Malpractice Risks in Cardiac Arrest Are Rising.* Dallas: American Heart Association, 1970.
35. Hyman, A. S. Resuscitation of the stopped heart by intracardiac therapy: II. Experimental use of an artificial pacemaker. *Arch. Intern. Med.* 50:283, 1932.
36. Kaplan, B. C., Civetta, J. M., Nagel, E. L., et al. The military anti-shock trousers in civilian pre-hospital emergency care. *J. Trauma* 13:843, 1973.
37. Koch-Weser, J. Drug therapy: Bretylium. *N. Engl. J. Med.* 300:473, 1979.
38. Lang, T. W., Bernstein, H., Barbieri, F. F., et al. Digitalis toxicity. Treatment with diphenylhydantoin. *Arch. Intern. Med.* 116:573, 1965.
39. Lemire, J. G., and Johnson, A. L. Is cardiac resuscitation worthwhile? *N. Engl. J. Med.* 286:970, 1972.
40. Lown, B., Crampton, R. S., DeSilva, R. A., et al. The energy for ventricular defibrillation—too little or too much. *N. Engl. J. Med.* 298:1252, 1978.
41. Mikulic, E., Cohn, J. N., and Franciosa, J. A. Compara-

tive hemodynamic effects of inotropic and vasodilator drugs in severe heart failure. *Circulation* 56:528, 1977.

42. National Safety Council. *Accident Facts.* Washington, D.C., 1977.

43. O'Rourke, G. W., and Greene, N. M. Autonomic blockade and the resting heart rate in man. *Am. Heart J.* 80:469, 1970.

44. Palmer, R. F., and Lasseter, K. C. Drug therapy: Sodium nitroprusside. *N. Engl. J. Med.* 292:294, 1975.

45. Pribble, A. H., and Tyler, M. L. Emergency! *Nurs. '75* 5:45, 1975.

46. Robertson, K. J., and Guzzetta, C. E. Arterial blood-gas interpretations in the respiratory intensive-care unit. *Heart Lung* 5:256, 1976.

47. Rosenberg, A. S., Grossman, J. I., Escher, D. J., et al. Bedside transvenous cardiac pacing. *Am. Heart J.* 77:697, 1969.

48. Schnitzler, R. N., Caracta, A. R., and Damato, A. N. "Floating" catheter for temporary transvenous ventricular pacing. *Am. J. Cardiol.* 31:351, 1973.

49. Sonnenblick, E. H., Frishman, W. H., and LeJemtel, T. H. Dobutamine: A new synthetic cardioactive sympathetic amine. *N. Engl. J. Med.* 300:17, 1979.

50. Spann, J. F., Moellering, R. C., Haber, E., et al. Arrhythmias in acute myocardial infarction: A study utilizing an electrocardiographic monitor for automatic detection and recording of arrhythmias. *N. Engl. J. Med.* 271:427, 1964.

51. Starmer, C. F., McIntosh, H. D., and Whalen, R. E. Electrical hazards and cardiovascular function. *N. Engl. J. Med.* 284:181, 1971.

52. Stone, E. W., and Zuckerman, S. The esophageal obturator airway. *Am. J. Nurs.* 75:1148, 1975.

53. Steen, P. A., Tinker, J. H., Pluth, J. R., et al. Efficacy of dopamine, dobutamine, and epinephrine during emergence from cardiopulmonary bypass in man. *Circulation* 57:378, 1978.

54. Subcommittee on Emergency Cardiac Care Task Force on CPR—ECC Learning Program. *Manual for Instructors of Basic Cardiac Life Support.* Dallas: American Heart Association, 1977.

55. Thalen, H. J. The artificial cardiac pacemaker. *Am. Heart J.* 81:583, 1971.

56. Ungvarski, P. J., Argondizzo, N. T., and Boos, P. K. CPR: Current practice revised. *Am. J. Nurs.* 75:236, 1975.

57. Vera, Z., Awan, N. A., Amsterdam, E. A., et al. Cardiac pacemakers: Indications and complications. *Heart Lung* 4:444, 1975.

58. Winslow, E. H., and Marino, L. B. Temporary cardiac pacemakers. *Am. J. Nurs.* 75:586, 1975.

59. Ziesche, S., and Franciosa, J. A. Clinical application of sodium nitroprusside. *Heart Lung* 6:99, 1977.

60. Zoll, P. M. Resuscitation of the heart in ventricular standstill by external electric stimulation. *N. Engl. J. Med.* 274:768, 1952.

Acute Myocardial Infarction

Barbara Montgomery Dossey

Coronary artery disease—myocardial infarction specifically—is the leading cause of death in the United States. The physical signs of acute myocardial infarction depend on the presence or absence of complications of the acute infarction. Nurses who care for patients who have had an acute myocardial infarction must understand the disease process and must be able to assess symptoms and complications, to relate the complications to the physiological or psychological causes, and to initiate or anticipate the appropriate treatment. Nursing care must focus on the prevention of complications. When complications occur, nurses must be able to make the decisions needed to carry out the appropriate nursing actions.

Objective

When a patient has the most commonly occurring symptoms of acute myocardial infarction, the nurse should be able to (1) evaluate the problem (using the nursing process), (2) do a systematic assessment, (3) help relieve pain and anxiety, (4) determine whether she has alleviated the pain and anxiety, and (5) anticipate the possible life-threatening complications.

19

Achieving the Objective

To achieve the objective, the nurse should be able to:

1. Identify the urgent problems. (The nurse should not use time for history taking until the urgent problems are alleviated.)
2. Describe the pathological changes in acute myocardial infarction and be aware of the specific complications.
3. List the most common complications of acute myocardial infarction.
4. Carry out rapidly the nursing care for each complication as it occurs.

How to Proceed

To develop an approach to acute myocardial infarction, the nurse should:

1. Read the case study that follows and then study it in detail.
2. Analyze the symptoms of acute myocardial infarction that the patient in the case study shows.
   a. List the patient's urgent problems and specific nursing actions.
   b. Describe the pathological changes that occur during acute myocardial infarction.
3. Outline the steps for her initial assessment of the patient.
4. Explain her plan for assessing the patient and why it is useful for the particular patient.
5. State the physiological and psychological problems that she anticipates for the patient.
6. Outline the major objectives for patient care and management before reading the discussion of Nursing Orders found later in the chapter.

Case Study

Mr. C. V., aged 44, was admitted to the coronary care unit. He was wearing tennis clothes. In the initial assessment, the nurse described Mr. V. as an anxious man of medium build who was in acute distress. Mr. V. stated, "I have chest pain going down my left arm and up into my left jaw. I'm short of breath."

Mr. V.'s wife stated that Mr. V. had been playing tennis and had complained of a dull, pressing heaviness in his chest that forced him to stop his tennis game. His tennis partner called an ambulance and Mr. V. was taken to the hospital. Mr. V.'s wife stated that Mr. V. had been very healthy and that he had no history of heart disease. Two weeks before his

admission, the patient had had a routine health examination.

The patient's profile and social history stated that Mr. V. was an attorney, that he was 6'2" tall, and that he weighed 185 lbs. His wife, aged 40, was well. She seemed very apprehensive and spoke of her fear that her husband would die. Mr. and Mrs. V. had three children, aged 17, 18, and 20; they were alive and well. The oldest son was with his mother at the hospital; the other children were away at school. The wife stated that her husband was active in community, church, and professional organizations. She said that this was an unfortunate time for him to be sick because he had several lawsuits pending in which he was the trial lawyer. Mr. V. did not smoke. He drank socially, consuming three drinks at the most at parties.

Mr. V.'s past medical history stated that he had no heart disease, hypertension, or diabetes mellitus. He had never been hospitalized. He had no known allergies, and he was not taking any medications.

Mr. V.'s family history stated that his father died of a heart attack at the age of 54 and that his two brothers, aged 46 and 50, were taking antihypertensive medication. His mother, aged 72, was alive and well.

A physical examination showed that Mr. V.'s blood pressure was 80/50 mm Hg, his pulse 140 and irregular, his respirations 28, and his temperature 98.6°F. Lateral motion of his chest wall showed that he used accessory muscles for respiration. His breath sounds were normal. His skin was warm and moist. An examination of his cardiovascular system showed the point of maximal impulse at the fifth intercostal space in the left midclavicular line. He had no murmurs or thrills. His peripheral pulses were full and equal. He had no abdominal tenderness or masses. The bedside monitor showed that he had tachycardia (140 beats/min), with multifocal premature ventricular contractions and elevated ST segments.

Mr. V.'s initial diagnostic tests (see assessment sheet), which were done about three hours after his chest pain began, showed that his creatinine phosphokinase level was 323 μ/ml (normal for a man is 5–35 μ/ml), his serum glutamic-oxaloacetic transaminase level was 120 μ/100 ml (normal is 15–40 μ/ml), his lactic dehydrogenase level was 140 μ/ml (normal is 130 μ/ml), and that his electrolytes, blood, and urine were normal. The ECG showed sinus tachycardia (140 beats/min), with multifocal premature ventricular contractions, and elevated ST segments in leads V_1 through V_4 (Fig. 19-1). Those leads reflect the electrical activity of the anterior wall of the left ventricle. The involvement was most probably in the anterior descending branch of the left coronary artery.

Mr. V.'s cardiac enzyme levels were grossly elevated because of cardiac muscle damage. (Enzymes released from damaged or infarcted muscle can elevate the serum levels.)

Mr. V. was first given intravenous morphine sulfate (5 mg/5 ml sterile H_2O) for his chest pain, then lidocaine (a 50 mg/2.5 ml intravenous bolus), and then a continuous intra-

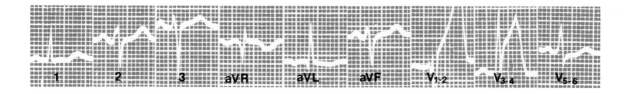

Figure 19-1

The ECG reveals elevated ST segments of acute anterior wall myocardial infarction, illustrating infarction of the anterior wall of the left ventricle.

venous infusion of lidocaine (4 mg/ml) for his persistent multifocal premature ventricular contractions. He continued to complain of chest pain after the initial dose of morphine, and he was given morphine sulfate (2 mg/5 ml sterile H_2O) every 30 minutes for the next two hours.

Eight hours after Mr. V.'s admission, on cardiac auscultation his physician found a third heart sound that suggested early left ventricular failure. Mr. V.'s pulse was 110. His apparent congestive heart failure was treated initially with intravenous furosemide (40 mg/4 ml).

Pulmonary auscultation showed moderate congestion of both lungs, with bilateral basilar rales. Radiological examination confirmed the presence of moderate bilateral congestion and Kerly B lines at each base.

The congestion in his lungs was the result of transudation of fluid into the interstitial spaces and the alveoli caused by acute left ventricular failure.

About 24 hours after Mr. V.'s admission, his condition changed suddenly. His skin became cool and clammy. His blood pressure dropped to 50/0 mm Hg, and his pulse was rapid (140) and thready. Mr. V.'s physician ordered that Mr. V. be given levarterenol (16 mg in 1 L of a 5% dextrose in water solution) and that intermittent positive pressure breathing be begun. Arterial blood gases were measured. A Foley catheter was inserted as ordered, and 50 ml of urine was drained. The physician inserted a Swan-Ganz catheter with an initial pulmonary capillary wedge pressure of 25 mm Hg (normal is 5–12 mm Hg). Intravenous furosemide (80 mg) was given.

Cardiogenic shock occurred due to widespread necrosis of the anterior surface of the left ventricle that caused left ventricular dysfunction. Mr. V. developed third-degree heart block (35 beats/min), as shown on the bedside monitor.

To treat the heart block, a temporary demand pacemaker was inserted at Mr. V.'s bedside using a flow-directed, balloon-tipped catheter. Intermittent positive pressure breathing was begun.

The following additions to the problem list were made:

7. Cardiogenic shock.
8. Third-degree heart block.

Mr. V. showed no clinical improvement over the next hour, and his physician decided to use intraaortic balloon counterpulsation (Fig. 19-2).

Intraaortic balloon counterpulsation was begun to reduce the work load of the left ventricle and thus restore the balance between the myocardial oxygen supply and demand and improve peripheral tissue perfusion. The balloon was inserted into Mr. V.'s descending thoracic aorta through the femoral artery to a position just distal to the left subclavian artery.

After about 36 hours, Mr. V.'s condition had stabilized, and he was weaned from balloon support. His vital signs and urine output were normal. He had no evidence of congestive heart failure or dysrhythmia.

Mr. V. continued to make steady progress for the next four days. However, on day 5, while talking to his physician and the coronary care nurse he became dyspneic. His blood pressure suddenly went from 110/70 mm Hg to 80/50 mm Hg. Within minutes, Mr. V. developed acute florid pulmonary edema and ventricular fibrillation. Despite immediate medical and nursing management, he did not respond to cardiac emergency resuscitative efforts. A staff nurse summoned the hospital chaplain to be with the family while the health team was treating him.

Reflections

The staff's brief involvement in Mr. V.'s life caused them much stress. Each member of the staff present at the time of Mr. V.'s death was affected. As the day went on, one of the nurses realized that the strain was depressing the staff and that the staff needed to ventilate their feelings. With the guidance of the head nurse, the staff decided that for their own mental health they should:

1. Meet weekly for 30 minutes or longer in the critical care unit.
2. Discuss their feelings about unexpected death.
3. Announce early the topic of the weekly meeting so that the nurses who are off duty or who are on another shift the day of the meeting can arrange to attend the meeting.

Critical Care Nursing Admission Assessment

Head to Toe Approach

Date	Time	
		Pt. Name: *Mr. C.V.* Age: *44* Allergies: *NKA*
11-1-	*1³⁰PM*	Admitted Bed No: *4* Via: *stretcher* Ad. Dx.: *Acute Myocardial Infarction*
		T.: *98°F(o)* A.P.: *140* R.P.: *140* R.: *28* B.P. Supine R: *80/50* L: *80/50* Sitting: ——
		Wt. (unit scale): *185 lbs* Ht.: *6'2"* ECG Rhythm: *Sinus Tach* Ectopy: *multifocal PVC's*
		Informant: *pt. and wife* Last meal: *breakfast at 8 AM*
	1.	Chief complaint: *severe chest pain radiating down left arm; SOB*
	2.	Hx. of present illness: *dull, pressing heaviness in ant. chest while playing tennis; had to stop tennis game - came to hospital*
	3.	Past medical Hx. (include all surgeries, hosp., diseases, injuries, blood trans.): *none*
	4.	Family Hx.: *father died of MI at 54; brothers 50 and 46 hypertensive and on medication; mother alive and well*
	5.	Current drugs: *none*
	6.	Alcohol and tobacco habits: *occasionally drinks socially; does not smoke*
	7.	Dietary and fluid needs: *eats 3 meals a day*
	8.	Sleep and rest patterns: *sleeps average 7 hrs. per night*
	9.	Bowel and bladder habits: *daily BM; does not use laxatives*
	10.	Hygienic needs: *none*
	11.	Psychosocial needs: *poor comprehension of information at present; revaluate*
	12.	Occupation and education: *Trial lawyer c̄ large law firm*
	13.	Exercise habits: *plays tennis 4-5 x a week*
	14.	Spiritual needs: *active Baptist church*
	15.	Personal interests: *community and professional organizations - very active committee member*
	16.	Family member interaction and availability: *wife and 20 y.o. son at hospital; wife apprehensive, verbalizing fear of husband's death.*
	17.	Attitude towards illness and hospitalization: *pt. very anxious as demonstrated by being afraid to move in bed for fear of "making chest pain come back." Concerned about many pressures of job that need to be done.*

Physical Examination

Date	Time	
	18.	Gen. appearance: *well developed male c̄ no visible abnormalities* color: *dark from sun* skin: *warm + moist*
	19.	Neurological:
		a) level of consciousness: *alert, cooperative, anxious*
		b) cerebellar: posture: *deferred* gait: *deferred*
		c) motor function: upper: *normal* lower: *normal*
		d) sensory function: upper: *normal* lower: *normal*
		e) reflexes: *deferred*
	20.	Head and face: *no abnormalities*
	21.	Eyes: *no diplopia; uses glasses for reading*
	22.	Ears: *no discharge; no difficulty hearing*
	23.	Nose: *negative*
	24.	Mouth/throat: *upper left dental plate*
	25.	Neck: *no neck vein distention*
	26.	Chest: *equal excursion*
	27.	Breast: *negative*
	28.	Respiratory: *normal vesicular breath sounds*
	29.	Cardiac: *tachycardia - frequent ectopy - PMI 5th ICS in left MCL; heart sounds normal; no S3, S4, or murmurs*
	30.	Abdomen: *normal; bowel sounds: normal*
	31.	Genitourinary: *no bladder distention; voided 4 hrs. prior to admission*
	32.	Extremities (all pulses): *all pulses strong and equal*
	33.	Back: *no sacral edema, scars.*
	34.	Problems requiring possible referral service: *none*
	35.	Teaching needs: *cardiac rehabilitation c̄ pt. and family*
	36.	Other:

11-1		PROBLEM LIST: **ACTIVE**	**INACTIVE**
		1. *chest pain*	
		2. *multifocal PVCS*	
		3. *↓ cardiac output*	
		4. *anxiety*	
		5. *SOB*	

Barbara Dossey RN, CCRN
NURSE'S SIGNATURE

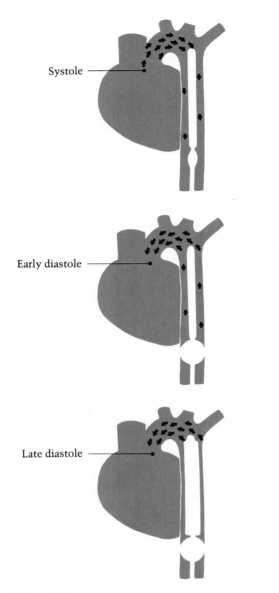

Systole

Early diastole

Late diastole

Figure 19-2
During *systole*, the aortic pressure decreases, thus reducing the work load of the left ventricle. During *diastole*, the aortic pressure increases, causing an increase in the coronary perfusion pressure, with the end results of increased coronary and cerebral blood flow.

The meetings were held as planned. One meeting was devoted entirely to a discussion of risk factors for atherosclerotic heart disease. The nurses discussed the risk factors—smoking, obesity, sedentary habits, and stress and anxiety—as reflections of life-style. The nurses asked, "Don't those risk factors reflect how a patient thinks and feels about himself? Don't they involve decisions on the part of a patient about how he should structure his life? Can't a patient take responsibility for changing his life-style and thus reduce those risk factors?"

One critical care nurse said that she considered those risk factors psychological because they were produced by the patient's attitude toward his life. Another nurse said that although those risk factors might be psychological, they could affect the heart just as seriously as nonpsychological risk factors, such as elevation of the serum cholesterol level. In the discussion that followed, the nurses came to the conclusions that a patient's attitudes toward himself and his life affect his health and that the state of a patient's health reflects his thoughts and actions.

The Anatomy and Physiology of the Heart

Normally the heart is located in the lower anterior mediastinal space of the thoracic cavity. When one is standing, the left ventricle of his heart lies on the superior aspect of the diaphragm, anterior to the trachea, esophagus, and thoracic aorta and posterior to the sternum. The heart is surrounded by the inferior and middle (right) lobes of the lungs, and it is separated from the lungs by the pericardium. Since the right and the left sides of the heart differ in musculature, vascular structure, and function, the left side and the right side are discussed separately in the material that follows.

The heart is a complex muscle whose sole function is to pump blood. The heart is composed of four chambers, which act as a double pump with four one-way valves (Fig. 19-3). The function of the right atrium and the right ventricle is to pump venous blood to the lungs. The function of the left side of the heart is to pump oxygenated blood into the systemic circulation. The pumps operate simultaneously. In the normal heart, the atria are separated by the thin, muscular interatrial septum, and the ventricles are separated by the interventricular septum. Those structures prevent communication between the right and the left sides of the heart. The movement of blood

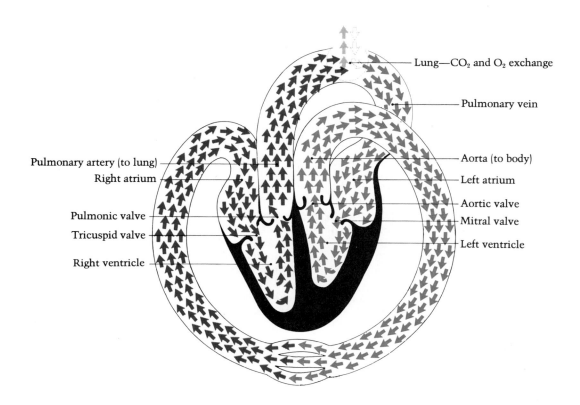

Lung—CO₂ and O₂ exchange

Pulmonary vein

Pulmonary artery (to lung)
Right atrium

Pulmonic valve
Tricuspid valve

Right ventricle

Aorta (to body)
Left atrium
Aortic valve
Mitral valve
Left ventricle

Figure 19-3
Normal circulation.

in and out of each chamber of the heart is related to the cardiac cycle. Systole is the time during which the ventricles contract. Diastole is the time during which the ventricles relax.

Blood from the superior vena cava, inferior vena cava, coronary sinus, and thebesian veins enters the right atrium, a thin-walled, muscular structure. Blood enters the right atrium under low pressure. It then goes through the tricuspid valve (the three-leaflet atrioventricular valve).

The right ventricle is a crescent-shaped, thin-walled, muscular structure. A slightly greater pressure in the right atrium moves blood into the right ventricle during diastole. During atrial contraction and right ventricular relaxation, additional blood enters the ventricle because of a pressure gradient. The right ventricle receives about 85 percent of its un-oxygenated blood through the tricuspid valve during diastole. Atrial contraction contributes the remaining

15 percent of unoxygenated blood. Blood leaves the right ventricle under low pressure through the pulmonic semilunar valve and the pulmonary artery to the lungs. Contraction of the right ventricle is a bellows-like action. A healthy tricuspid valve keeps blood from regurgitating into the right atrium; a healthy pulmonic valve keeps blood from regurgitating into the right ventricle.

Within the right ventricle are papillary muscles that are attached to the ventricular wall. The chordae tendineae are attached at their one end to the apex of the papillary muscles and at their other end to the free edges of the three leaflets of the tricuspid valve. As venous blood enters the right atrium, the leaflets of the tricuspid valve move downward; during right ventricular contraction, the chordae pull on the tricuspid valve, causing the valve to close. During closure of the tricuspid valve, pressure exerted in the contracting right ventricle exerts pressure on the three semilunar leaflets of the pulmonic valve, causing the leaflets to flap open and back against the pulmonary artery wall as blood is sent to the lungs.

The main pulmonary artery bifurcates into the

right and left branches, which go to the right and left lungs, respectively. The right pulmonary artery has branches that supply the three lobes of the right lung, and the left pulmonary artery has branches that supply the two lobes of the left lung. Unoxygenated blood in the lungs becomes oxygenated due to the pulmonary circulatory system. Carbon dioxide is exchanged for oxygen at the alveolar capillary level. Oxygenated blood is returned to the left side of the heart through the four pulmonary veins to the left atrium.

The left atrium has a thicker musculature than the right atrium. During ventricular systole, the major portion of oxygenated blood enters the left atrium. This occurs at the same time as the onset of atrial diastole, during which the left atrium expands to accept blood from the pulmonary circulation. The pressure difference between the blood-filled left atrium and the relaxed left ventricle in diastole forces the oxygenated blood through the mitral valve (the two-cusp atrioventricular valve), which opens during the filling of the left ventricle.

The left ventricle is approximately two to three times thicker than the right ventricle owing to the difference in work load. Greater force is required to move blood from the left ventricle to the systemic circulation than to move blood from the right ventricle to the lungs. The left ventricle, a high-pressure chamber, contracts in a corkscrew action as it propels blood through the outflow tract and the aortic valve to the aorta.

At the beginning of ventricular systole, the mitral valve begins to close. As ventricular pressure increases, the only exit for blood is through the ascending aorta, which originates at the outflow tract of the left ventricle. The aortic valve, a three-leaflet valve, opens as a result of increased ventricular pressure during systole, just as does the pulmonic valve on the right side. At the end of systole, the pressure in the aorta exceeds the pressure in the left ventricle. The aortic valve closes, preventing regurgitation of blood into the left ventricle. The two papillary muscles on the left side of the heart help to close the mitral valve during systole.

The Anatomy of the Coronary Arteries

The critical care nurse can anticipate the complications of acute myocardial infarction more often and more accurately if she knows the anatomy of the

coronary arteries (Fig. 19-4). Knowledge of the standard anatomy of the coronary arteries is useful to the nurse even though the anatomy of the arteries may vary in each of her patients.

THE LEFT CORONARY ARTERY

The main left coronary artery originates in the left sinus of Valsalva and branches into the left anterior descending artery and the circumflex artery immediately below the level of the pulmonary artery. The left anterior descending artery travels in the anterior interventricular sulcus to the apex, and, typically, wraps around it. It terminates in the inferior third of the posterior interventricular sulcus. Branches of the anterior descending artery perforate into the right half of the interventricular septum toward the posterior interventricular sulcus. The first large branch is referred to as the major septal branch. The other branches supplying the anterior left ventricular wall are referred to as the diagonal branches because of their position on the free wall of the left ventricle.

The left anterior descending artery has five segments: (1) the proximal segment, the portion from its origin to the beginning of the first major septal branch, (2) the midsegment, the portion from the first major septal branch to the midpoint of the midsegment and the apex, (3) the apical segment, the portion from the midsegment to the apex of the heart, (4) the first diagonal branch, and (5) the second diagonal branch.

THE CIRCUMFLEX ARTERY

The left circumflex artery runs along the left posterior atrioventricular groove to the crux of the heart (the crossing of the interatrial and the interventricular septa in the atrioventricular plane). In about 10 percent of people the circumflex artery continues past the crux of the heart and then turns downward to form the posterior descending artery. In those people, the left coronary artery supplies the entire left ventricle and the interventricular septum. The circumflex artery supplies parts of the left ventricle, the anterior, lateral, and, in some cases, the posterior parts. The largest branch of the circumflex artery is the obtuse marginal branch. The posterolateral branch supplies a part of the posterior part of the left ventricular wall. The circumflex artery has branches to the atria, called the atrial circumflex branches. (Forty-one to 45 percent of people have a branch of the

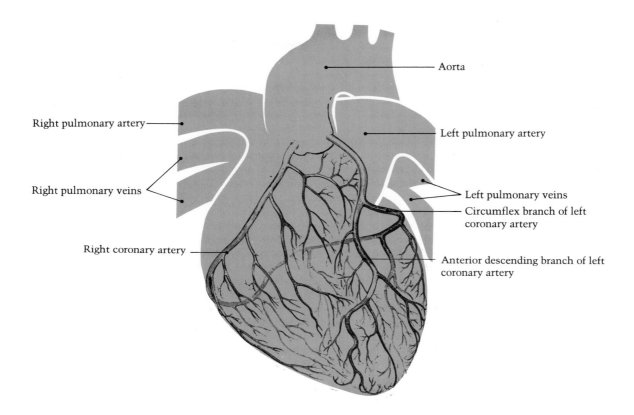

Right pulmonary artery

Right pulmonary veins

Right coronary artery

Aorta

Left pulmonary artery

Left pulmonary veins

Circumflex branch of left coronary artery

Anterior descending branch of left coronary artery

Figure 19-4
Anatomy of the coronary arteries.

circumflex artery that goes to the sinus node; 12 percent of people have a branch of the circumflex artery that goes to the atrioventricular node.)

The circumflex artery also has five segments: (1) the proximal segment, the portion from the artery's origin to the beginning of the obtuse marginal branch; (2) the obtuse marginal branch; (3) the distal segment, the portion between the origin of the obtuse margin and the posterior descending artery; (4) the posterior descending artery (not always present); and (5) the posterolateral branch.

THE RIGHT CORONARY ARTERY

As the right coronary artery leaves the wall of the ascending aorta in the right anterior sinus of Valsalva, it enters the right atrioventricular sulcus toward the diaphragmatic surface of the heart. At that point, the posterior portions of the interatrial and interventricular septa meet, forming the crux of the heart.

The right coronary artery has anterior branches that spread to the right ventricle. It has branches that spread superiorly and posteriorly and supply the atria. The anterior branches of the right coronary artery are (1) the conus branch, (2) the sinus node branch, (3) two or more right ventricular branches, (4) the posterior descending branch, and (5) a branch or branches to the left ventricle. The important superior and posterior branches of the right coronary artery are those to the sinus node. The right coronary artery provides blood supply to the sinus node in about 55 percent of people. In 45 percent of people, the branch to the sinus node originates in the circumflex artery, the intermediate atrial artery, or the atrioventricular (AV) node branch [28]. It can also originate in the right coronary artery. The right coronary artery has three segments that are important for surgical purposes: (1) the proximal segment, the portion from the ostium to the right ventricular branch; (2) the midsegment, the portion from the right ventricular branch to the acute margin of the heart; and (3) the distal segment, the portion from the acute margin to the crux of the heart. The right coronary artery has a fourth segment, the posterior descending artery.

Coronary Artery Circulation

The heart receives its blood supply from the coronary arteries, which are perfused primarily during ventricular diastole. Decreased blood flow to coronary arteries may produce ischemia of the conduction system, causing certain types of problems. (Diseases such as polyarteritis nodosa, lupus erythematosus, and hereditary disorders associated with myocardiopathies also affect the small arteries and can cause many dysrhythmias and conduction disturbances. Those diseases are not discussed here.)

The left coronary artery supplies the right bundle branch, the anterosuperior division of the left bundle branch, part of the posteroinferior division of the left bundle branch, and the anterior two-thirds of the ventricular septum. The critical care nurse who knows the relevant anatomy can anticipate the most common complications of anterior wall myocardial infarction; namely, pump failure, atrial and ventricular dysrhythmias, and intraventricular conduction disturbances (Mobitz type II, bundle branch blocks, and hemiblocks) [11, 14, 46, 52].

Patients with inferior wall myocardial infarction usually have occlusion of the right coronary artery. In most people, the right coronary artery supplies the sinoatrial node, the atrioventricular junctional tissue, the His bundle, the posterior one-third of the ventricular septum, and the posteroinferior division of the left bundle branch. People who have had acute inferior wall myocardial infarctions often have either bradydysrhythmias caused by an ischemic sinus node or AV node, and Wenckebach phenomenon (Mobitz type I heart block).

Collateral Circulation

There are few connections between the large coronary arteries, but there are many anastomoses between the small coronary arteries. When coronary arteries occlude progressively, a collateral blood supply can develop that functions when the coronary arteries are completely occluded. Usually the collateral blood supply becomes well developed only after complete occlusion. At the time of occlusion, the arterioles reach their maximum diameters within seconds. Blood flow at that time is only half of that which is needed to keep cardiac muscle alive. Over the next 8 to 24 hours, the collateral vessels enlarge further, and collateral flow begins to increase over the next several days, sometimes reaching a near normal coronary supply within a month. Collateral intercoronary anastomoses increase the patient's chances of surviving a coronary occlusion.

The Cardiac Veins

The cardiac veins generally follow the branches of the major coronary arteries. There are three dominant coronary vein systems: (1) the coronary sinus and its tributaries, (2) the anterior cardiac veins, and (3) the thebesian veins. Those veins join in the coronary sinus and empty into the right atrium between the opening of the inferior vena cava and the atrioventricular opening.

The coronary sinus and its tributaries are the largest system. They drain blood primarily from the left ventricle. The anterior cardiac veins have several large trunks over the anterior wall, and they provide most of the draining of the right ventricle.

The thebesian veins are the smallest system. They are found primarily in the right atrium and right ventricle; occasionally they are found in the left side of the heart.

Compensatory Mechanisms

According to the Starling law, within normal physiological limits, the heart can pump all the blood that comes into it in diastole without allowing blood to back up into the veins [22]. The cardiac muscle has a normal reserve mechanism that allows it to stretch even when extra blood enters the chambers; it contracts with greater force to move blood into the arteries. As end-diastolic fiber length increases, so does cardiac output. The compensatory mechanism is seen not in patients with acute heart failure but in patients with chronic heart failure because it takes some time for hypertrophy to develop.

In aortic or pulmonic stenosis and pulmonary or systemic hypertension, too much stress is placed on the chambers of the heart that pump against resistance. Hypertrophy compensates temporarily until the chambers expand to such a size that the heart does not receive enough blood and ischemia exists.

An increase in stroke volume, the amount of blood ejected into circulation with each heart beat, is another compensatory mechanism of the heart. It works by increasing the venous return to the heart or by increasing the ejection fraction (the amount of blood ejected with each heart beat). Venous tone is increased by the increased reflex activity of the sympathetic nervous system. When venous pressure is increased, the venous return to the heart is also increased and the amount of blood returned to the heart is increased.

An increase in heart rate is also a compensatory mechanism. During exercise, the heart rate of a healthy person increases. The increased heart rate increases cardiac output and the body's demand for blood. In acute myocardial infarction, an increased heart rate may not be a useful compensatory mechanism. Diastolic ventricular filling decreases with tachyarrhythmias; heart rates above 160 beats per minute decrease ventricular filling, and decrease the cardiac output. It can precipitate angina, congestive heart failure, and dysrhythmias. Since the coronary vessels fill primarily during diastole, increased heart rate can be a dangerous event after acute myocardial infarction.

The Pathophysiology of Coronary Artery Disease

The exact cause of atherosclerosis is as yet unknown. Atherosclerosis is a disease with many causes that affects different people in different ways regardless of the number of known risk factors present in any person. There are two theories about the beginning of intimal plaque development in atherosclerosis. One theory is that of plasma lipid infiltration; and the other is that of mural thrombosis [7, 55].

The theory of plasma lipid infiltration suggests that hyperlipidemia from dietary or endogenous factors causes the infiltration of plasma lipids at the level of the intima and that the infiltration is the beginning of the development of atherosclerotic plaque. Analysis and identification of serum lipoprotein constituents reveal that serum low density lipoprotein (LDL) is the major cholesterol-carrying lipoprotein in plasma. The chemical characteristics of LDL and other factors related to the permeability of the vessel endothelium seem to cause selective trapping. Particles as large as those of LDL cannot pass between the endothelial cells. They are transported to the intima through the endothelial vesicles. The rate of vesicular transport is 10 times greater than that necessary to account for the observed accumulation of cholesterol in atherosclerotic intima in men.

The theory of mural thrombosis suggests that mural thrombosis (fibrin and platelet deposition) on the arterial intima with endothelialization is the beginning of the development of atherosclerotic plaque.

Atherosclerosis appears to involve the arterial system and spare the systemic veins and pulmonary arteries. However, thrombi are often found in the systemic veins without any evidence of atherosclerosis, suggesting that still other factors are important. While the blood flow is about the same in the systemic circulation, the pressure is only about one-fifth as high as in the arterial circulation. Researchers feel that the pressure difference in the venous circulation is probably not enough to cause the infiltration of circulating lipoproteins into the intima of the pulmonary arteries and systemic veins. However, in the presence of pulmonary hypertension, atherosclerotic plaques can develop in the pulmonary arterial system.

Important experimental data that contradict the theory of mural thrombosis have been demonstrated. The composition of atherosclerotic lesions has been analyzed using immunohistochemical techniques.

With the use of anti-LDL antibodies, marked fluorescence appeared in areas where lipid deposition was present. Fluorescence in the thickened intima and sometimes in the media was seen when antifibrinogen gamma globulin was used. Those results did not prove that fibrin accumulation is evidence of an organized or a recent thrombus [55]. Other studies indicated that platelets may enter the arterial wall and start the development of plaque [16].

Intraarterial Complications

Although the pathogenesis of atherosclerosis is controversial, there is information from necropsic examination about the varying types and degrees of atherosclerotic narrowing or occlusion at the level of the intima of the coronary vessels [55]. Within the intima are cells that begin to ingest cholesterol, forming tiny plaques. Cholesterol acts as an irritant, causing a reaction in which fibrotic tissue forms around the plaques and involves the media. As in any healing wound, capillaries grow into the plaques and become

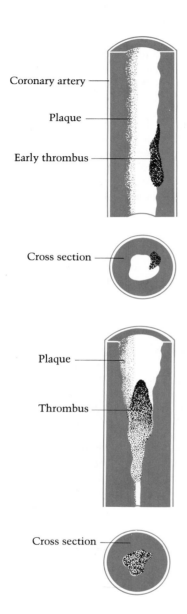

Coronary artery

Plaque

Early thrombus

Cross section

Plaque

Thrombus

Cross section

Figure 19-5
The arterial thrombus most frequently begins at the areas of luminal narrowing caused by atherosclerotic plaques. The chief thrombus components are platelets and then platelets and fibrin.

larger and larger. At some point, there may be hemorrhage into the plaques. Hemorrhage can be localized and resorbed within the plaques, and the damage may be minimal. However, the hemorrhage can dissect through the plaque into the lumen of the coronary artery, occasionally leading to the development of a clot, or thrombus. A thrombus can drastically and suddenly occlude the artery, and, depending on the size of the thrombus, the patient may or may not have symptoms associated with it, such as the pain of myocardial ischemia (Fig. 19-5). Arterial thrombus most often begins at the areas of luminal narrowing caused by atherosclerotic plaques. The chief thrombus components are platelets, followed by platelets and fibrin. Sooner or later, if the patient survives the thrombus, other phenomena follow. Calcification eventually occurs around the whole plaque, causing the lumen of the artery to become smaller.

The process usually occurs near the origin and bifurcation of the main coronary vessels, not throughout the vessels. Local mechanical factors, such as the turbulence of blood flow at and near the bifurcation, may help to retard or stimulate atherogenesis.

Risk Factors

The data that have accumulated over the last decade on multiple risk factors for coronary atherosclerosis are impressive [56]. The American Heart Association has identified the following nine factors that have commonly been found among people who have had a myocardial infarction: (1) a family history of atherosclerosis, (2) hypertension, (3) diabetes, (4) a sedentary life-style, (5) cigarette smoking, (6) obesity, (7) hypercholesterolemia, (8) a high intake of saturated fat, and (9) excessive stress. Three major risk factors have been found more often than others in many epidemiological studies; namely, hypercholesterolemia, hypertension, and cigarette smoking. A disturbing fact that emerged from the data on risk factors is that acute myocardial infarction can occur in people who have no risk factors.

However, the data reveal also that much can be done to reduce the risk and that people who have one or more risk factors have a greater chance of developing atherosclerosis than do people without risk factors [45].

Table 19-1
Familial Disorders of Lipoprotein Metabolism

	Possible Mechanism	Age of Detection	Clinical Presentation	Cholesterol	Triglyceride
Type I	Genetic recessive; deficiency in lipoprotein lipase	Early childhood	Lipemia retinalis, eruptive xanthomas, hepatosplenomegaly, abdominal pain	Normal or elevated	Markedly elevated
Type II	When genetic, dominant, sporadic; decreased catabolism of beta-lipoprotein	Early childhood (in severe cases)	Accelerated atherosclerosis, xanthelasma, tendon and tuberous xanthomas, juvenile corneal arcus	Elevated	Normal
Type III	When genetic, recessive, sporadic	Adulthood (over age 20)	Accelerated atherosclerosis of coronary and peripheral vessels, xanthoma planum, eruptive, tuberous, and tendon xanthomas	Elevated	Usually elevated
Type IV	When genetic, dominant, sporadic, excessive endogenous glyceride synthesis or deficient glyceride clearance	Adulthood	Accelerated coronary vessel disease, abnormal glucose tolerance, hyperuricemia	Normal or elevated	Elevated
Type V	Probably genetic and sporadic	Early adulthood	Lipemia retinalis, eruptive xanthomas, hepatosplenomegaly, abdominal pain, hyperglycemia, hyperuricemia	Elevated	Elevated to markedly elevated

Familial Hyperlipidemias

People with familial hyperlipidemias, which are hereditary disorders, have a higher rate of coronary atherosclerosis than do people who do not have those disorders. The familial disorders of lipoprotein metabolism have been classified (Table 19-1).

In one study (known as the Framingham study), the incidence of coronary disease in people with arterial pressures higher than 160/95 mm Hg was shown to be significantly higher than in people with lower pressures. Hypertension increases the turbulence of blood flow. Because of the extreme force that is exerted with each heart beat, the coronary arteries seem to be more susceptible to the formation of atheroma [36]. Hypertensive patients have more severe and frequent atherosclerosis, perhaps due to the increased pressure on the arterial walls.

Cigarette smoking is associated statistically with accelerated atherosclerosis. Although the exact mechanism of acceleration is not known, the relationships are probably between the direct and the indirect effects of nicotine levels [35]. Catecholamines are liberated in response to nicotine, and thus systolic blood pressure, heart rate, and cardiac output are increased.

Diabetes

It appears that diabetics have a higher incidence of atherosclerosis than have nondiabetics. Insulin modifies lipid metabolism. Diabetics often have increased levels of cholesterol and other circulating fats. The vascular changes common to diabetes increase one's chances of developing atherosclerosis.

Obesity

Although it has not been proved that obesity causes atherosclerosis, atherosclerosis appears to be slightly more prevalent among obese persons than among people of normal weight. And as a group, obese people have hypertension and hypercholesterolemia more often, as epidemiological studies show. People who wish to lose weight should avoid fad diets. Most fad diets focus on combinations of food groups rather than on how many calories are eaten. However, fad diets are frequently high in protein and fat. The biggest problem with these diets is an increase in hyperlipidemia. Behavior modification techniques have been recommended to accompany a sound nutritional approach to weight loss and weight maintenance. With behavior modification techniques, a person becomes aware of how to increase the frequency of desired behavior and to decrease undesirable behavior. Modification of eating habits is accomplished by altering events prior to eating and the different events of eating [21].

High Intake of Saturated Fats

The theory that a high intake of saturated fats and refined sugar is a risk factor is controversial. Saturated fats are the solid animal fats found in meat and dairy products. The polyunsaturated fats are the liquid (at room temperature) vegetable oils found in safflowers, soybeans, corn, and cottonseeds. Poultry and fish are also high in polyunsaturated fats. A high intake of polyunsaturated fats lowers cholesterol levels.

In normal subjects, low-fat–high-carbohydrate diets decrease serum cholesterol but increase lipoproteins (including triglycerides). Since such extreme variations occur in diets, the results of sound research on diets suggest that in the general population 90 percent of the cases of ordinary hyperlipidemias will respond to simple diets that have a 10:10:10 ratio of saturated, unsaturated, and polyunsaturated fats.

Sedentary Life-Style

The role of physical activity in atherosclerosis is not clearly understood. Several studies show a small reduction in mortality among people who have active jobs rather than sedentary ones. A study of British civil service employees that compared clerks with postmen and active bus conductors with sedentary bus drivers showed a negative correlation between physical exercise and angina pectoris, acute coronary occlusion, and the degree of myocardial fibrosis. The Framingham study showed that the incidence of coronary heart disease among men who were extremely sedentary was double that found among men who were not extremely sedentary.

Behavior, Personality, and Stress

Medical investigators think that there is a relationship between coronary disease and emotions and be-

havior [5, 16]. Two major personality types have been described, type A and type B. Type A people feel a sense of urgency about most areas of their lives. They are extremely competitive, ambitious, and preoccupied with achievement. People with type A personalities are more likely to develop coronary disease than are people with type B personalities [18].

At the opposite end of the spectrum are the cardiologists who believe that factors other than personality type and stress promote coronary disease. Those cardiologists point out the Japanese, who have an extremely low rate of coronary disease despite the crowding, turmoil, and competition of Japanese society. Those cardiologists point out also the rural Finns, who do manual labor, who, as a group, have calm dispositions, whose diet is high in saturated fat—and whose mortality from coronary disease is the highest in the world [31]. How and to what degree stress and personality affect immunity, circulation, lipid metabolism, and coagulation are not fully understood. Some people respond to stressful situations by overeating and by becoming frustrated, whereas other people turn stressful situations into positive experiences. The relationship of stress and coronary artery disease is also not fully understood and is currently being widely investigated.

Hereditary Predisposition

Many people in the third and fourth decades whose parents lived to old age are found to have coronary disease. Nevertheless, many investigators think that longevity is determined largely by genes. For that reason, people who have inherited a tendency toward heart disease should try to reduce the other primary risk factors and thus decrease their chances of having a myocardial infarction.

Sex

Women of childbearing age have a lower incidence of atherosclerosis than have men of corresponding age. Estrogen is thought to cause a decrease in the ratio of beta- to alpha-lipoprotein at given serum cholesterol levels. Estrogen also appears to stimulate the resistance of the coronary arteries to atheroma formation. The incidence of atherosclerosis in women after the menopause approaches that in men.

Age

Two factors seem to be involved in aging. One is the effect of time and exposure to the concentration of beta-lipoproteins within the arteries, and the other is aging itself. Although atherosclerosis is more prevalent in older persons, it does occur in younger persons. Children known to have hyperlipidemias of type II or III can have severe atherosclerosis. It is thought that in each person the flexibility of the artery and the effect of aging on metabolism affect the rate of atheroma formation.

Risk Factors for Sudden Death

Attempts are being made to specify certain risk factors for sudden death as well as for nonfatal illnesses. For example, frequent premature ventricular contractions associated with myocardial disease are accompanied by an increased risk of sudden death.

Treatment of Major Risk Factors

Until more concrete information about all the risk factors is available, from epidemiological studies it seems advisable that everyone modify his diet according to the recommendations of the Inter-Society Commission for Heart Disease Resources [56]. Those recommendations include reducing saturated fat (substituting polyunsaturated fat) and keeping caloric intake to the level needed to maintain one's optimum weight [37].

Smokers should be encouraged to stop smoking, and children should be taught about the dangers of smoking. Intensive education should be given to people with hypertension. People should be told— through television and the other media—about the importance of having their blood pressure checked annually. Primary prevention of atherosclerosis through the control of hypertension, cigarette smoking, and hypercholesterolemia (factors implicated in epidemiological studies) should be pursued by medical professionals and by laymen.

Metabolic Response to Acute Myocardial Infarction

The basis for most acute myocardial infarctions is a decrease in blood flow or an acute obstruction of blood flow in a coronary artery that damages the myocardium. The classic symptoms and severe pain frequently associated with acute myocardial infarction can cause extreme anxiety and complications that lead to changes in metabolites and hormones throughout the body.

During the first hour after an acute myocardial infarction, very little in the myocardium is static. In the acutely insulted myocardium, there is probably a great reduction in the amount of available oxygen rather than total deprivation of oxygen. The portion of the myocardium that lies beyond the occlusion undergoes rapid changes: blood flow and pressure decrease in some areas and collateral vessels open under metabolic stimuli or close as thrombi form in them. Potentially viable tissue can be perfused by changes in cardiac output and in left ventricular pressure.

The ischemic myocardium gets its energy from stored glucose, glycogen, and fatty acids. In order for nutrients to contribute to energy production in the heart, the heart must have enough oxygen, adequate concentrations of nutrients in arterial blood, and control of those nutrients for uptake, utilization, and storage by myocardial cells. Glucose, lactate, and free fatty acids are the main nutrients in the blood that the heart can use. Normally, blood glucose and insulin concentrations are high; glucose is the principal source of energy. Free fatty acids are the main source of energy, with glucose and lactate providing small but necessary amounts in the fasting state. In the fasting state, myocardial oxidation is normal and concentrations of free fatty acids in blood are high. The utilization of free fatty acids is determined by the plasma concentration; the utilization of glucose is determined by the availability of usable insulin.

After an experimental coronary occlusion, blood flow to dependent areas is immediately reduced to approximately one-third of normal [42]. Stored glucose and glycogen are released, and the utilization of fatty acids is reduced. There is a loss of cell integrity in anoxic areas, as well as a loss of calcium, potassium, and magnesium ions. (Cellular viability depends on a critical concentration of those ions.)

Acidosis and the release of myocardial catecholamines also occur in the cells at an early stage of acute myocardial infarction. Acidosis suppresses pacemaker activity and contractility. The release of catecholamines, which occurs soon after coronary occlusion, is caused by hypoxia and stimulation of the

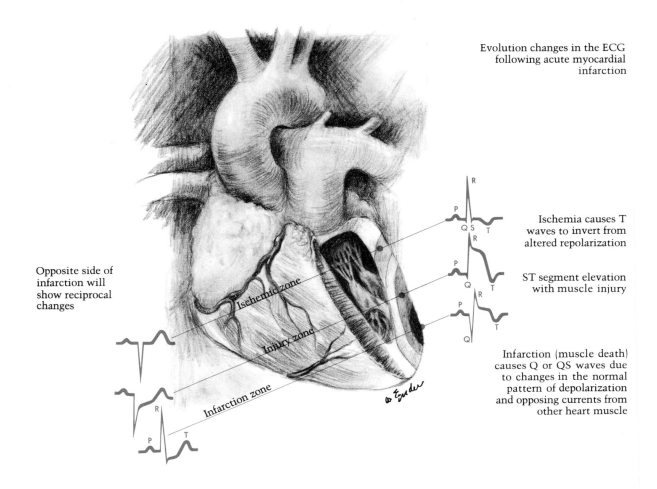

Evolution changes in the ECG following acute myocardial infarction

Ischemia causes T waves to invert from altered repolarization

ST segment elevation with muscle injury

Opposite side of infarction will show reciprocal changes

Ischemic zone

Injury zone

Infarction zone

Infarction (muscle death) causes Q or QS waves due to changes in the normal pattern of depolarization and opposing currents from other heart muscle

Figure 19-6
The effects of cardiac ischemia, injury, and infarction.

sympathetic nerves. Evidence exists that links catecholamine activity with serious dysrhythmias in experimental animals as well as in man.

SYSTEMIC METABOLIC RESPONSE

Systemic metabolic response is determined primarily by plasma catecholamine activity. During the first 24 to 48 hours after an acute coronary occlusion, the catecholamines norepinephrine and epinephrine are found in high concentrations in the plasma and urine. Norepinephrine causes the release of free fatty acids by acting directly on the beta-adrenergic receptors of adipose tissue. Epinephrine stimulates the liver and skeletal muscles and thus elevates the blood glucose level. Epinephrine affects the pancreas by suppressing beta-cell activity, which decreases insulin secretion and thus leads to increased blood sugar levels for sev-

eral days after an acute myocardial infarction. Increases of growth hormone and plasma cortisol levels after an acute myocardial infarction also contribute to a decrease in the production of insulin.

In acute myocardial infarction, an ischemic pattern is the earliest ECG change (Fig. 19-6). The next change in the ECG may be an injury pattern, an ST segment elevation in the leads that correspond to the injured area. The next change in the ECG is the appearance of abnormal Q waves over the area of infarction (that must last at least 0.04 sec), which is indicative of necrosis of the involved myocardial muscle tissue. In that phase there is still evidence of myocardial injury and ischemia. Myocardial necrosis means

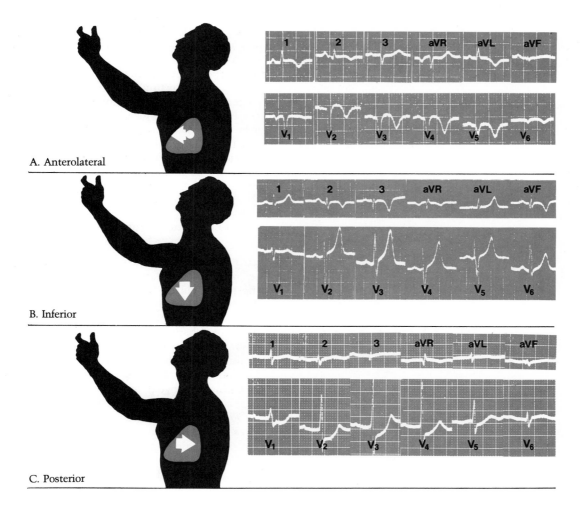

A. Anterolateral

B. Inferior

C. Posterior

Figure 19-7
A. Acute anterolateral myocardial infarction. Diagnostic Q waves and inverted T waves V_1 through V_6. Similar changes are seen in aVL, indicating lateral involvement. B. Acute inferior infarction. Diagnostic Q waves in leads 2, 3, aVF, with inverted T waves in those leads. Tall T waves are seen in the precordial leads, showing reciprocal changes. C. Acute posterior infarction. Prominent wide R waves are seen in V_1 and other precordial leads, with reciprocal ST-T wave changes in those leads.

that the cells in the affected area are electrically dead. Once the Q wave has evolved, it usually remains. ECG ischemia suggests that cellular metabolism is interrupted, thus causing the classic ECG pattern of electrical instability. The injury pattern records cell membrane damage, which indicates more serious electrical instability. The T wave and ST segment usually return to normal after the acute phase.

Since the left ventricle is the primary pumping chamber of the heart, an acute myocardial infarction affects primarily the left ventricle. The left ventricle is divided into anterior, inferior, lateral, and posterior walls (Fig. 19-7A–C). Acute myocardial infarctions are classified according to the place in the left ventricular wall at which they occur. An insult can

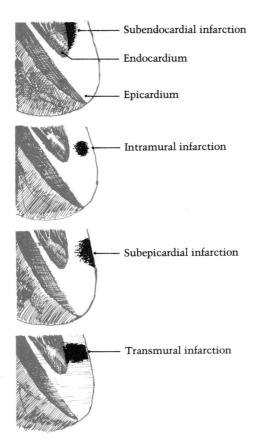

Figure 19-8
Location of various types of infarction in the ventricular wall.

involve several places in the wall, as shown in Figure 19-8.

Location of Infarction in the Ventricular Wall

An acute myocardial infarction can be subendocardial, subepicardial, intramural (confined to the interior of the myocardium), limited to the endocardium, limited to the layer below epicardial tissue, or transmural (involving the full thickness of the myocardium) (Fig. 19-8). A subendocardial infarction typically produces a depressed ST segment without a QRS complex alteration.

An infarction that destroys the entire thickness of the myocardium is called a transmural myocardial

infarction. A significant Q wave (one that lasts at least 0.04 sec) is produced in the lead overlying the infarction.

Because the shape of the chest and the position of the heart vary from person to person, it may be impossible to determine the exact location of an infarction from the ECG. Also, the location of the infarction may make it impossible to make a diagnosis. For example, a small intramural infarction that does not involve the endocardium or epicardium may not be seen on the ECG or the vectorcardiogram.

The Clinical Picture of Acute Myocardial Infarction

The appearance and behavior of people just after they suffer acute myocardial infarctions vary tremendously. Some people clutch their chests with pain. They may be pale, restless, diaphoretic, nauseous, or they may vomit. Most people are apprehensive and have pain. They may change their position or belch or walk to try to relieve the pain.

Angina pectoris usually lasts for three to five minutes. It can be relieved by removing the precipitating factor or by taking sublingual nitroglycerin, which should relieve the pain within minutes. However, the pain of acute myocardial infarction is continuous; it can radiate to the arms, fingers, shoulders, and jaws. The radiation of the pain suggests that the visceral afferent nerve fibers have central connections in common with the somatic afferent system. The persistence of the pain of acute myocardial infarction helps to differentiate it from angina pectoris. Narcotics are usually necessary to relieve the pain of the former. With luminal occlusion, a patient may die suddenly, apparently without pain. The usual cause of sudden death is thought to be a lethal dysrhythmia. Approximately 20 percent of the people with acute myocardial infarction have actual cardiac muscle damage without pain.

The Physical Signs of Acute Myocardial Infarction

The physical signs of acute myocardial infarction vary. Those seen most frequently are pallor, diaphoresis, tachydysrhythmia, bradydysrhythmia, extrasystoles, pulmonary rales, and gallop rhythm.

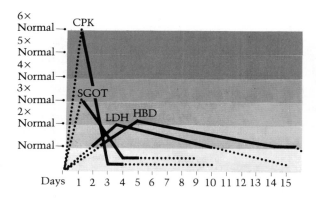

Figure 19-9
Time sequence of serum-enzyme elevations in acute myocardial infarction.

Diagnosis

Several diagnostic studies may be done to confirm the presence of acute mycocardial infarction. In some patients, the ECG may be negative, or the serum enzymes may be normal. However, if the history and physical examination suggest myocardial infarction, the patient should be observed for a period of time before myocardial infarction is ruled out.

A definitive diagnosis of acute myocardial infarction can be made when the signs of myocardial necrosis appear on the ECG. Those signs can appear within several days of the infarction or as late as a week after it [27]. Often, dysrhythmias and conduction disturbances distort the appearance of a diagnostic ECG. If that is the case, the diagnosis is based on the history, physical findings, and other laboratory data.

The serum enzyme measurements that are used to confirm the presence of acute myocardial infarction are the creatinine phosphokinase (CPK), serum glutamic oxaloacetic transaminase (SGOT), lactic dehydrogenase (LDH), and hydroxybutyrate dehydrogenase (HBD) levels (Fig. 19-9). The usual time sequence of serum enzyme changes after acute myocardial infarction is characteristic. Determination of the CPK-MB (the heart isoenzyme) level is thought to be the best laboratory parameter for the diagnosis of acute myocardial infarction, especially if no other muscle damage is present. Damage to many other tissues can elevate those serum enzymes. However, characteristic changes in the concentration at different rates help to pinpoint a myocardial source. The

sequence is due to the release of the CPK-MB from the damaged myocardial cells into the circulation.

As in other acute injuries, the leukocyte count and sedimentation rate are elevated in the early phase of an acute myocardial infarction [27]. The degree of elevation depends on the degree of damage sustained by the acute infarction and the associated inflammatory process.

Chest x rays are obtained routinely on admission to collect baseline information; the incidence of atelectasis and congestive heart failure after acute myocardial infarction is high. Other diagnostic studies may include serum electrolyte and blood sugar tests, clotting profiles, and a vectorcardiogram.

Hospital Care of the Patient with Acute Myocardial Infarction

Nursing and medical management in the coronary care unit after acute myocardial infarction is aimed at reducing the work load on the heart, anticipating and treating complications, treating emergencies, and promoting psychological support and optimal rehabilitation (see Nursing Orders for details). Coronary care unit nurses must determine what their patients find stressful, and the nurses should intervene effectively [26].

The medications most frequently given after acute myocardial infarction are analgesics, tranquilizers, oxygen, anticoagulants, cardiac glycosides, antidysrhythmia drugs, and stool softeners, as well as other medications for specific problems. Anticoagulant and digitalis therapy for the patient who has had a myocardial infarction is controversial.

Patients who had uncomplicated acute myocardial infarctions can be discharged 10 days to two weeks after the acute event. Patients who had significant complications following the infarction, such as frequent ventricular dysrhythmias, advanced heart block, symptomatic congestive heart failure, pulmonary edema associated with cardiogenic shock, or extension of the infarctions, may need to stay in the hospital for several more weeks.

Cardiac rehabilitation of the patients and their families after acute myocardial infarction [3, 23, 24, 29, 30] is useful. The best results are achieved by taking a multidisciplinary team approach. Rehabilitation begins as soon as the patient's condition is stable, and it continues throughout his hospital stay and after discharge. The level of activity following the patient's discharge from the hospital must be tailored to the individual patient. Patients who have had acute myocardial infarctions should be able to perform their daily activities at about three METs (metabolic equivalents). (One MET is the energy one expends sitting quietly in a chair, or about 3 to 4 ml O_2/kg/min [51].)

Common Complications of Acute Myocardial Infarction

A number of complications can occur after an acute myocardial infarction. The most common ones are:

1. Psychological complications.
2. Dysrhythmias.
3. Congestive heart failure.
4. Cardiogenic shock.
5. Pericarditis.
6. Pulmonary embolism.
7. Systemic embolism.
8. Papillary muscle dysfunction.
9. Interventricular septal rupture.
10. Ventricular aneurysm.

The treatment and care of each of those complications are discussed in the pages that follow immediately as well as in the Nursing Orders.

PSYCHOLOGICAL COMPLICATIONS

Patients in the coronary care unit often go through the stages of denial, anxiety, anger, and depression. Nurses must listen to and observe their patients and try to understand how their patients perceive what is happening to them. It appears that patients act in characteristic ways after an acute myocardial infarction, but the intensity of their responses as well as the duration of the stages varies with each patient [48]. The nurse who cares for a patient who has had an acute myocardial infarction must keep in mind that everyone is unique and that everyone responds differently to stress.

Because an acute myocardial infarction begins suddenly, patients at first go through a stage of disbelief and shock. That stage is usually brief. The behavior seen during that stage is characterized by denial and anxiety. Several days after the infarction occurs, the patient usually develops an awareness of what has occurred. Anger and depression are often his re-

sponses as he realizes that he has had a myocardial infarction. The third stage, that of resolution, usually begins after the patient has been discharged from the hospital. During the stage of resolution, all the behaviors just described may be seen. As the patient begins to assume responsibility during his recovery, his behavior may change from day to day.

The members of his family often react to the patient's illness with depression, fear, anxiety, hostility, and overprotective behavior. The physician and nurse must discuss any psychological problems that the patient and his family might have while the patient is in the hospital as well as during the rehabilitation phase, and try to help them through this stressful event [20].

DYSRHYTHMIAS

The increased use of electronic monitoring and portable tape-recording ECGs in coronary care units and the training in the recognition and treatment of dysrhythmias given the people who work in the units have revealed that cardiac dysrhythmias often occur after acute myocardial infarctions and often are serious [1]. Dysrhythmias occur in 90 percent of the patients who have had an acute myocardial infarction [27]. It is of the utmost importance that the nurse remember that she is observing and treating a person with a dysrhythmia, not the dysrhythmia itself, because each person responds differently to a dysrhythmia.

The following factors must be considered in the diagnosis and treatment of dysrhythmias and conduction disturbances: (1) the oxygen transport system, including the heart and the circulation; (2) the effect of the dysrhythmia on the individual patient; (3) the exact nature of the dysrhythmia; and (4) whether the patient had that dysrhythmia before and, if he had, how he responded to it. (See Chap. 10 for specific dysrhythmia details.)

If the heart is pumping effectively and the arteries and veins are serving as conduits for the blood, the heart and circulation can perform normally. Dysrhythmias that cause little difficulty in one setting can be lethal in another [34]. Ventricular premature beats in a healthy person are benign; however, when they occur frequently in a person with an acute myocardial infarction, they can lead to ventricular fibrillation.

If a dysrhythmia exists, one must observe the patient for signs of decreased cardiac output and decreased cerebral, coronary, or renal circulation. Close

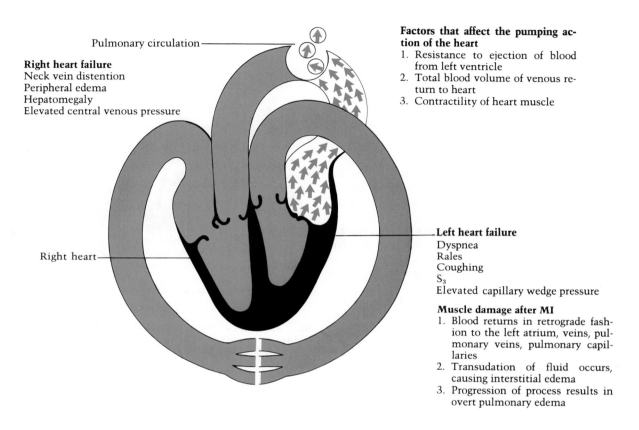

Pulmonary circulation

Right heart failure
Neck vein distention
Peripheral edema
Hepatomegaly
Elevated central venous pressure

Right heart

Factors that affect the pumping action of the heart
1. Resistance to ejection of blood from left ventricle
2. Total blood volume of venous return to heart
3. Contractility of heart muscle

Left heart failure
Dyspnea
Rales
Coughing
S_3
Elevated capillary wedge pressure

Muscle damage after MI
1. Blood returns in retrograde fashion to the left atrium, veins, pulmonary veins, pulmonary capillaries
2. Transudation of fluid occurs, causing interstitial edema
3. Progression of process results in overt pulmonary edema

Figure 19-10
Congestive heart failure.

observation of the patient's skin temperature and color is important. The nurse should watch for hypotension (which indicates decreased cardiac output), diaphoresis (which indicates peripheral arteriolar constriction), chest pain (which suggests myocardial ischemia), and mental dullness (which suggests cerebral ischemia). If those conditions occur, they must be recognized and treated.

The nurse must know the exact nature of a dysrhythmia. Ventricular fibrillation and cardiac standstill are lethal dysrhythmias, and in a patient with acute myocardial infarction they are always emergencies. The treatment of other dysrhythmias that occur in a patient with acute myocardial infarction must include a thorough assessment of the entire clinical setting—the patient, his oxygen transport system, and his clinical condition at the time the dysrhythmia occurred.

Patients should be encouraged to discuss their experiences with dysrhythmias. Often they can give valuable information to the physician and the nurse.

Congestive Heart Failure

Congestive heart failure is a common complication of acute myocardial infarction (Fig. 19-10). Heart failure causes one-third of the deaths of patients with myocardial infarction [27]. Heart failure usually involves the left ventricle. Because acute myocardial infarction involves the large muscle mass of the left ventricle, heart failure following an acute myocardial infarction is almost always left sided [7]. When the normal reserve mechanisms of the heart are exceeded, heart failure occurs.

It is common for a patient to have no early symptoms of left-sided heart failure. The patient may develop symptoms of decreased cardiac output when the heart fails to pump enough blood into systemic circulation. At that time, the pressure in the left ventricle increases, and it is transmitted in a retrograde path to the left atrium, the pulmonary veins, and the pulmonary capillaries. When pulmonary capillary pressure exceeds the oncotic pressure of plasma proteins, fluid transudates and causes interstitial edema. If fluid moves into the alveoli, dyspnea, frequent coughing, and rales may develop. If the condition progresses, the patient may develop overt pulmonary edema.

In pure left ventricular failure there is no peripheral edema or neck vein distention. Radiographically, the left ventricle may or may not be seen to increase in size. Third and fourth heart sounds in acute myocardial infarction are probably secondary to changes in ventricular compliance rather than to enlargement.

The insertion of a Swan-Ganz catheter to measure the pulmonary capillary filling pressure (which is an index of left ventricular filling pressure) is often done in coronary care units [9, 32].

Right ventricular failure is unusual in acute myocardial infarction. When it does occur, there is a rise in right ventricular pressure and right atrial pressure that can be measured by a central venous pressure catheter. One may see symptoms of systemic congestion, such as neck vein distention, peripheral edema, and hepatomegaly. Treatment of congestive heart failure is aimed at increasing cardiac output and decreasing pulmonary congestion and systemic congestion if it develops.

Cardiogenic Shock

Cardiogenic shock is another major complication of acute myocardial infarction (Fig. 19-11). In cardiogenic shock, the heart has failed to pump effectively, decreasing the stroke volume. Eventually, general tissue ischemia and hypoxia occur. A hypotensive state due to low cardiac output exists.

Statistics show that patients who die from cardiogenic shock have acute necrosis of at least 40 percent of the left ventricular myocardium [2, 41]. Cardiogenic shock is difficult to treat because the biochemical and physiological changes associated with shock change constantly and the exact mechanisms of shock are not fully understood. Owing to the inadequate tissue perfusion, anaerobic metabolism ensues, causing lactic acidosis. The physician aims his treatment at improving myocardial contractility without increasing the work load of the heart—at raising the mean arterial pressure to obtain adequate coronary blood flow and increasing peripheral vascu-

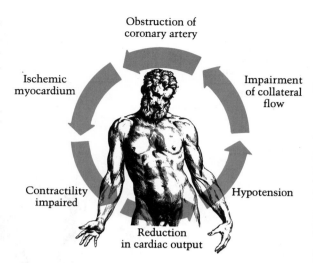

Figure 19-11
The vicious cycle of cardiogenic shock.

lar resistance without decreasing blood flow to the kidneys.

Pericarditis

Pericarditis is often a troublesome complication (see Fig. 19-12B). It occurs in about 15 percent of the patients who have just had myocardial infarctions [40]. The clinical hallmark of pericarditis is a friction rub. A friction rub may be a hallmark of transmural myocardial infarction in which damage to the entire myocardial wall has occurred. Bleeding from an inflamed pericardium may occur, leading to hemorrhagic tamponade and shock due to myocardial compression. This situation is much less common. Respiration may be painful if the surrounding pleura is involved. With splinting, atelectasis may occur and oxygen saturation may fall, predisposing the person to dysrhythmias or possible extension of the infarction. The most obvious symptom of inflammation of the pericardium is pain, and it is often aggravated by swallowing, coughing, inspiring, and rotating or moving the trunk. The treatment of pericarditis is aimed at relieving the pain and inflammation.

Pulmonary Embolism

Pulmonary embolism can be a major complication of acute myocardial infarction. Like most other pulmonary emboli, it usually originates in the deep veins of the lower extremities (see Chap. 16). Atrial fibrillation, transmural myocardial infarction, or subendocardial myocardial infarction involving the right ventricle may predispose one to thrombus formation and subsequent pulmonary embolus formation. The morbidity varies according to the size of the pulmonary embolus.

Systemic Embolism

Systemic embolism due to mural thrombus formation in the left ventricle may occur. One must observe the patient for any changes in his sensorium and specifically any changes in his extremities associated with a decreased or an absent pulse or a change in temperature in the involved extremity. When the nurse sees any of those changes, she must immediately bring them to the attention of the physician. Anticoagulant therapy with heparin may be instituted quickly if it is not contraindicated for some other reason. If the problem is not resolved by the medical treatment, the physician should consider surgical intervention.

Papillary Muscle Dysfunction

Many disease processes can cause left ventricular papillary muscle dysfunction (Fig. 19-12A). The most common ones are myocardial infarction and coronary insufficiency. The papillary muscles receive their blood supply from the terminal portions of the large penetrating branches of the coronary arteries. If the flow to the coronary arteries is impaired, the papillary muscles become very susceptible to injury. Papillary muscle dysfunction in the presence of acute myocardial infarction is suggested by the appearance or presence of an apical systolic murmur, which frequently radiates to the axilla and occasionally is associated with a thrill.

If acute myocardial infarction involves the papillary muscle to the point of necrosis, papillary muscle rupture may occur. However, rupture is uncommon. If papillary muscle rupture does occur, it usually does so within the first week after infarction. A pansystolic murmur can be heard, and a thrill is usually present. Typically, the patient has worsening of heart failure or sudden onset of heart failure, often with dysrhythmias and cyanosis; his condition deteriorates and he dies within hours or days. There have

been reports of people who survived for 11 and 14 months with ruptured papillary muscles, but those people had marked congestive heart failure until they died [27].

Rupture of the Interventricular Septum

Another complication of acute myocardial infarction is rupture of the interventricular septum (Fig. 19-12B). It occurs most commonly in the first week after acute myocardial infarction. Rupture of the interventricular septum can be identified during physical examination by a loud pansystolic murmur accompanied by a thrill [39]. It is loudest along the left sternal border in the fourth and fifth intercostal spaces. The rupture precipitates congestive heart failure and often shock. The degree of failure and shock depends on the size of the defect. A report of an emergency diagnostic catheterization using a Swan-Ganz catheter confirmed the bedside diagnosis of acute myocardial infarction and acute rupture of the interventricular septum complicated by cardiogenic shock [50]. The prognosis is usually poor when the condition is treated medically, although long-term survivals have been reported [10, 44]. In most cases, surgical repair should be considered. Right and left heart catheterization is done to look for evidence of a ruptured septum. An increased oxygen saturation in the right ventricle implies a left-to-right shunt secondary to interventricular septal rupture. Coronary arteriography is also done to study the coronary circulation; it helps the physician to decide whether coronary artery bypass can be performed.

Ventricular Aneurysm

The incidence of ventricular aneurysm accompanying acute myocardial infarction is not well established (Fig. 19-12C). The incidence of ventricular aneurysm accompanying coronary artery disease is different in different studies [13, 15]. The variations appear to be related to how aneurysm was defined in the study and whether the study was a clinical study or an autopsy study.

The term *aneurysm* is used to refer both to an area of the ventricle that does not move at all (the lack of motion is called akinesis) and to an expanding motion (dyskinesis) of the ventricular wall during systole. The dyskinesis varies from muscle of full thickness to scarred, thin muscle.

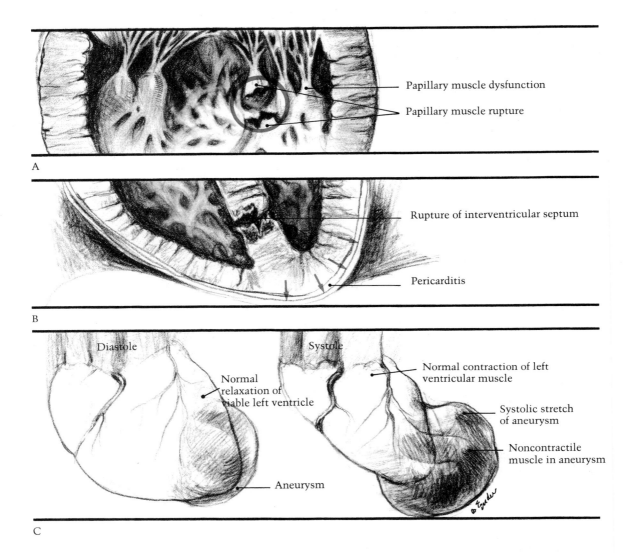

Figure 19-12
A. Papillary muscle dysfunction and rupture. B. Rupture of the interventricular septum and pericarditis. C. Ventricular aneurysm.

The paradoxical motion of the ventricular wall (systolic stretch) decreases the overall pumping action of the heart. As the normal portion of the ventricular muscle mass contracts, the area of aneurysm is forced outward by the increasing pressure inside the ventricle. Thus much of the pumping force of the ventricle is lost because of the ischemic or nonfunctional cardiac muscle. Ischemic bulges of the myocardium occur frequently during the clinical course of myocardial infarction. Many of those bulges disappear and cannot be identified at autopsy because systolic pressure is needed for their presence. Aneurysms involve the left ventricle in 95 percent of the cases and the right ventricle in 5 percent of the cases

[27]. Impaired ventricular function, arterial embolism, and ventricular tachycardia are complications of aneurysms [13].

Ventricular Rupture

Ventricular rupture rarely occurs unless reinfarction occurs at the aneurysmal border, where the tough fibrous sac of the aneurysm adjoins viable muscle. The patient so afflicted quickly develops intractable congestive heart failure and cardiogenic shock and usually dies.

Other Complications of Acute Myocardial Infarction

A list of other complications of acute myocardial infarction follows. The incidence of the complications listed here is not as high as the incidence of the complications already discussed.

1. Dressler's syndrome
2. Cerebral syndrome
3. Chest wall syndrome
4. Hiccoughing, nausea, and vomiting
5. Gastrointestinal problems
6. Genitourinary tract problems

DRESSLER'S SYNDROME

The exact cause of Dressler's syndrome, the post-myocardial infarction syndrome, occurs in 3 to 4 percent of the patients who have had acute myocardial infarctions. Typically, the syndrome causes pleuritic-type chest pain and fever. It begins 10 days to three months after the acute infarction. Dressler's syndrome is distinguished from a new myocardial infarction by the fact that the pain is pleuritic, and there are no changes in the ECG or the cardiac enzymes. Dressler's syndrome is usually benign and it lasts for one to two weeks.

CEREBRAL SYNDROME

Some patients experience some confusion, personality changes, and amnesia during their hospital stay. Those reactions are due to a variety of causes, such as drugs, hypotension, impaired cerebral blood flow, major complications of myocardial infarction, and isolation in the coronary care unit from one's normal environment and one's family.

CHEST WALL SYNDROME

The symptoms of chest wall syndrome are local tenderness and pain. It is often difficult to distinguish from anxiety neurosis.

HICCOUGHING, NAUSEA, AND VOMITING

Hiccoughing often accompanies an inferior wall myocardial infarction. It may keep a patient from sleeping. Nausea and vomiting can accompany acute mycardial infarction, but after the infarction has occurred they may be caused by opiates and other cardiac drugs. Retching often causes a dysrhythmia and therefore must be stopped.

GASTROINTESTINAL PROBLEMS

Abdominal distention, constipation, and fecal impaction are seen during the acute myocardial infarction. They are seen also after the acute stage owing to decreased exercise and roughage in the diet, to opiates, and to potassium depletion following diuresis. The stress reaction of myocardial infarction may precipitate gastrointestinal hemorrhage due to peptic ulcer.

GENITOURINARY TRACT PROBLEMS

Bladder distention is a common problem in the man who has prostatic hypertrophy after an acute myocardial infarction. Medications, such as atropine, sedatives, and opiates, and bed rest may aggravate the distention. Indwelling catheters may cause urinary tract infections and possibly lead to a Gram-negative septicemia.

Advances in Treating Ischemic Heart Disease

Despite the great strides that have been made since the early 1960s in the treatment of acute myocardial infarction, it continues to be the most common cause of in-hospital death in the United States. It is clear that nursing and medical treatment of the patient who has had an acute myocardial infarction is entering a new era. It is likely that in the near future there will be not just a single treatment for acute myocardial infarction. Rather, patients will be carefully categorized according to the ECG, clinical, hemodynamic, and coronary arteriographic findings.

New therapeutic interventions and diagnostic tests for acute myocardial infarction are being refined throughout the country. The critical care nurse must understand the implications of those new techniques for nursing care. The nurse must know about them so that she can give the appropriate nursing care and can anticipate the side effects or complications of the treatment.

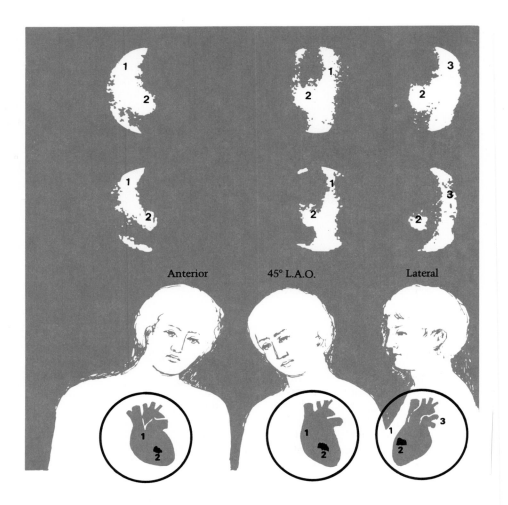

Diagnostic Tests for Acute Myocardial Infarction

The use of radionuclides for myocardial imaging in patients with acute myocardial infarction and coronary artery disease is an exciting research topic [43].

RADIONUCLIDE MYOCARDIAL SCINTIGRAMS

The scintigram (or myocardial scan) is a diagnostic tool capable of identifying the presence of myocardial infarction [Fig. 19-13]. Acute anteroseptal myocardial infarction is shown by the technetium 99m stannous pyrophosphate (^{99m}Tc-PYP) myocardial scintigram. The top three panels demonstrate "unprocessed views" of the ^{99m}Tc-PYP scintigram: (1) the sternum, (2) the site of infarction, and (3) the spine. The middle three panels demonstrate the helpfulness of the com-

Figure 19-13
Acute anteroseptal myocardial infarction as shown by the ^{99m}Tc-PYP myocardial scintigram. The top three panels demonstrate "unprocessed views" of the ^{99m}Tc-PYP scintigram: (1) sternum, (2) site of infarction, and (3) spine. The middle three panels demonstrate the helpfulness of computer processing of the images. The bottom three panels show a schematic representation of the site of the damage as the patient is rotated in the various views. L.A.O. = left anterior oblique.

puter processing of the images. The bottom three panels are schematic representations of the site of the damage as the patient is rotated to obtain the various views.

The scintigram visualizes acute transmural myocardial infarctions and pinpoints the areas involved. It also identifies acute subendocardial myocardial infarctions [54].

The procedure causes the patient no discomfort. It takes about 15 minutes, and it is done at the patient's bedside or in the x-ray department. When a radionuclide such as ^{99m}Tc-PYP is administered intravenously, the scintigram is done one to three hours after injection. Research shows that ^{99m}Tc-PYP scintigrams become positive as early as 12 hours after myocardial infarction and remain positive for at least six days. Authorities feel that the positive ^{99m}Tc-PYP scintigrams are a more sensitive technique of identifying myocardial necrosis than are enzymatic studies or the standard ECG.

Evaluation of Left Ventricular Function Using Radionuclides
Thallium appears to be ideal for imaging well-perfused areas of the myocardium. With the use of ^{99m}Tc-PYP to pinpoint the areas of irreversible myocardial damage and thallium to pinpoint the well-perfused areas of the myocardium, valuable information can be gained. The radionuclide combination can give the physician the information that he needs to care for patients. He can learn what portion of the myocardium has an adequate blood supply; that is, what part has irreversible damage and what part is underperfused but not yet irreversibly damaged.

Fractionation of Creatine Phosphokinase

The fractionation of the creatine phosphokinase (CPK) enzyme into its various enzymes provides additional information about the presence or absence of myocardial infarction [19]. CPK can be fractionated into the following different isoenzymes: BB, which is present in the brain; MB, which is specific for myocardial muscle; and MM, which is present in skeletal muscle and cardiac muscle. People who have had acute myocardial infarctions have elevated levels of MB, and people who have not had acute myocardial infarctions but who have other body areas of muscle damage (i.e., massive trauma, fractures) have elevated levels of either BB or MM. Research is currently being

done to develop techniques for detecting even small amounts of MB, knowledge of which might be useful in estimating the size of the myocardial infarction.

Measurement of Urine Myoglobin

People who have had acute myocardial infarctions develop myoglobinuria, which can be detected by radial diffusion immunoassay [47]. Myoglobin is a normal constituent of skeletal muscle. Owing to its small amount and lack of significant binding to serum protein, myoglobin is rapidly removed from the blood, filtered through the kidneys, and excreted in the urine. The myoglobin level does not appear to rise after the patient has been given a routine intramuscular injection.

Use of Sodium Nitroprusside

The heart's pumping ability is determined by preload (end-diastolic fiber length), afterload (resistance to left ventricular ejection), and contractility (inotropic state of the myocardium). Reduction in cardiac output after acute myocardial infarction is a result of reduced contractility in the ischemic border around the infarcted area and a loss of functioning myocardium.

Recently, the use of sodium nitroprusside (SNP), a vasodilator, has been reported to increase cardiac output in some patients with acute myocardial infarction [12]. The goal of SNP therapy is to decrease any impediment to left ventricular ejection, which permits more effective systolic emptying, rather than to decrease the arterial pressure. By decreasing any impediment to left ventricular ouflow and reducing systemic vascular resistance, SNP may increase left ventricular stroke volume and cardiac output, thus improving left ventricular pump performance.

Intraaortic Balloon Pump Counterpulsation; External Counterpulsation

Much experimental work continues on reducing the mortality in cardiogenic shock. Even with the latest advances in the treatment of cardiogenic shock, mortality in cardiogenic shock following acute myocardial infarction is 85 percent. Two new methods used in large medical centers to increase coronary perfusion and to reduce the work load of the left ventricle are intraaortic balloon pump (IABP) counterpulsation and external counterpulsation.

IABP COUNTERPULSATION

Counterpulsation reduces the ascending aortic pressure during ventricular systole and increases pressure during ventricular diastole [8, 53]. The balloon is inserted into the patient's descending thoracic aorta through the femoral artery to a position just distal to the left subclavian artery. The balloon is inflated during ventricular diastole, which displaces blood proximally and thus increases coronary perfusion during diastole. Deflation of the balloon at the onset of ventricular systole allows the ventricle to eject blood into the aorta at a lower systolic pressure [7].

The patient's hemodynamic status is monitored constantly. When the patient no longer requires vasopressors and when his blood pressure, urinary output, and sensorium are stable, he is weaned from balloon support.

EXTERNAL COUNTERPULSATION

External counterpulsation is accomplished by placing multichambered cuffs on both legs or on all four extremities. The cuffs are filled with compressed air or water. The system is activated by the patient's ECG as it is attached to a control device. The cuffs deflate during systole, which effects a decreased pressure that causes the ventricle to eject blood at a decreased aortic pressure. The cuffs reinflate during diastole, allowing perfusion of coronary arteries and other vital organs. The advantage of the procedure is that it is noninvasive. As soon as the patient's hemodynamic status improves the patient is weaned from the cuffs.

Nursing Orders

OBJECTIVE NO. 1

The patient should demonstrate signs of improvement following a myocardial infarction.

To achieve the objective, the nurse should:

1. Evaluate chest pain in regard to:
   a. Type (squeezing, constrictive, steady, intermittent, or crescendo)
   b. Location (midsternal, radiating, left precordial)
   c. Whether relieved by nitrates, meperidine hydrochloride, or morphine
   d. Severity (heavy or dull)
   e. Effects (diaphoresis, nausea and vomiting, or anxiety)
   (The nurse should assess all patients often to see whether they are in pain. Some patients may be reluctant to tell the nurse they are in pain.)
2. Watch for the signs and symptoms of the extension of myocardial infarction and early congestive heart failure:
   a. Chest pain
   b. Cardiac irritability
   c. Nausea and vomiting
   d. Dyspnea
   e. Frequent coughing with shortness of breath
3. Check the patient's vital signs before giving him narcotics (narcotics cause hypotension due to venous pooling of blood).
4. Reassure the patient often and help him during periods of pain. Those kinds of support will help him feel positively about recovery.
5. Be aware of the patient's ECG pattern and be on the alert for changes in the ST segment and for dysrhythmias [34, 46]. (The "emergency" dysrhythmias are ventricular fibrillation, ventricular tachycardia, asystole, and complete heart block. They should be treated according to the standing coronary care unit orders.)
6. With dysrhythmias, be alert to changes in the patient's vital signs.
7. Be able to distinguish the various dysrhythmias and treat them according to the standing coronary care unit orders.
8. Report any significant changes or persistent dysrhythmias to the physician.
9. Assess carefully every patient who has a dysrhythmia. The nurse should look for:
   a. A change in the patient's heart rate or respirations.
   b. A change in the patient's temperature and the color of his skin.
   c. A change in the patient's mental state.
   d. The development of hypotension.
   e. The development of left ventricular failure. (Tachyarrhythmias shorten ventricular filling time and thus decrease the cardiac output and coronary blood flow. Bradyarrhythmias decrease the cardiac output, and they can allow dangerous tachyarrhythmias to take over.)

10. Maintain a patent intravenous line at all times.
11. Know what antidysrhythmia drugs need to be given for specific dysrhythmias.
12. Know the effects that the antidysrhythmia drugs have on the patient and on the QRS complex, as shown on the ECG.
13. Give atropine for bradyarrhythmia—and treat it with a pacemaker if necessary.
14. Give medications for ventricular dysrhythmias as ordered (e.g., the most common ones are lidocaine, quinidine, digoxin, procainamide, diphenylhydantoin, and propranolol) and be prepared to assist with cardioversion if necessary.
15. If atrioventricular block appears first with anterior myocardial infarction, watch for first-degree heart block and Mobitz type II heart block or for the development of intraventricular conduction disturbances [11, 28, 49, 52].
16. If Mobitz type II heart block appears, have available a functioning temporary pacemaker and an isoproterenol drip.
17. Anticipate third-degree heart block if the patient has an idioventricular rhythm.
18. If a temporary pacemaker must be inserted:
    a. Explain the procedure to the patient.
    b. Have the procedure permit signed by the patient or a member of his family.
    c. After the insertion of a pacemaker, evaluate the pacemaker's functioning and the patient's rhythm.
19. Be aware of the common complications of using a pacemaker and of the appropriate nursing care should those complications occur:
    a. Pacemaker failure
    b. Improper stimulation
    c. Improper sensing
    d. Perforation of the heart
20. Be aware of electrical hazards and the possibility of microshock.
21. Record the rate, mode, and milliampere setting of the pacemaker on the patient's chart and on the care plan as ordered by the physician.
22. If cardioversion is necessary in an emergency or for a dysrhythmia not corrected by medication:
    a. Explain the procedure to the patient in simple terms.
    b. Prepare the patient for sedation or anesthesia.
    c. If possible, discontinue digoxin for one to two days before the procedure. Give quinidine or another antidysrhythmia drug as ordered.
    d. Have the procedure permit signed.

e. Make sure that the patient is fasting.
f. Have emergency drugs available.
23. When cardioversion is to be performed:
    a. Place the patient in a supine position.
    b. Remove the patient's dentures if he is wearing any.
    c. Secure the electrodes to the patient's chest and obtain a rhythm strip before cardioversion. (It is preferable to get a rhythm strip using a 12-lead ECG.)
    d. Apply conductive paste to the paddles.
    e. Set the cardiovertor on synchronization.
    f. Set the cardiovertor to the desired voltage.
    g. Charge the cardiovertor to the desired voltage.
    h. Position the paddles, using two anterior paddles or an anterior paddle and a posterior paddle.
    i. Apply firm pressure to the paddles.
    j. Avoid contact with wet areas and make sure no one is in contact with the patient or his bed while the physician performs the cardioversion.
    k. Obtain a 12-lead ECG after the cardioversion.
    l. Anticipate the possible complications—further instability and systemic or pulmonary embolism.
    m. Remain with the patient until he is stable and fully awake.
    n. Observe the patient closely for two to three hours after the cardioversion.
    o. Allow the patient to resume oral intake and drugs one hour after the cardioversion.
24. If defibrillation for ventricular dysrhythmia is necessary, follow the steps described in Nos. 22 and 23, except turn off the synchronizer circuit and turn on the defibrillator circuit. (Since the patient is unconscious, the procedure is not explained to him.)
25. Watch for the signs of congestive heart failure (CHF):
    a. Diminished first heart sound and second heart sound. (The development of a third heart sound is not always a sign of CHF.)
    b. The development of a murmur or a change in an existing murmur
    c. Gallop rhythms
    d. Coughing
    e. Dyspnea
26. Provide cardiac rest for the patient.
    a. Place him in the Fowler's or the semi-Fowler's position.

    b. Encourage him to rest in a chair.

    c. Encourage him to use a bedside commode.

    d. Relieve the psychological stress that accompanies CHF by explaining the procedures to the patient and his family and encouraging him to be as independent as possible.

    e. Give him sedatives as needed.

27. Give digoxin as ordered and watch for side effects:

    a. Nausea and vomiting

    b. Anorexia and malaise

    c. Headache

    d. Dysrhythmia

    (The patient's sensitivity to digoxin is increased in acute myocardial infarction. The following factors may aggravate digoxin intoxication: diuretic therapy, diarrhea, kidney disease, and low potassium levels.)

28. Give diuretics as ordered and watch for side effects:

    a. Weakness and muscle cramps

    b. Hypovolemia

    c. Electrolyte depletion, especially hypokalemia. (The nurse should weigh the patient at the same time each day, should keep an accurate record of his intake and output, and should watch his fluid restrictions.)

    d. Further complications of CHF and the onset of pulmonary edema. The nurse should:

       (1) Check the patient's vital signs.

       (2) Observe the patient for an increase in dyspnea or coughing.

       (3) Place the patient in a high Fowler's position. (Preload is reduced quickly by pooling blood peripherally without significantly reducing the stroke volume. Afterload is reduced by dilating the peripheral arteries and thus reducing the left ventricular end-diastolic pressure.)

       (4) Give oxygen via a face mask.

29. Anticipate the need for the following items and have them available:

    a. Digoxin

    b. Diuretics

    c. Positive pressure breathing equipment

    d. Morphine sulfate

    e. Aminophylline

    f. Rotating tourniquets

    g. Advanced life-support equipment

30. If rotating tourniquets must be applied, do the following:

    a. Explain the procedure carefully to reduce the patient's apprehension.

    b. Place the tourniquet cuffs high in the patient's axilla and groin.

    c. Take the patient's blood pressure before and during the procedure.

    d. Determine whether the patient's arterial pulses are adequate. (Venous flow only—not arterial flow—should be occluded.)

    e. Rotate one tourniquet at least every 10 minutes and occlude only three extremities at a time.

    f. When the procedure is to be discontinued, release the tourniquets one at a time every 10 to 15 minutes.

31. Before giving the patient oxygen, find out whether he has a history of chronic respiratory disease. If he has, give him the oxygen at low-flow rates.

32. If positive pressure breathing is given, explain the procedure to the patient and help him breathe at a normal rate (12–16 breaths/min).

33. Evaluate the effectiveness of the treatment by making a systematic assessment of the patient:

    a. Listen to his lungs.

    b. Assess his arterial blood gases.

    c. Assess his cardiac output.

    d. Assess his urinary output.

    e. Assess his mental state.

34. Put elastic stockings on the patient (they should be removed at least once every 8 hours for 5–10 minutes).

35. Use a footboard only to prevent foot drop. Do not use it as an exercise board. (Isometric exercises cause a marked rise in left ventricular and diastolic pressure, a rise that evokes or accentuates left ventricular dysfunction.)

36. Watch for signs of arterial thromboembolism:

    a. Loss of pulses in the lower extremities (if pulses were present when the patient was admitted)

    b. Pain in the calf on dorsiflexion (Homan's sign)

    c. Cold, mottled, painful extremities

37. Watch for signs of pulmonary embolism:

    a. Sudden onset of chest pain

    b. Coughing, bloody sputum

    c. Shortness of breath

38. Watch for signs of a cerebrovascular accident:

    a. Sudden weakness in one or more extremities

    b. Loss of consciousness

    c. Seizures (They may also be due to ventricular

fibrillation, occasional ventricular tachycardia, or a lidocaine reaction.)

39. Do the following to prevent the complications of pericarditis:
    a. Listen with the diaphragm of the stethoscope for an increase or a decrease in friction rub. The friction rub may be transitory. It is most easily heard on forced expiration while the patient leans forward or is in the left lateral position.
    b. Be aware of persistent clinical symptoms:
       (1) Pain in the precordial area (mild to sharp or severe). The pain may be relieved when the patient leans forward, and it may be increased when the patient deep breathes or rotates his chest.
       (2) Dyspnea or tachypnea
       (3) Fever, chills, sweating (Those symptoms are more significant if the patient has not been given salicylates to reduce his fever.)
40. Be alert to the possibility of cardiac tamponade. The nurse should:
    a. If cardiac tamponade is suspected, check for Kussmaul's sign (distention of the neck veins on inspiration; normally, the veins collapse on inspiration).
    b. Check for pulsus paradoxus (if it is greater than 10 mm Hg, pericardial tamponade should be suspected; 10 mm Hg or less is normal).
    c. If pericardial effusion develops rapidly, watch for signs of a decreased cardiac output.
    d. Watch for changes in the ECG (electrical alternans, tachycardia, or a decrease in QRS complex voltage).
    e. Watch for a decrease in heart sounds, hypotension, and orthopnea.
    f. Have emergency equipment at hand.

    c. A rapid, thready pulse or an imperceptible pulse
    d. Cool, clammy skin
    e. Collapsed, constricted peripheral veins
    f. Mental dullness, restlessness, agitation, confusion
    g. Decreased urinary output
    h. Oliguria (a urinary output of less than 400 ml/24 hrs)
    i. Anuria (no urinary output)
2. If cardiogenic shock is present:
    a. Provide adequate oxygenation and ventilation.
    b. Establish and maintain an airway.
    c. Give oxygen through a nasal cannula or face mask.
    d. Administer mechanical ventilation if necessary.
    e. Help relieve left ventricular failure. The nurse should:
       (1) Determine the central venous pressure or obtain a Swan-Ganz reading as ordered.
       (2) Give medications as ordered.
       (3) Maintain the patient's arterial blood pressure with vasopressors (levarterenol, metaraminol, or dopamine) as ordered.
       (4) Establish and maintain a fluid and electrolyte balance, using a crystalloid solution, volume expanders, or an electrolyte infusion.
       (5) Administer drugs to correct rhythm disturbances as ordered.
       (6) Anticipate the use of mechanical circulation assistance with IABP counterpulsation or external counterpulsation.
       (7) Anticipate the patient's needs by providing quiet and efficient care, by relieving his anxiety, and by positioning him comfortably.
       (8) Assess the patient's condition frequently.

OBJECTIVE NO. 2

The patient should demonstrate an adequate supply of oxygen to the myocardium.
    To achieve the objective, the nurse should:

1. Be aware of the patient's vital signs. The clinical signs of cardiogenic shock are:
    a. A systolic pressure below 90 mm hg (or unobtainable). (A drop of 20 to 40 points in systolic pressure in a patient who has been hypertensive is significant.)
    b. Pallor or cyanosis

OBJECTIVE NO. 3

The patient should develop an understanding of and a willingness to learn about the cardiac regimen in the coronary care unit (CCU).
    To achieve the objective, the nurse should:

1. Establish a good rapport with the patient.
2. Evaluate the patient's emotional response to his illness.
3. Engage the patient in the activities of daily living while he is in the CCU.

4. Help the patient to the bedside commode and warn him to avoid straining while defecating.
5. Have the patient avoid sudden physical effort.
6. Tell the patient how to turn from side to side in bed without overexerting himself.
7. Explain bed rest, monitoring, the use of intravenous lines, and diet to the patient.
8. Evaluate the patient's tolerance of activity (he should not be permitted to get overtired). The principles and methods of the progressive activity program should be discussed in the CCU.
9. Evaluate the patient's understanding of the information given him. Allow time for questions and feedback from the patient. As the patient improves, the nurse should explain to him the need for graduated, supervised levels of activity.

OBJECTIVE NO. 4

The patient should demonstrate the ability to cope with psychological problems caused by myocardial infarction.

To achieve the objective, the nurse should:

1. Show an interest in and patience with the patient.
2. Be aware of any distress or depression that the patient shows and respond to his feelings.
3. Answer the questions that the patient and his family ask about myocardial infarction.
4. Talk freely with the patient about his anxieties. The nurse should:
   a. Allow time for the patient to give the nurse information about his daily activities.
   b. Ask open-ended questions about the patient's knowledge of myocardial infarction.
   c. Be aware of what the patient reveals about his mental state as he expresses his concerns. The patient may reveal a state of:
      (1) Denial. He ignores his symptoms (e.g., he avoids discussing myocardial infarction).
      (2) Isolation or repression. He seems unafraid or unconcerned about his illness.
      (3) Displacement. He complains about relatively unimportant matters; e.g., the noise, food, or air conditioning.
      (4) Projection. He talks about the anxieties of his relatives but not about his own anxieties.
      (5) Rationalization. He blames the myocardial infarction on hard work rather than on smoking, obesity, high blood pressure, or known atherosclerotic heart disease.
      (6) Hallucinatory or delusional behavior. He shows symptoms of delirium, agitation, hallucination, delusion, or mania (e.g., he may accuse the CCU staff of trying to poison him).
5. Help the patient to develop trust in the nursing staff. The nurse should:
   a. Include the patient in routine decisions when appropriate.
   b. Give frequent explanations to the patient about his progress and give him specific information about his present condition. Do not make polite, evasive remarks (e.g., "You're okay").
   c. Spend some time alone with the patient during each day so that he can express his thoughts and feelings as soon as they occur. The extra time allows the nurse to learn more about the patient's concerns, both the concerns that he talks about and the concerns he expresses without words.
   d. Allow time to receive feedback from the patient.
   e. Allow the patient's spouse or significant others to help him perform some of his daily activities or to give him special instructions.
   f. Make sure that the patient understands the rehabilitation program. (Some patients at first react to rehabilitation with complaints; e.g., "They want me to rest, and now they tell me about an exercise program.")
6. Assess all the information that is given to the patient to make sure that he understands it. Unnecessary information that he does not understand may upset him.
7. Help the patient work through the following common responses to myocardial infarction (these time periods vary with each patient):
   a. Anxiety, which usually lasts for 24 to 48 hours after the patient's admission. When the patient feels very anxious, maintain continuous contact with him to help him develop trust in the staff so that the staff can assess his condition accurately. The nurse should learn about the patient's previous experiences with illness, hospitalization, and severe stress and how his previous experience relates to his present condition.
   b. Denial, which usually lasts for 24 to 48 hours after the patient's admission. The nurse should determine whether the patient's denial hinders his treatment. Is his denial verbal, or does he act it out? Assess the "threat" that has caused the

patient's denial. What does his illness mean to the patient?

c. Depression, which begins after the first 48 hours after the patient's admission. The nurse should ask for and listen to the patient's comments about his feelings, and she should respond when necessary. She should let the patient know that it is normal for him to feel depressed while he is ill.

d. Aggressive sexual behavior, which usually occurs (if it occurs at all) in the first 24 to 48 hours after the patient's admission. Find out what need or anxiety the patient expresses through his sexual aggressiveness. If the patient's aggressiveness makes the nurse uncomfortable, she should tell him so simply and directly.

Summary

Myocardial infarction is the single most important cause of death in the United States. The most accepted method of diagnosing acute myocardial infarction involves taking the patient's medical history, giving him a physical examination, and evaluating the results of laboratory tests performed on him. The clinical manifestations of acute myocardial infarction include chest pain and its variations, nausea and vomiting, diaphoresis, and characteristic physical findings. Laboratory data that suggest acute myocardial infarction are quantified by ECG cardiac enzyme tests and myocardial scans.

The most frequently occurring complications of acute myocardial infarction are psychological complications, congestive heart failure, cardiogenic shock, dysrhythmia, pericarditis, pulmonary embolism, systemic embolism, papillary muscle dysfunction, and intraventricular septal rupture. Nurses caring for patients who have had acute myocardial infarction must understand the disease process, be able to assess symptoms and complications, relate those complications to the physiological causes, and initiate or anticipate the appropriate treatment. The nurse's observation skills and care must focus on preventing complications. When complications occur, the nurse must be able to decide how to carry out the appropriate nursing actions. The progress of the condition of a patient who has had an acute myocardial infarction is most unpredictable, and care of the patient is a great challenge to the nurse.

Study Problems

1. Why are tachyarrhythmias after acute myocardial infarction dangerous?
2. What are some signs and symptoms that indicate that a myocardial infarction has extended?
3. What is cardiogenic shock? What are the signs and symptoms of cardiogenic shock?
4. Why are bradyarrhythmias after acute myocardial infarction dangerous?

Answers

1. Tachyarrhythmias shorten ventricular filling time and thus decrease cardiac output and coronary blood flow.
2. Chest pain, cardiac irritability, nausea and vomiting, dyspnea, and frequent coughing with shortness of breath.
3. a. Cardiogenic shock is a state in which the heart has failed to pump effectively. General tissue ischemia and hypoxia occur eventually if cardiogenic shock is not treated. The presence of normal or high left ventricular filling pressure distinguishes cardiogenic shock from hypovolemic shock. b. Systolic pressure below 90 mm Hg or an unobtainable systolic pressure (a drop in systolic pressure of 20 to 40 points in a person who was hypertensive is significant), pallor or cyanosis, a rapid, thready pulse, an imperceptible pulse, cool, clammy skin, collapsed, constricted peripheral veins, mental dullness, restlessness, agitation, confusion, semiconsciousness or coma, and decreased or absent urinary output.
4. Bradyarrhythmias result in a drop in cardiac output and the development of dangerous tachyarrhythmias.

References

1. Abdellah, F. G. The patient-nurse team approach to coronary care. *Nurs. Clin. North Am.* 7:423, 1972.
2. Amsterdam, E., Massumi, R. A., Zelis, R., et al. Evaluation and management of cardiogenic shock. *Heart Lung* 1:402, 1972.
3. Baden, C. A. Teaching the coronary patient and his family. *Nurs. Clin. North Am.* 7:563, 1972.
4. Benson, H., Kotch, J. B., and Crossweller, K. D. The usefulness of the relaxation response in the treatment of stress-related cardiovascular disease. *J. S.C. Med. Assoc.* (Suppl.) 72:50, 1976.

5. Blumenthal, J. A., Williams, R. B., King, Y., et al. Type A behavior pattern and coronary atherosclerosis. *Circulation* 4:634, 1978.

6. Brand, R. J., Rosenman, R. H., Scholtz, R. I., et al. Multivariate prediction of coronary heart disease in the Western Collaborative Group Study compared to the findings of the Framingham study. *Circulation* 53:348, 1976.

7. Braunwald, E. *The Myocardium: Failure and Infarction.* New York: H. P. Publishing, 1974.

8. Bregman, D. Management of patients undergoing intra-aortic balloon pumping. *Heart Lung* 3:916, 1974.

9. Bolognini, V. The Swan-Ganz pulmonary artery catheter: Implications for nursing. *Heart Lung* 3:976, 1974.

10. Campion, B. C., Harrison, C. E., Jr., and Guiliani, E. R. Ventricular septal defect after myocardial infarction. *Ann. Intern. Med.* 70:251, 1969.

11. Castellanos, A., Spence, M.I., and Chapell, D. E. Hemiblock and bundle branch block: A nursing approach. *Heart Lung* 1:36, 1972.

12. Chatterjee, K., Parmley, W. W., and Ganz, W. W. Hemodynamic and metabolic responses to vasodilator therapy in acute myocardial infarction. *Circulation* 43:1183, 1973.

13. Cheng, T. Incidence of ventricular aneurysm in coronary artery disease. *Am. J. Med.* 50:340, 1971.

14. Col, J., and Weinberg, S. Factors affecting prognosis in acute myocardial infarction. *Heart Lung* 1:74, 1972.

15. Davis, R. W., and Ebert, P. A. Ventricular aneurysm. *Am. J. Cardiol.* 29:1, 1972.

16. Eliot, R. S., and Forker, A. D. Emotional stress and cardiac disease. *J.A.M.A.* 236:2325, 1976.

17. Friedberg, C. *Diseases of the Heart* (3rd ed.). Philadelphia: Saunders, 1967.

18. Friedman, M., and Roseman, R. H. Association of specific overt behavior pattern with blood and cardiovascular findings. *J.A.M.A.* 169:1286, 1969.

19. Galen, R., Reiffel, J., and Gambino, R. Diagnosis of acute myocardial infarction. *J.A.M.A.* 232:145, 1975.

20. Gardner, D., and Stewart, N. Staff involvement with families of patients in critical care units. *Heart Lung* 1:105, 1978.

21. Gotto, A. M., Nichols, B. L., Scott, L. W., et al. Obesity-risk factor No. 1. *Heart Lung* 1:132, 1978.

22. Guyton, A. *Textbook of Medical Physiology* (5th ed.). Philadelphia: Saunders, 1976.

23. Guzzetta, C. Validation of Prescriptive Learning Outcomes for Patients with Acute Myocardial Infarction. Ph. D. dissertation, Texas Woman's University, 1977.

24. Guzzetta, C. *Heart attack: Taking Care of Yourself at Home.* Dallas: Medical City Dallas Hospital, 1977.

25. Harrison, T. R., Adams, R. D., Bennett, I. L., et al. *Principles of Internal Medicine* (8th ed.). New York: McGraw-Hill, 1977.

26. Hoffman, M., Donekers, S., and Hauser, M. The effect of nursing intervention on stress factors perceived by patients in a coronary care unit. *Heart Lung* 5:804, 1978.

27. Hurst, J. W., Logue, R. B., Schland, R. C., et al. *The Heart* (4th ed.). New York: McGraw-Hill, 1978.

28. James, T. N. Pathogenesis of arrhythmias in acute myocardial infarction. *Am. J. Cardiol.* 24:791, 1969.

29. Johnston, B. L., Cantwell, J. D., and Fletcher, G. F. Eight steps to inpatient cardiac rehabilitation: The team effort-methodology and preliminary results. *Heart Lung* 5:97, 1976.

30. Johnston, B., Cantwell, J. D., Watt, E. W., et al. Sexual activity in exercising patients after myocardial infarction and revascularization. *Heart Lung* 6:1026, 1978.

31. Keys, A. (ed.). Coronary heart disease in seven countries. *Circulation* (Suppl.) 41:1, 1970.

32. Lalli, S. The complete Swan-Ganz. *RN* 9:65, 1978.

33. Levinson, C. Thallium-201 myocardial imaging. *Heart Lung* 6:115, 1977.

34. Marriott, H., and Gozensky, C. Analysis of arrhythmias in coronary care—a plea for precision. *Heart Lung* 1:51, 1972.

35. McIntosh, H. D. Smoking as a risk factor. *Heart Lung* 1:145, 1978.

36. McIntosh, H. D., Eknoyan, G., and Jackson, D. Hypertension—a potent risk factor. *Heart Lung* 1:137, 1978.

37. McIntosh, H. D., Stamler, J., and Jackson, D. Introduction to risk factors in coronary artery disease. *Heart Lung* 1:126, 1978.

38. Maurer, B. J., Wray, R., and Shillingford, J. P. Frequency of venous thrombosis after myocardial infarction. *Lancet* 2:1385, 1971.

39. Meister, S. G., and Helfant, R. H. Rapid bedside differentiation of ruptured interventricular septum from acute mitral insufficiency. *N. Engl. J. Med.* 287:1024, 1972.

40. Niarchos, A. P., and McKendrick, J. Prognosis of pericarditis after acute myocardial infarction. *Br. Heart J.* 35:49, 1973.

41. O'Rourke, M. F. Cardiogenic shock following myocardial infarction. *Heart Lung* 3:252, 1974.

42. Oliver, M. F. The metabolic response to a heart attack. *Heart Lung* 4:57, 1975.

43. Parkey, R. W., Bonte, F., Meyer, S. L., et al. A new method of radionuclide imaging of acute myocardial infarction in humans. *Circulation* 50:540, 1974.

44. Payne, W. S., Hunt, J. C., and Kirklein, J. W. Surgical repair of ventricular septal defect due to myocardial infarction. *J.A.M.A.* 183:603, 1963.

45. Peery, T. M., and Miller, F. N. *Pathology: A Dynamic Introduction to Medicine and Surgery* (2nd ed.). Boston: Little, Brown, 1971.

46. Roos, J. C., and Dunning, A. J. Right bundle branch block and left axis deviation in acute myocardial infarction. *Br. Heart J.* 32:847, 1970.

47. Saranchak, H. J., and Bernstein, S. H. A new diagnostic test for acute myocardial infarction. *J.A.M.A.* 228:1251, 1974.

48. Scalzi, C. C. Nursing management of behavioral responses following acute myocardial infarction. *Heart Lung* 2:62, 1973.

49. Scanlon, P., Pryor, R., and Blount, G. Right bundle branch block associated with left superior or inferior intraventricular block: Associated with acute myocardial infarction. *Circulation* 62:1135, 1970.

50. Schwade, J., Pombo, J., Rea, W., et al. Emergency diagnosis and attempted therapy in post-infarction interventricular septal rupture. *Texas Med.* 68:74, 1972.

51. Sivorajan, E. S., Snydsman, A., Smith, B., et al. Low-level treadmill testing of 41 patients with acute myocardial infarction prior to discharge from the hospital. *Heart Lung* 6:975, 1977.

52. Vinsant, M., Spence, M., and Chapell, D. *A Common Sense Approach to Coronary Care: A Program* (2nd ed.). St. Louis: Mosby, 1975.

53. Whitman, G. Intra-aortic balloon pumping and cardiac mechanics: A programmed lesson. *Heart Lung* 6:1034, 1978.

54. Willerson, J. T., Parkey, R. W., Bonte, E., et al. Acute subendocardial myocardial infarction in patients. *Circulation* 51:436, 1975.

55. Wissler, R. W. Development of the Atherosclerotic Plaque. In E. Braunwald (ed.), *The Myocardium: Failure and Infarction.* New York: H. P. Publishing, 1974.

56. Yu, P. N., and Goodwin, J. F. *Progress in Cardiology.* London: Kempton, 1974.

Acute Pericarditis

Barbara Montgomery Dossey

Inflammation of the pericardium may occur under a variety of clinical circumstances. Many different disorders of many different organ systems may affect the pericardium either primarily or secondarily. They include disorders that have infectious, neoplastic, hemodynamic, autoimmune, and idiopathic causes. Acute pericarditis has a broad spectrum of clinical pictures, from a benign and self-limited disorder that seldom requires hospitalization to a serious and rapidly fatal disorder associated with cardiac tamponade that calls for the best possible emergency management. Nursing personnel must observe very carefully any patient who has a predisposition to acute pericarditis.

Objective

In regard to a patient with acute pericarditis, the nurse should be able to make a systematic assessment, evaluate the patient, write nursing orders, know the signs and symptoms of pericardial effusion and cardiac tamponade, and be prepared to assist in an emergency, lifesaving pericardiocentesis.

20

Achieving the Objective

To achieve the objective, the nurse should be able to:

1. State the pathophysiology of acute pericarditis.
2. List the symptoms of acute pericarditis.
3. State the serious complications of acute pericarditis.
4. Recognize the danger signals of pericardial effusion and cardiac tamponade.
5. Perform critical care nursing assessment and management of the patient with acute pericarditis, pericardial effusion, and cardiac tamponade.
6. Assemble the equipment needed for and give essential nursing care to the patient who is undergoing pericardiocentesis.

How to Proceed

To develop an approach to acute pericarditis, the nurse should:

1. Identify the characteristics of acute pericarditis and pericardial effusion that occur in the patient in the case study that follows. She should:
   a. Explain the pathophysiology.
   b. Identify the causative and/or precipitating factors.
2. Write a problem list immediately after reading the case study.
3. Make a written head-to-toe assessment using the information in the case study.
4. Plan a conference to discuss the nursing management for a patient with acute pericarditis, pericardial effusion, and cardiac tamponade.

Case Study

Mr. H. B., aged 38, was hospitalized with complaints of fever, severe shortness of breath, cough, and chest pain. His patient profile and social history described him as a 5'10", 175-lb Mexican-American farm worker from Laredo, Texas. His wife, aged 36, was also a farm worker.

Mr. B. was visiting relatives in Dallas when he became ill. He was taken to the city-county hospital, where he was hospitalized. His present and past medical histories were obtained with the help of Mr. B.'s sister; Mr. B. did not speak English.

Mr. B.'s sister said that Mr. B. had complained of recurrent chills and fever. At first Mr. B. was reluctant to cooperate in giving his history because he had been sick for more than a month without seeking medical help. Despite his illness, he took his vacation as planned because he felt that "getting away from work will make me feel better."

Through his sister, Mr. B. gave the following information. He had had a perforated gastric ulcer three years earlier that required an emergency gastrectomy. One year later, his epigastric distress recurred. At that time an upper gastrointestinal series revealed no new findings.

History of Mr. B.'s Present Illness

Four weeks before his present hospitalization, Mr. B. developed a nonproductive cough and a recurrent fever accompanied by nocturnal chills and drenching sweats. He had pain of the right lateral and substernal chest, as well as aching pain in many muscles and joints. He also described gnawing epigastric pain, and right upper quadrant fullness, but, he said, they were unlike the distress he had had with his gastric ulcer. He had had gradually increasing exertional dyspnea and orthopnea during the week before his admission. He had no history of cardiac murmur, jaundice, rheumatic fever, or tuberculosis. He was not taking any medications, and he had no known allergies.

Mr. B. was an orphan; he knew nothing of his family history. His wife and children, aged 12, 13, 15, and 16, were well. He and his family were Catholic. He smoked a pack of cigarettes each day, and he drank about six beers a day.

The physical examination showed Mr. B. to be a well-developed, well-nourished middle-aged man who was anxious, short of breath, and in pain. His temperature when he was admitted was 103°F, pulse 120, respiration 28, and blood pressure 120/70 mm Hg. During quiet respirations he had a pulsus paradoxus of 10 mm Hg; the systolic sound diminished as the cuff pressure was lowered to the diastolic level. His neck was supple. His cervical veins were distended to the angle of the mandible at 35 degrees of elevation. He had no palpable lymph nodes in his cervical and axillary regions. Diminished breath sounds and dullness to percussion were heard over the lower third of the right lung posteriorly. The point of maximum cardiac impulse was not palpable, the left border of cardiac dullness was 1 cm beyond the midclavicular line in the fifth intercostal space, and a grade 2/6 systolic murmur was audible at the apex. He had a loud to-and-fro pericardial friction rub, which was heard best at the lower left sternal border. The edge of his liver was felt 8 cm below the right costal margin, and it was moderately tender. His extremities were normal, without clubbing or edema. The initial diagnostic studies (see assessment sheet) revealed that Mr. B.'s hematocrit was 31%, his white cell count was 7400, and his differential count was normal. Blood cultures were done. A thoracentesis yielded 350 ml of serous fluid containing 175 red cells and 1250 white cells per cu mm, composed of 75% lymphocytes, 16% monocytes, and 9% neutrophils; his protein count was 4 gm per 100 ml. A cytological examination was negative for tumor cells, and a pathological examination revealed sheets of histiocytes with inflammatory cells. Examination of Mr. B.'s sputum revealed acid-fast bacilli. His urine was normal. The results of the tests of his renal and hepatic function were all normal.

An ECG showed sinus tachycardia; the QRS voltage was low, and the T waves were inverted in leads 2, 3, and V_1 through V_5. The chest x ray showed a large cardiopericardial silhouette, with diminished pulsations on fluoroscopic examination. A small right pleural effusion was present. A patchy, streaky infiltrate extended from the right hilum to the apex of the right lung. No hilar lymphadenopathy was present.

Clinical Diagnosis

On admission, Mr. B. had a febrile illness. The clinical diagnosis of tuberculous pericarditis was suggested by the recurrent fever, anemia, chills, drenching sweats, and associated radiographic findings, including apical lung infiltrates and pleural effusion.

The lack of pulsations and the large cardiac silhouette shown by fluoroscopic examination were thought to be due to a pericardial effusion. Mr. B.'s dyspnea, friction rub, elevated venous pressure, and ECG findings were consistent with the diagnosis of tuberculous pericarditis. The murmur was considered functional in origin and associated with the anemia. The high cervical venous pressure and the hepatomegaly were due to the pericardial disease, which impaired venous return and thereby produced the elevation of the central venous pressure.

Mr. B. was admitted to the critical care unit, and isolation precautions were instituted. Close observation of him was necessary because of possible pericardial effusion and cardiac tamponade. Appropriate antituberculosis chemotherapy was begun.

Late on the afternoon of his admission, Mr. B., who was resting in bed, felt short of breath. He called for help; when the nurse arrived, she found him in acute distress. She called for the immediate help of another critical care nurse and had an emergency call placed to the physician. Her immediate assessment showed a blood pressure of 70/50 mm Hg, a pulsus paradoxus of 20 mm Hg, faint heart sounds, a respiratory rate of 32, and a radial pulse of 150. Mr. B.'s neck veins were fully distended on inspiration, but they collapsed on expiration. The nurse placed Mr. B. in a semi-Fowler's position and prepared him for an emergency pericardiocentesis. She administered intravenous morphine sulfate and started an intravenous infusion as ordered.

When the physician arrived, he performed a pericardiocentesis immediately after he examined the patient. The pericardiocentesis yielded 575 ml of straw-colored fluid. Mr. B.'s condition improved immediately. By the end of the day, he was sitting beside his bed.

Mr. B.'s cardiac tamponade, which was due to a slow accumulation of fluid without early symptoms, was manifested by dyspnea and other characteristic signs that were quickly recognized.

Mr. B. was discharged 14 days after his admission. He and his family were given detailed information about his medication and diet.

Reflections

Mr. B. had been ill with recurrent chills and fever for a month before he was taken to the hospital. To the nurses caring for him, the delay was significant. Mr. B. seemed to them a stoic, a person who accepted illness as an unavoidable part of life. Mr. B. did not seek medical help for each trivial illness, as his history showed.

It began to seem to the nurses that Mr. B.'s pattern of not seeking medical care was not a matter of his denying that he was sick (as some of the nurses had postulated). Rather, Mr. B. seemed to be living according to a particular conviction about sickness and health. His conviction was an expression of his culture. Because health care was expensive, Mr. B. treated it as a luxury. He felt that people should be seriously ill before they asked for treatment.

At a weekly team conference, the nurses spoke of the significant mind-body aspects of Mr. B.'s illness. But those aspects were not seen as psychological in the usual sense. The nurses asked, "How did Mr. B.'s endurance of his illness for a month contribute to its seriousness and complications? How do one's convictions affect the outcome of one's illnesses? How is illness related to one's cultural milieu?"

The nurses realized that illness and beliefs about illness were intimately related. If Mr. B. had gone to a physician early in the course of his illness, he might not have developed pericardial infection and tamponade.

The effect of the relationship that exists between a patient's mind and his body on his illness became more evident to the staff after the team conference. Mr. B.'s illness became a more interesting event than a simple case of disseminated tuberculosis. His problems were seen as a complex of phenomena transcending the usual definition of disease as a simple "body" process.

Mr. B. presented a challenge to the nursing staff because of his acute illness as well as his inability to speak English. The language problem was solved by first making a list of the Spanish-speaking nurses in the hospital, what days and shifts they worked, and what times they could visit Mr. B. and his family and then arranging the visits. When they visited—and during the emergency procedure—the Spanish-

Critical Care Nursing Admission Assessment

Head to Toe Approach

Date 4-3	Time 1:00 pm	

Pt. Name: *Mr. H.B.*   Age: *38*   Allergies: *NKA*

Admitted Bed No: *8*   Via: *wheelchair* Ad. Dx.: *Acute Pericarditis / Active TB*

T.: *103°F(o)* A.P.: *120*   R.P.: *120*   R.: *28*   B.P. Supine R: *120/70* L: *120/70*   Sitting: *120/70*

Wt. (unit scale): *175 lbs.*   Ht.: *5'10"* ECG Rhythm: *NSR pulsus paradoxus -10 mm Hg.*   Ectopy: *none*

Informant: *pt's. sister*   Last meal: *yesterday 11 AM*

1. Chief complaint: *fever, SOB, cough, chest pain*
2. Hx. of present illness: *Temp, chills, fever for last month; pain in muscles increasing exertional dyspnea and orthopnea*
3. Past medical Hx. (include all surgeries, hosp., diseases, injuries, blood trans.): *Gastrectomy - 1975; recurrent gastric ulcer - 1976*
4. Family Hx.: *orphan - does not know history; wife 30 and well; children 16, 15, 13, 12 - all well*
5. Current drugs: *none*
6. Alcohol and tobacco habits: *likes to drink 6 beers daily; smokes 1 pk./day*
7. Dietary and fluid needs: *eats chili, tacos, and enchiladas daily*
8. Sleep and rest patterns: *sleeps 8 hrs./night; recent night sweats + fever interrupting sleep*
9. Bowel and bladder habits: *normal*
10. Hygienic needs: *needs oral hygiene; skin very dry*
11. Psychosocial needs: *primary language Spanish - evaluate pt's. understanding of all procedures*
12. Occupation and education: *farm worker - no formal education; does not read or speak English*
13. Exercise habits: *none*
14. Spiritual needs: *Catholic - would like to talk to Spanish-speaking priest*
15. Personal interests: *works hard at farm work - no hobbies*
16. Family member interaction and availability: *wife present and anxious; does not speak English; sister available - can interpret for pt.*
17. Attitude towards illness and hospitalization: *apprehensive; inability to understand English — stressful for pt.*

Physical Examination

Date	Time		
	18.	Gen. appearance: *well developed*	*well nourished, anxious, obvious stress* color: *dark Mexican* skin: *warm and dry* *no ecchymoses or lesions*
	19.	Neurological:	*American*
		a) level of consciousness: *L.O.C.: anxious and alert*	
		b) cerebellar: *posture: leaning forward to relieve pain; gait: deferred*	
		c) motor function: upper: *normal* lower: *normal*	
		d) sensory function: upper: *normal* lower: *normal*	
		e) reflexes: *deferred*	
	20.	Head and face: *normal*	
	21.	Eyes: *PERRLA; does not wear glasses*	
	22.	Ears: *no discharge; membranes intact; no hearing difficulties*	
	23.	Nose: *no discharge; flaring of nares c̄ inspiration*	
	24.	Mouth/throat: *dental care poor; evidence of many cavities*	
	25.	Neck: *neck vein distention to angle of mandible at 35° elevation* *no lymph nodes in cervical or axill. region*	
	26.	Chest: *chest pains c̄ deep inspirations; no retractions*	
	27.	Breast: *negative*	
	28.	Respiratory: *diminished breathing sounds; dullness to percussion lower ⅓ of rt.*	
	29.	Cardiac: *To + fro friction rub - lower left sternal border* *PMI - not palpable grade ⅔ SMPLLSB* *lung field posteriorly*	
	30.	Abdomen: *liver palpable 8 cm. below rt. costal margin; moderately tender*	
	31.	Genitourinary: *voided 200 cc. on admission* *UA to lab old midline abd. scar*	
	32.	Extremities (all pulses): *3+ and all equal; feet warm*	
	33.	Back: *no deviations noted; no scars or lesions*	
	34.	Problems requiring possible referral service: *dental care; assess health care facilities in home town for follow-up care*	
	35.	Teaching needs: *tuberculosis, diet, medications.*	
	36.	Other:	

4-3		PROBLEM LIST: **ACTIVE**	**INACTIVE**
		1. acute Pericarditis	1. Gastrectomy 1975 ⟶
		2. active TB	2. Recurrent gastric ulcer 1976 ⟶
		3. communication difficulty (does not speak English)	
		4. anxiety	
		5. dental caries	
		6. smoking	
		7. drinking	
		8. lack of knowledge of TB, diet, meds	*Barbara Dossey RN, CCRN*
			NURSE'S SIGNATURE

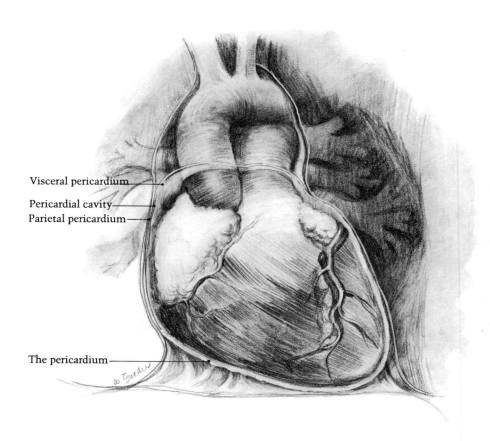

Visceral pericardium

Pericardial cavity

Parietal pericardium

The pericardium

Figure 20-1
A heart with a normal pericardium.

speaking nurses explained the procedures to Mr. B. and elicited questions from him.

During Mr. B.'s hospitalization, his wife was educated about tuberculosis and was tested to see if she also had tuberculosis. She was found to have an active case of tuberculosis, and she was placed under the care of a physician. The family was given information about the county health department in their hometown, about the need for follow-up medical care, and about nutrition and self-care.

Although the nurses had taken care of patients with acute pericarditis many times, their experience with Mr. B. illustrated the need to be prepared for the complications of the disease. The nurses learned that they must always carefully watch for signs of developing tamponade. During Mr. B.'s cardiac tamponade, they were made aware of the need for adequate preparation to assist with a pericardiocentesis in order to save a patient's life in an emergency.

Normal Physiology of the Pericardium

The space surrounding the heart is called the pericardial cavity. The dynamics in the pleural cavity are essentially the same as those in the pericardial cavity. The pressure within the pleural and the pericardial cavities is negative. During expiration and during filling of the heart, the pericardial pressure often rises intermittently to a positive value [5]. That phenomenon forces excess fluid into the lymphatic channels of the mediastinum.

The visceral pericardium is a serous membrane that is separated by a small amount of fluid from a fibrous sac, the parietal pericardium (Fig. 20-1). Normally, the pericardial sac contains less than 50 ml of fluid.

Functions of the Pericardium

The pericardium has several important functions. It holds the heart in a fixed position and minimizes friction between the heart and the surrounding structures [7]. It prevents sudden dilatation of the cardiac chambers during hypervolemia and exercise. It helps facilitate atrial filling during ventricular systole as the result of the development of negative intrapericardial pressure during ejection. The pericardium also probably retards the spread of infections from the pleural cavity and lungs to the heart [2, 5]. In some situations, however, the pericardium can be removed, and its absence does not lead to clinical disease.

Etiology and Precipitating Factors of Acute Pericarditis

Acute pericarditis is an inflammation of the pericardium. Pain is the most important symptom of acute pericarditis, and a pericardial friction rub is the most important physical finding.

The classification of pericarditis according to causes is as follows: (1) noninfectious pericarditis, (2) infectious pericarditis, and (3) pericarditis related to hypersensitivity or autoimmunity [1].

The causes of noninfectious pericarditis include myocardial infarction, uremia, neoplasia of benign or malignant origin, trauma, myxedema, irradiation, acute idiopathic causes, aortic aneurysm with leakage into the pericardial sac, and severe chronic anemia. The causes of infectious pericarditis are pyogenic, viral, tuberculous, and mycotic infections [11, 13]. Pericarditis that is related to hypersensitivity or autoimmunity can be caused by postcardiac injury, such as postpericardiotomy, Dressler's syndrome, drugs, rheumatic fever, and collagen vascular diseases, such as systemic lupus erythematosus.

Pathophysiology of Acute Pericarditis

The pathophysiological changes that occur in acute pericarditis include inflammation of the pericardium, the membranous sac that envelops the heart. A variety of inflammatory processes may involve the pericardium as secondary complications of acute pericarditis. Infection from bacteria, viruses, or other organisms usually occurs by way of the bloodstream; however, an infection from a nearby organ may also extend to the pericardium. Noninfectious pericardial inflammation may occur secondary to acute myocardial infarction, uremia, and collagen-vascular (autoimmune) disorders.

Diagnosis of Acute Pericarditis

The main signs and symptoms of many forms of acute pericarditis are pain, pericardial friction rub, ECG changes, and pericardial effusion with or without cardiac tamponade.

In her initial assessment and observations, the nurse should focus on the symptoms of the patient's illness and how the patient perceives his illness. Patients are extremely anxious with pain. Pain, the dominant symptom in most forms of acute pericarditis, is often aggravated by coughing, swallowing, inspiration, and rotation of the trunk. Most of the pain of acute pericarditis is caused by inflammation of the adjoining diaphragmatic pleura (Fig. 20-2). It has been shown that only the lower portion of the external surface of the parietal pericardium is pain-sensitive [5, 12]. The pain may be felt either in the precordium or in one or both shoulders, and it may be relieved by having the patient sit up and lean forward. The patient frequently complains of dyspnea, which results from compression of the bronchi or the parenchyma of the lung by the distended pericardium. The patient may also have pleuritic pain if the surrounding pleura becomes secondarily inflamed. The dyspnea and pleuritic pain can frighten the patient and he needs constant reassurance that the discomfort is temporary.

Pericardial Friction Rub

Probably the most important physical sign of acute pericarditis is the pericardial friction rub. The pericardial friction rub is heard most frequently during forced expiration while the patient leans forward or rests on his hands and knees (Mohammed's sign) [1] (Fig. 20-3). The friction rub can be inconsistent and transitory [16]. It may have up to three components per cardiac cycle. It is best heard with the diaphragm of the stethoscope, and it has been described as a to-and-fro leathery sound. One study—of 50 consecutive, prospectively studied patients with pericardial

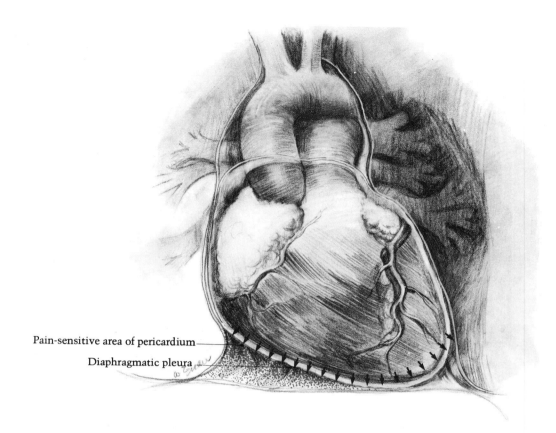

Pain-sensitive area of pericardium

Diaphragmatic pleura

friction rubs—showed that 24 percent of the rubs were of the to-and-fro type and of several biphasic patterns; 18 percent were monophasic and 58 percent were triphasic. The triphasic rub occurred in atrial systole, ventricular systole, and protodiastole [15]. The pericardial sound is thought to be due to the roughening of the two serous membranes by fibrin deposits. With the accumulation of fluid in the pericardial sac, the friction rub may disappear. The nurse must be aware that pericardial fluid can accumulate slowly in amounts up to 100 to 150 ml without producing noticeable symptoms. If the pericarditis is due to a bacterial infection, the fluid is likely to be purulent. If the effusion is due to a viral infection, the fluid is usually serous.

The physician should observe the ECG closely to distinguish the changes of acute pericarditis from those of acute myocardial infarction. In acute myocardial infarction, a distinctive pathological Q wave may develop that does not occur in acute pericarditis. In acute myocardial infarction, the T waves often be-

Figure 20-2
Sensitive area of the pericardium.

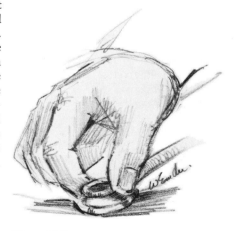

Figure 20-3
Listening for the pericardial friction rub, one of the most important physical findings in acute pericarditis.

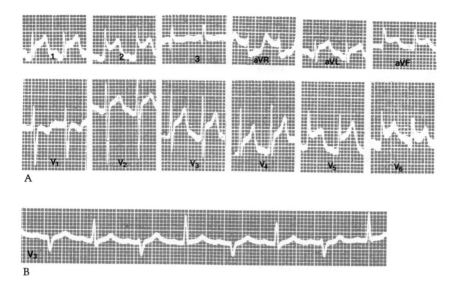

Figure 20-4

A. ECG of a patient with acute pericarditis. The ST segment shows a characteristic elevation in leads 1, 2, V_1, V_5, and V_6. B. Partial ECG of a patient with pericardial effusion and tamponade. The V_3 lead shows "total electrical alternans," with an every-other-beat variation in the amplitude of P, QRS, and T waves. That abnormality disappears as fluid is aspirated by pericardiocentesis.

come negative during periods of the ST-segment elevation. However, the ST-segment elevation in acute pericarditis lasts for a few days to a week. After that, the ST segments return to normal, and then the T waves may become negative as the subacute phase of pericarditis occurs.

The ECG in acute pericarditis without massive effusion may show elevation of the ST segment in two or three limb leads and the anterior precordial leads [5] (Fig. 20-4A). Reciprocal depression usually is seen only in aVR and V_1. The only change in the QRS complexes is an occasional lessening of voltage (called electrical alternans) which is usually found only when a considerable effusion is present (Fig. 20-4B). Total electrical alternans is an every-other-beat variation in the amplitude of P, QRS, and T waves. The abnormality disappears as fluid is aspirated by pericardiocentesis.

Pericardial Effusion

Pericardial effusion is usually associated with an enlargement of the cardiac silhouette as seen radiographically (Fig. 20-5). The rapid accumulation of effusion over a short period of time is especially ominous and may result in cardiac tamponade. With the rapid accumulation of effusion, the heart sounds become faint, the friction rub may or may not disappear, and the apical impulse may vanish. If the effusion is large, one may find Ewart's sign, probably caused by compression of the lung (tubular breath sounds and an area of dullness can be heard at the left scapular angle).

Clinical signs suggesting pericardial effusion are (1) dyspnea and diminished heart sounds due to distention of the pericardial sac, (2) hypotension and tachycardia resulting from reduced cardiac output, (3) pulsus paradoxus resulting from a rapid accumulation of pericardial fluid and increasing venous pressure, and (4) Kussmaul's sign, indicating impaired right-sided cardiac filling. Kussmaul's sign is increased neck vein distention on inspiration. Normally, neck vein distention disappears on inspiration.

Pulsus paradoxus is an exaggeration of the normal variation in systolic blood pressure usually associated with inspiration. The normal variation of systolic blood pressure during inspiration is 3 to 10 mm Hg in the healthy person. It is thought that the normal

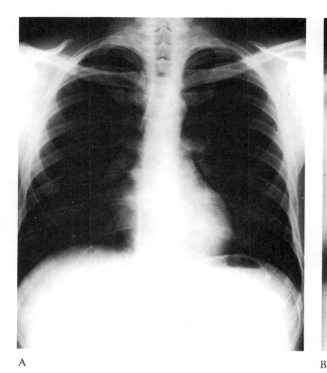

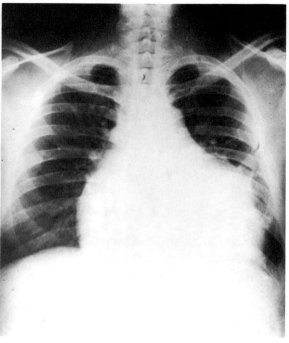

A

B

Figure 20-5
A. Normal chest x ray. B. Chest x ray of a patient with a large pericardial effusion that resulted in pericardial tamponade.

variation of blood pressure that accompanies respiration results from the pooling of blood during inspiration in the pulmonary vasculature because of lung expansion and increased negative intrathoracic pressure [6]. Pulmonary vascular pooling normally occurs during inspiration with a resultant decrease in blood return to the left side of the heart, causing decreased left ventricular output. The fall in systolic blood pressure is therefore exaggerated when venous return to the heart is impaired for any reason.

When pericardial fluid rapidly accumulates (Fig. 20-6) and when venous pressure rises (as it does in pericardial effusion or cardiac tamponade), the pericardial sac is distended and it becomes globular. During inspiration, the pericardium becomes elliptical because the diaphragm pulls the pericardium downward. That change is thought to increase intrapericardial pressure and thus hinder venous return to the right and left atria. Respiratory distress also seems to exaggerate the mechanism and increases intrathoracic pressure. The right atrium and right ventricle are also distended by the inspiratory increase, causing increased venous return. Increased

venous return interferes with left ventricular filling and thus the decrease in left ventricular stroke volume is much greater than normal.

To determine whether pulsus paradoxus is present, one must use a blood pressure cuff and stethoscope to observe the components of the patient's blood pressure. To try to elicit a pulsus paradoxus, the examiner asks the patient to breathe in a normal manner. As the examiner deflates the blood pressure cuff, he observes the level at which Korotkoff sounds are first noted. At this point Korotkoff sounds are heard only during expiration. The blood pressure cuff is deflated until Korotkoff sounds are heard throughout the respiratory cycle. The pulsus paradoxus is the difference in mm Hg between the first Korotkoff sounds heard and the continuous Korotkoff sounds. In patients whose breathing is normal and not obstructed,

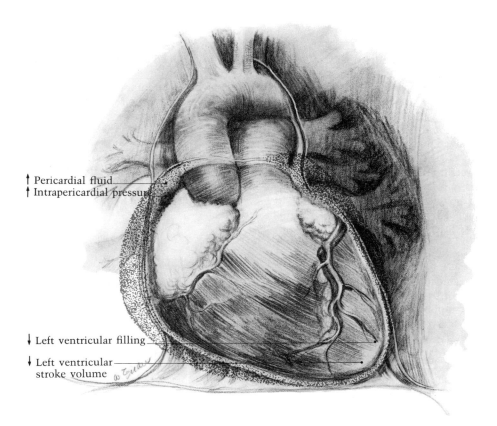

↑ Pericardial fluid
↑ Intrapericardial pressure

↓ Left ventricular filling

↓ Left ventricular
stroke volume

Figure 20-6
Pericardial effusion and cardiac tamponade. The following hemodynamic effects may result following pericardial effusion:

1. Accumulation of pericardial fluid resulting in intrapericardial pressure
2. Elevation of right atrial pressure
3. Elevation of left ventricular end-diastolic pressure
4. Reduction in left ventricular end-diastolic volume and cardiac output
5. Elevated venous pressure.

a difference in arterial pressure that exceeds 10 mm Hg usually indicates cardiac compression.

The presence of pulsus paradoxus, however, does not always mean the presence of pericardial disease. Pulsus paradoxus can be found occasionally in patients with congestive heart failure, specifically in patients whose congestive heart failure is due to chronic myocardial disease.

PROCEDURES USED TO DETECT PERICARDIAL EFFUSION

Echocardiography
Echocardiography is a method of outlining the borders of the cardiac chambers by directing sound waves across the heart and recording the reflections of the waves (echoes) off solid structures in their path [4, 8]. Pericardial fluid appears as a relatively echo-free space between the posterior left ventricular wall or anterior right ventricular wall and the parietal pericardium [18].

Cardiac Catheterization and Angiography
Catheterization of the right heart may support the diagnosis of pericardial effusion. As the catheter traverses the right atrium, its tip is pushed against the inner wall of the atrium; an abnormal widening of the distance between the catheter tip and the radiolucent lung (normally represented by the very thin atrial wall) suggests pericardial effusion. Contrast

material injected into the atrium can give a better idea of the increase in thickness of the pericardial shadow. In the presence of pericardial constriction by effusion, pressure recordings from the right ventricle show an abnormally rapid fall in pressure during diastole due to the impairment of filling [1, 5].

Carbon Dioxide Angiocardiography

Carbon dioxide injected intravenously into a patient who is on his left side collects as a "bubble" against the inner wall of the right atrium, affording an estimate of pericardial thickness similar to that obtained by angiography [5]. Carbon dioxide is used because it is absorbed much more rapidly from the circulation than is air, and thus it is less likely to obstruct blood flow.

Blood Pool Scanning

In blood pool scanning, a radioactive isotope (e.g., iodine 125 attached to albumin) is injected intravenously. It gives an image of the inner dimensions of the cardiac chambers as it traverses the heart [5]. Normally, owing to the relatively thin ventricular walls, the interior of the heart is only slightly smaller than the cardiac silhouette as seen on a chest roentgenogram. A greater-than-normal discrepancy in the relative sizes of the interior heart and the cardiac silhouette suggests pericardial effusion.

Cardiac Tamponade

Most often, cardiac tamponade results from bleeding into the pericardial space following cardiac surgery, trauma (including perforation of the heart during diagnostic procedures), tumor, pyogenic infections, and tuberculosis [17].

The major clinical manifestations of cardiac tamponade are (1) a fall in cardiac output and (2) systemic venous congestion. Both phenomena are caused by obstruction of the inflow of blood to the ventricles [6]. When tamponade develops slowly, the patient's condition resembles that seen in right-sided congestive heart failure. The patient has tachycardia, dyspnea, orthopnea, hepatic engorgement, and a positive hepatojugular reflex. When severe tamponade develops, such as in cardiac trauma, faint heart sounds, electrical alternans, and arterial hypotension occur. When a patient has acute cardiac trauma following direct cardiac trauma from gunshot or stab wounds his condition is critical (see Chap. 15). Since the rise in

the patient's intrapericardial pressure interferes with cardiac filling, his cardiac output quickly becomes inadequate to sustain life. Until cardiac tamponade can be relieved, the rapid administration of intravenous saline solution or blood may temporarily improve the patient's blood pressure by increasing the filling pressure and thus the cardiac output.

The accumulation of fluid in the pericardium necessary to produce a critical state may be as small as 250 ml when the fluid accumulates rapidly. However, when the pericardium has been able to stretch and adapt to a slowly increasing effusion, the amount of fluid may reach 1000 ml before hemodynamic impairment occurs [1].

Treatment of Acute Pericarditis

Patients with acute pericarditis need relief of their symptoms and treatment of the cause of the pericarditis. In patients with benign idiopathic acute pericarditis, salicylates are usually sufficient for the relief of pain. However, some patients require meperidine or morphine in the acute phase. The patient needs constant reassurance, and he must be encouraged to remain in bed as long as he has pain and fever. If the physician rules out tuberculosis as the cause and if the pain is not relieved by salicylates, corticosteroids may produce dramatic improvement [5, 10].

Tuberculous pericarditis requires long-term tuberculous therapy. It is believed that tuberculous therapy combined with corticosteroid therapy may reduce mortality and morbidity in patients who have recurrent pericardial effusion [13].

Rheumatic pericarditis requires bed rest and treatment of the rheumatic fever. Therapeutic dosages of penicillin are given and are followed with prophylactic penicillin. Steroids are considered when endocarditis or myocarditis occurs [13].

For patients with infectious pericarditis that is related to diseases of the left pleural space or to septicemia, the physician orders specific antibiotics or surgical treatment if the patient's clinical situation requires it [14].

Direct trauma to the heart from gunshot wounds, stab wounds, or wounds caused by other penetrating foreign objects can cause cardiac tamponade, a rapidly fatal condition that must be corrected immediately. Needle aspiration of the pericardial space must be done [9]. It is considered a lifesaving procedure. Complications of the aspiration are laceration of the myocardium or coronary arteries, vagovagal arrest, and ventricular fibrillation (see Chap. 15 for details). While the needle aspiration is being performed, the patient's blood pressure and ECG must be monitored constantly [17]. When a number of aspirations are required, surgical resection is usually indicated. However, most patients respond to pericardiocentesis. Only a small number of patients require a "pericardial window" procedure, the surgical removal of a segment of the pericardium to establish continuous decompression and drainage.

Assessment and Management of the Patient with Acute Pericarditis, Effusion, or Tamponade

OBJECTIVE NO. 1

The patient should not have more episodes of undue pain caused by pericarditis.
    To achieve the objective, the nurse should:

1. Give meperidine or morphine as ordered to relieve the pain.
2. Give salicylates as ordered to reduce fever and inflammation.
3. Give steroids as ordered to control the symptoms of pericarditis and to reduce the inflammatory process. The nurse should *watch* for the side effects of steroids:
    a. Weight gain due to sodium retention and fluid retention
    b. Decreased resistance to infection
    c. Hypertension
    d. Euphoria and excitability
    The steroid therapy should be terminated slowly as ordered by the physician. Abrupt withdrawal can cause a rebound of symptoms or acute adrenocortical insufficiency.
4. Assess anxiety level and use appropriate nursing interventions.

OBJECTIVE NO. 2

The patient should not have more complications of pericarditis.
    To achieve the objective, the nurse should:

1. Listen with the stethoscope for increasing or decreasing intensity of the friction rub. The friction rub may be transitory and may have a to-and-fro biphasic or triphasic pattern.
2. Be aware of persistent clinical symptoms:
    a. Pain in the precordial area (mild to sharp or severe)
    b. Dyspnea
    c. Fevers, chills, and sweating (more pronounced if salicylates have not been given to reduce the patient's fever)
3. Be alert for the signs of pericardial effusion and cardiac tamponade:
    a. Dyspnea
    b. Hypotension
    c. Diminished heart sounds
    d. Tachycardia
    e. Pulsus paradoxus greater than 10 mm Hg
    f. Distended neck veins
    g. Increased central venous pressure
    h. Kussmaul's sign
    i. ECG changes (dysrhythmias, decreased QRS voltage, or electrical alternans)
4. Be ready to infuse rapidly saline solution or blood intravenously in order to make the venous pressure greater than the pericardial pressure in cases of cardiac tamponade (medical treatment).
5. Be ready to assist with pericardiocentesis. On physical examination, the "rule of 20" is often invoked as a criterion for pericardiocentesis: pulsus paradoxus greater than 20, venous pressure greater than 20, and pulse pressure less than 20.
6. Prepare the patient for pericardial drainage if necessary.

OBJECTIVE NO. 3

The patient should understand the usual course of pericarditis.
    To achieve the objective, the nurse should:

1. Assure the patient that the pain of pericarditis is temporary and will decrease when pain medication, steroid and salicylate therapy, or other specific therapy is given.
2. Help the patient to increase his activity gradually.
3. Observe the patient for signs and symptoms of pain and determine what activity or position precipitates or alleviates his pain. His pain may be:
    a. Increased by breathing.
    b. Increased by coughing, swallowing, rotation of the trunk, and changes in the flexion, exten-

sion, or rotation of the spine (including the neck).
  c. Increased by lying on the back.
  d. Decreased by sitting up or leaning forward.
4. Give appropriate medications to relieve acute pericarditis when the cause is an infectious or immunological one (e.g., tuberculosis, rheumatic fever, or a fungus).

OBJECTIVE NO. 4

The diagnostic tests should be explained to the patient.

  In order to achieve the objective, the nurse should be able to assist with and inform the patient about the various laboratory techniques and procedures that can be used to establish the diagnosis of pericardial effusion. The nurse should have the patient sign the consent forms and so agree to the following special procedures:

1. Special cultures
2. ECG
3. Echocardiogram
4. Cardiac catheterization and angiogram
5. Carbon dioxide angiogram
6. Blood pool scanning

Summary

Acute pericarditis is painful, and the pain is often aggravated by coughing, swallowing, breathing, and lying supine. Dyspnea also occurs frequently. The diagnosis of acute pericarditis is confirmed by the patient's clinical history and physical examination; a pericardial friction rub is a significant finding. Specific diagnostic procedures that help confirm the diagnosis are the ECG, the echocardiogram, cardiac catheterization and angiography, carbon dioxide angiography, and isotopic blood pool scanning.

  Patients whose condition has been diagnosed as acute pericarditis must be closely observed so that any complications of the illness can be detected as soon as they occur. If the complications of the illness are not detected, pericardial effusion and cardiac tamponade can cause death in a short time.

Study Problems

1. What are the physical signs of acute pericarditis?
2. What is the clinical condition of a patient with acute pericarditis?
3. What are the major complications that the nurse must be aware of when caring for a patient with acute pericarditis?
4. What are the classic signs of cardiac tamponade?
5. What causes the clinical manifestations of cardiac tamponade?

Answers

1. Fever, friction rub, tachycardia.
2. Dyspnea, pleuritic chest pain, cough, mental confusion, pain that changes when the patient changes position.
3. Pericardial effusion, cardiac tamponade, and cardiac dysrhythmias.
4. Extreme dyspnea, orthopnea, tachycardia, hepatic engorgement, pulsus paradoxus, and electrical alternans.
5. A fall in cardiac output, and systemic venous congestion.

References

1. Braunwald, E. Pericardial Disease. In T. P. Harrison (ed.), *Principles of Internal Medicine* (8th ed.). New York: McGraw-Hill, 1977.
2. Cortes, F. M. (ed.). *The Pericardium and Its Disorders.* Springfield, Ill.: Thomas, 1971.
3. Dressler, W. Effect of respiration on pericardial friction rub. *Am. J. Cardiol.* 7:130, 1961.
4. Feigenbaum, H. Echocardiographic diagnosis of pericardial effusion. *Am. J. Cardiol.* 26:475, 1970.
5. Fowler, N. O. The Recognition and Management of Pericardial Disease and Its Complications. In J. W. Hurst and R. B. Logue (eds.), *The Heart* (4th ed.). New York: McGraw-Hill, 1978.
6. Guntheroth, W. G., Morgan, B. C., and Mullins, G. L. Effect of respiration on venous return and stroke volume in cardiac tamponade. *Circ. Res.* 20:381, 1967.
7. Holt, J. P. The normal pericardium. *Am. J. Cardiol.* 26:455, 1970.
8. Jacobs, W. R., Talano, J. V., and Loib, H. S. Echocar-

diographic interpretation of pericardial effusion. *Arch. Intern. Med.* 138:622, 1978.

9. Jones, E. W., and Helmsworth, J.   Penetrating wounds of the heart: Thirty years' experience. *Arch. Surg.* 96: 671, 1968.

10. Logue, R. B., Taylor, D. R., and Carter, L. Y.   Diagnosis and treatment of pericardial effusion without pericardiocentesis: Use of steroids and diuretics. *Circulation* (Suppl. II) 36:174, 1967.

11. Lyons, H. A., Rooney, J. J., and Crocco, J. A.   Tuberculous pericarditis. *Ann. Intern. Med.* 68:1175, 1968.

12. Moore, S. J.   Pericarditis after acute myocardial infarction. *Heart Lung* 8:551, 1979.

13. Pamukcoglu, T.   Endocardial tuberculosis. *N.Y. State J. Med.* 67:2868, 1967.

14. Shabetai, R. (ed).   Symposium on pericardial disease. *Am. J. Cardiol.* 26:445, 1970.

15. Spodick, D. H.   Pericardial function. *N. Engl. J. Med.* 278:1204, 1968.

16. Spodick, D. H.   Acoustic phenomena in pericardial disease. *Am. Heart J.* 81:114, 1971.

17. Stein, L., Shubin, H., and Weil, M. H.   Recognition and management of pericardial tamponade. *J.A.M.A.* 225:503, 1973.

18. Yu, P. N., and Goodwin, J. F.   *Progress in Cardiology.* Philadelphia: Lea & Febiger, 1974.

Cardiac Surgery

Cathie E. Guzzetta

Care of the cardiac surgical patient may be a stressful, challenging, and rewarding experience. It may be stressful because of the many skills, procedures, and responsibilities that are demanded of the critical care nurse. It may be challenging because the nurse plays an essential role in the preoperative and postoperative psychobiological assessment and management of her patient. The nurse must understand the pathophysiology of cardiac disease, diagnostic and surgical procedures, critical physiological changes, and complications. She is challenged to use her information to assess the patient, make nursing diagnoses, implement care, prevent and treat complications, and evaluate the results of the process. Caring for the cardiac surgical patient may also be rewarding because it gives the nurse an opportunity to demonstrate her understanding of psychobiological nursing care, to demonstrate her expert knowledge and skills, and to participate with the patient in achieving the desired outcomes of care.

This chapter discusses aspects of coronary artery disease and valvular disease as they are related to cardiac surgery. It discusses the pathophysiology, clinical manifestations, diagnostic procedures, surgical techniques, and nursing and medical management.

21

Objective

In caring for a patient who is to undergo cardiac surgery, the nurse should be able to assess and manage the patient preoperatively, postoperatively, and during his rehabilitation phase of care.

Achieving the Objective

To achieve the objective, the nurse should be able to:

1. Describe the pathophysiology of coronary artery disease and valvular heart disease.
2. Describe the major operative risk factors.
3. List the major indications for surgery.
4. Outline the steps involved with the patient's preparation for surgery.
5. Describe the management of the patient during the immediate postoperative phase.
6. Identify and describe the management of postoperative complications.
7. Describe the management of the patient during his rehabilitation phase.
8. Teach the patient and his family about preoperative, postoperative, and discharge care.

How to Proceed

To develop an approach to cardiac surgery, the nurse should:

1. Read the material that follows.
2. Using only the information in the case study, do a written head-to-toe systematic assessment of the patient in the immediate postoperative period, and make out a problem list.
3. As the primary care nurse, know the answers to the following questions about the patient in the case study:
   a. What are the objectives for his care?
   b. What other kinds of information would she want to know?
   c. What is her nursing care plan for the patient in
      (1) The preoperative phase?
      (2) The postoperative phase?
      (3) The rehabilitation phase?
   d. If the patient developed ICU psychosis while in the surgical intensive care unit, how would she organize patient grand rounds in an attempt to deal with the problem?
      (1) How would she organize the conference?
      (2) Whom would she invite?
      (3) What things would she include as factors leading to ICU psychosis?
      (4) What things could be done to solve the problem in her particular institution?
      (5) How would she change the patient's nursing care plan in view of this new problem, ICU psychosis?
4. Take the opportunity to care for a patient undergoing surgery. The nurse should:
   a. Care for the patient preoperatively.
   b. Observe him undergoing an exercise tolerance test and a cardiac catheterization.
   c. Observe him during cardiac surgery.
   d. Care for him in the ICU.
   e. Care for him during his rehabilitation phase.
5. For further information, read the articles listed in the references at the end of the chapter.

Case Study

Mr. G. H., a 55-year-old white shoemaker, was admitted to the telemetry unit for evaluation of chest pain. He was free of symptoms despite his moderately strenuous job until about six months ago, when he began experiencing chest pain during physical exertion (about one or two times a week). The dull, tight chest pain was retrosternal and radiated to his neck and left arm. The pain was relieved promptly by rest and nitroglycerin. It was not associated with dyspnea or diaphoresis, and it never lasted more than five minutes.

During the past two months, the pain had increased in frequency and severity, occurring three or four times a day with minimal exertion (e.g., walking short distances) or excitement. Occasionally it occurred when Mr. H. woke up or when he was at rest. He was given sublingual isosorbide dinitrate (5 mg every 6 hr) in addition to his usual nitroglycerin, but his condition did not improve. Because the attacks continued to become more frequent and severe, Mr. H. was hospitalized for further assessment and observation.

Mr. H. had a nervous, restless personality. Divorced once, he was currently married. He had a son, aged 26, from his first marriage. He had smoked two packs of cigarettes a day for 30 years, and he drank moderately on weekends (four or five cocktails). He usually drank a glass of wine before bedtime. His interests were bass fishing and bowling. He said that he was allergic to sulfa drugs. He was Catholic.

Mr. H.'s past medical history included an appendectomy in 1952 and a hemorrhoidectomy in 1960. He was deaf in his right ear, and he used a hearing aid to correct a moderately severe hearing impairment in his left ear. His mother had a history of diabetes mellitus, and his father died at age 60 of a myocardial infarction. His older brother, aged 62, had had an acute myocardial infarction two years ago. The rest of Mr. H.'s family history was not relevant.

Mr. H.'s physical examination showed that he was a well-developed, well-nourished, middle-aged man who was not in acute distress. His blood pressure was 160/110. He had grade II hypertensive changes in his fundi. Examination of his neck revealed symmetrical carotid pulses with normal upstroke and no bruits. He had no jugular venous distention. Examination of his lungs revealed bilateral rhonchi that cleared when he coughed. His heart was regular at 110 beats per minute. He had a normal first and second heart sound and no third heart sound, murmurs, or rubs. He had an atrial gallop at the fifth intercostal space, midclavicular line. His abdomen, back, genitourinary system, and extremities were normal.

Mr. H.'s ECG showed a regular sinus tachycardia. His chest x ray revealed that his heart was normal in size and configuration. His lung fields were clear. His electrolyte values were normal. His serum cholesterol level was 160 mg/100 ml and his triglyceride level was 130 mg/100 ml, both within normal limits. Other routine hematological studies were normal. A treadmill exercise tolerance test was performed. The results were clearly positive, with the simultaneous development of angina pectoris.

A left heart catheterization was performed via the right brachial artery, and a series of arteriograms were made. They showed that the proximal circumflex coronary artery was narrowed 80 to 85 percent. The anterior descending branch of the left coronary artery was narrowed 70 to 80 percent. Both arteries appeared to have good distal runoff. The right coronary artery was found to be normal. A left ventriculogram revealed a normal ejection fraction and normal contractility. There were no valvular defects or ventricular aneurysms.

Because of the information gathered from Mr. H.'s history, stress testing, and cardiac catheterization, aortocoronary saphenous vein bypass surgery was recommended. Discussion of the risk factors, surgery, and preoperative teaching were done by a nurse-physician team. The following day, Mr. H. was taken to surgery.

With Mr. H. under general anesthesia, the saphenous veins were taken from his groin and reversed. A median sternotomy incision was made and his heart was exposed; it had a normal appearance and no adhesions or scars suggestive of a previous myocardial infarction. The ventricles were normal in size.

Mr. H. was placed on cardiopulmonary bypass and a quiet operative field was obtained by electrically inducing ventricular fibrillation. To revascularize the left ventricle, the saphenous veins were placed to bypass the stenotic portions of the circumflex and anterior descending branches of the left coronary artery.

The surgical procedure lasted approximately four hours. Mr. H. was then taken to the ICU postoperatively (see the admission assessment sheet). He remained in the unit for 72 hours without complications and was discharged to the telemetry unit. There he continued to receive postoperative and discharge teaching concerning exercise, diet, and medications. After seven days without complications, he was discharged from the hospital.

Reflections

The care of the patient undergoing cardiac surgery must be managed by an interdisciplinary team. The primary care nurse provides for continuity of care throughout the preoperative, postoperative, and rehabilitation phases. She is the person to whom the patient can let his needs be known. During the admission assessment of the patient and throughout the patient's hospitalization, the nurse evaluates the patient's physical condition and mental status. She identifies the patient's and family's expectations, adaptation capabilities, anxieties, fears, and readiness for the teaching-learning process.

Cardiac surgery has a profound impact on the psychobiological unity of the patient. In many cultures, the heart is popularly regarded as the center of life. A disease of the heart can seriously disrupt one's adaptation capacity, perhaps more than can a disease of most other organs. The nurse and the patient participate together in an important role; together they work to help the patient achieve an acceptable level of psychobiological adaptation during the preoperative and postoperative phases. The teaching-learning process, when shared by both the patient and the nurse, is one method that can be used to help the patient adapt. The nurse might ask, "Why is that process beneficial in helping the patient to achieve psychobiological adaptation?" The following paragraphs discuss that issue [2].

The idea of the patient as a psychobiological unit (see Chap. 1) can be enormously fruitful when applied to patient education. As a psychobiological unit, the patient is not divisible into body and mind; he is inseparably both. Mind and body operate on a continuum. Thus if the mind is educable, so is the body. To educate the mind is to educate the body.

The idea of psychobiological unity increases the nurse's opportunities for providing effective care. Because of the body-mind continuum, therapy can be more than drugs, treatments, and surgical procedures. The nurse's contributions to patient education can result in "body effects" that are as real as those achieved by traditional forms of therapy. Because of

Critical Care Nursing Admission Assessment

Head-to-Toe Approach

Date	Time		
		Pt. Name: *Mr. G.H.* Age: *55* Allergies: *Sulfa drugs*	
1-3-		Admitted Bed No: *1* Via: *litter* Ad. Dx.: *CABG; LAD + Circumflex*	
		T. *96* ® A.P.: *110* R.P.: *110* R. *on MA @ 12/min.* B.P. Supine R: *104/80* L: *106/80* Sitting: *100/76*	
		Wt. *bed scale (unit scale)* *77 kg.* Ht.: *5'10"* ECG Rhythm: *Sinus Tach.* Ectopy: *none*	
		Informant: *Hx obtained from pt. noc before surgery* Last meal: *last evening*	
	1.	Chief complaint: *LAD narrowed 70-80%; circumflex narrowed 80-85%*	
	2.	Hx. of present illness: *Angina - onset 6 mo. ago brought on by physical exertion past 2 mo, angina ↑ in frequency + severity 3-4 times/day c̄ minimal exertion/excitement + occasionally upon waking or rest. Pain relieved c̄ NTG.*	
	3.	Past medical Hx. (include all surgeries, hosp., diseases, injuries, blood trans.): *deaf ® ear; hearing impairment ⓛ ear* *Appendectomy 1952, hemorrhoidectomy 1960; pre-op hypertension 160/110 no hx of valvular defects, arthritis, hyperthyroidism, gout, diabetes. No previous symptoms of palpitation, syncope, edema, dyspnea or fatigue. No previous transfusions*	
	4.	Family Hx: *Father died age 62 of M.I.; mother had history of diabetes, died age 70; older brother age 62 has hx of MI 2 yrs. ago*	
	5.	Current drugs: *s.l. NTG prn; s.l. isosorbide dinitrate 5mg. q6h.*	
	6.	Alcohol and tobacco habits: *drinks 4-5 cocktails/weekend; smokes 2 pkg. cigarettes/day x 30 yrs.*	
	7.	Dietary and fluid needs: *on low atherogenic diet; doesn't eat brkfast*	
	8.	Sleep and rest patterns: *sleeps 6-7 hr./noc; drinks glass of wine at bedtime; 30 min. nap after work*	
	9.	Bowel and bladder habits: *uses MOM for occasional constipation; no difficulty voiding*	
	10.	Hygienic needs: *showers daily in evening*	
	11.	Psychosocial needs: *began to verbalize that future lifestyle will need to be altered c̄ regard to CAD risk factors (smoking, exercise, stress).*	
	12.	Occupation and education: *H.S. graduate; owns own shoe repair store. works 6 days/wk.; 8-10 hrs./day*	
	13.	Exercise habits: *moderate strenuous activity at work.*	
	14.	Spiritual needs: *Catholic; Father Paul visited pt. prior to surgery; St. Ritas #368-1594*	
	15.	Personal interests: *enjoys bowling + bass fishing*	
	16.	Family member interaction and availability: *married for 7 yrs.; wife's name Joan; 26 y/o son John through 1st marriage (not living at home). Family members have supportive and calming influence on pt.*	
	17.	Attitude towards illness and hospitalization: *Has been anxious and restless during hospitalization. Pt. states he is anxious to have surgery so that he can return to normal lifestyle.*	

Physical Examination

Date	Time	
	18.	Gen. appearance: *intubated, well developed, well nourished* color: *pale, no cyanosis* skin: *no rashes, cool, dry, good turgor*
	19.	Neurological:
		a) level of consciousness: *remains under morphine anesthesia*
		b) cerebellar: *unable to evaluate*
		c) motor function: upper: *normal muscle size, symmetry; no fasciculations* lower: *normal size + symmetry; no fasciculations*
		d) sensory function: upper: *reacts to painful stim.* lower: *reacts to painful stim.*
		e) reflexes: *unable to evaluate*
	20.	Head and face: *normal hair distribution + symmetry; no scars or edema*
	21.	Eyes: *R+L eye react equally to direct + consensual light; pupils equal c̄ 1⁺ constriction*
	22.	Ears: *no drainage; deafness R ear; moderate hearing impairment L ear; wears hearing aid*
	23.	Nose: *no drainage; no septal deviation or deformities*
	24.	Mouth/throat: *dry mouth + lips; E.T. tube in place c̄ small leak; coated tongue; mod. amt. white thick sputum by suction*
	25.	Neck: *no JNVD; no rigidity; trachea midline; no scars or lymph enlargement*
	26.	Chest: *bilateral symmetrical expansion; median sternotomy c̄ dry dressing; 2 ant. drainage tubes to water seal bottles*
	27.	Breast: *normal appearance, size + shape*
	28.	Respiratory: *bilateral breath sounds c̄ rhonchi RUL; on MA, at 12/min; F_1O_2 60%; T_V 1200 cc*
	29.	Cardiac: *normal S_1 + S_2; no Ⓜ; no S_3 or S_4 or rubs*
	30.	Abdomen: *no distention; appendix scar; no bowel sounds*
	31.	Genitourinary: *Foley catheter in place; pink dilute urine; S.G. 1.009, 1⁺ sugar, trace acetone, trace blood*
	32.	Extremities (all pulses): *good bilateral pulses; ace bandages on both legs; all extremit. cool, peripherally constricted*
	33.	Back: *no scars or sacral edema; no spinal abnorm.; reddened coccyx*
	34.	Problems requiring possible referral service: *post-op physical therapy + recreational therapy + respiratory therapy*
	35.	Teaching needs: *Has received complete preoperative teaching program - asked many questions and appeared to comprehend well; will need post-op teaching*
	36.	Other: *be sure pt. has hearing aid inserted left ear; hearing aid in bedside drawer ICU rm. #1; after return to telemetry floor*

	PROBLEM LIST: ACTIVE	INACTIVE
1-3-	1. Post-op CABG (LAD + Circumflex)	Appendectomy 1952
	2. Sinus tachycardia	Hemorrhoidectomy 1960
	3. Pre-op hypertension	
	4. Pre-op anxiety	
	5. heavy smoker c̄ chronic bronchitis	
	6. deaf R ear; hearing impairment L ear.	

Cathie E. Guzzetta, R.N., CCRN
NURSE'S SIGNATURE

its importance in affecting the body-mind continuum, patient education should be viewed as a mandatory goal, not an elective one. The critical care nurse must come to view the teaching-learning process as an indispensable part of the therapeutic process, one that is applicable to all patients and all illnesses.

After the benefits of the teaching-learning process have been identified, the nurse might ask, "How do I begin? What should I teach?" A starting point for any type of patient education program is standardizing the information to be presented. The content should be developed and approved by nurses, physicians, dietitians, psychiatrists, and members of the clergy, and occupational, physical, and respiratory therapists. The input from the health team members helps in deciding what should be taught, prevents the omission of necessary information, and ensures that the material is presented consistently by everyone.

Standardization, however, does not imply formalization of patient education. The teaching-learning process is more than presenting well-chosen facts to the patient. The standardized material is an organizational guideline providing basic information that can be applied to patients with similar illnesses. The patient's needs, concerns, level of learning, and anxiety and other factors that inhibit or promote the teaching-learning process must be individually assessed and incorporated into the body-mind-spirit approach.

As mentioned, the standardization of information must be the work of all members of the health team. The content is based on the information that the health team believes to be important. During preoperative and postoperative teaching periods, the nurse must also identify and evaluate what areas the patient feels are important. She should encourage him to ask questions and to participate actively in the process. Nurses who are involved in the preparation of written teaching materials might also identify other areas of concern by sending the materials to patients who have been discharged and asking them for their recommendations and suggestions.

An important objective in educating cardiac surgical patients is reduction of their anxiety and fear. Descriptions of procedures, treatments, and methods of care are usually included in the teaching. Johnson's investigation [33], however, found that the usual practice of explaining the meaning or need for a test, procedure, or surgery in detail to a patient was not as effective in reducing his stress as was giving the patient accurate descriptions of how and what he will feel (i.e., during a cardiac catheterization, with an endotracheal tube, while on a ventilator, or when being suctioned). The findings of the study are important in guiding patient education programs and in assisting nurses to help the patient adapt. The patient wants to know the "how" and "what" of an experience before the "why."

Dealing with a patient undergoing cardiac surgery is never a neutral event. It is a stressful yet challenging and rewarding experience. The critical care nurse can scientifically, imaginatively, and humanely apply the concepts derived from a body-mind-spirit approach to assist the patient in achieving the desired outcomes and to help in defining the professional practice of nursing.

Myocardial Revascularization

Vineberg developed the first operative approach for myocardial revascularization in 1946 [79]. That approach involved tunneling the left ventricular wall and implanting the internal mammary artery in the myocardium (Fig. 21-1). Vineberg believed that the implanted artery would anastomose with the arteriolar network of the cardiac muscle and form channels supplying blood to the main coronary circulation. Vineberg's indirect revascularization approach was reported to have had excellent clinical results. But because methods to evaluate the approach objectively were lacking, it did not become popular until the early sixties.

In 1962, Sones developed a safe and reliable procedure for cardiac catheterization [73]. The procedure enabled the location and extent of the atherosclerotic obstruction to be visualized and it also provided a method to evaluate the results of cardiac surgery. Consequently, new interest was created in the Vineberg procedure, and several modifications of that procedure were attempted. In time, however, it was observed that many patients who initially found relief from angina pectoris after indirect myocardial revascularization later experienced a recurrence of symptoms. At present, the benefits of the Vineberg procedure, in terms of its ability to increase coronary blood flow and to improve survival, remains questionable [48].

Shortly after the introduction of selective coronary arteriography, the interest in developing techniques for direct myocardial revascularization [4, 68] was re-

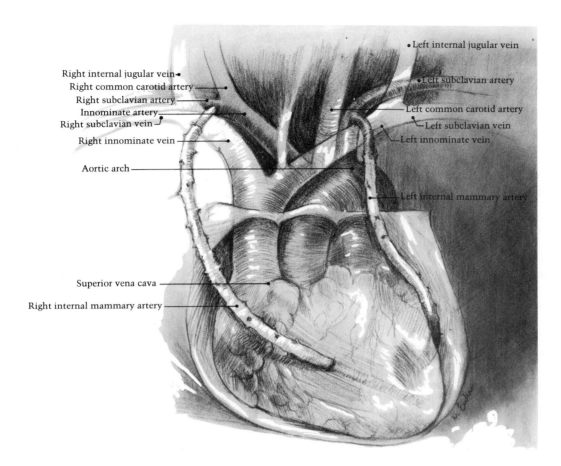

Right internal jugular vein
Right common carotid artery
Right subclavian artery
Innominate artery
Right subclavian vein
Right innominate vein
Aortic arch
Superior vena cava
Right internal mammary artery

Left internal jugular vein
Left subclavian artery
Left common carotid artery
Left subclavian vein
Left innominate vein
Left internal mammary artery

Figure 21-1
Internal mammary artery implant (Vineberg procedure). The Vineberg procedure is the older method of myocardial revascularization. It is still used for the occasional patient or in combination with a bypass procedure.

vived. Proximal coronary artery endarterectomy [16] and carbon dioxide gas endarterectomy [62] were among the earlier direct revascularization procedures.

Investigators also began exploring the feasibility of direct revascularization using the saphenous vein for grafts. Aortocoronary bypass surgery was first performed in 1965 [23], and the initial trials were reported on by Favalaro and his associates [21, 22], and Johnson and his associates [34]. Although there have been minor changes in the techniques of cardiopulmonary bypass, the basic procedure, aortocoronary saphenous vein bypass, has remained one of the primary methods of revascularization.

Indications for Myocardial Revascularization

In coronary artery disease, atherosclerotic plaques are primarily composed of cholesterol, other lipids, and fibrous tissue, which are deposited along the intimal wall of the coronary artery (see Chap. 19). Typically, the atherosclerotic plaques are found in the larger portions of an artery, resulting in proximal narrowing or occlusion with little involvement in the smaller distal sections. The amount of involvement of one or more branches of the coronary arteries depends on the patient's individual disease process. When the atherosclerotic process impairs the coronary blood flow to the myocardium, serious hemodynamic disturbances and clinical manifestations are observed.

The selection of a patient for aortocoronary bypass surgery is based on the belief that revascularizing the myocardium will improve the patient's symptoms. Not all patients with coronary artery disease are candidates for surgery. Aortocoronary bypass surgery is frequently recommended for patients with intractable or unstable angina pectoris; it may be considered for patients with acute myocardial infarction, congestive heart failure, cardiogenic shock, and refractory ventricular irritability. The following pages discuss the indications for aortocoronary bypass surgery.

INTRACTABLE ANGINA PECTORIS

Patients with severe, or intractable, angina pectoris find their lives greatly limited or crippled because their disease imposes great psychobiological and socioeconomic problems [17]. Medically the patients are first treated with propranolol, long-acting nitrates, and restriction of activity. If a patient continues to have intractable pain that is easily precipitated by emotional or physiological stressors despite adequate medical therapy, surgery is considered.

UNSTABLE ANGINA PECTORIS

Unstable angina pectoris, a second indication for myocardial revascularization, has been called a number of different names (Table 21-1). The term *unstable angina pectoris* is probably the best one to describe patients with a broad spectrum of disorders [11]. It is characterized by the following phenomena [16, 72]:

1. Recurring progressive episodes of angina pectoris lasting longer than 15 minutes and poorly relieved by rest or nitroglycerin
2. Deteriorating chronic angina pectoris (which was previously stable) that has become more easily provoked, increased in frequency, intensity, and duration, and less readily relieved by nitroglycerin or rest
3. No diagnostic evidence of serum enzyme changes
4. No ECG evidence that is consistent with acute myocardial infarction
5. ST- or T-wave changes associated with myocardial ischemia

Physiologically, the condition suggests that the coronary blood supply relative to the demand is deficient, even at rest. Hemodynamically, unstable angina pectoris is associated with a rise in heart rate and blood pressure that precedes the onset of pain. Since heart rate and blood pressure are the chief determinants of coronary blood flow demand, increasing those parameters can create a relative ischemia.

Table 21-1
Terms Used to Describe the Syndrome Between Stable Angina Pectoris and Acute Myocardial Infarction

Unstable angina pectoris
Intermediate coronary syndrome
Acute coronary insufficiency
Preinfarction angina pectoris
Crescendo angina pectoris
Accelerated angina pectoris
Impending myocardial infarction
Theatening myocardial infarction
Prethrombotic syndrome
Preocclusive syndrome
Coronary failure
Rest angina

As its name states, the condition is unstable and associated with a higher morbidity and mortality than is stable angina pectoris [81]. The rate of myocardial infarction and/or death is as high as 20 to 25 percent within a year of the onset of the syndrome [14, 41, 43, 50, 60].

Because unstable angina pectoris initially responds well to medical treatment, the patient is stabilized for several days to weeks with bedrest, a quiet environment, oxygen, sedation, nitroglycerin, long-acting nitrates, beta-adrenergic receptor-blocking drugs, and, perhaps, anticoagulation and mechanical circulatory assistance before coronary arteriography and elective surgery are performed [11, 15, 17, 19, 30, 32, 54, 67]. Control of the ischemia then allows the surgeon to operate on a stable patient who is at low risk. If the pain does not subside in 48 to 72 hours, however, emergency arteriography and aortocoronary bypass surgery are seriously considered [14, 24, 32, 74].

ACUTE MYOCARDIAL INFARCTION

Until recently, aortocoronary bypass surgery was contraindicated in the presence of acute myocardial infarction. Current evidence suggests that emergency revascularization performed on selected patients may be effective in interrupting the ischemic process or in reducing the size of the infarct [52].

It is known that infarcted muscle is surrounded by a "twilight zone" of ischemic tissue after an acute myocardial infarction. That zone, which is destined to become necrotic, remains viable for several hours after the acute infarct [18]. It can be salvaged if emergency revascularization is performed in three to six hours [10, 51]. Because preparing the patient for cardiac arteriography and surgery is generally time consuming, emergency surgery is generally not feasible.

Because the balance between myocardial oxygen demand and myocardial oxygen supply appears to determine the fate of the ischemic area, various pharmacological and mechanical interventions have been used to improve the relationship. The use of drugs such as propranolol or nitroprusside to reduce left ventricular afterload (systemic vascular resistance), in combination with mechanical circulatory assist devices, has also proved effective in decreasing the ischemic process in this group of patients [6, 19, 30]. The problem of determining what method of treatment is more successful will remain unanswered until more accurate methods of determining the size of the infarct are widely available [18] (see Chap. 19).

CONGESTIVE HEART FAILURE

The indications for myocardial revascularization in the treatment of congestive heart failure are controversial [50]. Surgery does not appear to be promising, because it is associated with a high mortality and uncertain clinical results [8]. Myocardial dysfunction is generally the result of an extensive area of infarcted myocardium, and it is reasonable to believe that revascularization may not be beneficial in reversing the damage. Surgery has been found to both improve and reduce ventricular wall segment function while not consistently affecting the overall resting ventricular function [8].

Candidates for surgery are those who have angina pectoris as their major symptom, an ejection fraction (ratio of stroke volume to end-diastolic volume) of greater than 25 percent, bypassable coronary arteries, not more than two dyskinetic left ventricular wall segments (i.e., segments that show paradoxical systolic expansion), a left ventricular aneurysm, a ventricular septal defect (postinfarction), or mitral regurgitation [50]. The use of early postoperative mechanical circulatory assistance has been helpful in this group of patients.

CARDIOGENIC SHOCK

Cardiogenic shock following acute myocardial infarction has an 85 to 95 percent mortality in patients treated medically [14, 50, 81]. Although diastolic aug-

mentation with intraaortic balloon counterpulsation has been effective in the reversal of the shock state for several hours or days, it has done little to alter the long-term survival in 75 percent of the patients [50]. The combination of mechanical circulatory assistance, immediate coronary arteriography, and myocardial revascularization has improved the survival rate when a capable diagnostic and surgical team is involved [10, 14, 52, 65, 81].

REFRACTORY VENTRICULAR IRRITABILITY

Myocardial revascularization has been indicated for other complications of acute myocardial infarction. Recurrent, symptomatic ventricular dysrhythmias that are refractory to medical management pose a serious problem. Myocardial revascularization and myocardial resection can be successful in treating patients with recurrent ventricular dysrhythmias and severe, well-localized left ventricular wall motion abnormalities if performed more than one month after the acute infarct [10, 32, 50, 59, 65]. Under those conditions, the operative mortality is modest, and the long-term survival is excellent.

Patient Selection

Several factors must be considered before a patient is selected as a candidate for aortocoronary bypass surgery.

A thorough history is taken and a complete physical examination is done to determine the physical problems as well as coexisting disease [55]. The history is especially important to determine the severity and frequency of the chest pain and to find out whether the patient had a previous myocardial infarction. The history includes information about the patient's general health, any preexisting pulmonary, dental, liver, or renal disease, any fluid and electrolyte imbalance, blood dyscrasias and clotting defects, or other vascular problems, such as hypertension and cerebrovascular disease. His saphenous veins must be evaluated and assessed in regard to phlebitis.

Besides the patient's general health, specific cardiac factors, such as the anatomical distribution of the coronary artery disease and left ventricular functioning, are considered. Evaluation of the left ventricle includes assessment of heart size and any gallop heart sounds, murmurs, and signs or symptoms of congestive heart failure. A normal resting ECG and an exer-

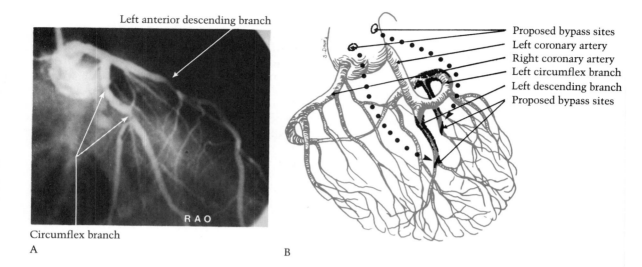

Left anterior descending branch

Circumflex branch

A   B

Proposed bypass sites
Left coronary artery
Right coronary artery
Left circumflex branch
Left descending branch
Proposed bypass sites

RAO

cise tolerance test are generally performed to determine the duration and intensity of exercise necessary to produce angina pectoris and/or ECG changes. Further information can be obtained from the echocardiogram to determine ventricular size and wall motion. The most important information, however, is obtained from cardiac catheterization (see Chap. 10).

Surgery is considered for the patient who has an atherosclerotic plaque that narrows the diameter of an artery more than 50 percent corresponding to a reduction in the cross-sectional area of greater than 75 percent (Fig. 21-2A, B). The patient must have good distal runoff in the vessel to be bypassed, which is visualized on coronary arteriography as a large segment of the artery that is minimally diseased beyond the site of major obstruction. Also, a ventriculogram is performed to determine the functioning of the left ventricle.

Operative Technique: Aortocoronary Bypass Surgery

In addition to the parameters usually monitored, most patients undergoing cardiac surgery have continuous monitoring of arterial and venous pressures, the ECG, and blood gas measurements. Depending on the hospital's policy and the availability of equipment, left atrial pressure monitoring may also be done. A number of anesthetic drugs are used (e.g., halothane, morphine sulfate, succinylcholine, and nitrous oxide).

Figure 21-2

A. Selective coronary angiography prior to surgery, showing a right anterior oblique projection of the left coronary artery and demonstrating significant occlusive lesions (> 50% narrowing of the luminal diameter) in the circumflex and anterior descending branches of the left coronary artery (arrows). B. Proposed aortocoronary bypass of severe stenosis of the circumflex and anterior descending branches of the left coronary artery. The arrows indicate the routes taken in placing saphenous vein grafts in the circumflex and left anterior descending branches.

The surgery is performed through a median sternotomy incision to allow good exposure of the heart and to avoid entering the pleural spaces. The pericardium is opened to expose the heart. The patient is prepared for cardiopulmonary bypass or extracorporeal circulation used to oxygenate the blood, remove carbon dioxide, and provide peripheral blood flow to meet the metabolic needs of the body. A cannula is placed in a vein and artery to direct blood flow from the heart to the bypass machine and then return it to the patient. Arterial cannulas can be placed in the femoral artery, iliac artery, or ascending aorta. Venous cannulas are placed in the venae cavae. The specific sites for vessel cannulation are determined by the type of surgery performed and the preference of the surgical team. Generally, the left ventricle is vented with a cannula to aspirate intracardiac blood and to avoid overdistention of the chamber.

The bypass machine is equipped with a mechanical pump that simulates left ventricular pumping action and an oxygenator that performs the work of the lungs by creating a blood-gas exchange. There are several kinds of good oxygenators. The rotating-disk oxygenator, the bubble oxygenator, and the membrane oxygenator are the ones most commonly used [42].

Before the patient is placed on cardiopulmonary bypass, the machine is completely primed with fluid (e.g., low-molecular-weight dextran, dextrose, or Ringer's lactate solution) to replace the venous blood that is diverted to the machine. The primer solution dilutes the patient's blood volume, a phenomenon that is advantageous because it reduces the need for additional units of blood and, it is believed, it decreases postoperative bleeding and respiratory problems [3].

The patient is given heparin for anticoagulation and cardiopulmonary bypass is begun. The venous reservoir is connected to the oxygenator, where venous blood is oxygenated and carbon dioxide is removed. The arterialized blood enters the heat exchanger, where it is cooled to hypothermic levels (30–32°C or 86–90°F) to reduce the metabolic rate and the oxygen demands of the tissues. Cooling further protects the major organ systems from the effects of anoxia and ischemia. The blood is returned to the patient via the arterial cannula. A filter or bubble trap is used to prevent clots, fat debris, air, or other particulate matter from entering the patient's blood.

The mean blood pressure is maintained at preoperative levels during bypass by adjusting the rate of perfusion and blood volume or by administering vasopressor drugs. Red blood cells are traumatized and hemolyzed by direct contact with oxygen, the mechanical action of the pump, turbulent flow, and intracardiac suction systems. The hemolyzed cells can generally be cleared from the blood by the use of mannitol or some other diuretic.

In preparing for a direct bypass procedure, a long segment of the saphenous vein is removed from the patient's thigh or lower leg—15 to 30 cm of vein for each graft to be performed. At the same time, aneurysms and plaques are excised. The veins are reversed before they are inserted because of the direction of the venous valves.

A quiet operative field is achieved by fibrillating the heart or by ischemic arrest produced by cross-clamping the aorta. During the insertion of several vein grafts, the heart is defibrillated and perfused for several minutes between periods of ischemia.

The coronary artery is dissected beyond the area of

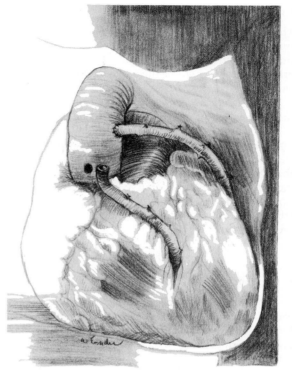

Figure 21-3
Nearly completed aortocoronary saphenous vein bypass of the circumflex and anterior descending branches of the left coronary artery.

obstruction, and a vein-coronary end-to-side anastomosis is performed. Following completion of the distal anastomosis, the vein is brought upward over the right ventricle and is then proximally connected to the aorta (Fig. 21-3). After the bypass grafts have been completed, the rate of blood flow is measured with a flowmeter.

Before removing the patient from bypass, anesthetics are discontinued, the patient is ventilated with 100% oxygen, he is suctioned, and the blood is rewarmed. Perfusion is discontinued slowly by reducing the venous flow over a period of several minutes. The cannulas are not removed until satisfactory arterial pressure and cardiac functioning are achieved. Atrial and ventricular pacing wires and mediastinal chest tubes are placed. Protamine sulfate is given to neutralize the effects of heparin. The sternum is sutured with wire, and the skin is closed.

Operative Mortality

The overall operative mortality for coronary bypass surgery is now under 5 percent. The percentage varies from institution to institution; and it depends primarily on the skill of the surgeon and the cardiology team, including the skill in selecting patients [1].

A number of risk factors have been found to affect the operative mortality. Undoubtedly, the most important factor is the patient's resting left ventricular function [1, 31, 35, 44, 48, 57, 65] as measured by the ejection fraction. A normal ejection fraction of greater than 55 percent as determined by ventriculography indicates an excellent operative risk, whereas an ejection fraction of 20 to 25 percent is often considered inoperable. Other factors that affect the operative mortality are listed in Table 21-2.

Postoperative Complications

Physiological and psychological complications may occur as a result of cardiopulmonary bypass, prolonged surgery time, and preoperative risk factors or disease. Perioperative myocardial infarction occurs in approximately 10 percent of patients undergoing coronary bypass surgery, and it is a common cause of death in the early postoperative period [14, 49, 63]. Other complications [78] are listed in Table 21-3 and are discussed under Nursing and/or Medical Management.

Table 21-2
Factors That Affect the Operative Mortality in Aortocoronary Bypass Surgery

Great Effect	Little Effect
Left ventricular function	Age (< 70 years)
Acute myocardial infarction	Diabetes mellitus
Other cardiac surgery in combination with revascularization	Number of diseased vessels
	Number of grafted vessels
Unstable angina without prior stabilization	Severity of the angina pectoris
Left main coronary disease	Old myocardial infarction (> 2 months with normal ventricular function)
Sudden withdrawal of propranolol	
Technical skills of the team	

Table 21-3
Postoperative Complications of Aortocoronary Bypass Surgery

Common Complications	Less Common Complications
Acute myocardial infarction	Renal failure
Vein graft closure	Stress ulcer
Dysrhythmias	Respiratory failure
Hemorrhage	Cardiac tamponade
Pneumonia	Cardiogenic shock
Pericarditis	Endocarditis
Embolism	
ICU psychosis	

Results of Myocardial Revascularization

The most impressive benefits of aortocoronary bypass surgery are related to the improvement of angina pectoris. Fifty to 72 percent of patients report complete relief of angina pectoris, and 60 to 94 percent have significant improvement [1, 5, 14, 17, 32, 39, 45, 49, 65]. Unfortunately, those statistics are extremely difficult to quantify because of the subjective criteria used to evaluate chest pain. The statistics may be further biased because of the placebo effect of major surgery or the patient's reluctance to admit the return of persistent pain.

Aortocoronary bypass surgery is capable of improving oxygenation of the myocardium and, in some instances, left ventricular wall segment function [45]. A patent bypass graft establishes a normal autoregulatory pattern of functioning. There are appropriate changes in coronary blood flow during exercise, for example, which are dictated by increases in peripheral coronary vascular resistance [37]. That mechanism can be objectively evaluated by means of stress testing; most patients show improvement of their exercise tolerance postoperatively [39, 49]. The risk factors (diabetes mellitus, hypertension, smoking, obesity, hyperlipidemia, and a family history of coronary artery disease) and the number of diseased vessels do not statistically affect the long-term symptomatic results [55].

Relief of angina pectoris may or may not correspond with the effectiveness of the bypass graft [32]. In some patients, one or more grafts may become occluded but they still have relief from angina pectoris while others may have patent grafts but no improvement in symptoms. The rate of vein graft occlusion varies from 8 to 30 percent within the first 12 months following surgery [12, 81]. Although the occlusion rate is high within the first year, it is considerably lower in subsequent years [25, 69]. Thus, if the graft remains patent during the first year (and looks normal angiographically), there is an excellent chance that it will remain open during the next two or three years [32, 66]. Early graft occlusion may be caused by stasis and thrombosis, whereas late occlusion may be caused by subintimal hyperplasia [25].

Competition between the bypass graft and the coronary artery occurs after revascularization. Competition may lead to progressive atherosclerotic obstruction in the proximal bypassed coronary artery. Therefore, if a partially occluded coronary artery becomes completely obstructed following bypass, late graft occlusion can be a dangerous situation because essentially the patient has less coronary blood flow than he had before surgery. That problem is a major drawback to aortocoronary bypass surgery.

Medical Versus Surgical Treatment of Coronary Artery Disease

Although aortocoronary bypass surgery has rapidly become one of the most common surgical procedures in the United States, very few studies show that surgical treatment of coronary artery disease is more effective than medical treatment (except in the case of left main coronary artery disease) [15, 31].

Probably the most important question that remains to be answered is the long-term survival in medically as opposed to surgically treated patients with coronary artery disease. Studies that have attempted to answer this question to date have been highly criticized because of the lack of controlled randomization when comparing those two groups. The data collected from patients treated medically before surgical intervention was available cannot be considered valid because the forms of medical treatment used today were not available then. When comparing the long-term survival of medical and surgical patients today in a nonrandomized study, the findings are not valid or reliable because patients with diffuse coronary artery disease and poor left ventricular function are most often selected for medical intervention. As a result, the data are biased because a significantly larger number of patients with less advanced disease and good left ventricular function (and thus a better prognosis) are selected for the surgical group.

It is important to realize the ethical dilemma inherent in a controlled randomized study comparing the results of surgical therapy with the results of medical therapy. If one mode of therapy (surgery) is known to be effective in the symptomatic relief of pain, is it ethically acceptable to deny that form of therapy (surgery) and continue with a form of therapy (medical) that has failed? Specifically, if medical treatment has failed to relieve the pain in a patient with severe but stable angina, can that patient be denied surgery (because he was randomly selected for medical therapy) knowing that the majority of patients have symptomatic improvement following revascularization?

The problem could be ethically and scientifically satisfied by designing a controlled, prospective, randomized investigation to study patients who have not yet been treated medically or those who have been successfully controlled by medical intervention with mild stable angina.

One such study has been conducted on a national basis by the Veterans Administration Hospital [31, 53, 70] to study the surgical versus medical mortality of patients with chronic stable angina pectoris. The results of the study to date show similar survival rates in both groups concluding that surgery cannot be justified as a means of reducing mortality (except in patients with left main coronary artery disease). Successful surgical intervention, however, was found to reduce angina pectoris symptoms better than medical therapy. The preliminary conclusions reported by the National Cooperative Study to Compare Medical Versus Surgical Therapy of Unstable Angina Pectoris sponsored by the National Heart, Lung, and Blood Institute [11] found comparable survival outcomes related to medical management versus urgent surgical treatment of unstable angina but a somewhat better quality of life in the surgical group. A great deal of controversy currently exists related to the methodology and results of those studies. It appears that before concluding that medical and surgical treatment are equally good (or equally bad) in terms of survival factors for patients with coronary artery disease, further investigation is needed to answer not only many of the medical but also the moral and ethical questions generated by previous research.

Acquired Valvular Disease

The steadily expanding scope of cardiac surgery requires that the nurse become familiar with the features of valvular disease. Valve replacement began in 1960 when Harken and Starr independently replaced the aortic valve with a ball-valve prosthesis [26, 76]. Since that time, advancement in the design and understanding of prosthetic valve replacements has been progressive. The development of valvular surgery has enabled many patients to lead active and useful lives. Valvular surgery is primarily recommended for adult patients with aortic stenosis or regurgitation and mitral stenosis or regurgitation. These conditions will be discussed in detail in the following pages.

Aortic Stenosis

ETIOLOGY

Approximately 25 percent of all patients with chronic valvular disease have aortic stenosis [5]. Of those symptomatic patients, about 80 percent are male. Aortic stenosis can be congenital in origin or secondary to rheumatic inflammation or calcification.

The congenitally affected valve may be stenotic at birth and become progressively calcified over the next three decades of life. Calcification produces valvular rigidity and hence increases the obstruction already present. A history of rheumatic fever is present in 30 to 50 percent of patients with aortic stenosis [75]. Rheumatic endocarditis of the aortic valve produces stenosis, which leads to calcification and further narrowing. Idiopathic calcific aortic stenosis occurs most frequently in the older patient. It is generally a mild physiological obstruction associated with "wear and tear" of the valve.

PATHOPHYSIOLOGY

Aortic stenosis is observed during systole when blood is being ejected from the left ventricle to the aorta across a narrowed aortic valve. It is a hemodynamic abnormality caused by an obstruction to the left ventricular outflow tract, causing a high pressure gradient between the left ventricle and the aorta during systolic ejection. Because of the increase in left ventricular systolic pressure over a period of time, the cardiac work load is increased, leading to a progressive ventricular hypertrophy and a rise in myocardial oxygen demands. Those compensatory mechanisms generally permit cardiac output and stroke volume to be maintained within normal limits at rest. During exercise, however, those variables may fail to rise.

The normal aortic valve has a cross-sectional area of 2.5 to 3.5 sq cm. Severe aortic stenosis exists if the cross-sectional area is reduced to 0.5 to 0.7 sq cm, requiring a systolic pressure gradient of over 50 mm Hg to produce a moderate cardiac output [5].

CLINICAL MANIFESTATIONS

Generally there is a prolonged latent period before the symptoms of aortic stenosis develop. Most patients do not become symptomatic until their forties or fifties. Cardiac output is generally maintained at rest until the late stages of the illness. Clinical disability depends on the patient's life-style, but generally it is not produced until the valve orifice has been narrowed to approximately one-third normal. The turning point in the disease is heralded by one or more of the three cardinal signs: angina pectoris, syncope, and/ or exertional dyspnea. During the late stages of the illness, fatigability, peripheral cyanosis, orthopnea, paroxysmal nocturnal dyspnea, pulmonary edema, and other symptoms of left ventricular failure appear.

Sudden death accounts for about 20 percent of the fatalities associated with the disease [75]. The average life expectancy for a patient with untreated aortic stenosis once angina pectoris or syncope appears is three to four years [5]. Left ventricular failure, a grave development, demands immediate treatment. Death following the development of left heart failure usually occurs within one to two years, but it may occur within a week. Although most patients do not survive long enough to develop associated pulmonary hypertension and right ventricular failure, the findings of systemic venous hypertension, hepatomegaly, atrial fibrillation, and tricuspid regurgitation point to a poor prognosis.

PHYSICAL FINDINGS

The systemic arterial pressure of a patient with aortic stenosis is usually normal. The arterial pulse tracing (for details, see Nursing and/or Medical Management) characteristically records a delayed systolic peak and an anacrotic notch (a small, abnormal, extra wave in the ascending limb of the pulse tracing).

A classic finding in aortic stenosis is a systolic diamond-shaped ejection murmur caused by the forced flow of blood through a stenotic orifice. The low-pitched, harsh murmur is best heard in the aortic region (the second intercostal space to the right of the sternum), and it is generally transmitted up to the neck and carotid vessels. It begins shortly after the first heart sound, increasing in intensity toward the middle of the ejection period and decreasing until aortic valve closure (see Chap. 10).

A systolic thrill is generally present at the base of the heart. The jugular venous pulse is normal in pure aortic stenosis. The cardiac rhythm is usually regular. In advanced stages, left ventricular systole may become so delayed that aortic valve closure comes after pulmonic valve closure (P_2A_2). The phenomenon is known as paradoxical splitting of the second heart sound. An atrial gallop (S_4) may be audible at the apex, signifying the presence of left ventricular hypertrophy. A ventricular gallop (S_3) frequently reflects left ventricular dilatation and failure (see Chap. 10).

The ECG reveals left ventricular hypertrophy. In advanced stages of the illness, there may be a "strain" pattern, with ST-segment depression and T-wave inversion in leads 1, aVL, V_5, and V_6. The chest x ray may show enlargement of the left ventricle and, in advanced cases, pulmonary congestion; aortic valve calcification may be noted, but it usually requires fluoroscopy to be defined.

A cardiac catheterization is performed to determine the pressure gradient between the left ventricle and aorta in order to estimate the severity of the stenosis. The cross-sectional area of the valve is also determined by the measurement of the pressure gradient and the cardiac output. The presence of aortic regurgitation or mitral valvular disease is also assessed. Coronary arteriography is generally performed on patients having anginal symptoms and on all patients over age 40, regardless of symptoms.

TREATMENT

The management of the patient depends on the symptoms and the degree of stenosis and cardiac hypertrophy. The patient with associated cardiac failure is treated with digitalis glycosides, a low-sodium diet, and diuretics. Once the patient develops symptoms of heart failure, angina pectoris, or syncope, however, the mortality is high despite medical therapy. The outlook and symptomatic relief for such a patient is significantly improved by surgical replacement of the aortic valve [38]. In a patient who has both aortic stenosis and coronary artery disease, aortic valve replacement and aortocoronary bypass surgery frequently result in a striking hemodynamic improvement.

The anesthetic drugs, monitoring lines, surgical incision, and cardiopulmonary bypass techniques used in aortocoronary bypass surgery (described under Operative Technique: Aortocoronary Bypass Surgery) are also used in aortic valve replacement. In that operation, the ascending aorta is clamped and an incision is made in the aorta above the right coronary artery. The right and left coronary arteries are cannulated and perfused (although many surgeons avoid that step and simply cool and arrest the heart). After the removal of the entire aortic valve, an appropriate size valve is sutured into place. The aorta is closed, the heart is filled with blood to expel air, and the patient is removed from bypass.

The average operative mortality for aortic valve replacement is 5 to 8 percent; it may be lower in patients without long-standing heart failure. A major factor in mortality (if the surgeon has elected to cannulate the coronary arteries) is effective perfusion of the coronary arteries during surgery. Most patients show a significant clinical improvement following surgery and little or no limitations in their physical activities.

Anticoagulant therapy is frequently begun after surgery. In some cases (e.g., when a tissue valve, porcine valve, or homograft is used), it is discontinued approximately four weeks after surgery. Anticoagulants are recommended for life when a disk valve, ball-in-cage valve, or similar mechanical prosthesis is used [46]. Postoperative complications include prosthetic leaking, infection of the replaced valve, thromboembolism, mechanical problems with the prosthesis, and sudden death due to dysrhythmias. The patient is particularly susceptible to infective endocarditis, and he must be instructed about prevention (see Chap. 23).

Aortic Regurgitation (Insufficiency)

ETIOLOGY

Approximately 75 percent of all patients suffering from aortic regurgitation are men. Rheumatic fever is a common cause of aortic regurgitation. Infective endocarditis, dissecting aortic aneurysm, and dilatation of the aortic annulus can also produce the disease. It may also be congenital in origin, or it can be produced by rheumatoid arthritis or connective tissue degeneration, resulting in the "floppy valve" syndrome (see Mitral Regurgitation [Insufficiency]).

PATHOPHYSIOLOGY

Aortic regurgitation is observed during diastole when the aortic valve is closed. Because the aortic valve is incompetent, blood is ejected forward in the aorta to the body but it also leaks back through the closed aortic valve into the left ventricle.

There is an increase in the total stroke volume ejected by the left ventricle in aortic regurgitation. Total stroke volume is the sum of the forward stroke volume and the volume of blood that regurgitates into the left ventricle. An increase in left ventricular end-diastolic volume (see Nursing and/or Medical Management) is the major hemodynamic compensation in the disease. Progressive dilatation of the left ventricle occurs. A normal forward stroke volume may be observed even in patients with moderately severe aortic regurgitation and elevated left ventricular end-diastolic pressure and volume [9]. The cardiac output may be normal at rest but often fails to rise during exercise. Tachycardia may have a beneficial effect because the period of diastole is shortened and thus allows less time for the blood to regurgitate into the ventricle. Peripheral vasodilatation plays a compensatory role by reducing peripheral vascular resistance and the amount of regurgitant flow.

In advanced stages of the illness, left ventricular failure ensues, lowering cardiac output and bringing an associated rise in left atrial, pulmonary capillary, and right ventricular pressures. Because most coronary blood flow occurs during diastole, coronary perfusion may be markedly impaired due to reduced diastolic perfusion pressures, which, coupled with tachycardia and augmented myocardial oxygen demands, may result in myocardial ischemia.

CLINICAL MANIFESTATIONS

A person who has severe aortic regurgitation may be asymptomatic for many years. The earliest symptom may be palpitations produced by the forceful contractions of a dilated left ventricle. Sinus tachycardia or premature ventricular contraction may contribute to the uncomfortable phenomenon. Dyspnea on exertion is generally the first indication of diminished cardiac reserve. Symptoms of left ventricular failure or angina pectoris frequently follow.

PHYSICAL FINDINGS

The patient with severe aortic regurgitation can be observed to have a bobbing motion of the head (de Musset's sign) or jarring of the body with each systole. A water-hammer (Corrigan's) pulse, which collapses

suddenly during late systole as arterial pressure rapidly falls, is characteristic of the disease. Capillary pulsations (Quincke's pulse) may be demonstrated by applying pressure to the tip of the nail and observing alternate flushing and blanching of the skin. A "pistol-shot" sound (Traube's sign) is heard with the bell of the stethoscope over the femoral arteries. A to-and-fro murmur (Duroziez's sign) can frequently be heard over the femoral artery. A diastolic thrill is often palpated along the left sternal border.

The arterial pulse is widened with an elevated systolic pressure. The diastolic arterial pressure is lowered and may even be heard when the sphygmomanometer cuff is completely deflated. The sound of aortic valve closure is generally reduced or absent. An atrial or ventricular gallop is commonly heard.

Three types of murmurs may be associated with aortic regurgitation [9]:

1. The classic murmur of aortic regurgitation, produced by the backflow of blood from the aorta to the left ventricle, which is a blowing, high-pitched, decrescendo, diastolic murmur that is heard best in the third left intercostal space (see Chap. 10). When the murmur is soft, the diaphragm of the stethoscope should be applied to the chest with the patient holding his breath in forced expiration while sitting up or leaning forward. The murmur may radiate widely, especially to the lower sternal border.
2. The systolic ejection murmur, which is caused by the increased volume of blood across the aortic valve. It has the following salient characteristics:
   a. It does not necessarily signify the presence of aortic stenosis
   b. It is heard best at the base of the heart
   c. It may radiate to the carotid arteries
   d. It is generally higher pitched than the murmur of aortic stenosis
3. The Austin Flint murmur, which is a low-pitched, soft, diastolic bruit heard best at the cardiac apex. It is probably caused by the regurgitant blood flow passing the anterior mitral valve leaflet and preventing it from fully opening [51].

The ECG may show left ventricular hypertrophy and ST-segment depression and T-wave inversion in leads 1, aVL, V_5, and V_6. The chest x ray frequently shows left ventricular enlargement; it is probably the single best noninvasive procedure for measuring the severity of chronic aortic regurgitation. The best invasive method of measuring the severity of the disease is aortography, in which dye is injected into the aorta and the degree of reflux into the left ventricle is estimated. Cardiac catheterization is usually performed on patients suspected of having other associated valvular lesions or coronary artery disease.

TREATMENT

Because prolonged aortic regurgitation frequently leads to irreversible ventricular damage, aortic valve replacement is recommended for asymptomatic patients before the development of heart failure or angina pectoris [9, 38]. Cardiac dysrhythmias or infection is not well tolerated and must be treated promptly.

The surgery has a hospital mortality of approximately 5 percent. (The details of aortic valve replacement were discussed under Aortic Stenosis.)

Mitral Stenosis

ETIOLOGY

Mitral stenosis is frequently caused by rheumatic fever, which produces ulceration, fusion, and calcification of the mitral valve. Approximately two-thirds of the patients are women [5]. Congenital mitral stenosis is rare. It is called the parachute mitral valve because all the chordae are inserted into a single papillary muscle.

PATHOPHYSIOLOGY

Mitral stenosis is observed during diastole when blood is being ejected from the left atrium across a narrowed mitral valve to the left ventricle.

The mitral valve orifice is approximately 5 sq cm in the normal adult. When the orifice is less than one-half normal, significant obstruction is present. Mitral stenosis produces three significant events: (1) an increase in left atrial mean pressure, (2) an increase in pulmonary vascular resistance, and (3) a decrease in cardiac output.

When the orifice is significantly narrowed, blood can flow from the left atrium to the left ventricle only as a result of a high left atrioventricular pressure gradient. The high left atrial mean pressure (normally less than 10–12 mm Hg) that develops is an important compensatory mechanism to maintain cardiac output

despite the stenotic valvular lesion. The left ventricular diastolic pressure generally is maintained at normal levels.

A rise in left atrial mean pressure, however, is also accompanied by a rise in the pulmonary venous, capillary, and arterial pressures. When the pulmonary capillary pressure exceeds the oncotic pressure of the blood, pulmonary transudation occurs. If pulmonary transudation exceeds the rate of pulmonary lymphatic drainage, pulmonary congestion and edema develop.

The degree of pulmonary vascular resistance varies from patient to patient. Pulmonary hypertension is caused by the backward transmission of the elevated left atrial pressure, arteriolar constriction, and degenerative changes in the pulmonary vascular bed. Severe pulmonary hypertension is a serious complication of mitral stenosis; it produces tricuspid and pulmonic regurgitation and right heart failure.

There is also considerable variation in cardiac output in patients with mitral stenosis. Exercise tends to increase left atrial, pulmonary venous, pulmonary capillary, pulmonary arterial, and right ventricular pressures. Patients with mild stenosis are usually able to maintain an effective cardiac output at rest that increases with exercise. Generally, however, the cardiac output is fixed at a low level by the rigid stenotic valve. In people who have severe mitral stenosis, the cardiac output may be normal at rest, but exercise may produce no change in or even a decrease in cardiac output. Right heart failure and tricuspid regurgitation may further reduce cardiac output during exercise. Despite an associated rise in left atrial pressure, cardiac output may be lowered as a result of tachycardia. Accelerated heart rates shorten the period of diastole more than the period of systole. In mitral stenosis, the accelerated rate reduces the time available for blood flow across the mitral valve (the flow occurring from atrium to ventricle during ventricular diastole), thereby decreasing left ventricular filling and cardiac output.

CLINICAL MANIFESTATIONS

The symptoms of mitral stenosis are related to the degree of valvular dysfunction and to disturbances in the cardiac rhythm. The most characteristic symptom is dyspnea. Dyspnea generally is precipitated by extreme exertion, excitement, severe anemia, sexual intercourse, pregnancy, fever, thyrotoxicosis, or paroxysmal tachycardia. As the stenosis becomes more severe, dyspnea is produced by lesser degrees of exertion or stressors, and the patient becomes progressively limited in daily activities.

Several other symptoms develop as a result of recurrent pulmonary congestion. Complaints of orthopnea, paroxysmal nocturnal dyspnea, or cough may be elicited. Those problems are aggravated by recumbency or exercise. The degenerative pulmonary changes that occur in association with pulmonary hypertension include a reduction in vital capacity, diffusion capacity, and pulmonary compliance.

Hemoptysis that is not associated with pulmonary edema is a frequent complication. It is alarming, but it is almost never fatal. It is caused by the rupture of a pulmonary bronchial connection, and it may vary from a small amount of blood-tinged sputum to a large amount of bright-red blood.

Atrial dysrhythmias, such as premature atrial contractions, paroxysmal atrial tachycardia, and atrial flutter or fibrillation occur frequently in mitral stenosis. Arterial embolism associated with ineffective left atrial contractions and with thrombus formation in atrial fibrillation occurs to the brain, kidney, spleen, and extremities.

PHYSICAL FINDINGS

On physical examination, the patient may be found to have peripheral cyanosis and a classic malar flush. The jugular venous pulse may reveal a prominent *a* wave due to the powerful atrial systole in a person who has a normal sinus rhythm and pulmonary hypertension. In atrial fibrillation, the jugular pulse may be only a single pulsation (a *c-v* wave).

The size of the heart is generally normal; the apical impulse is normal but diminished in intensity. A diastolic thrill can be felt at the cardiac apex, particularly when the patient is turned on his left side. A right ventricular "lift" may be present along the left sternal border, resulting from a hypertrophied right ventricle.

The three significant auscultatory findings in mitral stenosis are a loud first heart sound, an opening snap (OS), and a diastolic murmur [9]. The loud first heart sound is generally accentuated because mitral valve closure is often delayed until the left ventricular pressure reaches the level of the elevated left atrial pressure.

The OS of the stenotic mitral valve (not heard when the valve is normal) is audible early in diastole along the lower left sternal border and apex (see Chap. 10). In mitral stenosis with an elevated left atrial pressure, the rigid valve snaps open during the period of diastole to allow blood to flow from the atrium to the ventricle. The OS is produced by a sudden stop in the opening movement of the stenotic valve. The higher the left atrial pressure, the more rapidly the valve is opened to produce the sound. Also, the more severe the mitral stenosis, the closer the OS is to the second heart sound. The OS is frequently mistaken for a ventricular gallop.

Following the OS, a low-pitched, rumbling diastolic murmur is heard best at the apex with the patient turned on his left side (see Chap. 10). The murmur is produced by the flow of blood passing through the stenotic mitral valve. The intensity of the murmur does not correlate with the severity of the stenosis. A soft systolic murmur is commonly heard at the apex, but it does not necessarily signify mitral regurgitation.

The ECG may show bifid P waves in leads 1, 2, and V_5 that are consistent with left atrial enlargement, right axis deviation, and right ventricular hypertrophy. Atrial fibrillation is common. The chest x ray may show dilatation of the left atrium with calcification of the mitral valve. The echocardiogram is useful in determining abnormal movement of the valve; it is the most specific noninvasive test. Cardiac catheterization is an important procedure used to evaluate the severity of the disease in regard to the transvalvular pressure gradient, the cardiac output, and the cross-sectional area of the mitral valve. Coronary arteriography is often indicated.

TREATMENT

Symptomatic patients are treated medically with avoidance of strenuous activity, restriction of sodium intake, and diuretics. Although digitalis glycosides do not necessarily improve the hemodynamic functioning, they are indicated to slow the ventricular rate in patients with rapid atrial fibrillation [9]. Attention is directed toward the correction of anemia or infection and conversion of atrial fibrillation to sinus rhythm.

Surgery is recommended for patients who are symptomatic or who have minimal symptoms and evidence of pulmonary vascular disease. There are three major surgical approaches to correct mitral stenosis: closed commissurotomy, open commissurotomy, and mitral valve replacement.

A closed commissurotomy is indicated for patients who have good valvular mobility, who have not had previous mitral valve surgery, and who show no evidence of valvular calcification, regurgitation, or left atrial thrombosis [75]. An incision is made into the left atrium, and the valve is blindly opened by a finger or by a dilator. The cardiopulmonary bypass machine is placed on a "standby" basis. If the closed commissurotomy does not open the orifice, the patient is put on cardiopulmonary bypass, and an "open" repair is carried out [75]. The hospital mortality is approximately 2 percent.

Some surgeons prefer the open techniques for all cases of mitral stenosis. Open commissurotomy and cardiopulmonary bypass are particularly indicated for patients with more severe mitral valve obstruction, mitral regurgitation, valvular calcification, or left atrial thrombi [5]. The heart is fibrillated, and an incision is made over the left atrium after cardiopulmonary bypass has been established. The aorta is clamped intermittently to attain a dry, quiet operative field. The fused commissures are exposed and carefully separated with a knife. Following commissurotomy, the atrium is partially closed. The heart is defibrillated, and a finger is introduced into the left atrium to palpate the mitral valve for insufficiency. Correction of the mitral stenosis is confirmed by measurement of the left atrial and ventricular pressures. The operative mortality is about 2 percent.

Replacement of the mitral valve with a prosthetic valve is particularly indicated for patients with both mitral stenosis and regurgitation or for patients with extensively calcified valves [13, 38]. The patient is put on cardiopulmonary bypass and an incision is made into the left atrium to expose the mitral valve. Ischemic arrest is attained by occluding the aorta. The mitral valve and papillary muscles are excised. The prosthetic valve is inserted using a series of sutures. Care is taken not to injure the conduction system or the circumflex coronary artery. The motion of the valvular prosthesis is determined. The ventricle and aorta are vented to remove air, and the patient is removed from cardiopulmonary bypass. The hospital mortality is about 5 percent. Many patients show symptomatic improvement after valve replacement, and they are able to resume their normal daily activities. Unless a tissue valve is used, oral anticoagulant therapy is continued indefinitely. (The postop-erative complications of mitral valve replacement are the same as those discussed under Aortic Stenosis.)

Mitral Regurgitation (Insufficiency)

ETIOLOGY

Rheumatic fever is the cause of mitral regurgitation in about 50 percent of the patients suffering from it [5]. Unlike mitral stenosis, rheumatic mitral regurgitation occurs more frequently in men than in women. Mitral regurgitation is also caused by myocardial ischemia or infarction. It may be congenital, or it may be the result of the "floppy valve" syndrome, a connective tissue degenerative disease in which the valve leaflets and chordae are thin and elongated and permit prolapse of the leaflets during systole.

PATHOPHYSIOLOGY

Mitral regurgitation is observed during ventricular systole when the mitral valve is closed and the ventricle is ejecting blood to the aorta. Because the mitral valve is incompetent, blood is ejected not only forward to the aorta but also backward to the left atrium.

The regurgitant volume may be nearly as large as the forward stroke volume. The left ventricle attempts to compensate for the regurgitant blood flow by emptying more completely during systole to maintain an effective cardiac output. Progressively, the left ventricle dilates, producing a rise in left ventricular end-diastolic pressure until eventually left ventricular failure appears. The regurgitant blood produces a rise in left atrial pressure and enlargement of the left atrium. Left atrial hypertension may eventually be the cause of increased pulmonary vascular resistance and right heart failure.

CLINICAL MANIFESTATIONS

Some patients with mitral regurgitation never have any symptoms or any loss of cardiac reserve. Symptomatic patients, however, experience fatigue, exertional dyspnea, orthopnea, nocturnal dyspnea, palpitations, and, less commonly, pulmonary congestion and edema.

PHYSICAL FINDINGS

In patients with mitral regurgitation the arterial pressure is normal, but the arterial pulse is characterized by a sharp upstroke. The jugular venous pulse may show an abnormally prominent *a* wave. A systolic thrill usually is palpable at the apex. A characteristic rocking motion of the chest during each cardiac cycle may be observed as a result of both left ventricular contraction and left atrial expansion during systole.

The first heart sound is soft or absent. The second heart sound is normal, but it may be widely split in a patient with severe regurgitation. Occasionally, both third and fourth heart sounds are present.

The characteristic feature of mitral regurgitation is a high-pitched blowing, holosystolic (throughout systole) murmur (see Chap. 10) heard best at the apex and radiating to the axilla. It is produced by the regurgitation of blood from the left ventricle to the left atrium after mitral valve closure. In patients with ruptured chordae tendineae, the murmur may have a "sea gull," or cooing, sound. A short rumbling diastolic murmur may also be present, resulting from increased blood flow across the mitral valve.

The chest x ray usually shows enlargement of the left ventricle and atrium. Left ventricular hypertrophy and left atrial enlargement are frequently shown on the ECG. Atrial fibrillation is associated with chronic severe regurgitation.

Mitral regurgitation is best assessed by cardiac catheterization. The degree of insufficiency is estimated by injecting dye into the left ventricle and evaluating the amount of reflux into the left atrium.

TREATMENT

The management of the patient with mitral regurgitation depends on his symptoms and the severity of his valvular incompetence. Medical management of dyspnea and fatigue include limiting physical activity, administering digitalis glycosides and diuretics, and restricting sodium. Atrial fibrillation should be converted to a sinus rhythm.

Mitral valve replacement, already discussed, has provided symptomatic improvement in patients with mitral regurgitation. The hospital mortality ranges from 10 to 15 percent, but it may be as low as 5 percent for patients who do not have long-standing heart failure [13]. Patients with progressive symptoms or with mild symptoms but an enlarging heart are urged to undergo surgery in an attempt to prevent irreversible ventricular failure [13, 38].

Nursing and/or Medical Management

Preoperative Phase

OBJECTIVE

The patient should maintain physiological and psychological stability in preparation for surgery [53].

To achieve the objective, the nurse should:

1. Perform a thorough nursing assessment of the patient before surgery to gather information that will serve as a baseline. The information collected is sent with the patient to the ICU. Pertinent information is written on the patient's care plan and communicated to all the ICU personnel.
2. Order a low atherogenic diet (as directed by the physician)—one that is low in cholesterol and saturated fat and high in polyunsaturated fat. The nurse should also assess the need for restriction of the patient's salt and caloric intake.
3. Weigh the patient daily—and at the same time each day. Information about the patient's preoperative weight can be used to interpret any postoperative fluctuation in weight. The evening before surgery, weigh the patient on the ICU scales so that his postoperative weight can be assessed accurately.
4. Order the following preoperative tests as directed by the physician:
   a. Posteroanterior, lateral, right oblique, and left oblique chest x rays
   b. Portable upright chest x ray (to be used as a baseline for postoperative evaluations)
   c. ECG
   d. Complete blood count
   e. Electrolyte panel
   f. Serum creatinine and blood urea nitrogen levels
   g. Urinalysis
   h. Sedimentation rate
   i. Serum glutamic oxaloacetic transaminase level
   j. Lactic dehydrogenase level
   k. Creatine phosphokinase
   l. Alkaline phosphatase level
   m. Bilirubin level
   n. Coagulation panel (platelet count, prothrombin time, partial thromboplastin time, bleeding time, thrombin time, and clotting time)
   o. Fasting blood sugar level
   p. Typing and crossmatching for blood and blood components
   q. Arterial blood gas analyses

r. Pulmonary function tests

s. Sputum tests

5. Assess the patient's readiness to learn

6. Teach the patient and family about the preoperative information the patient will need to prepare for his surgery. The teaching should include information related to:

a. The surgical operation—the physician is responsible for explaining the type of surgery, risk factors, operative mortality, and complications. The nurse must also know those facts so that she can reinforce them or further explain them to the patient. The nurse can use heart models and drawings to explain the procedure to the patient and his family.

b. Coughing and deep breathing exercises.

c. Using intermittent positive pressure breathing.

d. The how, what, and why of tests: ECG, bloodwork, chest x ray, pulmonary function.

e. How to take pHisoHex showers and why the shower is needed.

f. Restricting smoking.

g. The type of diet and the reason for the diet.

h. Preparing the patient and his family for the patient's admission to the ICU. Before surgery, the ICU nurse should visit the patient and his family to explain to them what will happen to the patient in the immediate postoperative period. The patient and family should be shown the ICU, the patient's room, and the family waiting area. Also, they should be told about noises, alarms, lights, visiting hours, approximate length of surgery and stay in ICU, and what items the patient may bring to the ICU.

i. What the patient will experience when he awakens from surgery. Preoperative teaching dolls (Fig. 21-4) can be used as an aid in describing the endotracheal tube, ventilator, median sternotomy incision, chest tubes (and bloody drainage), cardiac monitor, intravenous lines, arterial and central venous pressure lines, Foley catheter, and elastic stockings. Often the first postoperative visit is a terrifying experience for the family, despite the best explanations. I have found the teaching dolls useful in preparing members of the patient's family for their first visit.

j. When the physician will report the results of the surgery and the patient's immediate postoperative condition to the family.

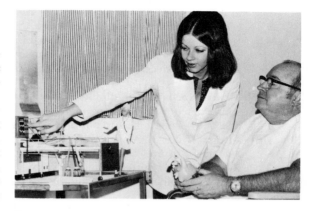

Figure 21-4

A cardiovascular clinical nurse specialist using teaching dolls and a heart model to explain to the patient what he can expect in the immediate postoperative period.

k. When the family can make their first postoperative visit to the patient.

l. When the patient will be allowed to eat postoperatively.

m. When the patient will return to the floor.

n. What things the patient can do to assist in his recovery.

o. The name and type of medications the patient will receive. The nurse should know that:

(1) Nitroglycerin should be placed at the patient's bedside preoperatively and he should be told to tell the nurse when and how often he needs to take the medication.

(2) Prophylactic antibiotics, such as cephalexin (Keflex), are usually started a day before surgery.

(3) Digitalis is generally discontinued several days before surgery to reduce the possibility of ventricular irritability during surgery, but it may be continued in patients with atrial fibrillation or in those with severe cardiac failure.

(4) Diuretics are stopped several days before surgery to avoid serious fluid and electrolyte disturbances as well as dysrhythmias postoperatively.

(5) In view of the recent reports that propranolol withdrawal can cause acute coronary insufficiency and death when the

drug is stopped abruptly [56], patients are generally kept on propranolol until the time of surgery. (In the past, propranolol was discontinued 24 hours before surgery to allow its negative inotropic effects to abate.)

(6) Monoamineoxidase inhibitors increase the action of fentanyl and droperidol (Innovar), and they should be discontinued before surgery when Innovar is used as an anesthetic agent.

(7) Reserpine is omitted before surgery to allow norepinephrine stores to be replenished.

(8) Diabetic patients should omit their usual dose of insulin the morning of surgery, and they should be given 10 units of regular insulin with each 500 ml of a 5% dextrose in water solution.

(9) Patients who have been taking steroids must be given supplemental doses to prevent the complications induced by the stress of surgery.

(10) The use of other drugs, such as stool softeners, hypnotics, and tranquilizers, is recommended before surgery.

Immediate Postoperative Phase

OBJECTIVE

The patient's condition should be stabilized during the immediate postoperative period.

To achieve the objective, the nurse should be aware of the following:

1. Because many technical steps must be taken in the immediate postoperative period, the systematic assessment made when the patient enters the ICU may be neglected. A thorough admission assessment, however, provides the essential framework for nursing care, and it must be done as soon as possible after the patient arrives in the unit. The process of assessment, problem identification, management, and evaluation must be based on an understanding of the patient's preoperative status, the surgical procedure, the normal recovery stages, and the potential complications.

2. Immediately after surgery, the patient is admitted to the ICU. He is accompanied by the anes-

thesiologist, the cardiovascular surgeon, and the monitoring technician. The critical care nurse, the respiratory therapist, and the x-ray technician generally are present when the patient returns from surgery. The surgeon and the anesthesiologist discuss the operation with the ICU staff and give them any information that could affect the patient's postoperative care.

3. The initial management of the patient is done by a team, and it is done according to priorities. The nurse determines the patient's mental status. If the patient can be aroused, he is told that the surgery is over and that he has been admitted to the ICU. A respiratory therapist connects the patient's endotracheal tube to the ventilator and rechecks the ventilator settings in regard to oxygen concentration, respiratory rate, amount of volume, and/or pressure. The patient's tidal volume is evaluated.

The nurse connects the patient to the cardiac monitor, records the admission rhythm, and sets the alarms. The patient's blood pressure is taken with a cuff, and it is compared to the arterial monitored pressure. The patient's apical and radial pulse is taken, and his peripheral pulses are palpated. His heart and bilateral breath sounds are assessed. His dressings are assessed in regard to the amount and type of drainage. The atrial and ventricular pacing wires are covered with gauze, placed in a plastic covering (rubber glove), and taped to his chest (see Chap. 18).

The monitoring technician recalibrates the transducer, connects the arterial, central venous, and left atrial pressure lines to the monitor, and records baseline pressures. The intravenous lines and solutions are assessed in regard to type, drugs used, flow rate, patency, and stability. The nurse connects the chest tubes to water-sealed drainage if that was not done in surgery. All connections are checked again and taped. The water level should have been marked on the chest tube bottle. A chest x ray is taken to check the positioning of the endotracheal tube, the width of the mediastinum, the positioning of the central venous catheters and chest tubes, the condition of the lungs, and the size of the heart.

The Foley catheter is checked for patency, taped to the patient's inner thigh, and connected to a urometer to measure the patient's hourly urine output. The color and amount of urine are noted. A 12-lead ECG is made. The patient's temperature is taken rectally with a glass thermometer. The reading is compared to that made by a rectal probe which is used for continuous temperature monitoring. Blood is drawn for a hemoglobin, hematocrit, arterial blood gases, and electrolyte and coagulation profiles. After the physician has talked with the patient's family and the patient's condition has stabilized, the family, accompanied by the nurse, should be allowed to visit the patient.

Postoperative Phase

The postoperative medical and nursing management of the patient is based on three major goals:

1. Maintenance of the patient's physiological and psychological stability.
2. Prevention, identification, and correction of complications.
3. Promotion of a physically and psychologically therapeutic environment.

OBJECTIVE NO. 1

The stability of the patient's cardiovascular status should be maintained and cardiovascular complications should be prevented.

To achieve the objective, the nurse should:

1. Prevent dysrhythmias or identify any existing dysrhythmias. The nurse must:
   a. Know the causes of dysrhythmias, which may be produced:
      (1) Iatrogenically; that is, as a result of the surgery itself because of injury, ischemia, or transient edema involving the electrical conduction mechanisms of the myocardial tissue during surgery.
      (2) By ischemia due to acute myocardial infarction, hypotension, or hypoxemia.
      (3) By respiratory acidosis, alkalosis, metabolic acidosis, electrolyte imbalance (especially hypokalemia), and pain and fear that cause sympathetic nervous system overactivity.
   b. Assess the patient's cardiovascular status in regard to:
      (1) Heart rate, rhythm, and regularity; heart sounds, murmurs or rubs; apical and radial pulses (for deficits); and ECG.

      (2) Blood pressure (cuff and arterial monitor pressures).
      (3) Respiratory status, arterial blood gas measurements, and ventilator settings.
      (4) Color; cerebral, renal, and peripheral perfusion.
      (5) Serum electrolyte (potassium, sodium, chloride, calcium, magnesium, and bicarbonate) levels.
      (6) Verbal and behavioral manifestations of pain, anxiety, or apprehension.
   c. Identify the cause of the dysrhythmia and treat the patient appropriately. The treatment is aimed primarily at prevention (see Chaps. 10 and 18).
2. Maintain the patient's arterial blood pressure at 80 to 90 mm Hg or at the level ordered by the physician to prevent irreversible shock to vital tissues. The nurse should check the patient's blood pressure every 15 minutes until the patient's condition is stable. She should periodically check the cuff pressure in the right and left arms and compare those readings to the arterial monitor readings.
3. Prevent hypotension. The nurse should:
   a. Know the causes of hypotension: hypovolemia, hemorrhage, hypoxemia, pain, cardiac tamponade, low-cardiac-output syndrome, dysrhythmias.
   b. Assess the patient in regard to:
      (1) Heart rate, rhythm, regularity, and sounds and ECG.
      (2) Respiratory status and ventilator settings.
      (3) Volume status. The patient's fluid intake and output, central venous pressure, and left atrial pressure should be checked and signs and symptoms of hemorrhage should be looked for.
      (4) Cerebral status. The nurse should look for signs of disorientation, confusion, or restlessness.
      (5) Cuff and arterial monitor pressures.
      (6) Arterial pressure curve. The arterial curve consists of two waves separated by the dicrotic notch. The upstroke of the pressure curve ascends steeply, corresponding with the QRS complex of the ECG, and it represents ventricular systole. The dicrotic notch indicates closure of the aortic valve. The final downstroke represents diastole; it is characterized by a fall in pressure. The

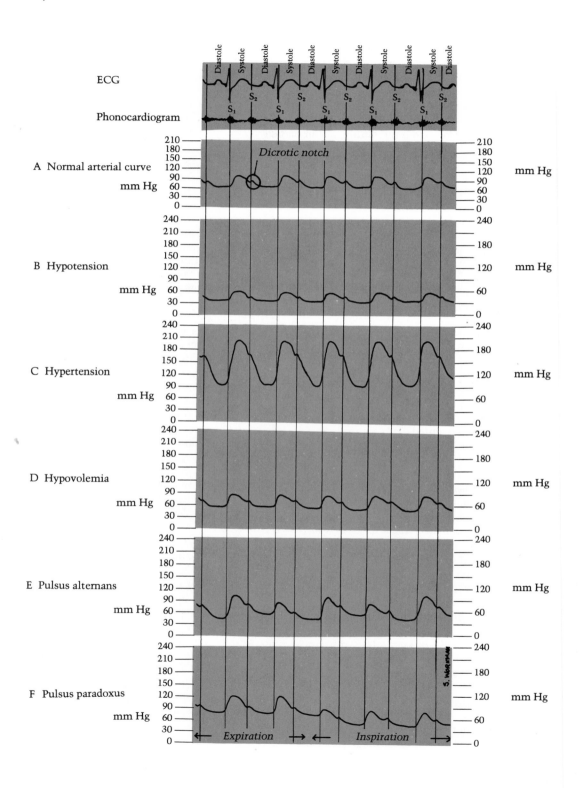

highest point of the arterial pressure curve is the systolic pressure. The lowest point just before the next upstroke is the diastolic pressure (Fig. 21-5A). Hypotension is indicated by a low rounded curve (Fig. 21-5B).

c. Depending on the cause of the hypotension, treat the patient by:

(1) Fluid and colloid replacement.

(2) Adequate ventilation and oxygenation.

(3) Administration of intravenous levarterenol, metaraminol, isoproterenol, dopamine, epinephrine, phenylephrine, methoxamine, calcium chloride, and analgesics.

(4) Correct dysrhythmias and/or assist with artificial cardiac pacing.

4. Prevent hypertension. The nurse should:

a. Know the cause of hypertension, which is frequently observed during the first six postoperative hours. Hypertension is present when the patient has a blood pressure greater than 160 mm Hg systolic and/or 100 mm Hg diastolic. Hypertension is caused by increased peripheral vascular resistance [61, 77].

b. Assess the patient (using the approach described for hypotension). Hypertension is indicated by a high, peaked arterial pressure curve (Fig. 21-5C).

c. Treat the patient's hypertension by:

(1) Lowering the patient's arterial pressure to reduce outflow impedance to left ventricular ejection or systolic wall stress (afterload). Reducing afterload improves left ventricular performance and thus improves stroke volume and cardiac output.

(2) Administering sodium nitroprusside, chlorpromazine, trimethaphan camsylate, and/or analgesics, sedatives, and diuretics.

d. Know the complications of immediate postoperative hypertension: (1) hemorrhage and suture line disruption, (2) myocardial ischemia, and (3) low cardiac output.

5. Evaluate the patient's central venous pressure (CVP), which reflects the ability of the heart to pump the volume of blood being returned to it.

The CVP measurement is used to assess hemoconcentration (hypovolemia) or hemodilution (hypervolemia). It is also used to determine complications, such as right heart failure and cardiac tamponade [29]. The CVP or the right atrial pressure does not, however, necessarily indicate how well the left heart functions. It does not therefore differentiate hypovolemia from poor venous return or hypervolemia from left heart failure.

The normal CVP ranges from 4 to 15 cm H_2O or 3 to 11 mm Hg. In the patient who has undergone open heart surgery, the CVP is allowed to be elevated, on the basis of the Frank-Starling law, which states that the greater the stretch of the muscle (the more volume), the greater the strength of contraction.

The CVP may be measured in centimeters of water by a water manometer or in millimeters of mercury by a transducer. An understanding of the conversion factor is important. Mercury is 13.4 times heavier than water. To convert millimeters of mercury (from a transducer) to centimeters of water, the number of millimeters of mercury should be multiplied by the conversion factor 1.34 (e.g., 8 mm Hg × 1.34 = 10.72 cm H_2O).

The transducer or the zero of the water manometer must be positioned at the level of the right atrium. An isolated CVP reading generally is not significant; serial CVP readings provide essential information about the patient's response to therapy (to intravenous fluids, diuretics, and cardiovascular medications). The patient must be in the same position for each reading. The patient is removed from the ventilator before his CVP is determined because the increased intrathoracic pressure (the intrapulmonic and intramediastinal pressures) will elevate the reading falsely. If the patient cannot be removed from the ventilator, that variable must be taken into consideration.

6. Prevent hypovolemia. The nurse should:

a. Know the causes of hypovolemia: inadequate replacement of fluid or blood, hemorrhage from an active bleeder in the chest, coagulopathy, sequestration of fluid or blood, vasodilatation from rewarming after surgery.

b. Assess the patient in regard to:

(1) The clinical manifestations of hypovolemia: dry mucous membranes, poor tissue turgor, sunken eyeballs, a decreased level of consciousness, restlessness, a pro-

Figure 21-5
Arterial curves. A. Normal arterial curve. B. Hypotension. C. Hypertension. D. Hypovolemia. E. Pulsus alternans. F. Pulsus paradoxus.

longed peripheral filling time, a low arterial pressure, a low arterial pressure curve (indicated when the notch is less than one-third the height of the curve) (Fig. 21-5D) and a rapid, weak pulse.

(2) His volume status, measuring the fluid intake and output, the amount of blood lost from the chest tubes and dressings, a low CVP, and a rise in systolic pressure without a significant increase in CVP when physiological saline solution is administered.

(3) Hemoglobin, hematocrit, and coagulation and electrolyte profile.

c. Depending on the cause of the hypovolemia, treat the patient by:

(1) Replacement with fluids, fresh blood, fresh frozen plasma, platelets, aminocaproic acid, protamine, or vitamin K as ordered.

(2) Surgical intervention if the patient's coagulation profile is normal and the bleeding continues.

7. Prevent hypervolemia. The nurse should:

a. Know the cause of hypervolemia; namely, fluid overload in the early postoperative period.

b. Assess the patient in regard to:

(1) His volume status, measuring his fluid intake and output.

(2) Any neck vein distention when he is in a semi-Fowler's position, a high CVP, dyspnea, tachycardia, third or fourth heart sounds, bilateral rales, coughing, and pulmonary edema.

(3) Poor oxygenation.

(4) His hemoglobin, hematocrit, and electrolyte (potassium) levels.

c. Treat the hypervolemia by limiting fluids, giving fast-acting diuretics (furosemide, ethacrynic acid) and inotropic drugs (digitalis), and using rotating tourniquets.

8. Evaluate the patient's cardiac output and his left heart functioning. The nurse should:

a. Assess the patient's arterial pressure curve in regard to:

(1) Pulsus alternans, a sign of left ventricular failure, which is present when every other arterial curve is low (Fig. 21-5E).

(2) Pulsus paradoxus, a sign of cardiac tamponade (see Chap. 20), which is present

when the curve varies with the patient's respirations (Fig. 21-5F).

b. Assess the patient's cardiac output, which may be measured by the following techniques [61, 71, 80]:

(1) The indicator dilution technique, which involves injecting a measured quantity of some indicator (an isotope or a dye) into the right atrium or pulmonary artery and drawing a blood sample from the peripheral arterial circulation. The cardiac output is calculated by an indicator dilution curve that measures the passage of the indicator over time from the venous blood to the arterial blood.

(2) The thermodilution technique, which involves injecting a cold saline solution into the right atrium and measuring the temperature change of the blood in the pulmonary artery by means of a thermistor-tipped catheter.

(3) The oxygen consumption technique, which is carried out by calculating the arteriovenous oxygen difference using systemic and pulmonary arterial samples.

c. Assess the patient's left atrial pressure (LAP), which directly reflects the filling pressure of the left ventricle just before contraction (commonly referred to as the left ventricular end-diastolic pressure—LVEDP). The LAP reflects the cardiac output and the capacity of the left ventricle to accept a volume load. The normal LAP is 4 to 12 mm Hg.

If a left atrial line is not inserted during the surgical procedure, a Swan-Ganz flow-directed, balloon-tipped catheter can be inserted into a vein and passed through the vena cava, the right atrium, the tricuspid valve, the right ventricle, and the pulmonary valve and positioned in the pulmonary artery. The passage of the catheter through the heart can be observed by watching the coded distance markings on the catheter and the changes in the pressure wave forms displayed on the cardiac monitor [64].

The Swan-Ganz catheter is capable of measuring the pulmonary artery (PA) pressures, which represent left atrial and ventricular activity. The PA systolic pressure represents the peak pressure of the right ventricle. It ranges from 20 to 30 mm Hg. The lowest pressure generated in the pulmonary artery is the PA diastolic pressure (PADP), which ranges from 10 to 15 mm Hg. It indicates the LVEDP. The PA mean pressure represents the averages of the systolic and diastolic pulmonary artery pressures. It ranges from 10 to 20 mm Hg.

The pulmonary artery wedge pressure (PAWP; pulmonary artery capillary pressure) is measured by inflating the balloon on the catheter to wedge it tightly in the small distal branch of the pulmonary artery. The pressures exerted distal to the inflated balloon are blocked so that the proximal tip of the catheter measures only the pressure in the pulmonary capillary system. The PAWP is used to adjust left ventricular volume. It indirectly reflects the left atrial pressure and the LVEDP. The normal mean PAWP is 4 to 12 mm Hg. It should be noted that the LAP, the PAWP, and the PADP all normally reflect the LVEDP.

To ensure maximal filling pressure (hence maximal stroke volume) postoperatively, the LVEDP is generally maintained at 15 to 25 mm Hg.

d. Correlate the LAP and CVP. The nurse should be aware that:
   (1) During the early postoperative period, both the CVP and the LAP must be assessed.
   (2) If both the CVP and the LAP are elevated, the patient is relatively or absolutely hypervolemic. He should be treated with vasodilators (to reduce afterload) or diuretics—or with vasopressors if he is hypotensive.
   (3) If both the CVP and the LAP are low, the patient is relatively or absolutely hypovolemic. He should be treated with fluids to increase the preload.
   (4) If the CVP is normal and the LAP is elevated, the patient has left ventricular failure. He should be treated with positive inotropic drugs, such as digitalis in combination with diuretics, or with vasodilators to reduce the afterload.

e. Assess the stability of the patient's peripheral perfusion, noting his temperature, color, and blanching of his extremities, the strength of his carotid, radial, femoral, pedal, popliteal,

dorsalis pedis, and posterior tibial pulses. The nurse may evaluate venous filling by having the patient elevate his hand above the level of the apex. The venous blood should empty in three to five seconds when the patient's hand is elevated, and it should refill in three to five seconds when the patient's hand is lowered.

9. Identify acute myocardial infarction. The nurse should:
   a. Know the causes of acute myocardial infarction. Myocardial revascularization is often performed to prevent the development of acute myocardial infarction. Unfortunately, 10 to 15 percent of patients so treated can be expected to develop an intraoperative or an early postoperative acute myocardial infarction [14, 49, 63].

      Although the development of acute myocardial infarction probably affects the patient's long-term survival and the functional results of the surgery, it has been suggested that the development of a small infarction during or shortly after surgery contributes to the symptomatic relief of angina pectoris by "sealing off" an unstable area of ischemic myocardium [12, 13].
   b. Assess the patient for acute myocardial infarction by looking for ECG evidence of new Q waves; a significant rise in the serum glutamic oxaloacetic transaminase, creatine phosphokinase, and lactic dehydrogenase levels [2]; sinus tachycardia; and signs of heart failure. Myocardial scintigraphy should be performed if it is available (see Chap. 19).
   c. Treat the patient as indicated. Patients who develop postoperative infarctions should be mobilized early. Their discharge from the hospital is generally not delayed [7].

10. Prevent cardiogenic shock or identify existing cardiogenic shock. The nurse should:
    a. Know the causes of cardiogenic shock: myocardial ischemia or infarction, dysrhythmias, cardiac trauma, malfunctioning of prosthetic valves, myocardial depression by anesthesia and hypothermia, reduced left ventricular compliance or contractility.
    b. Assess the patient for the following manifestations of cardiogenic shock:
       (1) A systolic blood pressure of less than 80 mm Hg

(2) A urinary output of less than 20 ml per hour

(3) A diminished cerebral perfusion; confusion and lethargy

(4) Tachycardia

(5) Cyanosis

(6) Hypoxemia and acidosis

(7) Rapid, shallow respirations

(8) Cold, clammy, mottled skin

c. Treat the patient in cardiogenic shock by:

(1) Measuring his cardiac output.

(2) Providing adequate oxygenation and ventilation.

(3) Correcting his acidosis.

(4) Administering digitalis.

(5) Determining his volume status. If the patient's PAWP is less than 18 mm Hg or his CVP is less than 15 cm H_2O, fluids should be infused.

(6) Administering norepinephrine, glucagon, dopamine, dobutamine, or nitroprusside.

(7) Inserting an intraaortic balloon pump or using an external counterpulsation device to augment intraaortic pressure during diastole, thereby increasing coronary perfusion without increasing myocardial work or oxygen demands. Those devices also lower intraaortic pressure during systole to reduce afterload (and hence myocardial oxygen requirements) and promote larger stroke volumes by decreasing resistance to left ventricular ejection.

11. Prevent thromboembolic complications or identify existing thromboembolic complications. The nurse should:

a. Know the causes of thromboembolism: venous stasis from inactivity, cardiopulmonary bypass, and coagulation abnormalities.

b. Assess the patient for clinical manifestations of cerebral, pulmonary, peripheral, renal, splenic, or mesenteric embolism. The patient's coagulation panel should be evaluated.

c. Treat the patient's condition by promoting:

(1) Performance of active and passive exercises.

(2) Early ambulation and progressive activity.

(3) The use of antiembolism stockings or leg wraps.

(4) The administration of anticoagulants or fibrinolytic drugs.

OBJECTIVE NO. 2

The stability of the patient's respiratory status should be maintained and respiratory complications should be prevented.

To achieve the objective, the nurse should:

1. Evaluate the patient's respiratory status. The nurse should:

a. Assess the patient in regard to his level of consciousness, color, rate, depth, and type of respirations, adequacy of oxygenation and ventilator settings, expired minute volume, and arterial blood gas measurements. Bilateral auscultation should be done to evaluate the patient's breath sound. If breath sounds are not audible on the patient's left side when the endotracheal tube is in place, it can be assumed that the tube has slipped into the right bronchus. A chest x ray should be taken, and the tube should be repositioned.

b. Treat the patient's respiratory status by:

(1) Keeping the endotracheal tube and tubing secure and adequately supported.

(2) Using an oral airway to prevent the patient from clamping down on the endotracheal tube.

(3) Identifying and correcting any sudden abnormal functioning of the ventilator. The ventilator should provide an adequate minute volume, oxygenation, and humidification of inspired gases.

(4) Using sterile deep tracheal suctioning as needed.

(5) Repositioning the patient frequently.

(6) Determining the patient's psychological response to the ventilator.

(7) Providing information and care to reduce the patient's anxiety and fear.

(8) Frequently reminding the patient that the ventilator has taken over the work of breathing but only temporarily.

(9) Giving the patient a pencil and paper or a Magic Slate so that he can communicate.

(10) Determining whether the patient is "fighting" the ventilator. The nurse should provide reassurance and sedation as necessary.

2. Help wean the patient from the ventilator. The nurse should:

a. Assess the patient in regard to his arterial blood gases, chest x ray, breath sounds, neuromuscular functioning, level of consciousness, and cardiovascular functioning.
b. Treat the patient by:
  (1) Explaining the weaning process to him.
  (2) Increasing the length of time he is off the ventilator (and breathing on the T bar with humidified oxygen or intermittent mandatory ventilation).
  (3) Assessing his blood gases when he is off the ventilator.
  (4) Measuring his minute volume inspiratory force (should be greater than 25 cm H_2O) and his vital capacity (should be greater than 15 cc/kg).
  (5) Observing his physiological and psychological tolerance to weaning; staying with the patient while he is off the ventilator and reassuring him.
3. Assist with extubation of the patient. The nurse should:
  a. Know that the decision to extubate the patient is based on his clinical assessment during the weaning period.
  b. Several hours before extubation, discontinue giving the patient narcotics that depress respiration.
  c. Observe the patient after extubation for laryngeal edema and spasm.
  d. Administer a high-humidity mixture of air and oxygen.
  e. Help the patient to hyperinflate his lungs every one to two hours.
    (1) Have the patient cough and deep breathe; help him to turn while supporting the incision area.
    (2) Have the patient use blow bottles, incentive spirometry, and/or intermittent positive pressure breathing.
  f. Use chest physiotherapy and tracheal suctioning as needed.
  g. Encourage the patient to engage in progressive activities. Continue to assess his respiratory status.
4. Evaluate the patient's chest tube drainage. The nurse should:
  a. Connect the chest tubes to water-sealed drainage (they may be connected to 20 cm of suction). Most chest tubes are placed not in the pleural space but in the mediastinum to facilitate intrathoracic drainage after surgery. It is the responsibility of the nurse to know what tubes are mediastinal and what tubes are pleural.
  Generally, two intercostal tubes and a right-angle precordial mediastinal tube are used to prevent cardiac tamponade and facilitate drainage.
  b. Treat the patient's condition by:
    (1) Measuring and recording the amount and color of the drainage every hour. The blood lost is generally replaced with an equal amount of intravenous blood.
    (2) Observing the patient for hemorrhage (> 200 cc/hr or > 500 cc in the first eight hours).
    (3) Maintaining the patency of the tubes; stripping the chest tubes every hour.
    (4) Removing the chest tubes, using Vaseline gauze or sterile sponges.

OBJECTIVE NO. 3

The stability of the patient's gastrointestinal status should be maintained and gastrointestinal complications should be prevented.
  To achieve the objective, the nurse should:

1. Prevent gastric distention. The nurse should:
  a. Know that gulping air may (1) cause pulmonary complications due to pressure on the diaphragm, (2) compromise venous return or cardiac output by exerting pressure on the venae cavae, or (3) cause dysrhythmias.
  b. Assess the patient by (1) percussing his left upper abdomen, (2) measuring his abdomen to check for abdominal distention, (3) determining the degree of nausea and vomiting, and (4) noting the size of the gastric air bubble shown on the chest x ray.
  c. Treat the patient's gastric distention by sedation and by the use of a nasogastric tube attached to low intermittent suction.
2. Prevent stress ulcers. The nurse should:
  a. Know the causes of stress ulcers: stress of surgery, respiratory failure, sepsis, peritonitis, burns, renal failure, and hypotension [28].
  b. Assess the patient in regard to the clinical manifestations of stress ulcers: abdominal pain,

red or coffee-ground-colored gastric secretions, black or tarry stools, and an unexplained drop in hematocrit.

c. Treat the patient's potential stress ulcer by titrating his gastric contents with antacids to a pH greater than 3.5 [28] and avoiding drugs known to cause ulceration.

OBJECTIVE NO. 4

The stability of the patient's renal status should be maintained and renal complications should be prevented.

To achieve the objective, the nurse should:

1. Evaluate the patient's renal status. The nurse should:
   a. Assess the patient in regard to his urine output, color, odor, and pH, the presence of blood, protein, sugar, or acetone in his urine, his daily weight, his tissue turgor, his hydration status, his CVP, and his blood urea nitrogen, creatinine, and serum electrolyte levels. The nurse should evaluate the specific gravity of the patient's urine (normal is 1.015–1.020). (The specific gravity of urine may be low owing to overhydration, diuretics, or the inability of the kidneys to filter the waste products. The specific gravity of urine may be high owing to a decreased urinary output, dehydration, or the presence of fragmented red cells or of large molecular substances, such as glucose or proteins, in the urine.)
   b. Treat the patient's condition by maintaining an indwelling Foley catheter connected to a closed dependent drainage system. The patient's urinary output should be measured and recorded every hour. A urinary output of at least 30 ml per hour should be maintained.
2. Maintain an adequate urinary output and identify any existing reduction in urinary output. The nurse should:
   a. Know the causes of a reduction in urinary output: hypovolemia, hypotension, renal damage due to cardiac failure, hemolysis of red blood cells from cardiopulmonary bypass (bypass may cause hypotension during surgery, increased renal vascular resistance, and fragment red cells that liberate free hemoglobin).
   b. Know the clinical manifestations of reduced urinary output: low urine output, peripheral

edema, weight gain, high CVP with right heart failure, low CVP with hypovolemia, elevated blood urea nitrogen and creatinine levels, electrolyte imbalance, and confusion and disorientation.

c. Treat the patient's reduced urinary output by:
   (1) Measuring the patient's fluid intake and output.
   (2) Weighing the patient every day.
   (3) Ordering the patient a low-sodium diet if indicated.
   (4) Helping correct any electrolyte imbalance.
   (5) Increasing the fluid volume (if the patient's central venous pressure is low).
   (6) Increasing the blood pressure (if it is low).
   (7) Administering diuretics as ordered.

OBJECTIVE NO. 5

The stability of the patient's fluid and electrolyte balance should be maintained and fluid and electrolyte complications should be prevented.

To achieve the objective, the nurse should:

1. Evaluate the patient's fluid and electrolyte balance. The nurse should:
   a. Assess the patient's circulating blood volume, which is reflected by his urinary output, hydration and electrolyte status, blood pressure, and CVP. (See the discussion of hypovolemia and hypervolemia in this chapter.)
   b. Treat the patient's condition by:
      (1) Restricting fluids to 1500 to 2500 ml during the first 24 hours, depending on the patient's hydration status. (Fluids are generally restricted because antidiuretic hormone and aldosterone are released in response to the stress of surgery and because fluids are sequestered into the interstitial spaces.)
      (2) Replacing fluids and blood products.
      (3) Recording the patient's hourly fluid intake. (The patient's intravenous crystalloid and oral fluid intake should be measured separately from his intake of blood, plasma, and albumin.)
      (4) Correcting any imbalance of the patient's serum electrolytes (sodium, potassium, chloride, calcium, bicarbonate, magnesium, and phosphate).
      (5) Carefully labeling all intravenous solutions

and additives, with the date and time of administration. (Each intravenous bottle should be labeled with a strip of tape on which is written the hourly times of infusions. An infusion pump and a microdrip administration chamber should be used in the administration of intravenous fluids.)

(6) Putting the patient on a clear-liquid diet after extubation. (The diet should be advanced to a low-sodium, low-atherogenic one as tolerated by the patient.)

2. Prevent hypokalemia. The nurse should:
   a. Know the causes of hypokalemia: forced diuresis during bypass and after surgery and by metabolic alkalosis. (Potassium ions are excreted in the urine in exchange for hydrogen ions in the setting of metabolic alkalosis.)
   b. Know the clinical manifestations of hypokalemia:
      (1) Ventricular irritability
      (2) Low serum potassium levels; pH above 7.45
      (3) ECG changes consistent with hypokalemia: prolongation of the QT interval (a low T wave merging with a taller U wave), T-wave inversion, ST-segment depression
      (4) Acid urine (pH below 5) due to excessive excretion of hydrogen ions (will depend on degree of hypokalemia and/or metabolic alkalosis)
      (5) Anxiety, tremors, weakness, ileus, confusion, seizures
   c. Treat the patient's hypokalemia by:
      (1) Replacing potassium intravenously.
      (2) Using G.I.K. solution (10% glucose in water solution, 10 units of regular insulin, 20–60 mEq of potassium chloride per liter of solution).
      (3) Monitoring the patient's electrolyte panel.
      (4) Using an oral potassium supplement when indicated.

OBJECTIVE NO. 6

The stability of the patient's neurological status should be maintained and neurological complications should be prevented.

To achieve the objective, the nurse should:

1. Evaluate the patient's neurological status. The nurse should:
   a. Assess the patient's condition by giving him neurological checks every hour. The patient should be observed for the signs and symptoms of cerebral hypoxia or edema: seizures, disorientation, extreme weakness, and communication problems.

2. Prevent the development of ICU psychosis. The nurse should:
   a. Know the causes of ICU psychosis: prolonged cardiopulmonary bypass (postperfusion delirium), prolonged and deep hypothermia, cerebral microembolism or hypoxia, metabolic acidosis, dysrhythmias resulting in diminished cardiac output, febrile reactions, overwhelming psychophysiological stress, inadequate psychological preparation for surgery, sleep deprivation, sensory deprivation/overload, loss of orientation to time and date, immobilization, limitations on visiting by family members, and impersonal attitude of staff [36, 40].
   b. Treat the patient's condition by:
      (1) Giving preoperative teaching to the patient and his family.
      (2) Making sure the patient has a preoperative visit from his critical care nurses.
      (3) Putting the patient in a separate room that has a window, a large clock, and a calendar.
      (4) Making sure that all monitoring equipment is outside the patient's room when possible.
      (5) Eliminating monotonous sounds (e.g., those from air conditioning units).
      (6) Modifying nursing procedures to allow the patient as much uninterrupted sleep as possible.
      (7) Orienting the patient to time, place, person, weather, and news events often throughout the day.
      (8) Promoting early mobilization and other activities, helping the patient in self-care, reducing environmental stimulation, and placing responsibility for recovery on the patient.
      (9) Establishing and encouraging sufficient and flexible visiting times.
      (10) Communicating to the patient a caring, empathetic approach expressed by interest in and concern for him (not his tubes).

3. Reduce anxiety and fear postoperatively. The nurse should:
   a. Assess the patient's verbal and nonverbal behavior.

b. Accept the patient.

c. Provide care that allows the patient to maintain a sense of dignity and value.

d. Describe how the patient will feel, what he will experience physically and emotionally, and why the procedures are being done.

e. Promote a humanistic, caring environment.

f. Establish a means of communication.

g. Alleviate pain.

h. Communicate with the patient's family members and recognize their importance.

4. Prevent fever. The nurse should:

a. Know the causes of fever: cardiopulmonary bypass, systemic or local infection, and hemolysis of red blood cells.

b. Treat the patient's condition by:

(1) Using careful aseptic techniques in regard to intravenous fluids, medication additives, invasive lines, and catheters. All intravenous tubing should be changed at least once every 24 hours; sterile dressings should be changed every 24 hours. The venipuncture site should be observed for signs of phlebitis, infection, and infiltration. The time, date, type, and needle size of each intravenous catheter inserted should be recorded. Indwelling catheters must be changed every 48 hours to prevent phlebitis and infection. The stopcock sidearms should be sealed with sterile caps to prevent contamination and infection.

(2) Maintaining a closed-seal drainage system for an indwelling Foley catheter. Catheter care must be given every eight hours. The catheter should be removed as soon as possible.

(3) Maintaining a closed system of chest drainage.

(4) Using aseptic technique for all dressing changes.

(5) Using sterile technique for tracheal suction.

(6) Sterilizing all oxygen equipment daily.

(7) Culturing and reporting any signs of infection.

(8) Administering appropriate antibiotics.

(9) Taking the patient's temperature every four hours.

(10) Administering antipyretic medications, hypothermia, ice packs, or alcohol sponges for fever.

Rehabilitation Phase

OBJECTIVE

The stability of the patient's physiological and psychological status should be maintained during rehabilitation.

To achieve the objective, the nurse should:

1. Teach the patient about the postoperative information he will need to prepare for his rehabilitation and his hospital discharge. The teaching should include information related to:

a. A progressive exercise program.

b. Restricting strenuous activities.

c. Coughing and deep breathing exercises.

d. Caring for his incision site.

e. Signs and symptoms of incisional infection.

f. Taking his temperature daily, weighing himself daily.

g. When the patient can return to work, resume sexual activities, and drive a car.

h. The name, dosage, actions, indications, and side effects of his discharge medications.

i. His diet.

j. Methods to reduce his cardiovascular risk factors.

k. When to return to his physician for a check-up.

l. Preventing systemic infection (patients having cardiovascular valve surgery need to know how to prevent endocarditis; see Nursing and Medical Management section in Chapter 23).

m. Methods of oral hygiene.

n. The name and telephone number of his primary care nurse and other hospital personnel who may be of assistance after the patient is discharged (e.g., dietitian, social worker, psychologist, physical therapist, primary care nurse).

Summary

To provide quality care to the cardiovascular surgical patient, the nurse needs a thorough knowledge of the pathophysiology, surgical indications, operative procedure, and complications. An interdisciplinary team approach is essential in coordinating the various phases of the patient's hospitalization. The nurse has the opportunity to demonstrate her expertise and skills in helping the patient achieve optimum health postoperatively.

Study Problems

1. The indications for myocardial revascularization are:
   a. Intractable angina.
   b. Unstable angina.
   c. Acute myocardial infarction.
   d. All the above.

2. The preoperative assessment of the patient who is to undergo myocardial revascularization comprises:
   a. A thorough history and physical examination.
   b. Coronary arteriography.
   c. A ventriculogram.
   d. All the above.

3. The overall operative mortality for aortocoronary bypass surgery is:
   a. 1%.
   b. 5%.
   c. 10%.
   d. 25%.

4. The most important operative risk factor in aortocoronary bypass surgery is:
   a. The number of diseased coronary vessels.
   b. The age of the patient.
   c. Left ventricular functioning.
   d. The severity of the angina.

5. A functioning aortocoronary bypass graft:
   a. Establishes an autoregulatory mechanism.
   b. Improves clinical symptoms in a large percentage of patients.
   c. Improves left ventricular function when the dysfunction is due to scar tissue.
   d. a and b.

6. Preoperative preparation of the cardiac surgical patient includes:
   a. Physiological and psychological stabilization.
   b. Reduction of anxiety.
   c. A thorough nursing assessment.
   d. Patient education.
   e. All the above.

7. The immediate postoperative care of the cardiac surgical patient includes:
   a. Maintaining the stability of the patient's physiological and psychological status.
   b. The prevention of complications.
   c. Educating the patient about home care.
   d. a and b.

8. Postoperative dysrhythmias may be the result of:
   a. Ischemia or trauma due to surgery.
   b. Hypotension.
   c. Pain.
   d. a and b.
   e. All the above.

9. The pulmonary artery wedge pressure measurement:
   a. Is accurately measured by a central venous catheter.
   b. Reflects the left ventricular end-diastolic pressure or the left ventricular filling pressure of the heart.
   c. a and b.

10. The classic physical findings in a patient with aortic stenosis include(s):
    a. A diastolic murmur.
    b. A systolic murmur.
    c. Atrial fibrillation.
    d. An Austin Flint murmur.

11. Anticoagulant therapy is usually continued for life when a patient's aortic or mitral valve is replaced with:
    a. A porcine valve.
    b. A tissue valve.
    c. A homograft.
    d. A disk valve.

12. Mitral stenosis produces:
    a. An increase in left atrial mean pressure.
    b. An increase in pulmonary vascular resistance.
    c. A decrease in cardiac output.
    d. All the above.

13. Atrial dysrhythmias are frequently associated with:
    a. Aortic stenosis.
    b. Mitral stenosis.
    c. Aortocoronary bypass surgery.

14. The murmur of mitral regurgitation is:
    a. A systolic murmur.
    b. A diastolic murmur.
    c. Likely to radiate to the axilla.
    d. a and c above.

15. Which of the following patients need special postoperative teaching in regard to preventing endocarditis after their surgery?
    a. Patients who have had open mitral commissurotomies.
    b. Patients who have had aortocoronary bypass surgery.
    c. Patients who have had mitral or aortic valve replacements.
    d. a and c above.

16. If the patient's CVP is normal and his LAP is elevated following aortocoronary bypass surgery, the patient may be:
    a. Hypervolemic.

b. Hypovolemic.
c. In right heart failure.
d. In left heart failure.
17. The complication(s) of cardiac surgery is (are):
   a. Acute myocardial infarction.
   b. Dysrhythmia.
   c. Pulmonary infection.
   d. All the above.
18. A decreased urinary output in the postoperative cardiac surgical patient may be caused by:
   a. Hypovolemia.
   b. Inhibition of antidiuretic hormone.
   c. Inhibition of aldosterone.
   d. All the above.
19. Postoperative hypokalemia is associated with:
   a. Metabolic acidosis.
   b. Ventricular irritability.
   c. Peaked T waves on the ECG.
   d. All the above.
20. ICU psychosis may be caused by:
   a. Prolonged cardiopulmonary bypass.
   b. Cerebral microembolism.
   c. Inadequate psychological preparation of the patient.
   d. All the above.

Answers

1. d.
2. d.
3. b.
4. c.
5. d.
6. e.
7. d.
8. e.
9. b.
10. b.
11. d.
12. d.
13. b.
14. d.
15. d.
16. d.
17. d.
18. a.
19. b.
20. d.

References

1. Alderman, E. L., Brown, C. R., Sanders, G. R., et al. Survival following bypass graft surgery. *Clev. Clin. Q.* 45:157, 1978.
2. Aspinall, M. J. *Nursing the Open Heart Surgery Patient.* New York: McGraw-Hill, 1973.
3. Behrendt, D. M., and Austen, W. G. *Patient Care in Cardiac Surgery.* Boston: Little, Brown, 1976.
4. Bloomer, W. E., Beland, A. S., and Cope, J. Clinical use of the splenic artery for myocardial revascularization: Technical considerations. *Ann. Thorac. Surg.* 5:419, 1968.
5. Braunwald, E. Valvular Heart Disease. In M. M. Wintrobe (ed.), *Principles of Internal Medicine* (7th ed.). New York: McGraw-Hill, 1974.
6. Bregman, D. Management of patients undergoing intraaortic balloon pumping. *Heart Lung* 3:916, 1974.
7. Brener, E. R. Surgery for coronary artery disease. *Am. J. Nurs.* 72:469, 1972.
8. Bristow, J. D., and Rahimtoola, S. H. Effect of coronary bypass surgery on left ventricular function. *Cardiovasc. Clin.* 8:97, 1977.
9. Cobbs, B. W. Clinical Recognition and Medical Management of Rheumatic Heart Disease and Other Acquired Valvular Disease. In J. W. Hurst (ed.), *The Heart* (3rd ed.). New York: McGraw-Hill, 1974.
10. Cohn, L. H. Selection of patients for emergency coronary revascularization. *Clev. Clin. Q.* 45:181, 1978.
11. Conti, C. R., Hutter, A., Rosati, R., et al. Unstable angina: A national cooperative study comparing medical and surgical therapy. *Cardiovasc. Clin.* 8:167, 1977.
12. Corday, E. Status of coronary bypass surgery. *J.A.M.A.* 231:1245, 1975.
13. Danielson, G. K. Surgical Treatment of Acquired Heart Disease. In H. L. Conn and O. Horwitz (eds.), *Cardiac and Vascular Diseases* (1st ed.). Philadelphia: Lea & Febiger, 1971.
14. Davidson, R. M., and Corday, E. Current status of coronary artery bypass surgery. *Primary Cardiol.* 1:30, 1975.
15. DeMots, H., Rosch, J., McAnulty, J. H., et al. Left main coronary artery disease. *Cardiovasc. Clin.* 8:201, 1977.
16. Effler, D. B., Groves, K., Suarez, E. L., et al. Direct coronary artery surgery with endarterectomy and patch graft reconstruction. *J. Thorac. Cardiovasc. Surg.* 53:93, 1967.
17. Ehrlich, I. B. Patient selection and preoperative evaluation. *Heart Lung* 4:373, 1975.
18. Engler, R. L. Is there a role for surgery in acute myocardial infarction? *Cardiovasc. Clin.* 8:213, 1977.
19. Epstein, S. E., Kent, K. M., Goldstein, R. E., et al. Reduction of ischemic injury by nitroglycerin during acute myocardial infarction. *N. Engl. J. Med.* 292:29, 1975.
20. Favalaro, R. G. Double internal mammary artery im-

plants: Operative technique. *J. Thorac. Cardiovasc. Surg.* 55:457, 1968.

21. Favalaro, R. G. Saphenous vein graft in the surgical treatment of coronary artery disease: Operative technique. *J. Thorac. Cardiovasc. Surg.* 58:178, 1969.

22. Favalaro, R. G., Effler, D. B., and Cheanvechai, C. Acute coronary insufficiency (impending myocardial infarction and myocardial infarction): Surgical treatment by the saphenous vein graft technique. *Am. J. Cardiol.* 28:598, 1971.

23. Garrett, H. E., Dennis, E. W., and DeBakey, M. E. Aortocoronary bypass with saphenous vein graft: Seven year follow-up. *J.A.M.A.* 223:792, 1973.

24. Goodin, R. R., Inglesby, T. V., and Lansing, A. M. Preinfarction angina pectoris: A surgical emergency. *J. Thorac. Cardiovasc. Surg.* 66:934, 1973.

25. Grondin, C. M. Factors influencing graft patency. *Clev. Clin. Q.* 45:107, 1978.

26. Harken, D. E., Soroff, H. S., Taylor, W. J., et al. Partial and complete prostheses in aortic insufficiency. *J. Thorac. Cardiovasc. Surg.* 40:744, 1960.

27. Harken, D. E. Postoperative care following heart-valve surgery. *Heart Lung* 3:893, 1974.

28. Hastings, P. R., Skillman, J. J., Bushnell, L. S., et al. Antacid titration in the prevention of acute gastrointestinal bleeding. *N. Engl. J. Med.* 298:1041, 1978.

29. Haughey, B. CVP lines: Monitoring and maintaining. *Am. J. Nurs.* 78:635, 1978.

30. Hillis, L. D., and Braunwald, E. Myocardial ischemia. *N. Engl. J. Med.* 296:1093, 1977.

31. Hultgren, H. N., Takaro, T., Detre, K., et al. Veterans Administration cooperative study of surgical treatment of stable angina: Preliminary results. *Cardiovasc. Clin.* 8:119, 1977.

32. Isom, O. W., and Spencer, F. C. The current status of bypass grafting for coronary artery disease. *South. Med. J.* 68:897, 1975.

33. Johnson, J. E. Effects of structuring patients' expectations on their reactions to threatening events. *Nurs. Res.* 21:499, 1972.

34. Johnson, W., Flemma, R. J., and Lepley, D. Extended treatment of severe coronary artery disease: A surgical approach. *Ann. Surg.* 170:460, 1969.

35. Johnson, W., and Lepley, D. An aggressive surgical approach to coronary disease. *J. Cardiovasc. Surg.* 59:128, 1970.

36. Kaplan, S., Achtel, R. A., and Callison, C. B. Psychiatric complications following open-heart surgery. *Heart Lung* 3:423, 1974.

37. Kent, K. M., Borer, J. S., and Green, M. V. Effects of coronary-artery bypass on global and regional left ventricular function during exercise. *N. Engl. J. Med.* 298:1434, 1978.

38. Kirklin, J. W., and Karp, R. B. Surgical treatment of acquired valvular heart disease. In J. W. Hurst (ed.), *The Heart* (3rd ed.). New York: McGraw-Hill, 1974.

39. Kloster, F. E., Rahimtoola, S. H., Ritzmann, L. W., et al. Prospective randomized study of coronary bypass surgery for chronic stable angina. *Cardiovasc. Clin.* 8:145, 1977.

40. Kornfeld, D. S., Zimberg, S., and Malm, J. P. Psychiatric complications of open heart surgery. *N. Engl. J. Med.* 273:291, 1965.

41. Krauss, K. R., Hutter, A. M., Jr., and DeSanctis, R. W. Acute coronary insufficiency: Cause and follow-up. *Arch. Intern. Med.* 129:808, 1972.

42. Long, M. L., Scheuhing, M. A., and Christian, J. L. Cardiopulmonary bypass. *Am. J. Nurs.* 74:860, 1974.

43. Lopes, M. G., Spivack, A. P., and Harrison, D. C. Prognosis of noninfarction coronary care patients. *Am. J. Cardiol.* 31:144, 1973.

44. Manley, J. C. Postoperative assessment of left ventricular function. *Clev. Clin. Q.* 45:116, 1978.

45. Miller, D. W., Bruce, R. A., and Dodge, H. T. Physiologic improvement following coronary artery bypass surgery. *Circulation* 57:832, 1978.

46. Miller, J. I., and Craver, J. M. Current status of prosthetic valve replacement. *J. Med. Assoc. Ga.* 64:282, 1975.

47. Mills, N. L., and Ochsner, J. L. Concepts of coronary bypass surgery. *Postgrad. Med.* 57:97, 1975.

48. Mundth, E. D., and Austen, W. G. Surgical measures for coronary heart disease: Part I. *N. Engl. J. Med.* 293:13, 1975.

49. Mundth, E. D., and Austen, W. G. Surgical measures for coronary heart disease: Part II. *N. Engl. J. Med.* 293:75, 1975.

50. Mundth, E. D., and Austen, W. G. Surgical measures for coronary heart disease: Part III. *N. Engl. J. Med.* 293:124, 1975.

51. Mundth, E. D., Buckley, J., and Daggett, W. M. Surgery for complications of acute myocardial infarction. *Circulation* 45:1279, 1972.

52. Mundth, E. D., Buckley, J., and Leinbach, R. C. Surgical intervention for the complications of acute myocardial ischemia. *Ann. Surg.* 178:397, 1973.

53. Murphy, M. L., Hultgren, H. N., and Detre, K. Treatment of chronic stable angina: A preliminary report of survival data of the randomized Veterans Administration cooperative study. *N. Engl. J. Med.* 297:622, 1977.

54. Neill, W. A., Ritzmann, L. W., Okies, J. E., et al. Medical vs. urgent surgical therapy for acute coronary insufficiency: A randomized study. *Cardiovasc. Clin.* 8:179, 1977.

55. Oldham, H. N., Kong, Y., and Bartel, A. G. Risk factors in coronary artery bypass surgery. *Arch. Surg.* 105:918, 1972.

56. Olson, H. G., Miller, R. R., Amsterdam, E. A., et al. The propranolol withdrawal rebound phenomenon: Acute and catastrophic exacerbation of symptoms and death following abrupt cessation of large doses of propranolol in coronary artery disease. *Am. J. Cardiol.* 35:126, 1975.

57. Parker, J. O. Prognosis in coronary artery disease. *Clev. Clin. Q.* 45:145, 1978.

58. Pitorak, E. F., Hudak, C., O'Gureck, J., et al. *Nurse's Guide to Cardiac Surgery and Nursing Care.* New York: McGraw-Hill, 1969.

59. Ricks, W. B., Winkle, R. A., Shumway, N. E., et al. Surgical management of life-threatening ventricular arrhythmias in patients with coronary artery disease. *Circulation* 56:38, 1977.

60. Robinson, W. A., Smith, R. F., and Stevens, T. W. Preinfarction syndrome: Evaluation and treatment. *Circulation* 46(Suppl. 2):212, 1972.

61. Russell, R. O., Kouchoukos, N. T., and Karp, R. B. Hemodynamic considerations in the postoperative management of the cardiovascular surgical patient. *Clev. Clin. Q.* 45:54, 1978.

62. Sawyer, P. N., Kaplitt, M., Sobel, S., et al. Experimental and clinical experience with coronary gas endarterectomy. *Arch. Surg.* 95:736, 1967.

63. Schrank, J. P., Slabaugh, T. K., and Beckwith, J. R. The incidence and clinical significance of ECG-VCG changes of myocardial infarction following aortocoronary saphenous vein bypass surgery. *Am. Heart J.* 87:46, 1974.

64. Schroeder, J. S., and Daily, E. K. Techniques in bedside hemodynamic monitoring. St. Louis: Mosby, 1976.

65. Segal, B. L., Kotler, M. N., Likoff, W., et al. Current status of aorto-coronary bypass graft surgery. *Cardiology* 59:277, 1974.

66. Seides, S. F., Borer, J. S., Kent, K. M., et al. Long-term anatomic fate of coronary-artery bypass grafts and functional status of patients five years after operation. *N. Engl. J. Med.* 298:1214, 1978.

67. Seldin, R., Neill, W. A., Ritzman, L. W., et al. Medical vs. surgical therapy for acute coronary insufficiency. *N. Engl. J. Med.* 293:1329, 1975.

68. Sewell, W. H. Results of 122 mammary pedicle implantations for angina pectoris. *Ann. Thorac. Surg.* 2:17, 1966.

69. Sheldon, W. C. Factors influencing patency of coronary bypass grafts. *Clev. Clin. Q.* 45:109, 1978.

70. Sheldon, W. C., Loop, F. D., and Proudfit, W. L. A critique of the VA cooperative study. *Clev. Clin. Q.* 45:225, 1978.

71. Smith, R. N. Invasive pressure monitoring. *Am. J. Nurs.* 78:1514, 1978.

72. Smitherman, T. C. Unstable Angina Pectoris. Presented at Medical Grand Rounds, Parkland Memorial Hospital, Dallas, Texas, June, 1975.

73. Sones, F. M., Jr., and Shirey, E. K. Cine coronary arteriography. *Mod. Concepts Cardiovasc. Dis.* 31:735, 1962.

74. Spencer, F. C. Bypass grafting for preinfarction angina. *Circulation* 45:1314, 1972.

75. Spencer, F. C. Acquired Heart Disease. In S. I. Schwartz (ed.), *Principles of Surgery* (2nd ed.). New York: McGraw-Hill, 1974.

76. Starr, A., and Edwards, M. L. Mitral replacement: Clinical experience with a ball valve prosthesis. *Ann. Surg.* 154:726, 1961.

77. Ullyot, D. J. Postoperative care. *Clev. Clin. Q.* 45:50, 1978.

78. Venderger, A. Cardiopulmonary bypass: Postoperative complications. *Am. J. Nurs.* 74:868, 1974.

79. Vineberg, A. M. Development of an anastomosis between the coronary vessels and a transplanted internal mammary artery. *Can. Med. Assoc. J.* 55:117, 1946.

80. Walinsky, P. Acute hemodynamic monitoring. *Heart Lung* 6:838, 1977.

81. Wilson, W. S. Aortocoronary bypass surgery II—an updated review. *Heart Lung* 3:435, 1974.

Dissecting Aortic Aneurysm

Joan B. Fitzmaurice

Dissecting aortic aneurysm is the most common catastrophe involving the aorta, occurring two to three times more often than rupture of an abdominal aneurysm. If the condition is untreated, it is predicted that 50 percent of people who have acute dissecting aneurysm will die within 48 hours of its onset. Recognition of the condition has increased in recent years because the condition has become more widely known and because increasingly sophisticated diagnostic techniques (notably angiography), that offer the opportunity to reduce mortality have been developed.

Two diagnostic clues that are of the utmost significance are the presence of chest pain and a history of hypertension. The single most important factor in altering the course of dissecting aneurysms is that the nurse, physician, and patient have a high index of suspicion.

Objective

The nurse should be able to recognize the common manifestations of dissecting aortic aneurysm, identify high-risk patients, understand the current modes of therapy, and be able to collect a data base, formulate nursing diagnoses, and carry out the appropriate nursing actions during the acute and the chronic phases of the illness.

22

Achieving the Objective

To achieve the objective, the nurse should be able to:

1. Describe the basic pathophysiological changes in dissecting aortic aneurysm.
2. Describe its characteristic pain.
3. List its common causes.
4. Outline the antihypertensive drug regimen recommended for the acute phase.
5. Anticipate the needs of patients and the interventions to be carried out during the critical phase.
6. Formulate approaches that increase the patient's compliance with therapy after his discharge from the hospital.

How to Proceed

To develop an approach to patients with dissecting aortic aneurysm, the nurse should:

1. Analyze the characteristics of dissecting aortic aneurysm that are present in the patient discussed in the following case study.
2. Anticipate the patient's physiological and psychological problems.
3. Develop a plan of care for the patient.
4. Plan a staff conference to discuss the major problems to be anticipated in the patient.
5. Read the pages that follow as well as the references listed at the end of the chapter.

Case Study

Mr. B., a 55-year-old black man, came to the hospital's emergency room with the complaints of persistent dull chest pain and dyspnea of two days' duration. He said that a severe, "sharp, hot" pain that shot from his sternal notch to below his umbilicus began suddenly while he was eating dinner. The pain, which lasted about two to three minutes, was associated with a burning sensation throughout his chest and a momentary feeling that he had no body below his hips. Mr. B. was markedly short of breath during the period of pain, but he did not become lightheaded or dizzy, nor did he experience any visual changes. For the next 24 hours, he had an ache in the muscles of his anterior chest, back, and arms that was affected by movement and pressure. He treated the ache with the local application of heat but got only slight relief. He also had difficulty sleeping supine because he had pain and respiratory distress.

Mr. B.'s patient profile and social history described him as a 6'2", 190-lb attractive black man who had a master's degree in biology, and who was currently employed as a jazz pianist.

His wife worked as an industrial technician. The couple had no children. Mr. B. was not an active member of any religious group. He did not drink or smoke (except, occasionally, a pipe), and he had no allergies. His main hobby was working with a local high school band.

Mr. B.'s current medical history was negative, except for infrequent attacks of gastric distress, which he treated successfully with an antacid. Although Mr. B. had no history of hypertension, he also had not had his blood pressure checked since his discharge from the army (more than 30 years ago). He said that since he had always been healthy he had had no reason to consult a doctor.

Mr. B.'s family history was significant in that his mother died at age 50 from "heart failure." His physical examination revealed a marked difference in blood pressure and pulse quality in both arms. Two murmurs were noted: a grade 2 systolic ejection murmur that was loudest at the second right intercostal space and a grade 4 early diastolic decrescendo murmur along the left sternal border. Mr. B. had both third and fourth heart sounds, as well as moist bilateral basilar rales. He had a visible pulsation in the right supraclavicular area.

The only significant laboratory findings were that his hematocrit was 30% and his hemoglobin level was 11 gm, indicating a slight anemia. The chest x ray showed borderline cardiomegaly, with a cardiothoracic ratio of 16 cm to 31 cm. Mr. B.'s aorta was prominent, widened, and tortuous. His ECG demonstrated left ventricular hypertrophy but no signs of ischemia.

Mr. B. was transferred to the intensive care unit, where central venous and arterial catheters were inserted for continuous monitoring of his vital signs. A Foley catheter was also inserted; a urine output of less than 25 ml per hour may indicate renal involvement and the need for immediate surgery.

Over the next two days, an antihypertensive drug regimen consisting of continuous intravenous infusion of trimethaphan, followed by reserpine and propranolol, reduced the blood pressure adequately and maintained it at 120/75 mm Hg. During that time Mr. B.'s pain also subsided completely, indicating that he had no further dissection.

Four days after his admission to the hospital, Mr. B. was taken to the cardiac catheterization laboratory, where fluoroscopic examination revealed an enlarged left ventricle with dilatation of the ascending aorta. An aortic angiogram showed a 4+ aortic regurgitation and a type I dissection beginning at the aortic root and extending into the abdominal aorta with occlusion of the left renal artery (Fig. 22-1). Mr. B.'s coronary angiograms were normal.

The next week, Mr. B.'s dissecting aneurysm was repaired surgically with Teflon felt that was inserted between the walls of the true lumen and the false lumen. The support thus given to the aortic ring obviated the need for replacement of the aortic valve.

Mr. B.'s recovery was uneventful. After his discharge from the hospital, he required maintenance antihypertensive

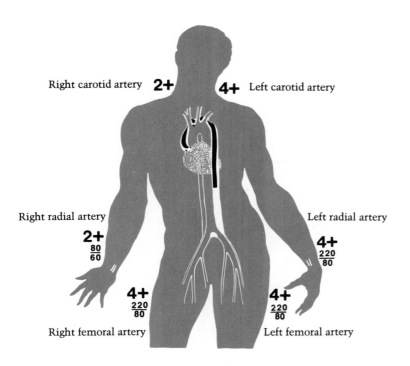

Right carotid artery **2+**   **4+** Left carotid artery

Right radial artery
2+
$\frac{80}{60}$

Left radial artery
4+
$\frac{220}{80}$

4+
$\frac{220}{80}$

4+
$\frac{220}{80}$

Right femoral artery   Left femoral artery

Figure 22-1
Sites of aortic dissection with resulting differences in blood pressure and pulse quality.

therapy with methyldopa (500 mg every four hours), and digoxin (0.375 mg a day) and furosemide (40 mg twice a day) for control of congestive heart failure. Mr. B.'s functional status was also good; he was able to climb two flights of stairs without symptoms or significant changes in blood pressure.

Reflections

The sudden onset and uncertain outcome of Mr. B.'s illness were foremost in his thoughts. Realistic reassurances, adequate information, and opportunities to ventilate his feelings were specific nursing interventions to help Mr. B. minimize the potentially deleterious effects of his internal stress. Carrying out those interventions while continuously monitoring Mr. B.'s blood pressure was not easy.

Modification of the environment of the surgical intensive care unit to reduce stress was a challenge to the nurses. Mr. B. had come to the emergency room because he had persistent dull chest pain and dyspnea

that had lasted two days. In a short time, his condition was diagnosed as an emergency one—hypertensive crisis and dissecting aortic aneurysm. Mr. B. was quickly taken to the critical care unit, where tubes, catheters, and devices for continuous monitoring of his vital signs were employed, and a continuous intravenous infusion was given to reduce and maintain his blood pressure. Those procedures, frightening to any patient, are common in critical care units. Nurses and physicians must continuously seek to diminish the stress caused by those and other procedures, which are lifesaving. Important in the healing process are the use of infusion pumps, frequent checking of vital signs, an atmosphere conducive to emotional support, and an alert health team. In the psychobiological view of the patient, emotional support is physical support. Interactions between the autonomic nervous system and the cardiovascular system are thought to be extremely sensitive to emotional stimuli.

Virtually all the sympathetic nervous system responses that are mediated by the central nervous system can be harmful to the patient who has hypertension and dissecting aortic aneurysm. The anxiety, stress, fear, and pain that are common in most critical care units are particularly harmful to the patient with a dissecting aortic aneurysm. Anxiety and stress elicit sympathetic responses, and specific therapy must be directed toward alleviating them. Elimination or diminution of stress and anxiety is an integral part of therapy; blocking the sympathetic responses is necessary.

Both pharmacological and psychological interventions to relieve stress and anxiety are useful, based on the concept that body and mind are interrelated.

Anatomy of the Aorta

The aorta extends from the aortic opening of the left ventricle to its bifurcation into the common iliac arteries. It is divided into (1) the ascending aorta, (2) the aortic arch, which extends to the left side of the fourth thoracic vertebra, (3) the thoracic aorta, which extends from the arch to the diaphragm, and (4) the abdominal aorta, which extends from the diaphragm. The aorta functions as a compression chamber or a reservoir for blood that has been rapidly ejected from the left ventricle. Its walls have many elastic fibers that permit it to be stretched and lengthened with every heart beat. Three layers of tissue make up the aortic wall: the intima, the media, and the adventitia. The intima, the inner layer, consists of the endothelium and the delicate elastic tissue beneath it that lies in coarser elastic tissue, which is condensed into a thick plate called the internal elastic lamina. The media, the middle layer, constitutes the bulk of the wall. It is composed of elastic connective tissue. The outermost portion of the middle layer is called the external elastic lamina. The adventitia, the outer layer of arteries, is composed of irregularly arranged connective tissue that contains both collagen and elastic fibers. The aorta does not reach the state just described until one is 25 years of age. That fact explains why dissecting aortic aneurysm is extremely rare in people under 30 years of age.

Aortic Aneurysms

Aortic aneurysms have been classified into the following three groups [8]:

1. True aneurysms, which are localized dilatations of arteries that result from atrophy of the media. They may be fusiform, in which case the aneurysms encompass the entire circumference of the aorta and assume a spindle shape, or they may be saccular, in which case the aneurysms are pouchlike protrusions from the aortic wall that have narrow necks.
2. False aneurysms, which result from the rupture of true aneurysms or from penetrating trauma to an artery. The appearance of false aneurysms is similar to that of true aneurysms; they are both expansile, pulsatile masses.
3. Dissecting aneurysms (dissecting hematomas) result when blood gains access to the media. The layers of the media are dissected so that a false channel is formed between the adventitia and the intima.

Prognosis; Incidence

Although uncommon, dissection of a thoracic aortic aneurysm is lethal if it is not treated. Its predicted incidence is 10 per 1,000,000 people per year. Among people 50 to 60 years of age, three times more men than women have dissecting aortic aneurysm. Among people younger than 40 years of age, 50 percent of the dissecting aortic aneurysms that occur in women occur in those who are pregnant. Acute dissecting aortic aneurysm is more common among blacks than among people of other races, perhaps because blacks have a higher incidence of hypertension.

Classifications of Dissecting Aortic Aneurysms

Systems of classifying dissecting aortic aneurysms are based on the anatomical and clinical manifestations of the disease. The simplest and the most commonly accepted anatomical classification is that of DeBakey et al. [3], who divided dissecting aortic aneurysms into:

1. Type I aneurysms, which extend from the ascending aorta to the arch and beyond. Type I aneurysms account for 60 to 90 percent of the cases of dissecting aortic aneurysm.
2. Type II aneurysms, which involve primarily the ascending arch. Type II aneurysms are rare.
3. Type III aneurysms, which originate beyond the subclavian artery and may or may not be confined to the thoracic aorta. They account for 20 to 30 percent of the cases of dissecting aortic aneurysm (Fig. 22-2).

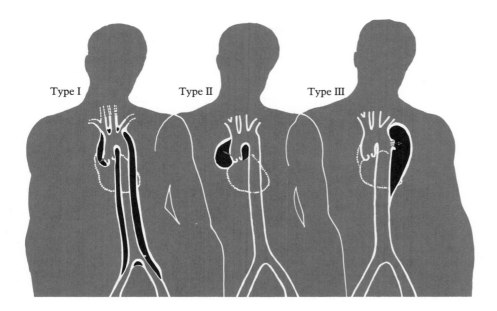

Type I   Type II   Type III

Figure 22-2
Classification of dissecting aneurysms of the aorta.

Aneurysms may also be classified as acute, sub-acute, or chronic. The basis for that type of clinical classification is how long the dissection has been present before the person seeks medical attention. Acute aortic dissection is characterized by the formation of a true (intimal) and a false (medial) lumen minutes to two to four weeks before the person seeks medical attention. The risk of sudden death is extremely high in people who have acute aortic dissecting aneurysm. Subacute aortic dissecting aneurysm is present in the person who seeks medical attention in two to six weeks, a span that indicated a slower progression of the dissection from the time of the intimal tear to the appearance of the medial dissection. Chronic aortic dissection is usually diagnosed by the second month, at which time healing of the false lumen with eventual fibrosis has occurred.

Pathology

Aortic dissections occur in aortas that have extensive medial disease or necrosis. Although exact cause of the necrosis is unknown, local hemodynamic and vasal supply characteristics are most crucial in determining the presence and location of these lesions.

The human aorta is particularly susceptible to dissection because of the high-amplitude pressure waves created by the flow of viscous blood. Pulsatile flow through the aorta presses outward and then (perhaps) sucks inward at the wall, requiring great elasticity of the aorta. The blood supply to the media of the aorta is through the vasa vasorum, the fine capillaries imbedded in the wall of the aorta. As the wall expands during systole, it becomes thinner, particularly the highly elastic ascending portion.

The vasa vasorum are squeezed down, temporarily decreasing or stopping the flow of blood through them and are maximally patent only during diastole. Moreover, in a person with diastolic hypertension or localized hypertension (e.g., a person who has coarctation of the aorta), the vasa vasorum may well have a decreased overall flow. The aortic wall may then undergo periods of stress that cause local degenerative changes over a short or (more likely) a long period of time.

The areas of the aorta most involved by dissection and medial degeneration are the ascending and transverse areas, precisely the areas with hemodynamic and capillary characteristics that, theoretically, make them more likely to degenerate [18]. They are the most elastic areas of the aorta, and they seem to have the most meager mural circulation. Although the exact mechanism of dissection is unclear, it appears either that the vasa vasorum of the aorta rupture and allow bleeding into the diseased media or the intima tears, owing to its weakened attachment to the medial structure, and allows blood to pass from the aortic lumen directly into the media. A second channel for blood to flow within the aortic wall itself is then created. If the aneurysm thus formed extends to the aortic root, aortic valve regurgitation often complicates the situation.

Etiology

Dissecting aortic aneurysm may be divided according to cause into (1) conditions that increase stress on the arterial wall, (2) conditions in which there is a defect in the vessel wall itself, and (3) conditions that are iatrogenic [8]. Hypertension, pregnancy with associated hypervolemia and hypertension, and coarctation of the aorta resulting in increased vascular pressures fall into the first category. Marfan's syndrome with cystic degeneration of the media is the most common cause of medial wall defect. Iatrogenic causes include subintimal dye injections following arteriographic procedures and extracorporeal circulation.

Clinical Picture

The clinical picture of aortic dissection includes pain, which, typically, begins suddenly and is excruciating or even unbearable from its inception. Often the patient describes the pain as ripping or tearing [14]. Classically, the pain is localized to the anterior chest, being most severe in the interscapular area, simulating a myocardial infarction. The pain may also be in the epigastric or midabdominal area, and, in fact, it may shift distally in the midline along the course of the dissection. Painless dissection is relatively uncommon, occurring in about 5 percent of cases [13]; it is associated with Marfan's syndrome. The location of pain is described according to the site of origin of the dissection. If the dissection is proximal to the innominate artery, central chest pain (rarely radiating to the back) is more common than abdominal chest pain radiating to the back, which is associated with a dissection originating distally to the innominate artery. The other presenting symptoms are variable.

A person with a proximal dissection frequently has neurological deficits, including cerebrovascular accidents, ischemic paraparesis, ischemic peripheral neuropathy, and disturbances of consciousness. Pulse deficits and differences between the blood pressure in both arms are also common. The murmur of aortic regurgitation is also present more frequently among people who have proximal dissections.

Hypertension is the predominant physical finding in distal dissection. In fact, if all dissections are considered, approximately 90 percent of people either are hypertensive on admission or have a history of hypertension [16].

Diagnostic Studies

The laboratory findings are not related to the location of the dissection. However, leukocytosis and an elevation in lactic dehydrogenase levels are the most frequent findings. The most significant ECG abnormalities are the presence of left ventricular hypertrophy with strain pattern and the absence of acute ischemic changes.

The chest x rays are important because the aortic contour is usually abnormally widened. Separation of intimal calcification from the outer border of the aortic knob is considered pathognomonic. The most definitive diagnostic study is contrast angiography to define the site of origin and the extent of the dissection and to evaluate the status of the renal, mesenteric, and iliac circulations.

Treatment

Dissecting aneurysms may be treated in two ways: (1) by intensive drug therapy and (2) by surgical therapy. Drug therapy is based on the premise that the medial dissection of the aorta may be arrested by reducing the contractility of the left ventricle and by lowering the mean arterial blood pressure. Surgical therapy means definitive surgical treatment of the main dissecting process or its complications through resection and graft replacement or end-to-end anastomosis of the aorta.

Intensive drug therapy as a treatment for acute dissecting aortic aneurysm was introduced by Wheat et al. in 1965 [17]. It is now an established treatment for certain types of dissecting aneurysm (Table 22-1). The initial objective of drug therapy is to reduce the systolic blood pressure to 100 to 120 mm Hg, using trimethaphan (1–2 mg/100 ml in an intravenous drip)

Table 22-1
Actions of Drugs Used to Treat Dissecting Aortic Aneurysm

Drug	Myocardial Contractility	Peripheral Resistance	Heart Rate	Other
Trimethaphan (Arfonad)	Decreased	Decreased	No change	Ileus Bladder distention
Reserpine (Serpasil)	Decreased	Decreased	Decreased	Gastric hyperacidity Drowsiness Depression
Guanethidine (Ismelin)	No change	Decreased	Decreased	Postural hypotension Diarrhea
Propranolol (Inderal)	Decreased	Increased	Decreased	Mild hypotension
Methyldopa (Aldomet)	No change	Decreased	Decreased slightly	Sedation Mild depression

if necessary for 24 to 48 hours to maintain the blood pressure at the desired level. Reserpine (1–2 mg) or propranolol (1 mg intramuscularly every 4–6 hours) is given to control the hypertension and reduce the force of the left ventricular contractions. Those drugs may also be given combined in lower doses to reduce the central nervous system side effects of reserpine. It is important to remember the two- to three-hour delay in the action of reserpine after administration. By the second to fifth day of therapy, methyldopa (250–500 mg every four hours) or guanethidine (25–50 mg twice a day orally) is given to maintain the lowered blood pressure. The use of nitroprusside has recently been suggested although its clinical applicability in dissecting aneurysm is controversial [10].

When the patient's blood pressure and pain are under control, indicating that the dissection of the aneurysm has been arrested and the patient's condition has stabilized, the next steps are to perform aortography and to choose the definitive therapy.

Surgical Therapy

Surgery aims at preventing rupture of the aorta, the most common cause of death in dissecting aortic aneurysm. It consists of removing the site of the intimal tear, obliterating the false lumen, and restoring aortic continuity by means of a synthetic tubular graft. It is often possible to restore integrity to the aortic valve by resuspending the aortic valve leaflets. That procedure is preferable to replacement of the aortic valve, although in Marfan's syndrome it is usually not possible [12]. The problems encountered during surgery are usually related to how extensive the dissection is and how fragile the aortic media is.

In general, the choice between medical therapy and surgical therapy has become easier to make [1, 2] since the clinical profile of patients with dissection of the ascending aorta has been shown to be different from that of patients with dissection of the descending aorta. Initially, intensive drug therapy is the treatment of choice in all dissections. That approach allows the reactive edema to clear and the healing fibrotic process to begin, with a resulting decrease in bleeding during a subsequent operation. If the aortogram shows dissection of the ascending aorta (types I and II), immediate surgical repair is undertaken. However, if the dissection is limited to the descending aorta (type III) and if there are no absolute contraindications to medical therapy (Table 22-2), the hypotensive regimen outlined is begun. It has been noted [11] that localized saccular aneurysms can develop in as many as 15 percent of patients with type III aneurysms in the chronic phase. Prompt resection is required to prevent rupture.

Management after the acute phase is similar for patients in both groups since the underlying process of cystic medial necrosis makes all patients prone to either a redissection or a second dissection. The aims of chronic antihypertensive drug therapy are maintenance of the systolic pressure at 130 mm Hg or lower and continued reduction of cardiac contractility through the administration of propranolol. The follow-up consists of checking the patient for absence of pain, presence of peripheral pulses, elevation of

Table 22-2
Contraindications to Medical Therapy in Dissecting Aneurysm

Congestive heart failure
Pericardial tamponade
New aortic insufficiency
Symptomatic coronary ischemia
Symptomatic cerebral ischemia
Failure to control pain
Failure to reduce blood pressure

blood pressure, and murmurs in the aortic area. Serial chest x rays are important for the evaluation of the size of the aneurysm and/or of the area of graft insertion or aortic anastomosis. The prognosis for patients in both groups is good.

Assessment and Management

The Acute Phase

OBJECTIVE NO. 1

The patient should exhibit a reduction in blood pressure.
   To achieve the objective, the nurse should:

1. Give emergency antihypertensive drugs as ordered.
2. Elevate the head of the patient's bed 30 to 40 degrees to increase the orthostatic effect of the medication.
3. Monitor the patient's blood pressure in both arms as ordered.
4. Observe the patient for symptoms of gastric distress due to the hyperacidic effect of reserpine.
5. Instruct the patient how to change his position without performing the Valsalva maneuver, which may increase the force of his cardiac contractions and elevate his systolic blood pressure.

OBJECTIVE NO. 2

The patient should exhibit a reduction in cardiac demand and in the degree of congestive heart failure [6].
   To achieve the objective, the nurse should:

1. Maintain the patient at bed rest with his head elevated.

2. Allow him frequent rest periods.
3. Assist him with his basic hygiene care.
4. Observe him for peripheral and sacral edema.
5. Auscultate his lungs for the presence and degree of severity of rales.
6. Auscultate his heart for a third heart sound.
7. Measure his jugular venous pressure and observe his neck veins for distention.
8. Measure his urine output hourly; report it if it is below 30 ml.
9. Make sure that his diet is in accordance with his sodium restriction.

OBJECTIVE NO. 3

The patient should be free of pain.
   To achieve the objective, the nurse should:

1. Observe the patient for signs and symptoms of pain: moaning, rigidity, clutching of a painful area, and withdrawal from social contact.
2. Carefully elicit from him a description of the pain: its location, degree, duration, and radiation. Immediately report the pain if it increases; an increase may indicate a progression in the dissection or the presence of myocardial ischemia due to dissection involving the coronary ostia.
3. Employ comfort measures and prescribed narcotics as indicated by the patient's condition.

OBJECTIVE NO. 4

The patient's sources of external and internal stress should be controlled.
   To achieve the objective, the nurse should:

1. Place the patient in an area that is as quiet and free from traffic as possible.
2. Maintain a calm, competent attitude when giving him care.
3. Assess his verbal and nonverbal behaviors as indexes of stress.
4. Acknowledge his concerns about the uncertain outcomes of the dissection.
5. Discuss with him the purpose of the therapy.
6. Evaluate the results of visits by his family and friends, and encourage those visits if they seem to help him.
7. Administer sedatives as ordered.

OBJECTIVE NO. 5

The patient should be protected from the complications of bed rest.

To achieve the objective, the nurse should:

1. Assess the patient's skin in regard to changes in color, temperature, and sensation, paying particular attention to the pressure areas.
2. Change his position every two to three hours.
3. Observe him in regard to elimination and discuss with the physician any need for intervention.
4. If authorized by the physician, initiate passive range-of-motion exercises of the lower extremities as prophylaxis against deep venous thrombosis.
5. Observe him for the development of pain, temperature changes, and swelling of the lower extremities, particularly the calf, and report any changes immediately.

The Immediate Postoperative Phase

OBJECTIVE

The patient should recover from cardiothoracic surgery without complications.

1. Know the material in Chapter 21.

The Convalescent Phase

OBJECTIVE NO. 1

The patient should progress to full activity.

To achieve the objective, the nurse should:

1. While the patient assumes a sitting and/or a standing position, observe him for the following signs of postural hypotension: dizziness, lightheadedness, and a drop in systolic blood pressure.
2. Plan a progressively more demanding activity schedule and discuss it with the patient.
3. Assess the patient's tolerance for activity and record the clinical data [7]. The nurse should assess the patient's performance of activities in regard to his:
   a. Heart rate. It should not increase more than 20 beats per minute above resting level; that increase indicates approximately a 25-percent increase in the cardiac output.
   b. Heart rhythm. It should not become irregular.
   c. Blood pressure. The systolic pressure may increase 20 mm Hg; it should not drop. The diastolic pressure should not change.
   d. Respiration. It may increase in rate and depth. It should not become irregular, nor should the patient complain of dyspnea.
   e. Skin. The patient should not become diaphoretic.

OBJECTIVE NO. 2

The patient should maintain a systolic blood pressure of 130 mm Hg or below.

To achieve the objective, the nurse should:

1. Evaluate the patient's knowledge of hypertension. The patient should be able to:
   a. Describe hypertension as an increase in the pressure in the arteries.
   b. Explain hypertension as an increase in the work load of the heart and arteries.
   c. State the expected actions and untoward side effects of each medication prescribed.
   d. Correctly identify his medications by sight.
   e. Identify activities that elevate blood pressure.
   f. Identify methods of dealing with the stress-producing factors in his life.
2. Develop an educational plan to correct any deficiencies in the patient's knowledge.
3. Identify the factors that are related to any noncompliance with the health care regimen and discuss with the patient methods to increase his compliance [4, 9] (Table 22-3).
4. Teach the patient how to take his blood pressure if it is appropriate for him to do so.

The Posthospitalization Phase

OBJECTIVE NO. 1

The patient should be able to list and describe the signs and symptoms that should be reported to his physician.

To achieve the objective, the nurse should alert the patient to the following:

1. Chest pain of any kind (except the pain expected because of the incision).

Table 22-3
Factors Increasing Patient's Noncompliance with Health Care Regimen in Dissecting Aortic Aneurysm

Multiple medications
Complex regimens
Extended time in therapy
Side effects of therapy
Family problems
Inaccessibility of health care
Patient's confusion
Poor relations with health care providers
Patient's mistaken conviction that he is well because he feels well

2. Signs of congestive heart failure; for example, the patient:
   a. Avoids lying flat or is restless at night.
   b. Voids more at night.
   c. Is generally more fatigued.
   d. Has a decreased tolerance for exercise.
   e. Has feelings of heaviness in his chest.
   f. Has swelling of both ankles.
   g. Has a sudden increase in weight.

OBJECTIVE NO. 2

The patient knows the guidelines for activity.
   To achieve the objective, the nurse should make sure the activities:

1. Are based on the patient's home situation.
2. Are prescribed exactly by the physician.
3. Include activities of daily living, recreational activities, and occupational activities.

OBJECTIVE NO. 3

The patient should understand his dietary restrictions and their relationship to his condition.
   To achieve the objective, the nurse should:

1. Have the patient consult the nutritionist.
2. Know the material in Chapter 36.

Summary

The patient with acute aortic dissection characteristically has severe chest pain accompanied by differences in the blood pressure and/or the quality of the pulses in both arms. Immediate intervention to reduce the systolic blood pressure and decrease the force of the myocardial contractions is required if the dissection is to be arrested. To provide expert care, the nurse must understand thoroughly the objectives of treatment and the antihypertensive drugs commonly used. After the acute episode, the primary goals are to help the patient adapt to living with chronic hypertension and to provide him with the information he needs to respond to another emergency if one occurs.

Study Problems

1. Describe the chest pain characteristic of dissecting aortic aneurysm.
2. Name the key antihypertensive drugs used in the acute phase of treatment.
3. According to the DeBakey classification, what type of aneurysm is most amenable to medical therapy?
4. List four factors that may explain any noncompliance of the patient with the health care regimen after his discharge from the hospital.

Answers

1. Abrupt onset, and excruciating ("tearing") pain in the anterior chest.
2. Trimethaphan, reserpine, guanethidine, and methyldopa.
3. Type III.
4. Many drugs, complex regimens, extended time in therapy, side effects of therapy, family problems, inaccessibility of health care, confusion of patient, patient's poor relations with health care providers, patient's mistaken conviction that he is well because he feels well.

References

1. Applebaum, A., Karp, R. B., and Kirklin, J. W. Ascending versus descending aortic dissections. *Ann. Surg.* 183:296, 1976.
2. Dalen, J. E., et al. Dissection of the thoracic aorta—medical or surgical therapy? *Am. J. Cardiol.* 34:803, 1974.

3. DeBakey, M. E., Henley, W. S., Cooley, D. A., et al. Surgical management of dissecting aneurysms of the aorta. *J. Thorac. Cardiovasc. Surg.* 49:130, 1965.

4. Finnerty, F. A., Mattie, E. C., and Finnerty, F. A., III. Hypertension in the inner city. I. Analysis of clinic dropouts. *Circulation* 47:73, 1973.

5. Gebbie, K. M. *Classification of Nursing Diagnoses.* Clearinghouse: National Group for Classification of Nursing Diagnoses, St. Louis, 1976.

6. Goldstrom, D. K. Cardiac rest. *Am. J. Nurs.* 72:1812, 1972.

7. Gordon, M. Assessing activity tolerance. *Am. J. Nurs.* 76:72, 1976.

8. Hurst, J. W., and Logue, R. B. *The Heart* (2nd ed.). New York: McGraw-Hill, 1970. Pp. 1454, 1527.

9. Marston, M. V. Compliance with medical regimens: A review of the literature. *Nurs. Res.* 19:312, 1970.

10. Palmer, R. F., and Lasseter, K. C. Nitroprusside and aortic dissecting aneurysms. *N. Engl. J. Med.* 294:1403, 1976.

11. Parker, F. B., et al. Management of acute aortic dissection. *Ann. Thorac. Surg.* 19:436, 1975.

12. Shumway, N. E., and Griepp, R. B. Surgical Therapy of Dissection of the Aorta. In C. E. Anagnostopoulos (ed.), *Diseases of the Ascending Aorta.* Baltimore: University Park Press, 1976.

13. Slater, E. E., and DeSanctis, R. W. The clinical recognition of dissecting aortic aneurysm. *Am. J. Med.* 60:625, 1976.

14. Strong, W. W., Moggio, R. A., and Stansel, H. C., Jr. Acute aortic dissection: Twelve year medical and surgical experience. *J. Thorac. Cardiovasc. Surg.* 68:815, 1974.

15. Talbot, S. Clinical features and prognosis of dissecting aneurysms and ruptured saccular aneurysms. *Chest* 66:252, 1974.

16. Wheat, M. W., Jr. Treatment of dissecting aneurysms of the aorta: Current status. *Prog. Cardiovasc. Dis.* 16:87, 1973.

17. Wheat, M. W., Jr., Palmer, R. F., Bartley, T. D., et al. Treatment of dissecting aneurysms of the aorta without surgery. *J. Thorac. Cardiovasc. Surg.* 50:364, 1965.

18. Wolinsky, H. Comparison of medial growth of human thoracic and abdominal aortas. *Circ. Res.* 27:531, 1970.

Subacute and Acute Infective Endocarditis

Cathie E. Guzzetta

23

Endocarditis is an infection of the endocardium that involves primarily the heart valves. It may also affect the endocardium of the heart or the intima of the great vessels or both. In 1885, Osler stated that there were few diseases that presented such insurmountable obstacles to diagnosis [18]. Today endocarditis continues to baffle the clinician who is unfamiliar with its clinical manifestations.

Endocarditis should no longer be termed *bacterial* endocarditis, because, in addition to bacteria, other organisms, such as fungi and rickettsia, are known to be causative factors. The term *infective* endocarditis is preferred [2, 15]; and even more descriptive is the use of the name of the particular microorganism followed by the term endocarditis [5] (e.g., *Streptococcus viridans* endocarditis).

Before the days of antimicrobial therapy, infective endocarditis was classified according to the length of the patient's survival, and it was therefore divided into subacute endocarditis and acute endocarditis. Nearly everyone who had either form of endocarditis eventually died from it. The person with subacute endocarditis followed a chronic course and died in six to eight months [2]. The patient with acute endocarditis, on the other hand, suffered a sudden, life-threatening episode and usually died in the first six weeks.

At present, infective endocarditis is classified according to the virulence of the infecting organism.

Subacute endocarditis is generally produced by organisms of low virulence that have become opportunistically engrafted on abnormal heart valves. People with subacute endocarditis usually do not show signs of toxemia, and cardiac damage is seen only as a late complication. In contrast, acute endocarditis is produced by a highly virulent organism. Normal heart valves are often involved, and the patients show early clinical manifestations of cardiac damage, septic embolism, and toxemia [2, 5]. To present a complete picture of endocarditis, this chapter discusses both the subacute and the acute forms of the disease.

Objective

The critical care nurse should be able to describe the etiology, pathophysiology, clinical manifestations, complications, and management of subacute and acute infective endocarditis.

Achieving the Objective

To achieve the objective, the nurse should be able to:

1. Write a paragraph discussing the causes of subacute and acute infective endocarditis.
2. Compare and contrast the differences in the pathophysiological mechanisms of subacute and acute infective endocarditis.
3. List the major clinical manifestations and complications of subacute and acute infective endocarditis.
4. Describe the basic principles involved in doing diagnostic blood cultures and list the precautions that must be taken.
5. Contrast the therapeutic management of a patient with subacute infective endocarditis with the management of a patient with acute infective endocarditis.
6. Teach the patient and his family about the signs, symptoms, and complications of endocarditis and about prophylactic care.

How to Proceed

To develop an approach to subacute and acute infective endocarditis, the nurse should:

1. Read the material that follows.
2. Plan a staff conference to discuss the major causative factors in subacute and acute endocarditis. The discussion should cover:
   a. Dental problems.
   b. Skin lesions.
   c. Infections.
   d. Surgical procedures.
   e. Invasive treatments or examinations.
3. Construct a written care plan that includes the major objectives of nursing management and care.
4. Develop a teaching program for patients with endocarditis that includes information on:
   a. The role of the interdisciplinary health team.
   b. The basic principles of patient education.
   c. The written teaching content and audiovisual aids.
   d. A teaching booklet.

Case Study
Admission Assessment
Mr. S. P., a 50-year-old male, was admitted to the coronary care unit with the chief complaint of chest pain without radiation. The pain began the evening before his admission, it lasted for 15 to 20 minutes, and it was associated with nausea and shortness of breath. The patient said that he had no history of chest pain. He complained also of chills, fatigue, headache, and a poor appetite. He said that those symptoms began two weeks ago, and he called them "flulike" symptoms.

Mr. P. had had rheumatic fever as a child and he subsequently developed a murmur of mitral regurgitation. One and a half months before admission, he had had an abscessed tooth extracted. He had not had antimicrobial prophylaxis before or after the extraction.

Mr. P.'s profile and social history described him as a well-developed, 5' 10", 165-lb man who was lethargic and depressed during the admission interview. He was also reluctant to discuss his past medical history. He made no eye contact with his primary care nurse during the interview. He was a high-school graduate, and he worked five days a week, eight hours a day as a manufacturer of metal pipes.

Mr. P. was married. He had two daughters, aged 16 and 18, who were well and who lived at home. He was a practicing Baptist, and he sang every week in the church choir. He enjoyed fishing, bowling, and yardwork. He said that he had smoked 15 cigarettes a day for the past 25 years and that he drank one or two beers a day.

As mentioned, Mr. P.'s past medical history included rheumatic fever and a tooth extraction. He said that he had never had diabetes mellitus, hypertension, angina pectoris, cardiac failure, or myocardial infarction. This hospitalization was his first since childhood. He said that he had no food or drug allergies and that he had not been taking any medications prior to admission, except antacids for occasional indigestion.

Mr. P.'s father had had rheumatic fever, and he had died at age 52 of a myocardial infarction. Mr. P.'s mother was alive and well. The rest of his family history was not relevant. (The accompanying admission assessment sheet outlines the interview, history, and physical findings.)

After the admission interview, Mr. P. was attached to a continuous bedside cardiac monitor, which revealed that he had a sinus tachycardia. An intravenous 5% dextrose and water solution was begun using an 18-gauge steel needle. Mr. P.'s initial diagnostic orders called for a check of his vital signs every two hours, auscultation for any change in his cardiac murmur, and observation for any signs and symptoms of myocardial ischemia, cardiac decompensation, and dysrhythmias. The nurses were instructed to observe the patient carefully throughout each shift for any other signs that were consistent with the diagnosis of endocarditis.

The initial ECG suggested that Mr. P. had anteroseptal myocardial ischemia. The posteroanterior and lateral chest x rays were normal. Laboratory studies were done, including aerobic and anaerobic blood cultures. Mr. P. was placed on bed rest, and he was put on a 2-gm sodium diet.

Second Day
By the end of Mr. P.'s second day, his temperature had risen to 101°F; his pulse was 110, his blood pressure was 124/86, and his respirations were 18. His lethargy and depression continued. He had refused all food except liquids since his admission. He slept through his wife's and daughters' visits, spoke only when asked a question, and refused his morning bath.

The critical care nurses noted that Mr. P. had a new splinter hemorrhage on the ring finger of his left hand and two new conjunctival petechiae in his left eye. There was no change in the intensity or quality of his heart murmur. There were no clinical manifestations of myocardial ischemia or cardiac decompensation.

Based on Mr. P.'s clinical history and assessment, the presumptive diagnosis of subacute infective endocarditis was made by his primary physician. Mr. P. was given intravenous potassium penicillin G (10 million units in a 5% dextrose in water solution daily in divided doses, with 2500 units of heparin added to each 1000 ml). He was also given intramuscular streptomycin (0.5 gm twice a day).

The primary care nurse was concerned about Mr. P.'s mental attitude, and she had a conference with his attending physician, wife, and daughters (see Reflections).

Third Day
The next day, Mr. P.'s blood cultures were found to be positive for *Streptococcus viridans*, and the diagnosis of *Streptococcus viridans* endocarditis was made and entered in the nursing care plan.

The significant laboratory findings were a low red blood cell count, a low hemoglobin and hematocrit, an elevated erythrocyte sedimentation rate, a positive rheumatoid factor, urine 2^+ for protein with broad, coarsely granular casts and white and red blood cells. The cardiac enzyme levels were normal.

Fourth Day
By the end of the fourth day, Mr. P.'s temperature and other vital signs had returned to normal. He was transferred to the telemetry unit, where his primary care nurse followed his progress until his discharge 26 days later. He was put on a 1200-calorie general diet, and he was allowed restricted activities. Throughout Mr. P.'s hospitalization, he received intravenous penicillin.

Discharge
Before Mr. P.'s discharge, the primary care nurse held sessions with the patient and his wife and daughters to discuss prophylactic care and the prevention of complications (see Nursing and Medical Management, Objective No. 5).

Reflections

The primary care nurse was concerned about Mr. P.'s withdrawal and depression. But the coronary care unit was filled with critically ill patients who were being treated with the intraaortic balloon pump, who had recurrent ventricular fibrillation, and who were in need of lifesaving procedures. And so, although the primary care nurse was aware of Mr. P.'s psychological problems, she had little time to investigate their causes.

The second afternoon after Mr. P.'s admission, the unit was still very busy. Because the primary care nurse regarded Mr. P.'s behavior as a complication of his illness, she assumed the responsibility of identifying his problems and discussing them with the patient's attending physician and family. She discussed Mr. P.'s withdrawal behavior—his unwillingness to talk, eat, or visit with his family.

Mrs. P. said that she also was very concerned about her husband's behavior. She said that he had always considered himself a healthy man who had assumed a strong leadership role in the family. Also, she was quite upset about the possibility that he had had a heart attack. She said that Mr. P.'s father also had had rheumatic fever and that he had died at age 52 of an acute myocardial infarction. Her concern about the similarities in the histories of Mr. P. and his father were realistic. While glancing at the admission nurs-

Critical Care Nursing Admission Assessment

Head-to-Toe Approach

Date	Time	
		Pt. Name: *Mr. S.P.*　　　　Age: *50* Allergies: *NKA*
2-4		Admitted Bed No: *10*　Via: *wheelch.* Ad. Dx.: *R/O MI*
		T.: *100.4°F* A.P.: *110*　R.P.: *110*　R.: *16*　B.P. Supine R: *126/80* L: *124/80* Sitting: *124/76*
		Wt. (unit-scale): *165*　Ht.: *5'10"* ECG Rhythm: *Sinus tach.* Ectopy: *none*
		Informant: *Pt. - reliable historian*　　Last meal: *yesterday evening*
	1.	Chief complaint: *chest pain assoc. c̄ nausea + S.O.B. lasting 15-20 min.*
	2.	Hx. of present illness: *no previous hx. of chest pain, hx. of mitral regurgitation. flu-like symptoms past 2 wks. (chills, fatigue, headache, + poor appetite); hx. of dental extraction 1½ mo. ago c̄ no prophylactic antibiotics given before or after procedure*
	3.	Past medical Hx. (include all surgeries, hosp., diseases, injuries, blood trans.): *1st hospitalization since childhood; rheumatic fever as child → murmur of mitral regurgitation; no hx. of diabetes, hypertension, angina, cardiac fail.*
	4.	Family Hx.: *mother, wife, + children alive + well; father had hx. MI of rheumatic fever + died at age 52 of MI*
	5.	Current drugs: *antacids for occasional indigestion*
	6.	Alcohol and tobacco habits: *15 cigarettes/day × 25 yrs.; 1-2 beers/day*
	7.	Dietary and fluid needs: *dislikes fish*
	8.	Sleep and rest patterns: *sleep 6-7 hours/night*
	9.	Bowel and bladder habits: *eats fruit (apples) for occasional constipation*
	10.	Hygienic needs: *takes morning showers*
	11.	Psychosocial needs: *has always assumed a strong leadership role within family*
	12.	Occupation and education: *H.S. graduate metal pipe manufacturer - works 5 days/wk. 8 hrs./day*
	13.	Exercise habits: *none*
	14.	Spiritual needs: *active Baptist*
	15.	Personal interests: *sings in church choir, fishing, bowling, + yardwork.*
	16.	Family member interaction and availability: *wife + children (2 daughters age 16+18) present on admission. Family very concerned about pts. health*
	17.	Attitude towards illness and hospitalization: *Pt. requested wife to call Baptist minister. Extremely anxious about reasons for hospitalization for "just the flu."*

Physical Examination

Date	Time		
	18.	Gen. appearance: *no acute distress, lethargic* color: *pale* skin: *normal tissue turgor warm + dry*	
	19.	Neurological:	
		a) level of consciousness: *lethargic + depressed, oriented to time, place, + person*	
		b) cerebellar: *unable to assess posture + gait*	
		c) motor function: upper: *normal strength, movement + symm. normal muscle size* lower: *normal muscle size, movement + strength,*	
		d) sensory function: upper: *normal pain, touch, vibratory, + positional* lower: *normal pain, touch, symmetry vibratory + positional sense sense*	
		e) reflexes: *normal symmetrical reflexes*	
	20.	Head and face: *normal hair distribution + symmetry; no abnormal movement*	
	21.	Eyes: *bilateral conjunctival petechiae; Roth spots 2mm in R fundus at 2:00 c̄ surround. hemorrhagic zone*	
	22.	Ears: *no hearing loss, discharge, lesions, or edema*	
	23.	Nose: *normal sense of smell, no drainage, obstruction, tenderness or deformities*	
	24.	Mouth/throat: *normal lips gums, + tongue; poor oral hygiene; no cough, hoarseness,*	
	25.	Neck: *supple; normal contour, symmetry, + movement; no JNVD or hemoptysis*	
	26.	Chest: *normal contour + symmetry; bilateral expansion, left vent. heave at 5 LICS, MCL.*	
	27.	Breast: *normal appearance, size, + shape*	
	28.	Respiratory: *bilateral rhonchi which clear c̄ cough*	
	29.	Cardiac: *apical pulse regular; normal $S_1 + S_2$; no S_3, S_4 or rubs, grade $\overline{III}/\overline{VI}$ holosystolic (m) at LLSB c̄ radiation to left axilla.*	
	30.	Abdomen: *no scars, distention pain or tenderness, liver edge spleen not palpable*	
	31.	Genitourinary: *no bladder, renal or genital abnorm. 2+ bowel sounds*	
	32.	Extremities (all pulses): *normal, bilateral arterial pulses; splinter hemorrhages on distal 1/3 of nail on index + ring finger of rt. hand; no edema or clubbing; joints - no pain, swelling or inflammation*	
	33.	Back: *no scars, edema, or spinal abnormalities*	
	34.	Problems requiring possible referral service: *deferred until dx. confirmed*	
	35.	Teaching needs: *deferred until dx. confirmed*	
	36.	Other:	

		PROBLEM LIST: **ACTIVE**	**INACTIVE**
2-4		1. *rheumatic fever → (m) mitral regurgitation chest pain fever, chills x 2 wks. fatigue x 2 wks. headache x 2 wks. ↓ appetite x 2 wks. left ventricular heave conjunctival petechiae Roth spots splinter hemorrhage*	
		2. *poor dental hygiene*	
		3. *depression - 1st hospitalization since childhood.*	

Cathie E. Guzzetta, RN, CCRN
NURSE'S SIGNATURE

ing assessment sheet, the primary care nurse remembered that this hospitalization was the patient's first since his childhood. Mrs. P. and the nurse discussed the psychological impact that fact had on Mr. P.'s response to illness.

The primary physician said that Mr. P. had probably not had a myocardial infarction. Rather, his illness was probably the result of an infected heart valve caused by an organism entering the blood during his tooth extraction.

The group concluded that Mr. P. was having trouble changing his role from that of the family provider to that of a dependent critically ill patient. They felt that he was quite concerned about his condition and prognosis but was having difficulty expressing that concern. Finally, they agreed to discuss their concerns with Mr. P. the following day.

The next morning, the blood culture was found to be positive for *Streptococcus viridans*, confirming the diagnosis of subacute endocarditis. The primary physician talked with Mr. P. about the diagnosis, its cause, the pathological mechanisms involved, and his plan of medical care. Mr. P. asked how long he would be hospitalized, what his prognosis was, and when he could go back to work.

Later that day, the patient seemed much more relaxed. He said that he was relieved to know that he had not had a heart attack. His wife and primary care nurse discussed with Mr. P. their concerns about him. They talked about the psychological impact of illness and hospitalization. Mr. P. had several concerns and questions of his own—about the cardiac monitor, the bath procedure, his restricted activities, and his boredom. The primary care nurse answered the patient's questions about the cardiac monitor and the CCU routine. She gave him a copy of the progressive activity schedule and asked that he and his family help make out the care plan. They agreed that Mr. P., with the assistance of his wife, would do his own morning care. They discussed various kinds of diversional activities, and the primary care nurse requested a consultation with the occupational therapist.

Mr. P.'s primary care nurse knew that his negative response to his illness could affect his recovery. She believed that the patient's response was a very "real" complication. Viewing a patient as a psychobiological unit, she understood that therapy directed toward a patient's psychological response could produce a body response that is just as real as that produced by penicillin and other traditional forms of therapy.

Subacute Infective Endocarditis

Etiology

The organism that causes most cases of subacute infective endocarditis is *Streptococcus viridans*, a bacterium found in the oral cavity [2, 5, 8, 16]. *Streptococcus viridans* is an α-hemolytic organism of low virulence that becomes opportunistically engrafted on abnormal heart valves. Other causative organisms include a nonhemolytic *Streptococcus* strain (gamma streptococcus) and microaerophilic strains, commonly found in the mouth and intestinal, female genital, and respiratory tracts. *Streptococcus faecalis* (enterococcus), a more virulent strain, is found in the gastrointestinal and genitourinary tracts. The α-hemolytic and nonhemolytic streptococci cause more than 90 percent of the cases of subacute infective endocarditis. The remaining 8 to 10 percent of the organisms causing the disease are of low virulence; they include *Staphylococcus albus* and *Haemophilus influenzae*. About 1 percent of the patients have a mixed infection. Fungi (e.g., *Candida, Histoplasma, Aspergillus, Coccidioides, Blastomyces,* and *Cryptococcus*) have also been identified as causative organisms [2, 5, 10].

Pathogenesis

Streptococcus viridans is a selective bacterium that generally causes only the heart to become infected. Four mechanisms explain the selectivity and localization of the subacute infection: (1) preexisting valvular damage or other cardiac defects that cause a unique hemodynamic situation, (2) the development of sterile platelet-fibrin thrombi, (3) the presence of a bacteremia, and (4) a high titer of agglutinating antibodies for the infecting organism [6, 28, 29]. Those factors are discussed in the following paragraphs.

VALVULAR DAMAGE OR OTHER CARDIAC DEFECTS

The first mechanism involves preexisting valvular damage or other cardiac defects produced by rheumatic, congenital, or degenerative heart disease. Mitral and aortic regurgitation are the most common deformities. Among the congenital defects associated with endocarditis are small intraventricular septal defects, bicuspid aortic valves, coarctation of the aorta, tetralogy of Fallot, patent ductus arteriosus,

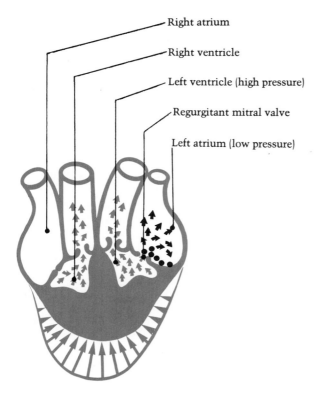

Right atrium

Right ventricle

Left ventricle (high pressure)

Regurgitant mitral valve

Left atrium (low pressure)

Figure 23-1
Hydrodynamic theory explaining the localization of lesions in subacute infective endocarditis. In the presence of mitral insufficiency, a regurgitant jet from the left ventricle to the left atrium during systole creates a reduction in the lateral pressure on the atrial side of the valve. The regurgitant flow causes a collection of particulate matter, an increase in local bacteria, and a reduction in nutrition in that area.

pulmonic stenosis, and idiopathic hypertrophic sub-aortic stenosis [2]. Prosthetic heart valves are also susceptible to infection [7, 8, 13, 16, 26].

Valvular damage or other cardiac defects can produce a hemodynamic situation that allows organisms to localize in the heart. Bacteria entering the body settle out of the bloodstream and localize around the irregularities of the valve [2]. The reason for that localization is not clearly understood although a hydrodynamic theory developed by Rodbard helps to explain it [21] (Fig. 23-1). According to Rodbard's theory,

the presence of valvular deformities creates a situation in which there is rapid blood flow, an incompetent valvular orifice, and a high pressure gradient. In mitral insufficiency, for example, the high left ventricular pressure observed during systole when the mitral valve is closed generates a high-velocity regurgitant jet from the left ventricle to the lower pressure of the left atrium [21]. The regurgitant jet produces a reduction in the lateral pressure on the atrial side of the valve, causing particulate matter to be deposited in the area because of a vortex-shedding effect, an increase in the local bacterial count, and a reduction in the endothelial nutrition. As a result, the atrium becomes highly susceptible to endocardial vegetation. Similar hemodynamic principles, relevant to the localization of bacteria may apply to other cardiac defects [28].

STERILE PLATELET-FIBRIN THROMBI

The second mechanism responsible for the localization of subacute endocarditis is the development of sterile platelet-fibrin thrombi [28]. The endothelial surface is traumatized as a result of turbulence and the Venturi effect produced by various cardiac defects. As a result of the trauma, sterile platelet-fibrin thrombi form on the injured heart leaflets. The sterile thrombi are foci for infection if an appropriate bacteria is introduced into the bloodstream.

BACTEREMIA

The third mechanism necessary for localization of the infection is the entry of the infecting organism into the body to produce bacteremia (fungemia or rickettsemia). In most cases, organisms entering the body are either of such low virulence or are few enough that they fail to implant on normal heart valves. Although transient bacteremia occurs frequently in normal people, it rarely produces valvular infection. People with valvular damage or other cardiac defects, however, are susceptible to those organisms owing to the factors just discussed.

Bacteremia is produced by organisms entering the blood during procedures that cause trauma to tissues. Because *Streptococcus viridans* is normally present in the oral cavity, dental disease or dental procedures may produce bacteremia. Surgical procedures or manipulations of the upper respiratory, genitourinary, and gastrointestinal tracts may also introduce organisms into the bloodstream [13] (see Nursing and Medical Management, Objective No. 1).

Fungal infections are frequently observed in patients whose physiological resistance is low. Fungemia may occur in people receiving long-term antibiotic or cytotoxic therapy, in those who are immunosuppressed as a result of an underlying disorder (malignant neoplasm, collagen vascular disease, hepatitis, or burns), or in those receiving steroid therapy [8]. It can develop also in people with diabetes mellitus, in those who have had cardiac surgery, in those who have transvenous plastic catheters, and in narcotic addicts who use unsterile equipment.

CIRCULATING ANTIBODIES

The fourth major mechanism responsible for the localization and production of subacute endocarditis is the development of a high titer of agglutinating antibodies for the infecting organism. The platelet-covered valvular lesions probably provide a favorable surface for the organism. Also, circulating antibodies permit large numbers of bacteria to adhere to the platelet-fibrin thrombi. By clumping the organisms, circulating antibodies enhance the localization and multiplication of the infection [12, 28, 30].

Pathology

The endocardial valvular lesions (called *vegetations*) develop slowly. They are orange, tan, or gray. When the lesions are studied microscopically, they are seen to contain an inner mass of necrotic collagen and elastin, with platelets, fibrin, neutrophils, lymphocytes, red blood cells, and bacteria. Their middle layer is composed primarily of bacteria. Their outer layer is composed of fibrin and bacteria. The superficial irregular lesions are easily torn away. The mitral valve lesions are usually located on the atrial side with growth that can extend into the atrial wall, but they can also involve the chordae tendineae on the ventricular side. Aortic lesions are generally found on the ventricular side of the valve although they may develop on either side of the leaflet. The aortic and mitral valves are the most common sites of endocardial infection; less common sites are the tricuspid and the pulmonic valves.

The infective process in subacute endocarditis can cause thinning or destruction of the valve, producing myocardial dysfunction and cardiac failure. In some instances, valvular thinning may also produce valvular aneurysms, which may rupture or perforate. Erosive complications, producing significant hemodynamic abnormalities, may result from the involvement of the chordae tendineae, papillary muscle, or conduction system [28].

After the lesions are treated with antimicrobial drugs, fibrin is deposited over the surface of the lesions, followed by the growth of granulation tissue that extends into the vegetations. Phagocytic cells ingest the bacteria and collagen is deposited while hyalinization and endothelialization take place. Calcification, scarring, and deformities of the valve are common during the healing process, which may take as long as two or three months [2].

Clinical Manifestations

The clinical signs and symptoms of subacute endocarditis are outlined in Table 23-1. They include those related to (1) a reaction to the infection, (2) cardiac involvement, (3) embolism, and (4) immunological disorders [23, 25]. Those four factors are discussed in the following paragraphs.

REACTION TO INFECTION

Generally 97 percent of the patients infected with a low-virulent organism (e.g., *Streptococcus viridans*) manifest subacute endocarditis by a persistent, low-grade fever (99°F–102°F) [6]. Although bacteria are continuously released from the vegetations and could produce other sites of infections, the immune and cellular defenses generally protect the rest of the body against the organisms involved in the subacute infection.

CARDIAC INVOLVEMENT

Often patients suffering from subacute endocarditis have some form of cardiac involvement (Table 23-1). About 90 to 95 percent of the patients have heart murmur(s) [2]. But murmurs may be absent, and occasionally they are heard only after several weeks of therapy [8]. "Changing" murmurs are rare although old murmurs frequently become louder. New murmurs may develop late in the course of the disease owing to some destructive cardiac complication, such as valve perforation or torn chordae tendineae.

Congestive heart failure is probably the most

Table 23-1
Clinical Findings in Subacute Infective Endocarditis

Reactions to infection
  Low-grade fever
  Chills, diaphoresis
  Cough
  Anorexia
  Muscle aching
  Malaise, fatigue
  Weight loss

Cardiac manifestations
  New murmur
  Change in the quality or intensity of an old murmur
  Congestive heart failure
  Myocardial ischemia or infarction
  Pericardial friction rub
  Clubbing of the fingers
  Conduction and/or rhythm disturbances

Embolic manifestations
  Confusion
  Psychotic behavior
  Visual field defects   *Central nervous system*
  Hemiplegia, hemiparesis   Cerebral vascular accident
  Aphasia, dysphasia   Mycotic cerebral aneurysm or rupture
  Convulsions   Transient ischemic attacks
  Coma

  Substernal chest pain with radiation to arms, neck, shoul-   *Cardiovascular system*
    der and associated with sweating, nausea, vomiting,   Myocardial ischemia
    shortness of breath   Myocardial infarction

  Sudden onset of abdominal pain with radiation to left
    axilla, shoulder, or precordium and associated with ele-   *Gastrointestinal system*
    vated temperature, chills, vomiting, leukocytosis,   Splenic infarction
    toxemia   Mesenteric infarction

  Flank pain with radiation to groin, associated with hema-   *Genitourinary system*
    turia, azotemia   Renal infarction

Immunological derangements producing hypersensitivity
    reactions
  Arthralgia
  Arthritis
  Petechiae
  Splinter hemorrhages
  Osler's nodes
  Janeway's lesions
  Roth's spots
  Focal glomerulitis, acute or chronic glomerulonephritis
  Mycotic aneurysm

Laboratory findings
  Positive blood culture
  Anemia
  Elevated erythrocyte sedimentation rate
  Normal or slightly elevated white blood count
  Positive rheumatoid factor (IgM anti-IgG antibodies)
  Elevated IgG and IgM levels
  Hematuria
  Albuminuria

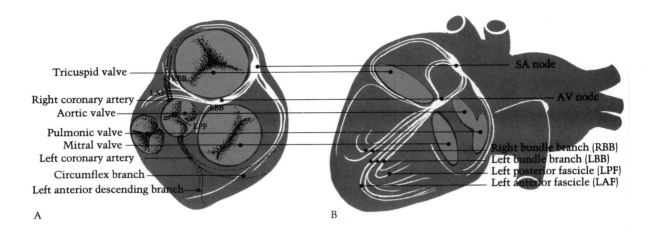

Tricuspid valve

Right coronary artery
Aortic valve

Pulmonic valve
Mitral valve
Left coronary artery

Circumflex branch
Left anterior descending branch

SA node

AV node

Right bundle branch (RBB)
Left bundle branch (LBB)
Left posterior fascicle (LPF)
Left anterior fascicle (LAF)

A

B

Figure 23-2
Anatomic relationships among heart valves, conduction system, and coronary arteries. A. Idealized superior view of a coronal section of the heart without the atria and the great vessels. B. Idealized anterior view of a sagittal section of the heart.

common complication of subacute endocarditis. It is produced by perforation, erosion, and/or rupture of the valves or other associated structures [8, 12]. The development of heart failure in a patient who has endocarditis carries a grave prognosis. The mortality is high despite effective antimicrobial therapy. Myocardial ischemia or infarction may be caused by obstructive lesions around the coronary ostia or by coronary embolism [2]. A pericardial friction rub occasionally develops.

Clubbed fingers may be seen in the late stages of endocarditis. Clubbing is diagnosed by a spongy feeling over the skin proximal to the nailbed. In some instances, there is flushing and pulsation of the ends of the fingers. The proximal nailbed becomes convex and rises above the plane of the finger. With successful antibiotic therapy, the nailbeds may return to their original shape.

Conduction abnormalities may occur in endocarditis [12, 29] because the noncoronary cusp and the right cusp of the aortic valve lie in close proximity to the conduction system (Figs. 23-2A,B). A prolonged PR interval, a new left bundle branch block, or a new right bundle branch block with or without left anterior hemiblock may indicate extension of the infection from the aortic valve into the myocardium with involvement of the conduction system. The mitral annulus, on the other hand, lies close to the atrioventricular node and to the bundle of His. Extension of the infection from the mitral valve to the atrioventricular node and bundle of His may cause junctional tachycardia, Mobitz type I (Wenckebach) second-degree atrioventricular block, or complete heart block. Ventricular dysrhythmias are occasionally ob-

served when myocardial infarction, abscess, or myocarditis is associated with endocarditis [8].

EMBOLISM

Arterial embolism is a common complication of endocarditis [5, 20] (Fig. 23-3). The friable vegetations, which are released continuously from the site of infection, produce changes in the arterioles. Occasionally larger embolic fragments detach to produce occlusion and small infarctions in the kidney, spleen, brain, or heart (Table 23-1). Pulmonary embolism and infarction develop occasionally in patients with right-sided endocarditis. Although embolic complications occur frequently in the early stage of the illness, embolization may continue for weeks, even after the institution of successful antimicrobial therapy.

IMMUNOLOGICAL DERANGEMENTS

Immunological derangements are also observed in subacute endocarditis. Agglutinating, complement-fixing, and opsonizing antibodies, specific for the infecting organism, are commonly found. The high titers of IgM anti-IgG antibodies (the rheumatoid factor) observed in many patients with subacute endocarditis inhibit the phagocytic action of the polymorphonu-

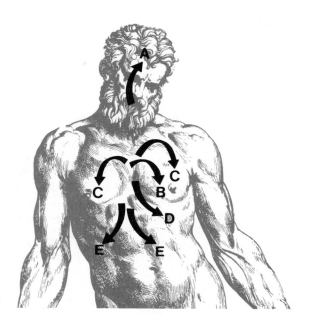

Figure 23-3
Common sites of arterial embolization in subacute infective endocarditis. A. Brain. B. Heart. C. Lungs. D. Spleen. E. Kidneys.

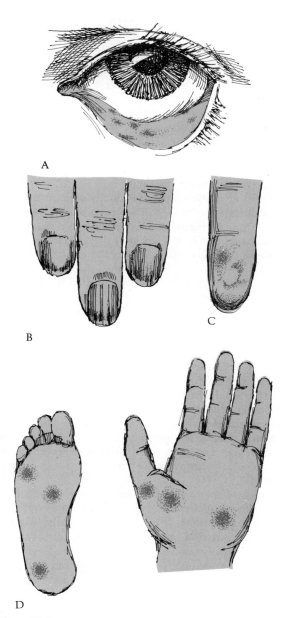

Figure 23-4
Findings in endocarditis. A. Conjunctival petechiae. B. Splinter hemorrhages. C. Osler's nodes. D. Janeway's lesions.

clear leukocytes. The high titers of IgM anti-IgG antibodies typically fall to low levels several weeks after effective antimicrobial therapy [29]. Other cryoglobulins representing circulating immune complexes and consisting of the IgG and IgM type are commonly found in patients with infective endocarditis [17].

Circulating immune complexes produce a hypersensitivity reaction manifested as an allergic vasculitis (Table 23-1). The arthralgia and arthritis associated with the disease are due to that allergic vasculitis. The classic peripheral manifestations of endocarditis, including petechiae, splinter hemorrhages, Osler's nodes, Janeway's lesions, and Roth's spots, are now also considered to be the results of the allergic vasculitis involving the arterioles rather than a result of embolic phenomena, as was believed [1, 25, 29].

Petechiae are commonly observed in the mucous membranes, conjunctiva (Fig. 23-4A) neck, wrist, and ankles. The petechiae are 1 to 2 mm in diameter, are flat, red, and nontender, and have white or gray centers. They appear in groups, and they fade away in a few days.

Splinter hemorrhages are frequently seen early in subacute infective endocarditis (Fig. 23-4B). They are black, longitudinal streaks generally found in the distal third of the nailbeds. The hemorrhages are not specific for endocarditis, however; they frequently are a result of trauma.

Osler's nodes are a major manifestation of endocarditis (Fig. 23-4C). They are cutaneous nodules that vary in size from 1 to 10 mm. They are reddish, tender lesions with a white center, and, classically, they are located on the pads of the distal fingers or toes, sides of the fingers, palms, or thighs.

Janeway's lesions are occasionally seen in subacute endocarditis (Fig. 23-4D). They are nontender, hemorrhagic, and erythematous lesions found on the palms, soles, arms, and legs. They are 1 to 5 mm in diameter, and they are accentuated when the extremity is elevated.

On funduscopic examination, Roth's spots are occasionally seen. They are boat-shaped retinal hemorrhages 3 to 10 mm in diameter, often have a pale or a white center, and are located near the optic nerve disk. They also occur in such diseases as leukemia, septicemia, and thrombotic thrombocytopenia.

Focal embolic glomerulitis and acute or chronic glomerulonephritis, previously thought to be the results of small embolisms, are now also believed to be due to an allergic vasculitis [23, 29]. The lesions may be associated with hematuria, acute renal failure, and uremia. The early administration of effective antimicrobial therapy is often helpful in reversing the pathological changes associated with the complications [1].

Mycotic aneurysm associated with both immunological abnormalities and embolism is a rare but serious complication of subacute endocarditis. Injury from deposition of immune complexes in the arterial wall may, in combination with microembolism, produce inflammation, necrosis, thinning, and dilatation of the artery. Mycotic aneurysms may rupture months or years after the subacute illness. Depending on their location, many mycotic aneurysms are potentially lethal.

Laboratory Findings

A normochromic, normocytic anemia occurs in 50 to 80 percent of patients with subacute endocarditis. Increased erythrocyte sedimentation rates are frequently observed. Other abnormal laboratory findings are described in Table 23-1 [2, 5, 28, 29].

Diagnosis

A high index of suspicion is the most important factor in the diagnosis of endocarditis [5]. Suspicion is warranted about any patient who presents with a heart murmur and a fever of unknown origin. He must be evaluated in regard to portals of entry of the infecting organism and whether he is undergoing chronic steroid, cytotoxic, or antibiotic therapy. The clinical diagnosis of subacute infective endocarditis depends on identifying the causative organism.

Antimicrobial therapy should not be instituted until an adequate number of blood cultures have been obtained. Approximately 15 percent of patients have negative blood cultures, even though they show clinical and pathological evidence of endocarditis [2, 5, 8]. Blood cultures may be negative because the culture techniques used are inappropriate for low levels of bacteria or for unusual organisms. Probably the most common cause of negative blood cultures, however, is the early administration of antibiotics that suppress bacteremia when the culture samples are taken [2]. Echocardiography, ECGs, gallium scans, and cardiac catheterization may occasionally be helpful in making the diagnosis [17].

Treatment

Management of the patient with subacute infective endocarditis entails: (1) identifying the portals of entry for the suspected infecting organism, (2) assessing the patient for clinical manifestation and complications of subacute infective endocarditis, (3) administering antimicrobial therapy to kill the causative organism for a long enough time to bring about sterilization of the vegetations, (4) preventing iatrogenic complications, and (5) teaching the patient about his illness (see Nursing and Medical Management).

The treatment of the disease depends on what the causative organism is. Streptococci (except enterococci) are very sensitive to penicillin. In most cases of *Streptococcus viridans* endocarditis, it is recommended that the patient receive 10 million units of potassium penicillin G daily, administered as a continuous intravenous infusion in a 5% dextrose and water solution. Heparin (2500 units/1000 ml) is added to reduce the incidence of postinfusion phlebitis, which occurs with high doses of penicillin. Streptomycin (0.5 gm by intramuscular injection twice a day) is also recommended. When combined with streptomycin or certain other aminoglycosides, penicillin has a higher potency and thus a greater bactericidal effect in regard to certain organisms. The treatment is continued for at least 28 days (generally four to six weeks) [5].

While he is treated with antimicrobial drugs, the patient is continually assessed for the signs and symptoms of ongoing infection. Persistent fever may indicate that the antimicrobial therapy is inadequate or inappropriate or that another infection, one caused by a different organism, has been superimposed on the original infection. It should be remembered, however, that embolism and petechiae may continue even after adequate therapy has been given.

After the treatment is completed, the patient is thoroughly evaluated for recurrent symptoms or other abnormal reactions. Blood cultures are done every other week for six weeks after the completion of treatment. A month of convalescence is recommended to promote the endocardial healing process [5]. The patient must be thoroughly educated about his disease and the need for prophylactic care (see Nursing and Medical Management).

Although the primary management of endocarditis involves the use of antibiotic therapy, valvular replacement (see Chap. 21) has recently been used to treat patients in whom antimicrobial therapy fails to eradicate the disease or in whom lethal complications develop [15, 27]. The indications for surgery are congestive heart failure due to valvular disruption that develops despite vigorous medical measures, resistant infection, or embolism [3, 6, 7, 14, 19]. Although active infection is not a contraindication to surgery, antimicrobial therapy must be continued throughout the preoperative and postoperative periods.

Acute Infective Endocarditis

Etiology

Typically acute infective endocarditis is produced by a highly virulent organism that localizes on normal heart valves and produces rapid and extensive cardiac damage. The primary infection site is generally remote from the heart.

Staphylococcus aureus causes 50 to 80 percent of the acute infections. Other organisms are *Diplococcus, Streptococcus pyogenes, Neisseria gonorrhoeae, Neisseria meningitidis, Escherichia coli, Proteus, Klebsiella, Pseudomonas, Salmonella, Hemophilus, Serratia, Listeria, Bacteroides, Candida*, and *Aspergillus*.

Pathogenesis

It appears that the only mechanism responsible for the pathogenesis of acute endocarditis is the presence of bacteremia produced by a highly virulent organism. Because the organisms involved in acute endocarditis are highly virulent, only a few are needed to establish the infection. Fifty to 60 percent of the acute infections involve normal heart valves [28]. The aortic valve is the one most commonly affected. Because the hemodynamic mechanisms (discussed under Subacute Infective Endocarditis) are not important in the pathogenesis of the infection, the right heart valves are more frequently involved in the acute form of the disease, particularly in the narcotic addict.

The portals of entry are septic foci from meningitis or pneumonia, minor skin infections, furuncles, contaminants during open heart surgery, arteriovenous cannulas used for hemodialysis, infected venipuncture sites (particularly those used for total parenteral nutrition therapy), indwelling transvenous electrodes used for cardiac pacemakers, and contaminants from unsterile, self-administered IV injections. Surgery, disease, or invasive procedures involving the genitourinary or gastrointestinal tract have also been found to introduce the infection [2, 5, 7, 13, 15, 26, 28].

Pathology

The vegetations in acute endocarditis develop rapidly; they appear to be larger and softer than those in subacute endocarditis. They also tend to be more hemorrhagic, with marked inflammatory changes, granulation tissue, and polymorphonuclear infiltration. As a result, there is a greater tendency for larger vegetations to break away, leaving ulcerated lesions on the valve leaflets. The inflammatory process may spread into underlying tissue, causing destruction of the papillary muscle, chordae tendineae, and conduction system [28].

Clinical Manifestations

The clinical manifestations of acute endocarditis depend on the causative organism and on the severity of the disease. The clinical picture in acute endocarditis, however, is generally more intense and serious than in subacute endocarditis.

REACTION TO INFECTION

A high-grade fever (103°F to 104°F), recurrent chills, prostration, and weight loss are common reactions to the infection. Leukocytosis, anemia, pyuria, hematuria, and proteinuria are commonly present.

CARDIAC INVOLVEMENT

Frequently, cardiac murmurs are not present when the person is admitted to the CCU; however, the rapid destruction of the valve in acute endocarditis may produce new murmurs or striking changes in the intensity or quality of an old murmur due to perforation of a valve or to functional hemodynamic changes [12]. Although endocarditis usually produces regurgitant murmurs, vegetations occasionally are large enough to cause stenosis of the valve and stenotic murmurs.

A variety of other destructive hemodynamic changes occur as a result of the large, friable lesions associated with acute infective endocarditis. The valves may develop an aneurysm, a tear, a perforation, or a rupture. Congestive heart failure, the most common cause of death in patients with endocarditis [8], often is a result of the degenerative process. Extension of the infection from the valve through the myocardial wall may lead to the formation of a fistula, abscess, ventricular septal defect, or a conduction or rhythm disturbance (see Fig. 23-2), pericarditis, and external rupture leading to cardiac tamponade.

EMBOLISM

Embolism and occlusion of major arterial vessels are serious problems that occur often. Fungal infections characteristically produce fragments large enough to block major vessels. The common sites of embolism are the coronary arteries, lungs, spleen, kidney, brain, and mesenteric arteries. The embolism produces ischemia and infarction of the affected organs.

IMMUNOLOGICAL DERANGEMENTS

Immunological derangements, producing hypersensitivity reactions, are observed in acute endocarditis also. Roth's spots, Janeway's lesions, and petechiae are commonly found (see Subacute Infective Endocarditis). Mycotic aneurysms, frequently seen in subacute endocarditis, are less common in acute endocarditis when the infecting agent is *Staphylococcus aureus*.

Diagnosis

Because the organisms involved are highly virulent, acute endocarditis is a medical emergency, and it demands immediate treatment. Death may occur in hours [2, 12].

A careful history is taken to evaluate the patient in regard to recent skin lesions, genitourinary or gastrointestinal disease or manipulation, narcotics use, and other septic factors. Any chronic steroid, cytotoxic, or antibiotic therapy must be identified. Murmurs (not usually present in the early stages of the disease) and embolic complications are late signs of severe valvular damage. Fever is an important sign but it is usually too general a sign to have diagnostic value. However, when a high-grade fever is observed in combination with acute hemodynamic impairment, acute endocarditis should be considered.

The single most important factor in the diagnosis of acute endocarditis is identification of the infecting organism. The need to do enough blood cultures before antimicrobial therapy is begun cannot be overemphasized (see Subacute Infective Endocarditis). The question arises, however, as to how long antimicrobial therapy should be delayed in order to complete the diagnostic studies. If the patient is acutely ill, with rigor, a spiking fever, and heart failure, three to five culture samples should be taken at 5- to 10-minute intervals. The administration of antimicrobial therapy should follow promptly. Assessment is made often to look for clinical manifestations, such as petechiae, embolic phenomena, and new or changing murmurs, that could confirm the diagnosis.

Treatment

Beyond the brief period of time required to do the blood cultures, there must be no delay in giving antimicrobial therapy to the patient who has acute endocarditis. Because the patient's condition is serious and the destructive process associated with the acute illness is rapid, the nurse must anticipate the objectives of care and be prepared to institute promptly the appropriate therapeutic measures. The choice of antimicrobial medication is frequently made before the results of the microbiological studies have been completed. The most active and potentially least dangerous drugs that will produce complete sterilization of the vegetations are selected. *Staphylococcus aureus* endocarditis is treated with 50 million units of potassium penicillin G in a continuous 24-hour intravenous drip [2]. Vancomycin is used for patients allergic to penicillin. Methicillin or oxacillin is used for penicillin-resistant strains of staphylococci; carbenicillin, ampicillin, kanamycin, colistin, and gentamicin are used for gram-negative organisms, and amphotericin B is used for fungi.

In addition, streptomycin and probenecid are often administered. Although the duration of treatment has not been clearly established, four to eight weeks is usually considered a sufficient period of time. The treatment of other infecting organisms depends on what organism is involved. Surgical valvular replacement is an important mode of therapy for the patient with acute endocarditis complicated by severe congestive failure (see Subacute Infective Endocarditis). The other objectives of care are the same as that for subacute infective endocarditis (see Nursing and Medical Management).

Endocarditis Complicating Cardiac Surgery

The remarkable advances of cardiac surgery have produced new opportunities for endocardial infection. Valvular infection has been associated with the use of prosthetic valves and patches, silk sutures, contamination of the membrane oxygenator and operating room equipment, postoperative wounds, lung and catheter complications, as well as bacteremia during the late convalescent period [2, 5, 7, 15, 22, 26]. It is recommended that required dental procedures be done several weeks before cardiac surgery whenever possible in an attempt to reduce the incidence of late postoperative endocarditis [13]. Fortunately, only a small percentage of patients develop infective endocarditis after cardiac surgery. The common infective organism in those patients is *Staphylococcus.*

Frequently, endocarditis that develops in the early postoperative period is not recognized because of the administration of prolonged, prophylactic antibiotic therapy. Since medication is generally continued during the patient's hospitalization, the blood cultures are usually negative within a few days after surgery. If a patient develops chills, marked toxemia, and a fever more than three days postoperatively, endocarditis should be suspected. Endocarditis is also suggested by fever, chills, leukocytosis, and a new murmur that occurs as late as 4 to 12 weeks or up to several years after surgery. If the infection develops on a prosthetic valve, it is extremely difficult to eradicate it without reoperation. After his discharge from the hospital, the patient who has a prosthetic valve must be educated about endocarditis and his need for prophylactic antibiotic care during dental and surgical procedures (see Nursing and Medical Management, Objective No. 5).

Marantic Endocarditis

Marantic endocarditis (known also as degenerative verrucous endocarditis, terminal endocarditis, and endocarditis simplex) is a nonbacterial form of endocarditis. It is characterized by the development of sterile thrombi on cardiac valves. Although marantic endocarditis is generally seen in patients with terminal malignant tumors or disease, it may be associated with a variety of disorders, such as acute pneumonia, pulmonary embolism, glomerulonephritis, peritonitis, and other acute illnesses [5, 29].

Previously scarred heart valves appear to be more susceptible to marantic endocarditis than are normal valves. The precipitating factor, however, is related to blood clotting derangements that are a part of the underlying disease [29].

The lesions of marantic endocarditis are important because they can cause peripheral arterial embolism that results in infarction of the brain, kidney, spleen, or myocardium. Although anticoagulation therapy may be useful in preventing recurrent embolic complications, there is no definitive therapy.

Libman-Sacks Endocarditis

Systemic lupus erythematosus (SLE) is the most common collagen disease that characteristically produces injury to the vascular system. Libman-Sacks endocarditis is a common manifestation of SLE, occurring in 50 percent of the cases. A nonbacterial form of endocarditis, it occurs as a late complication of SLE. The myocardium and pericardium may also be affected, producing cardiac conduction disturbances, pericarditis, pericardial effusion, and tamponade [5].

Nursing and Medical Management

OBJECTIVE NO. 1

The patient should be assessed for possible portals of entry for the suspected infecting organism.

To achieve the objective, the nurse should:

1. Assess the patient for a history of:
   a. Heart valve damage or other cardiac defects.
   b. Dental problems or dental procedures: poor dental hygiene, caries, periodontal or periapical disease, dental extractions, fillings, cleaning, root canal or bridge work, poorly fitting dentures, or trauma to gingivae.
   c. Skin lesions: trauma, lacerations, puncture sites from intravenous needles or intramuscular injections, or skin rash or eruptions.
   d. Infections of or from: the skin, lungs, urinary tract, a septic abortion, an incision and drainage of an abscess, endometritis, or tonsillitis.
   e. Surgical procedures:
      (1) Ears, nose, or throat (tonsil, adenoid) surgery.
      (2) Cardiac valve surgery.
      (3) Gastrointestinal tract (colon, rectal, hemorrhoidal) surgery.
      (4) Genitourinary tract surgery (and urethral or prostatic manipulations).
      (5) Obstetrical surgery.
   f. Invasive examinations or treatments: bronchoscopy, endoscopy, cystoscopy, sigmoidoscopy, indwelling urinary or venous catheterization, arteriovenous shunts for renal dialysis, indwelling transvenous electrodes for cardiac pacemakers.
2. Determine whether the patient has recently been taking antibiotics or cytotoxic medications.

3. Identify immunosuppression resulting from the administration of steroids or from an underlying disease (malignant neoplasm, collagen vascular disease, hepatitis, burns).

OBJECTIVE NO. 2

The patient should be assessed for the clinical manifestations and complications of infective endocarditis.

To achieve the objective, the nurse should:

1. Assess the patient frequently to help determine the severity of the disease and to help confirm the diagnosis.
2. Assess the patient for any clinical manifestations of:
   a. The infection (temperature, blood cultures, and laboratory studies; see Table 23-1).
   b. Cardiac involvement (heart rate, regularity, rhythm, blood pressure, respiration, and heart murmur (if any). Listen for new or changing murmur and note where it occurs in the cardiac cycle (i.e., is it systolic or diastolic?), and its pitch, intensity, duration, and radiation. Be alert for new organic murmurs due to rupture of a valve or the papillary muscle, torn chordae tendineae, fever, anemia, or hypermetabolism.
   c. Cardiac complications:
      (1) Signs and symptoms of congestive heart failure as a complication of perforation, erosion, or rupture of the valve.
      (2) Pericarditis or a pericardial friction rub.
      (3) Clubbing of the proximal nailbeds.
      (4) A conduction disturbance, such as a prolonged PR interval, new left bundle branch block, or new right bundle branch block with or without left anterior hemiblock.
      (5) A dysrhythmia, such as junctional tachycardia, Mobitz type I (Wenckebach) second-degree atrioventricular block, complete heart block, and ventricular dysrhythmias.
   d. Arterial embolism to the central nervous, cardiovascular, gastrointestinal, or genitourinary system (see Table 23-1).
   e. Immunological derangements producing hypersensitivity reactions (see Table 23-1).
3. Order and evaluate the laboratory studies prescribed by the physician (see Table 23-1).

OBJECTIVE NO. 3

The patient should receive treatment that aims at sterilizing the vegetations.

To achieve the objective, the nurse should:

1. Supervise the drawing of blood samples for culturing *before* antimicrobial therapy is administered. The nurse should explain the procedure to the patient.
   a. Clean the patient's skin and the rubber diaphragm on top of the culture tubes with a solution of 2% iodine in 70% alcohol. After a two-minute drying time, remove iodine with a 70% isopropyl alcohol solution before doing the venipuncture. Strict aseptic technique is essential to prevent contamination of the blood cultures.
   b. In the less acutely ill patient, draw five or six blood samples for culturing over the period of time specified by the physician. In acutely ill patients, draw three to five blood samples at 5- to 10-minute intervals. Each sample should be taken from a different venous site.
   c. Incubate each sample under both anaerobic and aerobic conditions.
   d. Label the blood culture tubes.
2. Determine whether the patient has a history of allergic reactions to antimicrobial medication.
3. When the organism is identified, write its name on the patient's care plan.
4. Explain to the patient the need for a 28-day (or longer) course of continuous intravenous antimicrobial therapy.
5. Administer antimicrobial therapy around the clock as ordered by the physician.
6. Be alert to any allergic reactions to penicillin or other antimicrobial drugs [4]. The nurse should know that:
   a. The allergic reactions to penicillin include mild skin rashes, hives, urticaria, fever, diarrhea, and anaphylactic shock (profound circulatory failure). If the patient has an allergic reaction, the nurse should assess the patient and consult with the physician before giving the next dose. Treatment for anaphylactic shock includes administering intravenous epinephrine (0.5 mg of a 1 : 10,000 solution). The dose should be repeated every 5 to 15 minutes until the patient responds. Other possible treatments are airway maintenance, cardiopulmonary resuscitation, use of a tourniquet above the injection site to delay absorption, and intravenous administration of fluids, aminophylline, or hydrocortisone.
   b. The adverse effects of streptomycin include possible irreversible damage to the eighth cranial nerve, causing dizziness, lack of balance, and hearing loss.

OBJECTIVE NO. 4

The patient should be protected against iatrogenic complications of intravenous therapy [9, 11].

To achieve the objective, the nurse should:

1. Wash her hands and maintain strict aseptic technique while preparing for and giving intravenous therapy.
2. Prepare the patient's skin for venipuncture using tincture of iodine (a solution of 2% iodine in 70% alcohol). After a two-minute drying time, the nurse should wash off the iodine solution with 70% isopropyl alcohol. She applies the solutions with friction, working from the center to the periphery. An iodophor skin preparation may be used for patients with skin sensitivities, but it should not be washed off with alcohol because its germicidal action depends on the sustained release of free iodine.
3. Use "scalp vein" (steel) needles when possible in an attempt to reduce the incidence of catheter-related infection and phlebitis. The nurse should record the needle or catheter size and the date, time, and site of the venipuncture.
4. Tape the needle securely to avoid to-and-fro motion, which could transport bacteria into the puncture site.
5. Apply a sterile dressing and a topical antibiotic preparation.
6. Make sure that the needle or catheter does not remain in place more than 24 to 48 hours.
7. During administration of continuous intravenous penicillin, add heparin (2500 units/1000 ml of a 5% dextrose and water solution) to reduce the incidence of postinfusion phlebitis associated with high-dose penicillin therapy.
8. Replace the intravenous solutions every 24 hours.
9. Change the intravenous tubing at least once every 24 hours (preferably when the intravenous solution is changed). The time and date of the change should be written on the tubing.

10. Using aseptic technique, clean the venipuncture site every 24 hours with iodine and alcohol and redress it. The time and date of the change should be written on the dressing.
11. Examine the venipuncture site at least every eight hours for signs and symptoms of phlebitis or infection (redness, drainage, swelling, pain, heat, or induration). If the catheter insertion is traumatic, the nurse should record that fact in the notes and observe the site according to the protocol just described.

OBJECTIVE NO. 5

The patient should be able to describe his illness and his prophylactic care.

To achieve the objective, the nurse should:

1. Teach the patient (and family) about endocarditis. The teaching should include information related to:
   a. The normal functioning of the heart and the heart valves (the nurse should use heart models and drawings).
   b. A definition of endocarditis and why the patient is susceptible to it. (Susceptible patients are those who have a history of endocarditis, cardiac surgery, prosthetic heart valves, or rheumatic, congenital, or degenerative heart disease that has produced valvular deformities or other cardiac defects.)
   c. The portals of entry for the infecting organism (see Objective No. 1):
      (1) Sites of dental problems.
      (2) Skin lesions.
      (3) Infections.
      (4) Sites of surgical procedures.
      (5) Sites of invasive tests or manipulations.
   d. The pathophysiologic changes in endocarditis and the patient's susceptibility to reinfection.
   e. The signs and symptoms of endocarditis such as chills, fever, sweating, fatigue, weight loss, and anorexia.
   f. Directions about taking one's own temperature.
   g. The necessity of contacting a physician at the first sign of fever or reinfection.
   h. The necessity of returning for follow-up blood culture studies every two weeks for six weeks after the completion of antimicrobial therapy.
   i. Restrictive activities (no strenuous activities, sports, or work) for one month to help the healing process.
   j. Good oral hygiene—brushing the teeth twice a day with a soft-bristled toothbrush, using a firm, gentle motion and avoiding trauma to the gums. The patient should also be told not to use a Water-Pik, dental floss, toothpicks, or any other devices that might cause the gums to bleed [1]. The patient should be told about the importance of regular dental examinations (even the patient who wears dentures).
   k. Birth control and pregnancy. Because birth control pills may enhance embolic activity in susceptible patients, they are generally not recommended. IUDs should also be avoided because they provide a portal of entry for infection. Other methods of birth control should be discussed with the patient. Pregnant women should be told about the need for antimicrobial prophylactic care during labor and delivery.
   l. The need for antimicrobial prophylactic care before and after the procedures listed in No. 1c. The patient must be told that although his physician and dentist are aware that people susceptible to endocarditis need prophylactic care before dental and some medical procedures, it is the patient's responsibility to tell his physician and dentist about his history of valvular heart disease and/or endocarditis.
2. Provide the patient with the information published by the American Heart Association in the booklet "Prevention of Endocarditis," which discusses what groups of people are susceptible to endocarditis, lists the dental and medical procedures and instrumentation that are associated with the development of bacteremia, and suggests dosages for prophylactic antimicrobial therapy.
3. Provide the patient with the name and phone number of the attending cardiologist and the primary care nurse.

Summary

Untreated infective endocarditis is potentially lethal. The possibility of error in making the diagnosis can be reduced by a thorough history taking, physical examination, and blood culture studies made before antimicrobial medications are administered. Long-term intravenous antimicrobial therapy is used to sterilize the vegetations. Occasionally, surgical intervention is needed to eradicate the infection and to replace the damaged valve.

Patient education is an important part of the therapeutic regimen. The critical care nurse must understand the etiology, pathophysiology, diagnosis, and treatment of infective endocarditis. A thorough understanding of the disease enables the nurse to play an independent, interdependent role in the assessment and management of infective endocarditis—and in its prevention.

Study Problems

1. The common causative organism in subacute infective endocarditis is:
   a. *Streptococcus faecalis.*
   b. *Streptococcus viridans.*
   c. *Staphylococcus aureus.*
   d. *Staphylococcus epidermidis.*
2. All of the following play a causative role in subacute infective endocarditis except:
   a. Abnormal heart valves that cause a unique hemodynamic situation.
   b. Sterile platelet-fibrin thrombi.
   c. Bacteremia.
   d. A high titer of agglutinating antibodies.
   e. A highly invasive and virulent infecting organism.
3. The destructive and infective process(es) in subacute endocarditis is (are):
   a. Eventual thinning of the valve.
   b. Rupture of the valve.
   c. Erosion of the chordae tendineae and papillary muscle.
   d. Cardiac failure.
   e. All the above.
4. The clinical manifestation(s) of subacute infective endocarditis is (are):
   a. Fever.
   b. Embolism.
   c. Immunological disorders.
   d. Cardiac complications.
   e. All the above.
5. The most common lethal complication in endocarditis is:
   a. Embolism.
   b. Septic shock.

c. Congestive heart failure.
d. Myocardial infarction.
6. Petechiae, splinter hemorrhages, Osler's nodes, Janeway's lesions, and Roth's spots are caused by:
   a. Embolic phenomena.
   b. An allergic vasculitis.
   c. Sterile platelet-fibrin thrombi.
   d. Bacteremia.
7. The treatment of endocarditis includes all of the following except:
   a. Antimicrobial therapy.
   b. Prevention of complications.
   c. Restricted activities.
   d. Prophylactic care.
   e. Steroid therapy.
8. Before the patient with endocarditis is discharged, he must be taught about:
   a. The signs and symptoms of endocarditis.
   b. His need for prophylactic care.
   c. The possible portals of entry for the infecting organism.
   d. All the above.

Answers

1. b.
2. e.
3. e.
4. e.
5. c.
6. b.
7. e.
8. d.

References

1. Bayer, A. S., Theofilopoulos, A. N., Eisenberg, R., et al. Circulating immune complexes in infective endocarditis. *N. Engl. J. Med.* 295:1500, 1976.
2. Bornstein, D. L. Bacterial Endocarditis. In H. L. Conn and O. Horwitz (eds.), *Cardiac and Vascular Diseases.* Philadelphia: Lea & Febiger, 1971.
3. DaLuz, P. L. Acute infection of the heart. *Heart Lung* 2:422, 1973.
4. Deliee, S., and Cardoni, A. A. Antimicrobials: Team effort helps keep wonder drugs wonderful. *Nurs. '75* 5:22, 1975.
5. Dorney, E. R. Endocarditis. In J. W. Hurst (ed.), *The Heart* (3rd ed.). New York: McGraw-Hill, 1974.

6. Everett, E. D. Infective endocarditis. *Mo. Med.* 75:167, 1978.

7. Finland, M. Current problems in infective endocarditis. *Mod. Concepts Cardiovasc. Dis.* 16:53, 1972.

8. Garvey, G. J., and Neu, H. C. Infective endocarditis: An evolving disease. *Medicine* 57:105, 1978.

9. Goldmann, D. A., Maki, D. G., Rhame, F. S., et al. Guidelines for infection control in intravenous therapy. *Ann. Intern. Med.* 79:848, 1973.

10. Grehl, T. M., Cohn, L. H., and Angell, W. W. Management of candida endocarditis. *J. Thorac. Cardiovasc. Surg.* 63:118, 1972.

11. Guzzetta, C. E. Effects of buffered glucose solutions on the incidence of postinfusion phlebitis. *Circulation* III:252, 1974.

12. Hutter, A. M., and Moellering, R. C. Assessment of the patient with suspected endocarditis. *J.A.M.A.* 235:1603, 1976.

13. Kaplan, E. L., Anthony, B. F., Bisno, A. L., et al. Prevention of bacterial endocarditis. (American Heart Association Committe Report) *Circulation* 56:139A, 1977.

14. Kinsley, R. H., Colsen, P. R., and Bakst, A. Emergency valve replacement for primary infective endocarditis. *South Afr. Med. J.* 53:86, 1978.

15. Maschak, B. J. Patient education and prevention of endocarditis. *Nurs. Clin. North Am.* 11:319, 1976.

16. McNeill, K. M., Strong, J. E., and Lockwood, W. R. Bacterial endocarditis: An analysis of factors affecting long-term survival. *Am. Heart J.* 95:448, 1978.

17. Miller, M. H., and Cassey, J. I. Infective endocarditis: New diagnostic techniques. *Am. Heart J.* 96:123, 1978.

18. Osler, W. Malignant endocarditis. *Lancet* 1:415, 1885.

19. Parrott, J. C., Hill, J. D., Kerth, W. J., et al. The surgical management of bacterial endocarditis: A review. *Ann. Surg.* 183:289, 1976.

20. Reagan, T. J. Cerebral ischemia in nonbacterial thrombotic endocarditis. *Curr. Concepts Cerebrovasc. Dis.* 10:13, 1975.

21. Rodbard, S. Blood velocity and endocarditis. *Circulation* 27:18, 1963.

22. Sande, M. A., Johnson, W. D., Hook, E. W., et al. Sustained bacteremia in patients with prosthetic cardiac valves. *N. Engl. J. Med.* 286:1067, 1972.

23. Scully, R., Galdabini, J. J., and McNeely, B. U. Weekly clinicopathological exercises. *N. Engl. J. Med.* 293:247, 1975.

24. Shanson, D. C. The prophylaxis of infective endocarditis. *J. Antimicrob. Chemother.* 1:2, 1978.

25. Tompsett, R. Infective endocarditis: Current topics. Paper presented at Medical Grand Rounds, University of Texas Health Science Center at Dallas. June, 1977.

26. Watanakunakorn, C. Infective endocarditis as a result of medical progress. *Am. J. Med.* 64:917, 1978.

27. Weinstein, L. Modern infective endocarditis. *J.A.M.A.* 233:260, 1975.

28. Weinstein, L., and Schlesinger, J. J. Pathoanatomic, pathophysiologic and clinical correlations in endocarditis: Part I. *N. Engl. J. Med.* 291:832, 1974.

29. Weinstein, L., and Schlesinger, J. J. Pathoanatomic, pathophysiologic and clinical correlation in endocarditis: Part II. *N. Engl. J. Med.* 291:1122, 1974.

30. Williams, R. C. Subacute bacterial endocarditis as an immune disease. *Hosp. Prac.* 6:111, 1971.

VII. The Critically Ill Adult with Metabolic Problems

To believe in many of the "new therapies"—biofeedback, relaxation techniques, meditation—is to be affected by them. The critical care nurse cannot merely say, "I believe," and leave the issue at that. To truly believe is to understand; and to understand is to experience personal change.

The emphasis is on *experience*, not *belief*.

Body-mind-spirit concepts are not "head trips." They are, first and last, *experiential*, not *intellectual*. They begin and end with feeling, not belief.

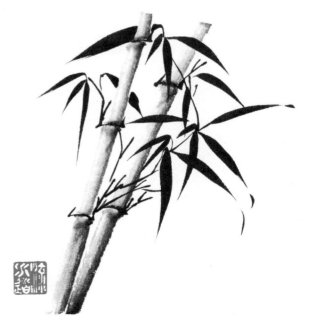

Diabetic Ketoacidosis

Angela Pruitt Clark

Diabetes mellitus is a major health problem that occurs in millions of people in the United States. Many physiological and pathological changes are present in the disorder. It can lead to several conditions that require emergency intervention and critical care nursing. One of the major complications the nurse may see is diabetic ketoacidosis (also known—less precisely—as diabetic coma). Diabetic ketoacidosis (DKA) is life threatening; it can lead rapidly to severe dehydration, electrolyte depletion, and death if it is not recognized and treated. The nurse must be able to assess the patient systematically and to implement the nursing plans that are based on a body of theoretical knowledge.

Objective

The critical care nurse should be able to state the most common causes and symptoms of DKA, perform a systematic assessment of the patient, including a physical examination, and anticipate and explain the medical and nursing management of the patient.

Achieving the Objective

To achieve the objective, the nurse should be able to:

1. List in the order of importance the primary patient care objectives for the patient with DKA.

2. List the most common causes of DKA.
3. List the subjective and objective symptoms of DKA.
4. State how the nursing process will be used.
5. Teach the patient and his family the essentials they need to know for safe and thorough self-care after the acute phase has passed.

How to Proceed

To develop an approach to DKA, the nurse should:

1. Study the physiological and pathological changes that occur in DKA.
2. Adapt a nursing assessment tool and apply it to the patient.
3. Read the case study that follows and immediately make a problem list.
4. Describe the main medical and nursing interventions that the patient needs.

Case Study

Mr. V. M., a 21-year-old college senior, was found unconscious in his apartment by his girlfriend. She called an ambulance. Mr. M. was taken to the emergency room of a nearby hospital, where he was immediately admitted to the intensive care unit.

The information obtained from Mr. M.'s girlfriend revealed that Mr. M. had complained of nausea and had been coughing for several days. She did not know whether he had had a fever or if he had notified his physician.

Mr. M.'s mother was notified. She arrived at the hospital within 15 minutes. Some additional information was obtained from her that was relevant to Mr. M.'s condition. Although Mrs. M. had not seen her son for about a week, she suspected that he might be ill because he had not attended his favorite sister's birthday party two nights earlier.

Mrs. M. said that her son had been a diabetic since he was 11 years old and that his condition was fairly well controlled. He had been taking one injection of Lente Insulin per day, and on the average he had four or five insulin reactions per month. He had not been following his diet well since he moved into his own apartment a year ago. He used to test his urine for sugar regularly, but lately, Mrs. M. suspected, he had not bothered.

Mr. M.'s girlfriend said that he drank alcohol at parties and that he had passed out about a month ago at a friend's house.

Mr. M.'s past medical history included many hospitalizations for diabetes-related conditions. His mother said that he had attended diabetic education classes held at a hospital when he was 17 years old. He had no history of surgery.

Mr. M.'s current medications included Lente Insulin. His mother said that her son was allergic to pork and thus must use insulin obtained from beef sources. He occasionally took medication for headaches and sinus problems. He had no other allergies.

Physical examination at the time of his admission to the critical care unit showed that Mr. M. was acutely ill. The following information was obtained (see assessment sheet):

General:	Acutely ill white male with rapid, deep respirations. Intravenous fluids: 0.9% normal saline solution given in the left antecubital vein (started by the emergency medical service)
Vital signs:	BP 96/70 supine position, right arm; heart rate 110; normal sinus rhythm; respirations 36/min and deep; temperature 101.8°F rectally; height 6'; weight 160 lbs
Integument:	Pale except for very flushed face, skin turgor poor; skin dry
Head:	No abnormalities noted. No lacerations
Eyes:	Pupils equal and reactive to light. Sclera clear; fundi grade I retinopathy; ocular pressure shown by palpation to be reduced
Ears:	Tympanic membrane intact and clear
Nose:	Flaring of nares
Mouth:	Mucous membranes dry and pink
Neck:	Supple; no neck vein distention; no bruits; no lymphadenopathy
Chest:	Vesicular breath sounds in left lung; right lung has bronchovesicular breath sounds; slight dullness in right lower lung; crepitant rales in anterior and posterior right lower lung
Cardiovascular system:	Normal sinus rhythm (110 beats/min); PMI fifth intercostal space at midclavicular line; poor capillary refill; extremities cool; first and second heart sounds normal; no murmurs
Abdomen:	Distended; bowel sounds absent; no palpable masses
Genitourinary system:	Bladder distended; genitals normal; testes descended with no masses
Extremities:	Intravenous line in left arm; full range-of-motion exercises possible; no edema or cyanosis; all pulses present
Neurological responses:	No response to commands; deep tendon reflexes 0 to 1+

The following laboratory data were obtained immediately.

Blood sugar:	650 mg/100 ml
Serum acetone:	Strong (4+ reaction at 1:16 dilution in plasma)
Complete blood count:	White blood cells 19,000/cu mm Neutrophils 70% Lymphocytes 26%

	Hemoglobin 16 gm/100 ml
	Hematocrit 58%
Arterial blood gases:	pH 6.9
	PO_2 98; O_2 saturation 95%
	PCO_2 20
	Calculated HCO_3 3.75
	Measured HCO_3 5
	Base excess −29
Electrolytes:	Na 129 mEq/L
	Cl 93 mEq/L
	CO_2 5 mM/L
	Potassium 5.1 mEq/L
Other:	Blood urea nitrogen 20 mg/100 ml
	Creatinine 0.8 mg/100 ml
	Cholesterol 186 mg/100 ml
Chest x ray:	Shows a diffuse infiltrate in the right lower lobe that appears to be pneumonia

Clinical Presentation of Case Study

Admitted to ICU Several actions were taken at once.

6:30 P.M. Mr. M. arrived with an intravenous route established. A 0.9% normal saline solution was given at 200 ml per hour. Hypotension (BP 96/70) was noted and check of Mr. M.'s vital signs every 30 minutes was ordered. The stat blood sugar on Mr. M.'s admission was 650 mg/100 ml and regular insulin (beef) (100 units by intravenous push) was given. Blood sugar checks every hour were ordered. An infusion pump was prepared with additional regular insulin, and it was piggybacked into the intravenous line. A rate of 6 units per hour was established. Monitor leads were attached to the patient; a continuing sinus tachycardia with no ectopic beats was noted. To relieve abdominal distention, a sump nasogastric tube was inserted and connected to low suction. A Foley catheter was inserted, and 870 ml of urine were obtained. The urinalysis revealed the following data: pH 5, specific gravity 1.036, sugar 5%, and acetone strong. A sputum specimen was obtained by tracheal suctioning, and sputum and urine cultures were requested.

7:30 P.M. No noticeable improvement in Mr. M.'s skin (2nd hour) turgor was seen. Bowel sounds continued to be absent. Aqueous penicillin G crystalline (1,000,000 units intravenously every six hours) was given for the pneumonia while results of the culture were awaited. A second blood sugar test showed 602 mg/100 ml. The electrolyte levels were: Na 130 mEq, K 5 mEq, Cl 93 mEq, CO_2 5 mM. The arterial blood

analysis showed: pH 6.9, PO_2 97, PCO_2 21, and HCO_3 5.

Because of Mr. M.'s pH and low PCO_2, sodium bicarbonate was given. (Caution should be used in administering sodium bicarbonate in metabolic acidosis because it may aggravate spinal fluid acidosis.) Currently, sodium bicarbonate is used only in severe acidosis (a pH of less than 7). A check of Mr. M.'s vital signs revealed a slight temperature decrease (to 101°F rectally) and a blood pressure increase (to 100/70). Mr. M.'s neurological responses continued to be depressed. His Kussmaul's respirations continued. Ultrasonic nebulizer mist therapy was administered every six hours for 20 minutes.

8:30 P.M. Potassium 4.2 mEq; blood sugar 542 mg/100 (3rd hour) ml; urine output for the last hour 320 ml; bowel sounds still absent; family members visited and asked whether they could see Mr. M. again. The nurse gave them a summary of Mr. M.'s condition. They seemed to be relieved but said they had been through similar experiences with Mr. M. many times before, and they did not worry about his dying in a coma as they used to. They asked to be allowed to return during the night, and were assured that they could.

11:30 P.M. Potassium 3 mEq, reflecting an intracellular (6th hour) potassium shift; potassium phosphate added to the intravenous fluids.

4:30 A.M. Blood sugar 402 mg/100 ml. BP 112/74. The (10th hour) regular insulin given via an infusion pump continued at the same rate. Intravenous infusion decreased to 130 ml/hr. Temperature 100.6°F rectally. Skin hydration state improved. Polyuria continued to a lesser degree. Arterial blood pH 7.1. Hourly check of vital signs continued.

10:30 A.M. Arterial blood pH 7.2. CO_2 (venous) rose to 13. (16th hour) Infusions continued.

12:30 P.M. Mr. M. slowly regained consciousness. Nurse (18th hour) told him where he was and why. Her explanation seemed to satisfy him. Family allowed to visit him. Blood sugar 355 mg/100 ml. Hourly urine checks continued; amount averaged about 100 ml/hr. BP 120/76. Sinus tachycardia continued. Bowel sounds still absent.

3:30 P.M. The patient was oriented to time and place. (21st hour) BP 122/76; HR 108; R 24; T 99.6°F orally. Arterial blood gas analysis showed pH 7.30 and serum PCO_2 18. Blood sugar 315 mg/100 ml.

Critical Care Nursing Admission Assessment
Major Systems Approach

PATIENT'S NAME: _Mr. V. M._   DATE: _10/14_   TIME: _4:30 pm_

DIAGNOSIS: _DKA_   T: _101.8 (R)_   A.P.: _110_   R.P.: _110_   R.: _36_

B.P.: _96/70_   E.C.G. RHYTHM: _Sinus Tach._   ECTOPY: _none_   WT: _160 lbs._   HT: _6'_

ADMITTED VIA: _stretcher_   INFORMANT: ___   LAST MEAL: _"4 days ago"?_

I. CHIEF COMPLAINT: _found in coma; known diabetic; had nausea + cough for several days_

II. PATIENT PROFILE:
1. Age _21_   2. Sex _male_
3. Marital Status M W D (S)
4. Race _caucas._   5. Religion _Lutheran-inactive_
6. Occupation _college student-hist.+ lit. major_
7. Availability of Family _mother + father in city; helpful-paying living + educ. exp. till out of school_
8. Dietary _ADA- 2000 cal.-lives alone doesn't stick to diet_
9. Sleeping _6-8 hrs./night; "night person" considered a "night person" by friends; occasional insomnia č anxiety_
10. Activities of Daily Living _college senior; many interests (athletics, photography); knows to supplement diet č exercise_

III. HISTORY OF PRESENT ILLNESS: _nausea + cough for several days - don't know if "Dr." called-found_

IV. PAST MEDICAL HISTORY:
1. Pediatric & Adult Illnesses _dx. Juvenile D.M. Feb. 67 - started on NPH + regular insulin_
2. Cardiac _no_
3. Hypertension _no_
4. Respiratory _no_
5. Diabetes Mellitus _Dx- 1967 (age 11) see below_
6. Renal _no_
7. Jaundice _no_
8. Infections _Sept. '67 - infect. (R) arm_
9. Other _attended diabetic educat. classes (17 y.o.)_
10. Hospitalizations & Surgeries _no surgeries; "many" hospitalizations for diabetes: 1967 Feb: Dx.; Sept. - Arm infection Nov. 68-Control of D.M.; Jan. 70 Insulin reaction; Jan. 71 DKA+ reaction to all pork insulin-switched to all beef 50u/day; Sept. 73 - Severe DKA č UTI (retinopathy noted); Feb. '76 abd. pain_

11. Current Medication _Lente (beef)_

12. Allergies _Pork + pork insulins_

13. Habits _doesn't smoke cigarettes- occas. marijuana; alcohol 2-3 x wk._

V. FAMILY HISTORY: _father-52-hypertension, mild angina; mother-45 D.M. diet controlled 2 sisters 11 + 15 alive + well_

VI. PSYCHOSOCIAL: _grandmother died of gangrene (DM)_
1. Behavior During Assessment _comatose_

2. Specific Problems _family feels he waits till situation acute to seek med. Rx_

VII. PHYSICAL EXAMINATION:
1. General _acutely ill, pale č flushed face_
arterial blood gases: pH 6.9 pO₂ 98 (pO_2 98)
pCO₂ 20, Δ base -29, (pCO_2 20, Δ base -29)
Cal HCO₃ 3.75 (HCO_3 3.75)
2. Respiratory System _measured HCO₃ 5_ (HCO_3 5)
Airway _patent_
Inspection _flaring of nares, configurat-ion normal_
Rate _36_
Rhythm _Kussmaul's_
Chest Wall _= expansion_
Palpation _trachea midline; unable to talk to patient_
Percussion _resonant and =_

Auscultation
Voice Sounds _____ (comatose)
Breath Sounds _____
 Normal ✓ Increased _____ Decreased _____
Adventitious Sounds crepitant rales in
RLL ant. + post.

3. Cardiovascular System
 A.P. 110 R.P. 110
 B.P. Supine R 94/68 L _____
 P.M.I. 5th i MCL
 Heart Sounds $S_1 S_2$ nml. - no $S_3 S_4$

 Thrills _____ no
 Peripheral Pulses _____ present
4. Neurological System
 Level of Consciousness _____ comatose

 Respiratory Pattern _____ Kussmaul's

 Cranial Nerves unable to assess all
 due to coma - no abnormalities
 noted

 Eyes retinopathy Grade I
 (1) Pupils   OD   OS
  Size   nml   nml
  Shape   nml   nml
  Light   reactive reactive > equal
  Consensual ok   ok
  Accommodation   (comatose)
 (2) Ocular Movements _____

 Motor _____
 Sensory _____ > comatose
 Coordination _____

 Reflexes no response to commands
 DTR 0 to 1+
5. Gastrointestinal System
 Nose & Mouth odor of emesis?
 acetone breath; no lesions
 Stomach _____ distended

 Abdomen _____ distended

 Bowel Sounds _____ absent
 Liver _____ > non-palpable
 Spleen _____

6. Renal & Genitourinary Systems
 I. _____ O. _____
 Urinary Bladder & Urethra Bladder
 distended
 Kidneys _____

7. Musculoskeletal System
 Spine _____ appears nml
 Extremities no edema, no
 dermopathy

 Sacral Edema _____ no
 Masses _____ no
8. Hematologic System
 Petechiae > none
 Ecchymosis
 Gingiva _____ no bleeding

9. Endocrine System
 Breath acetone; ? emesis
 Skin skin turgor poor; dehydrated;
 no lipodystrophy
VIII. LABORATORY:
 1. Hematology
  HGB 16 gm. HCT 58%
  W.B.C. 19,000 cu. mm. neutrophils 70%
  lymphocytes 26%
 2. Chemistry
  Na 129 meg. K 5.1 meg.
  CO₂ 5 mm. Cl 93 meg.
  Blood Sugar 650 mg. % Cholesterol 186 mgm.
  serum acetone strong Amylase
  BUN 20 mg. % Cr 0.8 mg. %
 3. Urinalysis sugar 5%; acetone - strong
  pH 5 spec. grav. 1.036
 4. Electrocardiogram
  Rate 112 Rhythm sinus tach.
  P-R .16 QRS .08 ST 0.11
  Interpretation sinus tachycardia
 5. Chest x-ray diffuse infiltrate in RLL -
 appears to be pneumonia

IX. PROBLEM LIST:
 ACTIVE   INACTIVE
1. severe diabetic ketoacidosis →
2. lack of knowledge re
 Diabetes Mellitus 4. DKA; infection (R)
3. immobility   arm 9/67
9. allergy to pork & 5. adm. for d.m. control
 pork insulins   6. insulin reaction 1/10 11/68
          7. DKA; reaction pork insulin
          8. severe DKA; UTI 1/77
           retinopathy 9/78

_____ A. Clark, R.N.
NURSE'S SIGNATURE

519

5:30 P.M. Blood sugar 266 mg/100 ml. Urine sugar 3%.
(24th hour) Urine acetone trace. Intravenous infusion of insulin discontinued to avoid a hypoglycemia reaction. Intravenous solution was changed to a 5% dextrose in 0.45% normal saline solution at 100 ml/hr.

6:30 P.M. Foley catheter removed. Urine sent for cul-
(25th hour) ture and sensitivity tests.

7:30 P.M. Blood sugar 230 mg/100 ml. Regular insulin
(26th hour) (25 units intramuscularly) given. A sliding-scale administration of regular insulin was ordered as follows: With the two-drop method and Clinitest tablets used, every six hours the patient should be given (1) 25 units of regular insulin for 5% (subcutaneously), (2) 20 units of regular insulin for 3%, (3) 10 units of regular insulin for 2% (4+), and (4) no units of regular insulin for 1%.

Bowel sounds present. Nasogastric tube removed. Clear liquids given by mouth and tolerated without nausea.

9:30 P.M. The intravenous infusion reduced to 50 ml/hr.
(28th hour) Clear liquids given to the patient on request. Rales still present in right lower lung, but the other areas of lungs still clear on auscultation. T 99.4°F orally. Penicillin continued. Chest x ray showed some clearing of the infiltrate. After 25 hours, sputum culture showed *Streptococcus pneumoniae* (pneumococcus), which was sensitive to the antibiotic being given. Intermittent positive pressure breathing treatments given every six hours. Mr. M. encouraged to cough and deep breathe every hour.

3:30 A.M. By the next morning, Mr. M. was well
(next day) oriented to his environment and could remember the events that led to his hospitalization. He had retained all the liquids he had been given, and he did not have any abdominal distention. The distention he had earlier was probably due to neuropathy or sodium loss. Mr. M. was put on an 1800-calorie ADA diet. Vital signs stable, except for an elevated temperature. Hydration state satisfactory as indicated by clinical signs. Blood sugar 154 mg/100 ml, with the infusion of a 5% dextrose in 0.45% normal saline solution only to keep a vein open for penicillin. Arterial blood gases normal. Sliding-scale administration of insulin continued.

11:00 A.M. Mr. M. transferred from the intensive care unit to a medical nursing unit. Vital signs: BP 130/78; HR 100; R 18; T 99.2°F orally. His mother was waiting for him in his new room.

4th Day Mr. M. again given Lente insulin (36 units every morning); sliding-scale administration of insulin stopped. Mr. M. was interviewed by member of diabetic teaching team, who assessed Mr. M.'s knowledge of diabetes and thus determined what Mr. M. needed to learn. Mr. M. said that he had become careless about checking his urine and did not understand significance of acetone in urine. He did not rotate injection sites systematically; in fact, he had never used abdomen as a site. Mr. M. and his teacher planned his teaching. He was to be instructed by a registered nurse, a pharmacist, and a dietitian during his hospitalization.

Mr. M. learned that drinking alcohol without eating carbohydrate food can predispose a diabetic to an insulin reaction. If a diabetic starves to the point of glycogen depletion, and he drinks alcohol, he will probably experience hypoglycemia since alcohol suppresses gluconeogenesis. Mr. M. was taught about the ADA diet that used the 1976 exchange list.

Mr. M. concerned about the relationship of impotence to diabetes. Had read about that complication but had hesitated to ask his physician about it. Was told that impotence occurs two to five times more often in the diabetic than in the general population. Mr. M. said he was not impotent at present but feared he might be in the future. Said that he now felt freer to discuss the subject with his physician if he needed to do so.

5th Day Mr. M. had achieved the learning goals planned for him, and he felt that he was ready to go home. The nurse told him that pneumonia was improving but that physician wanted him to remain in the hospital until it was completely gone. T 99°F orally. He was switched to oral penicillin (250 mg every six hours).

9th Day Mr. M. discharged from hospital. He was to take Lente Insulin (36 units subcutaneously every morning), and he was to follow a 2000-calorie ADA diet. He was to be contacted for follow-up care by a member of the diabetic teaching team within three days. He had an appointment to see his physician in five days.

Reflections

Nurses often care for people with a chronic disease. Do they really grasp the significance of the disease to the patient? An acute illness may cause the patient unexpected problems, but the illness is generally short in duration. A chronic illness like diabetes mellitus is a permanent one, and it affects many areas of a person's life.

The nurse must consider what having diabetes means to the patient. Often the diabetic may act in ways that reflect his feelings of guilt, anxiety, or fear. Many adult diabetics have said that they felt they had lost control over their bodies. One man with diabetes said that he lived in constant fear of having an insulin reaction when he was alone. One woman said that having diabetes meant to her that she might lose a leg or foot.

The physiological effect of stress on man is well known. It has been established that stress can elevate the blood sugar level and, in fact, can lead to a significant degree of hyperglycemia in some people. Stress is a high-risk factor in cardiovascular disease, one of the main complications of diabetes mellitus.

Diabetic persons sometimes use their disease to manipulate their families, friends, and environment. Some have threatened to commit suicide by taking an overdose of insulin or by overeating. More commonly, some diabetics manipulate others by not taking their insulin. The family of a diabetic and other people close to him may encourage the diabetic to become dependent because they fear for his well-being. That can create a serious conflict in the diabetic who is trying to adjust to his illness while maintaining some independence.

The diabetic must adhere to a regimen that may change his life-style. Testing urine several times a day, adhering to a special diet in different settings, and taking injections daily are a few of the possible restrictions.

The role of the critical care nurse in regard to the patient with a chronic disease is multifaceted. She must be knowledgeable and skillful in order to maintain life. However, she must remember that the patient must learn to cope with his disease and its complications for the rest of his life. She needs communication skills to help her counsel the patient and his family. The use of diabetic education teams for hospitalized patients and their families is highly recommended. The person with a chronic disease needs every possible opportunity to learn good self-care. Identifying what the patient needs to learn and using a nursing assessment tool before the teaching sessions are valuable.

Mr. M.'s case study illustrates how difficult it is to cope with a chronic disease. Mr. M.'s nurse explored with him the meaning of his condition and met his acute care needs, including his learning needs, and thus enabled him to care for himself better after his discharge.

Anatomy and Physiology

The pancreas is a fish-shaped organ that weighs 50 to 75 gm. It is located behind the stomach and toward the left side of the body. The pancreas is an exocrine gland and an endocrine gland. Its endocrine functions are carried out by the islets of Langerhans cells, which are found throughout the pancreas. Although there are about two million islet cells, they comprise only 1 percent of the weight of the organ [16].

The pancreas contains at least three types of cells: alpha cells, beta cells, and D cells. The alpha cells secrete glucagon, a substance that causes an elevation in the blood glucose levels. The beta cells produce insulin, a powerful hypoglycemic agent. The D cells appear to contain somatostatin, which can inhibit both insulin and glucagon secretion [15]. The islet cells are enclosed by a tissue known as the basement membrane. Since capillaries also have basement membranes, insulin must cross two membranes to go from the pancreas to the bloodstream [16].

The basement membrane is important in the physiology of insulin action as well as in the vascular complications of diabetes. Electron microscopy has shown that behind the endothelial cell layer of blood vessels is a homogenous membrane that appears to be made up of a glycoprotein. One theory (discussed later in the chapter) proposes that the basement-membrane thickening seen in diabetes is a cause of diabetes and of some of its vascular complications.

Insulin

Insulin, a protein, consists of 2 polypeptide chains and 51 amino acids. It is generally thought that about 50 units of insulin is produced daily and that about 200 units is stored in the pancreas most of the time [16]. The stored insulin awaits a stimulus for its release. Glucose is the major stimulus of insulin secretion and release. When the glucose level rises (as it does after a meal), the pancreas immediately begins to produce and secrete insulin.

Insulin acts primarily to facilitate the movement of glucose into the cell for use by the cell. It increases the rate of glucose transport from the bloodstream through the cell membrane. Since the glucose molecule is too large to enter the cell pores by simple diffusion, it must be carried in by a transport process. Some glucose can enter the cell without insulin, but only in small amounts. It is apparent that if insulin moves glucose intracellularly, it decreases the amount of glucose circulating in the bloodstream.

Some cells (e.g., the cells in the brain, liver, and nervous tissue) do not need insulin to transport glucose. Other cells that do not need insulin to transport glucose are the cells in the renal tubules and the erythrocytes. Those cells collectively make up a very small percentage of the total body mass.

Besides increasing the glucose metabolism rate and decreasing the blood glucose concentration, insulin increases glycogen storage in the tissues. The stored glycogen can be converted to glucose if it is needed for energy.

Carbohydrate Metabolism

Glucose is the body's primary source of energy. One obtains exogenous glucose by eating nutrients, principally carbohydrates. Endogenous glucose is obtained from the conversion of stored glycogen to glucose and by gluconeogenesis from amino acids.

When carbohydrates are eaten, they are broken down into monosaccharides, or simple sugars. The monosaccharides are absorbed from the small intestine into the intestinal capillaries and are transported to the liver via the portal vein.

The fate of nutrients is decided in the liver, and it depends on what the body needs at the time. Generally, about 50 percent of the glucose (the main monosaccharide) is used immediately to meet the body's energy needs. About 30 to 40 percent is stored in reserve as adipose tissue by conversion to fats. Usually about 5 percent is stored as glycogen in the muscles and the liver to be converted to glucose if needed.

Carbohydrate is the body's preferred source of energy—its active fuel. The proper utilization of fat and protein is dependent on an adequate intake of carbohydrate. The body can, however, use the fat and protein to provide energy if absolutely necessary.

Fats as a Source of Energy

Fats can become the major supplier of energy on demand by oxidation of the fatty acids and glycerol. Fats, a concentrated form of stored energy, provide nine calories per gm; proteins and carbohydrates provide four calories per gm.

A dangerous situation arises when large amounts of fat are used instead of carbohydrates. That situation results in the production of intermediate by-products—ketoacids—which are acidic. The primary acids—acetoacetic acid and beta-hydroxybutyric acid—accumulate in the bloodstream and are responsible for the metabolic acidosis that follows. Diabetic ketoacidosis is discussed further later in the chapter. Ketoacids are not totally undesirable. Although the body cannot tolerate large amounts of ketoacids, muscle and kidney cells can use them in reasonable amounts as nutrients.

Hormones

Besides insulin, several other hormones affect carbohydrate metabolism. They include glucagon, epinephrine, thyroid hormone, adrenocorticotropin, the corticosteroids, and growth hormone. Those hormones are able to elevate the blood sugar level by various means, and thus they may be considered antagonistic to insulin [2]. Hypoglycemia can cause the secretion of all those hormones, except thyroid hormone.

Insulin Resistance

It appears that obese people have some degree of insulin resistance. Surprisingly, many obese diabetics have been found to have high insulin levels (hyperinsulinemia). Researchers have closely studied the adipose tissue cell. It seems that the larger the cell, the less responsive it is to insulin [12].

Pathophysiology of Diabetes

Diabetes mellitus is a chronic, usually hereditary, disease characterized by an abnormally high blood glucose level and the urinary excretion of some of that glucose. All or part of the body's ability to use carbohydrates has been lost because of a deficiency in insulin or a decrease in the efficiency of insulin.

There are probably more than 10 million diabetics in the United States. The number is increasing rapidly; in 1973 there were 50 percent more known diabetics than there were in 1965. There are many explanations of the increase. Diagnostic screening has improved, and diabetes is discovered earlier in its course. Since people live longer, more people survive to develop diabetes in later life. Improved care for the pregnant woman with diabetes may be another factor.

The insulin deficiency in diabetes appears to be polygenic. The oldest theory is that of beta-cell dysfunction, with inadequate amounts of insulin being secreted. It is thought that one inherits the tendency through recessive genes. A decrease in insulin activity has been seen in children after viral infections. It is speculated that the virus destroys some of the beta cells in children, who may inherit an increased susceptibility to the virus. The basement membrane theory has been receiving much research attention. The basement membrane has been found to be abnormally thickened in diabetics, a phenomenon that may account for the decrease in available insulin. An excessive amount of glucagon, the hormone that is antagonistic to insulin in action, has been found in many juvenile-onset diabetics. Another theory proposes that insulin is destroyed by antibodies or by some of the body organs.

A system for classifying types of diabetes was developed in 1979. The new terms are type I (insulin-dependent diabetes mellitus, IDDM) and type II (non-insulin-dependent diabetes mellitus, NIDDM). Type I replaces the old category of *juvenile-onset diabetes* and is most common in children but may occur at any age. Type II consists of two subtypes that include obese NIDDM and nonobese NIDDM. Type II roughly replaces the term *maturity-onset diabetes.*

Complications of Diabetes

Diabetes has many serious complications. Diabetics who are admitted to the critical care unit may already have one or more of the complications. Generally, the duration of diabetes correlates with the extent of the complications, but there are exceptions.

Macrovascular or macroangiopathic disease is one of the major complications of diabetes. It is most frequently seen in the adult-onset diabetic. The arteriosclerotic process appears to be essentially the same as that in the nondiabetic, but it is accelerated in the diabetic. Lipid deposition and medical calcification of the vessel are common [16]. The complication may be manifested in coronary artery disease, arterial insufficiency to the central nervous system or extremities, or in other large vessels.

Atherosclerotic heart disease is the leading cause of death in diabetics [16]. Gangrene has been found to be 156 times more common in the diabetic in his fifties than in a nondiabetic of the same age [16]. It should be remembered that severe macrovascular disease is frequently present in patients with mild diabetes.

Microangiopathy is most often seen in the juvenile-onset diabetic. It is characterized by thickening of the vascular basement membrane. It is often manifested in the patient by the retinopathy or nephropathy. Retinopathy can involve numerous pathological changes, beginning with microaneurysms. Nephropathy can be manifested in many renal conditions (e.g., glomerulosclerosis, tubular nephrosis, or renal failure) [16]. Renal failure is the most common cause of death in the juvenile-onset diabetic.

Diabetics appear to have a greater predisposition for infections than have nondiabetics although the studies are limited. Common manifestations include acute pyelonephritis, skin infections with *Candida* and *Staphylococcus*, and vaginitis. Infection commonly triggers an episode of ketoacidosis and hence must be looked for when acidosis appears. Ketoacidosis alters the state of resistance in the diabetic. It appears to impair phagocytosis and to delay granulocyte activity. Leukocytosis commonly occurs in diabetic ketoacidosis *without* infection, making it an unreliable initial diagnostic index of infection. The latter type of leukocytosis is probably secondary to the dehydration state and caused by increased adrenocortical activity [9].

Many neurological symptoms may occur in the diabetic. Neuropathy can be seen in the visceral as well as the peripheral nerve degenerative processes. Defects in glucose and lipid metabolism in nerve tissue have been noted. There are numerous ways that neuropathy can be manifested; for example, diabetic neurogenic bladder, atrophy of the extremities, and neurotrophic foot ulcer. Impotence is probably the most common symptom of neuropathy in male diabetics. Possibly up to 60 percent of male patients who have had diabetes for five years are impotent [16].

Diabetic retinopathy is one of the leading causes of blindness in the United States. Diabetics also have a higher incidence of cataracts. Transient unilateral blindness can also occur in some diabetics. It is usually due to occlusion of an artery that supplies an optic nerve. Fluctuations in the blood sugar concentration can swell and shrink the lens, producing transient blurred vision.

Abnormal skin lesions can be a complication of diabetes. The term *diabetic dermopathy* is generally used to refer to the presence of reddish-brown papular spots on the shins. The spots may have an erythematous border. Crusts and scar tissue may form [4].

Another, more severe, skin lesion is necrobiosis lipoidica diabeticorum (NLD). It is an ulcerating and necrotic process, and it may be quite difficult to control.

Diabetic ketoacidosis (DKA) is an acute metabolic acidosis that occurs when the diabetic state of decreased insulin action leads to a significant degree of hyperglycemia and ketonemia.

The possible causes of DKA are:

1. Infection, a common cause, which increases the metabolic rate.
2. The omission of insulin, which can result in an imbalance between insulin and glucose.
3. An emotional crisis, which can cause hyperglycemia.
4. A decrease in the usual amount of exercise.
5. Increased food intake over a period of time, which can lead to DKA.

Pathophysiology of Diabetic Ketoacidosis

Insulin deficiency begins the process of ketoacidosis because insulin is not available to transport glucose into the cell through the cell membrane. The glucose concentration of the blood increases and will continue to do so if the condition is not treated. When the renal threshold for resorption of glucose is reached, some of the glucose is excreted in the urine. The threshold varies; in many people it is about 170 mg/100 ml. The hyperglycemic state initiates an osmotic diuresis, drawing fluid from intracellular and interstitial spaces into the intravascular compartment.

In search of energy from noncarbohydrate sources, the body begins to break down large amounts of fat to obtain glucose. Fat is broken down into glycerol and fatty acids. The glycerol is released and is converted to glucose. The fatty acids are converted to acetyl-coenzyme A (acetyl-CoA) by the liver. Acetyl-CoA unites with a substance called oxaloacetate before it is transferred to peripheral tissues to be used for energy production [5]. If the cycle were allowed to progress normally, the eventual outcome would be carbon

dioxide, water, and energy (stored as adenosine triphosphate and creatine phosphate).

Lipolysis increases, partly because insulin normally inhibits lipase. Free fatty acids are released and their oxidation results in excess amounts of acetyl-CoA. Acetyl-CoA accumulates because it is in excessive amounts relative to the available oxaloacetate. As mentioned, that situation increases the number of ketone bodies or ketoacids (acetoacetic acid, and beta-hydroxybutyric acid). Acetone is found in the patient's urine and is detectable on his breath; it is a spontaneous breakdown product of acetoacetic acid [5]. It has been noted that acetoacetic acid can suppress cerebral oxygenation [3].

Hyperglycemia and ketonemia can lead to a critical loss of water, electrolytes, and calories in the three body compartments. The osmotic diuresis is severe. Sodium, potassium, chloride, magnesium, and phosphate are apt to be lost, but the laboratory measurements may not show a decrease in those substances, primarily owing to the dehydration and hemoconcentration. Hemoconcentration can develop along with a decrease in the vascular volume and hence a decrease in the circulatory competence. Polyuria results from the large water loss because the tubular capacity to resorb glucose is exceeded; approximately 15 ml of water is needed to excrete 1 gm of glucose. If nausea and vomiting are present, they will contribute further to the loss of fluid and electrolytes.

A metabolic acidosis with excess hydrogen ion concentration results from the ketosis and death will occur if the condition is not treated. Some physicians think that the pH of the cerebrospinal fluid is a more accurate index of the degree of acidosis and coma. Mental confusion and coma occur when the cerebrospinal fluid falls below pH 7.15. Cerebral edema has been seen as a complication of the fluid therapy when treatment is started.

Compensatory mechanisms may be seen in buffering substances, the renal system, and the lungs. Acetoacetic acid unites with sodium acetoacetate. The respiratory center is stimulated, and the patient begins to breathe deeply and rapidly in an effort to blow off excess carbonic acid as water and carbon dioxide. (That type of respiration is called Kussmaul's respirations.) The kidneys increase their excretion of hydrogen ions by the secretion of ammonia, which is then excreted as ammonium chloride; the kidneys also excrete ketones (ketonuria).

Clinical Picture of Diabetic Ketoacidosis

The patient with DKA appears acutely ill. His significant degree of dehydration is manifested by dry skin with poor turgor, thirst, soft eyeballs, and possibly even wrinkled corneas. The mucous membranes in the conjunctival and oronasopharyngeal areas are dry. Polyuria, with bladder distention if the patient is comatose, is noted. Rales may be present (as in the case study), but they may not be heard because of the dehydration. A pleural friction rub may be present; it disappears on rehydration.

The signs of DKA that are related to the acidotic state are mental changes ranging from confusion to coma, an acetone odor to the breath, and a flushed face. The flush is probably due to superficial vasodilatation secondary to the increase in carbonic acid. Fever and dehydration may be other causes of the flush. Kussmaul's respirations occur in about 75 percent of patients [5].

Abdominal pain may result from sodium loss or possibly from a neuropathic occurrence. Fluid loss may also be a cause. Vomiting may be present; it has been seen in more than 75 percent of the cases studied [5].

Deep tendon reflexes may be diminished or absent. They return after treatment.

Diagnosis of Diabetic Ketoacidosis

The diagnosis of DKA is usually made without much difficulty. The patient is acutely ill, and he should be treated as soon as possible. If the patient is a known diabetic, the process is easier. Every patient in a coma should have a blood sugar test done. Unique causes of coma in diabetes are hypoglycemia (insulin reaction, insulin shock), hyperosmolar nonketotic coma, lactic acidosis, and DKA. A blood sugar test will quickly rule out hypoglycemia. Hyperosmolar coma is similar to DKA, but it lacks the acidotic phase. Hyperglycemia is present but not metabolic acidosis (see Chap. 25). Lactic acidosis may also be present in the patient with DKA and can cause a misreading of the serum and urine acetone tests. The lactic acid build-up causes a block in the conversion of beta-hydroxybutyrate to acetoacetate. Since acetoacetate is the only chemical detected by common laboratory tests, it may appear as though few or no ketones are present. As the lactic acidosis improves with the usual treatment for DKA, the patient's ketone levels

may increase dramatically even though the patient is getting better [7].

The diagnosis of DKA should be based on the patient's clinical picture, his history (if one is available), and the laboratory findings.

The clinical picture in DKA has been discussed. Often the nurse can tentatively diagnose DKA after making a few quick, astute observations. Kussmaul's respirations, acetone breath, and severe dehydration are important signs.

Diagnostic Tests

Many diagnostic tests are helpful. Obviously tests of the blood and urine sugar levels, the blood and urine ketone levels, and the arterial blood gases must be done immediately. Hyperglycemia up to 2000 mg/100 ml and glycosuria up to 5% may be seen. The usual blood sugar range is 400 to 800 mg/100 ml [16]. Arterial blood gases will reveal an acidotic arterial pH. As mentioned, some physicians prefer to rely on the cerebrospinal fluid pH as a more accurate reflection of the pH. There is no certain expected PO_2 reading. It varies with the individual and with other factors, such as the degree of hemoconcentration, preexisting lung disease, and other related pathology.

Leukocytosis is generally present. It may be as high as 30,000/cu mm. It reflects hemoconcentration and stress, but not necessarily infection.

The carbon dioxide combining power is expected to be low. It reflects the decrease in alkaline reserve.

Treatment of Diabetic Ketoacidosis

DKA must be treated if the patient is to survive. Because DKA is life threatening, early diagnosis and management are needed. The chief components of treatment are: (1) insulin therapy, (2) fluid replacement, (3) electrolyte replacement, (4) antiacidosis therapy, and (5) management of the symptoms. Use of a flow sheet (Table 24-1) to record and correlate the laboratory values and replacement factors is quite helpful.

Insulin Therapy

Insulin therapy is perhaps the cornerstone of treatment. Without it the pathological cycle cannot be

Table 24-1
Flow Sheet for Diabetic Ketoacidosis

Vital Signs								Laboratory Values									
Time	BP	HR	R	T	Urine Output	Level of Consciousness	Other	Time	Blood Glucose	Acetone Dilution	pH	PCO_2	HCO_3	Na	K	Cl	CO_2	Other

			Treatment					
	Time	Insulin	Type Intravenous Fluid	Amount	Cumulative Amount	K	Bicarbonate	Other

stopped. Insulin is given in intermittent doses or by continuous infusion. Research is active now to determine whether one method is significantly better than the other. Recent studies indicate that both methods are effective [11]. An immediate injection of insulin is recommended. It may even be given before the patient arrives at the hospital if that is possible.

When the intermittent method is used, large doses of a rapid-acting insulin (e.g., regular crystalline insulin) are given. Both regular crystalline and semilente insulin can be administered intravenously, but regular crystalline insulin appears to be the type most commonly used intravenously [16]. The amount of insulin given is determined by the blood sugar level. Initially about 100 units (1.5 units/kg) [16] is given intravenously and/or subcutaneously. The range for initial doses is 50 to 200 units [7]. The intravenous route is preferred if the patient has any degree of vascular collapse or shock since insulin cannot be absorbed adequately when the intramuscular or subcutaneous route is used. Some physicians prefer to give all insulin intravenously. Insulin is usually given every hour until the patient's blood sugar level has decreased to 250 to 300 mg. At that point, the danger

of hypoglycemia necessitates decreasing the insulin dose and monitoring the patient carefully. The amount of insulin given varies; the average is 50 to 100 units intravenously and/or subcutaneously. Most of the insulin is given in the first six hours of therapy.

The continuous infusion is usually given with an infusion pump piggybacked into an intravenous line. Generally about 5 to 6 units per hour of regular crystalline insulin is given. Some physicians will add insulin to a 500- or 1,000-ml intravenous bottle (instead of using an infusion pump) and will administer about 60 units per hour [7]. Albumin may be used to bind the insulin to it to keep it from adhering to the glass and tubing. Use of the infusion pump is more likely to ensure that the patient receives the prescribed dose, and it appears to result in a more predictable drop in blood sugar [11].

The biological half-life of insulin is about 10 minutes, a fact that should be considered in the administration of intravenous insulin. If 100 units is administered as an intravenous bolus, in 10 minutes, in the average patient, only 50 units will still be circulating [10]. Some clinicians feel the continuous infusion method best applies the concept of half-life [1].

Insulin resistance may be present in some patients. If insulin resistance is present, circulating antibodies counteract some of the effect of the insulin. Insulin must saturate the antibody before the effect of the insulin can be seen [14]. If insulin resistance is present, much higher doses of insulin are given, and the total amount may be in the thousands of units. Intravenous hydrocortisone (100 to 200 mg) can be given to decrease the antibody response [14].

The patient is carefully evaluated during the insulin therapy. Blood sugar evaluations are done every hour. After the first few hours of treatment, insulin may be given on a sliding scale, with the dosage based on the urine glucose level (e.g., 50 units for 4 + [2%] and 40 units for 3+). Knowing the patient's renal threshold is helpful since some people spill at much lower or much higher than normal levels. Insulin is inactivated when the pH is above 7.5 [8]. Thus some inactivation may be seen when bicarbonate therapy is used.

Hypoglycemia (insulin shock, insulin reaction) is one of the main complications of insulin therapy. It may follow rigorous treatment of diabetic ketoacidosis, and it can lead to permanent damage to the central nervous system. The clinical manifestations of hypoglycemia are a response to stimulation of the sympathetic nervous system. Vasomotor nerves lose their ability to maintain vessel tone and size, leading to vasodilatation and hypotension. A shock state can ensue if the hypoglycemia is untreated. Because the myocardium needs adequate amounts of glucose, cardiac functioning may be affected. The signs and symptoms of hypoglycemia include diaphoresis, excitability, dilated pupils, blurred vision, fall in blood pressure, weakness, pallor, and behavioral changes.

Hypoglycemia can usually be avoided by stopping the insulin therapy when the blood sugar level reaches 250 to 300 mg/100 ml. An intravenous solution containing 5% glucose should be administered at that point in the treatment.

Fluid Replacement

Rapid rehydration is needed to maintain vascular tone and metabolic functioning. Large amounts of fluids are given initially and as long as needed. A water deficit of 10 percent of the body weight may be lost in the average adult [5]. Isotonic normal saline solution (0.9%) is the initial fluid of choice in spite of its hyperosmolarity [11]. Normal saline solution (0.45%) may be given because it is less hyperosmolar for some patients. Generally 1000 to 2000 ml is given in the first two hours or so. Up to 10 liters of fluids is the average volume to be administered in the first 12 hours [7]. Some authorities calculate fluid losses and replace fluids accordingly. One formula estimates the average losses at 100 ml of water/kg of body weight [16]. Monitoring the central venous pressure is a useful guide for fluid replacement. After the first few hours, the fluid will probably be changed to 0.45% normal saline solution. Since more water than sodium is lost owing to osmotic diuresis, extra free water will be needed in the form of a 5% dextrose in water solution or a 0.45% normal saline solution. By that time, the extent of the patient's hyperosmolar state can be determined and the type of fluids selected with that in mind. A mixture of lactated Ringer's solution and distilled water is occasionally used. A 5% glucose solution should be given before hypoglycemia is likely to occur. After insulin therapy, glucose is metabolized and since there is no available glycogen, glucose is needed.

Alkalinizing solutions, such as sodium bicarbonate and sodium lactate, are occasionally used for severe acidosis. These solutions must be administered with caution because they can produce alkalosis or can contribute to the development of spinal fluid acidosis [5]. The use of sodium lactate can lead to lactic acidosis.

Cerebral edema can follow the too liberal use of insulin and fluids. The cause appears to be related to osmotic pull. The significance of the polyol pathway in the development of cerebral edema is a matter of controversy. Sorbitol synthesis is increased, but the extra sorbitol is not utilized. The sorbitol increases osmotic water pull. Water readily penetrates the blood brain barrier, but glucose does not. As insulin lowers the blood sugar level, osmotic pressure pulls water into the cerebrospinal fluid and, possibly, the brain cells to dilute the sugar in those cells. There may be an innate tendency for increased intracranial pressure to develop in DKA [17].

Electrolyte Replacement

Replacement of lost electrolytes is another major therapy. Losses of sodium, potassium, chloride, magnesium, phosphate, and calcium are seen in the patient with DKA. The primary concern of the clinician is generally the replacement of sodium, potassium, chloride, magnesium, phosphate, and calcium. These may be added to the intravenous solutions, but they are not always replaced.

Sodium and chloride are replaced with a 0.45% or 0.9% normal saline intravenous solution, given rapidly. The therapy is monitored by serum electrolyte studies.

Potassium replacement is the most difficult kind of electrolyte replacement. The serum potassium level does not reflect the patient's true status because most potassium is normally intracellular. In DKA, the total body amount of potassium is deficient. However, the patient may present with high, low, or even normal serum potassium levels. When insulin and fluid administration is instituted, potassium is rapidly moved back into the cell and a life-threatening hypokalemia can ensue. It usually occurs after four to six hours of treatment, but it may occur earlier [4]. Potassium replacement should be carefully evaluated using the serum potassium level. If the level is high initially, obviously no potassium is needed. In fact, to give the patient potassium would endanger him and make him susceptible to cardiac dysrhythmias. If the potassium level is normal, potassium chloride (20–40 mEq/L) may be given after the initial hydration therapy [7]. If the patient's potassium level is low on his admission (it is low extremely rarely), potassium replacement is begun immediately. Potassium phosphate may be given as a form of potassium replacement because it also treats phosphate depletion and may help in oxygen transport to tissue [2]. Recent data suggest potassium phosphate may lead to hypocalcemia [18].

The ECG is a useful guide to the patient's potassium level. Hyperkalemia is manifested by peaked T waves, a widened QRS complex, and sometimes the absence of P waves [7]. In hypokalemia, a prolonged QT interval, a depressed T wave, and prominent U waves may be seen.

The oral route of administering potassium is a safe one if the patient is able to tolerate liquids. Orange juice, beef broth, or other fluids high in potassium can be given.

Antiacidosis Therapy

Alkali therapy to counteract the metabolic acidosis is usually reserved for severe acidosis only. The carbon dioxide content can serve as a guide for the degree of acidosis. A pH of less than 7 indicates acidosis severe enough for sodium bicarbonate therapy [13].

Sodium bicarbonate therapy can lead to transient spinal fluid acidosis in which there is a decrease in the pH of the cerebrospinal fluid. Part of the bicarbonate is converted to carbon dioxide. That carbon dioxide diffuses into the cerebrospinal fluid readily while the bicarbonate is exchanged slowly. Some clinicians feel that the spinal fluid acidosis occurs even without bicarbonate replacement [7].

Management of Symptoms

Other medical treatments of DKA may be instituted, depending on the needs of the individual patient. The treatments include dextran, plasma, or whole blood replacement in severe hypovolemic shock. Vasopressors, such as metaraminol, may be used in peripheral vascular collapse. Catecholamines are not recommended because they can form lactic acid and inhibit the action of insulin on the muscles [16]. Antibiotics are prescribed if an infection is present. Gastric intubation is used if vomiting or distention is present.

Nursing Orders

Problem/Diagnosis

Diabetic ketoacidosis

OBJECTIVE NO. 1

The patient should demonstrate a degree of rehydration sufficient to maintain his vascular tone.

To achieve the objective, the nurse should:

1. Observe the patient and assess him in regard to his state of hydration. She should:
   a. Note his skin turgor and hydration status, eyeball tone, and the condition of his mucous membranes.
   b. Check his urine output every hour.
   c. Check and regulate his intravenous rate every hour.
   d. Note the status of his Kussmaul's respirations.
   e. Examine him for a pleural friction rub.
   f. Check the specific gravity of his urine.
2. Give the patient intravenous fluids as ordered. The nurse should:
   a. Give him a 0.9% or 0.45% normal saline solution.

b. Maintain the sterility of his intravenous line.

c. Check the infusion site every four hours for signs of phlebitis, infiltration, or infection.

3. Assess the patient's cardiovascular functioning. The nurse should:

a. Check his vital signs every 30 to 60 minutes or as needed.

b. Check his central venous pressure to help evaluate his venous tolerance of high volumes of fluids.

c. Evaluate his venous system. The nurse should check the patient's heart rate and look for distended neck veins and peripheral or sacral edema.

d. Carry out continuous cardiac monitoring.

e. Evaluate all the pulses every two hours.

f. Observe the patient for congestive heart failure, especially the elderly patient.

4. Record information about the patient's fluid intake and output and vital signs on the flow sheet. The nurse should:

a. Check the patient's hourly intake and output.

b. Check his vital signs every 30 to 60 minutes (more often if needed).

c. Check his intravenous line every hour.

5. Give the patient fluids by mouth when he can tolerate them. The nurse should:

a. Evaluate the patient in regard to peristalsis (check for presence of bowel sounds).

b. Offer him fluids that are high in potassium (e.g., beef broth, orange juice, and oatmeal gruel).

6. Monitor the patient for the signs of cerebral edema (namely, the patient begins to awaken from a coma and then slips into a coma again). The nurse should have available a lumbar puncture tray and an osmotic diuretic, such as urea or mannitol.

OBJECTIVE NO. 2

The patient should receive enough insulin to correct his hyperglycemia without causing hypoglycemia.

To achieve the objective, the nurse should:

1. Give the patient regular insulin as ordered (50–200 units intravenously and/or subcutaneously). She should:

a. For the intravenous push route, give 50 units or less every minute [8].

b. With the intravenous infusion pump, the nurse should:

(1) Check the dose carefully.

(2) Maintain a sterile technique.

(3) Check the pump periodically to make sure the proper dose is being delivered.

c. Be aware that as much as 20 percent of the insulin may be bound to the tubing and bottle or bag. More binding occurs when lower doses of insulin are used. In time, the equipment can become saturated with insulin. Therefore, changing the equipment decreases the amount of insulin the patient receives, and keeping the same equipment increases the amount of insulin the patient receives [6]. As much as 44 to 47 percent of the insulin may be bound [14].

d. To avoid inactivation, do not mix the insulin with sodium bicarbonate.

2. Evaluate the patient's blood sugar levels every 30 to 60 minutes. The nurse should:

a. Check the patient's urine every hour. She should:

(1) Use fresh urine—either a specimen obtained by the needle method from the catheter or a second voided specimen.

(2) Select a method of urine testing that is the most accurate one in view of the other medications the patient is taking.

(3) Use the two-drop Clinitest method if the blood sugar level is 2% (4+) when the five-drop Clinitest method is used.

(4) Watch carefully for the "pass through" phase, and record the maximum amount if that phase occurs.

(5) Be aware of the differences in the readings of various urine test methods in regard to the lack of equality in percentages (%) and pluses (+). (For example, 2+ with Testape = ¼%; 2+ with Clinitest = ¾%; and 2+ with Diastix = ½%.) This can greatly affect the sliding-scale administration of insulin if used.

b. Notify the physician if the patient's blood sugar levels are 250 to 300 mg/100 ml.

3. Observe and assess the patient for hypoglycemia. The nurse should:

a. Know the signs of hypoglycemia:

(1) Excitability

(2) Diaphoresis

(3) Tremors

(4) Increased heart rate

(5) Dilated pupils

(6) Headache

(7) Seizures

(8) Decreased blood pressure

b. Know that sympathetic nervous system signs may be diminished or absent in the long-term diabetic (e.g., one who had had diabetes for 20 years).

c. Give a 5% glucose solution in the intravenous infusion when the patient's blood sugar level reaches 250 mg/100 ml.

d. Determine the patient's blood sugar levels if hypoglycemia is suspected.

e. Treat hypoglycemia with a 50% dextrose in water solution.

f. Observe the patient for the Somogyi phenomenon—the rebound effect. The nurse should:
   (1) Suspect the Somogyi phenomenon when the patient has alternating periods of hyperglycemia and hypoglycemia.
   (2) Know that the Somogyi phenomenon occurs when hypoglycemia causes a physiological compensation that elevates the blood sugar levels (i.e., the release of growth hormone, ACTH, and glucagon) and thus causes hyperglycemia.
   (3) Know that with hyperglycemia, the cycle is made worse if the physician increases the dosage of insulin (as often happens). The treatment is to *decrease* the insulin.

4. Watch the patient for signs of insulin resistance. The nurse should:
   a. Compare the patient's blood sugar levels to the amount of insulin given.
   b. Take into consideration the patient's usual dose of insulin.
   c. Give him hydrocortisone if his insulin resistance is severe.

OBJECTIVE NO. 3

The patient should regain his normal electrolyte balance.

To achieve the objective, the nurse should:

1. Assess the patient's potassium status. She should:
   a. Know the signs of hypokalemia:
      (1) Muscle weakness
      (2) Decrease in peristalsis (evidenced by ileus or distention)
      (3) Decrease in blood pressure
      (4) Weak pulse
      (5) Dysrhythmia

      (6) Respiratory arrest
      (7) ECG changes: A prolonged QT interval, a depressed T wave, and prominent U waves
   b. Know the signs of hyperkalemia:
      (1) Dysrhythmias: Heart block, ventricular fibrillation, and cardiac arrest
      (2) Intestinal disturbances (diarrhea and nausea)
      (3) ECG changes: Peaked T waves, absence of P wave, and wide QRS interval
   c. If the initial potassium level is low (it rarely is), give potassium chloride (20–40 mEq/L) immediately.
   d. If the initial potassium level is normal, give potassium chloride (20–40 mEq/L) one to four hours after fluid therapy is begun.
   e. If the initial potassium level is high, withhold potassium.

2. Assess and treat any sodium deficiency. The nurse should:
   a. Look for the signs of hyponatremia:
      (1) Abdominal cramps
      (2) Diarrhea
      (3) Apprehension
      (4) Increased heart rate
      (5) Diaphoresis
      (6) Cyanosis
      (7) Seizures
   b. Give sodium chloride in the initial intravenous fluid replacement as ordered.

3. Evaluate the results of electrolyte studies and notify the physician of any significant or unexpected changes.

4. Give other electrolytes as ordered.

5. Carry out continuous cardiac monitoring.

6. Give the patient fluids high in potassium by mouth when he is able to tolerate them.

OBJECTIVE NO. 4

The patient's acidosis should be assessed and corrected.

To achieve the objective, the nurse should:

1. Observe the patient and assess his degree of acidosis. She should:
   a. Check the relevant serum laboratory data: pH, bicarbonate, base deficit, and/or presence of acetone.

b. Check the serum and urine every hour for the presence of acetone. (The urine should be taken from the catheter tubing with a sterile syringe.)

c. Assess the depth of the patient's coma.

2. Give sodium bicarbonate for severe acidosis. The nurse should:

a. Give the sodium bicarbonate by intravenous push or add it to the intravenous solution.

b. Give 50 to 150 mEq of sodium bicarbonate initially.

c. Monitor the patient's pH and CO_2 content.

d. Observe the patient for spinal fluid acidosis (evidenced by an increase in lethargy and by a cerebrospinal fluid pH that is more acidotic than the serum pH).

OBJECTIVE NO. 5

The patient should regain and maintain the functioning of the body systems that were affected by DKA.

To achieve the objective, the nurse should:

1. Assess the patient's pulmonary status. She should:

a. Assess the patient's respiratory status by:

(1) Noting any decrease in Kussmaul's respirations.

(2) Auscultating his lungs.

(3) Checking him for pulmonary edema and congestive heart failure, which may be manifested by an increased heart rate, a third or fourth heart sound, or rales.

b. Evaluate his gas exchange, noting his PO_2 and PCO_2.

c. Give him oxygen as needed.

d. Suction his oronasopharynx and/or trachea as needed.

2. Assess and evaluate the patient's urinary system. The nurse should:

a. If the patient is comatose, insert a Foley catheter under sterile conditions.

b. Give the patient catheter care every four hours.

3. Assess and evaluate the patient's gastrointestinal system. The nurse should:

a. Insert a nasogastric tube if the patient is vomiting or if his abdomen is distended.

b. Auscultate his abdomen for bowel sounds every two hours and use the information gathered to decide whether to give him fluids by mouth.

c. Check the patient's intake and output every hour.

d. Give the patient mouth care every four hours, using swabs or a mouthwash.

4. Assess and evaluate the patient's body defense systems. The nurse should:

a. Observe the patient for signs of infection.

b. If he has an infection, give him antibiotics as ordered.

c. Turn him every one to two hours.

d. Give him eye care if he is comatose.

5. Assess the patient's psychosocial integrity. The nurse should:

a. Listen to the patient.

b. Learn what having diabetes means to him.

c. Allow him to make some decisions about his care and thus to have some control over his illness.

d. Include the patient's family in the patient's care and education.

6. Assess and evaluate the patient's neurological system. The nurse should:

a. Note the degree of his coma.

b. Check his vital signs every 30 to 60 minutes or as needed.

c. Observe for signs of spinal fluid acidosis.

OBJECTIVE NO. 6

The patient should be educated about the prevention of DKA.

To achieve the objective, the nurse should:

1. Find out what the patient and his family know about preventing DKA.

2. Assess their readiness to learn more.

3. Discuss with them the causes of hyperglycemia:

a. Infections. The nurse should ensure that when the patient is at home he will be able to (1) determine the presence of an infectious process and (2) take proper care of any wound he might receive.

b. Increased food intake.

c. Emotional stress.

d. Inadequate amounts of insulin.

4. Evaluate the patient's self-care ability and his self-evaluation habits. The nurse should make sure the patient understands:

a. How to test his urine.

b. How to give himself insulin. The patient must understand:
   (1) The need to rotate the site of administration.
   (2) The onset, peak, and duration of the type(s) of insulin he is taking.
   (3) The complications of insulin therapy: (a) insulin reaction, (b) lipodystrophy (atrophy, hypertrophy), and (c) allergy.
5. Discuss the signs and symptoms of hyperglycemia and hypoglycemia with the patient:
   a. Hyperglycemia: thirst, weakness, flushed face, glycosuria, acetonuria, and polyuria
   b. Hypoglycemia: nervousness or excitability, weakness, headache, diaphoresis, and behavior changes
6. Discuss the relationship of illness to diabetes. The patient should be told to:
   a. Notify his physician if he consistently has sugar or acetone in his urine.
   b. Try to take liquids if he is unable to eat solid food.
   c. Not omit insulin. (The physician may change the dosage to regular insulin or to a sliding-scale administration of insulin if the patient has an infection. An infection increases the patient's need for insulin.)
7. Instruct the patient and his family about the ADA diet. The nurse should:
   a. Assess the patient's eating habits.
   b. Discuss with the patient the diet he should follow if he becomes ill.
8. Discuss with the patient the complications of diabetes mellitus:
   a. Macrovascular disease
   b. Microvascular disease
   c. Neuropathy
   d. Infections
   e. Visual problems

Summary

DKA is a life-threatening condition that can occur in the patient with diabetes mellitus. The mortality is 1.5 to 15 percent. The critical care nurse needs to be able to assess the patient quickly, using her knowledge of the pathophysiology, anticipated patient problems, and medical management. DKA leads to (1) severe dehydration, (2) metabolic acidosis, and (3)

electrolyte depletion. Treatment is aimed at correcting those disorders and giving and evaluating the discharge teaching, which aims at preventing the recurrence of DKA.

Study Problems

1. The primary action of insulin is to:
   a. Alleviate hypoglycemia.
   b. Facilitate the movement of glucose across the cell membrane.
   c. Decrease osmotic pressure inside the vascular system.
2. The signs of ketoacidosis include:
   a. Acetone breath, flushed face, dry skin.
   b. Bounding pulse, headache, diaphoresis.
   c. Excitability, soft eyeballs, decreased skin turgor.
3. Name the two main types of intravenous fluid commonly used in DKA for fluid replacement.
4. Spinal fluid acidosis is probably caused by:
   a. Insulin therapy.
   b. Bicarbonate therapy.
   c. Potassium administration.
5. Hyperkalemia may be detected on cardiac monitoring by the presence of U waves and peaked T waves.
   a. True.
   b. False.

Answers

1. b.
2. a.
3. 0.9% normal saline solution; 0.45% normal saline solution.
4. b.
5. b.

References

1. Alberti, K., and Nattrass, M. Severe diabetic ketoacidosis. *Med. Clin. North Am.* 62:799, 1978.
2. Boshell, B., and Chaudalia, H. B. Hormonal Interrelationships. In M. Ellenberg and H. Rifkin (eds.), *Diabetes Mellitus: Theory and Practice.* New York: McGraw-Hill, 1970.

3. Bradley, R. Diabetic Ketoacidosis and Coma. In A. Marble, P. White, R. Bradley, et al. (eds.), *Joslin's Diabetes Mellitus* (11th ed.). Philadelphia: Lea & Febiger, 1971.

4. Constam, G. R. The Pancreas. In A. Labhart (ed.), *Clinical Endocrinology: Theory and Practice.* New York: Springer-Verlag, 1974.

5. Danowski, T. Diabetic Acidosis and Coma. In M. Ellenberg and H. Rifkin (eds.), *Diabetes Mellitus: Theory and Practice.* New York: McGraw-Hill, 1970.

6. Eli Lilly Research Laboratories. *Diabetes Mellitus* (3rd ed.). Indianapolis: Eli Lilly, 1976.

7. Felts, P. *Coma in the Diabetic.* Kalamazoo, Mich.: Upjohn, 1974.

8. Gahart, B. *Intravenous Medications* (2nd ed.). St. Louis: Mosby, 1977.

9. Johnson, J. E. Infection and Diabetes. In M. Ellenberg and H. Rifkin (eds.), *Diabetes Mellitus: Theory and Practice.* New York: McGraw-Hill, 1970.

10. Larner, J., and Haynes, R. Insulin and Oral Hypoglycemic Drugs. In L. S. Goodman and A. Gilman (eds.), *The Pharmacological Basis of Therapeutics* (5th ed.). New York: Macmillan, 1975.

11. Lock, J. P., and Sussman, K. E. Diabetes Mellitus in the Adult. In H. F. Conn (ed.), *Current Therapy.* Philadelphia: Saunders, 1977.

12. Salans, L., Hirsch, J., and Knittle, J. Obesity, Carbohydrate Metabolism and Diabetes Mellitus. In M. Ellenberg and H. Rifkin (eds.), *Diabetes Mellitus: Theory and Practice.* New York: McGraw-Hill, 1970.

13. Skillman, T., and Thzagournis, M. *Diabetes Mellitus.* Kalamazoo, Mich.: Upjohn, 1973.

14. Weber, S., Wood, W., and Jackson, E. Availability of insulin from parenteral nutrient solutions. *Am. J. Hosp. Pharm.* 34:353, 1977.

15. Weir, G. C., Samels, E., Loo, S., et al. Somatostatin and pancreatic polypeptide secretion. *Diabetes* 28:35, 1979.

16. Williams, R., and Porte, D. The Pancreas. In R. H. Williams (ed.), *Textbook of Endocrinology* (5th ed.). Philadelphia: Saunders, 1974.

17. Winegrad, A., and Clements, R. Diabetic ketoacidosis. *Med. Clin. North Am.* 55:899, 1971.

18. Zipf, W., Bacon, G., Spencer, M., et al. Hypocalcemia, hypomagnesemia and transient hypoparathyroidism during therapy with potassium phosphate in diabetic ketoacidosis. *Diabetes Care* 2:265, 1979.

Bibliography

American Diabetes Association. Special report: Principles of nutrition and dietary recommendations for individuals with diabetes mellitus. *Diabetes* 28:1027, 1979.

Assal, J. Metabolic effects of sodium bicarbonate in management of diabetic ketoacidosis. *Diabetes* 23:405, 1974.

Blevins, D. *The Diabetic and Nursing Care.* New York: McGraw-Hill, 1979.

Breckbill, V. Physiological Alterations in Diabetes. In D. Blevins (ed.), *The Diabetic und Nursing Care.* New York: McGraw-Hill, 1979.

Colwell, J. *Clinical Recognition and Treatment of Diabetic Vascular Disease.* Springfield, Ill.: Thomas, 1975.

Desimone, B. Psychosocial Implications of Diabetes. In D. Guthrie and R. Guthrie (eds.), *Nursing Management of Diabetes Mellitus.* St. Louis: Mosby, 1977.

Elsberry, N., and Power, L. Metabolic Crisis. In L. Meltzer, F. Abdellah, and J. Ketchell (eds.), *Intensive Care for Nurse Specialists* (2nd ed.). Bowie, Md.: Charles, 1976.

Guthrie, D., and Guthrie, R. DKA: Breaking a Vicious Cycle. In P. Chaney (ed.), Nursing Skillbook, *Managing Diabetes Properly.* Horsham, Pa.: Intermed Communications, 1977.

Guthrie, D., and Guthrie, R. (eds.). *Nursing Management of Diabetes Mellitus.* St. Louis: Mosby, 1977.

Jackson, R., and Guthrie, R. *The Child with Diabetes Mellitus.* Kalamazoo, Mich.: Upjohn, 1975.

Jordan, J. Acute Care of Diabetes. In D. Guthrie and R. Guthrie (eds.), *Nursing Management of Diabetes Mellitus.* St. Louis: Mosby, 1977.

Labhart, A. (ed.). *Clinical Endocrinology: Theory and Practice.* New York: Springer-Verlag, 1974.

Martin, C. *Textbook of Endocrine Physiology.* Baltimore: Williams & Wilkins, 1976.

Schade, D., and Eaton, R. P. Pathogenesis of DKA: A reappraisal. *Diabetes Care* 2:296, 1979.

Scott, J. R., Espiner, E. A., Donald, R. A., et al. Antibody binding of insulin in diabetic ketoacidosis. *Diabetes* 27:1151, 1979.

Sherwin, R., and Felig, P. Pathophysiology of diabetes mellitus. *Med. Clin. North Am.* 62:695, 1978.

Stroot, V., Lee, C., and Schaper, C. *Fluids and Electrolytes* (2nd ed.). Philadelphia: Davis, 1977.

Vallance-Owen, J. (ed.). *Diabetes: Its Physiological and Biochemical Basis.* Lancaster, U.K.: MTP, 1975.

Hyperosmolar Coma

Angela Pruitt Clark

Hyperosmolar coma (hyperosmolar nonketotic coma) is a complication of diabetes mellitus that can be manifested as an acute illness. The mortality in hyperosmolar coma (HOC) is quite high; it is generally thought to be 40 to 60% [2]. Unfortunately, HOC is often not diagnosed early enough to be treated successfully. It occurs mainly in the maturity-onset diabetic, and it is an emergency condition. HOC occurs also in the nondiabetic. Like diabetic ketoacidosis (DKA), HOC can lead to severe dehydration with loss of electrolytes and, if untreated, to death. The critical care nurse must be familiar with HOC so that she can help to make a rapid assessment. She must be able to apply her theoretical knowledge of HOC to the acutely ill patient so that he can be treated promptly.

Objective

The critical care nurse should understand the common causes and symptoms of HOC, should be able to perform a systematic assessment of the patient, including a physical examination, and should be able to anticipate and explain the medical and nursing management of the patient with HOC.

25

Achieving the Objective

To achieve the objective, the nurse should be able to:

1. Describe the causative and precipitating factors in HOC.
2. Discuss the pathophysiology of HOC.
3. After reading Chapter 24 (Diabetic Ketoacidosis), differentiate the patient with HOC from the patient with DKA on the basis of the clinical manifestations and the expected laboratory data.
4. Identify and list (in the order of importance) the patient care objectives for the patient with HOC.
5. Teach the diabetic patient with HOC and his family what they need to know to prevent complications.

How to Proceed

To develop an approach to HOC, the nurse should:

1. Study the physiological and pathological changes that occur in HOC.
2. Draw up or adapt a nursing assessment tool and apply it to the patient with HOC.
3. Read the case study that follows and immediately make a problem list. The nurse should use all the data in the case study to justify her choice of problems.
4. Describe the main medical and nursing interventions that the patient needs.

Case Study

Mrs. S. W., a 66-year-old retired teacher, was taken on a stretcher from a nearby convalescent center to the hospital. The charge nurse in the convalescent center had noticed early that afternoon that Mrs. W., who had become more and more difficult to arouse, had become semicomatose.

Mrs. W. was examined by the physician in the emergency room. Using a report from the convalescent center, the results of his physical examination, and the laboratory data, the physician made a tentative diagnosis of HOC, and he ordered initial therapy. Mrs. W. was transferred to the critical care unit.

Mrs. W.'s daughter and son-in-law, who had been notified by the convalescent center of Mrs. W.'s transfer, arrived at the hospital soon after her admission. They were able to give information about Mrs. W. Also, Mrs. W.'s medical records from the convalescent center had been sent with her to the hospital.

Mrs. W. had recently been treated in the same hospital for coronary insufficiency and mild congestive heart failure. She had had cardiac problems for several years and a myocardial infarction six years before. Although she had been hypertensive in the past, she had some difficulty with "low blood pressure" during her last hospital stay. Her current medications were digoxin (Lanoxin), furosemide (Lasix), and propranolol (Inderal).

Mrs. W. was known to have had diabetes for 10 years. She controlled the disease by diet therapy alone. Her daughter said that she thought that her mother had taken the "pills for diabetes" many years ago but she was not taking them at present.

Two weeks ago, Mrs. W. had been discharged from the hospital and transferred to the convalescent center to regain her strength and ability to care for herself. Her family said that she had suggested the transfer and has seemed to accept the need for it (she lived alone). It was thought that she would need to stay at the center for about six weeks.

Mrs. W. had made good progress at the center. Until two days before her present hospitalization, she had been able to take short walks down the hall with assistance. But two weeks ago, she said that she was too tired to walk, and she complained also of a "head cold." She did not seem to have any respiratory difficulty.

Mrs. W.'s past medical history listed several hospitalizations for her cardiac condition. She had never had any education about diabetes.

Mrs. W. had no known allergies. In addition to the medications mentioned, she was taking a multivitamin compound and diazepam (Valium) as needed.

Physical Examination

As soon as Mrs. W. was admitted to the intensive care unit, she was given a physical examination. The information gathered was later combined with the other assessment information to form a rather complete data base.

The following information was gathered in the physical examination:

1. General observations: Acutely ill white female; no intravenous line; some dyspnea; when admitted, patient receiving oxygen by nasal cannula
2. Vital signs: BP 96/70 supine, left arm; HR 116; sinus rhythm normal with occasional ectopic beats, primarily PVCs; R 32 and deep; no acetone breath; T 100.2°F rectally; height 5'7"; weight 140 lbs
3. Integument: Skin tone and turgor poor; skin very dry to touch; no lacerations or breaks in skin; scar on left ankle
4. Head: No masses; no abnormalities
5. Eyes: Pupils equal and reactive to light; eyeballs soft; sclera clear; no retinopathy
6. Ears: Membranes clear; no discharge
7. Nose: Flaring of nostrils on inspiration; no discharge
8. Mouth: Pink; mucous membranes very dry; patient edentulous
9. Neck: No lymphadenopathy; no bruits or neck vein distention

10. Chest: Vesicular breath sounds; no rales or rhonchi
11. Cardiovascular system: Normal first and second heart sounds; no third or fourth heart sound; no murmur; apical thrust; poor capillary refill; patient pale
12. Abdomen: Distended; liver nonpalpable; bowel sounds absent
13. Genitourinary system: No discharge; bladder distended
14. Extremities: Pulses present; some pedal edema bilaterally; no cyanosis; scar on left ankle; no diabetic foot lesions
15. Neurological responses: Deep tendon reflexes grade 1; no response to verbal stimuli

Laboratory Data
The following laboratory data were obtained immediately:

1. Blood sugar level 1156 mg/100 ml
2. Plasma ketones negative
3. Serum osmolality 356 mM/L
4. Complete blood count: White blood cells 9000; hemoglobin 16.3 gm; hematocrit 60%
5. Electrolytes: Sodium 146 mEq; potassium 4.5 mEq; chlorides 103 mEq; carbon dioxide combining power 18
6. Arterial blood gases: pH 7.33; PO_2 90 mm Hg; PCO_2 33 mm Hg
7. Urinalysis negative except for 5% glucose
8. Other data: Blood urea nitrogen 70 mg; cholesterol 204 mg
9. Chest x ray: Negative; some cardiomegaly

Clinical Presentation of Case Study
When Mrs. W. was admitted to the intensive care unit, the nurse immediately began her assessment and examination (see assessment sheet). The following intravenous fluids were started: (1) a 0.45% normal saline solution infused in a left antecubital vein with an angiocath at a rate of 300 ml per hour and (2) regular insulin (25 units by intravenous push) for the elevated blood sugar level. Mrs. W.'s vital signs were checked every 15 minutes. It was felt that she was hypotensive because she was dehydrated but that she was not in hypovolemic shock. Continuous cardiac monitoring was initiated. It showed a normal sinus rhythm with about one premature ventricular contraction every two minutes. No T-wave changes were noted. A Foley catheter was inserted, and 1100 ml of urine was obtained.

3:15 P.M. BP 100/74. Apical HR increased to 128. No
(2nd hour) clinical signs of heart failure, except the sinus tachycardia. Observation continued. Intravenous fluid rate 300 ml per hour (no increase). Blood sugar 804 mg/100 ml. Regular insulin (25 units by intravenous push into tubing medication additive site). No improvement in skin turgor or mucous membranes.

5:15 P.M. Sinus tachycardia 140. Digoxin (0.25 mg by
(4th hour) intravenous push). Blood sugar 630 mg/100 ml.

Regular insulin (25 units by intravenous push). Urine glycosuria 3% when two-drop Clinitest method used.

6:15 P.M. HR decreased to 124. Electrolytes: sodium 134,
(5th hour) potassium 3.9. Blood sugar 501 mg/100 ml. Serum osmolality 338 mM/L.

9:15 P.M. Visit from family. Mrs. W. still unconscious. No signs of congestive heart failure. HR 100. Arterial blood gases: pH 7.34, PO_2 91, PCO_2 35. Potassium decreased to 3.6. Potassium chloride added to intravenous line. Regular insulin (20 units by intravenous push).

12:15 A.M. Blood sugar 379 mg/100 ml. Mrs. W. partly
(10th hour) aroused when spoken to. Hourly check of vital signs continued. BP 116/78; HR 98. Infusion of 0.45% normal saline solution continued but rate decreased to 200 ml per hour.

4:15 A.M. Mrs. W. awake and asking for daughter. Daugh-
(14th hour) ter not in family room; Mrs. W. assured by nurse that daughter had been present all evening. Patient seemed satisfied with that information.

5:15 A.M. Blood sugar 315 mg/100 ml. Regular insulin (10 units subcutaneously).

9:00 A.M. Patient taking fluids by mouth as tolerated.
(2nd day) Bowel sounds present. No distention. Saline infusion continued. Blood sugar 210 mg/100 ml. No insulin given. Intravenous therapy changed to 5% dextrose in water solution. Serum osmolality 308 mM/L.

3:00 P.M. Blood sugar 174 mg/100 ml. Regular insulin (8 units subcutaneously). Mrs. W. asked nurse if she would have to take insulin for the rest of her life. Nurse said that the physician thought Mrs. W. would not have to take insulin after she was discharged from the hospital and that the physician would discuss the question with Mrs. W. later. Mrs. W. tolerating liquids well. Intravenous infusion discontinued. Mrs. W. transferred from the intensive care unit to a nursing unit.

6:00 P.M. Sixteen-hundred calorie soft ADA diet taken without difficulty.

3rd Day Teaching about diabetes begun by teaching team made up of a nurse, a pharmacist, and a dietitian. Blood sugar 164 mg/100 ml. Patient told that she was to attempt to control her diabetes with diet and moderate exercise. If attempt not successful, patient would be given a "pill for your diabetes"—an oral hypoglycemic.

5th Day Patient still complaining of some weakness. Vital signs stable. Sugar level responding to diet.

Critical Care Nursing Admission Assessment
Major Systems Approach

PATIENT'S NAME: _Mrs. S.W._ DATE: _2/4_ TIME: _2^{15} pm_

DIAGNOSIS: _Diabetic coma; poss. CVA_ T: _100^2 (R)_ A.P.: _116_ R.P.: _116_ R.: _32_

B.P.: _96/70_ E.C.G. RHYTHM: _Sinus tach_ ECTOPY: _occas. PVC_ WT: _140 lbs._ HT: _5'7"_

ADMITTED VIA: _stretcher_ INFORMANT: _daughter; records from convalescent center_ LAST MEAL: _7pm yesterday_ _small amt._

I. CHIEF COMPLAINT: _found in somnolent state; came from convalescent center_

II. PATIENT PROFILE:
1. Age _66_ 2. Sex _female_
3. Marital Status M Ⓦ D S _attends church 2x week_
4. Race _Cauc._ 5. Religion _Baptist, "very religious"_
6. Occupation _retired school teacher; taught Freshman Eng. + Comp._
7. Availability of Family _daughter and son-in-law appear concerned + responsible_
8. Dietary _1800 cal. ADA; meals prepared at Conv. Ctr.; needs assistance to stay on diet; tends to eat less than she can_
9. Sleeping _5-6 hrs./night; 3-4 hr. nap every p.m.; severe insomnia after husband's death, but better now!_
10. Activities of Daily Living _recent discharge from hospital - dependent on staff at ctr. for most needs - ambulatory short distances (2 blocks twice a day c̄_

III. HISTORY OF PRESENT ILLNESS: _lethargic 2 days - too tired to walk last 2 days - unable to arouse all day today - known diabetic (diet controlled) - hospitalized for 9 days c̄ coronary insuff. - at ctr. for 2 weeks_

IV. PAST MEDICAL HISTORY:
1. Pediatric & Adult Illnesses _Pedi? adult - see below + childbirth 1945 (at home)_
2. Cardiac _1964 Chest pain   1973 CHF / 1970 Chest pain, cor. insuff.   1978 Coronary insuff. mild CHF / 1971 MI / 1972 CHF_
3. Hypertension _several years ago - last admission hypotensive_
4. Respiratory _1952 Pneumonia c̄ septic shock_
5. Diabetes Mellitus _dx 1967 diet controlled now_
6. Renal _____
7. Jaundice _1969 Cholecystitis s̄ jaundice_
8. Infections _occasional - not major problem_
9. Other _no diabetic education_
10. Hospitalizations & Surgeries _hospitalized c̄ all above cardiac problems + 1952 pneumonia_

11. Current Medication _Lanoxin, Lasix, Inderal, "a multivitamin"; (Valium prn)_
12. Allergies _NKA_
13. Habits _no alcohol or tobacco_

V. FAMILY HISTORY: _parents deceased; father had chest pain - no dx.; mother diabetic; 1 sister - hypertension, insul. dep. diabetic; 1 sister - nothing known_

VI. PSYCHOSOCIAL:
1. Behavior During Assessment _comatose_

2. Specific Problems _hx. of depression when husband died (40 yrs. together)_

VII. PHYSICAL EXAMINATION:
1. General _comatose, non-responsive, pale_

arterial blood gases: pH 7.33
2. Respiratory System _pO$_2$ 80mm Hg. pCO$_2$ 33mm Hg._
Airway _open_
Inspection _flaring nares; trachea midline; no retractions; 1:2;_
Rate _32_
Rhythm _tachypnea_
Chest Wall _no abnormalities noted_
Palpation _unable to elicit tenderness_
Percussion _resonant, equal_

Auscultation
Voice Sounds _unable to assess_
Breath Sounds _____
Normal ✓ Increased____ Decreased____
Adventitious Sounds _no rales, rhonchi,_
wheezing

3. Cardiovascular System
A.P. _116_ R.P. _116_
B.P. Supine R _96/70_ L _96/68_
P.M.I. _displaced left of MCL - approx 3cm. diam._
Heart Sounds _S₁ S₂ nml. - no S₃ or S₄_
heard - no murmurs heard
Thrills _no, but apical thrust present_
Peripheral Pulses _all present c̄ poor capillary_
refill

4. Neurological System
Level of Consciousness _comatose_

Respiratory Pattern _tachypnea_

Cranial Nerves _II, III, IV, VI_
grossly intact

Eyes _no retinopathy_
(1) Pupils   OD   OS
Size _nml_   _nml_
Shape _nml_   _nml_
Light _reactive, =_   _reactive, =_
Consensual _ok_   _ok_
Accommodation _(comatose)_
(2) Ocular Movements _____
Doll's eyes absent
Motor _comatose_

Sensory _comatose_
Coordination _comatose_

Reflexes _deep tendon reflexes grade_
_1+_

5. Gastrointestinal System
Nose & Mouth _no abnormalities; no_
acetone breath; needs oral care
Stomach _distended?_

Abdomen _____

Bowel Sounds _absent_
Liver _non-palpable_
Spleen _____ "_

6. Renal & Genitourinary Systems
I. _I.V. started / comatose all day_ O. _to be cathed_
Urinary Bladder & Urethra
bladder distended
Kidneys _unable to palpate_

7. Musculoskeletal System
Spine _nml_
Extremities _some pedal edema;_
scar on (L) ankle; no dermopathy
seen
Sacral Edema _no_
Masses _none noted_

8. Hematologic System
Petechiae _no_
Ecchymosis _no_
Gingiva _no bleeding_

9. Endocrine System
Breath _no acetone odor_
Skin _dry, dehydrated, poor turgor_

VIII. LABORATORY:
1. Hematology
HGB _16.3 gm._ HCT _60%_
W.B.C. _9000_
2. Chemistry
Na _146 meq._ K _4.5_
CO₂ _18_ CL _103_
Blood Sugar _1156 mg.%_ ~~Amylase~~ _plasma ketones neg._
BUN _70_ ~~C~~ _serum osmolarity 356 mM/L_
3. Urinalysis _neg. except glucose. 5%_

4. Electrocardiogram _sinus tachycardia_
Rate _114_ ~~Rhythm~~
P-R _.18_ QRS _.10_ Q wave in II, III, F
Interpretation _consistent c̄ old M.I., sinus tachycardia_
5. Chest x-ray _neg.; cardiomegaly_

IX. PROBLEM LIST:

ACTIVE	INACTIVE
1. comatose →	9. childbirth at home 1945
2. dehydration →	10. pneumonia c̄ septic shock 1952
3. ↑ BS →	
4. lack of knowledge, re diabetic and cardiac information	11. cholecystitis 1969
	12. MI 1971
5. self care deficit	13. CHF 1972, 1973, 1979
6. coronary insuff.	14. depression on death of husband 1977
7. immobility	

J. Clark, RN
NURSE'S SIGNATURE
8. Diabetes mellitus (dx. 1967)

6th Day Patient discharged to daughter's home. To see physician in two days for follow-up care. Patient and daughter encouraged to contact the teaching team if they had questions.

Reflections

HOC demonstrates vividly the interrelatedness of mind and body. One's mental acuity changes with changes in osmolality. As one's intellectual functioning deteriorates, a vicious cycle may become established. Thus the patient may forget to give himself insulin or take oral hypoglycemics, or he may become oblivious to his deteriorating physical condition. As his judgment fails, his self-care also fails. That failure is usually disastrous, because to prevent a diabetic crisis, the diabetic must pay close attention to detail. Thus in diabetes body and mind must function as a unit. In diabetes, what the patient thinks and perceives affects the course of the disease; and, as hyperosmolar coma demonstrates, the disease adversely affects the patient's thoughts and perceptions. Diabetes mellitus demonstrates the interrelatedness of mind and body, an essential concept for nurses to consider.

Pathophysiology of Hyperosmolar Coma

The principles of physiology discussed in Chapter 24 (Diabetic Ketoacidosis) are valid for HOC also. The pathophysiology discussed in Chapter 24 also helps one understand HOC better. (HOC and DKA are compared in Table 25-1.)

HOC is a comatose or near-comatose state that develops in (usually) an adult-onset diabetic. It is characterized by a significant degree of hyperglycemia, hyperosmolality, hypernatremia, and dehydration. If acidosis is present, it is due not to DKA but to an accompanying lactic or renal acidosis.

The incidence of HOC is the same in men and women, and it is one-sixth the incidence of DKA [2]. HOC is seen primarily in people 60 years of age and older [4]. Most people who develop HOC are adult-onset diabetics (as mentioned) or people who develop diabetes at the same time that they develop HOC. After the acute phase of HOC, the diabetes can usually be controlled by diet and oral hypoglycemic drugs [2]. In some cases, diabetes is not present, and it never develops [17]. Rarely, a child with juvenile-onset diabetes presents in HOC [3].

Numerous factors precipitate or accompany HOC. Those factors increase the person's need for insulin beyond the amount he can produce. The factors may be divided into three groups: (1) certain acute or chronic diseases, (2) the use of certain medical procedures, and (3) the use of certain drugs. The three groups are discussed in the following paragraphs.

Acute or Chronic Conditions

The following conditions have been noted to precipitate or accompany HOC:

1. Severe burns (often treated with large amounts of glucose) [17]
2. Diabetes insipidus [17]
3. Hyperthyroidism [17]
4. Dehydration [17]
5. Acute pancreatitis [17]
6. Central nervous system damage [13]
7. Gastrointestinal bleeding [13]
8. Protracted diarrhea [13]
9. Gram-negative pneumonia [2]
10. Uremia [2]
11. Acute pyelonephritis [3]
12. Acute myocardial infarction [2]
13. Subdural hematoma [2]
14. Arterial thrombosis [2]
15. Chronic renal insufficiency [4]

Most of the conditions that precipitate or accompany HOC are acute illnesses. However, many are chronic, such as renal disease. It is thought that about 85 percent of patients with HOC have renal and/or cardiovascular disease [2].

Medical Procedures

The following medical procedures are associated with HOC:

1. Peritoneal dialysis (involving the use of a hyperosmolar dialysate)
2. Hypothermia [17]
3. Nasogastric tube feedings with high-protein mixtures [13]
4. Intravenous hyperalimentation [2]

Table 25-1
Comparison of Hyperosmolar Coma (HOC) and Diabetic Ketoacidosis (DKA)

Factor	HOC	DKA
Age	Older adult, usually over 50	Any age
Diabetic status	Usually adult-onset diabetic—may be undiagnosed	Often a known diabetic, usually a juvenile-onset diabetic
Hyperglycemia	Frequently over 1000 mg/100 ml	Generally less than 1000 mg/100 ml
Ketosis; acidosis	No ketosis; if acidosis present, it is lactic or renal	Yes
Severe dehydration	Yes	Yes
Acetone breath	No	Yes
Serum sodium	Usually high (may be normal or low)	Usually low
Insulin as treatment	Not as much needed as in DKA, usually less than 100 units	Large amounts essential

Drugs

The following drugs have been known to cause or accompany HOC:

1. Diphenylhydantoin (Dilantin) [2]
2. Thiazide diuretics [2]
3. Steroids [17]
4. Mannitol [17]
5. Propranolol (Inderal) [2]
6. Immunosuppressive drugs [2]
7. Diazoxide [2]
8. Glucagon [4]
9. Furosemide (Lasix) [4]
10. Ethacrynic acid (Edecrin) [4]
11. Azathioprine [3]
12. Sodium bicarbonate (large amounts in infusion) [5]
13. Alcohol intoxication [5]

The stressors just listed increase the body's need for insulin. The person who develops HOC does not have enough insulin to cope with the stressor. Since insulin is not available to help transport glucose into the cell, the blood glucose concentration rises.

Hyperglycemia develops because of a decrease in the peripheral utilization of glucose by muscle and liver cells and also because the liver increases its glucose production as a result of glycogenolysis and glyconeogenesis [4]. The endogenous production of glucose by the liver in the adult-onset diabetic can reach large quantities—up to 1000 gm per day [2].

In the adult-onset diabetic the insulin reserve is decreased, whereas in the juvenile-onset diabetic significant amounts of insulin are not produced. The adult-onset diabetic usually has a progressively diminishing insulin release as his disease progresses.

The range of hyperglycemia is 800 to 2800 mg/100 ml or higher [10]. The normal renal threshold for glucose (about 170 mg/100 ml) is quickly exceeded, and glycosuria ensues, with a dramatic loss of water and electrolytes. The depletion causes severe dehydration and leads to hypovolemia and hemoconcentration [10]. With the decrease in volume, renal blood flow is decreased, and a prerenal azotemia [10] that leads to further hyperglycemia occurs. Renal insufficiency is probably present in all patients with HOC. The average blood urea nitrogen (BUN) level is 60 to 90 mg [2].

The osmolality of body fluids can be calculated with the use of an osmometer or one of several formulas. The normal range for serum osmolality is 280 to 300 mM/L. If an estimate of osmolality is desired, the following procedure can be followed:

1. Convert mg/100 ml to mM/L as follows:
   a. To get the number of mM/L of glucose, divide mg/100 ml by 18 (determined by the molecular weight of glucose).
   b. To get the number of mM/L of BUN, divide mg/ml by 2.8 (determined by the molecular weight of urea nitrogen).
   c. Sodium and potassium are already reported in mEq/L or mM/L.

To allow for the unmeasured anions, multiply the amount of sodium and potassium by 1.8.

2. The following formula can then be applied:

$$\text{Serum osmolality} = \frac{\text{glucose}}{18} + \frac{\text{BUN}}{2.8} + 1.8\,(\text{Na} + \text{K})$$

Example: $\frac{1200}{18} + \frac{60}{2.8} + 1.8 \times (150 + 5) = 367$ mM/L

When a patient's osmolality level is higher than 310 mM/L, he shows some signs of confusion. At a level of 325 mM/L and above, coma is likely to occur [5]. In HOC, the osmolality level is frequently higher than 360 mM/L [12].

Normally, variations in plasma osmolality regulate the amount of antidiuretic hormone (ADH). When a hypertonic osmolar state occurs, the hypothalamus is stimulated to release ADH, which renders the distal nephron and collecting tubules more permeable to water. Thus water can be resorbed. A decrease in plasma osmolality (hypotonicity) inhibits ADH secretion and thus renders the distal convoluted tubule and collecting ducts relatively impermeable to water. The result is excretion of a dilute urine so that water is lost but solutes are retained in order to establish a more normal plasma osmolality [1].

However, hyperglycemia and the osmotic diuresis it brings cause such an increased volume of urine through the distal convoluted tubules and collecting tubules that the kidney can no longer maintain a water balance. Severe dehydration in all three body compartments follows. People so affected lose water and electrolytes but they lose relatively more water than electrolytes [13].

The serum sodium levels in HOC are frequently high, averaging about 145 mEq/L, and they contribute to the hyperosmolar state [2]. Values as high as 200 mEq/L have been seen [3]. The serum sodium levels may be low or low normal, reflecting the dilution of serum sodium in the water osmotically obligated to glucose [13]. There is a decrease in the serum sodium of about 2.7 mEq/L for every 100 mg/100 ml of blood glucose.

The absence of ketosis distinguishes HOC from DKA. Although that absence is not entirely understood, it is theorized that sufficient amounts of insulin are produced to prevent or inhibit lipolysis. The ability of insulin to inhibit lipolysis is 10 times greater than its ability to promote glucose uptake [17]. Therefore greater amounts of insulin are needed to utilize the glucose than to keep pace with the free fatty acids in the liver [6]. In research studies, dehydration has been found to be antiketogenic [3].

Clinical Picture

The histories of patients with HOC usually note an insidious onset (a few days or weeks) of thirst and polyuria and no significant water replacement. Some patients have polyphagia, which they tried to satisfy by eating a high-carbohydrate diet [17]. Patients with HOC may be stuporous or comatose on admission [13], probably with severe dehydration, an altered state of consciousness, and other neurological disturbances [12].

Severe dehydration is shown by such clinical signs as decreased skin turgor, dry skin, thirst, and soft eyeballs. Hypotension is present and hypovolemic shock can be a complication of the dehydration. Vomiting and diarrhea are seen in many of the patients. Abdominal tenderness may be noted [16].

The respirations in HOC may be rapid but not acidotic as are the Kussmaul's respirations in DKA [17]. The breath does not smell of acetone [13].

The central nervous system dysfunction can be manifested in hallucinations or vestibular disturbances. Approximately 15 percent of patients have some seizures [2]. Dehydration accounts for the depressed state of consciousness [5].

Diagnosis

Prompt diagnosis of HOC is critically important. A delay can mean death for the patient. Because the symptoms may resemble those of many other conditions, HOC is often not suspected until it is too late. The most common misdiagnosis is cerebral vascular accident [2].

The diagnosis is based on a clinical assessment of the signs and symptoms and information obtained from the history (if one can be taken) and from laboratory tests. The nurse who understands HOC will be more apt to consider its presence in the acutely ill, dehydrated patient.

Laboratory Tests

Several diagnostic tests are indicated in HOC. The tests that should be done immediately are a blood sugar test, a urinalysis to test for the presence of sugar and ketones, and determinations of the blood ketone level (to rule out DKA), the arterial blood gas measurements, and the serum osmolality.

The blood sugar range in HOC is 800 to 2800 mg/100 ml [3]. (Rarely, a blood sugar up to 4800 may be seen [14].) It is higher than that in DKA. A high degree of glycosuria is present. If the blood sugar level is high and serum ketones are absent, HOC should be considered first.

The patient with pure HOC (no DKA or lactic acidosis) is not acidotic, but often he has a slight degree of metabolic acidosis. An average pH of 7.26 has been found in patients with pure HOC [2].

The serum osmolality test is the most important test. In HOC, a reading of over 350 mM/L is obtained [2].

Other helpful tests are the BUN and electrolyte levels and a white blood cell count. In HOC, the BUN level is elevated, averaging 60 to 90 mg [2]. Leukocytosis is marked and not particularly helpful in ruling out DKA. Electrolytes are lost in the osmotic diuresis, but the water imbalance may cause high, low, or normal electrolyte readings. Hypernatremia is usually seen, averaging 145 mEq [2]. A sodium range of 100 to 180 mg has been seen [17]. Serum potassium levels may be high, low, or normal, but there is a total body deficit [7]. The plasma bicarbonate level is usually greater than 15 mEq/L [9].

Treatment

It is obvious from the high mortality in HOC that prompt diagnosis and treatment are essential. The chief components of therapy are: (1) fluid replacement, (2) insulin therapy, (3) electrolyte replacement, and (4) management of other symptoms as needed. Since the treatment of HOC closely resembles that of DKA the reader will probably find it helpful to read the discussion of treatment in Chapter 24. The flow sheet in that chapter can be adapted to the patient with HOC and can be used as a record of treatment.

Fluid Replacement

Because patients with HOC are severely dehydrated, prompt initiation of rehydration therapy is of primary importance. There are wide variations of opinion regarding the best combinations of water and electrolytes for replacement. Usually more fluid replacement is needed for HOC than for DKA. Up to 20 percent of the total body water may have been lost in

HOC [2]. The volume replacement may range from 6 to 16 liters in 24 hours [9].

If the patient shows signs of hypovolemic shock or vascular collapse, a plasma expander (e.g., dextran) is used initially [2]. Isotonic normal saline solution may be used at the same time [7]. Albumin or whole blood is occasionally ordered [13]. After the blood pressure is stabilized, large volumes of hypotonic electrolyte solutions are administered. Most authorities prefer to use 0.45% normal saline solution, but some use full-strength saline solution. Dextrose solutions are not used early in the treatment, but they may be ordered later to provide more water [13].

Since most patients with HOC are elderly, their cardiovascular and renal tolerance of high-volume fluid replacement must be assessed. Monitoring the patient's central venous pressure and urinary output will help in managing rehydration.

Too rapid correction of the hyperglycemia and dehydration can lead to cerebral edema. The polyol pathway (glucose → sorbitol → fructose) is one of the possible factors in cerebral edema. The increased sorbitol formed in the cell tends to remain there because the membranes are not very permeable to sorbitol. The sorbitol then pulls in extracellular water by osmosis, increasing the edema potential [4]. Another cause of edema may be the correction of the extracellular high glucose levels without correction of the brain glucose levels [7]. Water readily penetrates the blood-brain barrier, but glucose does not.

Another complication of fluid therapy is a secondary or latent shock state of dehydration. As the hyperosmolar state improves and the blood glucose level falls rapidly, the intracellular spaces begin to pull in water, which leads to an intravascular hypotension [13].

Fluids are given by mouth when the patient is able to tolerate them and when bowel sounds are present.

Insulin Therapy

Chapter 24 discusses the methods of administering insulin and gives other information about insulin that is relevant to the treatment of HOC.

The amount of insulin needed in HOC is less than that needed in DKA (because acidemia and ketonemia are not present in HOC), but insulin is nevertheless essential. The blood glucose level will fall somewhat with rehydration alone, partly because hypertonicity inhibits the release of insulin from the pancreas. The goal of insulin therapy is a gradual decrease in hyperglycemia and hyperosmolality [10].

Patients with HOC have been shown to be more sensitive to insulin than are patients with DKA. Thus patients with HOC may respond to much smaller doses than would be expected. A total of 100 to 200 units may suffice [9]. An initial dose of 25 to 50 units of regular insulin is usual [16]. Further doses of regular insulin are based on continual blood sugar readings.

The biological half-life of regular insulin is about 10 minutes. When insulin is given intravenously, the response is immediate. If a bolus is given, in 10 minutes only one-half the total insulin remains. When insulin is given subcutaneously, it is absorbed more slowly and its half-life is about four hours. Intramuscular injections are absorbed faster than are subcutaneous injections, but obviously intramuscular injections are "slower" than are intravenous injections. The half-life of insulin given intramuscularly is about two hours [4].

After the acute phase of HOC, the patient usually does not require insulin to treat his diabetes; it can be controlled by diet. Some patients need oral hypoglycemics [16].

It is imperative to avoid hypoglycemia. Careful monitoring of the serum glucose levels and observation of the patient are also essential (see the discussion of insulin therapy in Chap. 24). Intravenous glucose should be administered and insulin stopped when the blood sugar level nears 250 mg/100 ml [2].

Electrolyte Replacement

Sodium replacement is done with a normal saline infusion. Parenteral replacement of potassium is considered after hydration begins to shift potassium back into the cells, lowering the serum potassium level. Potassium chloride or potassium phosphate may be added to the intravenous solution. Knowing the serum potassium levels and using cardiac monitoring should help the physician to decide about potassium replacement.

Other Factors

As discussed, many disease conditions may accompany HOC. Those conditions must be treated appropriately.

Nursing Orders

Problem/Diagnosis

Hyperosmolar coma

OBJECTIVE NO. 1

The patient should demonstrate a degree of rehydration sufficient to maintain his vascular tone.

To achieve the objective, the nurse should:

1. Observe the patient and assess him in regard to his state of hydration. The nurse should:
   a. Note his skin turgor, eyeball tone, and the condition of his mucous membranes.
   b. Check his urine output every hour.
   c. Check and regulate his intravenous rate every hour.
   d. Note his ventilation status.
   e. Examine him for a pleural friction rub.
   f. Check the specific gravity of his urine.
2. Give the patient intravenous fluids as ordered. The nurse should:
   a. Use a volume expander (e.g., dextran) for hypovolemic shock.
   b. Use a 0.45% normal saline solution (0.9% normal saline may be ordered).
   c. Maintain the sterility of his intravenous line.
   d. Check his infusion site every four hours for signs of phlebitis, infiltration, and infection.
   e. Check his intravenous line every hour.
3. Give fluids by mouth when the patient can tolerate them. The nurse should:
   a. Evaluate the patient in regard to peristalsis (check him for bowel sounds).
   b. Offer him fluids that are high in potassium (e.g., beef broth, orange juice, and oatmeal gruel).
4. Monitor the patient for signs of cerebral edema (e.g., the patient begins to awaken from a coma and then slips into a coma again). The nurse should have available a lumbar puncture tray and an osmotic diuretic, such as urea or mannitol.

OBJECTIVE NO. 2

The patient should receive enough insulin to correct his hyperglycemia without causing hypoglycemia.

To achieve the objective, the nurse should:

1. Give the patient regular insulin as ordered (25–50 units intravenously, subcutaneously, or intramuscularly). The nurse should:

a. For the intravenous push route, give 50 units or less over one minute [11].

b. With an intravenous infusion pump, the nurse should:
   (1) Check the dose carefully.
   (2) Maintain a sterile technique.
   (3) Check the pump periodically to make sure the proper dose is being delivered.

c. Be aware that as much as 20 percent of the insulin may be bound to the tubing and bottle or bag. More binding occurs when lower doses of insulin are used. In time, the equipment can become saturated with insulin. Therefore, changing the administration set decreases the insulin dose and keeping the same set can increase the amount of insulin the patient receives [8]. As much as 44 to 47 percent of the insulin may be bound [15].

d. To avoid inactivation, do not mix the insulin with sodium bicarbonate.

2. Evaluate the patient's blood sugar levels every 30 to 60 minutes. The nurse should:
   a. Check the patient's urine every hour. She should:
      (1) Use fresh urine—a specimen obtained by the needle method from the catheter or a second voided specimen.
      (2) Select a method of urine testing that is the most accurate in the light of the other medications the patient is receiving.
      (3) Use the two-drop Clinitest method if the blood sugar level is 2% (4+) when the five-drop Clinitest method is used.
      (4) Watch carefully for the "pass through" phase and record the maximum amount if that phase occurs.
      (5) Be aware of the differences in the readings of various urine test methods in regard to the lack of equality in percentages (%) and pluses (+). (For example, 2+ with Testape = ¼%; 2+ with Clinitest = ¾%; and 2+ with Diastix = ½%.) This can greatly affect the patient who is on a sliding scale.
   b. Monitor the patient's blood sugar levels.
   c. Notify the physician if the blood sugar levels are 250 to 300 mg/100 ml.

3. Observe the patient and assess him for hypoglycemia. The nurse should:
   a. Know the signs of hypoglycemia:
      (1) Excitability
      (2) Perspiration

      (3) Tremors
      (4) Increased heart rate
      (5) Dilated pupils
      (6) Headache
      (7) Seizures
      (8) Blood pressure that is normal initially and then decreases
      (9) Decreased blood pressure
   b. Know that sympathetic signs may be diminished or absent in the long-term diabetic (e.g., one who has had diabetes for 20 years).
   c. Give a 5% glucose solution intravenously when the patient's blood sugar reaches 250 mg/100 ml.
   d. Determine the patient's blood sugar levels if hypoglycemia is suspected.
   e. Treat hypoglycemia with a 50% dextrose in water solution.
   f. Observe the patient for the Somogyi phenomenon—the rebound effect. The nurse should:
      (1) Suspect the Somogyi effect when the patient has alternating periods of hyperglycemia and hypoglycemia.
      (2) Know that the Somogyi phenomenon occurs when hypoglycemia causes a physiological compensation that elevates the blood sugar levels (i.e., the release of growth hormone, ACTH, and glucagon) and thus causes hyperglycemia.
      (3) Know that with hyperglycemia the cycle is worse. The treatment is to decrease the insulin.

4. Remember that the person with HOC is sensitive to insulin.

OBJECTIVE NO. 3

The patient should regain a normal electrolyte balance.

To achieve the objective, the nurse should:

1. Assess the patient's potassium status. She should:
   a. Know the signs of hypokalemia:
      (1) Muscle weakness
      (2) Decrease in peristalsis (evidenced by ileus or distention)
      (3) Decrease in blood pressure
      (4) Weak pulse
      (5) Dysrhythmia
      (6) Respiratory arrest

(7) ECG changes: a prolonged QT interval, a depressed T wave, and U wave
b. Know the signs of hyperkalemia:
(1) Dysrhythmias: heart block, ventricular fibrillation, and cardiac arrest
(2) Intestinal disturbances (diarrhea and nausea)
(3) ECG changes: peaked T waves, absence of P wave, wide QRS interval
c. If the initial potassium level is low (it rarely is), give potassium chloride (20–40 mEq/L) immediately.
d. If the initial potassium level is normal, give potassium chloride (20–40 mEq/L) one to four hours after fluid therapy is begun.
e. If the initial potassium level is high, withhold potassium.
2. Assess and treat the patient for any sodium deficiency. The nurse should:
a. Know the signs of hyponatremia:
(1) Abdominal cramps
(2) Diarrhea
(3) Apprehension
(4) Increased heart rate
(5) Diaphoresis
(6) Cyanosis
(7) Seizures
b. Give sodium chloride in the initial intravenous fluid replacement as ordered.
3. Evaluate results of electrolyte studies and notify the physician of significant and unexpected changes.
4. Give other electrolytes as ordered.
5. Carry out continuous cardiac monitoring.
6. Give fluids high in potassium by mouth when the patient is able to tolerate them.

OBJECTIVE NO. 4

The patient should regain and maintain the functioning of the other body systems that were affected by HOC.
To achieve the objective, the nurse should:

1. Assess the patient's pulmonary status. The nurse should:
a. Assess his respiratory status. She should:
(1) Auscultate his lungs.
(2) Check him for pulmonary edema and congestive heart failure, which may be manifested by an increased heart rate, third and fourth heart sounds, or rales.
b. Evaluate his gas exchange, noting his PO_2 and PCO_2.
c. Give him oxygen as needed.
d. Suction his oronasopharynx and/or trachea as needed.
2. Assess and evaluate his urinary system. The nurse should:
a. Insert a Foley catheter under sterile conditions if the patient is comatose.
b. Give catheter care every four hours.
3. Assess and evaluate the patient's gastrointestinal system.
a. Insert a nasogastric tube if he is vomiting or his abdomen is distended.
b. Auscultate his abdomen for bowel sounds every two hours and use the information as gathered to decide whether to give him fluids by mouth.
c. Assess his hourly intake and output.
d. Give him oral hygiene care every four hours using swabs or a mouthwash.
4. Assess and evaluate the patient's body defense systems.
a. Observe him for signs of infection.
b. If an infection is present, give him antibiotics as ordered.
c. Turn him every 1 to 2 hours.
d. Give him eye care if he is comatose.
5. Assess the patient's psychosocial integrity. The nurse should:
a. Listen to him.
b. Learn what having diabetes means to him.
c. Allow the patient to have some control and make some decisions.
d. Include the patient's family in the patient's care and education.
6. Assess and evaluate the patient's neurological system.
a. Note the degree of his coma.
b. Check his vital signs every 30 to 60 minutes or as needed.

Summary

Nonketotic HOC, a comatose condition usually seen in the adult-onset diabetic, has a high mortality. It is very similar to DKA in regard to the physiological alterations, except for the acidosis seen in DKA. Some insulin reserve is present in the patient with HOC, preventing lipolysis and thus ketosis. The main problems of HOC are: (1) severe dehydration, (2) hyperosmolality from glucose and sodium, and (3) electrolyte alteration.

Treatment is focused on correcting those problems and thus restoring equilibrium.

Study Problems

1. HOC is characterized by which one(s) of the following conditions?
   a. Hyperglycemia.
   b. Hypernatremia.
   c. Acidosis from ketone bodies.
   d. Mild dehydration.
2. The mortality in HOC is:
   a. Less then 5 percent.
   b. 15 percent.
   c. 30 percent.
   d. 50 percent.
3. The most important component of treatment of HOC is:
   a. Large doses of insulin in Ringer's lactate solution.
   b. Small doses of insulin and initial fluid therapy of isotonic saline solution.
   c. Large doses of regular insulin given intravenously.
   d. Immediate replacement of electrolytes, especially potassium.
4. Put a check beside the laboratory values that are to be expected in HOC.
   a. A serum osmolality of 290 mM/L. _____
   b. A blood sugar level of 900 mg/100 ml. _____
   c. Positive ketones in the urine. _____
   d. A BUN level of 80 mg. _____
   e. A pH of 6.9. _____

Answers

1. a, b.
2. d.
3. b.
4. b, d.

References

1. Arieff, A., and Carol, H.   Cerebral edema and depression of sensorium in nonketotic hyperosmolar coma. *Diabetes* 23:525, 1974.
2. Arieff, A., and Felts, P.   *Hyperosmolar Coma.* Kalamazoo, Mich.: Upjohn, 1974.
3. Bradley, R.   Diabetic Ketoacidosis and Coma. In A. Marble, P. White, R. Bradley, et al. (eds.), *Joslin's Diabetes Mellitus* (11th ed.). Philadelphia: Lea & Febiger, 1971.
4. Boshell, B.   *Diabetes Mellitus Case Studies.* New York: Medical Examination, 1976.
5. Burrell, Z., and Burrell, L.   *Critical Care.* St. Louis: Mosby, 1977.
6. Constam, G. R.   The Pancreas. In A. Labhart (ed.), *Clinical Endocrinology: Theory and Practice.* New York: Springer-Verlag, 1974.
7. Danowski, T.   Hyperosmolar Coma and Other Non-Ketotic Comas in Diabetes. In J. Kryston and J. Shaw (eds.), *Endocrinology and Diabetes.* New York: Grune & Stratton, 1974.
8. Eli Lilly Research Laboratories.   *Diabetes Mellitus* (3rd ed.). Indianapolis, Ind.: Lilly, 1976.
9. Elsberry, N., and Power, I.   Metabolic Crisis. In L. Meltzer, F. Abdellah, and J. Ketchell (eds.), *Intensive Care for Nurse Specialists* (2nd ed.). Bowie: Charles, 1976.
10. Felts, P.   *Coma in the Diabetic.* Kalamazoo, Mich.: Upjohn, 1974.
11. Gahart, B.   *Intravenous Medications* (2nd ed.). St. Louis: Mosby, 1977.
12. Lock, J. P., and Sussman, K. E.   Diabetes Mellitus in the Adult. In H. F. Conn (ed.), *Current Therapy.* Philadelphia: Saunders, 1977.
13. Matz, R.   Coma in the Nonketotic Diabetic. In M. Ellenberg and H. Rifkin (eds.), *Diabetes Mellitus: Theory and Practice.* New York: McGraw-Hill, 1970.
14. Podolsky, S.   Hyperosmolar nonketotic coma in the elderly diabetic. *Med. Clin. North Am.* 62:815, 1978.
15. Weber, S., Wood, W., and Jackson, E.   Availability of insulin from parenteral nutrient solutions. *Am. J. Hosp. Pharm.* 34:3, 1977.
16. Whitehouse, F., and Kahkonen, D.   Diabetes Mellitus in Adults. In H. F. Conn (ed.), *Current Therapy.* Philadelphia: Saunders, 1976.
17. Williams, R., and Porte, D.   The Pancreas. In R. H. Williams (ed.), *Textbook of Endocrinology* (5th ed.). Philadelphia: Saunders, 1974.

Bibliography

Blevins, D.   *The Diabetic and Nursing Care.* New York: McGraw-Hill, 1979.
Boshell, B., and Chaudalia, H. B.   Hormonal Interrelationships. In M. Ellenberg and H. Rifkin (eds.), *Diabetes Mellitus: Theory and Practice.* New York: McGraw-Hill, 1970.
Cahill, G.   Diabetes Mellitus. In P. Beeson, W. McDermott, and J. Wyngaarden (eds.), *Textbook of Medicine* (15th ed.) Philadelphia: Saunders, 1979.
Danowski, T.   Non-ketotic coma and diabetes mellitus. *Med. Clin. North Am.* 55:913, 1971.

Desimone, B.   Psychosocial Implications of Diabetes. In D. Guthrie and R. Guthrie (eds.), *Nursing Management of Diabetes Mellitus.* St. Louis: Mosby, 1977.

Guthrie, D., and Guthrie, R.   The Adult. In D. Guthrie and R. Guthrie (eds.), *Nursing Management of Diabetes Mellitus.* St. Louis: Mosby, 1977.

Guthrie, D., and Guthrie, R. (eds.).   *Nursing Management of Diabetes Mellitus.* St. Louis: Mosby, 1977.

Jordan, J.   Acute Care of Diabetes. In D. Guthrie and R. Guthrie (eds.), *Nursing Management of Diabetes Mellitus.* St. Louis: Mosby, 1977.

Kravitz, A.   Emotional Factors in Diabetes Mellitus. In A. Marble, P. White, R. Bradley, et al. (eds.), *Joslin's Diabetes Mellitus* (11th ed.). Philadelphia: Lea & Febiger, 1971.

Labhart, A. (ed.).   *Clinical Endocrinology: Theory and Practice.* New York: Springer-Verlag, 1974.

Larner, J., and Haynes, R.   Insulin and Oral Hypoglycemia Drugs. In L. S. Goodman and A. Gilman (eds.), *The Pharmacological Basis of Therapeutics* (5th ed.). New York: Macmillan, 1975.

Martin, C.   *Textbook of Endocrine Physiology.* Baltimore: Williams & Wilkins, 1976.

Stroot, V., Lee, C., and Schaper, C.   *Fluids and Electrolytes* (2nd ed.). Philadelphia: Davis, 1977.

Vallance-Owen, J. (ed.).   *Diabetes: Its Physiological and Biochemical Basis.* Lancaster, U.K.: MTP Press, 1975.

Witt, K.   HHNK: Intercepting a New Hazard. In P. Chaney (ed.), Nursing Skillbook, *Managing Diabetics Properly.* Horsham, Pa.: Intermed Communications, 1977.

Hyperthyroidism and Thyroid Crisis

Cathie E. Guzzetta

Thyroid crisis is a syndrome characterized by severe thyrotoxic manifestations, such as fever and cardiovascular, gastrointestinal, and central nervous system disturbances. The clinical presentation of a patient in thyroid crisis is extremely variable, making the differential diagnosis difficult. Furthermore, the criteria used to distinguish the patient in thyroid crisis from the patient with hyperthyroidism are not clearly defined. An understanding of both normal thyroid functioning and hyperthyroid states is needed to fully comprehend the pathophysiology and clinical manifestations of thyroid crisis and the objectives of care in dealing with a patient in thyroid crisis.

Objective

The critical care nurse should be able to describe the basic pathophysiological problems, clinical manifestations, and complications of thyroid crisis and the management of the patient in thyroid crisis.

Achieving the Objective

To achieve the objective, the nurse should be able to:

1. Describe the normal synthesis and secretion of thyroid hormone.

26

2. Describe the transport and metabolism of thyroid hormone.
3. Describe the hypothalamic-pituitary-thyroid control system.
4. Identify the clinical manifestations of hyperthyroidism.
5. Describe the basic thyroid function tests used in the diagnosis of hyperthyroidism.
6. Contrast the major medical and surgical treatments of hyperthyroidism.
7. List the physiological and psychological stressors that may precipitate or accompany thyroid crisis.
8. List the modalities of treatment for thyroid crisis.
9. Describe the nursing care objectives for a patient in thyroid crisis.
10. Teach the patient and his family about discharge care and possible complications.

How to Proceed

To develop an approach to hyperthyroidism and thyroid crisis, the nurse should:

1. Read the material that follows.
2. Organize a patient conference to discuss the information given in the preceding section.
3. Do a written systems assessment using the information given in the case study.
4. Make out a problem list immediately after reading the case study.
5. Act as the primary care nurse for the patient described in the case study. The nurse should:
   a. List the patient care objectives.
   b. Write out a patient care plan that covers care (1) during thyroid crisis, (2) during ^{131}I therapy, and (3) before discharge.
6. For further information read the articles in the references listed at the end of the chapter.

Case Study

Mr. S. R., a 30-year-old grocery store stockclerk, was taken to the hospital by his mother because of progressive confusion, disorientation, and an elevated temperature. He was examined by the emergency room physician and immediately admitted to the intensive care unit.

Mr. R. had been well until age 28, when he was diagnosed as being hyperthyroid and was given methimazole (Tapazole). Three months later he underwent a subtotal thyroidectomy. Subsequently, his antithyroid medications were discontinued, and he did well.

Mr. R.'s mother said that her son had had a great deal of emotional trauma in the past two months; he was getting a divorce. He had been observed to be increasingly agitated, nervous, and generally not functioning at his normal level. Mr. R.'s mother had noticed a decrease in her son's weight, a dramatic swelling of his neck, and a trembling of his fingers.

During the past month, Mr. R. had moved back into his mother's house. He had refused to seek medical attention until he developed a severe sore throat. He consulted his family physician, who treated the sore throat with penicillin. His symptoms grew worse, and his mother sought additional medical help.

The patient's profile and social history were obtained from his mother. Two months ago, he and his wife had separated after a five-year marriage. He had a healthy 3-year-old daughter. He was a brown belt karate expert. He had no religious preferences. He did not smoke, and he drank alcohol only occasionally. He had no known drug or food allergies. He had been taking oral penicillin prior to admission. (His past medical history has already been mentioned.) His family history was not pertinent. The accompanying admission assessment sheet outlines the findings from the interview, history taking, and physical examination.

Admission diagnostic studies were ordered and done. A throat culture was also done. Blood gas samples were drawn while Mr. R. received oxygen through a face mask (6 L/min). The results of the blood gas studies which were corrected for the increase in temperature, were: PaO_2 121 mm Hg, O_2 saturation 98.4%, pH 7.45, $PaCO_2$ 32 mm Hg, plasma HCO_3^- 21 mEq/L, base deficit −1.

The chest film showed mild cardiomegaly without heart failure. The ECG showed a sinus tachycardia with frequent premature atrial contractions, junctional premature contractions with occasional aberration (lead 2), and left ventricular hypertrophy.

After the initial history taking, an assessment and an evaluation were made by the physician and primary care nurse, the presumptive diagnosis of acute thyroid crisis was made, and appropriate therapy was instituted (Fig. 26-1). Mr. R. was given crushed propylthiouracil (PTU) (200 mg through a nasogastric tube every four hours) to help reduce the overproduction of thyroid hormone. A few hours later, he was given intravenous sodium iodide (1 gm every eight hours) to prevent the release of thyroid hormone from the thyroid gland. He was given propranolol (Inderal) (20 mg every six hours) through a nasogastric tube to block sympathetic nervous system overactivity. Four liters per day of a 10% dextrose and normal saline solution (1600 calories) and multivitamins were given to combat the patient's dehydration and increased nutritional and metabolic needs. Because of the acute crisis and the probable reduction in adrenocortical reserve, Mr. R. was given intravenous hydrocortisone (50 mg every six hours). Intravenous potassium penicillin G (2.5 million units every six hours) was given to combat the infection. A hypothermia blanket was used to suppress the temperature. Continuous cardiac monitoring was begun.

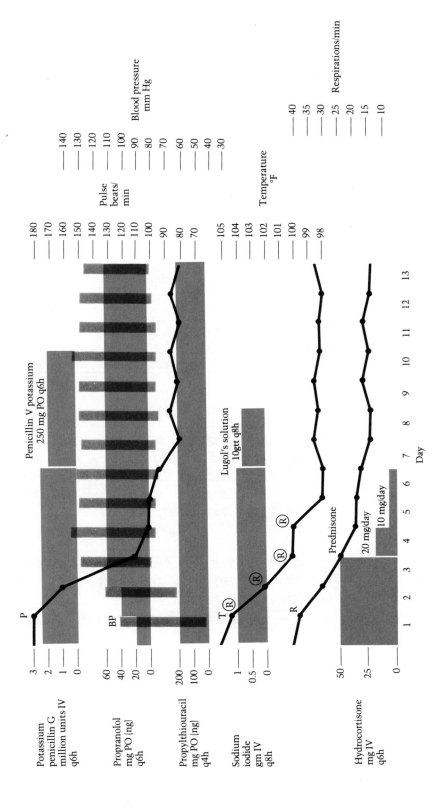

Figure 26-1
Thyroid crisis flow sheet.

Critical Care Nursing Admission Assessment
Head to Toe Approach

Date	Time	
		Pt. Name: *Mr. S.R.*　　　　Age: *30*　Allergies: *NKA*
1-16		Admitted Bed No: *4*　Via: *stretcher* Ad. Dx.: *Thyroid Crisis*
		T. *104.4°(R)* A.P. *180+ irreg* R.P. *180+ irreg* R. *40*　B.P. Supine R: *100/40* L: *102/40* Sitting: *96/40*
		Wt. *bed scale* *140*　Ht.: *5'11"* ECG Rhythm: *sinus tach* Ectopy: *PAC's, PJC's c̄ aberration*
		Informant: *mother-reliable historian* Last meal: *yesterday morning*
	1.	Chief complaint: *confusion, ↑ temp, vomiting + diarrhea × 2 days*
	2.	Hx. of present illness: *subtotal thyroidectomy at age 28; past 2 mo getting divorce, ↑ size of thyroid gland, ↑ hand tremor, ↑ nervousness + agitation; developed sore throat 2 days ago + placed on oral penicillin*
	3.	Past medical Hx. (include all surgeries, hosp., diseases, injuries, blood trans.): *hyperthyroidism 2 years ago; subtotal thyroidectomy 3 mo. later. Has not been on thyroid replacement medication; no other previous hx of diabetes,*
	4.	Family Hx.: *noncontributory*　｜ *adrenal disease, radiation therapy, trauma or surgery.*
	5.	Current drugs: *oral penicillin × 2 days for sore throat*
	6.	Alcohol and tobacco habits: *social drinking; does not smoke*
	7.	Dietary and fluid needs: *good appetite c̄ wt. loss last mo.; poorly hydrated;*
	8.	Sleep and rest patterns: *complaints of tiredness c̄ inability* ｜ *vomiting × 2 days*
	9.	Bowel and bladder habits: *diarrhea × 2 days*　*to sleep past mo.*
	10.	Hygienic needs: *showers daily in morning*
	11.	Psychosocial needs: *disruption of home + family life*
	12.	Occupation and education: *grocery store stockman; H.S. graduate*
	13.	Exercise habits: *gives karate lessons 5 nights / week*
	14.	Spiritual needs: *no religious preferences*
	15.	Personal interests: *brown belt karate expert; enjoys t.v. and cards*
	16.	Family member interaction and availability: *getting divorce, 3 y/o daughter lives c̄ wife; Pt. lives c̄ mother, mother appears concerned + supportive*
	17.	Attitude towards illness and hospitalization: *appears to have denied recurrence of illness over past month despite ↑ nervousness, wt. loss, tremor and "swollen neck"*

Physical Examination

Date	Time		
	18.	Gen. appearance: *acute distress, thin easily agitated*	color: *flushed* *no hyperpigmentation* skin: *warm, diaphoretic* *poor tissue turgor*
	19.	Neurological:	

thrill felt over upper lobes, bruits audible over entire gland, thyroidectomy scar

a) level of consciousness: *agitated, confused, disoriented to time, place, person*

b) cerebellar: *unable to evaluate*

c) motor function: upper: *prox. muscle weakness*   lower: *prox. muscle weakness*

d) sensory function: upper: *deferred*   lower: *deferred*

e) reflexes: *3+*

20. Head and face: *normal symmetry; no temporal hair loss, hair fine + silky*

21. Eyes: *round + equal, 3+/3+ dilation, react + accommodate light; infreq. blinking, lid lag*

22. Ears: *no redness, drainage, ringing, or hearing loss*

23. Nose: *no redness, drainage, or septal deviation*

24. Mouth/throat: *tongue dehydrated + erythematous; white tonsillar patches*   *pharyngeal erythema*

25. Neck: *supple, no JNVD, carotids brisk, trachea midline; large asymmetrical goiter c̄ lrg.*

26. Chest: *bilateral expansion, normal symm.+ contour*   *rt. lobe, goiter 5 × normal size (wt. approx. 100 gms.)*

27. Breast: *normal development*

28. Respiratory: *rate 40/min.; moist rales left base*

29. Cardiac: *irregularly irregular rhythm; PMI at 5 LICS, MCL; no S₃, S₄ (M) or rubs*

30. Abdomen: *no masses, pain, tenderness or hernias, 3+ bowel sounds; liver + spleen not palpable*

31. Genitourinary: *normal external genitalia*

32. Extremities (all pulses): *all pulses equal + full, no cyanosis, clubbing or edema, rhythmic finger tremor*

33. Back: *no deformities; no edema*

34. Problems requiring possible referral service: *defer until discharge decided*

35. Teaching needs: *educate pt./mother regarding signs + symptoms of recurrent disease, complications, medications + maintenance therapy*

36. Other:

PROBLEM LIST: **ACTIVE**	**INACTIVE**

1-16   ① *thyroid crisis:*
     sinus tachycardia c̄ ectopy
     fever
     dehydration
     wt. loss
     hyperactive bowel sounds
     lid lag
	subtotal thyroidectomy 2 years ago

    agitation + confusion
    goiter
② *throat infection*
③ *divorce pending*

Cathie E. Guzzetta, R. N. CCRN
NURSE'S SIGNATURE

Second Day

By the end of the second day after his admission, Mr. R. was combative and restless although less confused and disoriented. The results of the admission laboratory studies were: hemoglobin 15.2 gm, hematocrit 36%, white blood count 14,000 per cu mm, sodium 133 mEq/L, potassium 4.7 mEq/L, calcium 13.0 mg/100 ml, chloride 98 mEq/L, alkaline phosphatase 200, serum glutamic pyruvate transaminase 50, total bilirubin 2 mg/100 ml, fasting glucose 97 mg/100 ml, blood urea nitrogen 40 mg/100 ml, creatinine 2.1 mg/100 ml. The urinalysis showed three or four white cells per high-powered field and no red cells or bacteria. The thyroid function test results were abnormal: the serum thyroxine concentration (T_4 [D]) test was 20 μg/100 ml and the triiodothyronine radioimmunoassay (T_3 [RIA]) was 320 ng/100 ml. The throat culture showed β-hemolytic streptococci. The resting pulse was 160, respirations 30, blood pressure 110/60, and temperature 102°F rectally. The propranolol dosage was increased to 40 mg every six hours. Mr. R. continued to be given the intravenous and nasogastric medications mentioned (Fig. 26-1).

Third Day

The third day after Mr. R.'s admission, he was oriented to time, place, and person. He remained anxious, nervous, and combative, and he was abusive toward those caring for him. During his morning care, he lashed out physically at one of the nurses, striking her on her left shoulder. His resting pulse had decreased to 110, his respirations to 24, his rectal temperature to 100°F; his blood pressure rose to 126/78. His propranolol was increased to 60 mg every six hours.

The nursing staff became increasingly anxious about Mr. R.'s physical and verbal abuse. The primary care nurse held a short conference with the health team at which the problems, objectives, and plan of care were considered. The interrelatedness of the body and mind were discussed as the concept applied to Mr. R. (see Reflections). The emotional instability of patients in thyroid crisis was also discussed. It was decided that the primary care nurse would discuss Mr. R.'s behavior with him and that together they would plan his care.

Fourth Day

During the fourth day, Mr. R. was less anxious and more cooperative. One outcome of the planning of Mr. R. and his nurse was that his 3-year-old daughter was allowed to visit. Mr. R.'s spirits seemed to improve. His resting pulse was 100, rectal temperature 100°F, respirations 18, blood pressure 132/76. His nasogastric tube was removed, and he was put on a high-protein, 4000-calorie diet with supplemental feedings. His hydrocortisone therapy was discontinued, and he was given oral prednisone (20 mg per day). Oxygen therapy was discontinued.

Fifth Day

On the fifth day after his admission, Mr. R.'s oral temperature was 98°F, resting pulse 100, respirations 18, blood pressure 128/76. The prednisone dosage was reduced to 10 mg per day. He watched television and played cards with his mother. His daughter again visited him in his room. He began to ask questions about his illness and treatment. Mr. R.'s primary care nurse answered his questions honestly and in terms Mr. R. easily understood. Together Mr. R. and his nurse discussed his teaching care plan.

Seventh Day

During the seventh day, Mr. R. was transferred to a general medical floor. His medications were penicillin V potassium (Pen Vee K) (250 mg orally every six hours for four days), propranolol (60 mg orally every six hours), PTU (200 mg orally every four hours), Lugol's solution (10 drops by mouth every eight hours). His prednisone and intravenous infusion were discontinued. His resting pulse was 80, temperature 98.6°F orally, respirations 14, and blood pressure 126/76.

On Mr. R.'s transfer to the general medical floor, the primary physician told Mr. R. and his mother about the possible choices for therapeutic thyroid control. He did not recommend further thyroid surgery because of the high incidence of technical problems associated with reoperation. He recommended that Mr. R. be treated with radioactive iodine (^{131}I).

Eighth Day

On the eighth day, the therapy with Lugol's solution was discontinued. The nurse-physician team began discharge teaching that covered principles of home care and information about emotional stress, infection, and future ^{131}I therapy.

Discharge

The nurse explained to Mr. R. the indications for and dosage and side effects of his discharge medications (PTU and propranolol). On the thirteenth day, Mr. R. was discharged; he had had no further complications.

Readmission

Three months later, Mr. R. was readmitted to the hospital in a euthyroid state for ^{131}I therapy. An appropriate dose of ^{131}I was given seven days after PTU was discontinued. Seven days after Mr. R. had received ^{131}I therapy, he was again given PTU, which he was to take for two to three months. At the time of his discharge, Mr. R. had normal T_4 (D) and T_3 (RIA) levels and no symptoms of thyrotoxicosis.

Reflections

Physicians and nurses have long observed that during periods of psychological stress, the hyperthyroid patient may become clinically worse. If his disease had been undetected, during stress the patient may become symptomatic for the first time; or if his disease had been detected, during stress the patient may become more symptomatic. Thyroid crisis can also be precipitated by a psychological stressor.

On the other hand, it is well known that hyperthyroidism may itself cause marked psychological symptoms. Agitation, anxiety, paranoia, and depression are frequently observed during the course of illness.

Is the emotional instability associated with hyperthyroidism a cause or an effect? Does emotional stress worsen hyperthyroidism? Or does the hyperthyroid state itself result in psychological disturbances? And, in either case, what physiological mechanisms are involved?

There has been little systematic evidence that establishes emotional instability as either a precipitant or a result of thyroid disease. But it can be said with certainty that hyperthyroid states and emotional disturbances are frequently observed together.

Mr. R.'s case history clearly illustrates the body-mind-spirit continuum. One might speculate about whether Mr. R.'s hyperthyroid state affected his marriage or whether the emotional impact of his pending divorce affected his hyperthyroid state.

Depending on the severity of his disease and on his personality, the hyperthyroid patient is often hyperactive, tense, and restless. He tends to be extremely sensitive, crying at a slight provocation. He may be depressed and have feelings of impending disaster. His irritation and agitation may precipitate family quarrels and conflicts. His speech may be rapid, excitable, and high pitched. He may complain that he has lost control of his thoughts or that his ideas run together in a frightening way. His accelerated mental activity may lead to fears of insanity, disorientation, or delusions. He may have visual and auditory hallucinations.

It has been suggested that a product of excessive tissue breakdown in the patient with hyperthyroidism may affect the central nervous system and thus produce emotional instability. It may also be the result of a hypermetabolic state or excessive sympathetic nervous system activity. There are many physiological abnormalities that may produce psychological disturbances in the hyperthyroid patient.

It is well known that physiological stressors (e.g., infection, trauma, pregnancy, surgery, or prolonged exposure to cold) can increase the rate of thyrotropin secretion and can precipitate hyperthyroidism. Also, it is postulated that emotional stressors may precipitate or trigger the disease. Emotional shock during combat, prolonged worry, and loss of esteem, a loved one, or a job often occur before hyperthyroidism develops.

The preceding discussion of cause and effect leads to a discussion of the following popular assumptions about disease:

1. A disease is primarily either functional or organic in origin (i.e., either the mind or the body is the culprit, is at fault).
2. A disease is a process that affects primarily either the mind or the body.
3. Therapy should, therefore, be directed toward the mind (should be psychotherapeutic) or toward the body (should be traditionally medical or surgical), depending on whether mind or body is primarily at fault in the particular disease.

Those assumptions are so ingrained in people's thinking that they often escape attention. They operate unconsciously, but they determine in major ways people's attitudes toward patients and illness.

The concerns of the critical care nurse must, however, transcend the traditional assumptions of physiology, of how things happen. She must begin to question the basic assumptions about disease. Mainly, she must strive to see beyond the "either-or" of the assumptions. Disease is not a state of malfunction of *either* the mind *or* the body. The critical care nurse must try to discover the psychobiological unity that operates in every person in every disease process. Chapter 1 discussed the psychobiological point of view. The critical care nurse can implement that view not only with patients like Mr. R. but with every other patient with whom she is involved.

Anatomy of the Thyroid Gland

The thyroid gland, which has an average weight of 20 gm, is a relatively vascular organ. It is located below the larynx anteriorly and on either side of the trachea (Fig. 26-2). It comprises two lobes joined by an isthmus. The thyroid gland is made up of follicles whose walls are composed of cuboidal epithelium. Their lumina are filled with a colloid that contains thyroglobulin, a protein specific to the thyroid. The parathyroid glands are located on the posterior surface of the lateral lobes of the thyroid gland. The recurrent laryngeal nerves lie between the trachea and esophagus, just medial to the lateral lobes.

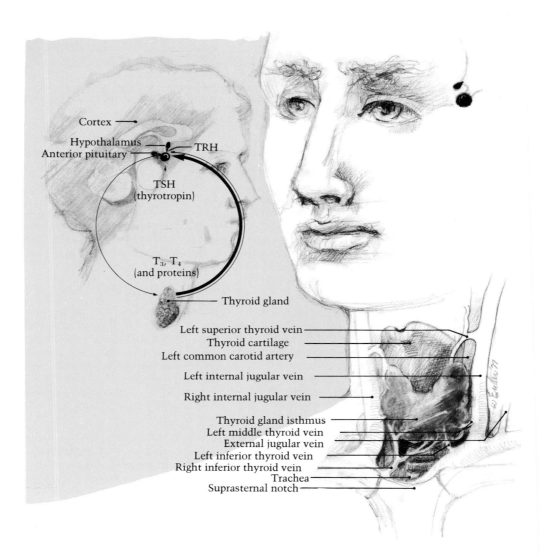

Cortex
Hypothalamus
Anterior pituitary
TRH
TSH
(thyrotropin)
T_3, T_4
(and proteins)
Thyroid gland

Left superior thyroid vein
Thyroid cartilage
Left common carotid artery
Left internal jugular vein
Right internal jugular vein
Thyroid gland isthmus
Left middle thyroid vein
External jugular vein
Left inferior thyroid vein
Right inferior thyroid vein
Trachea
Suprasternal notch

Synthesis and Secretion of Thyroid Hormone

The normal function of the thyroid gland is to secrete the thyroid hormones triiodothyronine (T_3) and thyroxine (T_4) into the circulatory system as a means of affecting and maintaining metabolic processes. T_4 and T_3 are needed for normal growth and maturation of the person, especially of the skeletal and central nervous systems.

The quantitative and qualitative synthesis of thyroid hormones depends on the entry of iodine into the thyroid. Iodine enters the thyroid from the bloodstream in an inorganic form that is derived primarily from iodine ingested from medications,

Figure 26-2
The thyroid gland and the hypothalamus-pituitary-thyroid control system.

water, and food. The average daily requirement of iodine is 0.1 mg. That amount is needed to replace the iodine lost in the urine. The principal dietary sources of iodine are bread, iodized salt, seafood, milk, and eggs. Because iodine is deficient in the soil of inland regions, the dairy products and eggs produced in those areas contain less iodine than do those in coastal regions [11]. Dietary iodine is rapidly converted to iodide in the stomach and upper small bowel. Iodide is then actively transported from the blood into the thyroid gland, where it is oxidized to elemental iodine in the follicular cells.

Iodide is removed from the blood primarily by the thyroid gland and the kidneys, which compete for plasma iodide. Because renal clearance depends largely on glomerular filtration and is not affected by plasma hormones or iodide concentrations, the kidneys are generally a passive competitor. Changes in the rate of iodide entry into the thyroid gland relative to the rate of urinary excretion are therefore controlled primarily by the thyroid gland.

Transport and Metabolism of Thyroid Hormone

The formation of thyroid hormone is described in Figure 26-3. Approximately 99 percent of the active thyroid hormone entering the circulatory system is in the form of T_4; the remainder is in the form of T_3 [11]. When T_3 and T_4 enter the blood, they are almost entirely bound by plasma proteins (i.e., mainly by thyroxin-binding globulin [TBG] and in small amounts by prealbumin and albumin).

Normally, less than 0.1 percent of the thyroid hormone is free or unbound in the plasma [4]. Only the unbound hormone is physiologically active and available to the tissues. The metabolic state of the patient, therefore, correlates more precisely with the concentration of free hormone than with the total concentration of hormone in the plasma (bound hormone plus unbound hormone).

The ability of TBG to combine with T_4 is much greater than its ability to combine with T_3. Also, T_3 is more potent than T_4. Because T_3 is less firmly bound to plasma proteins, it enters cells more rapidly. Moreover, since much of T_4 is converted to T_3, it is possible that T_3 may be the only active thyroid hormone [11].

Essentially all the metabolic activities of the tissues are increased under the influence of thyroid hormones. The overall metabolism of cells is accelerated. The mitochondria of most cells increase in size, and large numbers of intracellular enzymes are stimulated. As a result, the basal metabolic rate is increased, and the rate of utilization of foods for energy is increased. Carbohydrate and fat metabolism is increased. Protein synthesis and protein catabolism are increased. The growth rate is increased, and mental activities are excited.

Control Mechanism

The synthesis and release of T_3 and T_4 are controlled by the anterior pituitary hormone thyrotropin (also known as thyroid-stimulating hormone—TSH—and thyrotropic hormone). The main functions of thyrotropin are to:

1. Increase the size and secretory activity of the thyroid gland.
2. Increase the rate of iodine trapping into the thyroid gland.
3. Increase the number of thyroid cells.
4. Increase the proteolysis of the thyroglobulin in the follicles, resulting in the release of T_3 and T_4 into the blood.

Thyrotropin, like many other hormones, increases the quantity of cyclic 3′,5′-adenosine monophosphate (cyclic AMP) in the thyroid cell [9]. Cyclic AMP is an intracellular hormonal mediator. The hormone (thyrotropin) combines with a receptor specific for the particular type of stimulating hormone at the membrane of the target cell (the thyroid cell). Once combined with the receptor, the hormone activates the enzyme adenyl cyclase, which is found within the membrane. That enzyme catalyzes the chemical reaction, which results in the generation of cyclic AMP. Cyclic AMP is responsible for many cellular functions, such as altering the permeability of the cell membrane and initiating the synthesis of specific intracellular chemicals. The type of effect that occurs as a result of cyclic AMP depends on the character of the specific cell. An increase of cyclic AMP within a thyroid cell, for example, will result in an increase in thyroid hormone formation. A similar increase in the beta cells of the islets of Langerhans results in increased insulin secretion.

Both physiological and psychological stressors can increase the rate of thyrotropin secretion, which, in turn, increases the output of T_3 and T_4 (see Reflections). Likewise, altered concentrations of thyroid hormone in the blood can inhibit or stimulate the release of thyrotropin from the anterior pituitary. The hypothalamus also affects the rate of thyrotropin secretion through the release of thyrotropin-releasing hormone (TRH) (also known as thyrotropin-releasing factor—TRF). TRH acts on the anterior pituitary to increase the output of thyrotropin. The factors that regulate TRH are not fully understood. The regulation may be the result of influences from higher ner-

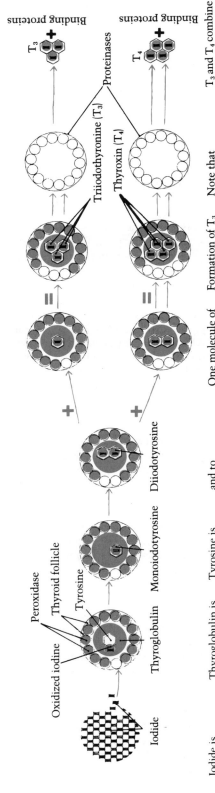

Iodide

Oxidized iodine · Peroxidase · Thyroid follicle · Tyrosine

Thyroglobulin

Monoiodotyrosine

Diiodotyrosine

Triiodothyronine (T_3)

Thyroxin (T_4)

Proteinases

T_3 + Binding proteins

T_4 + Binding proteins

Iodide is transported into the thyroid follicle and oxidized to elemental iodine by the peroxidase enzyme system.

Thyroglobulin is directly secreted into the thyroid follicle cells. Tyrosine, an amino acid, is found within the thyroglobulin molecule. The oxidized iodine combines with tyrosine within the thyroglobulin.

Tyrosine is oxidized to monoiodotyrosine . . .

and to diiodotyrosine.

One molecule of diiodotyrosine combines with one molecule of monoiodotyrosine; one molecule of diiodotyrosine combines with another molecule of diiodotyrosine.

Formation of T_3 and T_4. T_3 and T_4 may be stored within thyroglobulin molecule for several weeks before being released to the body.

Note that thyroglobulin is not directly released into the circulating blood. It is digested by proteinases that are secreted into the follicle by the thyroid cells. T_3 and T_4 are then split from the thyroglobulin molecule and diffuse through the cells.

T_3 and T_4 combine with binding proteins in the blood.

Figure 26-3
Formation of thyroid hormone.

vous centers or possibly the result of direct thyroid hormone stimulation, although the existence of that feedback mechanism has not been established.

Summary

To summarize the information about the negative feedback mechanism of the thyroid gland (see Fig. 26-1): Increased levels of T_3 and T_4 in the plasma reduce the secretion of thyrotropin from the anterior pituitary. When thyrotropin is reduced, there is a decreased stimulation of the thyroid gland, resulting in a decreased release of T_3 and T_4 that returns the thyroid hormone blood levels to normal. Conversely, when the plasma thyroid hormone levels fall below normal, thyrotropin secretion is stimulated, causing an increase in the secretion of T_3 and T_4.

Examination of the Thyroid Gland

The thyroid gland is evaluated by inspection, palpation, and auscultation. The gland is inspected for asymmetry and enlargement of one or both lobes. It is palpated from behind, from the front, and from beneath. The normal thyroid gland is barely palpable or not palpable by the examining fingers. Auscultation of the thyroid gland is accomplished by lightly placing the diaphragm of the stethoscope over the thyroid. Normally no sound is heard.

Hyperthyroidism

Hyperthyroidism (thyrotoxicosis) represents an excessive functional activity of the thyroid gland. Hyperthyroidism exists in three distinct forms. The first form, Graves's disease (also known as Parry's disease and Basedow's disease), is characterized by a diffuse enlargement of the thyroid gland (goiter). Graves's disease is manifested by a symptom complex that includes not only hyperthyroidism but also infiltrative ophthalmopathy, and occasionally infiltrative dermopathy.

Hyperthyroidism may also originate in the presence of a multinodular goiter, a syndrome that usually occurs in the older patient who has a history of a long-standing, previously inactive goiter [4]. The least common form of hyperthyroidism is the one that occurs when one hyperfunctioning nodule of the thy-

roid gland depresses the functioning of the rest of the gland.

Graves's Disease

Graves's disease occurs more often in women than in men, and often in people in their thirties and forties [11, 12]. It occurs relatively rarely in children. There is a distinct familial predisposition to the disease.

Etiology

The cause of Graves's disease is not known. It is likely that there is no one cause of the entire syndrome. In the 1950s, Graves's disease was believed to be the result of a hypersecretion of the pituitary gland that produced an excess of TSH. More recently, the cause of Graves's disease [4, 11] has been thought to be associated with a plasma protein that is demonstrated in approximately 60 percent of the patients who manifest all the symptoms described [19]. The protein, which is known as long-acting thyroid stimulator (LATS), is capable of stimulating the release of thyroid hormone and increasing the activity of cyclic AMP. LATS has been established as one immunoglobulin of the IgG class synthesized by the lymphocytes in patients with Graves's disease, and it is believed to be an antibody to some component of human thyroid tissue. Graves's disease may, therefore, be caused by an autoimmune phenomenon. Serum LATS titers, however, do not correlate well with the presence or absence or the severity of hyperthyroidism, and so it is unlikely that LATS alone plays a direct causative role.

Pathophysiology

A patient with Graves's disease has a diffusely enlarged, soft, and vascular thyroid gland. The parenchymal cells of his thyroid gland undergo hyperplasia and hypertrophy. The thyrotoxicosis of Graves's disease is caused by an abnormal rate of thyroid hormone synthesis and release. The disease is also associated with lymphatic hyperplasia and infiltration and occasionally with enlargement of the spleen and thymus. Also, fatty infiltration and fibrosis of the liver, loss of body tissue, decalcification of the skeleton, and degeneration of the skeletal muscles may be found.

The ophthalmopathic changes in Graves's disease are caused by inflammation and infiltration of the orbital contents with lymphocytes and mast and plasma cells. The orbital muscles are generally involved, causing the globe to protrude, the orbit to enlarge, and the muscle fibers to fibrose. The dermopathic changes are caused by lymphocytic infiltration and thickening of the skin.

Clinical Manifestations

The clinical picture of Graves's disease varies with the person, the severity of the disease, the age of the patient, and the presence of underlying disease. The diffuse toxic goiter may be lobular and asymmetrical. A bruit is often heard directly over the gland; it is caused by the increased blood flow. In severe cases, a thrill may be felt over the upper lobes. A thrill or bruit is highly suggestive of hyperthyroidism.

A stare or "frightened" facies is characteristic of Graves's disease. The person has wide eyes, exophthalmos (abnormal protrusion of the eyeballs) (Fig. 26-4), lid lag, infrequent blinking, and failure of the eyes to converge or the brow to wrinkle when the person looks up. Those signs are believed to be due to overstimulation of the sympathetic nervous system, muscle weakness, congestion, and edema.

The skin is velvety, moist, and warm as a result of cutaneous vasodilatation. There is excessive sweating and heat intolerance. The skin changes are usually seen in the legs or feet. They are commonly called localized myxedema, nonpitting myxedema, or pretibial myxedema. The affected area is usually raised and thickened, and it may be pruritic and nodular (Fig. 26-5). Excessive melanin pigmentation is frequent as a result of a hypersecretion of ACTH secondary to the accelerated metabolism of cortisol. The nails are soft and friable. Clubbing of the fingers and toes is occasionally noted. The hair is fine, silky, and easily broken; often it does not hold a curl. There may be hair loss on the temporal scalp.

The relationship of thyroid hormones and catecholamines has been studied. Hyperthyroidism is known to increase adrenergic activity. It was believed that thyroid hormones exerted their chronotropic and inotropic effects through the sympathetic nervous system by sensitizing the myocardium to catecholamines. It is now known, however, that thyroid hormones have a direct chronotropic and inotropic effect on the myocardium that is independent of sympa-

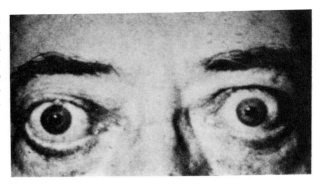

Figure 26-4
Exophthalmos.

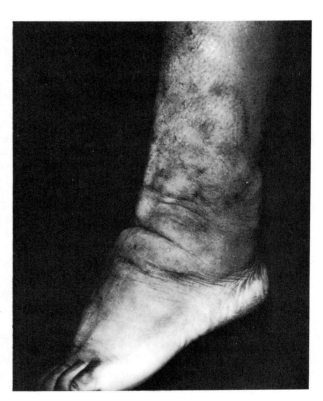

Figure 26-5
Localized myxedema.

thetic stimulation [13, 16]. Nevertheless, an increase in adrenergic activity does occur, and it appears that the effects of catecholamines and thyroid hormones are additive.

The hyperthyroidism of Graves's disease has a dramatic effect on the cardiovascular system. The hypermetabolism and the need to dissipate excess heat produce increased circulatory demands. There is an increase in stroke volume and heart rate associated with a decrease in peripheral vascular resistance and an increase in local blood flow to the tissues. Cardiac output may, therefore, be increased as much as two times normal. Clinically, tachycardias are generally observed. Palpitations, a frequent complaint, are caused by an increase in the force of contraction. Atrial fibrillation or other atrial dysrhythmias are common. Systolic heart murmurs, a loud first heart sound, and a widened pulse pressure due to a rise in the systolic pressure and a decrease in the diastolic pressure may be noted. Cardiac enlargement, mild edema, and high output cardiac failure are occasionally present [6].

Several other physiological effects may occur as a result of the presence of hyperthyroidism. They include an increased utilization of oxygen and the formation of carbon dioxide, causing an increase in the rate and depth of respirations. Although often the person has a great increase in appetite, both at and between meals, he does not eat enough to meet his increased demand for calories. Gastrointestinal motility and food absorption are increased. Occasionally, anorexia, nausea, vomiting, and abdominal pain are observed. Because the rate of protein catabolism is greater than the rate of protein synthesis, there is a net degradation of tissue protein that results in a negative nitrogen balance, weight loss, muscle wasting, and hypoalbuminemia. A rise in lipid catabolism produces an increase in free fatty acids and glycerol. Serum cholesterol levels and occasionally serum triglyceride levels may be reduced. Serum calcium levels may rise as a result of bone reabsorption, and large amounts of calcium and phosphorus may be lost in the urine and stool. Excessive losses may be associated with demineralization of the bone and pathological fractures.

The nervous system may be affected, producing accelerated mental activity (see Reflections). The person is likely to become extremely nervous, hyperactive, anxious, or paranoid. He may be chronically tired and yet unable to sleep. An important sign of hyperthyroidism is a fine, rhythmic muscle tremor of the hands, tongue, or eyelids (when the eyelids are slightly closed). Sexual development is frequently delayed although skeletal growth may be increased. Menstrual disturbances, particularly amenorrhea, are common.

Thyroid Tests

There are many tests of thyroid functioning and hormone homeostasis. Although many of the tests are sensitive and specific to thyroid disorders, each has its inherent limitations. No one test is completely reliable because of the exogenous and endogenous factors that can complicate the findings. The interpretation of each test is dependent on an understanding of the individual patient and the pathophysiological mechanisms and clinical manifestations of each disease state.

RADIOACTIVE IODINE UPTAKE TEST

The radioactive iodine uptake (RAIU) test is commonly used to assess thyroid functioning. Radioiodine (^{131}I) mixes with endogenous iodide and indicates the percentage of iodide entering and leaving the thyroid. A trace of ^{131}I is given orally (usually 5–10 μc) and the amount of ^{131}I taken up by the thyroid is measured with a gamma counter placed over the gland. The RAIU varies inversely with the amount of endogenous iodide, and it can be correlated with the functional state of the thyroid. In hyperthyroidism, for example, both the peak uptake and the rate of uptake of ^{131}I are greater than in the euthyroid person. The uptake of ^{131}I is reduced, however, when a high level of inorganic iodide is present in the plasma as a result of a large intake of iodide, which is found in high amounts in some foods, cough syrups, lozenges, gargles, vitamins, drugs, and various x-ray contrast media.

PROTEIN-BOUND IODINE TEST

The protein-bound iodine (PBI) test measures the amount of thyroid hormone bound to protein. The test is discussed here for the sake of completeness although it is infrequently used today. The amount of PBI changes as the amount of binding proteins changes. A variety of different circumstances may increase or decrease the binding capacity or the amount of binding proteins in the blood [35] (Table 26-1).

Table 26-1
Factors That Alter the Binding Capacity or Concentration of
Binding Proteins

Increased Concentration of Binding Proteins	Decreased Concentration of Binding Proteins
Pregnancy	Steroids
Newborn state	Acromegaly
Oral contraceptives	Nephrosis
Estrogens	Genetic defects
Hepatitis	Chronic liver disease with iodine deficiency
Genetic defects	Iodine starvation
Acute intermittent porphyria	Major illness
	Surgical stress

Those factors must be kept in mind when assessing the PBI test results. The normal PBI range is 4 to 8 μg/100 ml.

SERUM THYROXINE CONCENTRATION TEST

The serum thyroxine concentration—$T_4(D)$—test is used to assess the hormonal concentration and binding in the blood. It is measured by the ability of T_4 to displace labeled T_4 from a protein mixture containing TBG. The normal range for $T_4(D)$ is 4 to 11 μg/100 ml. The value may also be expressed in terms of its iodine content, which is derived by multiplying the serum $T_4(D)$ level and the proportion of iodine in T_4 (0.653). The value is known as $T_4I(D)$. Serum T_4 levels may be elevated by factors that increase the concentration of binding proteins without indicating hyperthyroidism. A depression of serum T_4 levels may also occur when the concentration of binding proteins is low (Table 26-1).

SERUM T_3 CONCENTRATION TEST

Serum T_3 concentrations may be measured by radioimmunoassay; they are abbreviated T_3 (RIA). Serum T_3 is measured by its ability to displace labeled T_3 from anti-T_3 antibodies when compared with that of a known quantity of T_3. Normal values are 100 to 170 ng/100 ml.

RESIN T_3-UPTAKE TEST

The resin T_3-uptake (RT$_3$U) test is used to measure the binding of thyroid hormone in the blood; it provides an index of the proportion of free T_3. RT$_3$U is measured by adding a known amount of T_3 labeled with ^{131}I to a certain volume of the patient's serum. The serum is then absorbed on a resin sponge, which binds free T_3 and is measured isotopically. Any free TBG in the serum will also bind the radioactive T_3. Thus when there is nearly complete binding of the proteins by endogenous thyroid hormones (as seen in the hyperthyroid person), there is little opportunity for the exogenous radioactive T_3 to bind with protein. The T_3 therefore remains free or unbound in the tested serum sample to be absorbed by the resin sponge. The result is a high level of RT$_3$U, indicating hyperthyroidism. Conversely, in the hypothyroid person, the RT$_3$U is low because the exogenous T_3 labeled with ^{131}I attaches to the large quantity of the patient's unbound serum TBG. Less labeled T_3 remains to be absorbed by the resin sponge because it is bound to the patient's own proteins. The RT$_3$U is also affected by factors that increase and decrease the concentration of binding proteins (Table 26-1). The normal range for the RT$_3$U is 25 to 35 percent.

FREE T_4 INDEX

The RT$_3$U test just described is capable of measuring the proportion of free hormone in the blood. It does not, however, differentiate primary alterations in the hormone concentration from primary alterations in hormone binding.

In hyperthyroidism, the concentration of binding proteins does not increase proportionately with the elevated thryoid hormone concentration. The concentration of both total (bound and free) thyroid hormone and free thyroid hormone increases, but the increase in free thyroid hormone is relatively much greater than the increase in the total hormone concentration so that the *proportion* of free hormone increases. When RT$_3$U is used to evaluate thyroid disorders, abnormal values are presumed to be the result of a primary alteration in the concentration of the hormone (i.e., a high level of RT$_3$U is presumed to be the result of a primary increase in the concentration of thyroid hormone). It is known, however, that abnormal RT$_3$U values, similar to those obtained in primary thyroid disease, may also be produced when the TBG concentration is abnormal (Table 26-1).

To distinguish primary alterations in hormone binding from hormone concentration, the absolute concentration of free thyroid hormone is calculated. The absolute concentration of free hormone is the product of the proportion of free hormone and the total concentration of the hormone. For example, the value of RT_3U can be expressed as a ratio of the RT_3U value of the patient's serum to the value obtained from the control specimen (the RT_3U ratio). The product of the RT_3U ratio and the serum T_4 concentration—$T_4(D)$—yields the absolute concentration of free T_4 (free T_4 index, or T_4–RT_3 index). If the concentration of TBG is altered, the T_4–RT_3 index remains normal. Conversely, primary alterations in thyroid hormone concentration produce an abnormal T_4–RT_3 index. As a result, the T_4–RT_3 index provides an important means of determining whether a change in the total concentration of the hormone is due to a change in the production rate of thyroid hormone or a change in hormone binding, and it plays an important role in differentiating hypothyroidism and hyperthyroidism from euthyroid states.

THYROID-STIMULATING HORMONE STIMULATION TEST

The TSH stimulation test is used to assess thyroid reserve. RAIU by the thyroid is measured by the response to intramuscular injections of TSH. Since serum TSH measurements are now generally available, the TSH stimulation test is used less frequently; it has been replaced by the thyrotropin-releasing hormone stimulation test.

THYROTROPIN-RELEASING HORMONE STIMULATION TEST

The TRH stimulation test is used to assess thyroid function. After the intravenous administration of TRH, the serum TSH rises in 10 minutes, peaks in 20 to 45 minutes, and then falls. The test may be useful in assessing pituitary reserve, hypothyroidism, and thyrotoxicosis.

RADIOACTIVE IODINE SUPPRESSION TEST

The RAI suppression test is another test of thyroid functioning. In the euthyroid person, RAIU is suppressed after the administration of exogenous thyroid hormones. The person receives T_3 or T_4 hormones orally and then is given ^{131}I. The RAIU by the thyroid gland is measured, and in all cases of hyperthyroidism, the decline in RAIU normally induced by the suppressive effects of the thyroid hormones does not occur. The test helps to differentiate patients with

hyperthyroidism from those with "high normal" RAIU levels.

BASAL METABOLIC RATE TEST

The basal metabolic rate (BMR) test assesses the metabolic processes of thyroid hormones in the peripheral tissues. It measures the amount of oxygen consumed in the basal state as an index of energy expenditure. The BMR is affected by age, sex, and body surface area. Those factors are taken into consideration in determining the BMR values. Because of the many factors that affect the measurement, the test has limited diagnostic value, and it is rarely used.

THYROID SCINTISCANNING

Thyroid imaging by scintiscanning localizes sites of technetium Tc 99m or RAI accumulation in the thyroid gland. The scintiscan is used to determine the overall size of the thyroid. It is also used to define areas of increased function ("hot" areas) and areas of decreased function ("cold" areas). A nodule that is palpable and appears cold on the scintiscan demonstrates a decreased uptake of the isotope and may be malignant. Conversely, a functioning nodule that is more active than the surrounding tissue and that appears hot on the scintiscan is not likely to be malignant.

Diagnosis

The patient suffering from Graves's disease with severe hyperthyroidism frequently has a history of many of the clinical manifestations previously discussed. Also, laboratory findings may reveal increases in RAIU, $T_4(D)$, $T_4I(D)$, T_3 (RIA), RT_3U, and the T_4–RT_3 index. Along with those findings, a high index of suspicion should be present in regard to any patient who presents with unexplained cardiac decompensation or atrial dysrhythmias [9, 11].

Treatment

Graves's disease is often characterized by periods of exacerbation and remission. There are no clinical criteria that are universally useful in predicting medical remission early in the course of treatment [13]. There is no way to treat the cause of the disease,

Table 26-2
Drugs Used in the Treatment of Hyperthyroidism

Drug	Function	Adverse Effects
Thionamides Propylthiouracil (PTU) Methimazole (Tapazole)	Block synthesis of thyroid hormones by inhibiting the coupling of iodotyrosines	Hypothyroidism resulting in goiter and ophthalmopathy, skin rash, gastrointestinal symptoms, arthralgias, fever, hepatitis, agranulocytosis, "physiological" leukopenia
Iodides Lugol's solution Sodium iodide	Inhibit release of thyroid hormone; cause involution and reduce vascularity of thyroid gland	Skin rash or skin lesions, salivary gland inflammation, conjunctivitis, rhinitis, eosinophilia Not recommended for long-term use Response unpredictable if given before administration of antithyroid drugs May delay the therapeutic response of subsequently administered antithyroid medication Iodine may accumulate in gland to be used for synthesis of additional thyroid hormone
Beta-adrenergic receptor-blocking drugs Propranolol (Inderal)	Control peripheral manifestations of sympathetic overactivity by blocking catecholamine response at receptor site	Cardiac arrest, cardiac failure, bradycardia, hypotension, acute respiratory problems

since the cause is not known with certainty. Because there is no ideal therapy, the treatment is controversial [36, 37].

There are, however, two basic approaches to the treatment of Graves's disease that are aimed primarily at reducing the overactivity of the thyroid gland. The first approach involves the use of long-term antithyroid medication that prevents the overproduction of thyroid hormone. The second approach attempts to ablate a portion of the thyroid by means of RAI or by subtotal thyroidectomy.

ANTITHYROID DRUGS

Antithyroid drugs inhibit one or more stages of hormone synthesis. Long-term medical therapy has been limited for the most part to patients under 40 years of age [36]. The major drugs used are the thionamide drugs, including propylthiouracil (PTU) and methimazole (Tapazole) (Table 26-2). They act primarily by inhibiting the coupling of iodotyrosines. The production of thyroid hormones is then reduced, and the patient can be made euthyroid until the natural course of the disease carries it into remission. The response to those drugs may take days to weeks to occur.

Because thionamide drugs inhibit the synthesis but not the release of thyroid hormone, the thyroid gland must first be depleted of its hormonal stores before there is a reduction in the supply of hormone at the tissue level. Once the patient becomes euthyroid, the antithyroid dosage is reduced to the lowest therapeutic level.

It is suggested that the patient should then be given daily thyroid hormone therapy to prevent the development of hypothyroidism, which may develop as a result of prolonged use of antithyroid medication [11, 36]. The undesirable consequences of hypothyroidism (e.g., ophthalmopathy and enlargement of the thyroid gland) may thus be avoided. Thyroid replacement therapy that involves the long-term use of antithyroid medication is, however, controversial. Some authorities [13, 37] believe that hypothyroidism is best prevented simply by adjusting the dosage of the antithyroid medication. Perhaps more important, medical follow-up is essential to carefully assess the patient's intent to take the appropriate drugs faithfully.

The length of therapy is difficult to predict; it may depend simply on the spontaneous course of the disease. Frequently the patient is treated from 12 to 24 months before his medications are discontinued. In general, patients who have been symptomatic less than one year or who have small goiters that quickly diminish in size during antithyroid therapy are more likely to have permanent remissions after adequate medical therapy [8, 36]. The overall rate of remission after prolonged antithyroid medication is about 15 to 50 percent [8, 32]. The recurrence rate of hyperthyroidism after medical treatment is increasing, however, probably because larger amounts of iodine have been added to daily foods [34].

The minor side effects of antithyroid drugs include skin rashes, gastrointestinal symptoms, arthralgias, fever, and hepatitis. Agranulocytosis, a rare but serious complication, is usually preceded by a sore throat or some other localized or generalized infection. The condition will disappear when the drug is withdrawn. A low-grade fever or "physiological" leukopenia is the principal side effect of both antithyroid medication and untreated Graves's disease, but it is not generally an indication for discontinuing the medication.

IODIDES

Iodides (see Table 26-2) inhibit the release of thyroid hormone and are more rapid acting than are antithyroid medications. Iodides are useful primarily in preparing patients for subtotal thyroidectomy or for acute surgical emergencies. They are often used to treat patients with impending or actual thyroid crisis. Their effects are transient, and they should be used only for short-term therapy (see Nursing Orders, Objective No. 2).

ADRENERGIC ANTAGONISTS

Because catecholamines contribute to the symptoms of hyperthyroidism, adrenergic antagonists, that block or deplete catecholamines, are used in the treatment of hyperthyroidism and thyroid crisis. Propranolol, a beta-adrenergic receptor-blocking drug (see Table 26-2), is used to control the manifestations of sympathetic overactivity, such as palpitations, sweating, heat intolerance, tremor, nervousness, and eyelid retraction [11, 13, 15, 16, 18, 35, 37] by blocking the catecholamine response at the receptor site. Propranolol is useful in decreasing the heart rate and the cardiac work. It has been found to control those factors dramatically and to abort early thyroid crisis [13, 15, 16, 18] when given in oral doses of 20 to 120 mg per 24 hours or intravenous doses of 2 to 10 mg. Propranolol must be used carefully, because adrener-

gic activity may be necessary in some patients for optimal cardiac functioning. Abolition of sympathetic drive may result in, or contribute to, cardiac decompensation. If propranolol is used to treat a patient who has cardiac failure, the patient must first be digitalized [13] (see Chap. 18).

The contraindications to propranolol therapy include asthma or other bronchoconstrictive disorders, cardiac failure (except when cardiac insufficiency is caused by sinus tachycardias), sinus bradycardia, atrioventricular heart block, pregnancy (because of propranolol's ability to increase uterine activity), and severe thyrocardiac disease. Other adrenergic antagonists that deplete tissues of their catecholamine content (e.g., reserpine and guanethidine sulfate) are used occasionally.

RADIOACTIVE IODINE

The second major approach to the treatment of hyperthyroidism is the destruction of functional thyroid tissue, which limits the amount of thyroid produced. The destruction is accomplished either by ^{131}I therapy or by surgery. [131]I, which was introduced in 1941, was considered to be the ideal treatment until long-term follow-up studies demonstrated hypothyroidism to be a serious complication [11, 36]. [131]I eliminates thyroid tissue by radiation necrosis of the thyroid follicle cells, replacing it with interstitial fibrosis.

The administration of ^{131}I is a simple, painless, bloodless, and inexpensive procedure. The early fears about the possible carcinogenic and harmful genetic effects of ^{131}I therapy have not been realized [25]. It now seems that bone marrow intoxication in the form of leukemias is not linked to the small doses of ^{131}I used to treat hyperthyroidism. Because a carcinogenic effect has not been demonstrated in adults [5], the only question which remains unanswered is, what are the genetic effects of ^{131}I on future generations? To date, a large number of women treated with therapeutic doses of ^{131}I have produced offspring without any increased incidence of congenital abnormalities [36]. But further investigation seems to be warranted since only one generation has been studied. [131]I therapy is not generally recommended for patients who are pregnant or who have childbearing potential [3, 32]. Nor is it recommended for patients who cannot be adequately followed medically throughout their life [11, 36, 37].

[131]I is effective in 100 percent of cases: 75 to 80 percent of patients become euthyroid after the initial

dose, and the remaining 20 to 25 percent become euthyroid after a second treatment [32, 36]. Because the patient should be euthyroid before the administration of ^{131}I, the patient is given antithyroid medication until his thyroid function tests are normal. Antithyroid therapy is then discontinued for several days before and after the administration of ^{131}I to allow ^{131}I to accumulate in the thyroid and then once again administered to maintain a eumetabolic state until ^{131}I exerts its effect (usually weeks to months).

The major side effect of ^{131}I therapy for hyperthyroidism is hypothyroidism [23]. Most patients treated with ^{131}I become hypothyroid at some time in their lives [36]. Since the incidence of that complication is so well documented, it is essential that the patient be educated about the problem and that thyroid replacement therapy be instituted as soon as the patient becomes euthyroid [21, 32, 36]. Because hypothyroidism may develop insidiously and cause irreversible damage, the use of thyroid medication following ^{131}I therapy cannot be overemphasized. The lifetime replacement of thyroid hormone in therapeutic doses is simple and inexpensive, and it is not associated with untoward metabolic or allergic effects.

SUBTOTAL THYROIDECTOMY

Before ^{131}I therapy was introduced, subtotal thyroidectomy was the treatment of choice for hyperthyroid patients. Surgery is still recommended for children, adults with childbearing potential, patients who refuse ^{131}I therapy, and pregnant women who do not respond to antithyroid medication.

Preoperatively, patients should be rendered euthyroid to prevent thyroid crisis. That is accomplished by use of adrenergic antagonists [30] and a two- to four-month course of a thionamide drug with the addition of iodides during the final two or three weeks before surgery. Iodide is an antithyroid compound when used for short-term therapy (see Nursing Orders, Objective No. 2), and it is useful in reducing the vascularity of the gland before surgery. The surgery involves removal of most of the thyroid tissue, leaving only a small remnant in place. The remnant left behind will, it is hoped, produce enough thyroid hormone to allow the patient to maintain a euthyroid state. The surgery eliminates both the hyperthyroidism and the goiter of Graves's disease.

In the hands of skilled surgeons, most patients achieve a euthyroid state after surgery. The mortality associated with the surgery is extremely low (less

than 0.1 percent) [26, 35]. Complications include wound infections, transient tetany, and hemorrhage leading to respiratory obstruction [11, 36]. Recurrent hyperthyroidism persists in 2 to 8 percent of patients, who will at some time require therapy with antithyroid medication or [131]I [35]. The complication of hypothyroidism can be expected to develop in 8 to 10 percent of all patients [1, 35]. Damage to the recurrent laryngeal nerve during surgery can produce permanent vocal cord paralysis in approximately 0.6 percent of patients [20, 21, 30, 35]. Permanent hypoparathyroidism is a severe complication, occurring in up to 3 percent of patients [1, 26, 35]. It is induced iatrogenically—by the inadvertent removal of parathyroid tissue or by impairment of the blood supply of the parathyroid gland during surgery.

Thyroid Crisis

Thyroid crisis is a syndrome characterized by exaggerated manifestations of hyperthyroidism, including fever and cardiovascular, gastrointestinal, metabolic, and central nervous system problems. The difference between severe hyperthyroidism and thyroid crisis is not clear. McArthur [17] says that thyroid crisis is a state in which the patient can no longer tolerate the strain imposed by thyrotoxicosis and finally reaches a point where hyperthyroidism is "life-endangering." To date, there are no universally accepted criteria to define thyroid crisis [13, 31].

Before 1930, 70 percent of all deaths from thyrotoxicosis were due to thyroid crisis (thyroid storm) following thyroidectomy [29]. But because the hyperthyroid patient is now given iodide, antithyroid, and beta-adrenergic receptor-blocking drugs before surgery, thyroid crisis following thyroidectomy is rare [22, 29, 35].

Although "surgical storm" following thyroidectomy is no longer a problem, "medical storm" is common. It occurs in patients with untreated or inadequately treated disease [11]. It is not uncommon for thyroid crisis to develop suddenly in a patient who has never been diagnosed as hyperthyroid [13].

Thyroid crisis is generally precipitated by or associated with psychological stressors or some concurrent pathophysiological process, such as infection, trauma, or surgery (see Reflections) [13]. It also may be precipitated by such physiological stressors as vascular accidents, diabetic ketoacidosis, adrenocortical insufficiency, pulmonary embolism, x-ray contrast studies, postirradiation thyroiditis, premature withdrawal of antithyroid drugs, ether anesthesia, or too vigorous palpation of the thyroid gland in the thyrotoxic patient [2, 7, 10, 16, 24, 27, 33]. The amount of TBG may also be reduced after surgery or stress, resulting in an increase in both the proportion and the absolute concentration of free T_3 and T_4 in the plasma.

Clinical Manifestations

The clinical picture of a patient in thyroid crisis is a result of an abrupt and life-threatening exacerbation of thyrotoxic manifestations and a marked increase in general cellular function.

The compensatory mechanism of peripheral vasodilatation and diaphoresis no longer is adequate to dissipate the excess heat production. As a result, fever, considered the sine qua non of thyroid crisis, usually ranges from 100°F to 103°F. Profuse sweating is frequent. The increased central nervous system metabolism may cause severe agitation, restlessness, anxiety, and psychotic behavior, and the patient's condition may progress to extreme weakness, disorientation, coma, and death.

The syndrome is further characterized by nausea, vomiting, diarrhea, abdominal pain, and hypotension due to dilatation of the blood vessels. Sinus or ectopic tachydysrhythmias or atrioventricular heart block may be accompanied by cardiac decompensation or pulmonary edema. Cardiac output may be increased to the point of high-output failure. A reduction of adrenocortical reserve may be observed [11]. The liver is frequently enlarged, and mild jaundice may be seen.

Diagnosis

Besides the clinical manifestations, many of the thyroid tests (discussed under Graves's Disease) can be used in the diagnosis of thyroid crisis. Although many of those tests may be helpful in the diagnosis, the seriousness of the situation demands that treatment be instituted even before the results of laboratory measurements are available. Furthermore, there are no criteria that clearly differentiate a patient in severe hyperthyroidism from a patient in crisis. But labeling the illness is not essential because the therapeutic management of hyperthyroidism and thyroid crisis is similar. The presumptive diagnosis is based on the history, the clinical findings, and sound medical judgment [13, 16, 22, 31].

Treatment

The treatment of thyroid crisis includes taking certain immediate measures to counteract the harmful effects of hypermetabolism. If the condition is not recognized, the illness is generally fatal. The therapy is directed toward [16, 31]: (1) diagnosing and treating any associated or precipitating disease or problem, (2) inhibiting the synthesis and release of excess quantities of thyroid hormone, (3) reducing the metabolic effects of excessive thyroid hormone and sympathetic overactivity, (4) providing general supportive therapy, and (5) preparing the patient to assume responsibility for his health maintenance.

Nursing Orders (for the thyroid crisis patient)

OBJECTIVE NO. 1

The patient's associated or precipitating disease or problems (stressors) should be identified and treated.

To achieve the objective, the nurse should:

1. Obtain information from the patient and his family about:
   a. The patient's thyroid history and medications.
   b. Physiological stressors (e.g., pregnancy, childbirth, diabetes mellitus, adrenal insufficiency, irradiation therapy, infection, trauma, and surgery).
   c. Psychosocial stressors (e.g., emotional stress, loss of self-esteem, loss of job, loss of loved one, and divorce) (see Reflections).
2. Identify and treat coexisting problems.

OBJECTIVE NO. 2

The patient should be treated to inhibit the synthesis and release of thyroid hormone.

To achieve the objective, the nurse should:

1. Assess the patient for:
   a. Diffuse toxic goiter, enlarged goiter, asymmetry of the thyroid gland, thyroid bruit or thrill, and hoarseness (thyroid compression symptom).
   b. Clinical manifestations of thyroid crisis.
2. Assess the thyroid function tests.

3. Treat the patient by:
   a. Administering medications that inhibit the synthesis of thyroid hormone immediately after the physician has made the diagnosis and ordered the drugs.
      (1) Give PTU (200 mg) or methimazole (20 to 30 mg) by mouth every four hours or as ordered by the physician. If the patient is unable to swallow or to cooperate, the nurse should crush the medications and administer them through a nasogastric tube.
      (2) Observe the patient for adverse reactions to antithyroid therapy (skin rashes, gastrointestinal symptoms, fever, arthralgias, hepatitis, leukopenia, and agranulocytosis).
   b. Administering medications that inhibit the release of thyroid hormone.
      (1) Do not administer iodide therapy until at least one hour after the administration of antithyroid medications. Iodides given in large doses transiently inhibit the synthesis of thyroid hormone. They are also useful in reducing the vascularity and causing involution of the thyroid gland. More important, they effectively inhibit the release of thyroid hormone by retarding the proteolysis of thyroglobulin, thereby preventing the release of T_3 and T_4. The response to iodide is usually rapid and dramatic, frequently occurring within the first 24 hours of therapy (as opposed to antithyroid medication, which may not show evidence of clinical benefit for days or weeks).

      Because iodides increase the storage of thyroid hormone within the gland, they may unfortunately delay the therapeutic response of subsequently administered antithyroid hormones and they may cause an accumulation of iodide in the thyroid that might be used to synthesize additional thyroid hormone. As a result, iodide must be given several hours after the administration of antithyroid hormones [11, 13, 16].

      Because its inhibitory effect on the thyroid gland is transient and unpredictable, long-term iodide therapy is not recommended. In the clinical setting of thyroid crisis, iodide may be given in the form of Lugol's solution (30 drops by mouth or nasogastric tube per day) or in the form of sodium iodide (1 gm intravenously every eight hours).
      (2) Observe the patient for any adverse reactions to iodide therapy (skin rash or skin lesions, salivary gland inflammation, conjunctivitis, rhinitis, and eosinophilia).

OBJECTIVE NO. 3

The patient should receive therapy directed at reducing the metabolic effects of excess thyroid hormone and sympathetic overactivity.

To achieve the objective, the nurse should:

1. Suppress adrenergic overactivity:
   a. Identify the contraindications to therapy with beta-adrenergic receptor-blocking drugs (asthma, other bronchoconstrictive disorders, cardiac failure, atrioventricular heart block, sinus bradycardia, pregnancy, and thyrocardiac disease).
   b. Administer propranolol in the following dosages to block beta-adrenergic activity:
      (1) Oral dosage: 20 to 120 mg per day (the effects last from 4 to 8 hours). The dosage should be divided throughout 24 hours.
      (2) Intravenous dosage: 2 to 10 mg diluted and titrated slowly in a 5% dextrose in water solution (the effects last 4 hours).
      The nurse should check the patient's blood pressure, pulse, and respiration and cardiac rhythm before, during, and after the administration of propranolol.
   c. Observe the patient for the adverse effects of propranolol: cardiac arrest, severe reduction in pulse rate, sudden drop in blood pressure, orthostatic hypotension, syncope, signs and symptoms of congestive heart failure, and symptoms of asthma or acute respiratory problems.
   d. Assess the patient for the signs of therapeutic control of sympathetic overactivity after the administration of propranolol: reduction of heart rate, palpitations, sweating, heat intolerance, tremor, tension, agitation, and psychomotor activity.

OBJECTIVE NO. 4

The patient should be given the general supportive therapy needed to counteract the harmful side effects of thyroid crisis.

To achieve the objective, the nurse should:

1. Evaluate and combat the fever caused by hypermetabolism:
   a. Assess the patient's rectal temperature, his degree of diaphoresis and dehydration, the temperature and condition of his skin, and his degree of peripheral vasodilatation.
   b. Treat the patient by:
      (1) Using a hypothermia blanket or ice packs to reduce his temperature.
      (2) Not using aspirin to reduce his fever (because aspirin can increase the metabolic rate of a patient with thyroid crisis) [14].
      (3) Giving the patient scrupulous skin care.
      (4) Giving the patient frequent sponge baths.
      (5) Making sure the patient's bed clothes are not too warm.
      (6) Turning the patient frequently (at least every two hours) to increase the blood circulation to the bony prominences and pressure areas.

2. Evaluate and reverse any dehydration:
   a. Assess the patient's fluid and electrolyte status and notify the physician of any abnormalities or signs and symptoms of dehydration or fluid overload.
   b. Treat the patient by:
      (1) Recording his daily intake and output.
      (2) Giving him parenteral electrolytes as ordered.
      (3) Giving him parenteral fluids as ordered.

3. Evaluate the patient's increased need for energy and provide nutrition and calories to supply the need:
   a. Assess the patient's signs and symptoms of gastrointestinal disturbances (e.g., anorexia, nausea, vomiting, diarrhea, increased hunger, and abdominal pain or tenderness). The patient's abdomen should be auscultated for hyperactive bowel sounds, a sign of increased gastrointestinal motility. The patient's ability to tolerate an oral diet should be evaluated. The patient's protein catabolism rate (manifested by fatigue, weak and/or wasted musculature, weight loss and hypoalbuminemia) should be determined.
   b. Treat the patient by:
      (1) Weighing him every day.
      (2) Giving him 10% dextrose in water as ordered by the physician because it has protective effects on the liver, replaces depleted glycogen reserves, and supplies calories.
      (3) Supplementing his diet with parenteral multivitamins.
      (4) Providing increased protein and calories and supplemental feedings when the patient can tolerate an oral diet.

4. Evaluate and treat his nervous system disturbances:
   a. Assess the patient's agitation, restlessness, anxiety, disorientation, degree of psychomotor activity (picking at sheets, thrashing or crawling out of bed), unusual or psychotic behavior, subtle changes in his level of consciousness, coma, and degree of insomnia. Determine the patient's degree of tremor of the tongue, eyelids (when they are slightly closed), and fingers (by placing a strip of thin paper over the patient's extended fingers and observing the degree of vibration of the paper).
   b. Treat the patient by:
      (1) Checking his neurological signs every four hours.
      (2) Orienting him in regard to time, place, and person.
      (3) Making sure that there is a clock and a calendar in his room.
      (4) Allowing supportive relatives to visit him frequently.
      (5) Restraining him only as necessary.
      (6) Reassuring him; explaining all procedures to him.
      (7) Confirming reality for him as necessary.
      (8) Giving him mild sedatives if necessary.
      (9) Administering total care to decrease his metabolic needs and oxygen consumption.
      (10) Assessing his degree of weakness and fatigability; allowing for frequent rest periods.
      (11) Considering the need for and the benefits of a body-mind-spirit approach to his care.

5. Evaluate and treat cardiovascular abnormalities:
   a. Assess the patient's heart rate, rhythm, regularity, quality of heart sounds (e.g., loud S_1, systolic murmurs, and S_3 or S_4 gallop rhythms). Tachydysrhythmias (atrial fibrillation, sinus tachycardia), ectopic or aberrant beats, and first-degree, second-degree, or third-degree atrioventricular heart block should be determined. The degree of hypotension, orthostatic hypotension, or widened pulse pressure should be determined. The patient should be observed for cardiac decompensation or increased cardiac

output beyond physiological limits as seen in "high-output" cardiac failure.

b. Treat the patient by:
   (1) Checking his vital signs often.
   (2) Carrying out continuous cardiac monitoring.
   (3) Having periodic chest films taken to observe for cardiac enlargement.
   (4) Administering propranolol to reduce adrenergic overactivity (see Objective No. 3).
   (5) Suppressing dysrhythmias.
   (6) Administering digitalis, bronchodilators, and sedatives.

6. Evaluate and treat the patient's respiratory disturbances:
   a. Assess the rate, depth, and regularity of his respirations; check his blood gases; auscultate his lungs for any abnormal breath sounds and congestion associated with cardiac failure; note the color of his extremities, as well as any cyanosis or clubbing.
   b. Treat the patient by administering oxygen therapy through a face mask or cannula as ordered to compensate for his increased metabolic demands.

7. Administer adrenocortical hormone replacement therapy [11, 13, 16, 22, 28, 29, 35] (the adrenocortical reserve has probably been reduced as a result of the acute crisis). The adrenal gland functions at maximum capacity and approaches a state of exhaustion during thyroid crisis, resulting in acute adrenal insufficiency. Adrenocortical hormone replacement therapy is, however, controversial. When hydrocortisone is used, the dosage (100 to 300 mg per day) should be calculated according to the amount the adrenal gland would be expected to produce under maximal stress.

OBJECTIVE NO. 5

The patient should be prepared to assume responsibility for his health maintenance after his discharge.
   To achieve the objective, the nurse should:

1. Explain the anatomy and physiology of the thyroid gland to the patient.
2. Discuss with him the pathophysiology of hyperthyroidism.
3. Discuss with him the physiological and psychological stressors that precipitate or are associated with thyrotoxicosis.

4. List the clinical manifestations of thyrotoxicosis.
5. Discuss with him the need for medical follow-up in the future.
6. Explain to him the indications for and the dosage, frequency, and adverse side effects of antithyroid medications. The patient must understand:
   a. The need for maintaining daily therapeutic blood levels.
   b. The importance of seeking medical attention at the first sign of any local or generalized infection, which may herald the approach of the serious complication of agranulocytosis.
7. Explain the indications for and the dosage, frequency, and adverse side effects of propranolol therapy.
8. Discuss with him his possible future treatment with ^{131}I therapy or subtotal thyroidectomy as appropriate.

Summary

Thyroid crisis is a life-threatening exacerbation of thyrotoxicosis, and it is an acute emergency condition. There are no universally accepted criteria for diagnosis. The survival of patients in thyroid crisis depends on the assessment, diagnosis, early institution of specific therapy, and alleviation of any underlying illness or problems. The critical care nurse who understands the pathophysiology, clinical manifestations, complications, and objectives of care is equipped to play an essential role in caring for the patient in thyroid crisis.

Study Problems

1. Thyroid hormone is stored:
   a. In the membrane of the thyroid gland.
   b. In a molecule called thyroglobulin.
   c. In the plasma-binding proteins.
2. The rate of thyroxine and triiodothyronine release is controlled by:
   a. Thyrotropin.
   b. TRH.
   c. The body's need for thyroid hormone.
   d. All the above.
3. What percentage of thyroid hormone is found free or unbound in the plasma?
   a. 99 percent.
   b. 0.1 percent.

c. 10 percent.

d. 80 percent.

4. Pregnancy, oral contraceptives, and steroids can change the concentration of binding proteins and affect the results of all the following thyroid tests except:

a. T_4 (D).

b. T_3 (RIA).

c. RT_3U.

d. T_4-RT_3 index.

5. Graves's disease is characterized by all of the following except:

a. Nonpitting myxedema.

b. Hyperthyroidism.

c. Diffuse goiter.

d. High-grade fever.

6. The most common complication of ^{131}I therapy is:

a. Congenital defects.

b. Recurrent hyperthyroidism.

c. Hypothyroidism.

d. Hypoparathyroidism.

7. Thyroid crisis may be associated with which one(s) of the following?

a. Trauma.

b. Infection.

c. Surgery.

d. Loss of a loved one.

e. All the above.

8. The clinical picture of a patient in thyroid crisis includes all of the following except:

a. Fever.

b. Severe agitation.

c. Tachydysrhythmias.

d. Hypertension.

9. The management of a patient in thyroid crisis includes all of the following except:

a. Antithyroid medications.

b. [131]I therapy.

c. Adrenergic blocking drugs.

d. Iodide.

10. Nursing care of the patient in thyroid crisis includes which of the following?

a. Administering iodine medications before antithyroid medication is begun.

b. Administering aspirin to reduce fever.

c. Providing a low-protein diet to reduce binding proteins.

d. Identifying psychological and physiological stressors that may disrupt psychobiological unity and recovery.

Answers

1. b.
2. d.
3. b.
4. d.
5. d.
6. c.
7. e.
8. d.
9. b.
10. d.

References

1. Beahrs, O. H., and Sakulsky, S. B. Surgical thyroidectomy in the management of exophthalmic goiter. *Arch. Surg.* 96:512, 1968.
2. Blum, M., Kranjac, T., Park, C., et al. Thyroid storm after cardiac angiography with iodinated contrast medium. *J.A.M.A.* 235:2324, 1976.
3. Burrow, G. N. Hyperthyroidism during pregnancy. *N. Engl. J. Med.* 298:150, 1978.
4. Davies, A. G. Thyroid physiology. *Br. Med. J.* 2:206, 1972.
5. Dobyns, B. M., Sheline, G. E., Workman, J. B., et al. Malignant and benign neoplasms of the thyroid in patients treated for hyperthyroidism: A report of the cooperative thyrotoxicosis therapy follow-up study. *J. Clin. Endocrinol. Metab.* 38:976, 1974.
6. Fowler, N. O. Hyperthyroidism: How to recognize it from circulatory signs. *Consultant* 4:25, 1976.
7. Freeman, M., Giuliani, M., Schwartz, E., et al. Acute thyroiditis, thyroid crisis and hypocalcemia following radioactive iodine therapy. *N.Y. State J. Med.* 69:2036, 1969.
8. Greer, M. A., Kammer, H., and Bouma, D. J. Short-term antithyroid drug therapy for the thyrotoxicosis of Graves' disease. *N. Engl. J. Med.* 297:173, 1977.
9. Guyton, A. C. *Textbook of Medical Physiology.* Philadelphia: Saunders, 1977.
10. Hanscom, D., and Ryan, R. J. Thyroid crisis and diabetic ketoacidosis. *N. Engl. J. Med.* 257:697, 1957.
11. Harrison, T. R., et al. (eds.). *Principles of Internal Medicine* (7th ed.). New York: McGraw-Hill, 1974. Pp. 465–484.
12. Ingbar, S. H. Management of emergencies: Thyrotoxic storm. *N. Engl. J. Med.* 274:1252, 1966.
13. Ingbar, S. H. When to hospitalize the patient with thyrotoxicosis. *Hosp. Prac.* 11:45, 1975.
14. Larsen, P. R. Salicylate-induced increase in free triiodothyronine in human serum. *J. Clin. Invest.* 51:1125, 1972.

15. Lee, T. C., Coffey, R. J., Mackin, J. F., et al. The use of propranolol in the surgical treatment of thyrotoxic patients. *Ann. Surg.* 177:643, 1973.

16. Mackin, J. F., Canary, J. J., and Pittman, C. S. Thyroid storm and its management. *N. Engl. J. Med.* 291:1396, 1974.

17. McArthur, J. W. Thyrotoxic crisis. *J.A.M.A.* 134:868, 1947.

18. McLarty, D. G., Brownlie, B. E. W., Alexander, W. D., et al. Remission of thyrotoxicosis during treatment with propranolol. *Br. Med. J.* 2:332, 1973.

19. Menendez, C. E., and Goldzieher, J. W. Modern laboratory diagnosis of thyroid disease. *Tex. Med.* 72:66, 1976.

20. Moosman, D. A., and DeWeese, M. S. The external laryngeal nerve as related to thyroidectomy. *Surg. Gynecol. Obstet.* 127:1011, 1968.

21. Mountain, J. C., Stewart, G. R., and Colcock, B. P. The recurrent laryngeal nerve in thyroid operations. *Surg. Gynecol. Obstet.* 133:978, 1971.

22. Nelson, N. C., and Becker, W. F. Thyroid crisis: Diagnosis and treatment. *Ann. Surg.* 170:263, 1969.

23. Nofal, M. M., Beierwaltes, W. H., and Patno, M. E. Treatment of hyperthyroidism with sodium iodide I[131]. *J.A.M.A.* 197:605, 1966.

24. Roizen, M., and Becker, C. Thyroid storm. *Calif. Med.* 115:5, 1971.

25. Safa, A. M., Schumacher, O. P., and Rodriquez-Antunez, A. Long term follow-up results in children and adolescents treated with radioactive iodine (^{131}I) for hyperthyroidism. *N. Engl. J. Med.* 292:167, 1975.

26. Schwartz, S. I., Hume, D. M., and Kaplan, E. L. Thyroid and Parathyroid. In S. I. Schwartz (ed.), *Principles of Surgery* (2nd ed.). New York: McGraw-Hill, 1974.

27. Shafer, R., and Nuttall, F. Acute changes in thyroid function in patients treated with radioactive iodine. *Lancet* 2:635, 1975.

28. Shires, G. T. (ed.). *Care of the Trauma Patient.* New York: McGraw-Hill, 1966. Pp. 173–174.

29. Thompson, N. W., and Fry, W. J. Thyroid crisis. *Arch. Surg.* 89:512, 1964.

30. Toft, A. D., Irvine, W. J., Sinclair, I., et al. Thyroid function after surgical treatment of thyrotoxicosis. *N. Engl. J. Med.* 298:643, 1978.

31. Urbanic, R. C., and Mazzaferri, E. L. Thyrotoxic crisis and myxedema coma. *Heart Lung* 7:435, 1978.

32. Utiger, R. D. Treatment of Graves' disease. *N. Engl. J. Med.* 298:681, 1978.

33. Waldstein, S. S., Slodki, S. J., Kaganiec, I., et al. A clinical study of thyroid storm. *Ann. Intern. Med.* 52:626, 1960.

34. Wartofsky, L. Low remission after therapy for Graves' disease: Possible relation of dietary iodine with antithyroid therapy results. *J.A.M.A.* 226:1083, 1973.

35. Werner, S. C., and Ingbar, S. H. (eds.). *The Thyroid* (3rd ed.). New York: Harper & Row, 1971.

36. Wool, M. S. The investigation and treatment of hyperthyroidism. *Surg. Clin. North Am.* 50:545, 1970.

37. Zellmann, H. E. Hyperthyroidism. *Med. Clin. North Am.* 56:717, 1972.

Acute Adrenal Insufficiency

Barbara Montgomery Dossey

Acute adrenal insufficiency (Addison's disease or addisonian crisis) is a life-threatening event in which a person's normal physiological requirement for mineralocorticoid and glucocorticoid hormones exceeds his supply. The patient can present in a state of shock and follow a rapidly deteriorating clinical course. It is of the utmost importance that the nurse understand the etiology, pathology, and treatment of acute adrenal insufficiency in order to help reverse the process.

Objective

In regard to the adult patient with acute adrenal insufficiency, the nurse should be able to identify the clinical manifestations of the disease, perform a systematic assessment of the patient, and write nursing orders for the management of the patient.

Achieving the Objective

To achieve the objective, the nurse should be able to:

1. Identify the subjective and objective manifestations of acute adrenal insufficiency.
2. Know in what clinical setting acute adrenal insufficiency is most likely to occur.

27

3. List the effects mineralocorticoids and glucocorticoids have on the body.
4. Explain the therapeutic management of the patient with acute adrenal insufficiency.
5. Educate the patient about self-care during the intercritical phase of acute adrenal insufficiency.

How to Proceed

To develop an approach to a patient with acute adrenal insufficiency, the nurse should:

1. State the characteristics of acute adrenal insufficiency that are seen in the patient described in the case study that follows.
2. Make out a problem list immediately after reading the case study.
3. Write a nursing care plan for the patient in the acute, intermediate, and intercritical phases of acute adrenal insufficiency.
4. Know what physiological and psychological problems are to be anticipated for the patient described in the case study.

Case Study

Mr. B. L., aged 70, was admitted to the medical intensive care unit on a stretcher. He had come from the emergency room. The initial assessment by the primary care nurse described him as a confused, deeply pigmented Caucasian man who was unable to answer questions. Before he was taken off the emergency room cart, Mr. L. vomited about 200 ml of greenish matter and he was incontinent (he passed about 300 ml of diarrheic stool and urine).

Mr. L.'s wife said that two days before his admission, Mr. L. had complained of feeling tired and urinating frequently. He also complained of a chest cold. Mrs. L. said also that over the past few weeks her husband's skin seemed to get darker although he had not had excessive exposure to the sun. Mr. L. had unintentionally lost 20 pounds over the last six months. He had not sought medical help.

Mr. L.'s patient profile and social history described him as a 5'5'', 105-lb retired printer. He had little formal education; he had learned the printing trade from his father. His wife, aged 68, was a retired high-school teacher who did needlework and sold it at a small profit. Mr. L. was active in the Baptist church. His hobbies were collecting and trading old printing press equipment and repairing antique clocks, at which he made a small profit. He did not smoke or drink alcohol.

Mr. L.'s past medical history listed active tuberculosis (1947 to 1949) that had required medical management through 1950 and acute anterior wall myocardial infarction (1965) with no complications. He had a history of peptic ulcers (1966) with no complications. He was not taking any medications, and he had no known allergies.

A review of Mr. L.'s family history revealed that both parents died of "old age" at the age of 99. He had four brothers (aged 62, 64, 65, and 68), who were well. He also had two sisters (aged 72 and 74), who took antihypertensive medication.

Mr. L.'s admission vital signs were temperature 101°F rectally, pulse 60, respirations 12, and blood pressure 90/70 mm Hg (see accompanying assessment sheet).

Within the first hour of his hospitalization, Mr. L. became comatose, extremely hypotensive (50/0 mm Hg), and cold and clammy. He had three episodes of ventricular fibrillation that was converted to normal sinus rhythm. He was intubated, attached to a volume ventilator, and his nasogastric tube was connected to intermittent suction. Intravenous physiological saline solution and glucocorticoids were administered rapidly.

Mr. L.'s initial laboratory values were sodium 124 mEq per liter (normal is 132–142 mEq/L), potassium 6.7 mEq per liter (normal is 3.5–5 mEq/L), chlorides 90 mEq per liter (normal is 98–106 mEq/L), bicarbonate 20 mEq per liter (normal is 22–26 mEq/L), 8:00 A.M. plasma cortisol level 0.6 μgm per 100 ml (normal is 5–25 μgm/100 ml), blood urea nitrogen 35 mg per 100 ml (normal is 10–20 mg/100 ml), creatinine 2 mg per 100 ml (normal is 1–1.5 mg/100 ml), and serum pH 7.30 (normal is 7.35–7.45). A complete blood count showed 10% eosinophils (normal is 1–4%).

A thyroid function test showed a T_3 resin uptake of 30% (normal is 22–35%) and a T_4 of 7.6 μgm per 100 ml (normal is 4–11 μgm/100 ml).

The x rays of the skull and sella turcica were normal. The chest x ray showed previous apical scarring and calcific granulomas that appeared to be inactive.

The presumptive diagnosis of acute adrenal insufficiency was made. It was based on the history; physical examination; the patient's signs and symptoms, which were classic; the initial laboratory data; and the patient's response to therapy. The physician's therapy was empirical; because Mr. L.'s condition was deteriorating rapidly, the physician had no time to confirm his clinical impression with further diagnostic studies.

Mr. L. had only one known predisposing factor to acute adrenal insufficiency—the tuberculosis mentioned earlier. Conceivably, the tuberculosis had damaged his adrenal cortex significantly. A viral infection may have been a precipitating factor.

Treatment and further attempts at diagnosis began simultaneously. Mr. L. received 2 liters of normal saline solution during the first two hours. A single dose of intravenous hydrocortisone sodium succinate (100 mg) was given initially. During the next 24 hours, Mr. L. received 8 liters of a 5% dextrose in normal saline solution, and glucocorticoid replacement continued.

Eighteen hours after his admission, Mr. L. was extubated. He was very weak, but he began to talk and to respond accurately to simple questions. During the next 14 days, Mr. L. regained his strength. His steroid therapy was maintained with hydrocortisone (30 mg/day) and fludrocortisone (0.1 mg/day). He was discharged 17 days after the initial crisis. He was given specific information by the physician and nurses about self-care after hospitalization (see the nursing orders for the intercritical phase of adrenal insufficiency).

In Mr. L.'s state of acute primary adrenal insufficiency, he had a significant degree of aldosterone deficiency that caused the absorption of sodium by the kidney to be severely altered. Mr. L. was hyponatremic because he had lost a tremendous amount of sodium in his urine. Sodium loss is almost always associated with diuresis. Also, the renal sodium loss caused an increased renal loss of hydrogen ion. The loss of sodium and water was associated with a decreased blood perfusion to the kidney that increased the blood urea nitrogen level (prerenal azotemia). The decreased sodium levels and the increased potassium levels were due to the aldosterone deficiency and acidosis. The increased potassium levels may have helped produce the severe bouts of cardiac dysrhythmias. Mr. L.'s potassium level initially was 6.7 mEq per liter. Because he had frequent premature ventricular contractions and an acidotic serum pH, he was given two ampules of sodium bicarbonate (44.5 mEq/L) during the first two hours. His potassium level dropped to normal and his cardiac dysrhythmias were corrected. The hyponatremia and hyperkalemia had contributed to severe muscle weakness, confusion, and gastrointestinal irritability (vomiting and diarrhea with resultant weight loss). Mr. L.'s increased pigmentation was due to an increase in the deposition of melanin in his skin. The lack of cortisol secretion had a positive feedback effect on the anterior pituitary; it stimulated the secretion of increased amounts of adrenocorticotropin (ACTH) and melanocyte-stimulating hormone (MSH). The increase in MSH caused Mr. L.'s increased pigmentation.

Reflections

Although immediate lifesaving measures were the first steps in Mr. L.'s nursing and medical management, the critical care nurses felt the need to discuss their experiences with him with the nurses in the other parts of the hospital. They felt also that Mr. L. should understand his problem as well as the nurses did. Thus a few of Mr. L.'s critical care nurses organized and presented a workshop on the management of the patient during the acute, intermediate, and intercritical phases of adrenal insufficiency. The workshop emphasized the nurses' responsibility for understanding and being aware of the pathophysiological processes, the nursing diagnosis, the nursing process, and patient education. Like diabetic patients, patients with adrenal insufficiency, in-

cluding those who have had bilateral adrenalectomies, need careful education about their disease for the rest of their life.

The following is an outline of the workshop:

1. Management of the patient during the acute phase of adrenal insufficiency
   a. Pathophysiology
   b. Causative and precipitating factors
   c. Nursing and medical management
2. Management of the patient during the intermediate phase of adrenal insufficiency
   a. Pathophysiology
   b. Nursing and medical management
3. Management of the patient during the intercritical phase of adrenal insufficiency
   a. Pathophysiology
   b. Self-care after hospitalization

One is tempted to view certain "classic" diseases as disturbances or failures of specific organ systems. The more complicated the pathophysiology and the more pervasive the illness, the more tempting it is to define the illness in organic terms. One views it as a "body problem."

That seems true of adrenal disease, including adrenal insufficiency. One tends to view it as a specific somatic event that has specific physiological consequences. The pituitary gland and the adrenal glands, although they act in concert, are viewed as isolated in a purely physiological sense.

The reality is otherwise, as observations from neuroanatomy show. Neurological pathways in the spinal cord and sympathetic chain connect the cerebral cortex, the conscious brain, and the adrenal glands. Because of those connections, what one thinks can literally stimulate one's adrenal glands. Those connections illustrate vividly the concept of mind-body interrelatedness, as Mr. L.'s case shows.

The nurse who cares for critically ill patients must strive to maintain the view that mind and body are interrelated. Adrenal disease shows that mind-body interrelatedness is not a matter of poetic metaphor or sentimentality. It is a matter of neurophysiological fact.

Anatomy and Physiology of the Adrenal Glands

The two adrenal glands lie at the superior poles of the kidneys (Fig. 27-1). Each adrenal gland is composed of

Critical Care Nursing Admission Assessment

Head to Toe Approach

Date	Time		
10-8	10³⁰ am	Pt. Name: *Mr. B.L.* Age: *70* Allergies: *NKA*	

Admitted Bed No: *2*   Via: *ER cart* Ad. Dx.: *Acute Adrenal Insufficiency*

T.: *101°F(R)* A.P.: *60*   R.P.: *60*   R.: *12*   B.P. Supine R: *90/70* L: *90/70* Sitting: *—*

Wt. (unit scale): *105*   Ht.: *5'5"* ECG Rhythm: *NSR*   Ectopy: *occ PVC*

Informant: *wife*   Last meal: *breakfast yesterday - 8 a.m.*

1. Chief complaint: *confused, lethargic*

2. Hx. of present illness: *2 days PTA tired, urinating frequently; complains of "chest cold". skin getting dark last 2 wks. s̄ sun; 20 lb. weight loss last 6 mo.*

3. Past medical Hx. (include all surgeries, hosp., diseases, injuries, blood trans.): *TB 1947-1948 c̄ medical management through 1950; AWMI c̄ complications - 1965; history of peptic ulcer - 1966.*

4. Family Hx.: *Both parents died of "old age" at 99; 4 brothers ages 62, 64, 65, 68 alive + well; 2 sisters, age 72 and 74 alive - have hypertension + are on medication*

5. Current drugs: *none*

6. Alcohol and tobacco habits: *none*

7. Dietary and fluid needs: *dehydrated at present; eats poorly*

8. Sleep and rest patterns: *usually sleeps 10 hrs./night; has slept more last 2 wks.*

9. Bowel and bladder habits: *takes occasional laxative; BM every other day*

10. Hygienic needs: *needs mouth care*

11. Psychosocial needs: *impaired thought processes - re-evaluate*

12. Occupation and education: *retired male printer - self-educated*

13. Exercise habits: *working in yard; walks 1 block a day when well.*

14. Spiritual needs: *active Baptist church*

15. Personal interests: *trading printing press equipment; repairs antique clocks*

16. Family member interaction and availability: *wife extremely anxious; 2 brothers and 1 sister live near pt. - wife + pt. appear very close*

17. Attitude towards illness and hospitalization: *pt. confused; wife states pt. is a "cooperative and kind man."*

Physical Examination

Date	Time			
	18.	Gen. appearance: *very thin*	(wife states this has occurred last 2 wks. & sun) color: *dark tan* skin: *dehydrated* *turgor-poor*	
	19.	Neurological:		
		a) level of consciousness: *confused*		
		b) cerebellar: *posture: too weak to stand gait: too weak to walk*		
		c) motor function: upper: *generalized weakness moves extremities appropr.* lower: *generalized weakness*		
		d) sensory function: upper: *normal* lower: *normal*		
		e) reflexes: *diminished*		
	20.	Head and face: *normal except increased pigmentation*		
	21.	Eyes: *PERRLA*		
	22.	Ears: *no drainage; membranes intact*		
	23.	Nose: *dry mucous membrane*		
	24.	Mouth/throat: *dry mucous membranes and tongue*		
	25.	Neck: *no scars, lymph nodes, or neck vein distention*		
	26.	Chest: *bilateral and equal excursion*		
	27.	Breast: *negative*		
	28.	Respiratory: *decreased vesicular breath sounds; no adventitious sounds*		
	29.	Cardiac: *PMI 5th left ICS-* MCL; *normal heart sounds*		
	30.	Abdomen: *no distention; vomited 200cc greenish emesis on admission*		
	31.	Genitourinary: *incontinent of urine on adm.* approx. 300cc *bowel sounds: decreased; incont. of diarrheal stool*		
	32.	Extremities (all pulses): *weak 2+, equal on both extremities*		
	33.	Back: *no scars or deformities*		
	34.	Problems requiring possible referral service: *have social worker talk c̄ wife about finances*		
	35.	Teaching needs: *Dietary, medication, self-care in regard to disease*		
	36.	Other:		

	PROBLEM LIST: **ACTIVE**	**INACTIVE**
10-8-78	1. *anorexia*	7. *TB* 1947-1950 →
	2. *weight loss - 20 lbs.*	8. *AWMI* 1965 →
	3. *weakness*	9. *peptic ulcer* 1966 →
	4. *increased pigmentation*	
	5. *hypotension*	
	6. *impaired thought process*	

Barbara Hossey, RN, CCRN
NURSE'S SIGNATURE

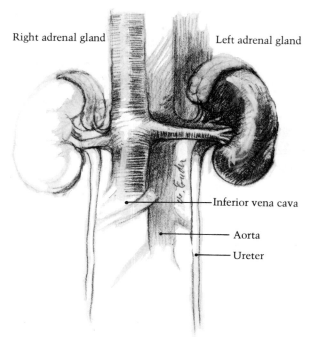

Right adrenal gland

Left adrenal gland

Inferior vena cava

Aorta

Ureter

Figure 27-1
The location of the adrenal glands.

two distinct parts, the adrenal medulla and the adrenal cortex. As far as is known, there is no direct functional relationship between the adrenal medulla and the adrenal cortex. The adrenal medulla secretes the hormones epinephrine and norepinephrine in response to sympathetic stimulation. The adrenal medulla is not involved in adrenal cortical insufficiency. However, it is important to understand the normal effects of epinephrine as well as its effects during periods of hypoglycemia, hypotension, mild hypoxia, and emotional stress [5]. Epinephrine causes constriction of the arterioles, except those in the heart and the skeletal muscles. Epinephrine increases the cardiac rate, the force of contraction, and the cardiac oxygen consumption, and it dilates the bronchioles by relaxing the smooth muscles. Epinephrine also causes glycogen breakdown in the liver, thus elevating blood glucose. There is also a decrease in insulin secretion because epinephrine affects carbohydrate metabolism by inhibiting the release of insulin from the pancreas. Epinephrine stimulates the production of ACTH, which in turn stimulates the pro-

duction of adrenal cortical hormones. Norepinephrine is secreted both directly from the sympathetic postganglionic nerve endings during periods of stress and from the adrenal medulla. Both hormones are able to stimulate structures that are not directly innervated by sympathetic fibers.

Regulation of the Adrenal Cortex by the Pituitary Gland

The pituitary gland plays an important role in regulating the outer layer of the adrenal gland, the adrenal cortex. The pituitary gland lies at the base of the brain, in the concave superior surface of the body of the sphenoid bone, the sella turcica. The pituitary gland is divided into two distinct parts: (1) the anterior pituitary, which secretes ACTH, growth hormone, thyroid-stimulating hormone, luteinizing hormone, and follicle-stimulating hormone; and (2) the posterior pituitary, which secretes antidiuretic hormone and oxytocin [5].

The anterior pituitary plays an important role during stress as well as in the absence of stress. The following sequences occur with stress (Fig. 27-2): corticotropin-releasing hormone (CRH) is transmitted from the hypothalamus to the anterior pituitary, causing the release of ACTH. ACTH stimulates the receptor sites in the adrenal cortex, causing the secretion of adrenal hormones. Those secretions have two major effects: (1) the mineralocorticoid effect, the regulation of the electrolytes of the extracellular fluid, especially sodium, potassium, and chlorides; and (2) the glucocorticoid effect, the regulation of carbohydrate, protein, and fat metabolism and increased blood glucose concentration during stress [5, 12, 13, 15].

ACTH secretion is also present in the absence of stress. Characteristically, cortisol secretion is increased in the early morning and inactive in the late evening. The central nervous system appears to cause the diurnal pattern, since both ACTH and CRH are secreted in a diurnal pattern. If one has a sudden change in his sleep-awake patterns, his diurnal pattern is not affected. However, a permanent change in one's daily sleeping habits causes a gradual change in his diurnal pattern [18, 20]. ACTH and cortisol secretion is episodic. Those hormones are released only in short bursts. Most of the bursts occur in the early morning, accounting for the diurnal pattern [17, 19].

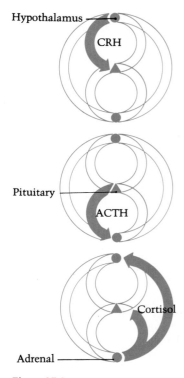

Hypothalamus

CRH

Pituitary

ACTH

Cortisol

Adrenal

Figure 27-2

Normal hypothalamus-pituitary-adrenal axis with cortisol feedback loop (CRH = corticotropin-releasing hormone; ACTH = adrenocorticotropic hormone).

The Adrenal Cortex

The two most significant of the 30 different steroids that have been isolated from the adrenal cortex are aldosterone, the chief mineralocorticoid, and cortisol, the major glucocorticoid [5].

ALDOSTERONE

Fluid and electrolyte balance is dependent largely on the regulation of aldosterone, which controls 95 percent of the body's mineralocorticoid activity. Aldosterone reduces the loss of urinary sodium. It acts by increasing the rate of tubular reabsorption of sodium in exchange for potassium and hydrogen ions in the loop of Henle and in the distal and collecting tubules [5, 8].

Aldosterone increases the resorption of chloride ions and plays a significant role in the mainte-nance of acid-base balance. In response to aldosterone secretion, hydrogen ions are secreted into the tubules in exchange for sodium ions, which are then resorbed. When the hydrogen ions are secreted in the urine as a result of sodium resorption in response to aldosterone, the hydrogen content of the blood is reduced, promoting a metabolic alkalosis [5].

A similar mechanism occurs with the regulation of potassium in response to the presence of aldosterone. As sodium is resorbed, potassium ions are exchanged and excreted into the urine in exchange for sodium ions [3, 5].

The combined resorption of sodium and chloride in response to aldosterone secretion affects another important system. This increased serum electrolyte concentration of sodium and chloride stimulates the production of antidiuretic hormone (ADH), which produces an osmotic gradient across the renal tubular membrane, resulting in water resorption. This produces increases in cardiac output and arterial pressure because of the increased extracellular fluid volume.

ADH, which is secreted by the posterior pituitary, also plays a significant role in fluid and electrolyte balance. It inhibits the excretion of water by the kidneys, thus causing stimulation in the response to an increase in the osmolality of the extracellular fluids via the osmoreceptors, which are specialized cells in the anterior hypothalamus. When a hypotonic state exists, or as osmolality decreases, the osmoreceptors swell because of the osmosis of water into them. If hypertonicity or increased osmolality is present, the osmoreceptors shrink, thus sensing a decrease in body fluid, and thereby increase their rate of discharge. Those impulses are transmitted to the posterior pituitary, where ADH is released [2, 4]. Therefore ADH secretion leads to water resorption, and inhibition of ADH secretion causes a diuresis.

CORTISOL

Cortisol, the major glucocorticoid produced by the adrenal cortex, controls gluconeogenesis, the formation of glucose from amino acids by the liver. The exact mechanisms are not fully understood, but the following theories have been offered [2, 3, 5, 9]:

1. Cortisol increases the active transport of amino acids from the extracellular fluids into the liver cells. The increased amino acids can be converted by the liver to glucose.

2. The liver contains enzymes that convert amino acids to glucose. It is thought that glucocorticoids may activate the enzymes involved in gluconeogenesis.

Cortisol slightly decreases the rate of glucose utilization by cells. Due to decreased glucose utilization by the cell and an increase in glucose concentration, the blood glucose levels rise. Cortisol can decrease amino acid transport into the muscle cells while increasing amino acid transport to liver cells.

Cortisol affects both fat and protein metabolism. As fatty acids are mobilized, their plasma concentration increases, resulting in another source of available energy.

Although the exact benefit of increased cortisol secretion by the adrenal cortex during stress is not understood, it is thought that glucocorticoids cause a fast mobilization of fats and amino acids from cellular stores for tissues that need energy.

ACTH affects the production of cortisol, corticosterone, and (to a lesser degree) aldosterone and adrenal androgens [4, 5, 9]. In response to stress, impulses are transmitted to the hypothalamus causing corticotropin-releasing hormone (CRH) production. CRH stimulates the cells of the anterior pituitary, causing the release of ACTH, which regulates the control of cortisol, corticosterone, and, to some extent, aldosterone. The resulting elevated blood cortisol levels cause a negative feedback stimulus to the anterior pituitary, reducing the production of ACTH and thus lowering the circulating ACTH levels.

Tests of Adrenocortical Function

The plasma cortisol levels can be measured by fluorimetric, radioimmunoassay, and protein-binding assay techniques. Those techniques measure total blood cortisol levels and are affected by changes in the amount of binding protein. An 8:00 A.M. cortisol level normally ranges from 5 to 30 μg per 100 ml; by 8:00 P.M., the level normally declines by at least 50 percent.

Plasma aldosterone determination can be obtained by radioimmunoassay techniques. The level varies, depending on the patient's sodium intake and posture. If the patient's salt intake is normal, the average normal value when he is supine is 8 ng per 100 ml. If the patient assumes an upright position for four hours, the values will rise to an average of 22 ng per 100 ml.

The secretion rates of cortisol and aldosterone can be determined over a 24-hour period. A tracer dose of ^{3}H-labeled steroid is injected intravenously and is then followed with a 24-hour urine collection. The cortisol secretion rate is 10 to 20 mg per 24 hours in women and 12 to 25 mg per 24 hours in men. The normal aldosterone secretion rate is 50 to 150 μg per 24 hours.

The urinary 17-hydroxysteroid (17-OHCS) levels reflect fairly closely the secretory rate of cortisol during a 24-hour period. The metabolism of increased amounts of cortisol results in a rise in urinary 17-OHCS excretion even though the plasma cortisol levels may be normal. The normal range of urinary 17-OHCS is 3 to 10 mg per 24 hours. Women usually have lower rates than do men.

Manifestations of Acute Adrenal Insufficiency

Acute adrenal insufficiency is the life-threatening event that is manifested clinically when the adrenal cortex fails to produce normal amounts of mineralocorticoid and glucocorticoid hormones. The manifestations of acute adrenal insufficiency depend on the extent of destruction of the adrenal gland.

Etiology and Precipitating Factors

Many factors may precipitate acute adrenal insufficiency. Formerly, the principal cause was destruction of the adrenal glands by tuberculosis [10]. Although the incidence of tuberculosis has declined in the United States in recent years, it is still a common cause of adrenal insufficiency in other parts of the world. The most common cause of adrenal insufficiency today is idiopathic atrophy of the adrenal glands. There is evidence that idiopathic atrophy may represent autoimmune destruction of the adrenal cortex [21]. Some studies show that patients with idiopathic adrenal atrophy have antibodies to adrenal tissue, as well as antibodies to other tissues, such as the parathyroid glands and the gastric mucosa [21]. Acute adrenal insufficiency may also be caused by amyloidosis, infection, histoplasmosis, and other fungal diseases.

Drug therapy can provoke acute adrenal crisis. Long-term heparin therapy may result in structural changes in the zona glomerulosa of the adrenal cortex, causing reversible aldosterone deficiency. Abrupt cessation of corticosteroids in patients receiving therapeutic doses for extended periods is the most common cause of relative adrenal insufficiency. A two-week period of steroid therapy may make a patient susceptible to acute adrenal insufficiency for up to a year. During periods of stress, supplemental cortisone should be given.

The stress of surgery can also precipitate acute adrenal insufficiency. Conditions that cause adrenal hemorrhage, such as metastatic carcinoma, trauma, sepsis, and leukemia, are other important causes of acute adrenal insufficiency. A bilateral adrenalectomy can also produce it.

Acute Pathophysiology

Acute adrenal insufficiency does not occur until more than 90 percent of the adrenal cortex has been destroyed, regardless of the cause of the destruction [4]. Total absence of adrenal cortical secretion will cause death in three to seven days unless extensive mineralocorticoid and salt therapy is administered. The mineralocorticoids are referred to as the lifesaving portion of the adrenal cortical hormones. If the patient is totally lacking in mineralocorticoids, the extracellular sodium concentrations and water plasma volume decrease, and the total extracellular fluid volume is greatly reduced. The pathophysiological mechanism in acute adrenal insufficiency involves the urinary loss of sodium, which causes concomitant water loss. The hyponatremia is due to the loss of sodium from the vascular compartments into the bones, tendons, and cartilage; it also results from the urinary sodium loss that follows aldosterone deficiency. That sodium loss depletes the extracellular fluid volume and accentuates hypotension. The hyperkalemia seen in adrenal insufficiency is caused by several factors. The most significant causes are an impaired glomerular filtration rate, an aldosterone deficiency, and acidosis. The patient develops acidosis primarily because of the failure of hydrogen ions to be excreted in exchange for sodium ions in the renal tubule resorption.

Primary and Secondary Adrenal Insufficiency

Primary and secondary adrenal insufficiency must be differentiated. Primary adrenal insufficiency is by definition due to disease originating in the adrenal glands themselves, and implies cortisol deficiency, usually accompanied by aldosterone deficiency [21]. Secondary adrenal insufficiency is due to disease originating in the anterior pituitary gland. The aldosterone mechanism in this situation is usually intact, and no mineralocorticoid therapy is required.

Pituitary ACTH deficiency will produce secondary adrenal insufficiency. Patients with secondary adrenal hypofunction may have many signs and symptoms of primary adrenal insufficiency, but characteristically they are not hyperpigmented. Another feature that distinguishes primary from secondary adrenal insufficiency is the near-normal levels of aldosterone in secondary adrenal insufficiency.

The reason for differentiating primary and secondary adrenal insufficiency is that primary adrenal insufficiency should alert the physician to the possible coexistence of autoimmune disorders, tuberculosis, amyloidosis, or histoplasmosis. Secondary adrenal insufficiency should alert the physician to the possibility of deficiencies of multiple pituitary trophic hormones, as well as to the possibility that the disease leading to pituitary destruction might endanger neighboring neural structures. Early recognition and treatment of a pituitary tumor or cyst may prevent its encroachment on the optic chiasm or the surrounding vascular structures.

Diagnosis

The diagnosis of acute adrenal insufficiency should be considered when a patient presents with nausea and vomiting, anorexia, weight loss, weakness associated with hypotension, or severe hypotension-to-shock states. If hyperpigmentation is present, acute adrenal insufficiency should be seriously considered (but it is not excluded because of lack of hyperpigmentation). Laboratory data often reveal hyponatremia, hyperkalemia, and fasting hypoglycemia. Radiographic studies may show characteristics of primary adrenal insufficiency, among them a small heart, calcification in the ear cartilages, occasionally adrenal calcification, and no changes in the area of the sella turcica.

In patients with primary adrenal insufficiency, the levels of plasma ACTH and MSH are elevated owing to the disturbance of the usual hypothalamus-pituitary-adrenal feedback mechanism [1]. However, patients with secondary adrenal insufficiency have low plasma ACTH levels. The diagnosis of adrenal insufficiency also depends on evidence of insufficient adrenal cortical function. The 24-hour urinary 17-OHCS levels may be low or even in low normal, especially if the patient is physiologically stressed [7]. The plasma cortisol and cortisol secretion rates may be low or low normal. When the baseline plasma or urinary steroid levels are low, ACTH stimulation tests should be done to demonstrate adrenal insufficiency.

Measurement of Adrenal Reserve

The diagnosis of adrenal insufficiency must be made by demonstrating low plasma levels of cortisol. The distinction between primary and secondary forms of adrenal insufficiency is made by observing the responsiveness of the adrenal gland to injections of exogenous ACTH. Plasma cortisol samples taken before and one hour after injections of ACTH should normally show a threefold increase. In primary adrenal insufficiency, there is either no rise or a subnormal rise in the cortisol levels following the injection of ACTH. In secondary adrenal insufficiency, because the pituitary gland fails to produce ACTH, the adrenal gland is usually capable of functioning normally when stimulated with ACTH. Therefore, a normal rise in the plasma cortisol levels may be seen following ACTH injection in secondary forms of adrenal cortisol insufficiency [21].

When the physician combines the diagnostic-therapeutic protocol that follows, it is imperative that no hydrocortisone or cortisone be administered. Dexamethasone, which is used therapeutically, will not interfere with the diagnostic studies that will be done since it is not detected in the assays for plasma cortisol or urinary 17-OHCS. When dexamethasone is not available, the physician has to decide whether to follow a modified therapeutic diagnostic protocol—giving saline solution and hydrocortisone and deferring the diagnostic studies—or to give ACTH with saline solution and measure the plasma and urine steroid responses. If the patient does have adrenal insufficiency, whether primary or secondary, his clinical condition should improve significantly in response to treatment with saline solution and dexamethasone. In primary and secondary adrenal insufficiency, the initial plasma cortisol value should be less than 5 μg per 100 ml and the urinary 17-OHCS value should be less than 2 mg per 24 hours. Those values hold for blood and urine samples that are obtained after the administration of corticotropin for the treatment of primary adrenal failure [6, 11, 21].

To help the physician measure adrenal reserve, the following medical protocol is listed. The nurse should make sure that the measurement protocol is followed correctly and thoroughly.

1. Obtain 10 ml of blood for plasma cortisol assay.
2. As ordered by the physician, administer rapidly an intravenous infusion of physiological saline solution and give dexamethasone phosphate (4 mg) and ACTH (25 IU). The first liter of saline solution with dexamethasone and corticotropin should be infused within one hour.
3. Obtain another 10 ml of blood for plasma cortisol assay at the completion of the first infusion.
4. Administer more 5% dextrose in saline solution as rapidly as necessary to treat dehydration and hypotension (specific orders will be given by physician).
5. Begin to collect a 24-hour urine specimen for a 17-OHCS assay.
6. Administer an intramuscular injection of corticotropin (80 IU); or add corticotropin to each liter of intravenous saline so that at least 3 IU is infused every hour for at least eight hours.
7. Obtain a third 10-ml blood specimen for plasma cortisol assay between the sixth and eighth hours of treatment with ACTH.
8. Analyze the results according to the criteria given earlier.

Treatment

The first step in the treatment of acute adrenal insufficiency is the administration of salt, water, and glucocorticoids. Then the cause of the adrenal insufficiency is treated [6, 21].

Replacement of Glucocorticoids

Hydrocortisone sodium succinate should be given in a 100-mg intravenous bolus once the diagnosis of acute adrenal insufficiency is considered. But if a combined therapeutic diagnostic protocol is being followed, dexamethasone is used initially. After the initial administration of intravenous hydrocortisone (100 mg), the same dosage should be given every 8 hours in a continuous intravenous infusion for a total of 300 mg during the first 24 hours. That dosage should protect the patient against the results of the stressful situation that may have caused the crisis.

Once the patient's condition has been stabilized, oral glucocorticoids can be given (hydrocortisone, 5 mg every six hours). In cases of poor gastrointestinal absorption of oral doses, intramuscular cortisone acetate should be given (50 mg every 12 hours) to maintain a continuous supply of glucocorticoids. If the patient is hypotensive, cortisone acetate should not be given intramuscularly because of its variability of absorption. Due to the slow absorption rate following intramuscular injection, cortisone acetate should never be the only therapy during acute adrenal insufficiency.

As soon as the physician is certain that the acute episode has passed, the glucocorticoid dosage is reduced about 20 to 30% daily until the maintenance dose has been achieved.

Since hydrocortisone (200 mg/24 hr) will provide sufficient mineralocorticoid activity, mineralocorticoid therapy is not needed during acute adrenal insufficiency. However, once the patient's condition has been stabilized and the total glucocorticoid dose has been reduced to below 100 mg per 24 hours, supplementary mineralocorticoids are usually required (e.g., deoxycorticosterone acetate, 2.5–5 mg intramuscularly every 24 hours, or fludrocortisone acetate [Florinef] 0.1 mg orally every 24 hours).

Correction of Fluid and Electrolyte Abnormalities

In the first hour or two of acute adrenal insufficiency, one liter of a 5% dextrose in physiological saline solution should be administered. Most patients require one liter or more of physiological saline solution every 3 to 6 hours for the first 24 hours. The patient's clinical response determines how much fluid he requires.

During the acute phase, hyperkalemia usually does not require therapy. Following rapid hydration with saline solution and treatment with glucocorticoids, the serum potassium level will promptly return to normal. If the serum potassium level does not return to normal (e.g., if it stays above 6.5 mEq/L) and if cardiac dysrhythmias occur, the physician may order intravenous sodium bicarbonate given every one to two hours until the potassium level is lowered and the cardiac dysrhythmias are corrected.

Hypoglycemia

Although hypoglycemia is usually not a problem in acute adrenal insufficiency, it can be troublesome if the patient is a diabetic and is taking insulin. In particular, hypopituitary patients and children may have hypoglycemia. If hypoglycemia is present, saline infusions with glucose are ordered early in the therapy. When the patient is a diabetic requiring insulin, the insulin dosage must be adjusted carefully according to his blood glucose levels.

Miscellaneous Considerations

The patient's blood pressure usually responds to rapid hydration with physiological saline solution and glucocorticoids. Vasopressors are usually not indicated, but if they are, phenylephrine hydrochloride (0.25 mg–0.5 mg) may be given in an intravenous bolus. It can also be given as a continuous infusion in a concentration of 4 mg per 1000 ml of physiological saline solution at a rate of 4 μg per minute.

Fever usually subsides with glucocorticoid therapy. Alcohol sponge baths or ice blankets may be needed if the patient has an extremely high temperature.

The physician also evaluates the patient for coexisting infection. Appropriate cultures are done, and antibiotic therapy is initiated early if an infection is suspected.

Long-Term Treatment

The long-term treatments of primary adrenal insufficiency are glucocorticoid replacement therapy, usually for the rest of the patient's life, and mineralocorticoid replacement therapy if necessary. Patients with adrenal insufficiency, including those who have undergone adrenalectomy, should be encouraged to have on their person a medical identification card or bracelet. Those patients need careful and continuing education in regard to their medication and disease. They must be taught how to administer intramuscular injections of dexamethasone in emergencies, and they must be encouraged to do so. They need information about special therapeutic situations they may encounter, such as dental extractions, upper respiratory tract infections, and other localized infections that cause physiological stress. Emotional stress is as significant as physiological stress. The special therapeutic situations may call for an increase in the maintenance steroid dosage. Patients may need to increase their steroid dosage and add salt to their diet when they exercise in extremely hot weather or when they vomit or have diarrhea. If a patient with adrenal insufficiency is to undergo surgery, his steroid dosage will be increased by his physician.

The primary goals of treatment of secondary adrenal insufficiency are to provide the exogenous glucocorticoids in quantities similar to those secreted by people with normal adrenal functioning and, if possible, to eradicate the inciting cause of the secondary adrenal failure.

Nursing Orders

Problem/Diagnosis

Acute phase of adrenal insufficiency.

OBJECTIVE NO. 1

The patient should show improvement of his extracellular volume depletion and electrolyte abnormalities.

To achieve the objective, the nurse should:

1. Be alert to the following clinical manifestations of disease, which are due to (1) depletion of sodium and water, intracellular and extracellular dehydration, (2) disturbances in sodium and potassium metabolism, and (3) infection:
   a. Fatigue, weight loss, and weakness.
   b. Gastrointestinal symptoms—vague abdominal pain, nausea, vomiting, diarrhea, and anorexia.
   c. Low serum sodium levels.
   d. Low serum chloride levels.
   e. Increased serum potassium levels.
   f. Hypotension.
   g. Mental dullness and confusion.
2. Complete the specific medical orders: obtain complete blood count and electrolyte, blood urea nitrogen, blood glucose, plasma cortisol, and arterial blood gas measurements.
3. Have the appropriate cultures done when infection is suspected.
4. Help with insertion of a large-gauge intravenous line.
5. Correct any fluid and electrolyte abnormalities. The nurse should:
   a. Determine the patient's serum, sodium, potassium, chloride, bicarbonate, and blood urea nitrogen levels and pH. (The discussion of the assessment and management of acute renal failure in Chapter 32 lists the signs and symptoms of electrolyte abnormalities.)
   b. Give the patient 1 liter of a 5% dextrose in physiological saline solution rapidly within 1 or 2 hours.
   c. For subsequent fluid therapy, give a 5% dextrose in physiological saline solution (1 liter every 3 to 6 hours for 24 hours).
   d. Correct any hypotension. Rapid hydration of the patient with saline solution and glucocorticoid replacement therapy is usually effective. If the hypotension does not respond to those measures, give phenylephrine (Neo-Synephrine) hydrochloride (0.25–0.5 mg intravenous bolus) or phenylephrine (0.4 mg/100 ml) administered as an intravenous infusion at 4 μg per minute—or some other vasopressor as ordered by the physician. The salt and water depletion is usually corrected during the first 24 hours.
   e. Correct hyperkalemia. Rapid hydration with physiological saline solution and glucocorticoid therapy usually lowers the patient's serum potassium level. One or two ampules of sodium bicarbonate should be given intravenously if the serum potassium level is greater than 6.5 mEq per liter in the presence of cardiac dysrhythmias and if the serum pH indicates acidosis.
6. Monitor the patient's vital signs and watch for cardiac dysrhythmias.

OBJECTIVE NO. 2

The patient's glucocorticoid and mineralocorticoid deficiencies should improve.

If patient is known to have acute adrenal insufficiency:

1. Give intravenous hydrocortisone sodium succinate (100 mg) as ordered by the physician.
2. Give a continuous intravenous infusion of hydrocortisone (100 mg every 8 hours for a total of 300 mg in the first 8 hours).
3. Once the patient's condition has stabilized, give oral cortisone acetate or hydrocortisone (50 mg every 6 hours). Add cortisone acetate (50 mg intramuscularly every 12 hours) to ensure a continuous parenteral supply.
4. If the intravenous line is not patent, start another intravenous line immediately to avoid further complications.
5. After an acute episode, glucocorticoid therapy should be reduced by 20 to 30% daily until the maintenance does is reached.

6. While the glucocorticoid dosage is being tapered to below 100 mg per 24 hours, many patients require supplementary mineralocorticoid therapy (intramuscular deoxycorticosterone, 2.5–5 mg every 24 hours, or oral fludrocortisone, 0.1 mg every 24 hours).
7. Watch for the side effects of mineralocorticoid therapy:
   a. Potassium depletion (evidenced by tiredness, alkalosis, and weakness)
   b. Sodium and water retention (evidenced by elevated blood pressure, weight gain, and edema)
8. If patient is not known to have adrenal disease, be prepared to help measure his *adrenal reserve* while his acute adrenal crisis is being treated.
9. Monitor carefully the patient who is undergoing corticosteroid therapy.
   a. Observe frequently the catheter site, flow rate, and patient's clinical response. Know the exact flow rates of the fluids so that precise amounts of the medication can be given.
   b. Be aware of the signs and symptoms of adrenal crisis—weakness, nausea and vomiting, restlessness, headache, and hypotension.
10. Know that the pharmacological action of the particular steroids must be understood before the scheduled doses can be planned.
11. Treat hypothermia or hyperthermia with routine measures as ordered by the physician.
12. Delay unnecessary procedures until the patient's condition has stabilized.
13. Give the patient the best possible nursing care. The nurse should assist the patient in all phases of his care. She should not allow him to do anything for himself during the period of acute adrenal insufficiency (and she should tell him why). She should be aware that the patient tires easily and she should allow him periods of rest during his nursing care.
14. Record the intravenous intake and urinary output so that the amount needed for replacement can be determined. All urine should be saved for the 24-hour urinalysis.
15. Be aware of the effects emotional stress has on the patient and his family; begin patient education when appropriate.

Problem/Diagnosis

Intermediate phase of adrenal insufficiency.

OBJECTIVE

The patient should show no further signs of acute adrenal crisis.

To achieve the objective, the nurse should:

1. Be alert to the early signs of acute adrenal insufficiency:
   a. Sudden drop in blood pressure
   b. Weak pulse
   c. Tachycardia
   d. Hypothermia or hyperthermia
   e. Cyanosis
   f. Nausea and vomiting
   g. Confusion
2. Be aware that circulatory collapse may result from the following (and may precipitate another adrenal crisis):
   a. Acute infection
   b. Decrease in salt intake
   c. Diarrhea, nausea, and vomiting
   d. Overexertion
   e. Physiological and psychological stressors
3. Check the patient's vital signs often. The nurse should:
   a. Take the patient's temperature every hour, because a change in temperature may be significant.
   b. Know that a sudden decrease in blood pressure or pulse may indicate an impending crisis.
4. Be thoroughly familiar with the patient's hormone replacement therapy and with the side effects of steroid therapy.
5. Be aware of the problems encountered during the periods when the steroid dosage is being lowered. The nurse should:
   a. Report any stress situations.
   b. Associate the symptoms of muscular weakness, lethargy, and tiredness with drug withdrawal.
6. Begin to teach the patient about the lifelong steroid therapy he will need for his adrenal insufficiency.
7. After the patient has begun to take food by mouth, assess closely what he eats. The nurse should be aware that:
   a. Patients under stress usually cannot be relied on to follow a full diet.
   b. Because the patient does not have normal adrenal function, he may become dangerously depleted of sodium if he does not take oral sodium. (Some patients are given 1 liter of sa-

line solution daily during the intermediate stage until they demonstrate a hearty appetite.)

Problem/Diagnosis

Intercritical phase of adrenal insufficiency.

OBJECTIVE

The patient should understand his self-care after his discharge.
To achieve the objective, the nurse should:

1. Educate the patient about adrenal insufficiency and long-term therapy.
2. Educate the patient about the signs and symptoms of adrenal insufficiency or crisis.
3. Educate the patient about self-care between the onset of the crisis and the institution of long-term therapy.
4. Understand that hydrocortisone is the mainstay of treatment. Supplemental doses are usually necessary. The dosage varies from 12.5 to 50 mg a day. Some studies indicate that dexamethasone does not reduce the patient's resistance to infection as does hydrocortisone; dexamethasone may therefore become widely used for maintenance therapy in chronic adrenal insufficiency instead of the glucocorticoids (e.g., prednisone, prednisolone, and hydrocortisone) [14]. The larger portion (25 mg) of the medication is taken in the morning and the rest (12.5 mg) is taken in the late afternoon to simulate the normal diurnal adrenal rhythm.
5. Educate the patient about giving himself steroids. The nurse should:
   a. Teach him how to give himself injections.
   b. Tell the patient to carry a sterile syringe containing 4 mg of dexamethasone for emergency intramuscular injection.
   c. Tell the patient to wear a Medic-Alert bracelet or to carry a card that gives his name, his physician's name, an emergency phone number, and the following information: "I have Addison's disease. In an emergency involving vomiting, loss of consciousness, or injury, I should immediately be given an intramuscular injection of dexamethasone phosphate (with the syringe that I am carrying). A physician should be summoned without delay."
6. Educate the patient about the proper time to take steroids. The steroids have a direct local effect on gastric mucosa. The patient should be encouraged to take his steroids with his meals, or, if that is impractical, to take them with milk or an antacid preparation. The common side effects that occur soon after the initiation of cortisone therapy are:
   a. Irritability
   b. Mental excitement
   c. Euphoria
   d. Insomnia
   e. Frank psychosis
   f. Gastric distress
7. Educate the patient about steroid side effects and when he should notify the physician. (Problems that may be precipitated by steroids are congestive heart failure, hypertension, cardiac enlargement, or hypokalemia.) He should notify his physician:
   a. When he becomes short of breath while exercising or while at rest.
   b. When he experiences extreme weakness.
8. Educate the patient about special therapeutic problems that may require an increase of cortisone therapy:
   a. Dental extractions
   b. Acute illness or injury
   c. Minor or major surgery
   d. Physiological or psychological stress
9. Educate the patient about his diet. He should know to:
   a. Take liberal amounts of sodium (at least 150 mEq a day).
   b. Take supplemental sodium chloride if he has diarrhea, nausea, or vomiting, or if he is exposed to extremely hot weather or is sweating profusely.
10. Educate the patient about routine tests and measurements, including when they should be done:
    a. Weight checks
    b. Serum electrolyte studies
    c. Blood pressure checks
    d. ECGs
    e. Chest x rays
11. Educate the patient about the basics of long-term

therapy for adrenal insufficiency. The patient must understand his need for:

a. *Lifelong* therapy.
b. Adequate rest.
c. Adequate warmth.
d. Avoidance of overexertion.
e. Adequate diet.
f. Avoidance of cathartics.
g. Avoidance of psychological stressors.
h. Regular medical check-ups.
i. Calling his physician whenever he has questions about his medication, symptoms, or illness.
j. Increased hormone when he is under stress.

Summary

Acute adrenal insufficiency is usually characterized by severe weakness, nausea and vomiting, hypotension, hypoglycemia, hyponatremia, and hyperkalemia. The diagnosis is usually considered in any patient in shock of undetermined cause whose clinical condition is deteriorating rapidly. The picture of acute adrenal insufficiency results when more than 90 percent of the adrenal cortex has been destroyed. The immediate treatment is correction of fluid and electrolyte imbalance, replacement of glucocorticoids, and removal of the precipitating cause if possible. After the crisis is over and the patient enters the recovery phase, the nurse and the physician must give him specific guidelines for self-care. The guidelines should be explained thoroughly and clearly, and the patient should realize that he must follow them for the rest of his life.

Study Problems

1. Acute adrenal insufficiency is caused by:
   a. Aldosterone deficiency.
   b. Extracellular volume depletion.
   c. Cortisol deficiency.
   d. A precipitating cause.
   e. All the above.
2. Name two causes of primary deficiency of adrenal cortical hormones.
3. During an acute adrenal crisis, the patient should

be encouraged to be more independent so that he can adjust more quickly to his chronic disease.
a. True.
b. False.
4. What are the three most important events in acute adrenal insufficiency that must be corrected?

Answers

1. e.
2. Destruction of the adrenal cortex and idiopathic adrenal atrophy.
3. False.
4. Replacement of glucocorticoids, correction of fluid and electrolyte imbalances, and specific treatment of any recognizable precipitating cause.

References

1. Abe, K., Nicholson, W. E., Liddle, G. W., et al. Normal and abnormal regulation of beta MSH in man. *J. Clin. Invest.* 48:1580, 1969.
2. Baxter, J. D., and Forsham, P. H. Tissue effects of glucocorticoids. *Am. J. Med.* 53:573, 1972.
3. Forsham, P. H. The Adrenal Cortex. In R. H. Williams (ed.), *Textbook of Endocrinology* (5th ed.). Philadelphia: Saunders, 1974.
4. Ganong, W. F., Alpert, L. C., and Ler, T. C. ACTH and the regulation of adrenocortical secretion. *N. Engl. J. Med.* 290:1006, 1974.
5. Guyton, A. *Textbook of Medical Physiology* (5th ed.). Philadelphia: Saunders, 1976.
6. Hemathong Kam, T. Acute adrenal insufficiency. *J.A.M.A.* 230:1317, 1974.
7. Irvine, W. J., and Barnes, E. W. Adrenocortical insufficiency. *J. Clin. Endocrinol. Metab.* 1:549, 1972.
8. Laragh, J. H., and Stoerk, H. C. A study of the mechanism of secretion of the sodium-retaining hormone (aldosterone). *J. Clin. Invest.* 36:383, 1957.
9. Liddle, G. W. Pathogenesis of glucocorticoid disorders. *Am. J. Med.* 53:638, 1972.
10. Mason, S., Meads, T. W., Lee, J. A. H., et al. Epidemiological and clinical picture of Addison's disease. *Lancet* 2:744, 1968.
11. Musa, B. U., and Dowling, J. Rapid intravenous administration of corticotropin as a test of adrenocortical insufficiency. *J.A.M.A.* 201:633, 1967.
12. Nelson, D. H. Regulation of glucocorticoid release. *Am. J. Med.* 53:590, 1972.
13. Newton, D. W., Nichols, A. O., and Newton, M. N. Corticosteroids. *Nurs. '77* 6:26, 1977.

14. Peters, W. P. Corticosteroid administration and localized leukocyte mobilization in man. *N. Engl. J. Med.* 282:342, 1972.
15. Samuels, L. T., and Uchikawa, T. Biosynthesis of Adrenal Steroids. In A. B. Eisenstein (ed.), *The Adrenal Cortex.* Boston: Little, Brown, 1967.
16. Tzagournis, M. Acute adrenal insufficiency. *Heart Lung* 4:603, 1978.
17. Weitzman, E. D. Neuro-endocrine pattern of secretion during the sleep-wake cycle of man. *Proj. Brain Res.* 42:93, 1975.
18. Weitzman, E. D. Biologic rhythms and hormone secretion patterns. *Hosp. Pract.* 11:79, 1976.
19. Weitzman, E. D. Circadian rhythms and episodic hormone secretion in man. *Ann. Rev. Med.* 27:225, 1976.
20. Weitzman, E. D., et al. The twenty-four hour pattern of episodic secretion of cortisol in normal subjects. *J. Clin. Endocrinol. Metab.* 33:14, 1971.
21. Williams, G. H., Dluhy, R. B., and Thorn, G. W. Diseases of the Adrenal Cortex. In T. R. Harrison (ed.), *Principles of Internal Medicine* (8th ed.). New York: McGraw-Hill, 1977.

VIII. The Critically Ill Adult with Neurological/Neurosurgical Problems

We have received messages from modern science that say, "Do not dismiss your ideas merely because they do not make sense." We have learned mathematical proofs which show us that we can use apparently contradictory ways of describing something, if this is necessary to obtain a complete description of the thing itself. This observation from modern physics is called the Principle of Complementarity.

If body-mind-spirit concepts seem to contradict traditional ways of viewing the patient, perhaps it is possible to accept both views. Can we say that these views are not contradictory, but complementary?

Do I contradict myself?
Very well then I contradict myself,
(I am large, I contain multitudes).

Walt Whitman
"Song of Myself"

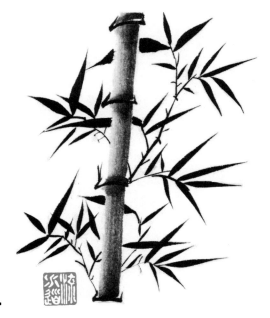

Guillain-Barré Syndrome

Diane Turbin Ender

Guillain-Barré syndrome, a disease of the peripheral nerves, is one of the most feared acute paralytic diseases known to man. Pathologically, it is inflammatory, but its cause is essentially unknown. It generally follows a mild infection. Approximately 5 to 21 days after the infection, an ascending paralysis involving the peripheral and cranial nerves may be observed. The need for ventilatory assistance may occur quite rapidly as a result of respiratory failure secondary to the muscular paralysis. Although Guillain-Barré syndrome is potentially completely reversible, the mortality is greater if the complication of respiratory failure develops. Treatment of Guillain-Barré syndrome is limited to the alleviation of the symptoms. Therefore, the critical care nurse must be a keen observer and be able to assess and carefully manage the symptoms as they arise.

Objective

In regard to a patient with Guillain-Barré syndrome, the nurse should be able to assess his condition systematically, write nursing orders for him, implement his care, evaluate his symptoms, and be prepared for the development of life-threatening complications.

28

Achieving the Objective

To achieve the objective the nurse should be able to:

1. Understand and discuss the pathophysiologic changes in Guillain-Barré syndrome.
2. List its cardinal manifestations.
3. Explain its precipitating factors.
4. List the diagnostic criteria.
5. Recognize its life-threatening complications.
6. Observe and assess the regression of symptoms and adjust the treatment accordingly.
7. Perform the necessary nursing care.
8. Evaluate the nursing care being given.
9. Teach the patient and his family about the disease process and the plans for his rehabilitation.

How to Proceed

To develop an approach to Guillain-Barré syndrome, the nurse should:

1. Analyze the characteristics of Guillain-Barré syndrome that occur in the patient in the case study that follows.
2. Anticipate the patient's physiological and psychological problems.
3. Develop an assessment tool for the patient.
4. Outline the short-range and long-range goals for the management of the patient's care.
5. Design a flow sheet to be used for the patient.

Case Study

Ms. M. W., 28 years of age, was hospitalized with an admitting diagnosis of Guillain-Barré syndrome. Her chief complaint was increasing weakness of her upper and lower extremities and a difficulty in breathing that had become more severe in the past week. She reported that she had numbness of her feet and hands and legs and back pains. The pains persisted although she had taken analgesics and muscle relaxants.

Her patient profile and social history described her as a 5'4", 130-lb, right-handed Caucasian woman from Dallas, Texas. She was married, and she had two daughters, 3 and 5 years old. Her husband, 30 years old, was a traveling salesman for a well-known insurance company. Ms. W. worked full time as a legal secretary. She was a Baptist, and she attended church regularly with her family. Her hobbies were needlepoint and reading. She did not smoke, and she drank only moderately (at social events).

Her past medical history revealed the usual childhood diseases: measles, mumps, and chickenpox. Surgical procedures included a tonsillectomy at 6 years, an appendectomy at 14 years, and a cholecystectomy at 22 years. The operations were without complications. Ms. W. said that three years ago she had been hospitalized for two weeks for a "bleeding" ulcer that was controlled with medication and dieting. Also, she said that two years ago she had been hospitalized for a "rapid heart" problem.

Her medications were stool softeners (daily), multivitamins (daily), digoxin (0.25 mg a day), a potassium chloride elixir (20 mEq twice a day), and a sedative for sleep (nightly). She said that she had an allergy to penicillin that was manifested by a rash. She had no other known drug allergies. She was not using oral contraceptives.

Ms. W. had been visiting friends in another city when she developed flulike symptoms, including a sore throat, aching, an elevated temperature, a headache, and a general feeling of malaise. Those symptoms, which had begun about 30 days before her present hospitalization, lasted seven days and required no treatment. Ms. W. returned to Dallas. Two weeks after her flu attack, she developed leg pains that lasted three days. She described them as "deep shooting pains" in her calves. Her leg and back pains developed two weeks later, and they persisted. Those pains were unrelieved by medication. Six days later Ms. W. fell. She consulted a physician, and she was hospitalized the next day.

Ms. W.'s family history revealed coronary disease, cerebrovascular disease, and cancer of the bowel. Her father, 84 years old, had heart disease. She had two sisters, and they were well. Her husband and children were well.

The results of a review of Ms. W.'s body systems were unremarkable. She wore glasses for reading. Two years ago, she had been hospitalized for a "rapid heart rate" (160 beats per minute), and she was treated with digoxin. The review of Ms. W.'s gastrointestinal system revealed a bleeding ulcer of three years' duration that was managed by careful dieting, including the avoidance of spicy foods. No abnormalities of her pulmonary and renal systems were disclosed. Ms. W.'s menstrual cycles were regular, occurring every 28 to 30 days and lasting 5 days. The results of her last Pap smear (a year ago) were negative.

The results of Ms. W.'s physical examination are shown on the accompanying assessment sheet.

Clinical Presentation

Ms. W.'s initial laboratory studies were a complete blood count and blood chemistry studies, including tests for hepatic and renal functioning. Arterial blood gas analyses were made. The results of the tests were normal. The results of a chest x ray and a myelogram were negative.

A lumbar puncture that was done three days after Ms. W.'s admission showed an elevated protein level and no leukocytes. Based on the clinical findings and the results of an examination of the cerebrospinal fluid, the diagnosis of Guillain-Barré syndrome was made.

Ms. W.'s condition continued to progress in an ascending manner to include a flaccid paralysis of both upper extremities and a loss of deep tendon reflexes. Ms. W. also exhibited dysphagia and laryngeal paralysis. It was felt that her seventh, ninth, tenth, and eleventh cranial nerves were becoming involved. A program of passive range of motion exercises of the extremities was begun.

Because of Ms. W.'s increasing respiratory difficulty, she underwent a tracheostomy on her fourth hospital day. An analysis of her arterial blood gas showed that she had a severe hypoxemia with a mild respiratory alkalosis. She was given respiratory therapy with a volume-type ventilator (MA-1); the inspired oxygen concentration was 40%. Strict ventilatory support became necessary when further arterial blood gas analyses showed that she had a more severe alkalosis. After 24 hours of ventilatory support, her arterial blood gas measurements improved; she continued to be given ventilatory support, but she was able to assist ventilation on a 28% oxygen concentration despite her muscle paralysis. Frequent suctioning produced thick, tenacious secretions. A chest physiotherapy program was begun. Also, serial tests of vital capacities, including tidal volume and inspiratory force, were done every four hours to assess Ms. W.'s ventilatory efforts and to detect any worsening of her muscle paralysis.

Ms. W.'s nutritional status was maintained through nasogastric tube feedings. It was estimated that she needed 2500 calories per day. She was given 1900 calories in the tube feedings and 600 calories in 2500 ml of intravenous fluids that were administered daily. Vitamins were added daily to the intravenous fluids. An antacid and her daily dose of digoxin were also given in the tube feedings.

On Ms. W.'s tenth hospital day, her temperature rose. Her breath sounds demonstrated the presence of rales over the left lower lobe of her lungs. A diagnosis of pneumonia was made. The disorder responded to antibiotic therapy, suctioning, and chest physiotherapy. Penicillin was not used because she was allergic to it.

Continuous catheterization by gravity drainage was employed during Ms. W.'s hospital stay because she had poor bladder tone. Her urinary output continued to be adequate; she showed no signs of urinary tract infections. She did not have fecal incontinence. She had constipation, which was relieved by the use of stool softeners and enemas.

By Ms. W.'s thirty-third hospital day, her condition had begun to improve slowly. The gross motor functioning in her upper extremities improved, and she continued to assist in her ventilatory support. X rays of her chest showed that the pneumonia was completely resolved. After she had achieved adequate ventilation, she was able to be weaned from the ventilator in two days. She was extubated after 48 hours, during which time a T bar with 40% oxygen and mist was used.

Ms. W.'s tube and intravenous feedings could be discontinued by hospital day 42 because she had gradually increased her oral intake from clear liquids to a soft diet. She needed to take liquids through a straw, and she needed assistance with each feeding.

Ms. W.'s physical therapy program continued and by her fiftieth hospital day, Ms. W. was able to walk with the help of a walker for short periods each day. Her tracheostomy incision appeared to be healing without complication.

Sixty-five days after her admission, Ms. W. was transferred to a rehabilitation institute for continuation of her physical and occupational therapy programs.

Reflections

Ms. W.'s primary care nurse, as well as all the nurses, were challenged physically and emotionally by Ms. W.'s condition. Ms. W. had complex physical needs that had to be met, and she was totally dependent psychologically on her health care team. Her body-mind-spirit were involved in coping.

Ms. W. was not only dealing with her hospital situation, she was also worried about what was happening at home. When her unemployment and sick pay ended, it was a strain on her family to meet expenses. Because her husband traveled, he had had to hire a housekeeper to care for their two children. Also, Ms. W. missed her children tremendously. A definite problem was a lack of "significant others" in her life at that time.

In addition, any patient who has an idiopathic illness (an illness of unknown cause) presents a unique challenge to the critical care nurse. And as the illness becomes more serious, the likelihood increases that more serious problems will arise.

An idiopathic illness is more than a mere symptom complex. An idiopathic illness may be interpreted by the patient in symbolic and personal ways. For example, the patient may see it as a punishment or retribution. The more mysterious the illness, the more the patient is drawn to symbolic interpretations of the illness.

The patient with Guillain-Barré syndrome may have those painful reactions. The paralysis and the helplessness accompanying the syndrome can be devastating psychologically. Depression, perhaps accompanied by feelings of guilt if the patient views the illness as a punishment, is the rule.

The idiopathic nature of the illness also takes a psychological toll on the patient that is translated into physical terms, illustrating the mind-body continuum. Thus, the patient with an idiopathic illness who interprets it as a deserved punishment may not want to participate in his care; he may act as though he wants and needs to be punished. Symbolically he admits his guilt by making his illness worse through

Critical Care Nursing Admission Assessment
Major Systems Approach

PATIENT'S NAME: _Ms. M.W._   DATE: _6/23_   TIME: _2:00 p.m._

DIAGNOSIS: _Guillain-Barré Synd._ T: _98⁸_ A.P.: _96_ R.P.: _100_ R.: _20_

B.P.: _114/84_ E.C.G. RHYTHM: _NSR_ ECTOPY: _none_ WT: _130 lbs._ HT: _5'4"_

ADMITTED VIA: _stretcher_ INFORMANT: _patient_ LAST MEAL: _9:00 a.m._

I. CHIEF COMPLAINT: _"I have pains in my legs and hands and difficulty in swallowing."_

II. PATIENT PROFILE: _right-handed_
1. Age _28 y/o_ 2. Sex _Female_
3. Marital Status (M) W D S
4. Race _Caucas._ 5. Religion _Baptist_
6. Occupation _Legal Secretary_
7. Availability of Family _husband and children at home_
8. Dietary _3 meals/day; bland, no spicy foods_
9. Sleeping _needs med. each night - reg. 8 hrs._
10. Activities of Daily Living _works 5 days/wk. 8:30 am - 5:00 p.m.; cooks dinner each evening; spends quiet weekends at home_

III. HISTORY OF PRESENT ILLNESS: _Approx. 4 wks. ago, flu-like symptoms for 5 days → pain + tingling arms + legs for 2 wks - weakness + a fall c̄ some difficulty in breathing_

IV. PAST MEDICAL HISTORY:
1. Pediatric & Adult Illnesses _measles, mumps, chickenpox_
2. Cardiac _"rapid heart," 1973_
3. Hypertension _none_
4. Respiratory _no difficulty_
5. Diabetes Mellitus _no_
6. Renal _no difficulty_
7. Jaundice _no_
8. Infections _none significant_
9. Other _gall bladder disease - 6 yrs. ago_
10. Hospitalizations & Surgeries
tonsillectomy - age 6 y/o
appendectomy - age 14 y/o
cholecystectomy - age 22 y/o
"bleeding ulcer" - 2 wk. hosp.; age 25 y/o
"rapid heart rate" (160) hosp.; age 26 y/o

11. Current Medication _stool softeners, digoxin, KCl elixir multivits, sedative for sleep_
12. Allergies _penicillin - gives history of rash_
13. Habits _early riser; dislikes smoking; likes activities such as reading + needlepoint_

V. FAMILY HISTORY: _coronary, cerebrovasc. disease and ca bowel on mother's side; father had heart disease._

VI. PSYCHOSOCIAL:
1. Behavior During Assessment _appeared anxious and answered questions c̄ brief communication; wanted her husband to visit; fearful of outcome_

2. Specific Problems _pain in her thighs and arms during interview; related some difficulty in swallowing_

VII. PHYSICAL EXAMINATION:
1. General _well developed, well nourished, skull, head, neck normal_

2. Respiratory System _nose - midline_
Airway _normal - no obstruction_
Inspection _no respiratory restriction, no retraction_
Rate _16-20/min._
Rhythm _regular_
Chest Wall _equal bilateral movements_
Palpation _no tenderness; symmetrical excursion_
Percussion _resonant bilaterally_

594

Auscultation
Voice Sounds _normal "99" (muffled)_
Breath Sounds _bilaterally_
Normal ✓ Increased____ Decreased _____
Adventitious Sounds _____
negative bilaterally,
no rales or rhonchi

3. Cardiovascular System
A.P. _96_ R.P. _100_
B.P. Supine R _111/84_ L _110/80_
P.M.I. _5th I.C.S. @ M.C.L._
Heart Sounds _normal S_1 + S_2_

Thrills _none_
Peripheral Pulses _strong_

4. Neurological System
Level of Consciousness _alert + awake_
oriented x3
Respiratory Pattern _regular_

Cranial Nerves _CN I - not tested_
CN II → XII tested + intact

ears - tympanic membrane intact - can hear
Eyes _wears glasses - hyperopia - last exam whisp_
_1971_
(1) Pupils   OD   OS
Size _4mm_   _4mm_
Shape _round_   _round_
Light _react briskly_   _react briskly_
Consensual _normal_   _normal_
Accommodation _normal_   _normal_
(2) Ocular Movements _E O M's intact_

Motor _normal muscle mass; flaccid_
paralysis upper + lower prox. only
Sensory _int ; T-10 pinprick_
Coordination _unable to test_

Reflexes _negative Babinski_
DTR's decreased

5. Gastrointestinal System
Nose & Mouth _some fillings in mouth;_
uvula midline
Stomach _no distention or pain_

Abdomen _flat - 5 cm. midline scar_

Bowel Sounds _decreased_
Liver _normal - non palpable_
Spleen _non-palpable_

6. Renal & Genitourinary Systems
I. _I.V.R.L._ _1000 cc._ O. _Foley_
18 hrs.
Urinary Bladder & Urethra _no distention or_
pain; catheter in place
Kidneys _no pain on percussion_

7. Musculoskeletal System
Spine _normal curvature; no tenderness_
Extremities _flaccid paralysis_

Sacral Edema _none present_
Masses _none present_

8. Hematologic System
Petechiae _negative_
Ecchymosis _none noted_
Gingiva _negative, no redness or_
swelling

9. Endocrine System
Breath _normal_
Skin _good color_

VIII. LABORATORY: _CSF clear, protein 230_
1. Hematology _sugar 16, WBC 3, RBC 250_
lymph 100
HGB _13.0_   HCT _39.7_
W.B.C. _10,000_
2. Chemistry
Na _142_   K _4.4_
CO_2 _31_   CL _101_
Blood Sugar _120_   Amylase _—_
BUN _14_   Cr _—_
3. Urinalysis _clear yellow; rare casts_
Spec. gravity: 1.022, pH = 5, WBC 2-4
RBC 0-4
4. Electrocardiogram
Rate _100_   Rhythm _regular_
P-R _.12_   QRS _.04_ ST _0.08_
Interpretation _normal sinus rhythm_
5. Chest x-ray _negative_

IX. PROBLEM LIST:

ACTIVE	INACTIVE
1. Guillain-Barré Syndrome	6. status post
A. Quadriplegia 2° to 1	tonsillectomy
B. Dysesthesia 2° to 1	7. post-appendectomy
2. constipation	8. post-bleeding ulcer
3. financial difficulty	9. post-cholecystectomy
4. dependency role	10. post-"increased
5. penicillin allergy	heart rate"

Diane Ender, RN
NURSE'S SIGNATURE

595

neglecting self-care. The patient may dwell on his illness. He may become extremely negative, hostile, or dependent. It is rare that such a patient has any significant degree of psychological insight into his feelings.

The clinical course of an idiopathic illness can be profoundly affected by the mind-spirit component of the illness. Indeed, it is wise to view an idiopathic illness as a body-mind-spirit complex in which causes and effects blend indistinguishably.

In Ms. W.'s case, the staff's frustrations increased as the days became weeks. Ms. W.'s tracheostomy made verbal communication between her and the nurses impossible. That complication increased Ms. W.'s dependency and increased the staff's frustration. Knowing that they had to allow Ms. W. to be completely dependent on them tried the nurses' patience. Periodically they held multidisciplinary team conferences and staff–family conferences to discuss Ms. W.'s care and changing condition. Ms. W. definitely needed a total team approach.

Ms. W.'s depression and overt hostile behavior after extubation sometimes irritated the staff. Since Ms. W. and the nurses were close in age, the nurses identified with her and thus they felt guilty because of their irritability. Those feelings were discussed in the conferences, and everyone was helped to work through their feelings, which were natural ones.

When the goal of increasing Ms. W.'s independence was established and positive steps were taken toward decreasing Ms. W.'s feeling of depression, the nurses' negative feelings were resolved or at least alleviated. After Ms. W. was transferred from the critical care unit, special arrangements were made to allow her to visit in the lobby with her children. The nurses also arranged for her to attend services in the chapel.

The occupational therapist provided diversion by lending Ms. W. books and by planning crafts that Ms. W. might try. The therapy reflected the staff's awareness of the body-mind-spirit concept.

Clinical Description

Guillain-Barré syndrome was first described in 1859 in France by John Batiste Octabe Landry. Guillain, Barré, and Strohl described it again in 1916 in the French literature and in 1936 in the American literature. It is named after these four scientists—the Landry-Guillain-Barré-Strohl syndrome. The condition is called a syndrome because it is characterized by a set of symptoms that contribute to the diagnosis of the disease. The syndrome has been known by many other names, among them acute postinfectious polyneuritis, infectious neuronitis, polyneuritis with facial diplegia, and idiopathic polyneuritis. The syndrome's outstanding characteristic is an ascending flaccid quadriplegia. Occasionally it may affect first the upper extremities and then the lower extremities. A variant known as Fischer's syndrome has also been described [12], whose symptoms include ophthalmoplegia, ataxia, and areflexia [12].

There is often cranial nerve involvement in Guillain-Barré syndrome. About 25 percent of patients hospitalized with the syndrome have respiratory failure [12]. A major life-threatening complication is pulmonary embolism secondary to stasis in leg veins from immobility. Under ideal conditions, the mortality is less than 5% [21]. The mortality has decreased because critical care nursing has improved; the pulmonary, cardiac, and other complications are identified sooner; antibiotics are used for treatment; and tracheostomy is performed earlier in the course of the disease.

Etiology

There is still much disagreement among physicians and other scientists about the exact cause of Guillain-Barré syndrome. It is often considered idiopathic. Since the neuritic symptoms in many cases follow an upper respiratory tract infection, many have assumed that the causative agent is a filtrable virus [7]. Attempts to isolate the virus from the cerebrospinal fluid, blood, or spinal cord have been essentially futile. The theory most often put forth is that the neuritis is of allergic origin. That theory has been supported by the fact that the polyneuritis has been produced in animals by the injection of extracts of peripheral nerves [7].

The theory of the allergic origin of Guillain-Barre syndrome states that first the person becomes sensitized to his peripheral nerve myelin and then sensitized lymphocytes attack the myelin. The axon is usually spared unless it is coincidentally damaged with the myelin. The syndrome shows many of the findings of autoimmune diseases [16]. The later investigations of Sheremata and his associates [14] have attempted to identify the antigen in the peripheral nerve that is responsible for the production of experimental allergic polyneuritis.

Precipitating Factors

A viral infection usually precedes the appearance of the symptoms of Guillain-Barré syndrome. Most often, a respiratory or gastrointestinal tract infection precipitates the motor or sensory symptoms. Fever is often absent or slight [16]. Other causative factors that have been reported are herpes simplex virus [8], herpes zoster [14], rubella, rubeola, atypical pneumonia, and infectious mononucleosis [17]. Cases of Guillain-Barré syndrome were reported after the 1976 swine flu immunization in the United States. The syndrome was also reported to have occurred in a group of patients who did not seem to have precipitating factors [14].

The Peripheral Nervous System

The nervous system comprises three interrelated subsystems, one of which is the peripheral nervous system. The peripheral nervous system comprises the spinal nerves and some of the cranial nerves. (The first and second cranial nerves are not considered to be peripheral nerves.) The cranial nerves arise from or travel to the brain stem, and the spinal nerves travel to or from the spinal cord. Figure 28-1 illustrates the normal anatomy of a peripheral nerve with a microscopic enlargement of the components. Some peripheral nerves are purely motor; that is, they are concerned with the movement of muscles. Others are purely sensory; that is, they carry sensations inward to the central nervous system. Most of the peripheral nerves are mixed; that is, they have both motor and sensory fibers. Those peripheral nerves repeatedly branch, carrying their fibers to all parts of every organ [2]; they seem to be especially vulnerable to attack.

The term mononeuritis refers to an inflammation of one nerve, and the term polyneuritis refers to an inflammation of many nerves. Since nerves themselves do not become inflamed in the true sense of the meaning of the word *inflamed*, which is redness, pain, heat and swelling of some part of the body, caused by injury or disease, Guillain-Barré syndrome has been termed a polyneuropathic disorder by its investigators. The term polyneuropathic refers to the

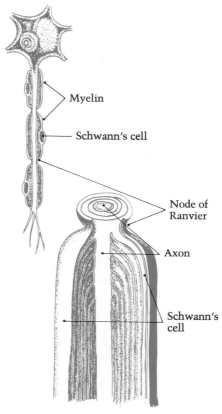

Figure 28-1
Microscopic enlargement of the anatomical components of a normal peripheral nerve.

changes that result from the involvement of multiple nerves [21].

Acute Pathophysiology

The following paragraphs discuss the acute pathophysiological process in Guillain-Barré syndrome. As mentioned, all motor axons and most sensory axons are covered by individual myelin sheaths. The myelin sheaths occur at gaps (or intervals), termed nodes of Ranvier. The axon is normally myelinated by Schwann's cells that are interspersed with the nodes of Ranvier. Some sensory axons do not have myelin sheaths. Those that do not have myelin

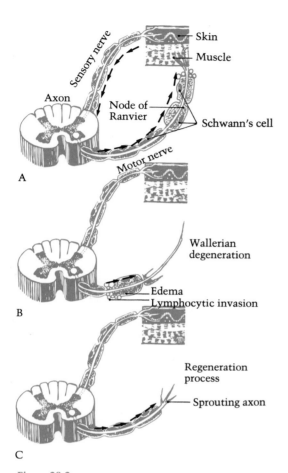

Skin

Muscle

Sensory nerve

Axon

Node of Ranvier

Schwann's cell

Motor nerve

A

Wallerian degeneration

Edema

Lymphocytic invasion

B

Regeneration process

Sprouting axon

C

Figure 28-2

Cross section of the spinal cord illustrating the pathophysiological changes of the Guillain-Barré syndrome. A. The anatomy of a motor and sensory peripheral nerve; the innervation of a muscle fiber with the sensory receptors displayed. B. Response of a neuron to injury, with wallerian degeneration. C. Regeneration with the sprouting axon.

sheaths conduct impulses more slowly than do those that have myelin sheaths [12].

In Figure 28-2, the spinal cord is shown in cross section. The motor neuron is located in the ventral or anterior horn of the cord. The axon is displayed as innervating a muscle fiber. The sensory neuron is located in the posterior or dorsal horn of the cord. As shown, it transmits signals from receptor end organs, such as the skin.

Pathological changes in the response of the neuron to injury or disease can be seen in Figure 28-2B. Those

changes include (1) an early inflammatory response with phagocytosis of myelin by the macrophages and the lymphocytes, (2) the resulting edema of the myelin, and (3) segmental demyelination (the loss of the Schwann's cells and its myelin sheath, resulting in a widened node of Ranvier).

If a myelinated axon loses its myelin, the nerve conducts impulses less rapidly. The interaction between the axon and its Schwann's cells is not clearly known. However, remyelination occurs rapidly if the axon remains intact. If the axon degenerates, the myelin disintegrates. This process of axonal damage is termed wallerian degeneration. The process of repair is extremely slow because both the axon and the myelin must regenerate.

However, it is possible to recover the integrity of a peripheral nerve. The numerous Schwann's cells are able to remyelinate the sprouting axon. Figure 28-2C shows the regeneration sequence that occurs as the patient shows improvement from a demyelinating neuropathy.

Figure 28-3 is a microscopic enlargement of an axon in the process of becoming myelinated. The Schwann's cells are shown; the growth of myelin in a circular fashion is also illustrated.

Guillain-Barré syndrome, a true postinfection idiopathic polyneuropathic disorder, is a classic example of a demyelinating neuropathy.

Clinical Manifestations

The clinical manifestations of Guillain-Barré are ascending paralysis occurring approximately 21 days after the onset of infection. The paralysis may be preceded by numbness or pain. A "normal" cerebrospinal fluid (CSF) white cell count (one that is approximately 5/cu mm) and an increase in the protein level are present. A white cell or lymphocyte count of up to 10/cu mm is acceptable in Guillain-Barré syndrome. The CSF protein level may not be elevated for one to two weeks after the onset of the weakness. The CSF findings merely support the diagnosis, which is made on clinical grounds. The reversibility of the disease process is a characteristic of the syndrome [16].

Guillain-Barré syndrome may occur at any age, but it has been reported to be most common between the ages of 30 and 50 [17]. It has been reported to occur in early childhood and as late as the ninth decade. Both sexes seem to be affected equally.

Neuritic symptoms usually follow the various in-

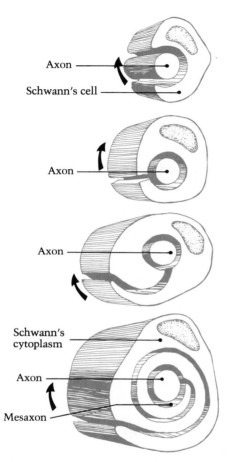

Axon

Schwann's cell

Axon

Axon

Schwann's
cytoplasm

Axon

Mesaxon

Figure 28-3
Microscopic enlargement of an axon undergoing myeliniza-
tion.

fectious processes in 4 to 21 days. The diagnostic
criteria are early polyneuritic symptoms of an ascending symmetric sensory and motor disturbance in
the extremities. Motor deficits are generally more apparent than are sensory deficits.

The sensory disturbances frequently reported by
patients are pain and numbness (paresthesias). Neurological tests may give evidence of a decrease in position sense and vibratory sense.

Muscle weakness, which is the first observable
motor disturbance, develops suddenly. Initially, it involves the lower extremities. It progresses to the
muscles of the trunk and upper extremities and the
muscles supplied by specific cranial nerves. Complete

paralysis may follow according to the extent of the
disease process.

If any cranial nerve involvement is evident, it is
usually paresis of the seventh cranial nerve. The other
cranial nerves that might be involved are, in the order
of frequency, the sixth, third, twelfth, fifth, and ninth
cranial nerves. Since the origins of many of the cranial nerves are in close proximity, several different
nerves may be involved. Cranial nerve dysfunctions
may lead to difficulty in swallowing, talking, and
chewing.

As early as the fourth or fifth day of the illness,
signs of impending respiratory failure may appear. As
the paralysis ascends, the intercostal and phrenic
nerves may become involved, as evidenced by shallow and irregular respirations. The patient may seem
short of breath while he is resting and he may use accessory respiratory muscles.

Neurological tests of reflexes reveal diminished or
absent deep tendon reflexes and the absence of plantar and abdominal reflexes. When muscle mass is palpated, many patients complain of tenderness on deep
pressure or squeezing of the leg or arm muscles.

Except when pneumonitis is present, the patient's
temperature generally remains "normal." However,
the blood pressure may vary considerably from patient to patient [16] and severe hypertensive and
hypotensive crises may occur as a result of autonomic
dysfunction. Also, it is very important to monitor the
patient's pulse since episodes of bradycardia and ECG
changes (e.g., dysrhythmias), leading to cardiac arrest,
have been reported [3]. Those phenomena could also
be due to the hypoxia and hypercapnea [12].

Laboratory Findings

Generally, the results of the laboratory studies, including urinalysis, are within normal limits.

The spinal tap findings are very helpful in confirming the diagnosis of Guillain-Barré syndrome.
The classic phenomenon occurring in the CSF is
known as albuminocytologic dissociation; i.e., the CSF
has an abnormal number of white cells and an increased protein level. In a classic case, the patient's
CSF will have less than 10 white cells/cu mm of fluid
and a protein level greater than 45 mg/100 ml (usually
75–1000 mg/100 ml). But the protein level is not always increased; values below 75 mg/100 ml are often
present [7]. The increase in the protein level may not
appear in the first four or five days, but it almost

always appears during the first one or two weeks. The diagnosis of Guillain-Barré syndrome is made only when the CSF white cell count is normal, with or without an increase in the protein level.

Differential Diagnosis

Other diseases that also have those findings are diphtheritic and diabetic forms of polyneuritis, acute encephalitis, and, in a high percentage of cases, acute poliomyelitis after the second week of infection. However, the symptoms of those diseases point to their diagnosis. Other differential diagnoses are hypokalemic paralysis, botulism, and acute intermittent porphyria.

There is no specific diagnostic test for Guillain-Barré syndrome. The diagnosis is based entirely on the clinical picture, especially the acute onset of paralysis. However, electromyography and tests of nerve conduction velocities may be useful in the diagnosis. Great care must be taken not to label all cases of widespread paralysis and increased CSF protein levels as Guillain-Barré syndrome [7]. Other diseases must be considered carefully and ruled out.

Treatment

If the muscles of respiration become paralyzed, pulmonary support is required. An elective tracheostomy may be performed if the vital capacity falls below 800 to 1000 ml (in some cases, less than 2000 ml) [12], especially if the patient has difficulty in removing secretions from his pharynx and tracheobronchial tree [21]. Maintenance on a positive pressure ventilator may also be necessary. Frequent monitoring of the patient's forced vital capacity and tidal volume is essential.

There is no specific medical therapy. The use of corticosteroids as an anti-inflammatory medication for the treatment of Guillain-Barré syndrome remains controversial. Harrison [21] reports that a therapeutic trial of prednisone (45-60 mg/day) in conjunction with a low-salt diet has in some cases had good results. Precautions must be taken against the development of peptic ulcer of the stomach and duodenum. Prednisone therapy should be discontinued if a definite improvement is not seen in one week. The drug can be tapered off and discontinued. In mild cases, steroids may prolong the time needed for recovery. However,

steroids are indicated in recurrent Guillain-Barré syndrome, which is chronic and relapsing.

The treatment of Guillain-Barré syndrome is basically supportive. Nonnarcotic analgesics may be necessary for limb pain, and hypnotics are useful to ensure sleep. If the patient is agitated, tranquilizers are prescribed. However, the most common cause of agitation in the patient with paralysis is respiratory failure.

If bronchial or pulmonary infections occur, appropriate antibiotic therapy should be instituted. Otherwise, antibiotics are to be avoided [12]. If hypotension develops, the blood pressure must be supported by the use of vasopressor drugs if respiratory failure is not the cause.

Many experimental treatments are still under investigation. They include the use of antimetabolites, such as methotrexate [1], an immunosuppressive drug. There is some controversy about whether the outcome of the methotrexate treatment was due to its administration during the natural remitting phase of the disease [12]. Also, the use of heparin was accompanied by a serendipitous decrease in the antileukocytic factor.

Complications

Respiratory paralysis and the resultant inadequate respiratory ventilation were reported to have occurred in about 25 percent of hospitalized patients [11]. Since respiratory embarrassment occurs rapidly, frequent monitoring of vital capacity and tidal volume is essential. Other pulmonary complications are pulmonary embolism, atelectasis, and pneumonia.

Other complications that have been observed are thrombophlebitis, ileus, gastric dilatation, gastrointestinal bleeding, septicemia, and septic shock. Standard methods of therapies may overcome many of those complications.

The complication of fatigue and depression must never be underestimated.

Prognosis

The symptoms of Guillain-Barré syndrome usually reach their peak within a week of onset, but sometimes they intensify for three weeks or more. The syndrome is self-limited, and the paralysis is potentially completely reversible.

The average hospital stay is 75 days. Seventy-five percent of patients have no residual neurological deficit [12]. Rosenberg [12] states that 20 percent have a minor neurological impairment and 5 percent have a significant neurological impairment. The best predictor of recovery is the interval between the time of greatest weakness and the time the patient begins to improve. An interval of more than 18 days indicates that the recovery will be incomplete.

With meticulous respiratory care and excellent critical care nursing for the patient's ventilatory difficulties and other complications, mortality is 2 to 5 percent [12]. The maintenance of adequate ventilation and cerebral circulation is of primary importance in keeping the mortality low. If death occurs, most commonly it does so within three weeks of the onset [7]. The absolute rate of recovery is variable. It may be quite rapid, with complete recovery occurring in days or weeks.

Generally, recovery takes months. It is often 80 percent complete within six months of onset. If nerves have degenerated, regeneration may require 6 to 18 months [21]. Residual problems that may be observed are weakness of the facial muscles or weakness and atrophy of the muscles of the extremities.

Nursing Orders

OBJECTIVE NO. 1

The patient will demonstrate a patent airway, adequate ventilation, and circulation.

To achieve the objective, the nurse should:

1. Assess the patient's airway.
2. Monitor and assess the patient's vital signs every 15 to 30 minutes until they are stable and then every hour while the patient is in the critical care unit, especially during the acute phase of the illness.
3. Draw arterial blood gas samples as ordered, evaluate the results, and record and report on them.
4. Perform spirometric techniques to measure vital capacities as ordered.
5. Critically assess the motor-sensory levels every 30 to 60 minutes; evaluate, record, and report on them; and fill out the flow sheet (Table 28-1).
6. Assess any increase or decrease in respiratory functioning by inspecting, palpating, and auscultating the patient every hour.
7. Help to perform intubation or tracheotomy as needed in a respiratory crisis.

Table 28-1

Sample Flow Sheet for Guillain-Barré Syndrome

Date	Time	Motor Findings	Sensory Findings	Temperature	Pulse	Respiration	Psychological Assessment	Other (e.g., physical and occupational therapy, intake and output)

8. Assess patient to see that his ventilatory assistance is adequate.
9. Meticulously care for the tracheostomy (i.e., change the dressing each shift or as required and suction every hour, using sterile technique).
10. Monitor the volume-cycled ventilator closely.
11. Administer pulmonary hygiene care (suction as required, turn the patient every two hours, perform postural drainage and clapping four times a day).
12. Assess the patient for readiness for extubation and assist in extubation as ordered.

OBJECTIVE NO. 2

The patient will demonstrate a return of neurological functioning and a maintenance of cerebral circulation.

To achieve the objective, the nurse should:

1. Assess the patient's neurological status each time she visits him and record and report on the serial findings.
2. Administer corticosteroids as ordered; be aware of the possible complications:
   a. Gastric irritation and hemorrhage
   b. Insomnia
   c. Irritability
   d. Hypokalemia
   e. Hypertension
   f. Edema

As mentioned, steroids are generally given in recurrent Guillain-Barré syndrome.

OBJECTIVE NO. 3

The patient will demonstrate an awareness of the disease process.

To achieve the objective, the nurse should:

1. Develop rapport with the patient by visiting him at predetermined times.
2. Using easily understood terms, discuss the progression of the disease and concurrent therapies with the patient and his family.
3. Allow the patient and his family to ask questions about the disease.
4. Discuss the ICU routine and any hemodynamic techniques being used.
5. Discuss with the patient and his family the reasons for his long stay in the ICU and in the hospital.
6. Discuss the rehabilitation programs he can embark on after his discharge.

OBJECTIVE NO. 4

The patient will demonstrate no complications from the use of hemodynamic techniques.

To achieve the objective, the nurse should:

1. Understand and explain the importance of cardiac monitoring to the patient and the other staff members.
2. Understand ventilatory and cardiac alarm systems and maintain their functioning.
3. Interpret, record, and report ECG tracings each shift and observe the monitor continuously for signs of dysrhythmias that need immediate intervention.
4. Be aware that some dysrhythmias may occur during suctioning.
5. Change the ECG lead probes each shift or whenever they become dislodged (see Chap. 10).
6. Understand the rationale for the use of transvenous demand pacemakers (their insertion, care, settings, and possible complications of their use—embolism and infection) (see Chap. 18).

OBJECTIVE NO. 5

The patient will demonstrate no development of complications due to immobility.

To achieve the objective, the nurse should:

1. Turn the patient every two hours or more frequently if he requests it.
2. Do not allow his bed linen to be wrinkled or wet.
3. Bathe him completely once each day; perform perineal care more frequently.
4. Give the patient a vigorous back massage each time he is turned and apply lotion to the pressure points.
5. Keep the bedrails up at all times when the patient is unattended.
6. As ordered, put antiembolic hose on the patient to promote venous return and thus prevent stasis and subsequent thromboembolism.
7. See that he is given intermittent positive pressure breathing treatments daily by the respiratory therapist or critical care nursing staff as ordered.

8. Encourage him to cough and deep breathe every one or two hours.

OBJECTIVE NO. 6

The patient will demonstrate the return of strength, coordination, and muscle tone throughout his recovery.

To achieve the objective, the nurse should:

1. Visit the patient often; he may not be strong enough to use the call bell.
2. Make sure that she and the other staff members encourage the patient to exercise the muscles that are recovering.
3. To prevent contracture, make sure that passive range-of-motion exercises involving all joints are performed every four hours.
4. Make sure that mild resistant exercises follow passive range-of-motion exercises as ordered by the physician.
5. Request physical and occupational therapy consultations for the patient as ordered.
6. Make sure that a footboard is used throughout the acute phase.
7. Be alert to the signs and symptoms of returning motor function, (e.g., sensations of itching).

OBJECTIVE NO. 7

The patient will have no adverse effects from possible complications.

To achieve the objective, the nurse should:

1. Make sure that eye care, including the use of methylcellulose drops, is given every four hours as ordered.
2. Make sure that complete bed baths and detailed skin care are given.
3. Assess the patient for signs and symptoms of complications (e.g., ileus) and record and report on the findings.
4. Assess the patient's urinary output and change the catheter every 24 to 48 hours (or whenever necessary or as ordered). A closed drainage system should be maintained, and specimens should be obtained as ordered.
5. Observe the patient's intravenous catheters for signs of infiltration or irritation and change the catheters every 24 hours.
6. Assess the patient for signs of autonomic nervous system dysfunction (e.g., tachycardia, fluctuations in blood pressure, vasomotor flushes, attacks of sweating, and bronchial and salivary hypersecretion) and record and report on them.

OBJECTIVE NO. 8

The patient will demonstrate good bowel and bladder functioning.

To achieve the objective, the nurse should:

1. Assess the patient's bladder functioning daily. The nurse should:
   a. Change the catheter and maintain a closed drainage system as ordered.
   b. Irrigate the catheter as necessary or as ordered.
   c. Obtain urine specimens for laboratory studies as ordered.
   d. Assess the color, odor, and amount of urine and investigate any complaints of urinary tract discomfort.
   e. Maintain the patient's fluid intake as ordered (i.e., by intravenous, oral, or tube feedings).
   f. Record and report on the patient's fluid intake and output.
2. Assess his bowel functioning daily. The nurse should:
   a. Administer cathartics (stool softeners) as ordered.
   b. Administer enemas as ordered (Fleet enemas if the cathartics do not produce a bowel movement every other day).
   c. Record and report on the findings accurately.

OBJECTIVE NO. 9

The patient will demonstrate nutritional and electrolyte balance.

To achieve the objective, the nurse should:

1. Encourage the patient to take at least 2000 ml of fluid every day by offering him 200 ml every two hours (if he is able to take fluids by mouth).
2. Maintain his intravenous therapy as needed.
3. Perform oral hygiene care, including brushing his teeth, rinsing his mouth, or cleansing his mouth with lemon-glycerin swabs at least once each shift or at the patient's request.
4. Maintain the patency and placement of his nasogastric tube and irrigate the tube as necessary.
5. Administer tube feedings at a slow rate.

6. Assess him for abdominal distention and bowel sounds at least once each shift—more often if needed.
7. Obtain and assess a blood sample for any electrolyte imbalance and record and report on the results.
8. Record and report on his fluid intake and output.

OBJECTIVE NO. 10

The patient will demonstrate adequate coping.
  To achieve the objective, the nurse should:

1. Be supportive in all her contacts with the patient and his family.
2. Allow the patient to be dependent in the acute stage of his illness but encourage him to look forward to being independent and achieving the highest level of functioning.
3. Allow the patient to verbalize his anger and depression and his feelings about being dependent.
4. Perform the activities of daily living willingly and unhurriedly and thus reassure the patient that he is not a burden.
5. Allow the patient to demonstrate his increasing ability to perform the activities of daily living.
6. Begin an occupational therapy program as early as possible.
7. Allow the patient to ask for help when he needs it.
8. Allow the patient as much rest and sleep as needed to prevent ICU psychosis.
9. Teach the patient a way to communicate while he is intubated (e.g., by blinking his eyes to indicate yes and no).
10. Plan the discharge teaching sessions with patient and his family at which the patient's follow-up rehabilitation care will be discussed.

Summary

The Guillain-Barré syndrome is manifested strikingly—by an ascending quadriplegia and weakness of the intercostal muscles, the muscles of swallowing, and the facial muscles. Although ascending quadriplegia is typical, an atypical quadriplegia may also occur (e.g., one giving rise to a descending pattern of weakness). Ascending quadriplegia begins with weakness and progresses to a flaccid paralysis of the lower extremities upward to the upper extremities. It is also characterized by diffuse areflexia.

The patient may require ventilatory support. If he has respiratory failure, he needs a tracheotomy and mechanical ventilation. Pneumonia is a major complication of respiratory problems.

The immediate treatment is to alleviate symptoms and to provide emotional support for the patient and his family. After the initial phase of the illness, the attempts to restore muscular strength and coordination are continued, as is a program of physical and occupational therapy. The patient and his family must be constantly aware of the disease process.

The patient's initial dependence must be linked to the long-range goal of achieving independence in regard to the activities of daily living. The patient must always be made to feel worthwhile. Thus it is important to begin the process of rehabilitation from the day of his admission. The patient must always be treated as a physical, psychological, and spiritual being.

Study Problems

1. Guillain-Barré syndrome is a disease of
   a. Cranial nerves.
   b. Sensory nerves.
   c. Peripheral nerves.
   d. All the above.
   e. None of the above.
2. What is the cause of Guillain-Barré syndrome?
3. The major complication of Guillain-Barré syndrome is urinary tract infection.
   a. True.
   b. False
4. The onset of neuritic symptoms may follow
   a. Swine flu immunization.
   b. Gastrointestinal tract infection.
   c. Herpes simplex infection.
   d. None of the above.
   e. All the above.
5. Guillain-Barré syndrome is reversible.
   a. True.
   b. False.

Answers

1. d.
2. Essentially unknown (idiopathic).
3. b.
4. e.
5. a.

References

1. Asbury, A. K., Arnason, B. G., and Adams, R. D. The inflammatory lesion in idiopathic polyneuritis. *Medicine* 48:173, 1969.
2. Bickerstaff, E. *Neurology* (3rd ed.). London: Hodder and Stroughton, 1978.
3. Emmons, P., Blume, W. E., and DuShane, J. W. Cardiac monitoring and demand pacemaker in Guillain-Barré syndrome. *Arch. Neurol.* 32:59, 1975.
4. Glenn, J. D., and Karels, Sister R. G. Pediatric paralysis in Bogota. *Am. J. Nurs.* 73:299, 1973.
5. Guyton, A. *Textbook of Medical Physiology* (5th ed.). Philadelphia: Saunders, 1979.
6. Marshall, J. The Landry-Guillain-Barré syndrome. *Brain* 86:55, 1963.
7. Merritt, H. H. *A Textbook of Neurology* (6th ed.). Philadelphia: Lea & Febiger, 1979.
8. Olivarius, B. D., and Buhl, M. Herpes simplex virus and Guillain-Barré polyradiculitis. *Br. Med. J.* 1:192, 1975.
9. Osler, L. D., and Sidel, A. D. The Guillain-Barré syndrome. *N. Engl. J. Med.* 262:964, 1960.
10. Polk, B. V. Cardiopulmonary complications of Guillain-Barré syndrome. *Heart Lung* 5:967, 1976.
11. Rosenberg, R. N. Idiopathic Acute Polyradiculoneuritis. Neurology-Neurosurgery Combined Conference. Parkland Memorial Hospital, Dallas, January 8, 1975.
12. Rosenberg, R. N. Idiopathic Acute Polyradiculoneuritis. Department of Internal Medicine Grand Rounds. Parkland Memorial Hospital, Dallas, May 29, 1975.
13. Schaumberg, H. H. Diagnosis, prognoses and treatment of peripheral neuropathies. *Resident Staff Phys.* 18:53, 1972.
14. Shermata, W., Colby, S., Lusky, G., et al. Peripheral nervous antigens in the Guillain-Barré syndrome. *Neurology* 25:833, 1975.
15. Smith, W. R., and Wilson, A. F. Guillain-Barré syndrome in heroin addiction. *J.A.M.A.* 231:1367, 1975.
16. Sodaro, E., and Perlick, Sister N. Guillain-Barré: The syndrome, patient care and some case findings. *J. Neurosurg. Nurs.* 6:97, 1975.
17. Tweed, G. G. Guillain-Barré syndrome. *Am. J. Nurs.* 66:2222, 1966.
18. Vonk, H. Guillain-Barré syndrome—what to tell your patients. *Nurs. '74* 4:27, 1974.
19. Wehr, K. L., and Masferrer, R. Respiratory care in neuromuscular disease. *Respir. Care* 17:324, 1972.
20. Whitehouse, A. C., and Petty, T. L. Recovery in Landry-Guillain-Barré syndrome after prolonged respiratory support. *Lancet* 1:1029, 1969.
21. Wintrobe, M. W., Thorn, G. W., Adams, R. D., et al. *Harrison's Principles of Internal Medicine* (8th ed.). New York: McGraw-Hill, 1977.

Ruptured Intracranial Aneurysm

Carol Lipin Speyerer

Intracranial aneurysms account for 51 percent of all subarachnoid hemorrhage. Those aneurysms usually occur in persons 50 to 54 years of age. However, the incidence of initial subarachnoid hemorrhage is also high in persons 40 years of age and younger. The possible modes of treatment are conservative medical management and surgical intervention. The decision about treatment is made on the basis of the risk factors each method holds for the individual patient.

Objective

In regard to a patient who shows signs of a subarachnoid hemorrhage due to the rupture of an intracranial aneurysm, the nurse should be able to monitor the patient for signs of increased intracranial pressure, observe him for signs of further hemorrhage or rupture, and facilitate his preoperative and postoperative nursing management.

Achieving the Objective

To achieve the objective, the nurse should be able to:

1. Perform a systematic assessment of the patient's neurological status.

29

2. Describe the anatomy and physiology of the cerebrovascular system.
3. Describe the different signs and symptoms of stroke.
4. Describe the major motor, sensory, and perceptual deficits of stroke.
5. Differentiate between aphasia, dysarthria, and apraxia.
6. List the signs of aneurysmal rebleeding.
7. Discuss the methods of managing a ruptured intracranial aneurysm.
8. Define the nursing care objectives for a patient with a ruptured intracranial aneurysm.

How to Proceed

To develop an approach to ruptured intracranial aneurysm, the nurse should:

1. Read the case study and the physical assessment that follow.
2. Formulate a problem list for the patient.
3. Review the other information in this chapter about ruptured intracranial aneurysm.
4. Write an initial plan of care using patient care objectives.
5. Plan a staff conference to discuss the major problems to be anticipated in a patient with a ruptured intracranial aneurysm.

Case Study
Mrs. B. C., a 58-year-old housewife, was admitted to a community hospital with complaints of severe headache and unspecified "blackout spells." On Mrs. C.'s admission to the emergency room, her blood pressure was 160/90, she was confused in regard to place and person, and she complained of a severe frontal headache and a stiff neck. She had been brought to the hospital by her daughter, who confirmed the existence of those symptoms over the past two days. Mrs. C.'s husband, who was away on a business trip, was expected home that same evening.

The patient profile described Mrs. C. as a somewhat obese (5'7", 170-lb) woman with a past medical history that included a hiatal hernia that had been treated medically during the past year. Mrs. C. was a cigarette smoker; she had a total of 35 pack years. She drank alcohol occasionally. She had no known drug allergies, but she took diazepam (5 mg three times a day) for "nervousness" and esophageal reflux. She had a family history of heart disease and arthritis. She had no known history of hypertension.

Mrs. C.'s physical examination showed that she had a right hemiparesis with confusion progressing to obtundation. Mrs. C.'s daughter gave her consent to two diagnostic tests, a lumbar puncture and arteriograms of the carotid arteries. The results were as follows:

1. The lumbar puncture showed an opening pressure of 280 mm H_2O and xanthochromic cerebrospinal fluid with a protein level of 144 mg per 100 ml.
2. The bilateral carotid arteriograms showed a large aneurysm of the left internal carotid artery just distal to the posterior communicating artery and proximal to the bifurcation into the anterior and middle cerebral arteries.

Mrs. C. underwent surgery two days after admission. Under general anesthesia, a left frontal craniotomy was performed with ligation of the aneurysm of the left internal carotid artery. There was evidence at surgery of the subarachnoid hemorrhage and extension of the hemorrhage into the inferior medial temporal lobe. A 3-cm intracranial hematoma was evacuated (see assessment sheet).

Clinical Presentation of the Case Study
After surgery, Mrs. C. was kept in the intensive care unit for several days. Her right hemiparesis had progressed to a right-sided hemiplegia, and she had aphasia. Her level of consciousness gradually improved. Mrs. C. was able to carry out some simple directions but she remained aphasic. Her speech disorder was Wernicke's or expressive aphasia. She had fluent, spontaneous speech but poor comprehension, she spoke repetitively, and her ability to name things was impaired. Unlike the prognosis of hemiparesis, which can be made within a few weeks of its onset, the outcome of aphasia may not be predictable for two or three months.

Reflections

Communicating with the patient with expressive aphasia is a special challenge for the critical care nurse. When language, the ordinary means of communication, is no longer available to the patient, the nurse is tempted to regard communication with him as difficult, if not impossible. A person who cannot speak is often disregarded. Nurses may regard the patient with expressive aphasia in a negative, prejudiced way. That negative attitude often reflects the nurse's own feelings of inadequacy about nonverbal communication.

But language is not the only form of communication. Just as the blind patient may develop an acute sense of hearing and touch, the patient with expressive aphasia learns alternative methods of communication. But the development of those alternative methods is not automatic. It requires encouragement, stimulation, and understanding from the nurses involved with the patient's care.

In this instance, "care" is more akin to "caring." Body-mind-spirit concepts foster the attitude of caring. The patient with expressive aphasia is seen as more than a body with a malfunctioning speech center in his cerebral cortex. He is seen as an indivisible whole. The nurse who is able to view the patient in such a way can easily grasp what caring for him is all about. The nurse who is unable to view the patient as a whole is unable to communicate with him, because she regards the aphasic patient as a mere object and as unrelated to her. But the patient is a whole; and he and the nurse comprise a whole. If the nurse feels her relatedness to the aphasic patient, she knows that she can learn to communicate with him. She sees that alternate forms of communication are unifying acts. They are nonverbal extensions of herself. They are such simple acts as touching, making eye contact, posturing, gesturing, using a certain tone of voice, and otherwise expressing caring, which is the essence of nursing. Those nonverbal communications can have enormous meaning for the patient. Also they remind the nurse that in the nurse-patient relationship there is never a neutral event. Every event has meaning, and that meaning can be conveyed to the aphasic patient.

Interpretation

The case study is that of a person with a subarachnoid hemorrhage due to a ruptured intracranial aneurysm. Because the medical, surgical, and nursing management of strokes is complex, the discussion that follows covers the following topics: the classification of strokes in general, the symptoms of various types of lesions (grouped according to their location), the common signs of stroke, and the formation, detection, and management of aneurysms.

Cerebral Circulation

The nurse bases the assessment and management of the patient with a stroke on her knowledge of cerebral circulation. The clinical symptoms and signs of a stroke depend on the location of the infarct (and the surrounding edema), the arterial blood supply and its potential for collateralization, and other factors, such as blood pressure.

Two major arterial systems supply blood to the brain: the carotid system (the anterior circulation)

and the vertebrobasilar system (the posterior circulation) (Fig. 29-1). The internal carotid artery arises from the common carotid artery at the level of the thyroid cartilage, running upward to the neck to the base of the skull before it branches. After branching into the ophthalmic, posterior communicating, and anterior choroidal arteries, the internal carotid artery bifurcates into the anterior and middle cerebral arteries (Fig. 29-2). The anterior cerebral artery supplies the medial aspect of the anterior two-thirds of each cerebral hemisphere. The middle cerebral artery supplies the greater portion of the convexity of the cerebral hemisphere (Fig. 29-3). It is the largest branch of the internal carotid artery, and it lies deep within the fissure of Sylvius [15].

The vertebral artery, a branch of the subclavian artery, ascends through the foramina of the transverse processes of the upper six cervical vertebrae, winds behind the articular process of the atlas, and enters the skull through the foramen magnum (Fig. 29-1). It continues forward on the anterior surface of the medulla oblongata, uniting with the corresponding vessel on the opposite side at the lower border of the pons to become the basilar artery. The cranial branches of the vertebrobasilar artery are the posteroinferior cerebellar, the anteroinferior cerebellar, the superior cerebellar, the pontine rami, and the posterior cerebral arteries (see Fig. 29-2). The posterior cerebral artery supplies the posterior pole and the medial portion (posterior third) of the cerebral hemisphere and the inferior portion of the temporal lobe. The posteroinferior cerebellar artery supplies the posteroinferior portion of the cerebellum and the lateral portion of the medulla (Fig. 29-3) [22].

Each internal carotid artery supplies the ipsilateral cerebral hemisphere, whereas the basilar artery carries blood to structures within the posterior fossa as well as to the occipital lobe. The union between the branches of the internal carotid and basilar arteries forms the circle of Willis, which is of vital importance in providing collateral circulation to the brain when certain of the major vessels are occluded.

Classification of Stroke

The acute onset of stroke (apoplexy) is usually associated with disease of the intracranial vascular network or with trauma. Cerebral vascular lesions are the most common causes of a generalized or focal disturbance of brain function. The spontaneous stroke may

Critical Care Nursing Admission Assessment
Major Systems Approach

PATIENT'S NAME: _Mrs. B.C._ DATE: _9-15_ TIME: _10 °° a.m._

DIAGNOSIS: _Ⓛ internal carotid artery aneurysm_ T: _98⁶_ A.P.: _88_ R.P.: _88_ R.: _24_

B.P.: _160/90_ E.C.G. RHYTHM: _normal sinus rhythm_ ECTOPY: _—_ WT: _170_ HT: _5'7"_

ADMITTED VIA: _emergency room_ INFORMANT: _patient + her daughter_ LAST MEAL: _coffee 4 hrs. ago_

I. CHIEF COMPLAINT: _severe left frontal headache, stiff neck_

II. PATIENT PROFILE:
1. Age _58_ 2. Sex _female_
3. Marital Status Ⓜ W D S
4. Race _white_ 5. Religion _Protestant_
6. Occupation _housewife_
7. Availability of Family _daughter present, husband on a business trip_
8. Dietary _deferred_
9. Sleeping _deferred_
10. Activities of Daily Living _dependent due to present illness_

III. HISTORY OF PRESENT ILLNESS: _presenting symptoms over past two days_

IV. PAST MEDICAL HISTORY:
1. Pediatric & Adult Illnesses ⎫
2. Cardiac
3. Hypertension
4. Respiratory ⎬ _negative_
5. Diabetes Mellitus
6. Renal
7. Jaundice
8. Infections ⎭
9. Other _hiatal hernia_
10. Hospitalizations & Surgeries _none_

11. Current Medication _Valium 5mg. p.o. t.i.d._

12. Allergies _none_

13. Habits _cigarettes 35 pack years, occasional alcohol ingestion_

V. FAMILY HISTORY: _heart disease, arthritis, + diabetes_

VI. PSYCHOSOCIAL:
1. Behavior During Assessment _mentally confused to place + person_

2. Specific Problems _history of emotional upsets - treated c̄ Valium_

VII. PHYSICAL EXAMINATION:
1 General _pale obese middle-aged woman, lethargic in response to verbal +/or noxious stimuli_

2. Respiratory System
Airway _patent_
Inspection _normal expansion all lobes_
Rate _24_
Rhythm _regular_
Chest Wall _full excursion_

Palpation _deferred_

Percussion _deferred_

610

Auscultation
Voice Sounds _____
Breath Sounds ____*normal*_____
Normal ✓ Increased_____ Decreased _____
Adventitious Sounds ___*neg.*_____
_____
_____

3. Cardiovascular System
A.P. __*88*__ R.P. __*88*__
B.P. Supine R _*160/90*_ L _____
P.M.I. __*5th ICS at MCL*__
Heart Sounds ___*normal*_____
_____
Thrills ____*none*_____
Peripheral Pulses ___*present*_____

4. Neurological System
Level of Consciousness __*obtunded*___
_____
Respiratory Pattern __*regular*_____
_____
Cranial Nerves __*intact*_____
_____
_____
_____
Eyes _____
(1) Pupils   OD   OS
    Size ____*5 cm*____*.5cm*_____
    Shape ____*round*_____
    Light _*equal + brisk response*_
    Consensual _____*present*_____
    Accommodation _*unable to assess*_
(2) Ocular Movements *no nystagmus*
_____
Motor ___*right hemiparesis*_____
_____
Sensory ___*difficult to assess*_____
Coordination _*finger to nose normal*_
    on left
Reflexes _*decreased on the right*_

5. Gastrointestinal System
Nose & Mouth ___*negative*_____
_____
Stomach_____
_____
Abdomen ____*soft, nontender*_____
_____
Bowel Sounds ___*present*_____
Liver ____*not palpable*_____
Spleen ___*not palpable*_____

6. Renal & Genitourinary Systems
I. _____ O. *catheterized for 350ml.*
Urinary Bladder & Urethra _____
Foley catheter inserted
Kidneys __*not palpable*_____

7. Musculoskeletal System
Spine ____*straight*_____
Extremities *warm c̄ good bilateral*
pulses
Sacral Edema _____*none*_____
Masses _____*none*_____

8. Hematologic System
Petechiae _____*none*_____
Ecchymosis ___*none*_____
Gingiva_____*normal*_____

9. Endocrine System
Breath _____*neg.*_____
Skin _____*neg.*_____

VIII. LABORATORY:
1. Hematology
HGB ____*14.2*____ HCT ___*39*___
W.B.C. __*8,500*__
2. Chemistry
Na ___*143*___ K __*3.6*__
CO_2 __*23*__ CL __*104*__
Blood Sugar __*128*__ Amylase _*90*_
BUN____*15*____ Cr _*1.3*_
3. Urinalysis _____ *normal*
4. Electrocardiogram
Rate _*88*_ Rhythm _*regular*_
P-R *0.2 sec.* QRS *.12 sec* *0.11*
Interpretation __*NSR*__
5. Chest x-ray__*normal*_____
_____

IX. PROBLEM LIST:

ACTIVE	~~INACTIVE~~
1. *subarachnoid*	8. *variation in*
hemorrhage → ⓛ	*functional performance*
internal carotid artery	*c̄ total self-care*
aneurysm → ligation	*deficit*
2. *smoker - 35 pack yrs*	9. *impaired mobility*
3. *rt hemiplegia 2° to #1*	
4. *aphasia 2° to #1*	
5. *Hx. of hiatal hernia*	
6. *Hx. of emotional upsets*	
7. *altered level of consciousness*	

NURSE'S SIGNATURE
Carol Lipin Speyerer, R.N.

611

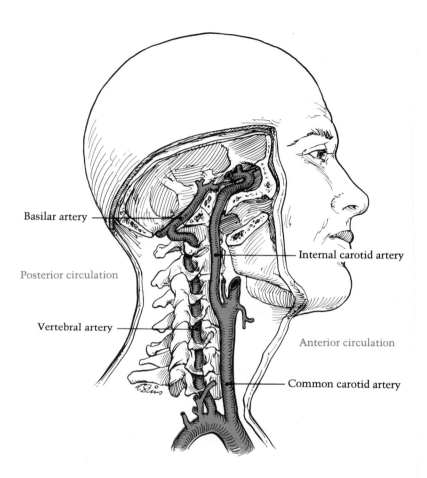

Basilar artery

Posterior circulation

Vertebral artery

Internal carotid artery

Anterior circulation

Common carotid artery

be classified according to cause as those due to (1) cerebral thrombosis, (2) cerebral embolism, (3) intracerebral hemorrhage, (4) subarachnoid hemorrhage, and (5) vascular malformation [5].

Figure 29-1
Major arterial supply to the brain.

Cerebral Thrombosis

A stroke (cerebrovascular insult) due to cerebral thrombosis can often be attributed to arteriosclerosis. Clotting occurs at a site where blood flow is impeded by a sclerotic plaque on the vessel wall. The area supplied by the occluded cerebral artery becomes ischemic and infarcted, with subsequent congestion and edema. As the edema subsides, the ischemic brain tissue becomes necrotic, is liquefied and removed by macrophages, and is replaced by a glial and vascular scar. Small multilocular cysts filled with clear fluid form in the affected area [14].

The symptoms of stroke caused by cerebral thrombosis progress over minutes to hours. Prodromal signs of dizziness, aphasia, or other focal neurological signs may occur with rapid improvement between episodes (so-called transient ischemic attacks—TIAs). Besides arteriosclerosis, hypertension may be an underlying cause of the thrombosis [14].

Cerebral Embolism

Cerebral embolism is manifested abruptly, without prodromal signs, owing to the sudden occlusion of a cerebral vessel by material arising elsewhere in the cardiovascular system. The heart is the usual source

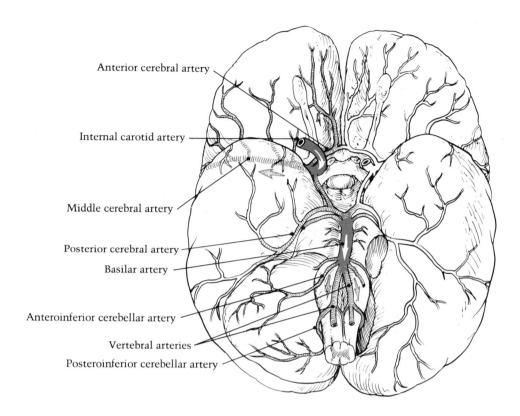

Anterior cerebral artery

Internal carotid artery

Middle cerebral artery

Posterior cerebral artery

Basilar artery

Anteroinferior cerebellar artery

Vertebral arteries

Posteroinferior cerebellar artery

Figure 29-2
Bifurcation of the internal carotid artery and the vertebrobasilar artery.

of embolization; other sources are blood clots,
tumors, bacteria, air from the lungs, and fat embolism
from a long bone fracture. The area of brain tissue
supplied by the occluded vessel becomes infarcted;
the infarction is resolved much as a thrombotic infarct is resolved [14].

Intracerebral Hemorrhage

Like a thromboembolic stroke, intracerebral hemorrhage is characterized by a severe headache, which
may progress rapidly to coma. How diseased vessels
rupture is not clearly understood. Hemorrhages may
be of arterial or venous origin; more usually they are
of arterial origin. Hypertension is a common precipitating factor in intracerebral hemorrhage. The
vessel (or vessels) involved becomes stretched and

displaced, and the resultant changes in the caliber and
tension of the vessel cause the rupture. The blood
clot that forms destroys and displaces the adjacent
brain tissue. If the hemorrhage is large, the site of the
ruptured vessel may not be apparent [14].

Blood and necrotic brain tissue are removed by
macrophages and are replaced by glia and new blood
vessels, thus producing a fluid-filled area. The basal
ganglia—internal capsular area is a common site of
intracerebral hemorrhage, which may rupture into
the lateral ventricles, where blood spreads throughout
the ventricular system and into the subarachnoid
space and base of the brain (Fig. 29-4).

Subarachnoid Hemorrhage

The most frequent cause of subarachnoid hemorrhage
in the adult is the rupture of a congenital or a saccular
aneurysm in a large artery of the circle of Willis (Fig.
29-5). Such an aneurysm is likely to form at an area of
bifurcation owing to either a congenital absence of
the media or a degeneration of the internal elastic

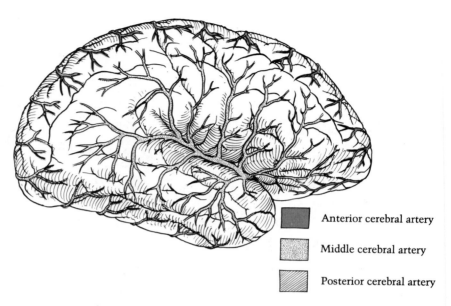

Anterior cerebral artery

Middle cerebral artery

Posterior cerebral artery

Figure 29-3
Vascular distribution to the cerebrum.

lamina that had contributed to the strength of the cerebral arterial wall. Although arteriosclerosis may destroy the elastic lamina, the plaques are not as common in aneurysms as are the irregular fibromuscular scars that form as a result of degeneration of musculoelastic pads. Further splitting of the elastica of the musculoelastic pads occurs with age and with the hemodynamic stresses from turbulent flow within the aneurysmal sac and increasing blood pressure [8].

Bleeding into the subarachnoid space is characterized by the sudden onset of a severe headache that is related to activity and by a brief interruption in consciousness. Focal neurological signs are frequently absent. Nuchal rigidity and preretinal hemorrhage may be present.

Vascular Malformation

Vascular malformation accounts for many of the sudden strokes seen in the younger patient. A history of repeated subarachnoid hemorrhages and seizures may be elicited (Fig. 29-6).

Comparison of Lesions

The focal signs of stroke are specifically associated with the occlusion of particular arteries. The effects of the occlusion vary, depending on collateral circulation, the size and position of the occluded vessel in the vascular network, and the duration and nature of the occlusion.

Occlusion of the common carotid artery and internal carotid artery may be manifested first by transient attacks of hemiplegia and then by persistent hemiparesis. Other manifestations are unilateral loss of vision due to involvement of the ophthalmic artery and, if the dominant hemisphere is affected, aphasia, contralateral sensory disturbance, and hemianopsia [9].

Occlusion of the anterior cerebral artery causes contralateral hemiplegia, particularly of the lower extremity, and mild sensory deficits, mental confusion, and clouded sensorium. Occlusion of the middle cerebral artery, which supplies the greater portion of the convexity of the cerebral hemisphere, is manifested by contralateral (initially flaccid) hemiplegia, hemianesthesia, hemianopsia, and aphasia if the dominant side is involved [9].

Occlusion of the posterior cerebral artery usually causes homonymous hemianopsia. Cerebellar signs, contralateral rigidity, tremors, and choreiform movements are less frequently seen.

Occlusion of the posteroinferior cerebellar artery causes ipsilateral facial analgesia, ipsilateral Horner's

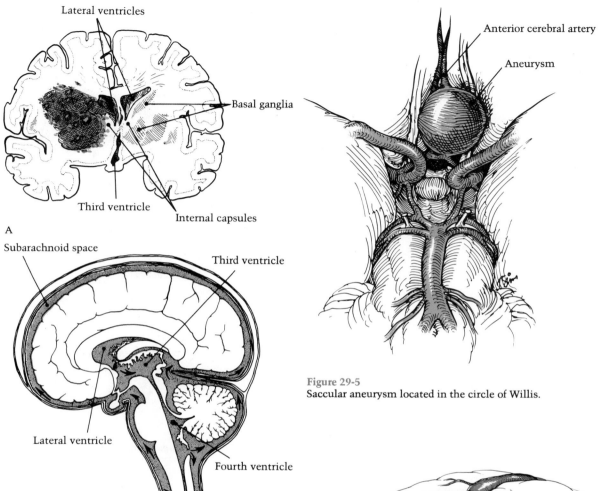

Lateral ventricles

Basal ganglia

Third ventricle

Internal capsules

A

Subarachnoid space

Third ventricle

Lateral ventricle

Fourth ventricle

B

Figure 29-4
A. Coronal section through the cerebrum showing hemorrhage with rupture into the lateral ventricle. B. Ventricular system showing cerebrospinal fluid circulation from the lateral ventricles to the subarachnoid space.

Anterior cerebral artery

Aneurysm

Figure 29-5
Saccular aneurysm located in the circle of Willis.

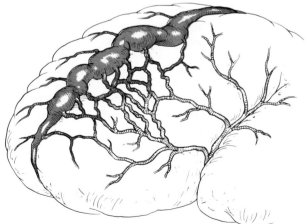

Figure 29-6
Arteriovenous malformation.

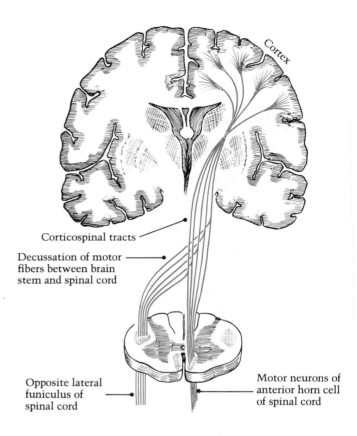

Corticospinal tracts

Decussation of motor
fibers between brain
stem and spinal cord

Opposite lateral
funiculus of
spinal cord

Motor neurons of
anterior horn cell
of spinal cord

Cortex

Figure 29-7
Decussation of the motor pathways to the spinal cord.

syndrome, ipsilateral ataxia, and ipsilateral weakness of the vocal cords and tongue with contralateral analgesia and hemiparesis. Occlusion of the superior cerebellar artery results in ipsilateral ataxia and contralateral hemianalgesia and hemianesthesia [9].

Occlusion of the basilar artery typically causes headache, dizziness, coma, flaccid quadriplegia, areflexia, complete anesthesia, pinpoint pupils, and hyperpyrexia [24]. Some of the more common clinical manifestations of strokes are described in greater detail in the following pages.

Motor Deficits

The pyramidal system consists of tracts connecting the cortical motor area with the motor neurons in the anterior horn cell of the spinal cord (Fig. 29-7). These corticospinal fibers decussate at the border between the brain stem and spinal cord to the opposite lateral funiculus of the spinal cord. Motor neurons that innervate muscles have their origin in the precentral gyrus of the cerebral cortex, where parts of the body (the larynx, tongue, lips, nares, eyelids, brow, neck, thumbs, fingers, wrists, elbows, shoulders, trunk, hips, knees, ankles, and toes) are represented topographically in a size that is proportionate to the amount of cortical area devoted to each (Fig. 29-8).

The pyramidal tract is sensitive to pressure from edema, which may cause paralysis when the motor areas are not affected. In such cases, motor return occurs as edema decreases.

Destructive lesions of the primary motor projection cortex (Brodmann's area 4) result in contralateral paresis or paralysis. The weakness is usually more pronounced in the distal portions of the extremities.

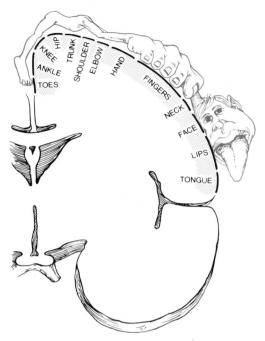

Figure 29-8
Precentral gyrus with localization of motor functions in the cortex.

In the upper extremities, it involves the extensors more than the flexors, and in the lower extremities, it involves the flexors more than the extensors. The trunk muscles are usually spared, but the abdominal muscles may be involved. The high incidence of strokes in the region of the Sylvian fissure and Rolandic area accounts for the predominance of upper extremity and facial involvement. Facial deficits are those of both the upper and lower face. If the lesion is above the brain stem, the face and extremities on the same side are affected. If the lesion is of the brain stem, the face on one side and the extremities of the opposite side are paretic [11].

Initially the motor deficit is diffuse, and some return of function usually occurs within the first month after the stroke. Strength returns first in the flexors of the upper extremity and the extensors of the lower extremity. Those muscles slowest to recover include the gluteus medius, the toe extensors, and the peroneals. Return of motor function may occur within a year.

Muscle tone in stroke is related to the length of time since the onset of the stroke. At first, muscle tone may be decreased (flaccidity). Within 48 hours after the stroke, hyperreflexia, especially on the affected side, and an increased resistance to passive stretch occur. Release of the reflex mechanism from control of the supraspinal inhibitory center accounts for the spasticity in hemiplegia. Spasticity results whenever the level of excitation exceeds the inhibitory capacity. Spasticity is characterized by a rapid increase in resistance to passive movement followed by a sudden loss of resistance (the clasp-knife effect). Typically it involves the flexors of the upper extremities and the extensors of the lower extremities. Spasticity in the lower extremities accounts for the characteristic "hemiplegic posture," in which there is increased tone in the hip and knee extensors and the hip adductors [11].

Sensory and Perceptual Deficits

The primary sensory area is arranged on the postcentral gyrus as a mirror image of the motor area. The cortical sensory deficits include impaired two-point discrimination, graphesthesia, stereognosis (the inability to accurately assess the size, shape, weight, and texture of objects), joint motion, joint position sense, and localization of light touch. The last deficit is demonstrated especially on simultaneous stimulation of both the involved and the uninvolved sides. The pin and temperature sensations seen or perceived at the thalamic level are relatively intact.

Perceptual impairment varies according to what side of the hemisphere the lesion affects. Lesions of the left hemisphere are characterized by alterations in language and perceptions of place and time. Lesions of the right hemisphere may impair spatial orientation and visual perception; they are characterized particularly by constructional apraxia and homonymous hemianopsia.

Cerebral functions (e.g., intelligence, memory, judgment, and abstract thinking) may be impaired. The psychological aspects of management of the stroke patient are increasingly important in view of the emotional disturbances that can accompany a stroke (lability, an altered body image, decreased self-esteem, impulsive behavior, a decreased attention span, depression, fear, anxiety, and hostility) [3].

Communication

Efficient and effective oral communication depends on [7]:

1. The organization of concepts and their symbolic formulation and expression.
2. The externalization of thought in speech through the use of the motor functions of respiration, phonation, resonance, articulation, and prosody.
3. Programming of these motor functions to produce speech sounds and to combine those sounds into words.

Impairment of those processes results in aphasia, dysarthria, or apraxia, respectively.

The term *aphasia* refers to a disturbance of language. Specific factors that should be assessed include fluency of spontaneous speech and conversational speech and abnormalities of comprehension, repetition, naming, reading, and writing.

Spontaneous speech is best evaluated by considering it in regard to its components: rate of output, press of speech, prosody or melody, content, phrase length, and paraphasia (the use of incorrect words). The presence or absence of those components of spontaneous speech will help to determine whether the aphasia is caused by an anterior or a posterior lesion of the dominant cerebral hemisphere (Fig. 29-9).

Lesions of Broca's area, which is located in the posterior portion of the third frontal gyrus just anterior to the face region of the motor strip, are characterized by a decreased rate of output and press of speech. The effort to speak is usually increased, and the content is limited to nouns and verbs. The phrase length is short, and the word usage is correct (telegraphic speech).

Lesions of Wernicke's area, the posterior portion of the superior temporal gyrus, result in an aphasia that has a normal or an increased rate of speech with normal effort. The person tends to ramble and to use extra words and phrases (circumlocutions). Paraphasia, the use of incorrect words, may be verbal (e.g., "The grass is blue"), phonemic (e.g., "I opened the door to the rouse"), or neologistic ("This is my quar" for "This is my mother"). Wernicke's area comprises the mid and posterior temporal lobe, the adjacent inferior parietal lobe, and the adjacent anterior occipital lobe.

Comprehension is intact in the anterior aphasias and impaired in the posterior aphasias. Comprehen-

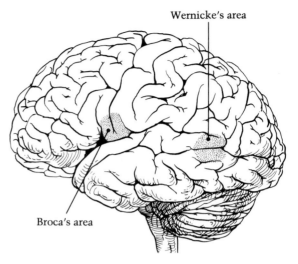

Figure 29-9
Speech centers affected by lesions of the cerebral hemisphere.

sion in the latter type may be intact for short simple commands (e.g., "eat," "walk," and "stand up"). The ability to name is usually impaired in all types of aphasia. Disorders of repetition occur in anterior aphasia because of the lack of fluency and in posterior aphasia because the command is not comprehended.

The term *global aphasia* refers to impairment in all four areas: spontaneous speech, comprehension, naming, and repetition.

Dysarthria and apraxia of speech are motor speech disorders, not language disorders. The term *dysarthria* refers to a group of speech disorders due to neurogenic dysfunction (i.e., impairment of the central or peripheral nervous system). All basic motor processes—respiration, phonation, resonance, articulation, and prosody—are variably involved in dysarthria. The most characteristic error made by the dysarthric person is the imprecise production of consonants, usually in the form of distortions and omissions.

Apraxia and aphasia may occur together. When they do, the person's speaking ability is significantly poorer than his ability to listen, read, or write. His difficulty is not in finding the proper words, but in positioning the speech muscles to produce phonemes and sequencing the muscle movements to produce words. The person may have fluent speech accompanied by stretches of poorly articulated speech. His automatic and reactive speech has fewer errors of articulation than has his volitional purposive speech.

Speech and language difficulties are common when the lesion is located in the dominant hemisphere, where the speech center is located. Handedness and dominance are related in that most right-handed people have a dominant left hemisphere. Left-handed and ambidextrous people have a less clearly differentiated dominance. Three to five percent of people are right-hemisphere dominant. Of those, 11 percent are left handed. Therefore, many left-handed people are left-hemisphere dominant. Representation of speech in one hemisphere is established at the time the brain achieves full weight—around puberty. Until then, lesions in the dominant hemisphere do not cause permanent aphasia, and they may be resolved. Dominance is determined by location of the speech centers rather than by handedness. Since most people are right handed and left-hemisphere dominant, lesions in the left hemisphere typically result in an aphasia.

Intracranial Aneurysms

Prior to rupture, aneurysms may be symptomatic or asymptomatic, depending on their size and location. While it is difficult to establish definite syndromes for aneurysms of the various intracranial arteries, there is sufficient difference in their biological characteristics to suggest the location and often the type of lesion [12].

Almost 50 percent of intracranial aneurysms arise from the internal carotid artery or the middle cerebral artery. Aneurysms of the internal carotid artery can be divided into those above or below the anterior clinoid process and those within the cavernous sinus. An unruptured infraclinoid aneurysm is characterized by visual disturbances as it enlarges and lifts up the optic nerve. The clinical diagnosis of such an aneurysm may often be suspected on the basis of a third nerve palsy (evidenced by ipsilateral dilated pupil and usually intact extraocular movements). Occasionally exophthalmos may be present.

Rupture of an intraclinoid aneurysm into the cavernous sinus produces the clinical picture of carotid cavernous fistula. It is uncommon. Most carotid cavernous fistulas are of traumatic origin, occurring soon after injury. A bruit in the head, often the first manifestation, may be present for weeks before exophthalmos is manifested. Exophthalmos is the cardinal sign of a cavernous carotid fistula. It is usually unilateral, and it occurs in the ipsilateral eye. The next most common sign is pulsation of the globe, often associated with a thrill on palpation of the orbit or the engorged vessels of the forehead. The bruit is heard as a crescendo systolic murmur, and it usually is more prominent over the eyeball and temporal regions. It is usually decreased or abolished by compression of the ipsilateral carotid artery. Involvement of the optic nerve or paresis of extraocular movements completes the syndrome of a carotid cavernous fistula.

A supraclinoid aneurysm is characterized by a headache, usually in the occipital region or behind the orbit. The aneurysm may be present for as long as 15 years before a frank rupture occurs. Failing vision in the form of a scotoma, hemianopsia, or unilateral blindness is commonly seen, as is hemiplegia. The hemiparesis is often associated with some degree of aphasia if the lesion is in the dominant hemisphere.

An aneurysm of the anterior cerebral artery or the anterior communicating artery may involve only one of those vessels, but more commonly it involves both. Focal symptoms are rare, but anosmia and involvement of the optic nerve and chiasm may occur. If circulation to the anterior cerebral artery is impaired, weakness of the contralateral leg or hemiplegia may occur. Seizures may occur. Hemorrhage from rupture of the aneurysm is often the first indication of its presence. Deep unconsciousness supervenes.

An aneurysm of the middle cerebral artery is usually saccular; it discloses its presence either by rupture or by symptoms of an expanding mass lesion. The common symptoms are seizures, contralateral hemiparesis, and aphasia if the circulation to the dominant hemisphere is compromised.

An aneurysm of the posterior communicating artery occurs most often at the junction of that artery with the carotid artery. Therefore, paralysis of the third cranial nerve may be present.

An aneurysm of the basilar and vertebral arteries may be saccular or atherosclerotic in origin. Occipital headache that occurs when the patient changes the position of his head is a symptom. The aneurysm tends to become very large before rupture and to simulate the signs of a tumor by causing intermittent pressure on the contiguous structures. The signs of involvement of the lower brain stem are vertigo, hemianesthesia, hemiparesis or paraparesis, dysphasia, dysarthria, paralysis of one side of the tongue, and respiratory disturbances.

Diagnostic Tests

The most useful diagnostic tests are cerebral angiography and CT scanning. Cerebral angiography may be carried out even before the patient's condition has stabilized or if an intracerebral clot is suspected. CT scanning is a noninvasive procedure and is therefore the more appropriate test for the unstable patient and for location of an intracerebral clot. But it does not show vasospasm nor the aneurysm itself because the blood vessels are minute. The other parts of the work-up are a history taking, a physical examination, a neurological examination, an ECG, a chest x ray, and a lumbar puncture. Radioisotope brain scanning may also be used to rule out a space-occupying lesion [10].

Warning Signs Prior to Rupture

Aneurysms are usually small, and they often have no symptoms until they rupture and produce a subarachnoid hemorrhage. A study undertaken by Okawara [17] analyzed the warning signs in patients with ruptured single aneurysms. Those signs were put in one of three categories on the basis of their presumed causes: (1) signs due to expansion of the aneurysm and the adjacent artery, (2) signs due to minor bleeding, and (3) signs due to a local ischemic lesion caused by vasospasm or occlusion. The most frequent warning signs were generalized headache, then localized headache, lethargy, impairment of extraocular movement, face and eye pain, and neck and back pain.

The average time between warning signs and major hemorrhage in the patients studied was 20.9 days. The study concluded that the survival rate was better for patients with warning signs than for those without warning signs. The incidence of warning signs also varied with the location of the aneurysm; it was highest with aneurysms of the internal carotid–posterior communicating arteries and lowest with aneurysms of the posterior fossa.

The symptoms of minor leakage are general headache, nausea, neck and back pain, lethargy, and photophobia. Minor leakage is usually intermittent and recurrent. Extravasated blood may create some fibrotic adhesions around the aneurysm, which then help prevent further extravasation and hemorrhage.

The patient with warning signs has a better chance to seek early treatment. Therefore, the knowledge of such signs and of their relationship to clinical course is vitally important.

Symptoms of subarachnoid hemorrhage due to ruptured intracranial aneurysm may be divided into two groups, the symptoms of slow or incomplete rupture and the symptoms of complete rupture. The symptoms of slow or incomplete rupture are recurrent retroorbital headaches, recurrent confusion or coma that persists for a few days, mild nuchal rigidity, and occasionally sudden frontal headaches followed by diffuse pain in the lumbar and gluteal regions bilaterally. Complete rupture occurs suddenly and is characterized by excruciating suboccipital pain, vertigo, and nausea. The patient is restless, confused, or comatose, his neck becomes rigid, he has a positive Kernig's sign and a slow pulse, and his spinal fluid is bloody and under increased pressure [2].

Grading Criteria for Intracranial Aneurysm

The grading criteria of Nishioka [16] are often used to categorize the patient with an intracranial aneurysm:

Grade 1. The patient is symptom free and has completely recovered from the effects of the last hemorrhage.

Grade 2. The patient is alert and responsive and complains of headache.

Grade 3. The patient is lethargic and has a headache or stiff neck, or he is alert, having recovered from the effects of the subarachnoid hemorrhage but has a hemispheric neurological deficit of hemiparesis and often dysphasia.

Grade 4. The patient is severely obtunded without a major neurological deficit, or he is lethargic and has a hemispheric deficit of hemiparesis, dysphasia, and mental confusion.

Grade 5. The patient is moribund, comatose, decerebrate, and unresponsive to all stimuli.

Only patients in grades 1 and 2 are ideal candidates for surgical intervention. Grade 3 patients are borderline candidates. One grade should be added for patients with complications (e.g., hypertension, diabetes, severe heart or kidney disease) [1].

Management of Subarachnoid Hemorrhage due to Ruptured Intracranial Aneurysm

In regard to a patient with intracranial aneurysm and recent subarachnoid hemorrhage who comes for diagnosis and treatment, the health team·care has two objectives: (1) helping the patient recover from the effects of the initial hemorrhage, and (2) helping prevent another, perhaps fatal, rupture of the aneurysm. Usually the patient has one hemorrhage; the danger of his having another hemorrhage is greatest between 14 and 21 days after the first hemorrhage occurred. His risk remains high until the sixth week; it returns to that of the normal population at one year [19].

Historically, four methods of treatment have been used, and numerous studies have been done on the efficacy of each method. Subarachnoid hemorrhage due to ruptured intracranial aneurysm was first treated by regulated bed rest (supportive therapy) and later by carotid artery ligation, craniotomy, and hypotension [20].

Bed Rest

Bed rest consists of symptomatic treatment and the avoidance of exertion over a period of about two months. As other methods have been perfected, that method has been used less commonly.

Surgical Management

Ligation of the common carotid artery is done for certain giant aneurysms involving the internal carotid–posterior communicating arteries. It can be done in a single procedure or by progressive occlusion using an adjustable clamp. The purpose of the procedure is to reduce the pressure in the aneurysm. Aneurysmal rebleeding is sometimes provoked by the procedure since surgery does not prevent refilling of the aneurysm by the collateral circulation. The possible operative complications are aphasia, hemiplegia, and generalized brain damage in the early period. Atherosclerosis at a later time may result in occlusion of the contralateral carotid and/or vertebral-basilar system.

Numerous variations of craniotomy have been done (e.g., the wrapping technique, body cooling, and the use of the dissecting microscope). The aneurysm may be ligated, excised, trapped, clipped, crushed, proximally occluded, sprayed with plastic, or thrombosed from electrical stimulation. The treatment of choice generally is clipping the aneurysmal neck or coating it with glue. Aminocaproic acid may be given intravenously to strengthen the aneurysmal seal and delay rebleeding. It works as an antifibrinolytic drug to counteract the natural lytic process that increases the chances of rebleeding one week after the aneurysmal hemorrhage.

In addition to the complications of carotid ligation already discussed, several more may occur: recurrent hemorrhage from iatrogenic aneurysms (those caused by clips applied to vessel walls with subsequent trauma, weakening, and ballooning that result in new aneurysms), intracerebral hematoma, subdural or epidural hematoma, meningoencephalitis, and hydrocephalus.

Hypotensive Therapy

Both carotid artery ligation and craniotomy have as their purpose the prevention of rebleeding. They do not help the patient recover from the initial hemorrhage. Hypotensive therapy was introduced to prevent early recurrent hemorrhages as well as to reduce current hemorrhage by diminishing blood pressure in the region of the circulatory break. The area of the aneurysm is relatively weak and does not require a hypertensive brachial blood pressure to rupture. The blood pressure is therefore reduced whether the patient is hypertensive or normotensive. At a lower blood pressure, there is less turbulence in the aneurysm and thus less vibration of its walls. That condition decreases the chances that the aneurysm would enlarge and rupture. Hypotensive drugs are used primarily to keep the blood pressure above the range of cerebrovascular insufficiency, which is determined by titration. Experimentation with a small number of hypotensive drugs may be needed until favorable results are achieved. If the patient has been taking any hypotensive drugs, the dosage of subsequent hypotensive drugs may be lower.

Nursing Orders

Problem/Diagnosis

Subarachnoid hemorrhage.

OBJECTIVE NO. 1

The patient should be free of the signs of increased intracranial pressure [18].

The nursing management is the same as that for head injury (see Chap. 30). The signs of increased intracranial pressure are likely to appear 24 to 48 hours after the hemorrhage. Since the symptoms of headache and altered levels of consciousness indicate either increased pressure or rebleeding, the differentiation is often made by means of a repeat lumbar puncture.

OBJECTIVE NO. 2

The patient should be free of the signs of further hemorrhage or rupture [13].

To achieve the objective, the nurse should:

1. Observe the patient for the signs of slow or incomplete rupture:
   a. Recurrent retroorbital headache
   b. Recurrent confusion and coma
   c. Mild nuchal rigidity
   d. Sudden frontal headaches followed by diffuse pain in the lumbar and gluteal regions
2. Observe the patient for the signs of complete rupture:
   a. Excruciating suboccipital pain
   b. Vertigo and nausea
   c. Restlessness, confusion, or coma
   d. Rigidity of the neck and positive Kernig's sign
   e. Slow pulse
   f. Cerebrospinal fluid that is bloody and under increased pressure
3. Administer antihypertensives as ordered.

OBJECTIVE NO. 3

The patient should be free of further neurological deficits [21].

To achieve the objective, the nurse should:

1. Observe the patient for seizure activity, a common occurrence with aneurysms of the anterior cerebral and anterior communicating arteries. She should:
   a. Have a plastic or rubber airway, a tongue depressor, and suction equipment at the patient's bedside.

b. If a seizure occurs she should:
   (1) Position the patient to maintain a patent airway and loosen any constricting clothing.
   (2) Note the character, duration, and pattern of the seizure and the patient's degree of strength and motor ability after the seizure, and give the information gathered to the physician.
   (3) Administer anticonvulsants as prescribed and observe their effects.
2. Assess the patient's neurological status hourly. She should record the information and report to the physician the following:
   a. Changes in the patient's mental status and level of consciousness (evidenced by his response to pain, his ability to carry out a command, and his orientation).
   b. Changes in pupillary response, especially a unilaterally enlarged pupil.
   c. Changes in motor function, especially contralateral weakness or hemiplegia. The nurse should:
      (1) Check the patient's hand grasp for strength, equality, and release.
      (2) Check the patient for paresis of the lower extremity (evidenced by the patient's leg being externally rotated in bed and by the leg falling easily when raised).
      (3) Note any weakness in the patient's facial musculature (evidenced by the patient's inability to close an eye completely, the drooping of one corner of his mouth, or drooling from one side of his mouth).
   d. Changes in vital signs, especially an increased blood pressure or a slowing pulse, a fever, or a change in the character of his respirations [6].

OBJECTIVE NO. 4

The patient should be free of postoperative wound infection.

To achieve the objective, the nurse should:

1. Observe the frontal surgical site for signs of swelling, bleeding, or infection and report any signs to physician.
2. Change surgical dressings as needed to maintain asepsis.
3. If continuous gentle suction is used, measure the drainage and make sure that the system is patent.

4. After the sutures are removed, provide a covering (a scarf or cap) for the patient's head.

OBJECTIVE NO. 5

The patient should be free of pulmonary complications.
   To achieve the objective, the nurse should:

1. Maintain a patent airway, using mechanical devices as needed to provide an adequate exchange and a balance of oxygen and carbon dioxide.
2. Rotate the patient's head laterally to help secretions drain and to decrease the possibility of aspiration. It is best to keep the patient's head to the side.
3. Do endotracheal suction as needed.
4. Observe and report signs of hypoxia (restlessness, airway obstruction, and cyanosis).
5. Assess the results of the blood gas studies and notify the physician of any change.
6. Help the patient deep breathe.
7. Examine the patient's extremities for signs of peripheral stasis (cyanosis, edema, and coldness) and report any to the physician.
8. Give the patient mouth care as needed to prevent drying of the secretions, which is uncomfortable for the patient.

OBJECTIVE NO. 6

The patient should be free of pressure areas.
   To achieve the objective, the nurse should:

1. Check the patient's bony prominences (the sacrum, foot, hip, knees, shoulders, elbows, and occiput) for signs of redness.
2. Lightly massage areas that are subjected to pressure.
3. Turn patient every one or two hours on his sides, his back and even his abdomen if he can tolerate the prone position. Positioning on the affected area should be limited to 30 minutes due to sensory loss.

OBJECTIVE NO. 7

The patient should be free of contractural deformities.

To achieve the objective, the nurse should:

1. Place a trochanter roll on the patient's side, from his iliac crest to his knee, to prevent external rotation.
2. Use a footboard. (The patient should be checked often for pressure formation due to the ensuing spasticity.)
3. Place a small pillow between the patient's trunk and right arm (on the hemiplegic side) to prevent adduction.
4. Use a handroll or splint to maintain the patient's involved extremity in a more functional position. If splinting is used, the patient should be watched for pressure areas. The patient should not squeeze a ball in his hand since in the upper arm the flexor muscles inherently override the extensor muscles.
5. Move the patient's joints through full range-of-motion exercises at least twice daily.
6. Maintain firm support under the patient's joints when handling his extremities.
7. Exercise slowly and smoothly, without going beyond the point of pain [23].

OBJECTIVE NO. 8

The patient should be free of postural hypotension.
   To achieve the objective, the nurse should:

1. Elevate the head of the patient's bed 20 to 30 degrees.
2. When the patient's level of activity is to be increased, have him dangle his legs at the bedside after he has gradually built up tolerance in bed to the Fowler's position.
3. Monitor the patient's blood pressure and pulse when increasing his activity. (The patient should be returned to the recumbent position if his blood pressure increases or his pulse decreases.)

OBJECTIVE NO. 9

The patient should be free of postoperative thrombophlebitis.
   To achieve the objective, the nurse should:

1. Apply elastic hose that reach to the groin. (The hose should be taken off for one hour each eight-hour shift.)

2. Avoid any pressure on the patient's popliteal fossae and heel. The patient's knees should be kept slightly flexed by putting padding or pillows over those areas.
3. See that the patient has range-of-motion exercises of his lower extremities once every eight-hour shift.
4. Record the patient's calf and thigh measurements weekly. (The areas 20 cm above and below the upper border of the patella should be measured.)
5. Observe the patient for unusual and/or severe pain in the chest or an extremity and ipsilateral edema of an extremity, calf tenderness, and respiratory distress.

OBJECTIVE NO. 10

The patient should demonstrate the best possible mental status [4].
To achieve the objective, the nurse should:

1. Frequently measure, record, analyze, and report alterations in the patient's central nervous system functioning. The nurse should observe the patient's responses to:
   a. Questions of orientation (time, place, person).
   b. Simple commands.
   c. Painful stimuli.
2. Orient the patient to his surroundings. The patient should have in his room a clock, a calendar, and small items that are familiar to the patient (e.g., a picture of his family).

OBJECTIVE NO. 11

The patient should exhibit a means of communication with staff and family.
To achieve the objective, the nurse should:

1. Evaluate the patient's communication problem if he has one. Obtain guidance from a speech pathologist.
2. Provide communication stimulation for the patient as soon as he regains consciousness.
3. Make communication with the patient frequent but short because of his decreased attention span.
4. Evaluate the patient's comprehension by asking him questions that require answers.
5. Allow time for the patient's answer.

6. Speak slowly and distinctly to the patient, using eye contact and gesturing as required.
7. Evaluate the patient's ability to respond.
8. Use a picture board if other forms of communication are impossible.
9. Coordinate the efforts of the team caring for the patient so that the approach taken is consistent and as little frustrating as possible.
10. Help the patient's family understand and cope with his disorder.

OBJECTIVE NO. 12

The patient should be free of emotional upsets.
To achieve the objective, the nurse should:

1. Elicit the cooperation of the patient's family in regard to their responses to the patient.
2. Encourage the patient's family to speak quietly and calmly to the patient.
3. Be supportive of the patient's emotional responses.
4. Establish rapport by assigning a primary care nurse to the patient.
5. Determine what the patient's personality traits and life-style were before he became ill and evaluate how they might affect his response.

Summary

Depending on their size and location, intracranial aneurysms may be asymptomatic or they may cause symptoms before they rupture. The symptoms of the subarachnoid hemorrhage that results from the aneurysm may be the symptoms of slow or incomplete rupture (i.e., recurrent retroorbital headaches, recurrent confusion and coma, and mild nuchal rigidity) or of complete rupture (suboccipital pain, nausea, decreased level of consciousness, positive Kernig's sign, slow pulse, and increased cerebrospinal fluid pressure).

The initial objectives of management are that the patient recover from the effects of the initial hemorrhage and that another, perhaps fatal, rupture of the aneurysm be prevented. Medical and/or surgical intervention may be undertaken.

The common signs of stroke may be present preoperatively or postoperatively; they include motor, sensory, perceptual, and communication deficits. The rehabilitaton period may be as long as two years.

Study Problems

1. Describe the configuration of cerebral circulation.
2. Contrast the presentation in stroke due to cerebral thrombosis with the presentation in stroke due to cerebral embolism.
3. What motor changes are seen in stroke at the onset? In what order may return of function be anticipated?
4. What is the cause of the spasticity that often accompanies stroke?
5. Name the more common sensory deficits in stroke.
6. What functions are impaired in an aphasia?
7. Differentiate dysarthria and apraxia.
8. What are the signs of aneurysmal rebleeding?
9. What is the purpose of management of a ruptured intracranial aneurysm?
10. Name the common types of surgical intervention for the treatment of aneurysms.

References

1. Alvord, E. C., Loeser, J. D., Bailey, W. L., et al. Subarachnoid hemorrhage due to ruptured aneurysms. *Arch. Neurol.* 27:273, 1972.
2. Baker, A. B., and Baker, L. H. (eds.). *Clinical Neurology.* Hagerstown, Md.: Harper & Row, 1974.
3. Burt, M. M. Perceptual deficits in hemiplegia. *Am. J. Nurs.* 70:1026, 1970.
4. Carini, E., and Owens, G. *Neurological and Neurosurgical Nursing* (5th ed.). St. Louis: Mosby, 1974.
5. Chusid, J. G. *Correlative Neuroanatomy and Functional Neurology.* Los Altos, Calif.: Lange, 1970.
6. Clipper, M. Nursing care of patients in a neurologic intensive care unit. *Nurs. Clin. North Am.* 4:211, 1969.
7. Darley, F. L., Aronson, A. E., and Brown, J. R. *Motor Speech Disorders.* Philadelphia: Saunders, 1975.
8. Eliasson, S. G., Prensky, A. L., and Hardin, W. B. (eds.). *Neurological Pathophysiology.* New York: Oxford, 1974.
9. Elliott, F. A. *Clinical Neurology* (2nd ed.). Philadelphia: Saunders, 1971.
10. Guyton, A. C. *Function of the Human Body* (3rd ed.). Philadelphia: Saunders, 1969.
11. Licht, S. (ed.). *Stroke and Its Rehabilitation.* Baltimore: Waverly, 1975.
12. Locksley, H. B. Natural history of subarachnoid hemorrhage, intracranial aneurysm, and arteriovenous malformation. Report on the cooperative study of intracranial aneurysm and SAH. *J. Neurosurg.* 25:219, 1966.
13. McQuillan, F. L. Proper care of stroke patients starts with recognition of danger signals. *Mod. Nurs. Home* 22:82, 1968.
14. Millikan, C. Eighth Princeton Conference on cerebral vascular disease. *Stroke* 3:105, 1972.
15. Netter, F. H. *Ciba Collection of Medical Illustrations—the Nervous System.* New York: Ciba, 1972.
16. Nishioka, H. Evaluation of the conservative management of ruptured intracranial aneurysms. *J. Neurosurg.* 25:574, 1966.
17. Okawara, S.-H. Warning signs prior to rupture of an intracranial aneurysm. *J. Neurosurg.* 38:575, 1973.
18. Plum, F., and Posner, J. B. *Diagnosis of Stupor and Coma* (2nd ed.). Philadelphia: Davis, 1972.
19. Sahs, A. L., Perret, G. E., Locksley, H. B., et al. (eds.). *Intracranial Aneurysms and Subarachnoid Hemorrhage—a Cooperative Study.* Philadelphia: Lippincott, 1969.
20. Slosberg, P. Treatment and prevention of stroke—subarachnoid hemorrhage due to ruptured intracranial aneurysm. *N.Y. State J. Med.* 73:679, 1973.
21. Spellman, G. G. Differential diagnosis—emergency care of the stroke patient. *J. Iowa Med. Soc.* 62:27, 1972.
22. Tobis, J. S. Pathophysiologic considerations in the evaluation of the stroke patient. *Bull. N.Y. Acad. Med.* 39:569, 1963.
23. Truscott, B. L., Kretschmann, C. M., Toole, J. F., et al. Early rehabilitative care in community hospitals: Effect on quality of survivorship following a stroke. *Stroke* 5:623, 1974.
24. Walker, A. E. Clinical localization of intracranial aneurysms and vascular anomalies. *Neurology* 6:79, 1956.

Head Injuries

Cornelia Vanderstaay Kenner

Head injuries are among the most devastating and lethal catastrophes that befall man. Nurses must monitor closely patients with head injuries and assess any subtle changes that could help them save patients' lives and improve the quality of those patients' lives.

Objective

In regard to head injuries, the nurse should be able to:

1. Describe the mechanism of head injury.
2. Differentiate among the types of head injury.
3. Compare and contrast uncal herniation and central herniation.
4. Compare and contrast the patient with increased intracranial pressure with the patient in shock.
5. Perform the initial assessment of a patient who has a head injury.
6. Monitor the physiological parameters that are relevant to patients with head injuries.
7. Observe and protect the patient who is having a seizure.

Achieving the Objective

To achieve the objective, the nurse should:

1. Review the basic anatomy and physiology of the nervous system, and memorize the functions of

30

the cerebrum, thalamus, hypothalamus, basal ganglia, pons, cerebellum, medulla, nerves, spinal cord, cerebrospinal fluid, meninges, myelin, and axons.

2. Study the material in this chapter.
3. Practice neurological assessment on a patient with residual problems several months after injury.
4. After acquiring basic skills, assess patients first on the neurological/neurosurgical floor and then in the neurological/neurosurgical critical care unit.
5. Develop a flow sheet for the neurosurgical critical care unit.
6. Practice psychomotor skills associated with intracranial pressure monitoring.

How to Proceed

To develop an approach to patients with head injuries, the nurse should:

1. Interpret the clinical course of several patients who have head injuries. The nurse should:
   a. Determine the patients' clinical signs and symptoms.
   b. Explain the pathophysiology of the injuries.
   c. Identify the precipitating factors of herniation.
2. Outline the steps of the initial patient assessment.
3. Determine what physiological and psychological problems should be anticipated.
4. Outline the major objectives for the patients' care and management.

Case Study

At a construction site where he was working, Mr. R. A., an 18-year-old man, fell down eight steps and struck his head. He was extremely difficult to arouse. The emergency medical technicians who came to help Mr. A. summoned the helicopter evacuation service, which quickly transferred him to the medical center.

Mr. A.'s previous health had been excellent. On arrival at the medical center, his blood pressure was 118/62 mm Hg, pulse 104, and respirations 22 and regular in rate and depth (see assessment sheet). A general physical examination revealed no gross abnormalities. Mr. A. was drowsy and displayed minimal spontaneous activity, his responses to verbal commands were sluggish and inconsistent, his pupils were 4 mm in diameter, they were equal, and they reacted to light. His ciliospinal and corneal reflexes were intact. He had spontaneous ocular movement with full lateral range. A funduscopic examination revealed no hemorrhages and no papilledema. He exhibited a flaccid left hemiplegia with no reflexes and a diminished sensitivity to pain. His arterial blood gas measurements were pH 7.4, PO_2 90 mm Hg, PCO_2 40 mm Hg, and delta base 0; CBC and SMA-12 results were normal and his skull, cervical spine, and chest x rays were normal.

Clinical Presentation of Case Study

Forty-five minutes later, Mr. A.'s level of consciousness had decreased; he had become extremely drowsy, and he displayed no spontaneous motor activity. He was aroused only by strong stimuli and his responses tended to be stereotyped and simplified. His Glasgow coma scale rating was 12. His eyes opened on command, he responded with inappropriate words, and he obeyed commands. His eye examination revealed the following: His right pupil was 6 mm in diameter, and it reacted sluggishly to light; on testing of his oculocephalic reflex, his right eye did not move entirely in the medial direction; his left pupil was 4 mm in diameter, and it reacted to light. One hour later, a CT scan was done that revealed a right-sided subdural hematoma; Mr. A. exhibited decorticate positioning in his left side. His respirations were 30 and regular and very deep. His right pupil was 8 mm in diameter, and it was fixed and dilated. He was immediately taken to the operating room for evacuation of the hematoma.

After surgery, Mr. A. returned to the neurosurgical critical care unit with an intracranial pressure monitor in place. On his first and second postoperative days, his level of consciousness consistently increased. He obeyed commands and displayed semipurposeful movements. His family, who were devoted to him, voiced their optimism. His primary care nurse asked the family liaison nurse and chaplain to help give the family support. The nurses, who never were without hope, participated even more in every positive occurrence. On the third postoperative day, Mr. A.'s level of consciousness decreased, and he exhibited semipurposeful movements only on deep pain stimulus. His intracranial pressure increased—from 20 mm Hg to 25 mm Hg; it was controlled with mannitol and hyperventilation. On Mr. A.'s fourth postoperative day, his intracranial pressure rose to 40 mm Hg, and it could not be controlled with mannitol and hyperventilation. On the fifth postoperative day, Mr. A. exhibited systolic hypertension and bradycardia. His pupils became fixed and dilated, and he had no corneal or oculocephalic reflexes. On sternal pain stimulation, his arms and legs assumed decerebrate posturing. On the sixth postoperative day, Mr. A. exhibited hypotension, tachycardia, and total flaccidity. He had a cardiopulmonary arrest, and he did not respond to resuscitation.

Reflections

Mr. A.'s family was grief-stricken over his accident and death. The health team tried to comfort the family, but they themselves felt uncomfortable in the situation. It was a particularly trying time for everyone because many of the patients in the unit had had catastrophes.

The interrelatedness and interconnectedness of nurse-patient emotions is nowhere more evident than in the neurosurgical critical care unit. Members of Mr. A.'s family grieved, and members of the health care team shared their grief. Grief had "crept into every crevice of the unit," and the members of the health team "felt uncomfortable."

The intense feelings patients experience are seldom isolated. All the people in a critical care unit—patients and nurses—seem to occupy a field in which emotions are more like processes and patterns than actual events. The reality of those feelings, which are shared by patients and nurses, is occasionally dramatic, as when every patient in the unit has experienced tragic illnesses. The ambience may be overwhelming. In an extreme situation, such as the one described in the case study, it is clear that the patient and the nurse interrelate in more than technical and perfunctory ways and that their interactions are never neutral events.

Nurse-patient interrelations are usually subtle and so might be ignored. Negative interactions can often be explained away as emotional aberrations on the part of the patient or as a failure of the patient's coping mechanisms. It is easy for the nurse to remain aloof or distant and to ignore the impact the patient's emotional state has on her. Indeed, she may use her own coping mechanisms (e.g., denial and repression) in an unconscious attempt to ignore the flux of feelings between her and the patient.

It is not only negative feelings that are shared. Positive feelings are also part of the emotional field, and the impact they have on patient and nurse depends on the "emotional charge" of the field. By seeing her interrelations with the patient as a dynamic process, the nurse can try to influence it in positive ways.

As the emotional field that exists between patient and nurse shows, the nurse is a participant in the patient's disease process. She is never a mere observer, as if the patient were somehow "out there," unaffected by her actions. To care for critically ill patients is to do more than observe their emotional and physical problems; it is to participate in them. The nurse-patient interchange has an awesome power.

Pathophysiology

Head injuries are caused by automobile accidents, gunshot wounds, stabbings, diving accidents, and falls or blows to the head—to name only a few causes. Most head injuries are caused by automobile accidents, in which the chances for serious injury are great since the speed is often high and the riders' heads are not supported.

Head injuries may be open (compound) or closed. They may be mild, moderate, severe, or lethal. In open head injuries, there is "communication" between the inside of the skull and the outside. Compound fractures of the skull, caused by both blunt and penetrating trauma, are open head injuries. They may result in different degrees of cerebral dysfunction. In open head injuries, the skull's contents have been exposed to the environment. Surgical debridement for cleansing and hemostasis is mandatory. Certain types of compound and penetrating injuries may be considered nonoperable under certain circumstances. Vigorous surgical management may not be indicated when vital signs show periods of apnea and bradycardia, when unconsciousness is profound, when pupils are fixed and dilated, and when reflexes are absent.

Immediate surgical intervention is usually not necessary in patients with a cerebrospinal fluid leak (rhinorrhea or otorrhea) since spontaneous closure is the usual course. In addition, prophylactic antibiotics are not indicated. If meningitis occurs, the infection is usually due to *Diplococcus pneumoniae* and it is responsive to methicillin and chloramphenicol.

In closed head injuries, there is no communication with the environment although a simple fracture may be present. In mild head injuries, retrograde amnesia may be present, but the loss of consciousness is brief. In moderate head injuries, unconsciousness is longer (hours to days) and is associated with abnormal neurological signs. In severe head injuries, unconsciousness is even longer and is commonly associated with a larger number of abnormal neurological signs. Death is inevitable in lethal injuries.

Formerly, the terms *concussion, contusion*, and *laceration* were commonly used to categorize injuries. Those terms are explained here although the terminology now used is mild head injury, moderate head injury, and severe head injury. In a concussion, the most common kind of head injury, the injury is less severe and the loss of consciousness is brief. Dizziness, loss of memory, and headache are of short duration. A contusion is much more serious; bruising and many small hemorrhages may be present, as may true laceration (tearing). There may be extensive permanent injury. On early evaluation, contusion is often clinically indistinguishable from laceration, but the difference can be seen on the CT scan.

Neurological Assessment

PATIENT'S NAME: _Mr. R.A._ DATE: _9/26_ TIME: _2 PM_

DIAGNOSIS: _Closed Head Injury_ T: _99°_ A.P.: _104_ R.P.: _104_ R.: _22_

B.P.: _118/62_ E.C.G. RHYTHM: _NSR_ ECTOPY: _—_ WT: _68 kg._ HT: _5'11_

ADMITTED VIA: _stretcher_ INFORMANT: _employer/mother_ LAST MEAL: _12 noon_

I. CHIEF COMPLAINT: _fell down stairs and struck head_

II. PATIENT PROFILE:
1. Age _18_ 2. Sex _m_
3. Marital Status M W D (S)
4. Race _B_ 5. Religion _Protestant_
6. Occupation _Construction worker_
7. Availability of family _In waiting room, live in city_
8. Dietary _deferred_
9. Sleeping _deferred_

III. HISTORY OF ILLNESS: _After striking head he was difficult to rouse_

IV. PAST MEDICAL HISTORY:
1. Pediatric & Adult Illnesses _usual childhood illness_
2. Cardiac
3. Hypertension
4. Respiratory
5. Diabetes Mellitus
6. Renal
7. Jaundice
8. Infections
9. Other
10. Hospitalizations & Surgeries _none_
11. Current Medication _none_
12. Allergies _penicillin_
13. Habits _none_

V. FAMILY HISTORY _Negative_

VI. PSYCHOSOCIAL
1. Behavior During Assessment _Unable to assess - obtunded_
2. Specific Problems _no previous problems_

VII. PHYSICAL EXAMINATION:
1. General _Well developed young male_

2. Respiratory System
Airway _patent_
Inspection _no gross abnormalities_
Rate _22_
Rhythm _regular_
Chest Wall _intact_
Palpation _no rubs_
Percission _no dullness or hyperresonance_
Auscultation
 Voice Sounds _deferred_
 Breath Sounds
 Increased ___ Decreased ___
Adventitious Sounds _no rales or rhonchi_

3. Cardiovascular System
A.P. _104_ R.P. _104_
B.P. Supine R ___ L ___
P.M.I. _5th ICS MCL_
Heart Sounds _normal S₁, S₂_
Thrills _none_
Peripheral Pulses _2+_

4. Gastrointestinal System
Nose & Mouth _Salem sump in place_
Stomach _no bleeding_
Abdomen _deferred_
Bowel Sounds _present_
Liver _not palpable_
Spleen _deferred_

5. Renal & Genitourinary Systems
I. ___ O. _catheter in place_
Urinary Bladder & Urethra _deferred_
Kidneys _deferred_

6. Musculoskeletal System
Skin Temperature & Color _cool_
Extremities _no fractures noted_
Spine _intact_
Sacral Edema _none_
Masses _none_

7. Neurological System
Handedness _right handed_
Consciousness _little spontaneous activity, follows commands inconsistently, Glasgow Coma Scale 14._

MENTATION:
1. Thinking
2. Remembering _____ *deferred*
3. Feeling
4. Language
MOTOR:
1. Seeing O.S.
          O.D. _____ *deferred*
   Confrontation fields
   Palpebral fissures _*normal*_
   Ptosis _*none noted*_
   Eye Position _*full lateral range*_
   Exophthalmos _*none*_
   Eye movements _*full lateral range*_
   *with spontaneous movement*
   Pupils:
   Size L_*4mm*_ R_*4mm*_ Shape _*round*_
   Reaction to light, direct
          L _*react*_ R _*react*_
   Consensual R to L _*react*_
          L to R _*react*_
   Reaction to near vision
          L _*def.*_ R _*def.*_
2. Eating _*deferred*_
3. Expressing _*deferred*_
4. Speaking _*confused*_
5. Moving
   a. Tone _*decreased*_
   b. Strength _*R + 2*_ _*Ⓛ hemiplegia*_
   c. Coordination: R   L
      Finger-nose
      Finger-finger
      Heel-shin
      Posture Holding _*deferred*_
      Rapid alternating
         movements
      Rebound
      Past-pointing
      Equilibrium _*deferred*_
      Gait
      Romberg
   d. Posture _*flaccid Ⓛ hemiplegia*_
   e. Involuntary movements
         (type and rate)
                *none*
   f. Reflexes:

	Right	Left
Biceps	+2	0
Brachioradials	+2	0
Triceps	+2	0
Patellar	+2	0
Achilles	+2	0
Plantar	+2	0

SENSORY:
1. Smelling _*deferred*_
2. Blinking _+_
3. Hearing _+_
4. Tasting _*deferred*_
5. Feeling _+_

VIII. LABORATORY:
   Hematology:
      HGB _*15 gm./100 ml.*_
      HCT _*45 %*_
      W.B.C. _*5.0/cu.cm.*_

   Chemistry:
      Na _*140*_ K _*4.2*_ CO$_2$ _*24*_
      CL _*100*_ Bl. Sug. _*150 mg%*_ BUN _*14 mg. %*_
      Urinalysis _*to lab*_

PROBLEM LIST:

          ACTIVE   ~~INACTIVE~~

9/26 1. *Incomplete data base*
3pm   2. *Closed head injury*
      3. *Altered level of consciousness*
      4. *Flaccid Ⓛ hemiplegia*
      5. *Diminished sensitivity to pain*
      6. *Respiratory dysfunction*
      7. *Self-care deficit*
          related to altered
          level of consciousness
          related to closed head
          injury
      8. *Allergic to penicillin*

Cornelia Kenner, RN,
          CCRN

Mechanism

There are many theories regarding the causes of brain damage. The factors mentioned include the transmission of waves of force, skull deformation, skull vibration, formation of a pressure gradient in the cranial cavity, brain displacement, brain rotation, and transient brain cavitation. No one theory has been generally accepted. Essentially, injuries to the head are caused by a force that is either focal or generalized or that is focal *and* general. All three types of force are serious, but the nursing observations and expectations are slightly different for each one. The types of force may be conceptualized by considering the difference between a moving object that strikes a stationary head and a moving head that strikes a stationary object. The former example involves a focal injury, and the latter example usually involves a generalized injury, a much more profound injury.

When the force is focal, the type of injury sustained depends on the local area involved and the extent of the injury. Symptoms will likely arise from the area injured, and observations for dysfunction would depend on what that area is. For example, a blow to the head by a blackjack is likely to cause a depressed skull fracture. Deformation and depression occur because the object has relatively low velocity. But in addition, the brain may strike the inner skull surface on the opposite side (in the contrecoup effect). If the blow is sufficiently intense, the dura is lacerated and the cerebral cortex extrudes through the laceration. That condition is usually associated with generalized cerebral edema and/or hemorrhage.

Several problems may result from a generalized force. First, the energy either dissipates into a fracture or is directly transmitted to the brain with resultant damage as the force is absorbed and the direction of force changes. Second, particularly during acceleration and deceleration, the brain strikes the skull and the dura and may even strike the inner skull surface on the opposite side. Linear stresses can cause bruising of the brain on the side opposite the impact. Third, generalized force is particularly dangerous if the direction of the blow is tangential and rotation occurs. The brain may strike the sphenoid ridges or falx (the brain stem may strike the edge of the tentorium at the tentorial notch); the brain stem may be compressed by rotation of the cerebrum. Vectoral force can be aimed at deep centers. For example, at the time of injury, the person may be traumatized to the point where no or only minimal linear skull fractures are observed on the x ray and the remaining energy is transmitted to the brain substance itself.

On postmortem examination, many patients are found to have a laceration of the corpus callosum that results from its being compressed against the falx. Cooper and Moody [8] observed that 90 percent of the patients shown by CT scanning to have a lacerated corpus callosum died.

Cineangiography

New light has been shed on the anatomical factors involved in brain damage following head injury. Cineangiographic studies that allowed 1000 frames per second have documented the existence of intracranial vascular movement during graded experimental trauma (a 4 m/sec blunt impact to the left temporoparietal region) in rhesus monkeys. Those studies indicated that most intracranial movement occurs in the first milliseconds following trauma [43]. Impacts that did not fracture the skull resulted in rapid transient movement of intracranial arteries. The most prominent change in such impacts was the rapid, transient, and reversible torsion displacement of the anterior cerebral artery across the midline. (Other cerebral parenchymal displacements were believed to be present, but they were not described.) Also, the horizontal segment of the ipsilateral middle cerebral artery had a distorted, interrupted appearance, and it was progressively displaced medially. The skull was compressed and bent inward. The authors suggested that those phenomena might represent a large transient mass movement and compression of blood vessels and brain parenchyma that might have caused coup injury. Occipital blows distorted the peripheral branches of the middle and posterior cerebral arteries and produced marked stretching of the extracranial vessels. The tension on the extracranial vessels was so severe that some have hypothesized that such tension is a cause of the extracranial arterial aneurysms that can occur after blunt head trauma.

Movement and Forces That Produce Injury

The mechanism of head injury depends on the mass and velocity of the type of injury. The brain is well protected by the scalp, the skull, and the cerebrospinal fluid. At the time of impact several things may occur. As the scalp moves across the skull, bleeding and/or a hematoma may result. The skull then may be fractured or may bend internally. The brain may be bruised locally. Also, gas bubbles (microcavitation) may be formed locally in the cerebral hemisphere and disrupt neural tissue. In turn, white matter may be lacerated. A significant problem may result from the movement of the brain across the many rough areas on the inside of the "bony box." The brain can move front to back or back to front so that the orbital surfaces are raked across the medial floor of the frontal fossa and the frontal lobes are contused (usually) or lacerated (occasionally). In particular, the temporal lobe is in a precarious position. The anterior part of the temporal lobe, which is bordered by the sphenoid bone, may become contused and edematous. Commonly, movement causes resonance cavitation, which is followed by movement in the temporal fossa and across the frontal fossa. Shearing forces result; they may be great enough to cause death. Significantly, the shearing force may cause injury at the spinal medullary junction since the brain is attached at the base of the skull and must rock back and forth. The rotary motion produces a vector of force toward deep midline structures. It probably is the cause of unconsciousness. In some instances, the motion is so intense that the brain stem strikes the tentorium and thus causes primary brain stem injury. Pressure waves follow the impact. They can injure the brain by compression and tension. Thus injury can occur anywhere and can be of any severity. The injury is then compounded by hypoxia and swelling, and the injured brain is far more susceptible to a second insult of any type.

Increased Intracranial Pressure

One of the consequences of head injury is an increase in the intracranial pressure (ICP). Increased ICP is a result of swelling (edema) and/or hemorrhage. The term *swelling* is preferred to the term *edema* because the probable mechanism is massive dilatation of blood vessels after injury and not true edema, as seen with tumors. Damage to the cerebral cells and their functioning is caused by the increased size or volume of the brain and by the intrinsic and extrinsic pressure. The fluid in the intracranial compartments (intracellular, cerebrospinal fluid, and intravascular compartments) is contained in a bony box that cannot expand. According to the Monro-Kellie doctrine, the volume of the cranium is equal to

the volume of the brain, blood, and cerebrospinal fluid. An alteration in the volume of any of the three components changes the cranial volume and leads to pressure changes. For example, increases in blood or fluid result in increases in volume. Therefore, increased ICP can result from hypoventilation, alterations in arterial carbon dioxide levels, and decreased venous return. In effect, hypoventilation produces increased carbon dioxide levels that produce vasodilatation and thus increased ICP.

Compensatory Mechanisms

Compensatory mechanisms are brought into play by the body in an effort to ensure adequate blood supply. In the presence of increased ICP, Cushing's reflex (increased blood pressure and decreased pulse, and respiratory abnormality) is activated in an attempt to decrease the amount of blood in the head without decreasing the perfusion of brain tissue.

Cerebral perfusion pressure =
$$\text{mean arterial pressure} - \text{ICP}$$

It is thought that compression of or interference with a small region in the medulla is critical for the production of arterial hypertension. If increased ICP is diffuse or if there are no pressure gradients along the craniospinal axis, the pressor response does not occur until the ICP equals or exceeds the diastolic blood pressure [22]. In contrast, a mass lesion that causes compression or distortion of the brain stem may produce a pressor response at relatively low levels of ICP. That increase in blood pressure is due to peripheral vasoconstriction from increased sympathetic activity and to increased cardiac output. Such compensatory mechanisms are not active with excessively increased levels of ICP; the patient exhibits a decreased blood pressure, and increased or decreased and irregular pulse and respirations shortly before death.

When the contents of the fluid compartments continue to expand and thereby increase pressure, shifts occur within the parenchyma of the brain. The shifts depend also on the rate of expansion. A rapid expansion of a small mass causes a larger increase in ICP and the degree of brain malfunctioning than does a slow expansion of a much larger mass, since the brain is able to accommodate a slowly growing mass without as much loss of functioning. Eventually, vascular problems and/or obstruction of the spinal fluid circulation becomes so great that compensation is no longer possible.

Pressure Transmission

Pressure is transmitted evenly and quickly to all intracranial compartments as long as there is fluid connection among the compartments (Pascal's law). In the event of obstruction, pressures in the various compartments are very different [21].

The intracranial space contains displaceable fluid (cerebrospinal fluid and blood) that can be expressed into the extracranial vascular system. A certain amount of cerebral or intracranial expansion is possible since cerebrospinal fluid is approximately 10% of the intracranial volume [3] and blood is approximately 2% to 11% of the intracranial volume. The entire normal ventricular system accounts for 35 ml, and part of that amount may be displaced. In order to accommodate an enlarging mass, the fluid is displaced, and the intracranial pressure does not change as long as the volume displaced equals the volume added. However, the volume of fluid that can be displaced is limited. If the mass continues to expand, the ICP increases monotonically. That is, increments in the mass produce an ever increasing rise in the ICP (Fig. 30-1). In fact, at the point when almost all the fluid has been displaced, an additional small increase in the mass produces a very large increase in the ICP.

Swelling develops gradually in the first hours after injury; the maximum development is usually reached in 36 to 48 hours. If the swelling reaches the point that the ICP equals the arterial blood pressure, circulation through the brain ceases and death results.

Types of Brain Swelling

Brain swelling may be vasogenic, cytotoxic, or interstitial [13]. Vasogenic swelling, the most common form, is characterized by an increased permeability of the capillary endothelial cells. The fluid is a plasma filtrate; it is composed of plasma proteins. Although the reason is not fully understood, cerebral white matter is known to be susceptible to vasogenic swelling. That susceptibility may be related to the fact that capillary density and blood flow are normally lower in white matter than in cortical and subcortical gray matter.

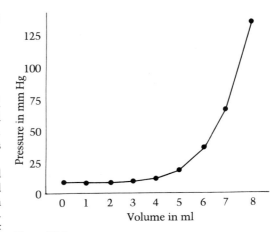

Figure 30-1

Volume and pressure relationship. The volume of fluid that can be displaced is limited, and if the volume continues to expand, the intracranial pressure elevates at an increasingly rapid rate.

Cytotoxic swelling is the result of intracellular fluid accumulation. It is characteristically seen after cardiac arrest with hypoxemia and in water intoxication. The fluid is composed of sodium and intracellular water and results from the failure of the adenosine triphosphate–dependent sodium pump. The neurons, glia, and endothelial cells swell, reducing the extracellular fluid space in the brain and markedly decreasing the size of the capillary lumen (mainly because of the swelling of the endothelial cells).

Interstitial swelling is the result of an increase in the sodium and water content of the periventricular white matter. It is characteristically seen in obstructive hydrocephalus. Cerebrospinal fluid moves across the ventricular walls, but the periventricular white matter decreases in size rather than increases. As the hydrostatic pressure within the white matter increases, the myelin lipids decrease rapidly, resulting in the decrease in periventricular white matter rather than in the anticipated increase.

The response within the cell depends on the blood brain barrier, the metabolism of cells, the osmolarity of water, and the free water. Surrounding each contused area is one or more of the following types of swelling: (1) anoxic, (2) hydrostatic, which is secondary to increased blood pressure or to the loss of autoregulation, and (3) necrotic, which is secondary to contusions or lacerations [3]. Ischemia and hypoxia compound the swelling. The small vessels become permeable to fluid. A change occurs even in the blood brain barrier, and fluid leaks from the vessels into the brain substances.

Autoregulation

Particularly significant are the impairments in pressure and metabolic autoregulation. Pressure autoregulation is a change in the diameter of blood vessels in the brain produced by a change in transmural pressure across the walls of the autoregulatory vessels, so as to maintain a constant blood flow during a change in perfusion pressure [23]. Normally, cerebral blood flow is kept constant at approximately 100 ml per gram per minute. The constancy is assured by the constriction or dilatation of the arteries, and it is only partly dependent on the systemic arterial blood pressure and the body posture. Following trauma, the autoregulatory capacity to change caliber and flow rate is decreased, producing swelling and the dilatation of intracranial vessels under the influence of the systemic blood pressure. Acute brain swelling may result.

Since vasoconstriction would decrease cerebral blood flow, the explanations offered for the phenomena include the Cushing reflex. In the presence of increased ICP, when there is a threat to the blood supply of the brain, increases in sympathetic vasoconstriction elevate the blood pressure (increased ICP→medullary vasomotor center ischemia→vasomotor inhibitory fibers are sensitive to the hypoxia resulting from ischemia while the sympathetic fibers are not→vasoconstriction→increased blood pressure). Once the systemic blood pressure rises in response to increasing ICP, the hydrostatic pressure in the arterial side of the cerebral circulation also rises, and the amount of hydrostatic edema increases.

Even more important in the person with a closed head injury is the compensatory change in blood flow to meet the altered metabolic demands of the tissue. Here the premise concerns chemical regulation dependent on local oxygen requirements and carbon dioxide production. The hydrogen ion concentration in the extravascular space is the key determinant of the diameter of the vessel. As more hydrogen ions are produced locally and diffuse to the vessels, the vessels dilate and increase the cerebral blood flow. Also, increased carbon dioxide levels decrease the extracellular pH and cause vasodilatation and increased cerebral blood flow [24].

Cerebral Blood Flow

Although cerebral blood flow (CBF) is an important consideration, assessment of brain functioning as well as brain damage in man and experimental animals cannot be accurately determined by measuring the CBF [3]. In injured people with severe neurological dysfunction and depressed brain metabolism, CBF may be normal. The converse can also be true. That is, the brain may be able to function normally with a decreased CBF as long as the decrease in metabolism is proportional to the decrease in CBF. The hypothermic patient exemplifies that concept in that his decreased temperature decreases his metabolism, which in turn decreases his CBF.

The addition of increased ICP makes the situation even more confusing. Several studies have found different correlations for increased ICP and survival [5, 32, 42]. Even in patients with intracranial hypertension, CBF has been observed to be normal (maintained by autoregulation). As a matter of fact, in some deeply comatose persons, CBF has been supranormal. One study in particular made an interesting observation. In patients with severe head injuries, regional blood flow values were high, and in patients who improved clinically, blood flow values tended to approach normal values [11].

Research studies on cerebral blood flow should be evaluated carefully [46]. Many studies do not truly simulate the pathophysiology of head injury. Usually the model includes rapid infusion of fluid into the subarachnoid space, resulting in a diffuse increase in the ICP. The clinical situation can be quite different in the case of the intracranial expansion of a supratentorial mass, which causes fluid obstruction and a difference in pressure gradients. Hence information about pressure from the subarachnoid space is not sufficient to evaluate the complex situation; knowledge of local tissue pressures is needed to establish a relationship between pressure and flow.

Furthermore, CBF is a function of the diameter of the cerebrovascular bed, blood viscosity, pressure, and vascular bed resistance. In the usual case, perfusion pressure across the brain is equal to the difference between internal carotid artery pressure and jugular vein pressure. However, the basic physiology is altered when the ICP is increased [23, 29]. Cerebral venous pressure (CVP) increases so that the jugular vein pressure approximates the internal carotid artery pressure. The following formula gives an estimate of CBF through the brain:

$$CBF = \frac{\text{Mean systemic arterial pressure (SAP)} - \text{mean ICP}}{CVP}$$

Thus cerebral perfusion pressure is elevated by increasing the SAP, and it is lowered by one of three mechanisms: (1) decreasing the SAP, (2) increasing the ICP, or (3) increasing the CVP.

Cerebral circulatory arrest (diffuse brain ischemia) occurs clinically when the ICP equals the SAP in patients with severe brain swelling and during cardiac arrest. The upper and lower limits of autoregulation to a change in SAP have been defined in baboons [3, 42]. CBF remained constant at a mean SAP of 125 to 140 mm Hg and then increased rapidly with any further rise in SAP (the upper limit of autoregulation). The lower limit was determined when the mean SAP was lowered to 65 mm Hg.

Xenon 133 is now used most frequently for measuring regional CBF. The procedure involves inserting a catheter into the internal carotid artery, injecting a bolus of ^{133}Xe, and recording the CBF from brain clearance curves using a multiple scintillation detector. Each curve is analyzed; the results give a mean flow value calculated from the flow in gray and white matter and from the weight. However, relatively little information has been gathered about normal values and about the reproducibility of the regional values in the same patient. Information about the clearance curves in normal patients is available. The techniques can also be used as an inhalation or intravenous method.

Hemorrhage

Another early potential complication is acute bleeding from an epidural (extradural), acute subdural, or intracerebral hemorrhage. Acute bleeding can cause unconsciousness, increasing abnormal neurological signs that indicate rostral-caudal deterioration or herniation and death. Those are signs of true surgical emergencies. A decrease in the level of consciousness

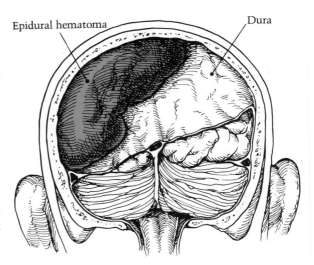

Figure 30-2
Epidural hematoma. Usually the bleeding is arterial in origin. The epidural hematoma tends to have a concave, localized formation since the dura is rather firmly affixed to the skull.

following head trauma is assumed to be caused by a hemorrhage. Further emergency neurodiagnostic tests may be indicated.

An epidural hematoma (Fig. 30-2) may be caused by arterial or venous bleeding in the frontal or temporal regions (very rarely in the posterior fossa). Most epidural hematomas are over the cerebral convexity, are usually related to the temporal lobe, and result from a laceration of the middle meningeal artery caused by a skull fracture [35]. The recovery rate for patients diagnosed and treated is extremely good—higher than 90 percent. Only a minority of individuals undergo the classic progression of symptoms—from unconsciousness to a conscious lucid interval and back to unconsciousness—but one must always look for the sequence. Although the clinical sequence apparent to the observer varies, the most common progression is as follows [12, 39]: As the hematoma expands, the brain is first pushed away from the skull, then it is compressed, and then herniation occurs. The signs and symptoms are headache, possibly followed by a subtle change in behavior, a decreased level of consciousness, and then a change in the ipsilateral pupil signs followed by contralateral motor paralysis. When the eye on the side of the hematoma is tested, first the pupil constricts, then it reacts more

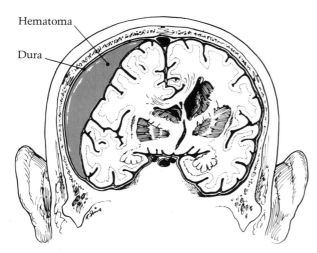

Hematoma

Dura

Figure 30-3
Subdural hematoma. Usually the bleeding is venous in origin. The subdural hematoma tends to have a convex, diffuse formation since the brain is not as firmly affixed to the dura as the dura is to the skull. The bleeding may encircle the hemisphere and have an elliptical, convex appearance.

slowly, and then it becomes fixed and dilated. Paralysis of the extraocular muscle follows quickly. The same sequence occurs in the contralateral pupil. If both pupils are fixed and dilated for more than 30 minutes, it is highly unlikely that the person will survive.

Acute subdural hematoma (Fig. 30-3) may be unilateral or bilateral as well as arterial or venous in origin. Arterial bleeding, although uncommon, is usually caused by a tear in the brain; the patient has a decreased level of consciousness and may demonstrate a focal neurological deficit. Venous bleeding commonly occurs from tearing of the veins that go from the brain to the dural sinuses. The mortality is extremely high because the hematoma develops suddenly and the brain is unable to withstand rapid compression. The shearing force that produces the intracranial shifting forces and venous tears also produces dramatic intracerebral shearing forces. It is those intracerebral forces that are probably so destructive. The expanding lesion compresses the midline structures to one side. The patient's death occurs in the same sequence; hemorrhage, compression, edema, and herniation. The pupil signs are ipsilateral, and the motor findings are contralateral. In adults under the age of 30, the survival rate is 50 percent. For those 30

to 50 years old, the survival rate is 20 percent. For those over the age of 50, the survival rate is extremely low.

Traumatic intracerebral hematoma in salvageable patients is less common than subdural hematoma but more common than epidural hematoma; often it mimics or accompanies one or both. The most common site is the temporal lobe. The occipital and frontal lobes are also common sites. Usually the hemorrhage is the result of acute contusion of the blood vessels in the brain. The symptoms are a decreased level of consciousness and a progressive focal neurological deficit.

CT scanning and arteriography are commonly used to help localize the lesion. They are done before surgery if time permits.

Herniation

Severe head trauma with symptoms of an expanding supratentorial mass resulting in herniation is a true surgical emergency. Unless treatment is instituted rapidly, the pressure and vascular injuries associated with herniation produce death by deterioration in a rostral-caudal progression. Accurate observations and recording are imperative to help determine whether the person is getting better or getting worse. Once the masses enlarge so that the skull is not large enough to hold its contents, the cerebral structures shift and compress other areas. Those areas then swell and shift. Volume and pressure increase progressively until the only exit is at the tentorial notch (the large, semioval opening in the center of the tentorium).

Herniation may be transfalcian, uncal, or central transtentorial. In rapidly expanding hematomas it is usually uncal. The process of herniation is well described by Plum and Posner [39].

Transfalcian Herniation

In transfalcian or cingulate herniation, cerebral ischemia and edema are increased by the compression of blood vessels (the anterior cerebral arteries) and tissues. The falx is a fold of dura mater that separates the two cerebral hemispheres and extends down into the interhemispheric fissure. Once the force produced by the enlarging mass is great enough, the hemisphere herniates under the falx. Also, ischemia in the distribution of the anterior cerebral artery can lead to paralysis of one or both legs.

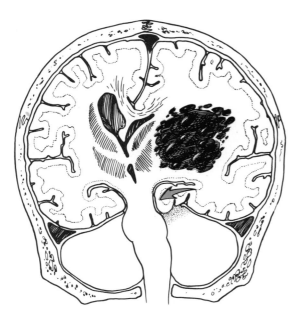

Figure 30-4
Uncal herniation.

Uncal Herniation

Uncal herniation (Fig. 30-4) occurs after a temporal mass has shifted the inner basal edge of the uncus and hippocampal gyrus over the lateral edge of the tentorium. Crowding at the tentorial notch compresses the midbrain and oculomotor nerve against the opposite edge. Classically, the uncus herniates over the free edge, pushes the posterior cerebral artery down, and compresses the oculomotor nerve. The temporal lobe then herniates into the notch. As the posterior cerebral artery is occluded, ischemia of the occipital lobe increases and infarction results. The aqueduct is compressed and spinal fluid circulation is blocked. The brain stem is damaged by ischemia and hemorrhage [39].

The signs of herniation may be described as those seen early and late. According to Plum and Posner [39], in uncal herniation a significant exception to the norm occurs in that theoretically the first sign is not a decreased level of consciousness but a sluggishly reactive pupil. However, as an important clinical finding that is not consistent with theory, a decreased level of consciousness precedes changes in the pupillary signs. In any event, the patient may arrive at the hospital with a subtle eye sign, such as a unilaterally

dilated pupil. Also, the classic signs of increased blood pressure and slowed pulse may not occur unless the posterior fossa is also involved. A progressive sequence of pupillary, respiratory, and motor signs is seen. Deterioration proceeds quickly once the signs of midbrain dysfunction occur [40].

The parameters used for assessment are described in Chapter 11 (Neurological Assessment). The evaluative criteria for early herniation are the following:

1. Level of consciousness: near wakefulness to coma
2. Respirations: eupnea
3. Eyes
    a. Pupil size: unequal, unilateral dilatation (6 mm in diameter)
    b. Pupil reaction: dilated pupil, sluggish reaction, opposite pupil reacts
    c. Ciliospinal reflex: intact
    d. Eye movements: unimpaired
    e. Oculocephalic reflex: unimpaired
    f. Oculovestibular reflex: unimpaired (the dilated pupil may not turn toward a cold stimulus)
4. Motor signs: no change
5. Pain: purposeful

The signs of late uncal herniation are those of midbrain dysfunction. They are the following:

1. Level of consciousness: stuporous or comatose
2. Respirations: Cheyne-Stokes or central neurogenic hyperventilation
3. Eyes
    a. Pupil size: unequal, unilaterally dilated (8 mm in diameter)
    b. Pupil reaction: direct response absent in dilated pupil, present in other pupil
    c. Ciliospinal reflex: intact but difficult to test in a fully blown pupil
    d. Eye movements: oculomotor paralysis
    e. Oculocephalic reflex: irregular
    f. Oculovestibular reflex: sluggish
4. Motor signs: frequently ipsilateral hemiplegia and contralateral decorticate posture or decerebrate posture
5. Pain: bilateral extensor plantar response, decerebrate posture

The signs of deterioration continue, and the signs of midbrain damage appear and progress caudally. The damage is due to secondary ischemia and necrosis. The patient's chances of full recovery are extremely poor. The portion of the midbrain compressed by the uncus is the cerebral peduncle [2]. Since that area is the carrier of motor fibers to the spinal cord, communication between the cerebrum and the midbrain is interrupted. Brain stem reflexes appear.

The signs of midbrain and upper pons damage are the following:

1. Level of consciousness: stuporous or comatose
2. Respirations: sustained central neurogenic hyperventilation
3. Eyes
   a. Pupil size: irregularly at midposition (4–6 mm in diameter)
   b. Pupil reactivity: fixed bilaterally
   c. Ciliospinal reflex: may disappear
   d. Eye movements: paralysis
   e. Oculocephalic reflex: absent or impaired (when the reflex is elicited, eye movements are dysconjugate and the medially moving eye does not move as far as the laterally moving eye) [41]
   f. Oculovestibular reflex: impaired
4. Motor: resting position or bilateral decerebrate rigidity
5. Pain: bilateral decerebrate rigidity

Without therapy, damage due to ischemia and necrosis continues down the brain stem. The following signs of the lower pons and upper medullary dysfunction appear:

1. Level of consciousness: comatose
2. Respirations: shallow, rapid eupnea (20–40 breaths) and apneustic
3. Eyes
   a. Pupil size: midposition
   b. Pupil reactivity: fixed
   c. Ciliospinal reflex: unobtainable
   d. Eye movements: unobtainable
   e. Oculocephalic reflex: unobtainable
   f. Oculovestibular reflex: unobtainable
4. Motor signs: flaccid, bilateral extensor plantar response
5. Pain: occasional flexion or perhaps response in lower extremity

Before death, the patient passes through a state exhibiting signs of medullary dysfunction. His respirations are slow, ataxic, and interrupted by deep sighs or gasps. His blood pressure drops, and his pulse is fast or slow.

Central Herniation

Following head injury, the patient may also herniate centrally (transtentorial). The diencephalon, the midbrain, the pons, and then the medulla are affected in an orderly progression. Preceding the sequence might have been a lateral shift and cingulate herniation that resulted in increased ischemia and edema from the compression of the cerebral artery and vein.

Downward pressure from the cerebral hemispheres then compresses the diencephalon and even the midbrain through the tentorial notch. Several brain stem changes occur (they are the same as those in uncal herniation): compression of the posterior cerebral artery, spinal fluid circulation blockage, brain stem ischemia, and then continued destruction. The early signs are different from those in uncal herniation but after the midbrain and upper pons stage, they are the same.

One of the most reliable early signs of central herniation is a decrease in the level of consciousness. Other early signs are as follows:

1. Level of consciousness: obtunded–stuporous–comatose
2. Respirations: Cheyne-Stokes with deep sighs or yawns
3. Eyes
   a. Pupil size: small (1–3 mm in diameter)
   b. Pupil reaction: brisk but hard to see
   c. Ciliospinal reflex: intact
   d. Eye movements: conjugate or roving and slightly divergent
   e. Oculocephalic reflex
      (1) If the eyes are conjugate at rest, they do not move when the head turns.
      (2) There is only a slight alteration from the resting eye movement.
      (3) Vertical movement may be impaired.
   f. Oculovestibular reflex: movement of eyes toward a cold stimulus
4. Motor signs
   a. If hemiplegia is present, it may worsen. The other side may develop paratonic resistance (that includes the whole body). Bilateral plantar extension.
   b. Later, grasp reflexes are present.
5. Pain:
   a. The nonhemiplegic side may respond appropriately to pain.
   b. In the hemiplegic limb, decorticate positioning appears, particularly in response to pain.

c. Occasionally, the hemiplegic side responds to pain with decerebrate posture, and the opposite side (ipsilateral to the mass) responds to pain with decorticate posture.

Associated Spinal Cord Injury

Injury to the spinal cord may be caused by several types of trauma. Penetrating injury caused by a stab wound, bullet, or other high-speed missile may result in direct damage to the spinal cord. In motor vehicle and motorcycle accidents, the head and spinal cord can move in any direction. Injuries caused by diving into shallow water are usually hyperextension injuries. Blows to the occiput and then to the vertex account for many compression fractures. A whiplash injury or a direct blow to the forehead results in sudden hyperextension. The areas of the body able to have the most movement sustain an even greater motion that then becomes abnormal. Application of a force continues until the ligaments and bones are involved. That is true of the C4 to C6 area (and of the T11 to L2 area), which is the most mobile.

The syndrome of swelling, hemorrhage, and transection occurs in cord injuries, but actual evaluation of spinal trauma is difficult since there is no way to determine the amount of damage. It has been known for 150 years that a weight of greater than 600 gm per square centimeter dropped on an animal's spine renders the animal permanently paralyzed. When the weight is less than 400 gm per square centimeter, the animal will recover from paralysis. It was learned much later that when a stainless steel wire was passed between the ligaments above and below the injury, the wire raised the weight needed to cause permanent paralysis from 600 to 800 gm per square centimeter. In other words, eliminating mobilization produced a decreased incidence of paralysis.

Nervous tissue withstands compression poorly; and the more rapid the compression, the poorer the tolerance. Even though the cord compression is transient, with sufficient force the result is total disruption of the cord. If the cord were viewed approximately 30 minutes after impact, a small amount of hemorrhage in the cord center would be seen. Two hours later, the hemorrhage would be bigger and the expanding hematoma would compress the cord and extend up and down the cord for several segments.

Mechanisms of Spinal Trauma

The most vulnerable part of the spine is the cervical area. The head is mobile, relatively heavy, and supported poorly—by rather weak muscles. So any head injury may well damage the spine. The mechanisms of spinal trauma must be analyzed to afford understanding of the clinical and pathological findings; the injuries are defined by the movement of the head in relationship to the spine: axial loading, flexion, and hyperextension (Fig. 30-5).

In an axial loading injury, the force is upward and downward with no posterior or lateral bending of the neck. Commonly a burst fracture of the vertebral body or a disk extrusion results. A typical axial loading injury is one that occurs in an automobile accident in which the person is thrown up against the roof and strikes the vertex of his head. The classic presentation is the fracture of the first cervical vertebra (Jefferson's fracture), in which the head is impacted from above and the ring at the first cervical vertebra bursts. It is unusual to have associated cord injury since the cervical space is relatively large at this site and the fracture site is not greatly displaced.

In a flexion injury, which is more common, the head is bent forward on the cervical spine. Flexion, both with and without rotation, produces a more complex injury. The person may have a residual compression fracture with more destruction anteriorly, posterior points of spinal dislocation, and a disk herniated posteriorly against the cord. If rotation accompanies the flexion, there may be more compression of one side of the body than the other. At the time of the flexion injury, one vertebral body moves forward and the cord is essentially totally compressed. Not a lot of force is required to produce a flexion injury. Characteristically, the type of spinal cord injury produced is complete paralysis with no functional segment of any kind below the transection. A typical flexion injury can occur to a football player who spears another player during a tackle.

When spinal flexion of the cervical spine occurs with disk extrusion (it occurs rarely), the anterior cervical spine syndrome is produced. Paralysis of all four limbs occurs, with loss of pain and temperature sense but with preservation of position sense and light touch since the posterior columns remain intact. Many surgeons consider the syndrome an indication for surgical decompression.

A hyperextension injury is the most common cause

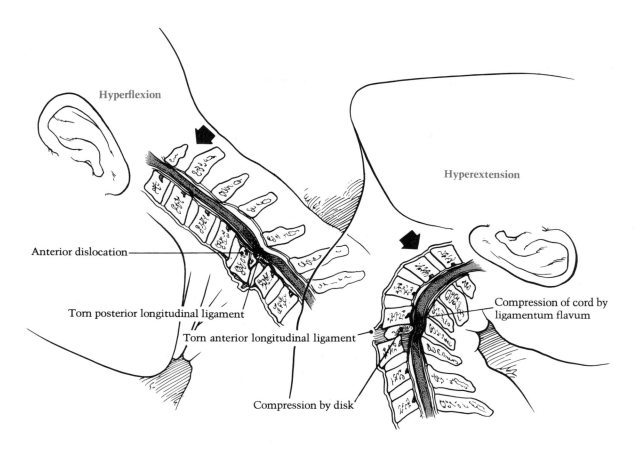

Hyperflexion

Hyperextension

Anterior dislocation

Torn posterior longitudinal ligament

Torn anterior longitudinal ligament

Compression of cord by ligamentum flavum

Compression by disk

Figure 30-5
Mechanism of spinal injury.

of cervical spinal cord injury. In a hyperextension injury, the cord is angulated acutely as the head is bent back sharply. If the direction of the force is significantly downward, varying degrees of compression of the vertebral bodies result. The wedging force may crush one of the adjacent vertebrae, and bony fragments may be driven posteriorly into the spinal canal. Depending on the direction and intensity of the force, there may also be a fracture of the pedicles or laminae. The fracture may be further complicated by forward dislocation of the upper vertebra on the lower if the posterior longitudinal ligament or the articular ligaments are torn. Hyperextension injuries caused by forces applied to the anterior skull or face result in a

stretched anterior longitudinal ligament. If the force is sufficient to carry the upper vertebra backward, the vertebral body above the break may separate from the one below, leaving the disk intact but stripping the posterior longitudinal ligament from the vertebra below. The spinal cord is carried backward with the vertebra above and may be contused against the lamina of the vertebra below. The alignment of the vertebra about the break depends on the type of injury and on how the patient is handled after his injury.

People who have spinal cord injuries often also have a narrow spinal canal and their spinal cord is essentially squeezed. The central cervical cord syndrome may result. Characteristically, the spinal cord lesion is incomplete; the arms, especially the hands, are more involved than are the legs. The loss of sensory function varies. A common injury occurs when the person falls and strikes his head, extending it backward; the hallmark is a bruise on the forehead.

Severity of Spinal Trauma

Cervical spine fractures do not necessarily cause a neurological deficit. The more severe and extensive the fracture, the more likely the person is to have a neurological deficit. Likewise, the greater the amount of subluxation, the more likely the person is to have a neurological deficit. In patients who have congenitally narrow spinal canals with or without spinal spondylosis, spinal cord injury and a neurological deficit may be present, even in the absence of fracture or subluxation. Relatively small degrees of subluxation in a narrowed area may cause severe and irreversible damage.

Fracture dislocations characterized by bony displacement in which the interarticular joints have been subluxed and the pedicles broken do not usually cause spinal cord compression. The presence of subluxations may be attributed to the facts that the spinal cord takes up a considerably smaller cross-sectional area than does its surrounding vertebral canal and that as the fracture separates, the canal may widen and take more room.

Thoracolumbar fractures are much less of a problem for the following reasons: (1) the cord becomes smaller as it approaches the end in the conus medullarus, and so the amount of free space is much larger, (2) the conus is more likely than the higher, more proximal areas of the spinal cord to recover, and (3) peripheral nerves are involved in the lumbar area.

The severity of the spinal injury varies according to the degree of pathology produced. The cord can look normal at surgery but the patient can have no function. There may be a simple contusion (bruising), laceration (tearing), and/or compression due to fracture dislocation and subluxation. If the cord has been contused, swelling occurs within the tough, inelastic pia with subsequent partial or complete interruption of conduction. Anatomical transection is exceedingly rare. The swelling increases for 48 hours and gradually subsides in a week.

Spinal cord compression abolishes all functions below the segment compressed. Ischemia to a cord segment that lasts for an hour produces irreversible infarctions, mainly in the gray matter. If the onset of the cord compression is slow, the deficit is seen first in the pyramidal tract and posterior columns. The deficit is manifested by loss of motor function and joint position; loss of pin sensation from spinothalamic dysfunction is temporally the last modality to be affected in spinal cord compression. Neurosurgical decompression can sometimes halt and even reverse the process.

Studies suggest that mechanical trauma severe enough to produce paralysis initiates a process in the spinal cord tissues that destroys the spinal cord parenchyma in 24 to 48 hours [4]. A biphasic phenomenon in blood flow to regions of the cord has been described in which perfusion to the center of the spinal cord is severely decreased while perfusion to the surrounding white matter is severely increased. Thus vessels and tissues that are unable to survive profound hypoxia become necrotic [37]. The microvasculature is the most trauma-sensitive tissue in the cord.

Spinal Shock

Spinal shock occurs with acute physiological or anatomical spinal cord transection; it results in sympathetic collapse, paralysis, anesthesia, areflexia, and the loss of sphincter function below the level of the lesion. Spinal shock may last up to six weeks; it ends when the reflexes are regained. At that point, the reflexes are generally hyperactive or spastic. The shock state appears to be due to loss of facilitation from descending tracts, inhibition of spinal segments, and degeneration of the axons. Corticospinal and reticulospinal stimuli no longer reach either the part of the trunk that is below the lesion or the extremities. The patient does not lose consciousness, but he displays a flaccid paralysis accompanied by a loss of sensation and reflexes in the involved parts. Vasomotor control is lost in the periphery since the reflex pathways in the spinal cord are cut. Blood then pools in the extremities.

In complete lesions of the spinal cord, neurological deficits below the level of the lesion include complete flaccid paralysis, total loss of sensation, loss of sweating below the level of the lesion, and paralysis of the bowel and bladder. The duration of spinal shock depends on the extent of injury to the spinal cord. If the cord is completely transected, spinal shock may last several weeks. After that period, the tendon reflexes become hyperactive, with marked clonus. Retention of urine is common when reflex activity returns because the sphincter recovers before the detrusor muscle. The leg muscles particularly show varying degrees of spasticity, mainly the extensors. Damage is considered to be functionally complete and permanent if the patient has an immediate motor and sensory paralysis that lasts for 24 hours. However, since reflexes below the injury are not operant in the presence of spinal shock, a complete lesion is not considered permanent until the return of the bulbocavernosus perineal reflex.

In incomplete spinal cord lesions, the period of spinal shock is shorter. The deep and superficial reflexes return in days or weeks. Sensation gradually returns. Motor function may return in varying degrees, and depending on the severity of the injury, it may be asymmetrical.

Determination of Spinal Cord Injury

Patients who have severe trauma are carefully assessed for spinal fracture and spinal cord injury. In particular, patients with chest and/or abdominal trauma, head injury, hematuria, and/or facial injuries are suspected of having sustained a cervical spinal injury.

The main symptom of spinal fracture is local pain that may radiate into the arms, thorax, abdomen, or legs. If the patient is in pain, he should not be moved until he is examined by the medical team. With the patient supine, the examiner should slip his hand underneath the patient and palpate the spine for displacement, crepitus, and abnormal mobility. Other examinations are done as indicated, and the appropriate x rays are then ordered by the physician.

Assessment of spinal cord damage entails examination for motor and sensory abnormalities, changes in reflexes, and autonomic alterations. Initially, the patient is observed for diaphragmatic breathing, flexion of his forearms across his chest, and a decreased blood pressure without other signs of shock. Spinal cord functioning is assessed by noting the patient's ability to move his extremities, his ability to respond to a pinprick on his hands and feet, his response to reflex stimulation, and the tone of his rectal sphincter. Muscle weakness may indicate cord damage. In the patient who has an altered level of consciousness, the presence of spinal cord injury is determined by a reduced or absent motor response to a deep pain stimulus. For example, facial grimaces may be noted when stimuli are applied above the clavicle but not when they are applied below the clavicle.

The key signs of damage to the various levels of the spinal cord are as follows [14, 15]:

1. C2-to-C3 vertebral level
   a. Respiratory paralysis (the outcome is probably death)
   b. Flaccid paralysis
   c. Areflexia (the patient who has complete areflexia that lasts longer than 24 hours has almost no chance of recovery)
   d. Loss of sensation below the level of the mandible
2. C5-to-C6 vertebral level
   a. Diaphragmatic breathing
   b. Paralysis of the intercostal and abdominal muscles
   c. Quadriplegia (shoulder girdle functioning and a minimal amount of deltoid, pectoral, and biceps functioning may remain, but motor power is essentially lost below the shoulder level)
   d. Anesthesia below the clavicle and anesthesia of the ulnar half of the arms
   e. Areflexia, with the possible exception of the biceps reflex
   f. Fecal and urinary retention
   g. Priapism
3. T12-to-L1 vertebral level
   a. Paraplegia
   b. Anesthesia in the legs
   c. Areflexia in the legs (the upper abdominal reflexes may be present)
   d. Fecal and urinary retention
   e. Priapism
4. L1-to-L5 vertebral level
   a. Flaccid paralysis to partial flaccid paralysis
   b. Abdominal and cremasteric reflexes present
   c. Ankle and plantar reflexes absent

The functional level is the level of the lowest nerve root that demonstrates muscle function. Muscle strength is graded on a scale of 0 to 4; grade 4 refers to good muscle strength manifested by complete motion against gravity and some resistance. Muscle innervations below the level of the injury are either paralyzed or weaker. The level of injury is determined by noting the lowest level of innervation that is functioning. In cervical spinal injury, the key muscles to determine particular functional levels are as follows:

1. C4 functional level: neck and upper trapezius
2. C5 functional level: weak deltoids and biceps

3. C6 functional level: strong deltoids and biceps, wrist extensors
4. C7 functional level: wrist flexors, pronators, and weak triceps
5. C8 functional level: finger flexors

The results of the assessment of spinal cord injury should be recorded in three ways:

1. At the fracture level, which is determined by x ray.
2. At the neurological level, or the lowest dermatome where there is impaired or intact sensation and/or where there is some degree of muscle function.
3. At the functional level (that is, at the level of the lowest key muscle in which there is a "good" grade). That applies only to complete injuries [25].

The x-ray examination is specific, and it is dictated by the findings. For example, with patients who are unconscious or who are suspected of having a cervical injury, the physician orders initial lateral x rays that include C7 and T1. (Taking anteroposterior x rays requires lifting and/or moving the patient, a dangerous undertaking unless the personnel are trained.) Following the lateral x rays, the neurosurgeon may order other x rays.

The changes found on both sides of the body at the level of the injury and below following hemisection of the cord above the midlumbar region have been named the Brown-Séquard syndrome. Incomplete forms of the syndrome also occur. Common findings below the level of injury are ipsilateral loss of motor ability, position, light touch, vibration, and contralateral loss of pain and temperature sensory modalities [16].

Treatment of Spinal Injury

In the presence of spinal damage, the patient is kept flat on a spinal board, handled carefully (to prevent undue motion), and lifted by at least three people. The patient who possibly has a thoracic or lumbar spinal injury is kept supine with a small pad under his spine at the site of injury. The patient who has a possible cervical spinal injury is immobilized by sand bags, neck bracing, or collar (to prevent flexion and rotation) or by cervical traction. Skeletal traction may be employed, using Crutchfield tongs or other modifications, such as Cone, Gardner-Wells, or Vinke skull

calipers. For stabilization in nondisplaced injuries, 5 to 10 lb of traction is used, and for reduction of a dislocation, 10 to 15 lb is used. Also, the head of the bed or turning frame may be elevated six inches to provide countertraction with the weight of the patient.

The traditional procedure for patients with penetrating wounds of the spine has been exploratory laminectomy. But because of the associated blood loss and increased potential for infection, many neurosurgeons have challenged that procedure. Those neurosurgeons think that exploration is not necessarily appropriate unless (1) the missile is near the site of an operation done for another reason, (2) the missile has gone through the bowel and is contaminated, (3) the missile is loose and can move within the spine and thus do additional damage, or (4) the missile is copper-jacketed and thus toxic to the nervous system. With blunt trauma, the neurosurgeon chooses the conservative approach under normal circumstances. A few medical centers use laminectomy with cooling in acute cord injury [6].

The outlook for recovery from spinal cord injury is very poor for patients who have complete paralysis that lasts longer than six hours. For patients with incomplete lesions, the prognosis varies. Generally sensory loss is recovered better than motor loss. Many people with the Brown-Séquard syndrome recover.

For patients with permanent cervical cord involvements, the outlook for a rewarding life is poor unless the rehabilitation program is successful. In particular, pulmonary problems are eminent. A patient who has a lesion above C4 is not likely to survive the initial stage because of breathing problems. Pulmonary embolism is common. Pneumonia is an ever-present threat; the higher the lesion, the more likely it is that the patient will develop pneumonia. Urinary tract infections are common, as are decubitus ulcers and bacteremia. (It is extremely rare for a paralyzed patient who develops a decubitus ulcer to be successfully rehabilitated.) Many patients die from kidney disease because their long-term urinary tract dysfunction requires urinary catheterization and results in infection and/or stones. Since such patients are unable to reverse their catabolic state, many die from malnutrition. Suicide is not infrequent since readjustment is extremely difficult and the divorce rate is high.

The challenges to the nurses are great. Nurses who incorporate rehabilitation principles into their patient care and who work in coordination with other health team members may bring the patient to his highest level of functioning, and thus help him become a contributing member of society.

Assessment

The outcome of severe head injury is determined primarily by the severity of the initial injury, and it is modified by the subsequent assessment and management of the neurosurgical team. Initially, whether at the scene of the accident or in the emergency room, the patient must be assessed for any life-threatening condition. He may have an obstructed airway, an open chest injury, or a severe hemorrhage. His level of consciousness may be decreased. A sign of neurological dysfunction, such as a dilated pupil or unconsciousness, also indicates an emergency. In a closed head injury, once the pupil dilates, herniation will soon follow (unless the patient has had a direct injury to the eye or a direct brain stem injury). The cause of unconsciousness must be ascertained (e.g., hypoxia, shock, drug or alcohol ingestion, hypoglycemia, or head injury). The cause is not always easy to determine, and the condition may have a number of causes. Often a patient is brought into the emergency room after having been drinking and then involved in an automobile accident. If the patient exhibits decreasing levels of consciousness, it is difficult to determine to what degree his condition is caused by alcohol and to what degree it is caused by the head injury (see Fig. 4-2).

History

The history is very important. The first details to be gathered are those of the accident. What happened in the accident? What caused it? What happened afterward? All the circumstances surrounding the accident may be vitally important. What was the person's state of consciousness before, during, and after the accident? (For example, was he unconscious and then conscious?) Did he hit his head? Did he have convulsions? Does his past history point to any significant preexisting problems?

Baseline Examination

The initial examination is the emergency examination (A, B, C, D—the basic approach of cardiopulmo-

nary resuscitation). The patient's respirations should be easy, even, and near a normal rate. If his respirations are deep, irregular, or slow, the team should be alert to the possibility of head injury. The patient's pulse should be regular and normal to fast. Hemorrhagic shock is not caused by intracranial bleeding since the amount of cerebral bleeding is not sufficient to cause the signs and symptoms of shock; it indicates another problem. Only rarely (and usually only in children) is hemorrhagic shock due to a scalp laceration. Most patients with head injuries who are in shock also have a thoracoabdominal injury or a fractured pelvis.

A spinal fracture, discussed earlier in the chapter, must always be considered. Examination of the head may reveal significant bleeding or an open skull fracture. Drainage from the nose or ear may be bloody. A bruise over the mastoid area (Battle's sign) should alert the team to a possible basilar fracture. Palpation must be done gently since further neurological damage can be caused by pressure on skull fragments.

The baseline neurological examination is like that for all neurosurgical patients (see Chap. 11). The patient's level of consciousness and respiratory pattern must be assessed and followed. The patient's respiratory pattern may be normal. The abnormal patterns are Cheyne-Stokes, central neurogenic hyperventilation, apneustic, or ataxic. Central neurogenic hyperventilation is not common and must often be differentiated from a similar pattern, one that is produced by a chest injury. That pattern is often not neurological but a response to a ventilatory problem. It must be monitored closely since overbreathing lowers the PCO_2 (respiratory alkalosis) and reflexly results in cerebral vasoconstriction (decreased cerebral blood flow). Although hyperventilation with the PCO_2 maintained at 20 to 30 mm Hg is the treatment of choice for increased ICP, arterial tension levels below 20 mm Hg are dangerous.

Examination of the eyes consists of noting pupillary size and reactivity, the ciliospinal reflex, eye movements, and the oculocephalic and oculovestibular reflexes. The pupillary signs are of utmost importance. Widely dilated pupils produced by third cranial nerve compression are an ominous sign and indicate impending brain stem injury. Funduscopic examination helps to assess hemorrhages and preexisting disease as well as to establish a baseline (papilledema is not usually apparent for 36 to 72 hours). Eye signs give valuable information about the person's status. A rule of thumb is, If there is a difference in eye signs and motor signs, rely on the eye signs.

Motor signs help one to focus on the neurological problems. Noting the movements of the face and extremities is followed by an appraisal of the reflexes. In addition, cranial nerve functioning must be evaluated and any focal problem must be thoroughly assessed.

In the event of increased ICP, serial determinations must be done to monitor the patient. Ninety to 95 percent of patients with closed head injuries do not require an intracranial procedure. The initial accurate neurological examination is only the first in a succession of examinations. The trend in the patient's condition is most important. The patient's level of consciousness is the best sign of his neurological status. Complete, concise, accurate, and descriptive standard terminology must be used in evaluating changes.

Emergency laboratory measurements commonly used are baseline blood tests (complete blood count, typing and crossmatching, blood sugar, blood urea nitrogen, and serum electrolyte tests) and urine tests (for sugar, acetone, protein, and formed elements). Arterial blood gas levels must be determined and monitored.

Additional Studies

Skull and chest x rays, radioactive brain scans, cerebral angiograms, echoencephalograms, electroencephalograms, CT scans, and/or monitoring of ICP may be done.

For head injuries, skull x rays and, perhaps, cervical spinal x rays are ordered by the physician. If the patient is unconscious, lateral cervical spinal x rays are mandatory. X rays of the skull are helpful if the pineal gland is calcified since a shift from its midline position signifies that a mass is present. However, the pineal gland is usually not calcified until after the age of 40, and most patients with head injury are younger than 40 years of age. Also, a depressed skull fracture (or fractures) that transverses the arterial vessel grooves in the skull (the middle meningeal artery), a foreign body, and/or air in the skull (resulting from a tear in the coverings of the brain) may be demonstrated on x rays. In the event of additional trauma, an x-ray evaluation of the appropriate area is made.

Carotid angiography, a very useful tool, is a specific neurodiagnostic technique. If time permits, the procedure is essential for accurate location of the prob-

lem. Although angiography has been largely superseded by CT scanning, it will certainly provide useful diagnostic information when CT scanning is not possible.

Echoencephalography can define the midline position; it is used by some physicians to indicate the presence of a localizing mass lesion [51]. It is hard to keep people on the staff who are properly trained to do the studies. The procedure is not considered consistently reliable. Also, there may be trauma to the scalp, particularly in the temporal region, which may disturb the echo midline. The procedure is rarely used, and many major neurosurgical units have abandoned it.

Electroencephalography is used only under rare circumstances and its primary value for comatose patients remains the evaluation of the coma.

CT scanning for head-injured patients, the newest noninvasive technique, is a breakthrough in radiological technology. In CT scanning the entire brain is routinely visualized. An antilog picture is obtained by the emission of x rays through the head to a densitometer. The scanner is moved in increments of two degrees, and the process is repeated again and again. The result is a digital computer printout of the x-ray densities of tissues that gives a picture of the part of the body through which the x-ray beam was passed. Anything that is in the way of the beam, such as blood (iron) or bone (calcium), alters the densities. Various lesions can be identified as a function of their densities, nature, and appearance (Fig. 30-6). Now commonly used in emergencies—and considered by many to be the procedure of choice—a CT scan series can be completed in a short time and with minimal radiation exposure. Also, the patient may be monitored before and after therapy and the densities can be measured to determine the effectiveness of the scanning and to visualize any new lesions.

Monitoring Intracranial Pressure

Detailed clinical observation is still the forte of assessment and management, but the development of the technique to measure ICP directly aids in diagnosing, prognosing, managing, and monitoring the patient's condition. Direct measurement of ICP is now possible. There are many measurement techniques, but there are also problems. The most important problem is the lack of consensus among authorities about the extent to which pressure is transmitted

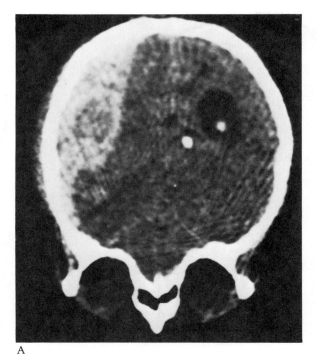

A

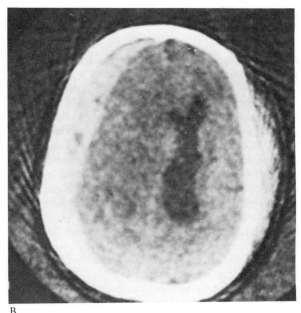

B

Figure 30-6
A. Epidural hematoma shown on a CT scan. B. Subdural hematoma shown on a CT scan.

across the dura and between the intracranial compartments.

MEASUREMENT

Monitoring systems are based on simple principles. Initially, a type of energy (pressure or electrical activity) must be evaluated. Some means is then developed to transmit and perhaps convert this energy so that it can be measured. ICP monitoring equipment consists of a transducer, a sensor (a moveable diaphragm, a balloon, a solid state probe, or a fluid column), and a recording device. It is particularly important that the system does not become even partly blocked, since the pressure recording will be damaged or lost.

The ICP can be monitored in several ways, often by ventricular catheterization or by a screw placed in the subarachnoid space. Ventricular catheterization involves the insertion of a catheter into the lateral cerebral ventricle through a small burr hole; it permits pressure monitoring, cerebrospinal fluid sampling and draining, ventriculography, and the administration of drugs [18] (Fig. 30-7). In trauma, it requires cannulation of a small, swollen, and possibly shifted ventricle. The procedure is particularly useful for monitoring during surgery since problems with ventilation or positioning can thus be quickly identified and assessed. Postoperatively, the catheter is useful for ventricular draining, detection of a hematoma, monitoring of the patency of a shunt, and identification of intracranial hypertension. The major disadvantage—threat of infection—is significantly reduced if the catheter does not remain in place longer than three days.

Mainly because of the problems with infection and with accurate stabilization of the ventricular catheter, the subarachnoid and epidural techniques have been developed. The subarachnoid technique using the Richmond screw (bolt) [48] is perhaps the more popular. In that technique, the ICP is monitored by means of a sensor and a transducer, and the output of the transducer is displayed on the oscilloscope or on a digital pressure-reading device. The tip of a hollow screw is placed in the subarachnoid space so that pressure recordings are obtained intermittently or continuously. The proximal end of the screw consists of a Luer-Lok and a hexagonal collar for insertion. The distal thread fits a 1/4-in. twist drill hole made through a 1-cm incision. The screw is connected to a stopcock assembly through a saline-filled extension tube. Then the transducer is opened to the subarachnoid space

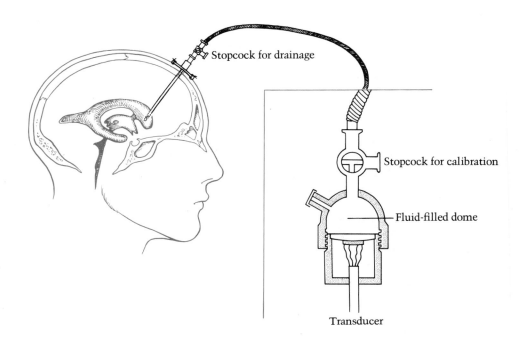

Stopcock for drainage

Stopcock for calibration

Fluid-filled dome

Transducer

and a calibrated ICP reading is taken. Isovolumetric measurements can be made because of the use of the transducer.

Figure 30-7
Ventricular catheterization.

EVALUATION OF ICP MEASUREMENTS

In regard to outcome criteria, the ICP levels are not as significant as are the clinical signs of severe cerebral and brain stem dysfunction. The ICP levels are of value in patients with diffuse brain damage; the higher the patient's ICP on his admission, the greater his risk of developing recurrent or persistent hypertension. In patients with purposeful motor responses, persistent ICP elevation is associated with a poorer outcome.

Intraventricular pressures between 0 and 10 mm Hg are generally regarded as normal. There is no agreement about whether 10 mm Hg, 15 mm Hg, or 20 mm Hg is the mean-level threshold for intracranial hypertension. The indication for treating increased ICP generally is a sustained increase to over 30 mm Hg or any increase that is associated with neurological deterioration. Unless arterial blood gas alterations or head and body position changes are determined to be the cause of the increase, the treatment usually consists of further hyperventilation by increasing the tidal volume, using closed drainage,

and/or administering intravenous mannitol intermittently or continuously.

Pressure waves (or fluctuations in the ICP) are spontaneous waves produced by systemic problems, such as an alteration in the arterial blood gases [27, 29]. Plateau (alpha) waves usually arise from an elevated ICP baseline and are probably caused by changes in cerebral blood volumes. They are rapid, spontaneous increases in pressure followed by rapid decreases accompanied by a temporary increase in neurological deficit. The plateau waves are more likely to occur when ICP is already elevated; they may increase to 50 to 115 mm Hg and usually last 5 to 20 minutes.

As pressure increases, blood circulation is eventually slowed and systemic blood pressure must be raised to maintain intracranial perfusion. The pulse slows, and the pulse pressure widens. The respirations are usually slow and deep. Breathing becomes irregular as the patient's condition worsens. The blood supply to the brain is finally cut off, and the respirations cease (Fig. 30-8). But although a rising systolic pressure, a widening pulse pressure, and a

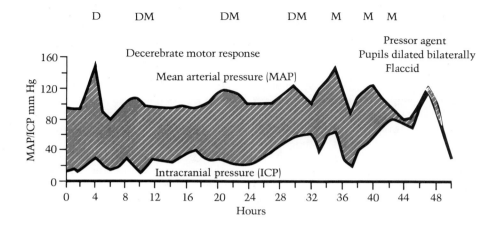

Figure 30-8
Progression of intracranial hypertension. Despite treatment with ventricular drainage and mannitol, cerebral perfusion decreased and the patient died. D = ventricular drainage; M = mannitol.

slow, pounding pulse are important indicators of increasing ICP, they do not necessarily correlate with the actual measurements of increased ICP. The only way to assess the intracranial pressure accurately is to measure it directly.

Management

A significant percentage of all patients admitted with head injuries also have systemic injuries, and so their management must include both their head injuries and their systemic injuries. Adequate perfusion of the injured brain is needed both to minimize morbidity and to increase the patient's chances of surviving. If the mean arterial pressure declines or if the ICP rises, the cerebral perfusion pressure falls. Thus the mean arterial pressure must be maintained at normotensive levels in patients who have multiple injuries. The morbidity and mortality of patients with head injuries who are hypotensive on admission are two to three times higher than the morbidity and mortality of patients with head injuries who are not hypotensive on admission. All possible measures must be taken to prevent increased ICP as a result of intracranial hematomas or swollen brain tissue.

Since initially it is not possible to determine clini-

cally whether a patient with a severe head injury has an increased ICP, it is assumed that he has, and he is managed accordingly. The neurosurgical resuscitation measures are described in the following paragraphs.

Intubation is often performed and hyperventilation measures are taken so that the patient does not become hypoxic or hypercarbic. Hypercarbia is a potent cerebral vasodilator, and when the intracranial blood vessels are dilated, the ICP can increase markedly. Conversely, with hypocarbia induced by hyperventilation, cerebral vasoconstriction will occur with a rapid decrease in the ICP. Hyperventilation increases the cerebral metabolic rate of oxygen. Thus intubation and hyperventilation are used to maintain the patient's arterial carbon dioxide levels at about 25 mm Hg (the range is 20–30 mm Hg).

To decrease brain water and thus brain volume in patients suspected of having increased ICP, 500 ml of a 20% mannitol solution is given intravenously for 30 minutes. ICP decreases rapidly, and a patient who has a dilated pupil frequently has constriction of that pupil as his brain is dehydrated and his ICP returns to more normal levels. Mannitol is contraindicated in a patient who is hypotensive on admission since his intravascular volume must be maintained.

Efforts are made to keep the ICP levels below 15 mm Hg. Often mannitol must be infused in 25-to-50-gm boluses every 4 to 6 hours as indicated. Since mannitol can cause renal failure when serum osmolality is elevated significantly (usually to levels above 340–350 mOsm), the serum sodium levels and the indices of renal function have to be monitored. Mannitol is customarily not administered to any patient whose serum sodium level is greater than 155 mEq per liter.

Also, spinal fluid is drained to decrease the ICP. The stopcock attached to the monitoring system is turned so that the spinal fluid drains into a closed system.

The patient is best positioned with his neck in a neutral position and the head of his bed elevated 30 to 45 degrees. The jugular venous pressure and, in turn, the ICP are thus reduced.

Control of temperature is important since the patient is thermolabile because he has a brain stem injury, blood in his subarachnoid space, increased heat production with decerebration, and/or a central nervous system infection. Hyperthermia greatly increases the cerebral edema and thus the ICP, and it increases the cerebral metabolism at a time when the tissue viability is borderline. Hyperthermia control should be instituted whenever the temperature rises to 38°C (101°F) or greater. If hyperthermia control is not instituted until the temperature has reached higher levels, the hyperthermia is much more difficult to control. The use of aspirin or Tylenol in appropriate doses and a hypothermia blanket is effective. Hyperthermic patients should have their temperatures lowered to normothermic (not hypothermic) levels. Injections of intramuscular thorazine (10 mg) may help to lower an elevated temperature. Thorazine, an alpha-adrenergic blocking drug, causes peripheral vasodilatation, which helps dissipate heat and prevents or reduces the shivering sometimes seen in hypothermia. (The shivering tends to retard the lowering of body temperature.)

Patients with severe decerebrate spasms accompanied by a significantly increased ICP may be helped by the administration of muscle relaxants. Intravenous morphine or drugs that exert a blocking effect at the myoneural junction (e.g., pancuronium bromide) are the drugs of choice.

The administration of steroids to patients with severe head injuries is controversial. Many studies of the effectiveness or noneffectiveness of steroid therapy are being done.

Complications

PULMONARY PROBLEMS

Pulmonary problems occur often, and frequently are lethal. Monitoring of arterial blood gas levels and of the other pulmonary parameters is very important. Decreased consciousness brings the threat of hypoxemia and hypercapnia. Aspiration is always possible.

Alterations in respiratory function may be caused by cerebral or pulmonary injury. Loss of the sighing mechanism leads to microatelectasis (secondary to a decrease in pulmonary surfactant). Patients so affected tend to breathe at the same tidal volume, and atelectasis results in nonventilated portions of the lung that continue to be perfused so that ventilation-perfusion abnormalities arise. The venous admixture results in right-to-left shunts, systemic hypoxemia, and an increased PCO_2. A problem that can compound the situation is a rapid reduction in PCO_2 since the cerebral vessel will constrict and decreased amounts of oxygen will be available.

Another cause of alterations in respiratory function is that neurogenic stimuli open pulmonary arteriovenous shunts that bypass the alveoli. In animal studies, following a head injury, prophylaxis with various sympatholytic antiepinephrine and general anesthetics (but not isoproterenol or atropine) prevents pulmonary complications and thus suggests that there is a neuroendocrine influence on pulmonary surfactant and compliance [1]. Also, increased ICP and brain compression, although uncommon, may cause acute pulmonary edema [26]. The cause has not been identified, but it may be pulmonary vein constriction or left heart failure. The two most critical periods are the admission period and the first two postoperative days. As a rule of thumb, a decrease in PO_2 to below 70 mm Hg is an indication for endotracheal intubation [45].

FLUID AND ELECTROLYTE PROBLEMS

Fluid and electrolyte problems are potential complications [19]. Usually only maintenance fluids are required, and the patient is kept dry. With the breakdown of the blood brain barrier at the capillary endothelial level, edema fluid passes into the brain parenchyma. Excess intravenous fluid enhances edema formation, negates the effects of mannitol, and produces increases in the ICP. If the 24-hour urinary output and the laboratory values (serum electrolytes, blood urea nitrogen, and creatinine levels, and the hematocrit) are normal, 1500 to 2000 ml of fluid is usually administered (Ringer's lactate solution or half-normal saline solution). Patients who have a fever, third space loss, and/or excessive movement require increased fluids. The use of dehydrating drugs to control cerebral swelling has not been well defined. Although a rebound effect may occur after administration of hyperosmotic agents, the immediate situation must be considered a critical event. The use of hyperosmotic agents is based on the idea that if the osmolarity of the blood is increased to a higher level than that of the tissues, fluid will move out of the brain tissue into the blood and subsequently be excreted in the urine. However, some of the hypertonic agent enters the brain parenchyma. As the blood is cleared of the hypertonic agent, the hypertonic agent that has entered the brain cells causes the cells to be hypertonic relative to the brain. The result is that fluid moves into the cells, producing cellular swelling (i.e., rebound swelling). Agents such as mannitol or glycerol are used, and they are supplemented with furosemide [38].

The hypothalamus and the posterior pituitary may be damaged, causing a decreased secretion of antidiuretic hormone and resulting in diabetes insipidus. The urinary output is quite high, even several liters per hour, and the specific gravity and osmolar concentration are low. Diabetes insipidus is considered to be the diagnosis when the urine cannot be concentrated to greater than 1.005 and the 24-hour urinary output is more than 4000 ml. Since the water loss is great, hypernatremia is a threat.

Since polyuria may result from many conditions (i.e., sodium loss, adrenal insufficiency, water diuresis, fluid overload, osmotic diuresis, or elevated blood glucose levels), a dehydration test is often done [8]. The patient is not permitted fluids during the night, and blood and urine specimens are obtained from 3 A.M. to 6 A.M. The patient with antidiuretic hormone insufficiency exhibits a low urine osmolality and is evaluated as follows: If he is alert and thirsty and has mild polyuria, he can probably maintain his fluid balance by drinking. If he is alert but his urinary output is greater than 250 ml per hour or if the patient is not alert and is not thirsty, aqueous pitressin (2–5 units subcutaneously) is usually ordered [44]. Fluid replacement matches urinary output, and 700 to 1000 ml additional replacement is given for insensible water loss. The fluids are replaced with a 5% dextrose in water solution (1000 ml/24 hr) given with Ringer's lactate solution since the urine is low in electrolytes. Fluid balance and electrolyte levels must be assessed serially.

On the other hand, antidiuretic hormone secretion may be inappropriately increased, resulting in water retention and dilutional hypovolemia. The mechanisms involved are an increased glomerular filtration rate, volume expansion, suppression of renin-angiotensin-aldosterone secretion, and decreased distal tubular sodium reabsorption, all of which result in increased sodium excretion. Clinically, the patient has renal sodium excretion associated with hypovolemia, normal thyroid-renal-adrenal functioning, a lack of peripheral edema, a lack of the signs of volume depletion, and an increased urine osmolality that is inconsistent with the plasma hypotonicity. If the serum sodium levels are below 120 mEq per liter, the patient may exhibit the cerebral signs of irritability, confusion, lethargy, or even psychosis. If the serum sodium levels are below 110 mEq per liter, the patient may have convulsions. Therapy usually is water restriction or administration of 500 ml normal saline daily. If convulsions occur or if severe hyponatremia is present, the therapy usually is the administration of a 3% to 5% hypertonic saline solution and mannitol or furosemide for free-water clearance. If the condition becomes chronic, the physician may order demeclocycline to inhibit antidiuretic action at the renal tubular site.

GASTRIC BLEEDING

Cushing's ulcers are probably caused by marked hypersecretion of gastric acid [8, 20]. In patients with severe head injuries resulting in coma and (particularly) in decerebrate rigidity, the degree of gastric hyperacidity correlates roughly with the amount of gastric bleeding, approximating the levels attained in the Zollinger-Ellison syndrome [30, 49]. The hypothesis that the hyperacidity is the result of direct stimulation of the vagal nuclei by increased ICP has been supported by the fact that the routine administration of parenteral anticholinergics blocked and reduced gastric acid secretion and essentially prevented the syndrome [34, 50]. Also, with the advent of prophylactic antacid therapy and cimetidine therapy, bleeding rarely occurs. It is considered almost a complication of the past.

EPILEPSY

Early (i.e., a seizure occurring in the first week after injury) traumatic epilepsy occurs in approximately five percent of patients who have head injuries that are not caused by missiles [19]. Even a mild seizure indicates that the patient will probably have more seizures and that he has significant brain damage. A consistent finding reported in the literature is that one of the most important contributing factors in traumatic epilepsy is a depressed skull fracture. In a series of 1000 patients who had depressed skull fractures not caused by missiles, the incidence of late (i.e., occurring after the first week after the injury) epilepsy was 15% with a wide variance in risk of onset in individual patients [18]. Yet identification of the high-risk group is extremely important since the seizures tend to recur. In the study, the risk tended to be greatest in patients with posttraumatic amnesia (the interval between the injury and the return of continuous memory prolonged more than 24 hours) and was associated with extensive local damage (tearing of the dura or focal signs) and early epilepsy. If the injury was missile-induced, prolonged coma was an important criterion for determining the extent of local damage. The prophylactic use of anticonvulsants for traumatic epilepsy seems to be beneficial.

ADDITIONAL PROBLEMS

A carotid cavernous sinus fistula can form. The carotid artery itself can be torn, resulting in an arteriovenous fistula. A particular danger is an increase in intraocular pressure leading to narrow angle glaucoma and blindness.

Other possible problems, particularly for the unconscious patient, are pulmonary complications, thrombi, pulmonary embolism, decubitus ulcer, and urinary tract infections.

Many problems occur after the initial danger is past. The Glasgow outcome score may be used for assessment. With it, the patient is classified as having made a good recovery, being moderately disabled, being severely disabled, being vegetative, or as dead [18]. Personality changes may occur. Sexual dysfunction (e.g., impotence) and dysmenorrhea occur often. It is hypothesized that those problems are secondary to energy forces directed toward deep midline structures, such as the hypothalamus [10]. Focal neurological deficits are dependent on the site of the injury and on the nerve involvement. Intelligence can be decreased, depending on the severity of the injury. For example, it is not unusual that an engineer resumes his working life as a draftsman.

Often postconcussion syndrome occurs for up to two years, and even for the rest of the patient's life. It is characterized by the loss of memory, dizziness, headaches, decreased concentration, and insomnia. Some authorities think that postconcussion syndrome has a psychological element while others think that it is purely physical.

Nursing Orders

Problem/Diagnosis

Closed head injury due to significant head trauma due to fall.

OBJECTIVE NO. 1

The patient should demonstrate stable vital signs, his intracranial or intraspinal swelling should be reduced, and any further injury to him should be prevented during his prehospital phase.

To achieve the objective, the nurse should be able to:

1. Perform the primary survey.
2. Obtain and maintain a patent airway. The nurse should:
   a. Since the incidence of associated spinal injury is significant, use the jaw thrust–chin lift maneuver.
   b. Use an oral airway and an esophageal airway as indicated.
   c. Ventilate the patient with 24 breaths per minute with a bag mask to decrease his arterial carbon dioxide tension and thus his intracerebral pressure.
3. Maintain the patient's circulation. The nurse should:
   a. Unless near an acute care unit, establish an intravenous route with a large-bore catheter.
   b. Monitor the patient's vital signs.
4. If the patient is unconscious, assume that he has a spinal injury.
5. Perform the secondary survey.
6. Take a history of the accident, noting the length of time the patient was unconscious, the presence or absence of seizures, hemiparesis, and urinary incontinence, and the pertinent past medical details.
7. Perform a baseline assessment, and continue to monitor:
   a. Level of consciousness (including Glasgow coma scale).

b. Pupillary size, equality, reaction to light, and position.
c. Motor responses (to pain, command, reflexes).
d. Protective reflexes (cough, gag, lash).
e. Respiratory pattern.
f. Vital signs.
g. Extraocular movements (doll's eyes and calorics).

8. Institute the appropriate protocols for associated trauma.
9. Start an intravenous infusion of Ringer's lactate solution if the patient is hypotensive or if there is not a hospital within 30 minutes' traveling time.
10. Cover any open wounds with sterile pressure dressings.
11. Not attempt to stop rhinorrhea or otorrhea.
12. Assume that a spinal injury is present if the patient has any problem moving his extremities and perceiving pain and/or touch sensations. The nurse should:
   a. Monitor the patient's vital signs.
   b. Have a high index of suspicion of associated injury.
   c. Record the baseline data.
   d. Immobilize the patient so that he can be taken to the hospital in the position of injury.
   e. Prevent any motion of his spine.
   f. Stabilize his neck and his head by the use of a backboard.
   g. Avoid hypoventilation.
13. En route to the hospital, monitor his vital signs often and take measures to prevent aspiration.

OBJECTIVE NO. 2

The initial assessment and management should include obtaining baseline data, listing priorities, and beginning treatment.

To achieve the objective, the nurse, in association with other health team members, should:

1. Initially assess the patient for any type of life-threatening trauma, such as an obstructed airway or a hemorrhage, perform oral or nasotracheal intubation as needed, assess the patient's cardiopulmonary status, and consider the possibility of a spinal injury.
2. If a respiratory abnormality or the Cushing triad is present, notify the physician. If the symptoms of shock are present and persist, the cause is probably a hemorrhage (a head injury rarely produces shock) [7].
3. Maintain the arterial oxygen tension at greater than 80 mm Hg.
4. Maintain the arterial carbon dioxide level at 20 to 30 mm Hg.
5. Assume that the patient has a cervical or other type of spinal fracture and treat him accordingly.
6. Determine the serial values and assess the trends.
7. Monitor the vital signs, use the Glasgow coma scale, and note the pupillary responses.
8. Look for open head wounds, bloody drainage from the ears, nose, or posterior pharyngeal wall, blood in the middle ear with an intact eardrum, or Battle's sign. (Manage the patient who has those signs as though he has a basilar or an open skull fracture.)
9. Obtain the relevant historical information about the patient and the accident. Find out about his state of consciousness before, during, and after the accident (especially note any period of unconsciousness), the circumstances surrounding the accident (clues to the amount of force transmitted to the brain and the severity of the injury are often given in a description of the accident), the treatment rendered plus any history of preexisting disease (e.g., cardiovascular or cerebrovascular disease, diabetes, chronic alcoholism, or epilepsy), and any medicine the patient has been taking (e.g., an anticoagulant). While obtaining those data, the nurse should also assess the patient's use of language, his memory, his orientation, and his clarity of speech.
10. Assess the chest and abdomen.
11. Look for fractures, especially of the pelvis, since fractures are the most common cause of shock.
12. Ascertain the level of consciousness (see Chap. 11), taking into account the patient's (a) ability to cooperate, (b) awareness of his environment, and (c) response to questions. The nurse should also take into account the following:
   a. The patient's depth of consciousness can be judged by his reactions to external stimuli on various levels [10].
   b. The patient may be completely unconscious and not respond to external or internal stimuli. Urinary retention is common. Corneal reflexes, the swallowing reflex, and/or some of the tendon reflexes may be present, but they are usually absent in deep coma, which is in-

dicative of severe damage to the brain stem. The patient makes no meaningful response to questions. His bladder empties reflexly when it is distended.

   c. A patient can respond to painful stimuli by:
     (1) Purposeful movements (e.g., grimacing or hand movements to push away the examiner's hand). Purposeful movements are considered defensive.
     (2) Nonpurposeful movements (e.g., a thrust toward the stimulus or some aberrant behavior). Nonpurposeful movements are considered defenseless.
   d. The patient's level of consciousness can be evaluated by describing his behavior, including his spontaneous activity and responses.
   e. The patient's orientation must be determined. The patient may be disoriented in regard to time, place, or person. His thoughts may be suddenly interrupted by inappropriate statements or behavior. In addition to the Glasgow coma scale and a description of consciousness, the following classification [47] is helpful:
     (1) Mild confusion. The patient is capable of coherent conversation, and his behavior is appropriate.
     (2) Moderate confusion. The patient is out of touch with his environment but on some insistence he may respond to simple questions (e.g., about his age or where he lives).
     (3) Severe confusion. The patient is out of touch with his environment, but he is able to follow simple and repeated commands (e.g., "Open your eyes," "Put out your tongue").

13. Assess the patient's respiratory rate, depth, and pattern.

14. Using the following guidelines, assess the pupillary size and reactivity and the eye movements:
   a. Pupils: size, position, reactivity, and consensual response
   b. Eye movements: spontaneous movements and doll's head response
   c. Mild injury: pupils equal, react to light, conjugate gaze, resistant to forced opening
   d. More serious injury: absent or deviant reactivity, fixed gaze with dilatation, lack of response

15. Assess the patient's skeletal responses. The nurse should compare the strength in the patient's right side to the strength in his left side and the strength in his arms to the strength in his legs. The following comparison should also be made on both sides of the body:
   a. Arms: patient's ability to hold his arms at a right angle to his body (watch for drift).
   b. Legs: patient's ability to hold his legs 10° off bed and ability to dorsiflex his feet against the pressure of the nurse's hands
   c. Reflexes
   d. Pain response
   e. The nurse should observe any failure of a body part to move, focal or generalized seizures, responses to verbal or noxious stimuli, decerebrate spasms, and/or lateralization of neurological signs (mainly evident in facial grimacing, movements of the extremities, absent deep tendon reflexes or superficial abdominal reflex and a Babinski response).

16. Check the patient's vital signs—temperature, pulse, respiration, blood pressure—every hour (more often if indicated).

17. Obtain baseline laboratory data. The clear nasal drainage should be tested for glucose.

18. Place a Salem sump nasogastric tube for acute gastric distention. Insertion is contraindicated in patients with gunshot wounds to the head if the nasopharynx or the tissues surrounding it have been removed by the blast, or if there is any danger of disrupting a hematoma at the base of the neck. Antacids, anticholinergics, or antihistamines are given as ordered.

19. Place a Foley catheter if the patient is unconscious.

20. Be aware that restlessness can be caused by the head injury, hypoxia, shock, pain, gastric dilatation, and/or a full urinary bladder.

21. Be aware that a lumbar puncture is usually not done since it provides little useful information and it is potentially disastrous. The risk is great that intracranial fluid pressures will be altered so that the temporal lobes and the cerebellum will herniate through the foramen magnum and thus compress the lower brain stem.

22. Ascertain that the patient has had a cervical spine series with negative results before a CT scan is done. One percent of patients who have head injuries also have fractures of the cervical spine, and positioning the patient for the CT scan requires considerable manipulation.

23. Before a CT scan of an agitated patient is done, administer intravenous diazepam if ordered, to minimize artifact movement.
24. Be aware that the patient who is being transported to the hospital must be accompanied by medical personnel who can clear his nasopharynx and assist his respirations. (The safest position for transport is with the patient's head elevated 15 to 30 degrees. In an airplane, the patient should lie facing the cockpit and with his head elevated, to minimize the effects of G forces.)

OBJECTIVE NO. 3

The patient should maintain pulmonary stability and his oxygenation should be ensured (see Chap. 17).
  To achieve the objective, the nurse should:

1. Assess and maintain the patency of the upper airway.
2. Give 40% oxygen through a mask as ordered.
3. Observe and record the pattern of respirations.
4. Draw arterial blood gas samples as ordered and send them for analysis.
5. Notify the physician of any decrease in PO_2 or pH, or any increase in PCO_2. Arterial carbon dioxide levels above 42 mm Hg or arterial oxygen levels below 50 mm Hg may produce vasodilatation and a sustained increase in the ICP.
6. If respiratory distress is noted, notify the physician; observe the patient closely, and do not leave him unattended.
7. Prepare the patient for endotracheal intubation if his PO_2 decreases to 70 mm Hg.
8. Monitor vital capacity, blood gases, and respiratory effort to assess respiratory status.
9. Maintain pulmonary hygiene and suctioning as indicated by the arterial blood gas measurements and the chest examination. Give the patient 100% oxygen for one to two minutes before and after suctioning, and limit the suctioning to 15 seconds.
10. Have equipment for suctioning and endotracheal intubation at the patient's bedside.
11. If hyperventilation measures and the use of a paralyzing drug are ordered, monitor the ICP closely.
12. Turn the patient onto his side and change sides every hour.

OBJECTIVE NO. 4

The patient should be free of the symptoms of increased cerebral edema in order to sustain neural cell metabolism.
  To achieve the objective, the nurse should:

1. Assess and record the patient's level of consciousness every 15 minutes. The nurse should not confuse progressive restlessness and agitation with an improvement in the level of consciousness; those signs may indicate increased ICP.
2. For serial determinations, use the Glasgow coma scale for patients who do not have lateralizing signs. Three assessment parameters are used: eye opening, best verbal response, and best motor response. The patient who is completely awake will score 15. The patient who scores 10 or less usually needs to be intubated and hyperventilated (20–22 breaths/min). Deterioration of the neurological and/or lateralizing signs is an indication for CT scanning. The following values are assigned to the assessment parameters:
  a. Eye opening
     Eyes do not open at all 1
     Eyes open after pain stimulation 2
     Eyes open on command 3
     Eyes open spontaneously 4
  b. Best verbal response
     Patient intubated 0
     Patient mute 1
     Patient makes
       incomprehensible sounds 2
     Patient uses
       inappropriate words 3
     Patients's conversation confused 4
     Patient's response appropriate and
       oriented 5
  c. Best motor response
     Flaccid 1
     Extensor response 2
     Flexor response 3
     Semi-purposeful 4
     Localized to pain 5
     Obedient to command 6
3. Observe the patient for changes in levels of responsiveness, restlessness, and bilateral motor response, as well as for changes in his pupils and respirations; any changes should be reported to the physician immediately. Serial assessments will identify trends (Fig. 30-9).

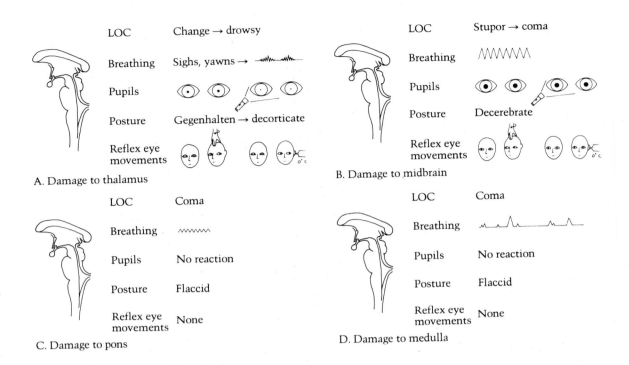

A. Damage to thalamus

LOC	Change → drowsy
Breathing	Sighs, yawns →
Pupils	
Posture	Gegenhalten → decorticate
Reflex eye movements	

B. Damage to midbrain

LOC	Stupor → coma
Breathing	
Pupils	
Posture	Decerebrate
Reflex eye movements	

C. Damage to pons

LOC	Coma
Breathing	
Pupils	No reaction
Posture	Flaccid
Reflex eye movements	None

D. Damage to medulla

LOC	Coma
Breathing	
Pupils	No reaction
Posture	Flaccid
Reflex eye movements	None

Figure 30-9

Progression of central herniation. Serial assessments will identify trends. The nurse may observe signs, beginning with diencephalic compression and progressing to lower brain stem involvement.

4. Check the vital signs every 15 minutes. If they are stable for two hours, the nurse should check them every 30 minutes for two hours, and then every 60 minutes. Although there is not a definite correlation between vital signs and progressive increases in the ICP, in many instances there is a certain relationship. Four stages have been described as the ICP increases gradually: two compensatory stages, in which the vital signs are affected little, the third (preterminal) stage, and the fourth (terminal) stage. In the third and fourth stages, classic changes are seen: increased blood pressure, widened pulse pressure, bradycardia, dysrhythmias, and slow, shallow respirations. Irregular respirations herald the beginning of stage four. Because the classic changes are late ones, clinical monitoring must cover all the parameters.

5. Every hour, observe for, report, and record:
   a. Pupillary changes (in size, equality, position, direct response, and consensual response).
   b. Respiratory irregularity (a decreased rate, an increased rate, or periods of apnea). One of the most important changes in respiration is from normal respirations to Cheyne-Stokes respirations or central neurogenic hyperventilation, which indicates actual or impending central herniation.
   c. Motor changes (movement and pain on the right side should be compared with movement and pain on the left side).
   d. Vomiting or incontinence.
   e. Increased blood pressure with widened pulse pressure. When the mean arterial pressure is 60 to 170 mm Hg, the cerebral blood flow remains within normal limits. However, arterial pressures below 90 mm Hg that are associated with an increased ICP and that peak to 60 to 90 mm Hg may produce a low perfusion pressure and cerebral hypoxia.
   f. Pulse <60 or >100.
   g. A moderately elevated temperature.

6. Maintain controlled hyperventilation and induced hypocarbia by keeping the arterial carbon dioxide levels at about 25 mm Hg (the range is

20–30 mm Hg). Adjust the minute ventilation. The arterial carbon dioxide tension level should not be allowed to drop below 20 mm Hg since further arterial constriction may result in tissue hypoxia and acidosis.

7. Use ventricular drainage via a closed system to vent and remove cerebrospinal fluid so that the ICP is kept below 25 mm Hg. Since the cerebrospinal fluid is produced at a rate of 20 ml per minute and since the amount that can be obtained is small, the patient should be monitored closely; the ICP may rise rapidly. The nurse should remember that just as the addition of one to two ml aliquot of cerebrospinal fluid to the total brain volume can at times increase the ICP exponentially (see Fig. 30-1), so the removal of 1 to 2 ml can make a vast difference; the same process works in reverse.

8. Elevate the head of the bed 30 to 45 degrees. Maintain the patient's neck in a neutral position using pillows wrapped in sheets. To prevent jugular vein compression, the patient's head should not be allowed to rest on a pillow.

9. Keep the patient's temperature below 38°C (101°F).

10. Administer intravenous furosemide as ordered. Normally 40 mg is the initial dose, and the repeat dose is 20 mg. An effective management of acute decompensation is the use of intravenous furosemide associated with mannitol.

11. Administer intravenous mannitol as ordered. Normally 0.18 to 2.5 gm per kilogram (in a 20% solution) is administered as a bolus for 2 to 20 minutes. Mannitol, a complex hypertonic osmotic diuretic, increases osmolar pressure in the blood and decreases cerebral volume, and therefore decreases edema. It is particularly valuable before emergency surgery. If it is used to help control intracranial volume, close observation is mandatory because the initial response is followed by a rebound phenomenon in several hours. During rehydration the pressure is sometimes even greater than it was before mannitol was given. For that reason, mannitol is often followed by an isotonic solution rather than by a 5% dextrose in water solution. Also, the following may be ordered: urea (30% as 1–1.5 gm/kg: 60 drops/min); glycerol (a 50% solution orally or by tube: 0.5–2 gm/kg) or 20% intravenously (1 gm/kg).

12. Avoid sedation.

13. Monitor the patient for headaches (they occur rarely). A headache that is severe and is associated with agitation indicates an epidural hematoma. Since opiates (e.g., morphine) mask neurological signs, they are not used.

14. Administer dexamethasone sodium phosphate as ordered. Normally 4 to 10 mg is given intravenously as the initial dose; then 4 to 6 mg is given every 4 to 6 hours for 5 to 10 days.

15. After arteriography, monitor the pedal pulses.

16. Monitor the ICP. ICPs of 4 to 10 mm Hg with an upper limit of 15 mm Hg (or torr) are considered normal; ICPs of 15 to 30 mm Hg are considered to be moderately elevated; and ICPs of 30 to 40 mm Hg are considered to be elevated. Autoregulation is impaired when the ICP is more than 30 to 35 mm Hg. A patient whose ICP is higher than 40 mm Hg for more than two to three days rarely survives [28]. In order to maintain the pressure below 20 mm Hg, therapies such as cerebrospinal fluid drainage or the use of osmotic diuretics, hyperventilation, and hypothermia and/or steroids may be instituted [9, 17]. The physician should be notified immediately of any clinical changes associated with an abrupt increase in ICP above the baseline, especially an altered state of consciousness, emesis, headache, irregular respirations, or purposeless movement during the peak pressure of waves, all of which indicate hypoxia of neural cells.

17. Avoid anything that might produce an abrupt rise in the ICP, such as neck flexion, Valsalva's maneuver (e.g., while straining at stool or turning abruptly), extremes of hip flexion, a prone position, painful stimuli, and waking the patient from sleep. To prevent jugular compression, the patient's head should not rest on a pillow. The nurse should use caution when changing the patient's bed linens, she should assist during procedures, and she should teach the patient to exhale during turning and not to push against the footboard. Passive range-of-motion exercises should be employed. The patient should be given time to rest between procedures since the additive effect may increase the ICP.

18. Measure the ICP. For example, with a subarachnoid screw, read and record hourly pressures concurrent with the neuro vital signs using the following protocol. The nurse should:
   a. Prepare the sterile equipment as needed.
   b. Assemble the transducer, dome, Luer-Lok

syringes, and stopcocks, and place them in the holder at the appropriate angle.

c. Use a venous monitor capable of measuring low pressures.

d. Fill the transducer from the bottom syringe upward into the top, being certain that all the air is removed.

e. Turn off the stopcocks to the transducer.

f. Connect the transducer to the pressure section of the monitor.

g. Elevate the head of the bed 30 degrees.

h. Level the transducer with the screw.

i. Open the line for calibration, and turn off the line to the patient; make certain the patient's line to the transducer is turned off. With the module in the systolic mode and using the zero dial, turn the dial until the digital display shows 0. Calibrate to 20 (turn the outer ring while depressing the calibrating button until 20 is reached).

j. Check the transducer's internal calibration, and close the Cobe stopcock to the transducer. Open the top end of the stopcock. Attach the wall unit and cuff to the side outlet (folding the cuff up).

k. Pump the cuff to 20 mm Hg pressure and turn off the cuff. Note the pressure readings. They should be within 2 to 3 mm of each other.

l. Turn the transducer off, release the cuff pressure, and turn the cuff off. Make certain the 0 on the wall unit matches that on the digital display.

m. Turn the transducer off. Remove the blood pressure equipment and cap the exposed ends. This side is never to be used for anything except checking, and it *must always* be turned off to the transducer.

n. Fill the manometer and turn the stopcock to get a pressure reading. Use sterile saline solution and maintain sterility since infection is a possibility.

o. Make sure the base of the manometer is level with the screw and the transducer.

p. Flush the manometer (use a small amount of normal saline solution).

q. Balance the transducer to the water manometer.

r. Open the lines so that direct communication is present.

s. Watch the manometer as the level falls; the lowest level that is reached is the ICP. Fluctu-

ations occur when the patient coughs, moves, and breathes (decreases occur on inspiration, and increases occur on expiration; if the reading is dampened, usually a slow leak is present).

OBJECTIVE NO. 5

The patient should be free from further complications.

To achieve the objective, the nurse should:

1. Observe all safety precautions: the patient is particularly susceptible to a second insult.

2. Report blood pressures of less than 100 and pulse rates of greater than 100. Head injury in itself rarely causes the symptoms of shock. Early bleeding is commonly caused by an abdominal injury or a fracture. Later, gastrointestinal bleeding may occur.

3. Administer an anticholinergic, antacid, or cimetidine as ordered to prevent GI bleeding.

4. If otorrhea or rhinorrhea occurs, notify the physician and lightly place cotton balls in the patient's ears or a drip pad under his nose. Tell the patient not to blow his nose or sneeze. Use a commercially prepared pH-sensitive tape to determine whether glucose is present (a gross test for cerebrospinal fluid). Do not suction nasally if the anterior fossa is fractured.

5. If bleeding starts from the ear or the nose, notify the physician and collect some blood in a test tube and on a tissue. The presence of cerebrospinal fluid is indicated by nonclotting blood and by blood with a ring about it.

6. If the patient becomes combative, pad his siderails, put mittens on him, and assess his need for a chest restraint. Mechanical restraints increase restlessness. Support the patient and stay with him.

7. Determine the cause of any restless behavior.

8. Have a padded tongue blade and suctioning equipment in the patient's room.

9. Protect the patient's eyes from corneal irritation.
   a. Inspect his eyes with a flashlight.
   b. Irrigate the patient's eyes with sterile saline solution and put drops in his eyes every eight hours as ordered.
   c. Report any corneal drying, irritation, or ulceration to the physician.

10. Observe the patient for bulging eyes or red vessels

in the sclera. Ask him whether he hears noise in his head (signs and symptoms of a carotid cavernous sinus fistula).

11. Observe for signs of the postconcussion syndrome (forgetfulness, insomnia, dizziness, and/or an inability to calculate).

12. If the patient develops a cranial nerve deficit, observe him carefully. A patient with a cranial nerve deficit is particularly prone to residual injuries.

13. Observe the patient for endocrine abnormalities.

OBJECTIVE NO. 6

The patient should maintain fluid and electrolyte balance.

To achieve the objective, the nurse should:

1. Administer intravenous fluid (Ringer's lactate solution, normal saline solution, or one-half strength normal saline solution) as ordered.
2. Record the fluid intake. Weigh the patient daily.
3. Place a Foley catheter.
4. Measure and record the hourly and daily urinary output (normal is 1200 ml–1800 ml/24 hr).
5. Obtain baseline data about the urinary output and report any change in the amount or appearance of the urine.
6. Monitor the patient's serum and urine electrolyte levels every 8 hours. Measure serum and urine osmolarity.
7. Administer potassium as ordered.
8. Check the hematocrit and the blood urea nitrogen levels daily.
9. Observe the patient for symptoms of hyponatremia.
10. If urine output is greater than 250 ml per hour for 2 hours in a row, or greater than 6000 ml per day, alert the physician.

OBJECTIVE NO. 7

The patient should attain a positive caloric balance.

To achieve the objective, the nurse should:

1. Administer intravenous fluids as ordered. Since caloric support during the first few days is not a major priority, treatment usually includes intravenous feedings. Parenteral nutrition may be added.
2. Initiate oral feedings (or nasogastric feedings) later after return of bowel sounds, as ordered. (For ex-

ample, nasogastric feedings may be ordered, perhaps a 150-ml blenderized diet every three hours followed by 200 ml of water.) Aspirate before giving the feeding and record the character and amount of the aspirate. Withhold feeding if the aspirate is greater than 100 ml. Report to the physician any coffee ground material or an aspirate of more than 100 ml. Keep head elevated.

3. If the patient is obtunded, nasogastric feedings will probably be withheld because of the danger of aspiration; a Dobhoff tube may be placed or a feeding jejunostomy may be performed.

OBJECTIVE NO. 8

The patient should receive sensory stimulation.

To achieve the objective, the nurse should:

1. Talk to the patient while caring for him.
2. Record exactly his reaction to touch, visual, and voice or other auditory stimuli.
3. Ask the patient to perform certain activities every four hours (e.g., raising his arm or protruding his tongue).
4. Encourage the patient's family to talk to him during their visits with him. Ask them to bring in family pictures or tape recordings of family messages, and involve them in ways to stimulate the patient in their absence (e.g., through poster boards or telephone conversations).
5. See that the patient has a clock and a calendar.
6. Keep a radio in the patient's room. Play music and change stations for him, even if he is unconscious.
7. Employ reality therapy.
8. If the patient has a speech impairment, consult with a neurologist, a clinical specialist, and a speech therapist. Patients whose speech centers are injured have many rehabilitation problems that require a thoughtful innovative approach on the part of the nurse.

OBJECTIVE NO. 9

The patient should maintain a normal temperature range or mild hypothermia (32°C–36°C; 90°F–97°F) or moderate hypothermia (27°C–31°C; 81°F–89°F).

To achieve the objective, the nurse should:

1. Take the patient's temperature every 2 hours with a tympanic membrane, or an esophageal or a rectal sensor.

2. Administer aspirin (1.2 6m rectally) or Tylenol every 4 hours as ordered for increased temperature. Observe the patient for gastrointestinal bleeding.
3. When the temperature is elevated, bathe the patient with tepid water sponges rather than alcohol sponges.
4. Make sure the patient's fluid intake is at least 3000 ml/day as ordered.
5. Keep the room temperature at 20°C (68°F). Keep the amount of bed clothes at a minimum.
6. Put a hypothermia blanket on the patient's bed before he arrives in the critical care unit.
7. Determine the mechanism of cooling to be ordered and make preparations for its institution: surface cooling, bloodstream cooling, barbiturate hypothermia, or administration of medications.
8. Use a cooling blanket when the patient's temperature elevates as ordered.
   a. Avoid temperature drops of more than 1°C each 15 minutes.
   b. Maintain the patient's temperature at normothermic levels unless otherwise ordered. Monitor the temperature by a continuous probe.
   c. Administer chlorpromazine hydrochloride as ordered to control shivering by peripheral dilatation.
   d. Monitor the patient with ECG (when the patient's temperature is below 31°C [89°F], the incidence of ventricular fibrillation increases).
   e. Take the patient's apical pulse for one full minute to note any irregularities and reduced rate.
   f. If ice bags are applied, observe the patient's skin carefully.
   g. Put a sheet on top of the hypothermic blanket.
   h. Observe the patient's skin every time he is turned, checking especially the bony prominences.
   i. Massage the patient's bony prominences each time he is turned. Protect elbows, feet, and other bony prominences with coverings such as socks or Kling bandages.
   j. Bathe the patient daily. Use lanolin or oil after bathing.
   k. Since medications are detoxified and excreted slowly with hypothermia, observe the patient for a cumulative reaction.
   l. Monitor intake and output.
   m. Massage and warm the muscle prior to a medication injection.
   n. When cooling or rewarming the patient, watch his temperature closely. Stop the procedure before the desired temperature is reached. The temperature tends to continue to drift one-half to two-thirds the number of degrees the temperature has been lowered. Rewarm the patient slowly. As a rule of thumb, allow one hour for each degree rise in temperature.
   o. Support the patient during the rewarming process. Reassure him with such phrases as, "In a while, you won't be as cold."

OBJECTIVE NO. 10

The patient should be free of the complications of seizures.

To achieve the objective, the nurse should:

1. Take the patient's seizure history; determine whether his seizures are grand mal, petit mal, jacksonian, or psychomotor. Avoid circumstances that might precipitate seizures (e.g., stress, interference with his normal sleeping patterns, and irregular eating).
2. If a seizure occurs, screen the patient, remove his bed clothes, and stand at the foot of the bed to observe him closely while another health team member maintains safety precautions. Note and record the following:
   a. The patient's level of consciousness before, during, and after the seizure
   b. The presence or absence of an aura
   c. The progression and involvement of activity (how the seizure began and how it spread)
   d. The deviation of his head and eyes
   e. The length of the tonic and clonic phases
   f. The respiratory changes (depth and regularity)
   g. The pupillary reactions during and after the seizure
   h. Incontinence
   i. Tongue biting
   j. The patient's ability to handle salivation
   k. Muscle weakness
   l. Duration of seizure
   m. Character and duration of status after the seizure, and the presence of paralysis or dysphasia
3. During convulsion, observe all safety precautions. The nurse should:
   a. If possible, before the tonic phase place a soft object (e.g., a padded tongue blade, napkin, or oral airway) between the patient's teeth. (But

once his jaws are clenched, do not attempt to place anything between his teeth.)
b. Loosen any tight clothing.
c. Lower the padded siderail on the nurse's side of the bed to help guide the patient's movements.
d. Protect the patient's head and the rest of his body; do not try to stop his movements. The nurse should move with his body to help protect him.
e. Remain in the patient's room.
4. Anticipate that the physician will order medication such as intravenous diphenylhydantoin (5 mg/kg/day) (it is not given intramuscularly or through a central venous catheter). Unless the patient is elderly or has associated cardiovascular disease, a common protocol is 250 mg every 30 minutes until 2.5 times the daily maintenance dose is reached. The rate of administration should not exceed 50 mg per minute. Vital signs are monitored carefully, and the patient is placed on a cardiac monitor. Diphenylhydantoin infusion should be monitored carefully because ventricular dysrhythmias may occur with rapid administration.
5. Administer the medication ordered by the physician. Depending on the patient assessment, the physician may not order any medication after the first seizure. (He may order sodium phenobarbital or another medication.) If the seizures continue, sodium amobarbital, paraldehyde, phenobarbital, diazepam, or thiopental sodium may be ordered. Generalized persistent seizures may be treated with intravenous diazepam given in a dose necessary to stop the seizures (usually 3–10 mg for 5–10 minutes and repeated as necessary).
6. Take the patient's temperature rectally only.
7. Keep a padded tongue blade and airway and suctioning equipment at the patient's bedside.
8. Perform mouth care while the patient is taking diphenylhydantoin.
9. Pad the headboard and side rails; keep side rails up, except when the patient is having a seizure.
10. Observe the patient carefully, particularly during the night.
11. Plan patient education and family education.

Problem/Diagnosis

Traumatic fracture of the cervical vertebra with subluxation and cervical traction.

OBJECTIVE NO. 1

Traumatic fracture of the cervical vertebra should be prevented by educating the public about the dangers (in safety lectures and in other types of education).

If the objective is to be achieved, the public must be made aware of safety measures. Examples follow:

1. Someone should be present when a swimming pool is being drained (to prevent a diving injury).
2. Swimmers should test the depth of the water before diving into it.
3. A person who has had a diving accident should be maintained floating in the water until enough people are present to move him from the area safely.
4. Football players should not spear one another while tackling.
5. Wrestlers and trampoline athletes should be aware of the hazards of their sports.
6. Shoulder and lap belts should be used in motor vehicles.
7. At the scene of any accident, an injured person should not be moved until enough people are present to move him safely. (Ten to 15 percent of patients who sustain a cervical spinal cord injury become quadriplegic after the initial accident.)
8. Before an injured person is moved, he should be asked, "Does your neck hurt? Does your back hurt? Do your arms or legs feel heavy?" If he answers yes to any of those questions, he should be immobilized for transport.

OBJECTIVE NO. 2

The patient should not have further cord damage.
To achieve the objective, the nurse should:

1. Maintain a patent airway.
a. Avoid moving the neck. Treat the unconscious patient as if he had cervical injury.
b. Insert an airway.
c. Prepare the patient for endotracheal intubation or tracheostomy if he needs ventilatory assistance. Airway management has the highest priority. Cervical spinal damage is usually due to the initial injury, but extreme care must be used to avoid compounding whatever problem exists. If airway management is needed, a modified jaw-thrust maneuver or intubation via the nasal route is recommended.
2. Immobilize the patient. The attendant should:
a. Place the patient in the supine position on a

firm surface that can be used to transfer him to the hospital.

b. Immobilize his neck, using sandbags, rolled towels, blankets, or a carefully applied cervical collar, or fix his head on a backboard.

c. Keep his head and neck in a neutral position, avoiding flexion, extension, and rotation.

d. Place wide strips of adhesive tape (or a rope or belt if tape is not available) across the patient's forehead and under his chin and secure it to the side of the stretcher.

e. Secure the patient's hands and feet to prevent their falling off the stretcher.

3. Determine baseline information against which later estimates of the extent of injury can be compared. The attendant should:

a. Ask the patient to describe any pain—its site, quality, and duration. Do not ask the patient to move his back if he feels no pain.

b. Palpate the site of the suspected injury gently to detect any tenderness of the spinous processes.

c. Observe for any obvious spinal deformity.

d. Look for any lacerations and contusions.

e. Assess the motor functioning of the extremities: The nurse should:
   (1) Categorize the patient's hand grasp as stong, weak, or absent.
   (2) Ask the patient to dorsiflex his foot.

f. Assess the sensory level of the patient's trunk with a needle to determine where he begins to feel pain.

g. Monitor the patient's breathing pattern and vital signs.

h. Check for sweating or other autonomic signs.

i. Monitor bladder function.

j. Listen for bowel sounds.

4. Maintain the patient's PCO_2 level (by hyperventilation) at 20 to 30 mm Hg. Maintain the PO_2 at levels greater than 80 mm Hg.

5. Monitor the patient's respiratory status. Assess preexisting pulmonary problems, determine if diaphragmatic breathing is present and if intercostals are functioning, auscultate breath sounds frequently, and assess tidal volume and vital capacity every two hours.

6. Determine the serial values and assess the trends.

7. Monitor the vital signs, pupillary responses (size, position, and movements), and oculocephalic response and use the Glasgow coma scale.

8. Place a urethral catheter.

9. Place a nasogastric catheter unless the patient has sustained a gunshot wound to his head.

10. Administer tetanus prophylaxis as ordered.

11. Know that analgesics and sedatives are to be avoided.

12. Assess the presence or absence of movement and sensation (pain and touch). Report any progression of neurological deficit.

13. Categorize muscle strength as strong, weak, or absent.

14. Compare the left and right sides and the arms and legs. Assess and record any differences.

15. Categorize the reflexes as normal, increased, decreased, or absent.

16. Set up a reassessment schedule.

17. Communicate specifics concerning x rays ordered by the physician.

18. Use aseptic technique in cleansing the lacerations.

19. If a cervical spinal injury is present, prepare for Holter traction or another stable means of immobilization. Do not turn the patient until the fracture is reduced and stable, and the physician orders the patient turned.

20. Maintain the immobilization of a fracture or dislocation (whether or not the patient has a neurological deficit) using skeletal traction if ordered. Example: Gardner-Wells tongs. The nurse should:

a. If ordered by the neurosurgeon, shave the temporoparietal areas (just below the temporal ridges) for an area about 5 cm in diameter. Then cleanse the shaved area with an antiseptic solution. (The physician then anesthetizes the two areas with a local anesthetic.) Using either aseptic or clean technique, the physician applies the tips of the tongs to the prepared areas and advances them through the scalp and into the outer table of the skull by steadily turning the screws (the skin is stretched snugly about the points, effectively sealing the entry and preventing bleeding). When the proper amount of squeeze is exerted, a spring-loaded point protrudes 1 mm from one of the knobs.

b. Put a sterile dressing around each tong site.

c. Attach orthopedic rope to the top of the tongs and bring it over a pulley attached to the head of the bed. Keep knot at least 2 in. from pulley.

d. Attach weights and allow them to hang free (for the stabilization of nondisplaced injuries,

5–10 lb of traction is generally used, and for the reduction of a dislocation, 10–15 lb of traction is generally used).

e. Position the patient in a neutral, flexed, or hyperextended position as ordered.

f. Elevate the head of the turning frame 6 in.

g. Inspect the traction for:
   (1) Proper alignment.
   (2) Free-hanging weights.
   (3) Any interference with the rope.
   (4) A 1-mm protrusion of the spring-loaded indicator.

h. Clean the sites with hydrogen peroxide four times a day.

i. Inspect the sites daily for bleeding, infection, or erosion.

21. Observe the patient for progressive neurological damage.

22. If the symptoms of progressive cord compression occur, notify the physician.

23. Monitor the patient for spinal shock. Check him for decreased blood pressure, paralysis, and bladder and bowel distention.

24. Maintain body support (if complications arise, rehabilitation is rarely successful). The nurse should:

a. Maintain a patent airway.

b. Maintain circulation.

c. Maintain the patient's respiratory status and pulmonary hygiene. Assist the patient with deep breathing, quad coughing, mobilizing secretions, and using incentive spirometry. Obtain blood gases as ordered. Record vital capacity every eight hours.

d. Maintain sterile urine and a sterile urinary tract. Pay particular attention to the details of maintenance of a closed system with Foley catheterization and to details of medical asepsis with intermittent catheterization.

e. Prevent infection. The most likely sources are the respiratory and urinary systems, and wounds.

f. Prevent bowel distention. Teach the program to the patient and his family.

g. Prevent a break in the integrity of the patient's skin and thus prevent decubitus ulcers.
   (1) Establish and maintain a turning schedule, every two hours. Include the patient and his family in planning.
   (2) Give skin care and light massage every two hours. Keep skin dry.
   (3) Inspect the skin and bony prominences during turning.
   (4) Use aids such as alternating pressure mattresses, sheepskins, flotation pads, egg crate mattresses.
   (5) Before turning the patient to the prone position, check his respirations, pulse, blood pressure, and vital capacity.

h. Maintain the patient's body alignment and prevent contractures.
   (1) Use passive range-of-motion exercises to maintain range. Encourage family to help.
   (2) Consult with the physical therapist and the occupational therapist. Develop a plan for positioning, splinting, and exercising.
   (3) Maintain any residual muscle strength that the patient has by means of a planned program.
   (4) Prevent thrombophlebitis by institution of an exercise program. Assess the patient's extremities for changes in size and color, and measure his thighs daily. (Measure 6 cm between trochanter and patella. Notify physician if there is a difference of 3 cm or more between thighs.)

i. Maintain the patient's psychological equilibrium.
   (1) Anticipate grief reactions.
   (2) Work with the patient and his family as individuals. Set reasonable goals.
   (3) Employ body-mind-spirit concepts.
   (4) Consult with the psychologist, social worker, and psychiatric nurse.
   (5) Plan visits with former patients.
   (6) Focus on the positive aspects of what the patient will realistically be able to accomplish. Emphasize success.
   (7) Allow the patient some control over his environment.

References

1. Backman, D., Bean, J. W., and Baslock, D. R. Neurogenic influence on pulmonary compliance. *J. Trauma* 14(No. 2):111, 1974.
2. Berkovsky, D. Physiological effects of closed head injury. *J. Neurosurg. Nurs.* 4:125, 1972.
3. Brock, M., and Dietz, H. (eds.) *Intracranial Pressure: Experimental and Clinical Aspects.* New York: Springer-Verlag, 1972.

4. Brodner, R., Vengelder, J., and Collins, W. The effect of antifibrinolytic therapy in experimental spinal cord trauma. *J. Trauma* 17:48, 1977.

5. Bruce, D. A., Langfitt, T. W., Miller, J. D., et al. Regional cerebral blood flow, intracranial pressure, and brain metabolism in comatose patients. *J. Neurosurg.* 38:131, 1973.

6. Charney, K. J., Juler, G. L., and Comair, A. E. General surgery problems in patients with spinal cord injuries. *Arch. Surg.* 110:1083, 1975.

7. Clark, K. The incidence and mechanism of shock in head injury. *Southern Med. J.* 55:13, 1962.

8. Cooper, P. R., and Moody S. Neurodiagnostic studies and the management of head injury. *Comput. Tomogr.* 2:197, 1978.

9. Cushing, H. Peptic ulcers and the interbrain. *Surg. Gynecol. Obstet.* 55:1, 1932.

10. Elliott, F. A. *Clinical Neurology.* Philadelphia: Saunders, 1971.

11. Enevoldsen, E. M., Cold, G., Jensen, F. T., et al. Dynamic changes in regional CBF, intraventricular pressure, CSF pH and lactate levels during the acute phase of head injury. *J. Neurosurg.* 44:191, 1976.

12. Fisher, C. M. Some neuro-ophthalmological observations. *J. Neurol. Neurosurg. Psychiatry* 30:283, 1967.

13. Fishman, R. A. Brain edema. *N. Engl. J. Med.* 293:706, 1975.

14. Green, B. A., and Hall, W. Recognition and accident scene care for spinal cord injured patients. *Paraplegia Life* 3:15, 1976.

15. Haymaker, W. *Bing's Local Diagnosis in Neurologic Disease.* St. Louis: Mosby, 1969.

16. Hewer, R. L. Paraplegia-neurological assessment. *Physiotherapy* 60:78, 1974.

17. Jennett, B. Early traumatic epilepsy. *Arch. Neurol.* 30:394, 1974.

18. Jennett, B. Assessment of outcome after severe brain damage. *Lancet* 1:480, 1975.

19. Jennett, B., Miller, J. D., and Broakman, R. Epilepsy after nonmissile depressed skull fracture. *J. Neurosurg.* 41:208, 1974.

20. Kamada, T., Fusamoto, H., Kawano, S., et al. Gastrointestinal bleeding following head injury: A clinical study of 433 cases. *J. Trauma* 17:44, 1977.

21. Kaufmann, G. E., and Clark, L. Continuous simultaneous monitoring of intraventricular and cervical subarachnoid cerebrospinal fluid pressure to indicate development of cerebral or tonsillar herniation. *J. Neurosurg.* 33:145, 1970.

22. Kety, S. S., Shenkin, H. A., and Schmidt, C. F. The effects of increased intracranial pressure on cerebral circulatory functions in man. *J. Clin. Invest.* 27:493, 1948.

23. Langfitt, T. W. Increased intracranial pressure. *Clin. Neurosurg.* 16:436, 1968.

24. Langfitt, T. W. Cerebral circulation and metabolism. *J. Neurosurg.* 40:461, 1974.

25. Long, C., and Lawton, E. B. Functional significance of spinal cord lesion level. *Arch. Phys. Med. Rehabil.* 36:249, 1955.

26. Luisada, A. A. Mechanism of neurogenic pulmonary edema. *Am. J. Cardiol.* 20:66, 1967.

27. Lundberg, N. Continuous recording and control of ventricular fluid pressure in neurosurgical practice. *Acta Psychiatr. Neurol. Scand.* 36 (Suppl. 149):1, 1960.

28. Lundberg, N. Clinical investigations of interrelationships between intracranial pressure and intracranial hemodynamics. *Prog. Brain Res.* 30:69, 1968.

29. Lundberg, N. Clinical Indications for Measurement of ICP. In M. Brock and H. Dietz (eds.), *Intracranial Pressure: Experimental and Clinical Aspects.* New York: Springer-Verlag, 1972.

30. Maravilla, K. R., Cooper, P. R., and Sklar, F. The influence of thin-section tomography on the treatment of cervical spine injuries. *Radiology* 127:131, 1978.

31. McClelland, R. N., Shires, G. T., and Pryer, M. Gastric secretory and splanchnic blood flow studies in man after severe trauma and hemorrhagic shock. *Am. J. Surg.* 121:134, 1971.

32. Merritt, H. *Textbook of Neurology* (5th ed.). Philadelphia: Lea & Febiger, 1973.

33. Miller, J. D., Becker, D. P., Ward, J. D., et al. Significance of intracranial hypertension in severe head injury. *J. Neurosurg.* 47:503, 1977.

34. Miller, J. D., Garibi, J., North, J. B., et al. Effects of increased arterial pressure on blood flow in the damaged brain. *J. Neurol. Neurosurg. Psychiatry* 38:657, 1975.

35. Miller, D., and Leech, P. Effects of mannitol and steroid therapy on intracranial volume-pressure relationship in patients. *J. Neurosurg.* 42:274, 1975.

36. Norton, L., Grier, J., and Eiseman, B. Gastric secretory response to head injury. *Arch. Surg.* 101:200, 1970.

37. O'Brien, P. K., Norris, J. W., and Tator, C. H. Acute subdural hematomas of arterial origin. *Neurosurgery* 4:435, 1974.

38. Osterholm, J. L. The Vascular and Cellular Basis for Spinal Cord Hemorrhagic Necrosis. In T. P. Moreley (ed.), *Current Controversies in Neurosurgery.* Philadelphia: Saunders, 1976.

39. Plum, F., and Posner, J. *Diagnosis of Stupor and Coma.* Philadelphia: Davis, 1972.

40. Rimel, R. W. Emergency management of the patient with central nervous system trauma. *J. Neurosurg. Nurs.* 10:185, 1978.

41. Sabin, T. D. The differential diagnosis of coma. *N. Engl. J. Med.* 290:1062, 1974.

42. Schutta, H. S., Kassell, N. F., and Langfitt, T. W. Brain swelling produced by injury and aggravated by arterial hypertension. *Brain* 91:281, 1968.

43. Shatsky, S., Evans, D., Miller, F., et al. High-speed angiography of experimental head injury. *J. Neurosurg.* 41:523, 1974.

44. Shucart, W. A., and Jackson, I. Management of diabe-

tes insipidus in neurosurgical patients. *J. Neurosurg.* 44:65, 1976.

45. Simmons, R. L., Ducher, T. B., and Anderson, R. W. Pathogenesis of pulmonary edema following head trauma. *J. Trauma* 8:800, 1968.

46. Sullivan, H. S., Martinez, J., Becher, D. P., et al. Fluid percussion model of mechanical brain injury in the cat. *J. Neurosurg.* 45:520, 1976.

47. Teasdale, G. Assessment of coma and impaired consciousness: A practical scale. *Lancet* 2:81, 1974.

48. Vries, J., Becher, D., and Young, H. A subarachnoid screw for monitoring intracranial pressure. *J. Neurosurg.* 39:416, 1973.

49. Watts, C., and Clark, K. Gastric acidity in the comatose patient. *J. Neurosurg.* 30:107, 1969.

50. Watts, C., and Clark, K. Effects of an anticholinergic drug on gastric acid secretion in the comatose patient. *Surg. Gynecol. Obstet.* 130:61, 1970.

51. White, R. J. Programmed management of severe head injuries revisited. *J. Trauma* 15:779, 1975.

Myasthenia Gravis

Mary Blount
Anna Belle Kinney

Myasthenia gravis is an autoimmune disease that causes weakness and abnormal fatigability of the voluntary muscles. The muscles involved and the severity of weakness form the basis of a clinical classification system. Myasthenia gravis is not a rare disease. The incidence has been estimated to be between 3 and 6 per 100,000 people. Although more women than men are affected (approximately six women to four men), the disease does not seem to have any environmental or racial predilection.

The danger of respiratory failure in severely affected myasthenic patients demands astute nursing management of the hospitalized patient. The patient in crisis requires constant monitoring and expert care. Thorough patient teaching and discharge planning are essential before the patient goes home. The degree to which the patient is able to function within the limitations of the disease is determined by the quality of the nursing care received.

Objective

In a situation involving a patient with myasthenia gravis, the nurse should be able to make initial and periodic assessments of the patient's status, evaluate the developing signs and symptoms, anticipate the potential complications of the disease and of its ther-

31

apy, and make appropriate interventions to prevent their occurrence.

Achieving the Objective

To achieve the objective, the nurse should be able to:

1. Perform a systematic assessment.
2. Construct a problem list for the patient.
3. Monitor fluctuations in the patient's swallowing ability and respiratory status.
4. List the nursing actions that maximize the patient's safety.
5. Discuss the rationales for thymectomy, anticholinesterase therapy, ACTH therapy, chronic steroid therapy, and plasma exchange.
6. Describe the nursing management of the myasthenic patient in crisis.
7. Differentiate myasthenic crisis from cholinergic crisis.
8. Evaluate the results of an edrophonium hydrochloride (Tensilon) test.
9. List the components of a teaching program for a patient with myasthenia gravis who is receiving chronic steroid therapy.

How to Proceed

To develop an approach to myasthenia gravis, the nurse should:

1. Analyze the clinical features of myasthenia gravis in the patient described in the case study that follows.
2. Outline the steps of the initial assessment of a patient with myasthenia gravis.
3. Discuss the methods of periodic monitoring of a patient with myasthenia gravis.
4. Develop a care plan for a patient with myasthenia gravis.
5. Develop a teaching program for a patient with myasthenia gravis.

Case Study

Sandy M., a 21-year-old white female who was diagnosed as having myasthenia gravis when she was 15 years old, was admitted to a university medical center hospital for an elective thymectomy. She was taking pyridostigmine bromide (Mestinon) every four hours and prednisone every other day.

This was her second admission to the medical center hospital.

Ms. M.'s initial assessment elicited the following history. At the age of 14, she began to experience diplopia, nasal regurgitation of food, and proximal muscle extremity weakness—all exacerbated by exercise. In addition, she noticed that her facial expression was less animated, her smile resembled a snarl, and her voice was very nasal. The changes caused Sandy much embarrassment, and when her friends began to comment on them, she retreated from social activities and spoke only rarely. She refused to be photographed. Her parents attributed her withdrawn behavior to a "phase." When she was 15 years old, she was admitted to a local community hospital to be treated for pneumonia. At the time she was seen by an ophthalmologist for evaluation of the diplopia. A Tensilon test was done. The results were positive and a diagnosis of myasthenia gravis was made. She was discharged three weeks later under the care of her local physician, who prescribed neostigmine bromide (Prostigmin) every four hours. The treatment reduced her symptoms considerably but did not totally alleviate them. Sandy continued to be extremely withdrawn.

For the next five years, her symptoms increased and decreased unpredictably and her neostigmine therapy was altered according to the severity of her symptoms. She was treated three times in her local community hospital for pneumonia. During her last admission, when she was 20 years old, she had a respiratory arrest, was intubated, and later had a tracheostomy. She required mechanical ventilatory support for nine days. At that time, her local physician referred her to a neurologist at the university medical center hospital.

The evaluation at the time of her first admission to the medical center hospital included an electromyogram, a muscle biopsy, a gallium scan, and Tensilon testing. The evaluation confirmed the diagnosis of myasthenia gravis. The physical examination revealed no other significant problems. The nursing evaluation described Sandy as having the following problems: social withdrawal, depression, and poor understanding of the disease and its treatment. The initial nursing management centered on: (1) ensuring the patient's safety (by giving her a room near the nurses' desk, by assessing her respiratory and swallowing abilities often, and by giving her the anticholinesterase exactly on time); and (2) teaching her about her disease and its treatment. To provide continuity of care, the head nurse limited the number of nurses assigned to Sandy.

After the initial diagnostic studies were completed, Sandy's drug therapy was changed from neostigmine to pyridostigmine every four hours. Chronic steroid therapy was instituted with the daily administration of prednisone (at 8 A.M.). Antacid therapy was begun at the same time. The nursing management included daily testing of the urine for sugar and acetone and testing each stool for occult blood. Since exacerbation of myasthenia gravis is common with the initiation of chronic steroid therapy, suctioning equipment was placed in Sandy's room, and she was given a tap bell to use in an emergency. As the anticipated exacerbation developed and her swallowing ability decreased, her meals were ordered to coincide with the peak pyridostigmine effect. Seven days after the initiation of chronic steroid therapy, her swallowing ability and vital capacity decreased rapidly. She was intubated before she went into respiratory failure, and she was given mechanical ventilatory support. An elective tracheostomy was performed two days later. Clinical improvement was apparent 12 days later, and Sandy was able to breathe unassisted. Shortly thereafter, an Olympic button which maintains the tracheostomy was put in place to ensure rapid provision of respiratory support in emergencies. By this time, her prednisone dosage had been changed to an every-other-day schedule. She also continued to receive pyridostigmine every four hours. Three weeks later Sandy was discharged; her case was to be followed by the hospital neurologists and by her local physician.

Prior to discharge the nursing staff taught her about her disease, its treatment, discharge plans, and self-care. A Medic-Alert bracelet identifying her as a myasthenic patient receiving chronic steroid therapy was obtained. Sandy and the nurses discussed her feelings of self-consciousness, and she expressed an interest in resuming some social activities. Arrangements were made to have a telephone installed in her home.

After discharge, Sandy was treated on an outpatient basis. Her steroid dosage was slowly tapered. Each time she returned to the center, a unit nurse met with her to discuss her progress and to review patient teaching. Sandy said that she felt well enough to visit her friends, and she was talking without embarrassment. She seemed happier and more relaxed. Shortly after her twenty-first birthday, she was scheduled to enter the university medical center hospital for a thymectomy.

Nursing management during Sandy's second admission was basically the same as that during her first admission; it centered on frequent evaluation of her status. She was instructed in preoperative and postoperative thymectomy management. She did well postoperatively and did not require ventilatory assistance, but her respiratory functioning was observed closely. After her discharge, Sandy was again followed closely as an outpatient. For the next year her symptoms slowly improved, and she is now receiving a maintenance dose of prednisone every other day and no anticholinesterase therapy. She works as a salesperson in a department store, and she has a more active social life.

Reflections

The patient with myasthenia gravis has the same problems that all patients with chronic illnesses face, and as a result must make many changes in life-style. Those enforced changes cause stress to the patient and the family. Therapeutic support from the health care team can do much to reduce the stress.

Unlike most people with chronic illnesses, the myasthenic patient must do more than adjust to a static disability or even to a steadily progressive illness. The person with myastheia gravis must adapt to a disease that has remissions and exacerbations that often occur with almost no warning. The exacerbations may be so severe as to make the patient unable to breathe, swallow, or talk and also dependent on others for even the most basic functions. Even in a period of relatively good muscle strength, the myasthenic patient may be too weak to participate in many activities, and may look and sound "different" to others. Finally, the therapy for myasthenia gravis makes it essential that the patient thoroughly understand the disease and therapy.

Through excellent physical management, psychological support, discharge planning, and patient teaching, the health care team, particularly the nurses, can do much to help the myasthenia gravis patient adjust to the illness.

Anatomy and Physiology

A knowledge of the following three aspects of normal anatomy and physiology helps the nurse better understand the pathophysiological basis of myasthenia gravis: (1) neuromuscular transmission, (2) the immune system, and (3) the thymus gland. Those topics are discussed briefly in the following paragraphs.

Neuromuscular Transmission

The chemical transmitter at the neuromuscular junction is acetylcholine (ACh). ACh is synthesized from choline and acetylcoenzyme A by the enzyme choline O-acetyltransferase (choline acetylase) in the axon terminal of the lower motor neuron. ACh is stored in vesicles (quanta) for release later. Each quantum contains about 5000 to 10,000 molecules of ACh.

Neuromuscular transmission begins with a motor nerve impulse traveling down the axon and releasing about 150 to 200 quanta of ACh from the motor endplate. ACh is released by fusion of the vesicle membrane with the nerve terminal membrane (exocytosis). The nerve transmitter diffuses across the synaptic cleft and interacts with ACh receptors, which are concentrated on the postsynaptic muscle membrane. When ACh combines with ACh receptors, a transient increase occurs in the permeability of the end-plate region to sodium and potassium. That increase generates an electrical potential that is sufficient to trigger an action potential. The action potential is propagated along the muscle membrane, and it initiates the events of muscle contraction.

Quanta of ACh are released spontaneously, giving rise to localized end-plate depolarizations of very small amplitudes. The depolarizations are termed miniature end-plate potentials (MEPPs).

There are between 30 and 40 million ACh receptors in the muscle end-plate, but only a very small number of them need to be activated at one time to produce an action potential sufficient to result in muscle contraction. Since each lower motor neuron releases 150 to 200 quanta from its motor end-plate (and each quantum contains 5000 to 10,000 ACh molecules), more molecules of ACh are released than are needed to interact with the ACh receptors to result in muscle contraction. The excess has been termed "the safety margin of neuromuscular contraction" [7]. The safety margin concept is important in understanding the present and past theories of the pathophysiology of myasthenia gravis.

Neuromuscular transmission occurs very rapidly (in milliseconds), and it is terminated by the hydrolization of ACh by the enzyme acetylcholinesterase (AChE)—located in the clefts of the muscle end-plate—by re-uptake of ACh into the presynaptic nerve terminal and by diffusion of ACh away from the muscle end-plate.

Immune System

The immune system is the body's major defense against foreign proteins. The lymphocyte precursors of the immune system originate in the yolk sac and migrate into the fetus, primarily to the thymus, liver, and spleen. After having been transformed from the precursors, the lymphocytes migrate to the lymph nodes and bone marrow.

The immune system has two subsystems, the cellular immune system and the humoral immune system. Lymphocytes transformed from precursors in the thymus are known as T-lymphocytes; they are responsible for cellular immunity. Cellular immunity is associated with delayed hypersensitivity. Examples of cellular immune activity are the rejection of transplanted tissue, antitumor activity, and the immune response to slowly developing diseases, such as tuberculosis. Lymphocytes transformed from precursors in the fetal liver and spleen are known as B-lymphocytes (a term derived from the bursa of Fabricius, the organ where similar lymphocytes were first identified in chickens). B-lymphocytes are responsible for humoral immunity. Humoral immunity involves at least two separate systems: the antibody system and the complement system. Clones of B-lymphocytes secrete large quantities of antibodies, known as immunoglobulins, into the systemic circulation. Immunoglobulin G (IgG) is the most common immunoglobulin. When antibodies combine with antigens, a system of plasma enzymes (the complement system) mediates the lysis of cells, opsonization of bacteria, release of histamine, and attraction of leukocytes to the area.

Although the immune system has two subsystems, those systems frequently interact with the complement system and thus join cellular immunity and humoral immunity. An interaction between T-lymphocytes and B-lymphocytes increases antibody production.

Thymus

The thymus is a two-lobed, triangular organ located in the anterior mediastinum between the trachea and the sternothyroid and sternohyoid muscles. Its apex is at the lower border of the thyroid, and its base reaches to the level of the fourth costal cartilage. It is the first lymphoid organ to develop in the embryo.

The embryonic and newborn thymus is essential to the development of the peripheral lymphoid tissue. If the thymus is absent in the newborn, lymphoid aplasia, lymphopenia, and the lack of cellular immunity lead to death from infection. By adolescence, the lymphoid system is fully developed, and the thymus directs its own involution via a humoral factor and undergoes gradual fibrosis and shrinkage. The function of the involuted thymus in the adult is one of maintenance. It ensures the supply of fresh, immunologically uncommitted T-lymphocytes able to react to new antigens. Removal of the thymus in an adult does not result in death as it would in the newborn, but only in a decreased response to new antigens.

In myasthenia gravis, the thymus often shows proliferative changes, such as germinal centers, hyperplasia, thymomas, or benign thymic tumors.

Pathophysiology

The pathophysiological basis of myasthenia gravis is not completely understood. In general, however, research is directed toward two major areas: (1) neuromuscular transmission and (2) the immune system. The following is a brief discussion of the current understanding of the pathophysiological basis of myasthenia gravis.

Numerous hypotheses have been proposed to explain the etiology and pathophysiology of myasthenia gravis, a disorder of neuromuscular transmission. Previously, investigators, by studying the amplitude and frequency of miniature end-plate potentials, concluded that the basic defect was presynaptic. It was postulated that either the quantum of ACh was small in each vesicle or there was a false chemical transmitter which could not interact with the postsynaptic ACh receptor (AChR) site.

The rapidly accumulating body of evidence does not support those postulates. It is now felt that myasthenia gravis is an autoimmune disorder in which an IgG antibody is directed against the postsynaptic AChR site or adjacent area. The result is a reduction in the available AChR sites producing a functional block of neuromuscular transmission. That hypothesis is supported by several kinds of experimental research. An animal model of experimental autoimmune myasthenia gravis (EAMG) has been developed by immunizing the animal with purified AChR protein from the electric organs of eels and rays. EAMG is clinically, pharmacologically, and electrophysiologically very similar to the myasthenia gravis seen in humans.

The evidence to support the autoimmune theory of the pathogenesis of myasthenia gravis includes the facts that:

1. Myasthenia gravis can be passively transferred to animals after injection of serum and IgG fractions from humans with myasthenia gravis.
2. IgG, C3, and C9 complement fractions have been demonstrated on the postsynaptic membrane of the AChR on muscles of patients with myasthenia gravis and of animals with EAMG.
3. Antibodies directed against the AChR protein have been found in up to 95 percent of myasthenic patients.
4. Myasthenia gravis is frequently associated with other autoimmune diseases, such as rheumatoid arthritis, systemic lupus erythematosus, thyroiditis, and polymyositis.

5. Thymus gland abnormalities occur often.
6. Transient neonatal myasthenia gravis occurs.
7. Myasthenia gravis improves after treatment with corticosteroids, antimetabolites, thoracic duct drainage, and plasma exchange.

To recapitulate, the most widely accepted hypothesis to explain the pathophysiological basis of myasthenia gravis is that it is an autoimmune disease in which the ACh receptor site or an adjacent area in the muscle membrane is erroneously "perceived" as "non-self" and so becomes an antigen. There is ultrastructural evidence that the synaptic cleft is structurally simplified. The autoantibody involved is immunoglobin G, and the plasma enzyme involved is probably a C3 complement. The autoimmune reaction results in diminished transmission of impulses across the neuromuscular synapse, producing the clinical weakness. With the exception of the use of cholinesterase inhibitors, the clinical and experimental therapy is aimed at immunosuppression.

Diagnosis

In the vast majority of cases, the diagnosis of myasthenia gravis can be established by the patient's history, physical examination, and one or more of the several low-risk tests that can be done. In a few cases, confirmation of the tentative diagnosis is based on the results of a more hazardous provocative test, the curare (d-tubocurarine chloride) test. Perhaps the most important element in the successful diagnosis of myasthenia gravis is that the examiner have a high degree of suspicion; only if myasthenia gravis is included in the differential diagnosis will the appropriate tests be done. In a significant number of cases, the weakness associated with mild myasthenia gravis is mistakenly attributed to an emotional disturbance.

The following is a clinical classification system of myasthenia gravis that was developed by Mann [18]. It is based on the particular muscles involved and the severity of the muscle weakness.

I. Ocular myasthenia gravis.
II. Predominately ocular plus mild limb-girdle myasthenia gravis.
III. Predominately faciopharyngeal plus mild limb-girdle and/or ocular myasthenia gravis.
IV. Moderate generalized myasthenia gravis.
V. Severe generalized myasthenia gravis.

Patient History and Physical Examination

Most patients with myasthenia gravis seek medical assistance for the evaluation of symptoms produced by weakness. Most commonly the symptoms are caused by weakness of the muscles supplied by the bulbar nuclei in the brain stem. The symptoms may include diplopia, ptosis, dysphagia, dyspnea, a high-pitched, nasal voice, a characteristic drooping, almost expressionless face (myasthenic facies), and an inability to hold the head erect or the jaw closed. However, any voluntary muscle may be affected. Most patients report that the weakness is worse in the evening than in the morning and that it is exacerbated by exercise and partially relieved by rest. The results of the physical examination are usually normal. The neurological examination demonstrates weakness and abnormal fatigability that may be restricted to specific muscle groups or that may be generalized, symmetrical or asymmetrical, proximal or distal.

Tests

Testing with an ergograph (a machine that makes a line on paper that corresponds in height to the strength of the patient's hand grip) demonstrates an abnormal fatigability of grip strength by the rapid decrement in the line height. A rapid but brief improvement in the signs and symptoms of untreated myasthenia can be achieved by an injection of neostigmine (Prostigmin) or Tensilon, making tests using those drugs valuable diagnostic tools. Positive results are almost always diagnostic of myasthenia gravis; the major exception is cases in which negative results are secondary to involvement limited to the ocular muscles.

Electromyography [26] is usually conducted with *repetitive*, rapid, supramaximal stimulation of a motor nerve. The muscle response decreases progressively, indicating that fewer muscle fibers are responding to each successive stimulation. Tensilon or neostigmine injections will partly or completely alleviate the defect. Another technique which measures neuromuscular blocking in a more sensitive way is single fiber electromyography (SFEMG). This method allows recordings to be made either with voluntary activation or with electrical stimulation. In voluntary activation, an electrode is positioned in the muscle to record activity from two individual muscle fibers (cells) innervated by the same motor neuron.

The temporal variability in the recorded muscle action potential from the two fibers is known as jitter. When neuromuscular transmission is disturbed, jitter increases; in more severe transmission defects blocking occurs. The equipment necessary for SFEMG is expensive and the specificity of the test is not yet well understood. However, it is expected that SFEMG will become increasingly more important in neuromuscular research and diagnosis. Until that time, activation of a muscle by repetitive, supramaximal stimulation of its motor nerve will remain the electrophysiological test of choice for confirming the clinical diagnosis of myasthenia gravis.

Diagnosis of patients with class I (ocular) myasthenia gravis is the most difficult to make because of the limited muscle involvement. Occasionally, a definitive diagnosis depends on the use of provocative tests; that is, drugs known to exacerbate myasthenia gravis are used to accentuate the symptoms of the disease. Examples of provocative tests are the curare and quinine stimulation tests. Those tests are rarely used because of the danger of respiratory failure if the patient does have myasthenia gravis and has a severe exacerbation. If provocative tests are used, the patient must be closely supervised and the personnel and equipment for emergency resuscitation must be quickly available.

Treatment

The most common treatments of myasthenia gravis can be divided into four general categories: (1) anticholinesterase drug therapy, (2) steroid therapy, (3) thymectomy, and (4) plasma exchange. While any one of those modes of therapy may be used singly in the management of a particular patient, most myasthenic patients are managed by a combination of two or more of those therapies.

Anticholinesterase Drug Therapy

Anticholinesterase drug therapy is directed toward treatment of the defect in neuromuscular transmission rather than the suspected underlying autoimmune process. It is therefore symptomatic treatment. The anticholinesterase drugs prolong the action of acetylcholine (ACh) by inhibiting its hydrolysis by acetylcholinesterase (AChE), thus permitting greater activity of the ACh in the depolarization of skeletal

Table 31-1
Differentiation of Myasthenic State and Cholinergic State

Types of Symptoms	Signs and Symptoms of Myasthenic State (patient undermedicated)	Signs and Symptoms of Cholinergic State (patient overmedicated)
Ocular symptoms	*Ptosis* *Diplopia*	*Ptosis* *Diplopia*
Bulbar symptoms	*Dyspnea* *Difficulty speaking* *Dysphagia* *Difficulty chewing*	*Dyspnea* *Difficulty speaking* *Dysphagia* *Difficulty chewing*
Gastrointestinal symptoms		Increased salivation Nausea Vomiting Abdominal cramps Diarrhea
General muscle symptoms	*Generalized muscle weakness*	*Generalized muscle weakness* Fasciculations (fine tremors or jerking movements of groups of muscle fibers) especially in eyelids, face, neck, and legs
Psychic symptoms	*Restlessness* *Anxiety* *Irritability*	*Restlessness* *Anxiety* *Irritability*
Miscellaneous symptoms		Increased bronchial secretions Tears Perspiration

Note: It is often difficult to distinguish myasthenic and cholinergic states because of their similar clinical pictures. The signs and symptoms common to both are indicated in italic type.

muscle. The most commonly used anticholinesterase drugs are neostigmine (Prostigmin), ambenonium chloride (Mytelase), and pyridostigmine (Mestinon). Those drugs are relatively long-acting; they have a duration of about four hours. Their peak effect is usually achieved in one hour. The use of anticholinesterase drugs significantly decreases the weakness associated with myasthenia gravis but it does not completely relieve it.

The major clinical problem in anticholinesterase therapy is how to determine and maintain a dosage that produces the most beneficial effects and the least adverse effects. Unfortunately, a balance between underdosage (a myasthenic state) and overdosage (a cholinergic state) is sometimes difficult to strike and maintain, particularly in more severely ill patients. The side effects of anticholinesterase overdosage are at least as harmful as those of anticholinesterase underdosage. Compounding the dosage problem is the fact that the myasthenic patient's anticholinesterase need may change suddenly. Stresses such as an infection, an emotional upset, a trauma, and the initiation

of or alteration in other therapies may alter the patient's optimal dose. Thus the hospitalized myasthenic patient is at particular risk in regard to dosage regulation.

Anticholinesterase overdosage and underdosage can be difficult to differentiate because the signs and symptoms of the cholinergic state and the myasthenic state are very similar (Table 31-1). The most obvious clinically recognizable difference between the two states is the parasympathetic effects (e.g., increased salivation, abdominal cramping, diarrhea, and increased bronchial secretions) associated with anticholinesterase overdosage, but even the presence of parasympathetic side effects is not absolutely diagnostic of a cholinergic state. To base adjustments in anticholinesterase dosages solely on clinical observations could obviously be hazardous, particularly if an already overdosed patient was mistakenly given an increased dosage of anticholinesterase.

Fortunately, another method of differentiating myasthenic and cholinergic states is available, the use of the Tensilon test. Tensilon is a very short-acting

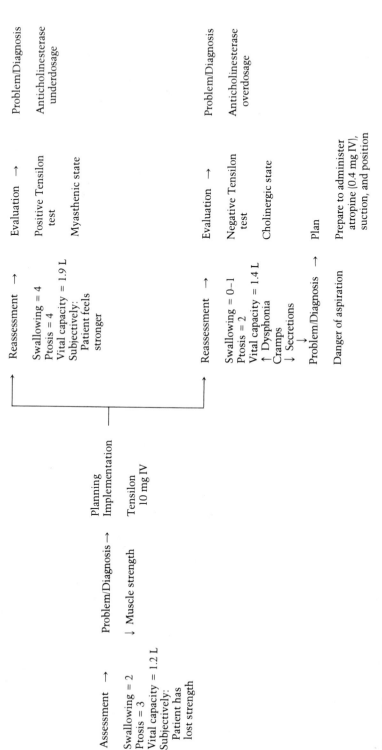

Figure 31-1

Two reactions to Tensilon testing. Swallowing is measured on a subjective scale: what the patient thinks he/she is able to swallow (0 = nothing, 1 = saliva, 2 = liquids, 3 = pureed diet, 4 = soft diet, 5 = regular diet). Ptosis is measured according to the following scale with the patient looking straight ahead attempting maximum eye opening: 1 = unable to open eye, 2 = none of pupil visible but lid not shut, 3 = lower half of the pupil visible, 4 = all of the pupil visible but none of the upper iris visible, 5 = all of the pupil visible and some of the upper part of the iris visible.

anticholinesterase drug that when injected intravenously has its peak effect in approximately 30 seconds and a duration of only several minutes. In myasthenic states, the intravenous injection of 10 mg of Tensilon produces a brief amelioration of weakness. That result signifies a positive Tensilon test. In cholinergic states, the same type of injection of Tensilon causes an exacerbation of weakness. That result signifies a negative Tensilon test. If parasympathetic side effects develop, the association of dysphagia with increased secretions and nausea and vomiting make aspiration a possibility. Intravenous atropine sulfate will minimize those parasympathetic side effects, but it will not affect the weakness associated with overdosage. Figure 31-1 summarizes those two outcomes of Tensilon testing.

Unfortunately, the results of the Tensilon test are not always so clear-cut. In an equivocal Tensilon test, some of the indices of patient status may improve while others worsen. Adjustments in the anticholinesterase dosage are made according to the effect the Tensilon has on the vital functions of respiration and swallowing.

Steroid Therapy

Steroid therapy, whether in the form of adrenocorticotrophic hormone (ACTH) or chronic steroid therapy, is becoming more and more important in the management of patients with myasthenia gravis. Steroid therapy is directed toward the suspected underlying autoimmune process. Two of the most common forms of steroid therapy are discussed briefly in the following paragraphs.

Short courses of ACTH are usually administered in doses of 100 IU per day for 10 days. In the majority of cases, an exacerbation of the disease occurs during the first three to four days of the therapy. The exacerbation may be severe enough to require respiratory support and tube feedings. An increase in muscle strength usually begins within days of the completion of the ACTH therapy, but the improvement usually lasts for only three months. A greater benefit is often obtained with paired courses of ACTH therapy given 14 days apart. In some cases, weekly ACTH injections prolong the patient's improvement between courses.

The most promising form of drug treatment of myasthenia gravis is chronic steroid therapy (CST). CST is directed toward the suppression of the autoimmune response associated with myasthenia gravis. CST is usually initiated with daily, high doses (up to 100 mg or more) of prednisone. Clinical improvement usually begins within days to three or four weeks. As sustained improvement is demonstrated, the patient is converted to alternate-day therapy; that is, if the patient was receiving "X" amount of corticosteroid daily, he receives "2X" amount every other day. That method of drug administration has been demonstrated to reduce the incidence of side effects and the complications of CST. As the improvement continues, the dosage of corticosteroid is very gradually decreased until an effective maintenance dose (maximum benefit with minimum side effects) is reached. Most patients receiving CST experience a significant improvement in their symptoms. In a large number of cases, the disease goes into remission.

The use of CST to treat myasthenia gravis is not without risk. As with short courses of ACTH, exacerbation (often severe) is common early in the course of the therapy. In addition, CST is associated with a variety of side effects and complications. Patients receiving CST must be closely observed for the development of these side effects and complications and must be thoroughly instructed in what signs and symptoms to observe for and report.

Thymectomy

Thymectomy has long been a valuable method of treating myasthenia gravis. Like steroid therapy, thymectomy is directed at the immunological disturbance thought to be basic to the pathogenesis of the disease. It has been especially effective in the treatment of young female myasthenic patients. In general, patients with thymomas have fewer beneficial effects from thymectomy than do patients with thymic hypertrophy. A sternal-splitting approach to thymectomy provides better operative visualization, but the transcervical approach seems to have a lowered morbidity. Remissions produced by thymectomy develop slowly, over many months.

Investigators at Mount Sinai Hospital in New York City have established the following clinical-pathological correlations and have identified the following therapeutic benefits of thymectomy [11]:

1. Younger myasthenics are more prone than older myasthenics to the development of thymic germinal centers.

2. The severity of the disease correlates directly with the presence of germinal centers.

3. Thymuses from patients operated on early in the course of the disease have fewer germinal centers than do thymuses of patients of the same age with long-standing symptoms.

4. Early thymectomy, particularly in patients without germinal centers, is often followed by early remission.

5. The longer the duration of disease before thymectomy, the greater is the risk of progression to more severe myasthenia and the more delayed is the onset of clinical improvement after thymectomy.

6. Fewer myasthenic patients who have thymectomies progress to severe myasthenia gravis with respiratory involvement than myasthenic patients who do not have thymectomies.

Plasma Exchange

Plasma exchange [3] is a relatively new method of treating myasthenia gravis. The procedure is based on the belief that the mechanical removal of circulating autoantibodies and immune complexes (which produce receptor damage) from the plasma should result in clinical improvement. In this procedure venous blood is removed from the patient, centrifuged, and the plasma removed. The remaining blood components and replacement fluids are returned to the patient. Concomitant immunosuppression is usually necessary to prevent a rebound elevation of antibody levels. The frequency at which plasma exchange is required and the results produced vary from patient to patient.

Plasma exchange is a very expensive and time-consuming procedure which is not without risks. It is usually reserved for patients who do not receive satisfactory results from more conventional therapy. It is also used, on occasion, to control an acute exacerbation or to improve patient condition prior to a surgical procedure such as thymectomy.

Other Therapies

Although anticholinesterase drug therapy, steroid therapy, thymectomy, and plasma exchange are the most commonly used methods of treating myasthenia gravis, other methods of treatment exist. However, most of those other forms of treatment have not had large-scale clinical trials, and they are generally considered only when the methods of treatment discussed have not been successful. Included in this category of alternative treatment options are: antimetabolite drugs, antithymocyte serum therapy, therapy with theophylline compounds, germaine monoacetate and diacetate therapy, and thoracic duct drainage. Of these alternative therapies the most promising seems to be the use of antimetabolites such as azathioprine (Imuran), cyclophosphamide (Cytoxan) and methotrexate.

Nursing Management

It is difficult to distinguish the critical care phase of myasthenia gravis from the noncritical care phase. Patients who are not critically ill may be admitted to a critical care unit when they are at particular risk of acute exacerbation of their myasthenia (e.g., after surgery or prior to a major change in therapy).

Thorough patient teaching in the critical care unit or in the general medical unit is essential to avoid the preventable acute exacerbations of myasthenia gravis.

Myasthenic patients are usually admitted to an acute care unit for one of three reasons: (1) the disease has worsened, (2) a particular kind of treatment (e.g., thymectomy, anticholinesterase therapy, steroid therapy or plasma exchange therapy) must be begun or changed, and (3) a diagnosis must be made. Since hospitalization puts the patient at greater risk of exacerbation, the hospitalized myasthenic patient should be monitored closely and carefully. The following paragraphs discuss the most common components of nursing assessment.

The swallowing ability of the myasthenic patient must be routinely assessed. A variety of methods of evaluating swallowing ability have been suggested. Some of the methods require that the patient demonstrate ability by swallowing liquids or solids of various consistencies. Those methods entail the risk of aspiration if swallowing ability is overestimated. A much safer, although subjective, method requires that the patient swallow (or attempt to swallow) with nothing but saliva in the mouth. The patient is asked to rate swallowing ability according to a prearranged scale. The following is an example of such a scale.

Nothing 0
Saliva 1
Liquids 2
Pureed diet 3
Soft diet 4
Regular diet 5

With a little experience, the patient can become adept at evaluating swallowing ability. The danger of aspiration when this method of evaluation is used is minimal. Decreases in swallowing ability should be reported immediately.

Poor swallowing ability has many implications for nursing management. Often the patient's swallowing ability changes according to anticholinesterase therapy. If that is the case, the nurse should arrange for the patient's meals to be served at times of the peak effect of the drugs. The consistency of the diet should be determined according to swallowing ability. Patients whose swallowing ability is poor or fluctuating should have suctioning equipment in their rooms and should be supervised while they eat or take medications. If the patient is unable to swallow for a long time, it may be necessary to insert a nasogastric tube. The position of the distal end of the tube should be checked before anything is administered through it.

Respiratory ability also must be assessed. Measurement of both tidal volume and vital capacity gives an indication of the patient's respiratory ability but vital capacity is usually preferred because it indicates the upper limit of respiratory capacity. Myasthenic patients who are weak may need help in taking those measurements to prevent air leakage around the mouthpiece of the spirometer. The validity of the results is somewhat dependent on the patient's position. When tidal volume or vital capacity is measured, the patient should sit up straight or should stand. The patient's position should be documented in addition to the respiratory volumes. In cases where respiratory ability is borderline, measurement of inspiratory and expiratory pressures may be more indicative of respiratory status than is vital capacity.

Downward trends in the patient's respiratory status should be reported immediately. The physician should also set a lower limit of function below which notification should occur. Patients who have severe decreases in their respiratory status should have one-to-one supervision. Emergency intubation and oxygen administration equipment should be quickly available.

The presence or absence of diplopia is another factor to be assessed. The nurse should indicate whether or not diplopia is present, and, if it is, in what direction (or directions) of gaze it exists.

Nursing responsibility in the evaluation of muscle strength is generally limited to observation of the patient's functioning. Precise and detailed testing of muscle strength is usually done by the physician. Many testing systems have been proposed. Most in-

volve counting the number of times and how long the patient can do such things as arm raising, leg crossing, eye blinking, or step climbing. The tests themselves may fatigue the patient. Other tests of muscle function evaluate strength by assessing strength against resistance. Usually numbers are assigned to different levels of strengths, ranging from absent strength to normal strength. Obviously this type of testing is rather subjective. For that reason, detailed testing should not be done more often than is necessary and it should be done by as few people as possible. In general, the nursing evaluation of muscle strength consists of comments on what the patient has been observed to be able to do.

When and how often muscle strength is tested depends on the patient's status. The minimum frequency is usually decided by the physician, but the members of the nursing staff should be encouraged and expected to use their judgment in deciding to make additional assessments when the patient's condition indicates the need to do so. If the patient is taking an anticholinesterase drug, the assessments should be made when the drug is administered; that is, when the drug's effect and the patient's abilities are lowest.

The major determinant of activity is the patient's general condition. Every effort should be made to avoid fatigue. If the patient is taking an anticholinesterase drug, activities may need to be planned to coincide with the peak effect of the drug. Once the patient's condition has stabilized at an acceptable level, activity should be increased until it is comparable to that required for independent living at home.

Crisis Management

The term *crisis* is used in myasthenia gravis to describe profound weakness and an inadequate respiratory ability. Cholinergic crisis is an exacerbation of myasthenia gravis that is caused by an overdose of an anticholinesterase drug. Myasthenic crisis is a sudden exacerbation of the disease process that occurs either from an anticholinesterase underdosage or in the absence of treatment with an anticholinesterase drug. Factors that may produce an exacerbation include pregnancy, menstruation, the initiation of steroid therapy, an emotional upset, surgical procedures, trauma, and infections (particularly infections of the respiratory and urinary tracts).

Frequent and consistent assessment of the myasthenic patient usually provides sufficient warning of an impending crisis to prepare for it adequately. One-to-one nursing supervision should begin as soon as a crisis is anticipated, and emergency respiratory support and suctioning equipment should be close at hand. Assessments should be made more often, but not to the point of fatiguing the patient. Special attention should be paid to respiratory status and swallowing ability.

Unlike the majority of patients receiving respiratory support, most myasthenic patients in crisis do not have pulmonary disease; rather, they have a problem with ventilation. That is, they have a problem with the mechanical movement of air into and (to a lesser extent) out of the lungs. The primary concerns in the respiratory management of myasthenic patients in crisis are to assist ventilation and to prevent the complications of intervention and/or inactivity.

There is usually some warning that respiratory failure is probable or imminent. Whenever possible, elective tracheotomy or intubation with a nasotracheal or orotracheal tube should be accomplished in a well-controlled environment with good lighting and proper equipment *before* the emergency arises; the patient's ability to understand and cooperate during these procedures is greater then. In addition, patient anxiety is decreased if the need for the respiratory support procedures is explained before rather than after they are instituted. The nursing management of the myasthenic patient requiring ventilatory assistance is basically the same as that of the patient who requires ventilatory assistance for some other reason (see Chap. 17). Patients subject to frequent respiratory failure may benefit from the permanent placement of an Olympic button.

All patients in crisis should be under the constant supervision of another person, preferably someone the patient can see at all times. The profound weakness associated with crisis may make it impossible for the patient to summon assistance if an emergency develops, such as a malfunctioning of the respiratory support equipment. Leaving the myasthenic patient in crisis alone in these circumstances may cause anxiety of such a degree as to cause further exacerbation of the disease.

The myasthenic patient in crisis is usually so weak that immobility is a problem. The patient should be helped to change position at least every two hours, to avoid prolonged pressure on any one area. Range-of-motion exercises, either passive or assisted, should be done at least daily to prevent loss of function. An-

tiembolic stockings may be indicated for some patients on bedrest. The patient should be encouraged to keep as active as possible. Activity should be encouraged, but the patient should not be permitted to do anything that would be unsafe or fatiguing.

The myasthenic patient in crisis usually cannot speak because of the presence of an endotracheal or a tracheostomy tube. A system of nonverbal communication between the patient and the health team members should be established—before the onset of the crisis if possible. The system of communication decided on should be described in the patient's care plan. Some of the possible communication systems are:

1. Use of a paper and pencil or a Magic Slate on which the patient can write.
2. Lip reading.
3. Use of a letter–number board on which the patient can spell out the communication. If the patient is very weak or is illiterate, a board with pictures of such things as a nurse, a physician, a bedpan, a urinal, and a suction catheter may be used.
4. "Writing" messages with a finger of the hand of the person the patient wishes to communicate with.

If severe weakness precludes the use of any of the methods just described, it may be necessary to ask a series of questions to which the patient can respond yes and no by nodding or shaking head, by moving eyes vertically or horizontally, by blinking eyes once or twice, or by using some other method of indicating agreement or disagreement. Whatever method of communication is chosen, the health team member communicating with the myasthenic patient should remember that the patient often has a great deal of frustration in trying to convey a message.

A myasthenic patient in crisis is under a tremendous amount of psychological stress. Nursing intervention can do much to minimize the stress and to facilitate the patient's adjustment. One of the most common fears the patient has is that of not being able to breathe because something has gone wrong with the ventilator. Constant supervision does much to alleviate that fear, as does the confidence of the nurses. A thorough explanation before each procedure also helps.

A certain amount of depression is to be expected. Reassurance that the crisis is temporary is helpful. The progress the patient has made should be emphasized. Most patients resent the dependency caused by their weakness. Some measure of independence can be retained by allowing the patient a voice in deciding when the necessary treatments should be done. The patient should be reassured that depression and feelings of resentment about dependency are normal.

Urinary elimination is rarely affected by a crisis but careful records should be kept of the patient's urinary output. Diarrhea and (to a much lesser extent) constipation are the most common problems of elimination encountered. Diarrhea is usually caused by anticholinesterase therapy, by tube feeding, or by a combination of both. The use of Lomotil (diphenoxylate hydrochloride with atropine sulfate), kaolin-pectin mixtures, or other antidiarrheal drugs usually controls the problem. Consultation with the dietitian about changes in the composition of the tube feeding may also help, as may administering the feeding over a longer period of time. Scrupulous skin care is essential for the patient who has diarrhea. Constipation is rare; it is best avoided or treated with stool softeners or other mild laxatives. Enemas should be avoided if possible because if the constipated patient is having problems with the regulation of anticholinesterase medication, enemas may overtax the already stressed parasympathetic nervous system. Anticholinesterase medications present the most serious challenge to the nurse.

No matter how acutely ill the myasthenic patient is, the demands of critical care should not cause neglect of basic needs. The basic needs include range-of-motion exercises, skin care, including frequent changes of position, mouth care, and eye care.

Medications

Anticholinesterase medications are administered to myasthenic patients on either a demand schedule or a fixed schedule. Most patients are put on a demand schedule when they are at home. They regulate their anticholinesterase intake (within specified limits) according to their need. For example, the dose may be slightly increased if an activity more strenuous than usual (e.g., shopping) is planned. Other patients, usually those with a more severe form of the disease, are on a fixed anticholinesterase schedule; that is, both the dosage and the time of administration are prescribed and inflexible.

Whatever their anticholinesterase schedule at home, the majority of myasthenic patients are put on a fixed schedule when they are hospitalized. The reason for the hospitalization has already put the patient at risk of exacerbation, and the fixed schedule permits the earlier detection and correction of any problems of regulation and puts the control of the medication in the hands of the health team. The physician should make certain that both the patient and the nursing staff know what type of anticholinesterase schedule is to be used.

The nurse should *always* administer the anticholinesterase medications *exactly* on schedule. Although a leeway of five or 10 minutes is rarely of consequence, the mild anxiety an inflexible rule produces in the nursing staff increases their awareness of the importance of the anticholinesterase therapy and reduces the possibility that a dose will be inadvertently omitted. The patient also should be aware of the medication schedule and retain some responsibility for medication administration.

The most important component of the nursing management of the patient undergoing anticholinesterase therapy is the nurse's observation. The nurse should be on the alert for any signs and symptoms of anticholinesterase overdosage or underdosage. Any signs and symptoms should be reported to the physician. The nurse may also identify more subtle indications of poor regulation, particularly if the relationship of the development of mild and equivocal signs and symptoms to the time of drug administration is kept in mind. For example, mild weakness that consistently occurs 30 to 40 minutes before each every-four-hour anticholinesterase dose should lead the nurse to suspect that the dosage is low and the patient slightly underdosed. On the other hand, weakness that consistently occurs one hour after each every-four-hour dose should lead the nurse to suspect that the dosage is high and the patient slightly overdosed. Although a precise diagnosis cannot be based on such observations, the nurse should be encouraged to make them and to speculate on the causes of any change. Such an approach may lead to the early detection of subtle but significant problems.

Patients undergoing anticholinesterase therapy usually have at least one Tensilon test done during their hospital stay. Much time can be saved if the unit has a Tensilon tray prepared and available. The tray should contain:

1. Intravenous Tensilon.
2. Intravenous neostigmine.

3. Intravenous atropine.
4. Tuberculin syringes and needles.
5. Alcohol swabs.
6. A tourniquet.

Steroid therapy in various forms is being used more and more to treat myasthenia gravis. Steroid therapy has many implications for nursing management. The therapy must be individualized to the patient. Some of the things to be considered in steroid therapy are:

1. The patient's room should be near the nurses' desk.
2. Frequent assessment is necessary.
3. The times the steroids are to be given. (If the steroids are to be given once a day, it is preferable to give them between 6 A.M. and 9 A.M., to coincide with the time of the peak endogenous steroid levels.)
4. The stools must be routinely tested for occult blood.
5. Oral steroids should be given at meals.
6. Antacids should be administered routinely between meals.
7. Urine should be tested routinely for sugar and acetone.

The most important thing for the nurse to remember about the nursing management of the patient undergoing steroid therapy is that the disease is exacerbated, perhaps critically, after initiation of the therapy. Generally, the exacerbation occurs within two weeks of initiation, and the patient is at particular risk on days four through 10. During that time, the nursing staff should be especially observant of the patient's status. Respiratory status and swallowing ability may need to be assessed more often. Decreases in status should be reported to the physician immediately.

Patients receiving chronic alternate-day steroid therapy may have fluctuations in status that vary according to the administration of the steroids. Nursing management should take these fluctuations into account. For example, the patient may be able to take a tub bath with assistance on "on" days but only a sponge bath with assistance on "off" days.

Other medications that are of concern are the drugs that are contraindicated for or should be used with caution with myasthenic patients. Some of those drugs are discussed in the following paragraphs.

The drugs that can be administered to the myasthenic patient only after double checking with a physician who knows the patient has myasthenia gravis are ACTH, steroids, thyroid compounds, respiratory depressants, sedatives, phenothiazines (e.g., prochlorperazine edisylate, prochlorperazine maleate [Compazine], chlorpromazine hydrochloride [Thorazine], promazine hydrochloride [Sparine]), -mycin antibiotics (e.g., neomycin, streptomycin, kanamycin, gentamicin, colistin [polymyxin E]), vasodilating drugs, and morphine sulfate. Some of the medications that should be administered only with extreme caution (because of the great potential for producing an exacerbation) include curare, quinine, quinidine, and succinylcholine.

Many drugs are potentially dangerous to a patient with myasthenia gravis. Many "harmless" drugs may exacerbate myasthenia gravis. Dangerous oversights may be avoided by tagging the front of the patient's chart with the diagnosis and a list of potentially dangerous drugs. A nurse asked to give any of the drugs just mentioned to a patient with myasthenia gravis would be wise to check the order before giving the drug. (That advice does not mean that the drugs are not used in treating patients with myasthenia gravis; it means only that they should be used with caution.)

Thymectomy

Thymectomy is a common treatment of myasthenia gravis. The nurse plays an important role in the preoperative and postoperative management of the patient undergoing thymectomy.

Patient teaching is the major component of the preoperative management. The teaching is planned and carried out by the health team, which includes the physician, the primary care nurse, the surgeon, the anesthesiologist, and the operating room nurse. The patient should understand the reason for the operation as well as what will be done during it. The patient should be told that symptoms will not disappear after surgery but that whatever benefits are received from the thymectomy will develop gradually over a period of months or years. It should be explained that it is impossible to predict exactly the degree of improvement that the individual patient will experience.

What will be done to and expected of the patient before and after the surgery should be explained in detail according to individual learning needs. It is often difficult for a patient to assimilate the information in one session. Other sessions should be planned in which the patient can ask questions and review any topics not yet mastered. A visit from a person with myasthenia gravis who has successfully undergone thymectomy may be beneficial for the patient.

The major concern in the postoperative management is the patient's respiratory status. The stress of surgery may decrease the patient's respiratory reserve. Pain from the incision may compromise respiratory ability. If the patient is breathing unassisted after surgery, constant one-to-one supervision and frequent monitoring of respiratory status (e.g., tidal volume, vital capacity, arterial blood gases, pulse, and respiratory rate) are necessary. Any sign or symptom of a worsening respiratory status should be reported immediately. The personnel and equipment needed for rapid intubation should be readily available. Oral intake should not be permitted until the patient's swallowing ability indicates that it is safe.

The patient who must have respiratory assistance should have one-to-one nursing supervision at all times. The patient should be weaned from the ventilator and activity increased to normal levels as soon as possible.

The patient who is receiving anticholinesterase medications after a thymectomy should be closely watched for the signs and symptoms of overdosage or underdosage. The stress of surgery and the improvement the thymectomy has brought may make regulation of the medications difficult.

Careful attention should be paid to the site of the incision. Any signs of infection and any elevation of temperature should be reported to the physician. The site of the incision usually heals without complication if the health team adheres to the principles of asepsis.

Psychological Support

Myasthenia gravis, because of its potential or actual severity and its variability, requires the patient to make a difficult adjustment. Hospitalization is an additional stress. Psychological support is necessary, particularly for the hospitalized patient; it is an important part of the nursing management. Time should be set aside regularly for empathetic listening to and reassurance of the patient. To help the patient cope with limitations imposed by the disease, the nurse should emphasize what the patient *can* do and what

can be done to compensate for the activities which can no longer be performed. Psychiatric help may be needed for those few patients whose adjustment is poor and whose mental health is compromised.

Safety

The myasthenic patient is subject to rapid and serious worsening in condition. Unfortunately, the resultant weakness frequently makes it difficult for the patient to summon help. The risk to the patient is decreased if the room is close to the nurses' station. The risk is also decreased if the patient is given a small tap bell besides the regular room call bell. The patient should be told to use the call bell for routine communication with the nursing staff and to use the tap bell only in an emergency. Since the sound of the tap bell is recognized easily, the nurses can respond quickly.

Documentation

Hospitalized patients with myasthenia gravis must be assessed frequently and monitored closely. Respiratory status and swallowing ability, muscle strength, and diplopia are among the parameters most commonly monitored. It is also important to relate assessment to other factors (e.g., the administration of medication, Tensilon testing, and activity). Other factors to be measured and commented on are indicated by the individual patient's needs.

Use of a flow sheet is the best way to record the results of periodic assessments of a number of parameters (Table 31-2). In the case of the myasthenic patient, a flow sheet is valuable for alerting those caring for the patient to changes in status. A flow sheet is also valuable for evaluating therapy.

Nursing Orders

Problem/Diagnosis

Dyspnea.

OBJECTIVE

The patient's arterial blood gas measurements should remain normal.

Table 31-2
General Purpose Flow Sheet

Problem: Myasthenia Gravis									
Date	Time	VC	Sw	Dip.				Medication	Comment
8-12-77	1100	1.8	4	No				45 mg Prostigmin	
	1430	1.6	4	No					Complains of increasing weakness
	1432	1.9	4	No				10 mg IV Tensilon	
	1433	1.9	5	No					Positive Tensilon test

VC = vital capacity (measured in liters); Sw = swallowing ability (see scale on p. 676); Dip. = diplopia.

ACHIEVING THE OBJECTIVE

To achieve the objective, the nurse should:

1. Measure the patient's vital capacity every ——— hour(s) and/or when anticholinesterase medication is administered. Vital capacities of less than ——— liters should be reported. The nurse should note the patient's position and the kind of spirometer used.
2. Measure the inspiratory and expiratory pressures every ——— hours; report inspiratory pressures of less than ——— and expiratory pressures of less than ———.

Problem/Diagnosis

Dysphagia.

OBJECTIVE

The patient should not aspirate and should not have nontherapeutic weight loss.

ACHIEVING THE OBJECTIVE

To achieve the objective, the nurse should:

1. Have the patient subjectively evaluate swallowing ability every ——— hours and/or when anti-

cholinesterase medication is administered. The following scale should be used to record the evaluation:

Nothing	.0
Saliva	.1
Liquids	.2
Pureed diet	.3
Soft diet	.4
Normal diet	.5

2. If the patient often has significant fluctuations in swallowing ability:
   a. Order meals to be delivered to coincide with the peak anticholinesterase effect.
   b. Order meals of the proper consistency (as indicated by evaluations of the patient's swallowing ability, which may have to be made on a meal-by-meal basis).
   c. Have suctioning equipment on standby in the patient's room.
   d. Stay with the patient during meals.

Problem/Diagnosis

Diplopia.

OBJECTIVE

The patient will have maximum benefit of vision.

ACHIEVING THE OBJECTIVE

To achieve the objective, the nurse should:

1. Evaluate the patient for the presence of diplopia every _____ hours and/or when administering anticholinesterase medication. (Slight degrees of diplopia may be elicited by having the patient turn eyes to the extreme in any direction.)
2. Record the results of the evaluation.
3. If diplopia is a major problem, confer with the physician about the advisability of using an eye patch alternately on both eyes.

Problem/Diagnosis

Generalized weakness.

OBJECTIVE

Before the patient is discharged, activities should approximate those which will be engaged in at home.

ACHIEVING THE OBJECTIVE

To achieve the objective, the nurse should:

1. Encourage maximal activity within the limits of strength and fatigue to determine adequacy of disease control.
2. If the patient is very weak, space activities throughout the day.

Problem/Diagnosis

Adverse psychological reactions.

OBJECTIVE

The patient should adjust to the condition in a positive manner as demonstrated by: (1) talking about the disease as being real and belonging to him/her; (2) verbalizing anger and bargaining attempts; (3) verbalizing acceptance of the disease; and (4) reformulating life goals.

ACHIEVING THE OBJECTIVE

To achieve the objective, the nurse should:

1. Be honest with the patient about the limitations in life-style the disease imposes but point out the adaptations which can be made.

2. Give the patient an adequate opportunity to discuss concerns.
3. If the patient's psychological reactions become a significant problem, consider a consultation with the psychiatric liaison clinical nurse specialist or other resource in psychiatric management.

Problem/Diagnosis

Fluctuating physical condition.

OBJECTIVE

The patient should not aspirate and arterial blood gas measurements should remain normal.

ACHIEVING THE OBJECTIVE

To achieve the objective, the nurse should:

1. See that the patient has a room that is near the nurse's station.
2. Give the patient a tap bell to use in emergencies.
3. Label the patient's chart with a list of drugs contraindicated in and/or to be used with caution in myasthenia gravis.
4. Have a Tensilon tray in the patient's room.

Problem/Diagnosis

Anticholinesterase drug therapy.

OBJECTIVE

The patient should not aspirate and arterial blood gas measurements should remain normal.

ACHIEVING THE OBJECTIVE

To achieve the objective, the nurse should:

1. *Always* administer the anticholinesterase medication *exactly* on time.
2. Report any signs and symptoms of anticholinesterase overdosage or underdosage.

Problem/Diagnosis

Ptosis.

OBJECTIVE

The patient will have maximum benefit of vision.

ACHIEVING THE OBJECTIVE

To achieve the objective, the nurse should:

Evaluate the patient (and record the results of the evaluation) for the presence of ptosis every ——— hours and/or when anticholinesterase medication is administered. (Both eyes should be checked while the patient is facing straight ahead while attempting maximum eye opening.) The following scale should be used to record the results:

Unable to open his eye 1
None of the pupil visible but lid not shut 2
Lower half of the pupil visible 3
All of the pupil visible but none of the upper iris visible 4
All of the pupil visible and some of the upper iris visible 5

Problem/Diagnosis

Potential adverse problems due to chronic steroid therapy.

OBJECTIVE

The patient should not aspirate and arterial blood gas measurements should remain normal.

ACHIEVING THE OBJECTIVE

To achieve the objective, the nurse should:

1. Be alert to changes in the patient's strength that correlate with steroid dosage.
2. Be alert for the exacerbation of myasthenia gravis during the initiation of chronic steroid therapy.
3. See The Myasthenia Gravis Patient Who Is Receiving Chronic Steroid Therapy below.

Problem/Diagnosis

Patient teaching and discharge planning.

OBJECTIVE

The patient is able to state the rationale for each component of the discharge plan.

ACHIEVING THE OBJECTIVE

To achieve the objective, the nurse should:

1. Instruct the patient to report any significant changes in swallowing ability.
2. Arrange a dietary consultation for any diet modifications that are needed.
3. Instruct the patient about reporting severe or prolonged respiratory tract infections and any subjective or objective evidence of a decrease in respiratory status.
4. Instruct the patient to avoid people who have respiratory tract infections.
5. Instruct the patient who is on a fixed anticholinesterase schedule to take medication *exactly* on schedule.
6. Make certain that the patient who is on a fixed anticholinesterase schedule has a non-electric alarm clock at home.
7. For the patient who is on a demand anticholinesterase schedule, review the limits within which dosage may be self-regulated.
8. Review the signs and symptoms of anticholinesterase overdosage and underdosage.
9. Review the handbook *Help Is on the Way* [19] with the patient and family.
10. Review the signs and symptoms of myasthenia gravis with the patient.
11. Instruct the patient to tell the following people of the diagnosis of myasthenia gravis: local physician, dentist, pharmacist, and the local rescue squad or emergency room staff.
12. Tell the patient about the services of the Myasthenia Gravis Foundation (230 Park Avenue, New York, N.Y. 10007).
13. Review the disease, the treatment, and the emergency care with the patient's family.
14. Make sure the patient has a home telephone.
15. Give the patient the phone numbers of the critical care unit, the neurology outpatient unit, and the hospital.
16. Give the patient a list of the drugs that may be dangerous for the person who has myasthenia gravis and instructions to carry the list at all times.
17. Obtain a Medic-Alert identification for the patient.

Problem/Diagnosis

Chronic steroid therapy.

OBJECTIVE NO. 1

The patient should have no infection secondary to immunosuppression.

ACHIEVING THE OBJECTIVE

To achieve the objective, the nurse should:

1. Instruct the patient about the importance of avoiding people with infections (especially upper respiratory tract infections) and of reporting any severe or prolonged infections.
2. If possible, avoid assigning staff members who have signs and symptoms of infection to work with the patient. If that is necessary, the staff member should wear a mask when in the room with the patient and should practice careful handwashing techniques.
3. Report the signs and symptoms of patient infection to the physician.
4. Confer with the physician about the advisability of using prophylactic isoniazid (INH) and pyridoxine therapy.

OBJECTIVE NO. 2

The patient should not develop vertebral compression, a condition that is secondary to demineralization. (The risk of developing vertebral compression is increased among postmenopausal women, the elderly, and the immobilized.)

ACHIEVING THE OBJECTIVE

To achieve the objective, the nurse should:

1. Question the patient about symptoms of vertebral compression (e.g., pain, sensory changes, weakness) and report positive responses.
2. Encourage the patient to achieve the highest activity level within the limits of safety and fatigability.
3. If an increase of dietary calcium and vitamin D is indicated, schedule dietary consultation. Review dietary plan with patient.
4. Confer with the physician about giving the patient supplemental calcium and vitamin D.

OBJECTIVE NO. 3

The patient should not develop diabetes mellitus secondary to increased gluconeogenesis and to increased cellular glucose utilization.

ACHIEVING THE OBJECTIVE

To achieve the objective, the nurse should:

1. Measure the patient's urinary sugar and acetone levels _____ (frequency).
2. Confer with the physician about the signs and symptoms of hyperglycemia and hypoglycemia.
3. If the patient has diabetes or glycosuria, the nurse should:
   a. Teach the patient about the administration, dosage, and beneficial and adverse effects of the hypoglycemic drug that has been prescribed.
   b. Teach the patient about the signs and symptoms of hyperglycemia and hypoglycemia.
   c. Obtain a Medic-Alert identification that says the patient is a diabetic.
   d. Give the patient a supply of urine testing material before discharge. Instruct in how to test urine. Observe return demonstration. Instruct in prescribed frequency of testing.

OBJECTIVE NO. 4

The patient's blood pressure should remain normal.

ACHIEVING THE OBJECTIVE

To achieve the objective, the nurse should monitor the patient's blood pressure every ____ hours. If the patient has hypertension, the nurse should:

1. Instruct the patient about a sodium-restricted diet.
2. Teach the patient about any hypertensive drugs that have been prescribed.

OBJECTIVE NO. 5

The patient should not develop myopathy secondary to increased catabolism.

ACHIEVING THE OBJECTIVE

To achieve the objective, the nurse should:

1. Measure the patient's muscle strength and bulk periodically.
2. Question the patient about symptoms of weakness (e.g., trouble getting out of bed, rising from a low chair, or climbing stairs); report positive responses.

OBJECTIVE NO. 6

The patient should not develop melena secondary to decreased tissue integrity.

ACHIEVING THE OBJECTIVE

To achieve the objective, the nurse should:

1. Administer steroid medication with meals or snacks.
2. Test stools for occult blood —— (frequency).
3. Confer with the physician about the prophylactic administration of antacids.
4. Instruct the patient to observe for and report:
   a. Epigastric pain.
   b. Vomiting, especially "coffee-ground" vomitus.
   c. Any change in the color of the stool.

OBJECTIVE NO. 7

The patient's serum potassium levels should remain normal.

ACHIEVING THE OBJECTIVE

To achieve the objective, the nurse should:

1. Instruct the patient about the signs and symptoms of hypokalemia.
2. Instruct the patient about the foods that have a high potassium content.
3. Confer with the physician about giving the patient supplemental potassium.

OBJECTIVE NO. 8

The patient's family should talk about the fact that the patient may have emotional and behavioral changes.

ACHIEVING THE OBJECTIVE

To achieve the objective, the nurse should:

1. Observe the patient for any emotional changes.
2. Instruct the patient's family to report any changes in the patient's behavior.
3. Arrange for a consultation with a psychiatric liaison clinical nurse specialist or other resource in psychiatric management.

OBJECTIVE NO. 9

The patient should adjust to the possibility of developing cushingoid body changes.

ACHIEVING THE OBJECTIVE

To achieve the objective, the nurse should:

1. Give the patient emotional support and attempt to increase self-esteem.
2. Tell the patient of the changes that might occur in appearance (e.g., increased weight, puffiness of the face, and acne).
3. Arrange for a consultation with a psychiatric liaison clinical nurse specialist or other resource in psychiatric management if such a consultation is indicated.

OBJECTIVE NO. 10

In order to avoid an addisonian crisis, the patient's steroid therapy should not be terminated abruptly.

ACHIEVING THE OBJECTIVE

To achieve the objective, the nurse should:

1. Instruct the patient not to decrease or terminate steroid therapy without consulting the physician.
2. Obtain a Medic-Alert identification for the patient that notes that the patient is undergoing chronic steroid therapy.
3. If the patient is taking steroids once a day or on alternate days, confer with the physician about administering the steroids to correlate with the patient's sleep-wake cycle.

Problem/Diagnosis

Preoperative preparation for thymectomy.

OBJECTIVE

The patient should be able to state the rationale for thymectomy and the purpose of the preoperative preparation and, with the help of the staff, to express fears and anxieties.

ACHIEVING THE OBJECTIVE

To achieve the objective, the nurse should:

1. Discuss with the patient the purpose of thymectomy in the management of myasthenia gravis.
2. Discuss with the patient the expected results of thymectomy. The nurse should stress that:
   a. Thymectomy will not cure myasthenia gravis but it may cause a remission of symptoms.
   b. Any improvement will not occur immediately; it will occur slowly—over a period of months or years.
3. Discuss what will happen to and be expected of the patient before, during, and after the thymectomy. The nurse should tell the patient about:
   a. The preoperative preparation (e.g., scrubs and medications).
   b. The surgical approach to be used.
   c. The postoperative management (e.g., the different hospital units where the patient will be treated, monitoring, the types and frequency of monitoring, the methods used to control pain).
4. Arrange to have another person with myasthenia gravis who has had a successful thymectomy visit the patient.
5. Discuss with the patient the importance of coughing and deep breathing postoperatively. The nurse should:
   a. Demonstrate the techniques of coughing and deep breathing to the patient; observe return demonstration of techniques.
   b. Instruct the patient about the techniques of splinting the incision site; observe return demonstration of techniques.
   c. Demonstrate the use of assistive devices (e.g., blow bottles, incentive spirometer); observe return demonstration.
6. Discuss the rationale of chest physiotherapy and demonstrate the techniques.
7. If it is anticipated that assisted ventilation will be needed:
   a. Discuss the rationale of assisted ventilation.
   b. Explain the equipment that may be used.
   c. Demonstrate suctioning techniques.
   d. Agree on and practice a method of nonverbal communication.
8. Include the patient's family and significant others in the preoperative preparation.
9. Give the patient an opportunity to discuss feelings about the impending operation. If the patient does not volunteer any information, ask the patient to describe feelings.

Problem/Diagnosis

Safety during thymectomy.

OBJECTIVE

The patient should not aspirate and arterial blood gas measurements should remain normal.

ACHIEVING THE OBJECTIVE

To achieve the objective, the nurse should make certain that the patient's chart cover and the medication record prominently display the myasthenic drug list (drugs to be avoided or to be used with caution in the management of the myasthenia gravis patient).

Problem/Diagnosis

Thymectomy while receiving chronic steroid therapy.

OBJECTIVE

The patient should not develop postoperative adrenal insufficiency.

ACHIEVING THE OBJECTIVE

To achieve the objective, the nurse should discuss with the physician the patient's need for supplemental steroids before, during, and after the surgery (supplemental steroids are necessary because the patient will be subjected to increased amounts of stress).

Problem/Diagnosis

Postthymectomy management.

OBJECTIVE NO. 1

The patient should not develop an infection.

ACHIEVING THE OBJECTIVE

To achieve the objective, the nurse should:

1. Monitor the patient's vital signs as ordered and as indicated by the patient's status.
2. After the chest dressing has been removed by the surgeon:
   a. Inspect the incision site every eight hours.
   b. Document and report any swelling, increased redness, or drainage.
3. Monitor and record the patient's breath sounds every eight hours.
4. Document and report any changes in the sputum that might indicate a respiratory infection (e.g., increased amount or thickness of the sputum and a darkening of the color of the sputum).
5. Assist the patient to turn, cough, and deep breathe every ＿＿ hours. Administer pain medication 30 minutes before the procedure if necessary to control pain.
6. Have the patient use the incentive spirometer every ＿＿ hours for ＿＿ minutes.
7. If a respiratory infection and/or pulmonary congestion develops, administer chest physical therapy every ＿＿ hours.

OBJECTIVE NO. 2

The patient should not aspirate and arterial blood gas measurements should remain normal.

ACHIEVING THE OBJECTIVE

To achieve the objective, the nurse should:

1. Monitor the patient's vital capacity every ＿＿ hours.
2. Monitor the patient's inspiratory and expiratory pressures every ＿＿ hours.
3. Be alert for the need to change the anticholinesterase dosage if either overdosage (secondary to the improvement in the patient's condition the thymectomy has brought) or underdosage (secondary to the stress of the operation) develops.

Preprocedure

Problem/Diagnosis

Preparation for plasma exchange.

OBJECTIVE

The patient should not aspirate and arterial blood gas measurements should remain normal.

ACHIEVING THE OBJECTIVE

To achieve the objective, the nurse should:

1. Measure and document the baseline and end of procedure data about the patient's vital capacity, swallowing ability, presence or absence of diplopia, and degree of ptosis.
2. Stay with the patient during the plasma exchange (the nurse should have had experience with myasthenia gravis patients).
3. Measure and document the patient's vital capacity during the plasma exchange procedure every 30 minutes and measure and document the other parameters listed in item 1 as indicated by the patient's status.
4. Administer the anticholinesterase medications as ordered at the scheduled times. If the patient is taking anticholinesterase medication, monitor closely for overdosage and underdosage.

Problem/Diagnosis

Anxiety.

OBJECTIVE

The patient should be able to state the rationale for the plasma exchange, to describe the plasma exchange procedure, and, with the help of the staff, to express feelings about the procedure.

ACHIEVING THE OBJECTIVE

To achieve the objective, the nurse should:

1. Describe to the patient the rationale for plasma exchange.
2. Describe what will happen to and be expected of the patient before, during, and after the procedure.
3. Arrange to have the patient observe an uncomplicated plasma exchange and/or arrange to have another patient who has had a successful plasma exchange visit the patient.
4. Describe to the patient the results that are expected from the plasma exchange, stressing that

the signs and symptoms may improve but the underlying disease will not be cured.

5. Provide opportunities for the patient to discuss feelings about the procedure. If the patient does not volunteer any information, ask about the feelings.
6. Be certain that the patient (or a family member) has signed the consent form for the procedure.

Problem/Diagnosis

Prevention of venous trauma secondary to the plasma exchange.

OBJECTIVE

Access to the patient's peripheral venous circulation should be maintained.

ACHIEVING THE OBJECTIVE

To achieve the objective, the nurse should:

1. Be certain that the veins to be used in the plasma exchange are not used for venipuncture, the administration of intravenous fluids, or for any other purpose.
2. Apply heat to the needle insertion sites 30 minutes before beginning the plasma exchange.
3. If an A-V shunt or fistula is present, check the patient for the presence of a bruit or thrill every —— hours.

Problem/Diagnosis

Loss of plasma-bound medications and electrolytes during plasma exchange.

OBJECTIVE

The patient should not develop complications secondary to undermedication, and/or electrolyte imbalance.

ACHIEVING THE OBJECTIVE

To achieve the objective, the nurse should:

1. Consult with the physician about whether plasma-bound medications (e.g., prednisone, im-

munosuppressive drugs, digitalis preparations, or thyroid preparations) should be given at the end of the procedure rather than before or during it.
2. If the medication must be given before or during the procedure (as is the case with insulin and heparin), monitor the patient for the signs and symptoms of underdosage.
3. Consult with the physician about the guidelines for potassium replacement.

During the Procedure

Problem/Diagnosis

Plasma exchange.

OBJECTIVE NO. 1

The patient's vital signs should remain stable.

ACHIEVING THE OBJECTIVE

To achieve the objective, the nurse should:

1. Measure and record baseline vital signs.
2. Measure and record vital signs every half hour, temperature every hour.

OBJECTIVE NO. 2

Access to peripheral circulation should be maintained.

ACHIEVING THE OBJECTIVE

To achieve the objective, the nurse should:

1. Measure blood pressure in an extremity *not* being utilized for plasma exchange.
2. Position the extremities to be used for plasma exchange securely on heating pads.
3. Observe needle insertion sites every half hour for bleeding or hematoma formation.
4. Document the presence of bruit every half hour, if the patient has an arteriovenous fistula or shunt.

OBJECTIVE NO. 3

The patient should not develop hypocalcemia (calcium is bound by ACD, the anticoagulant used during the procedure).

ACHIEVING THE OBJECTIVE

To achieve the objective, the nurse should:

1. Observe respirations carefully, because hypocalcemia may produce tetany of the respiratory muscles.
2. Be sure the patient receives continuous cardiac monitoring during the procedure (hypocalcemia causes slower ventricular conduction).
3. Document and report any cardiac arrhythmias, particularly lengthening QT intervals.
4. Document and report signs and symptoms of hypocalcemia, intermittent muscular contractions, fibrillations, paresthesias, and muscular pains (especially of the palatal and perioral areas, fingers, and toes).
5. Encourage the patient to drink milk before and during the procedure, if not contraindicated.
6. See that calcium gluconate for intravenous administration is available at the patient's bedside.

OBJECTIVE NO. 4

The patient should not develop hypercalcemia.

ACHIEVING THE OBJECTIVE

To achieve the objective, the nurse should (if hypocalcemia is treated with calcium gluconate) be alert for cardiac arrhythmias secondary to hypercalcemia; cardiac arrest is also a potential development.

OBJECTIVE NO. 5

The patient should not develop hypokalemia.

ACHIEVING THE OBJECTIVE

To achieve the objective, the nurse should:

1. Monitor the patient for and report weakening pulse, decrease in blood pressure, ECG changes (e.g., PVCs, prolonged QT interval, depressed T wave, prolonged PR interval, loss of P wave).
2. Document and report signs and symptoms of hypokalemia (nausea, vomiting, weakness, shallow respirations).
3. Be sure that potassium for intravenous administration is available at the patient's bedside.

OBJECTIVE NO. 6

The patient should not develop hyperkalemia.

ACHIEVING THE OBJECTIVE

To achieve the objective, the nurse should:

1. Monitor the patient for and report decreasing heart rate and ECG changes (A-V block, elevated T wave, depressed ST segment).
2. Document and report signs and symptoms of hyperkalemia (nausea, cramping, diarrhea, skeletal muscle weakness, neuromuscular irritability).

OBJECTIVE NO. 7

The patient should not develop fluid disequilibrium.

ACHIEVING THE OBJECTIVE

To achieve the objective, the nurse should:

1. Measure and record intake and output.
2. Document and report increasing or decreasing blood pressure or pulse.
3. Evaluate and document breath sounds every hour.

OBJECTIVE NO. 8

The patient should not develop transfusion reaction (rare complication).

ACHIEVING THE OBJECTIVE

To achieve the objective, the nurse should:

1. Be sure that epinephrine and diphenhydramine (Benadryl) for parenteral administration are easily accessible.
2. Document and report development of fever, chills, flushing, or urticaria.

OBJECTIVE NO. 9

The patient should be able to perform activities of daily living with assistance.

ACHIEVING THE OBJECTIVE

To achieve the objective, the nurse should:

1. Have the patient void immediately prior to needle insertion.
2. Provide privacy when the patient uses bedpan or urinal.
3. Feed the patient meals or order late trays.

4. Try to prevent boredom; attempt to find ways to occupy the patient's attention.
5. Be aware that the necessary extremity immobility can be very uncomfortable and provide necessary comfort measures.

Postprocedure

Problem/Diagnosis

Postplasma exchange management.

OBJECTIVE

The patient should have stable vital signs, should not hemorrhage from the needle insertion sites, and should not form hematomas at the needle insertion sites.

ACHIEVING THE OBJECTIVE

To achieve the objective, the nurse should:

1. Measure and record the patient's vital signs every hour for four hours and then revert to the schedule that was in effect before the plasma exchange was done.
2. If an artificial access to the patient's venous system is not present:
   a. Remove the source of heat.
   b. Apply digital pressure after the removal of the needle until the bleeding stops.
   c. Apply the pressure dressings.
3. If an artificial access to the patient's venous system is present, remove the source of heat and then consult the physician about what method of bleeding control should be used.
4. Check the needle insertion site for seepage of blood or hematoma formation every hour for four hours.
5. Educate the patient about monitoring the needle insertion sites.
6. Record and report any increases in pulse rate or decreases in blood pressure.

Summary

Myasthenia gravis is a chronic illness that often has acute exacerbations that require critical care. The management of the acute exacerbations is directed toward: (1) respiratory, nutritional, and emotional support, (2) assessment of the patient's condition and efficacy of the treatment, and (3) prevention of the complications of immobility. Patient teaching and discharge planning are extremely important. Prevention of unwitnessed acute exacerbations and of therapy complications depends in large part on the patient's understanding of the disease and treatment and on the successful preparation for discharge and self-care at home.

Study Problems

1. Myasthenic patients who are taking anticholinesterase medications may have myasthenic or cholinergic reactions to them. Nausea, vomiting, abdominal cramps, and diarrhea are almost always indicative of:
   a. A cholinergic reaction.
   b. A myasthenic reaction.
2. Curare is a frequently used diagnostic test for myasthenia gravis.
   a. True.
   b. False.
3. Thyroidectomy is commonly used in the management of myasthenia gravis.
   a. True.
   b. False.
4. When a myasthenic patient develops cramps and diarrhea following the administration of intravenous Tensilon, atropine is given intravenously to:
   a. Prevent a cholinergic crisis.
   b. Prevent a myasthenic crisis.
   c. Minimize the sympathetic side effects.
   d. Minimize the parasympathetic side effects.
5. Abnormal thymic involution is a common finding in patients with myasthenia gravis.
   a. True.
   b. False.

6.	Before Tensilon	After Tensilon
Vital capacity	1.4 L	0.9 L
Swallowing	4	2
Diplopia	None	Present

The before and after Tensilon test results listed in the table above are most indicative of:
a. A cholinergic state (a negative test).

b. A myasthenic state (a positive test).

c. An equivocal test.

7. A myasthenic patient was given 30 mg of neostigmine (Prostigmin) at 7 A.M. At 7:45, the patient complained of feeling weak and "nervous." Most probably, the patient was slightly:

   a. Overdosed.

   b. Underdosed.

8. Which of the following are common signs and symptoms of myasthenia gravis?

   a. Dysphasia, diplopia, ptosis, and dyspnea.

   b. Dysphagia, diplopia, ptosis, and dyspnea.

   c. Aphasia, dyspnea, bradycardia, and anisocoria.

   d. Dysphagia, cogwheel rigidity, ptosis, and diplopia.

9. Which of the following are common side effects of chronic steroid therapy?

   a. Gastrointestinal irritation.

   b. Hypoglycemia.

   c. Osteoporosis.

   d. Adrenal suppression.

   e. Gout.

   f. Rheumatoid arthritis.

   g. Hypertension.

   h. Hypokalemia.

Answers

1. a.
2. b.
3. b.
4. d.
5. b.
6. a.
7. a.
8. b.
9. a, c, d, g, h.

References

1. Armstrong, D. *Hang In There.* New York: Grossman, 1974. (Written by patients for patients)
2. Blount, M., and Kinney, A. B. Chronic steroid therapy. *Am. J. Nurs.* 74:1626, 1974.
3. Blount, M., Kinney, A. B., and Stone, M. Plasma exchange in the management of myasthenia gravis. *Nurs. Clin. North Am.* 14:173, 1979.
4. Cohen, S. L., et al. The pharmacokinetics of pyridostigmine. *Neurology* 26:536, 1976.
5. Dau, P. C. Plasma phoresis and immunosuppressive drug therapy in myasthenia gravis. *N. Engl. J. Med.* 9:1134, 1977.
6. DiMauro, S., Penn, A. S., and Rowland, L. P. Myopathies and Junctional Disorders. In D. B. Tower (ed.), *The Nervous System.* New York: Raven Press, 1975.
7. Drachman, D. B. Myasthenia gravis, Part 1. *N. Engl. J. Med.* 298:136, 1978.
8. Drachman, D. B. Myasthenia gravis, Part 2. *N. Engl. J. Med.* 298:186, 1978.
9. Engel, A. G., et al. Ultrastructural localization of the acetylcholine receptor in myasthenia gravis and in its experimental autoimmune model. *Neurology* 27:307, 1977.
10. Flacke, W. Treatment of myasthenia gravis. *N. Engl. J. Med.* 288:27, 1973.
11. Horowitz, S. H., et al. Electrophysiologic diagnosis of myasthenia gravis and the regional curare test. *Neurology* 26:410, 1976.
12. Horowitz, S. H., et al. Electrophysiologic evaluations of thymectomy in myasthenia gravis: Preliminary findings. *Neurology* 26:615, 1976.
13. Howard, J. F., Sanders, D. B., and Johns, T. R. The Role of Plasma Exchange Therapy in Myasthenia Gravis. In *The Proceedings of the Haemonetics Research Institute Advanced Component Seminar.* Boston, 1978.
14. Kempton, J. W. *Living with Myasthenia Gravis: A Bright New Tomorrow.* Springfield, Ill.: Thomas, 1972. (Written by patients for patients)
15. Kinney, A. B., and Blount, M. Systems approach to myasthenia gravis. *Nurs. Clin. North Am.* 6:435, 1971.
16. Lindstrom, J. M., et al. Antibody to acetylcholine in myasthenia gravis. *Neurology* 26:1054, 1976.
17. Liverani, L., and Osserman, R. S. Myasthenia gravis: A nursing care plan. *Nurs. Clin. North Am.* 7:185, 1972.
18. Mann, J. D., Johns, T. R., and Campa, J. F. Long-term administration of corticosteroids in myasthenia gravis. *Neurology* 26:729, 1976.
19. Myasthenia Gravis Foundation, Inc. *Help Is on the Way: A Handbook for Patients.* New York, 1972.
20. Myasthenia Gravis Foundation, Inc. *Myasthenia Gravis: A Manual for the Nurse.* New York, 1975.
21. Myasthenia Gravis Foundation, Inc. *Myasthenia Gravis: A Manual for the Physician.* New York, 1975.
22. Newsom-Davis, J., et al. Function of circulatory antibody to acetylcholine receptors in myasthenia gravis, investigated by plasma exchange. *Neurology* 28:266, 1978.
23. Nysather, J. O., Katz, A. E., and Lenth, J. L. The immune system: Its development and functions. *Am. J. Nurs.* 76:614, 1976.
24. Patten, B. M. Myasthenia Gravis. In H. R. Tyler and D. M. Dawson (eds.), *Current Neurology* (vol. 1). Boston: Houghton Mifflin, 1978.

25. Patten, B. M. Myasthenia Gravis Update. In H. R. Tyler and D. M. Dawson (eds.), *Current Neurology* (vol. 2). Boston: Houghton Mifflin, 1979.

26. Ross, A. J., Herr, B. E., Norwood, M. L., Donahoe, K. M., and Moxley, R. T. Neuromuscular diagnostic procedures. *Nurs. Clin. North Am.* 14:107, 1979.

27. Russo, L., Scoppetta, C., and Tonali, P. Shifting of the blood T-B lymphocyte ratio in myasthenia gravis patients after thymectomy. *Neurology* 27:642, 1977.

28. Sanders, D. B., Howard, J. F., Johns, T. R., et al. High Dose Day Prednisone in the Treatment of Myasthenia Gravis. In P. C. Dau (ed.), *Plasma Phoresis and the Immunobiology of Myasthenia Gravis.* Boston: Houghton Mifflin, 1979.

29. Sanders, D. B., Johns, T. R., Eldefrawi, M. E., et al. Experimental autoimmune myasthenia gravis in rats: Modification by thymectomy and prednisolone. *Arch. Neurol.* 34:75, 1977.

30. Smith, E., Hammarstrom, L., Moller, E., et al. The effect of ACTH treatment on lymphocyte subpopulations in patients with myasthenia gravis. *Neurology* 26:915, 1976.

31. Stackhouse, J. Myasthenia gravis. *Am. J. Nurs.* 73:1544, 1973.

IX. The Critically Ill Adult with Renal Problems

Because a patient's emotional states are reflected in physiological changes, could patients be taught to intentionally use their emotions to cause healthful changes in their own bodies? This is the primary idea underlying the clinical use of biofeedback.

The use of biofeedback facilitates a change in the usual doctor/patient relationship that appears to us to be quite unique, since the patient becomes his own therapist; the paradigm of the doctor/patient, parent/child relationship is pushed aside, and the doctor becomes more of a colleague.

The patient produces obvious changes in the functioning of his own autonomic nervous system and becomes aware, therefore, that malfunctioning is produced by himself. The concept that symptoms just happen, that the doctor will take care of them, is no longer feasible. Instead, he is responsible to himself for results. He is able to take the initiative in diminishing or eradicating symptoms.*

In many centers the nurse is already involved in teaching patients this new kind of therapy. In addition, the use of relaxation techniques has already invaded critical care areas. This invasion will modify the critical care nurse's role, perhaps as profoundly as her role was modified by the advent of modern coronary care units.

New skills will be needed. A thorough understanding of body-mind interrelations is the first step for the critical care nurse toward acquiring these new kinds of skills.

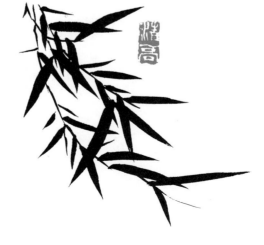

*Gladman, A. E., and Estrada, N. Biofeedback in Clinical Practice. In *Psychiatry and Mysticism.* Chicago: Nelson-Hall, 1975. Pp. 227–228.

Acute Renal Failure

Barbara Montgomery Dossey

Acute renal failure can occur in a variety of clinical circumstances to medical, surgical, and obstetrical patients. Acute renal failure involves an abrupt curtailment of renal function that produces renal insufficiency. It can rapidly become a life-threatening condition that must be recognized by the physician and the nurse. Even when careful attention is paid to the details of fluid and electrolyte balance and when peritoneal dialysis or hemodialysis is used, the mortality is still high. The associated illness that has led to the acute episode or the complications that occur during the acute episode determine the patient's outcome. The people who are responsible for the medical and nursing management of the patient must be on the alert for the high-risk clinical situations that are anticipated in acute renal failure, and they must recognize the early signs of acute renal failure if they are to reverse the process.

Objective

The nurse should know the signs of acute renal failure, do a systematic assessment of the patient who has acute renal failure and write nursing orders for his management.

32

Achieving the Objective

To achieve the objective, the nurse should be able to:

1. Describe the anatomy and physiology of the normal kidney.
2. Identify the categories of acute renal failure.
3. Identify the clinical manifestations of acute renal failure.
4. Describe the major medical therapies for acute renal failure.
5. Describe the basic diagnostic urine tests.
6. List the methods of reducing hyperkalemia.
7. Describe the nursing care objectives for a patient who has acute renal failure.

How to Proceed

To develop an approach to acute renal failure, the nurse should:

1. Read the chapter.
2. Make a problem list immediately after reading the case history that follows.
3. Act as the primary care nurse for the patient described in the case history. The nurse should:
   a. Make out a patient care plan.
   b. List the patient care objectives.
4. Plan a staff conference to discuss the major problems that are anticipated in a patient who has acute renal failure.

Case Study

Mr. R. M., aged 48, was admitted to the hospital emergency room with a chief complaint of nausea, vomiting, and persistent abdominal pain. He was accompanied by his wife, who said that Mr. M. had been depressed for the last few weeks about finances and had been drinking heavily for the last two days. She said that a year ago he had pancreatitis. (He had been treated for it in another city, from which he had recently moved.) The physician who admitted Mr. M. thought that Mr. M.'s abdominal pain was probably secondary to a recurrence of pancreatitis that was brought on by his heavy drinking. Mr. M. was admitted to the medical floor.

Mr. M.'s patient profile and social history described him as a well-developed 5'11", 170-lb man who had complained of persistent abdominal pain during the history taking.

Mr. M.'s wife gave the following information about Mr. M. He was a machine mechanic who worked eight hours a day, five days a week. He lived with his wife and two sons, aged 13 and 10. They were all well. Mr. M. was not active in a church. He enjoyed fishing and bowling, but had not done either in a long time. He had smoked two packs of cigarettes a day for the last 25 years, and he had drunk about four cases of beer a week for the last six months. Mr. M.'s wife said that she had warned Mr. M. that if he continued to drink he would get sick again. She seemed very concerned about her husband; she said that he drank too much.

Mr. M.'s past medical history noted the episode of pancreatitis mentioned earlier. Mr. M. had no history of hypertension, diabetes, or angina. He had no known food or drug allergies. He took daily antacids for indigestion.

Mr. M.'s father had died of alcoholic cirrhosis at the age of 64. His mother was alive and well. His other family history was unremarkable.

Mr. M.'s physical examination showed that his temperature was 101°F orally, his blood pressure was 130/80, his pulse was 110, and his respirations were 16.

He had bilateral rhonchi that cleared when he coughed. His heart sounds were normal. His abdomen was soft and showed rigidity in the epigastric region. The laboratory tests showed that his pancreatic enzyme levels were elevated, a finding that strongly supported acute pancreatitis.

During the first week of Mr. M.'s hospital stay, he had a persistent fever (103°F) that lasted for five days. He was given intravenous clindamycin (600 mg every 8 hours) and intramuscular gentamicin (80 mg every 8 hours). At the beginning of the antibiotic therapy, Mr. M.'s renal function was normal. After drainage of a pancreatic abscess on day 7, Mr. M. had a hypotensive episode that lasted 12 hours. It responded to a dopamine drip infusion.

After four days of dopamine therapy, Mr. M.'s urinary volume decreased to oliguric levels and his blood urea nitrogen and creatinine levels were elevated and rising. His temperature remained elevated until day 10, when it returned to normal. The urine studies that were done at this point showed numerous granular casts, trace proteinuria, a sodium concentration of 48 mEq per liter, and an osmolality of 300 mOsm per liter. Mr. M.'s antibiotic dosage was reduced when his azotemia was noted.

He was then transferred to the critical care unit for hemodialysis because he had signs of fluid overload and hyperkalemia (see the assessment sheet). Figure 32-1 shows the course of Mr. M.'s renal failure following combined therapy with gentamicin and clindamycin. He remained oliguric for seven days, and he required hemodialysis five more times.

While he was in the critical care unit, Mr. M. had wide mood swings. He went from being abusive to the nurses to being depressed and crying frequently. He referred to himself as an alcoholic. Everyone involved in his case considered him extremely unpredictable. He talked again about his financial problems and about the hospital costs that were not covered by his insurance. Mrs. M. became overbearing and anxious. She was rude to the nurses, did not observe the visiting hours, and seemed to bring out hostility in her husband.

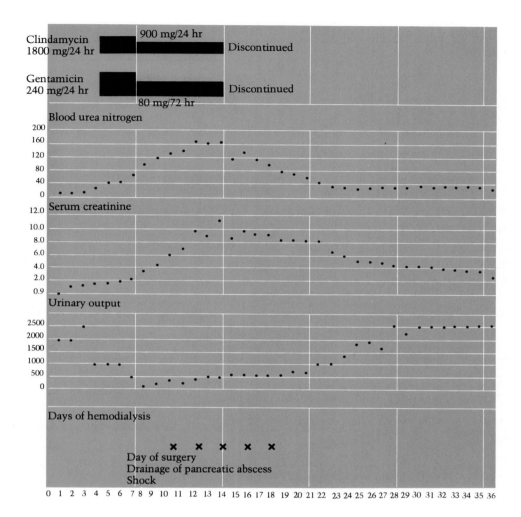

Figure 32-1
Renal failure following the use of gentamicin in combination with clindamycin.

Mr. M.'s physical condition began to improve; so did his and his wife's attitudes. Their case was referred to the hospital social worker and the psychologist, and Mr. and Mrs. M. were both grateful for the referral. Mr. M. received discharge teaching about his diet and his follow-up medical care. His renal function became stable and then gradually improved. His serum creatinine level was only slightly elevated (2.8 mg/100 ml) at the time of his discharge—36 days after his admission.

Reflections

Several team conferences were held to discuss Mr. M.'s difficult medical problem. One conference discussed the basic objectives and management of the patient with acute renal failure, with emphasis on the management of the clinical manifestations of the disease. Another conference, one given by three of the staff nurses, discussed Mr. M.'s management in particular. The nurses concluded that they needed a better understanding of the pharmacology of acute renal failure, and they decided to hold a conference every month at which they would discuss at least four of the drugs that are commonly used to treat

Critical Care Nursing Admission Assessment
Head to Toe Approach

Date	Time		
		Pt. Name: *Mr. R.M.* Age: *48* Allergies: *NKA*	
10-2-	11³⁰AM	Admitted Bed No: *4* Via: *bed* Ad. Dx.: *Acute Pancreatitis*	
		T.: *101°F (o)* A.P.: *120* R.P.: *120* R.: *20* B.P. Supine R: *⁸⁰⁄₀* L: *⁸⁰⁄₀* Sitting:	
7 days post-hospital admission		Wt. (unit scale): *174 lbs* Ht.: *5'11"* ECG Rhythm: *Sinus Tach* Ectopy: *multifocal PVC*	
		Informant: *floor nurse, wife, chart* Last meal: *NPO* Spiked T wave	

1. Chief complaint: *SOB, lethargic*
2. Hx. of present illness: *Acute pancreatitis due to alcohol; persistent temp. last 5 days, drainage pancreatic abscess followed by hypotensive episode requiring dopamine infusion, oliguric, ↑ BUN and creatinine*
3. Past medical Hx. (include all surgeries, hosp., diseases, injuries, blood trans.): *Acute pancreatitis 1 yr. ago - resolved c̄ medical treatment*
4. Family Hx.: *father died age 64 of alcoholic cirrhosis; mother alive + well*
5. Current drugs: *Clindamycin 600 mg. q 8h; gentamicin 80 mg. 1 mg 8h.*
6. Alcohol and tobacco habits: *4 cases of beer/wk. over last 6 mos.; 2 pkg./day cigarettes for 25 years*
7. Dietary and fluid needs: *poor last several months due to heavy drinking*
8. Sleep and rest patterns: *sleeping during day and missing some work over last month*
9. Bowel and bladder habits: *no problems*
10. Hygienic needs: *needs oral care; skin very dry*
11. Psychosocial needs: *very anxious - listen to pt. encourage pt. to participate in care*
12. Occupation and education: *machine mechanic - works 5 days/wk.*
13. Exercise habits: *none*
14. Spiritual needs: *does not attend church*
15. Personal interests: *fishing and bowling, but has not done any in a long time.*
16. Family member interaction and availability: *wife anxious and concerned about husband; two sons ages 13 and 10 anxious*
17. Attitude towards illness and hospitalization: *pt. depressed about illness and finances - communicates easily; demonstrates anxious behavior by frequent shift of positions and laughter about present situation.*

700

Physical Examination

Date	Time		
	18.	Gen. appearance: *well developed* color: *dark from sun expos.* skin: *warm, extremely dry*	
	19.	Neurological:	
		a) level of consciousness: *lethargic, somewhat confused-repeats same questions frequently.*	
		b) cerebellar: *posture: deferred, gait: deferred*	
		c) motor function: upper: *can move-weak* lower: *can move-weak*	
		d) sensory function: upper: *normal* lower: *normal*	
		e) reflexes: *deferred*	
	20.	Head and face: *no abnormalities*	
	21.	Eyes: *PERRLA; slight periorbital edema bilaterally*	
	22.	Ears: *no drainage; membranes intact*	
	23.	Nose: *no drainage*	
	24.	Mouth/throat: *dental care poor; no evidence of lesions*	
	25.	Neck: *no neck vein distention*	
	26.	Chest: *bilateral and equal excursion; use of accessory chest + neck muscles*	
	27.	Breast: *negative* *c̄ respiration*	
	28.	Respiratory: *bilateral rales; dyspneic*	
	29.	Cardiac: *gallop rhythm; PMI diffuse*	
	30.	Abdomen: *tender; bowel sounds decreased*	
	31.	Genitourinary: *oliguric -200 ml last 24 hrs.; admitted for hemodialysis*	
	32.	Extremities (all pulses):	
	33.	Back: *no sacral edema, scars, or deformities*	
	34.	Problems requiring possible referral service: *dietary instruction; have social worker and psychologist talk c̄ wife and pt. as soon as condition improves*	
	35.	Teaching needs: *follow up medical care; information in regard to smoking and alcohol reduction.*	
	36.	Other:	

	PROBLEM LIST: **ACTIVE**	**INACTIVE**
10-2-78	1. *Acute Pancreatitis*	9. *Pancreatitis 1977* ⟶
	2. *Oliguric*	
	3. *Hypervolemic*	
	4. *Hyperkalemic*	
	5. *Depressed*	
	6. *Concerned over finances*	
	7. *Excessive smoking*	
	8. *Excessive drinking*	

Barbara Dossey, RN, CCRN
NURSE'S SIGNATURE

acute renal failure. The nurses made a list of six drugs that they used in the critical care unit, and at the first conference they reviewed the pharmacology of each of those drugs.

Because so many patients in the critical care unit are candidates for or actually have acute renal failure, the nurses summed up their first conference by deciding that the following factors should be considered before medications are administered: (1) the susceptibility of the patient who has acute renal failure to a particular medication, (2) how the medication is metabolized and secreted, (3) the effect the medication has on the electrolyte balance, and (4) the effect an excessively high blood level of the medication has on the kidneys. Table 32-1 lists some of the drugs whose dosages need to be reduced in acute renal failure.

Mr. M.'s case challenged the critical care nursing staff. His medical and psychological problems were difficult. They demanded that all involved with his care use a systematic approach to his management and maintain open communication with the patient and among themselves.

As mentioned, Mr. M. was sometimes hostile, sometimes angry, and sometimes very aggressive. His mood swings were marked. He alternated from being calm to being abusive. The nurses directed their nursing interventions toward helping Mr. M. express his anger. Conferences with the physician and among themselves helped the nurses work through their anger at having to care for a critically ill, hostile patient who was emotionally unstable. Their involvement with Mr. M. reminded the nurses that nurses need to deal with their own frustrations and anxieties and that competent nursing care includes care of the patient's psychological needs.

One nurse commented that Mrs. M. "drove me out of my mind and made taking care of her husband difficult because she didn't observe the visiting hours." Another nurse said that the families of several other patients had also made it hard for the nursing staff. Her comment was, "The family is always in the way when I want to do something for the patient." Those comments led to an interesting conference in which the nurses discussed the fact that the family is a part of the patient's existence. Families become emotional when one of their members becomes ill. The nurses felt that visiting hours should be looked at as guides but that if the family needed to visit the patient, the nurse should be aware of that need, and find out whether the patient can tolerate

Table 32-1

Antibiotics That Must Be Given in Reduced Dosages in Acute Renal Failure

Antibiotics that need a major reduction in dosage
  Oxytetracycline
  Tetracycline
  Kanamycin
  Streptomycin
  Polymyxin
  Amoxicillin
  Carbenicillin
  Cephalosporins
  Vancomycin
  Colistimethate
  Sulfonamides
  Chloroquine
  Quinine
  Ethambutol

Antibiotics that need a slight reduction in dosage
  Penicillin G
  Ampicillin
  Lincomycin
  Isoniazid
  Amphotericin B

Antibiotics that need no reduction in dosage
  Oxacillin
  Methicillin
  Erythromycin
  Chloramphenicol
  Rifampin

the visit. The discussion led to interesting comments about how family members might perceive the individual critical care nurse. The nurses discussed the situation in which the wife had had a lot of family responsibility before her husband became ill. The wife is likely to feel helpless when she sees that the nurse has taken over her husband's care. The family feels concerned about their family member. They may turn their fears, hostility, or feelings of helplessness against the nurse, who seems to have taken over as if the patient belongs to her and as if the family had never been part of the patient's life. The nurses concluded that family life is a stabilizing force for the pa-

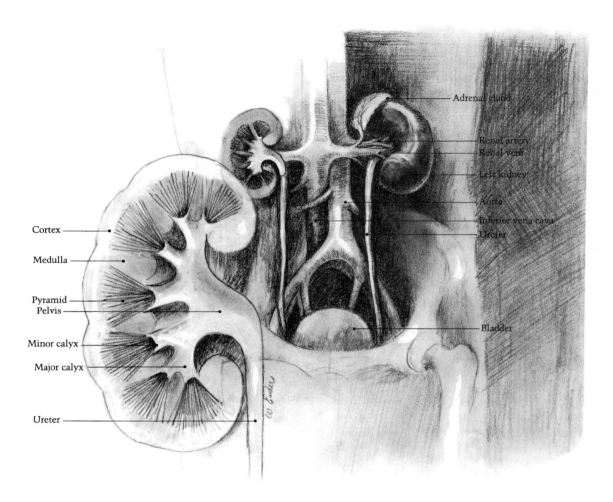

Cortex

Medulla

Pyramid
Pelvis

Minor calyx

Major calyx

Ureter

Adrenal gland

Renal artery
Renal vein

Left kidney

Aorta

Inferior vena cava
Ureter

Bladder

Figure 32-2
Location and internal structure of the kidney.

tient and that Mr. M.'s absence from his family created emotional turmoil for his wife and children. The nurses agreed that they could help family members by accepting them as people who are under stress and who are troubled.

The Kidney

The kidneys are two bean-shaped structures that have indented medial borders. The indented borders, which are called hila (*sing.* hilum), are the entrance

sites for the renal blood vessels and the renal pelvis. The kidneys lie in the retroperitoneal space, between the twelfth thoracic and the third lumbar vertebrae, behind the liver on the right side and behind the spleen on the left side. They are separated from the abdominal cavity anteriorly by layers of peritoneum; they are protected posteriorly by the lower thoracic wall. The kidney surface is a strong fibrous capsule that is covered by fat tissue.

Internal Structure of the Kidney

Internally each kidney is composed of a cortex, a medulla, and a pelvis (Fig. 32-2). The cortex, the outer layer of the kidney, contains the glomeruli and tubules. The medulla, the middle layer of the kidney, contains only tubules. The medulla is made up of pyramids. Along the bases of the pyramids, portions of the medulla penetrate the cortex. They are known as the medullary rays. The medullary rays contain the straight portions of the tubules, the loops of Henle, and the parts of the collecting system that pass directly down from the cortex to the papilla (or apex) of the pyramid.

The pyramids vary in number. They average about eight. A pyramid is made up of parallel tubules that form larger collecting ducts that penetrate the papilla. The large collecting ducts open into the minor calyx. The fornix, the portion of the minor calyx that faces upward around the papilla, is important because early signs of infection or obstruction such as increasing temperature and decreasing urinary output can occur at the fornix. Minor calyces form major calyces, which also vary in number (from two to four). Major calyces form the renal pelvis, which becomes the ureter, at a point called the ureteropelvic junction.

Renal Blood Flow

The total renal blood flow is about 1200 ml per minute, or about 20 percent of the cardiac output. Blood flow through the kidney is distributed differently. About 90 percent of the flow goes through the cortex, and the remaining 10 percent goes through the medulla. A low medullary flow results in concentrated urine (discussed under Countercurrent Mechanism).

Renal blood flow involves the renal arteries, capillaries, and veins. The two renal arteries, one on each side of the aorta, are located at the level of the second lumbar vertebrae (Fig. 32-2). The renal arteries carry waste products to the kidneys. Each of those large vessels divides into an anterior (ventral) and a posterior (dorsal) branch in the hilum and further divides into the interlobar branches, which divide into the arcuate arteries. The arcuate arteries form interlobular arteries.

AFFERENT AND EFFERENT ARTERIOLES

Afferent arterioles are made up of end branches of straight arteries. They give rise to many capillaries that supply the glomerulus. Those capillaries join to form efferent arterioles, which drain the glomerulus. They are found in the cortex.

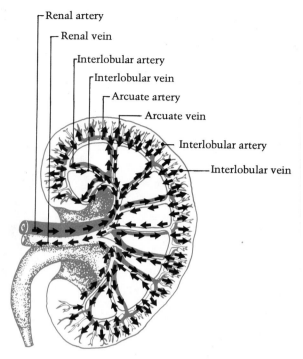

Figure 32-3
Renal blood flow.

The afferent arterioles, which supply blood to the glomeruli, are formed from the interlobular arteries; they divide, forming renal capillaries inside the glomeruli, and again come together to form the efferent arteriole (Fig. 32-3). The efferent arteriole leaves the glomerulus to form the arteriolae rectae (in the case of the juxtamedullary nephrons) or the peritubular capillaries (in the case of the cortical nephrons). Those wide capillary channels spread out between the loops of Henle, collecting ducts, and excretory ducts, and they are associated with resorption from the tubules. The efferent arteriole takes blood from the nephron back into the interlobular veins, which form arcuate veins at the corticomedullary junction. The arcuate veins then form the interlobular veins, which form near each kidney surface from the capillaries of the cortex. They carry more purified blood. The interlobular veins empty into tributaries that continue from the anterior and posterior sides of the renal pelvis, forming the right and left renal veins. Both renal veins empty into the inferior vena cava.

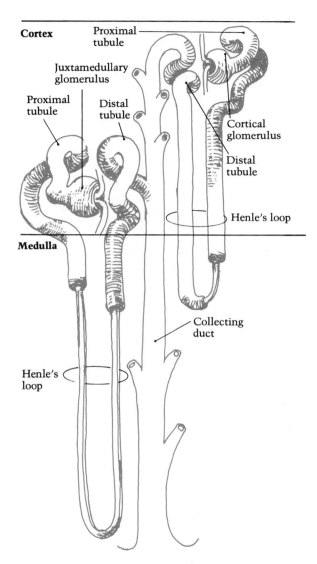

Cortex

Proximal tubule

Juxtamedullary glomerulus

Proximal tubule

Distal tubule

Cortical glomerulus

Distal tubule

Henle's loop

Medulla

Collecting duct

Henle's loop

Figure 32-4
Cortical and juxtamedullary nephrons.

The Nephron

The nephron is the functional unit of the kidney. Each kidney has about 1,000,000 nephrons, each of which is capable of forming urine [17]. About 75 percent of the nephrons can be destroyed before the patient has problems, because the remaining nephrons compensate.

The main functions of the nephrons are to excrete the waste products of metabolism and to maintain fluid balance by the regulation of sodium, water, and pH.

There are two different types of nephrons, cortical and juxtamedullary (Fig. 32-4). The cortical nephrons have a short, thin loop of Henle, while the juxtamedullary nephrons have a long loop of Henle that goes deep into the medulla of the kidney. Both types of nephrons have similar but not identical functions. The juxtamedullary nephrons have a greater ability to concentrate urine. (See Countercurrent Mechanism.)

NEPHRON STRUCTURE

Each nephron is composed of a glomerulus (Bowman's capsule and capillary tufts), a proximal tubule, a loop of Henle, a distal tubule, and a collecting duct system.

Glomerulus
The glomerulus has two openings. The first opening, the vascular pole, allows the afferent and efferent arterioles to enter and leave the glomerulus; the other opening, the urinary pole, begins with the lumen of the proximal tubule. The glomerulus has a visceral layer and a parietal layer. Between those two layers is Bowman's capsule.

Glomerular Filtration

The kidneys form about 180 liters of glomerular filtrate per day at the rate of 125 ml per minute, resulting in about 1 ml of urine per minute. The glomerular filtration rate is the rate at which fluid flows from the glomerulus into Bowman's capsule. Pressure is higher inside the glomerulus than it is in Bowman's capsule, causing fluid to constantly pass into Bowman's capsule. The glomerular filtrate that is collected in Bowman's capsule flows to the tubular system, where all but about one to two liters is resorbed into the blood. When blood passes through the glomerular capillaries, the balance of opposing physical forces determines the formation and passage of an almost protein-free ultrafiltrate of plasma across the glomerular filtration membrane. The ultrafiltrate constantly passes into Bowman's capsule and then enters the lumen of the proximal tubule of the tubular system.

The efferent arteriole that leaves the glomerulus twines around all parts of the tubule (Fig. 32-5). Re-

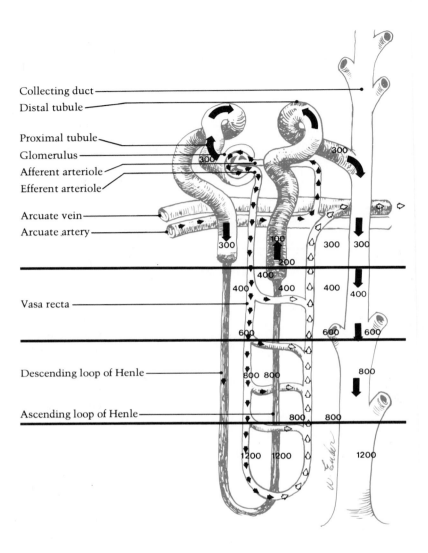

Collecting duct

Distal tubule

Proximal tubule

Glomerulus

Afferent arteriole

Efferent arteriole

Arcuate vein

Arcuate artery

Vasa recta

Descending loop of Henle

Ascending loop of Henle

Figure 32-5
The nephron and the countercurrent mechanism for urine concentration.

sorption from the tubule occurs in the arteriole. About 99 percent of filtrate and filtered water are resorbed into the peritubular capillaries and returned to the blood.

Proximal Tubule
The proximal tubule is contained within the cortex. It is easily damaged by disease and foreign material.

Loop of Henle
The loop of Henle is composed of the straight portion of the proximal tubule, the thin limb, and the straight portion of the distal tubule. One limb descends into the medulla as the other limb ascends to the cortex.

Distal Tubule
As the ascending thick limb of the distal tubule returns to the cortex, it passes between the afferent and efferent arterioles of its glomerulus and continues as a distal convoluted segment. In the area where the distal tubule passes near its arterioles, the macula densa is formed (the macula densa is discussed later). The distal convoluted tubule joins directly with a collecting tubule in the cortex.

Tubular System

The tubular system is composed of the proximal, distal, and collecting tubules (Fig. 32-5). Osmosis, diffusion, and active transport are the mechanisms responsible for the resorption of fluid and necessary products, such as sodium, potassium, magnesium, bicarbonate, chloride, and calcium, in the tubular system and from the interstitial spaces.

Collecting Duct System

The tubular system and the excretory ducts make up the excretory system. The excretory ducts are found in the medulla; they are formed by the collecting ducts. The collecting ducts open into the major calyces at the pyramid tips, which empty into the major calyces and then into the renal pelvis. From there urine is carried to the ureter and then to the urinary bladder.

Osmosis is the movement of permeable substances (usually water) in one direction across a membrane, passing from an area of lower concentration to one of higher concentration. The passage is caused by the presence of a larger concentration of nonpermeable molecules on one side of the membrane. Diffusion is the movement of molecules from an area of higher concentration to an area of lower concentration. In the kidney, water, sodium, urea and other materials pass through the tubular membranes into the interstitial spaces. Active transport is the transport of substances through the tubular walls into the interstitial spaces as a result of chemical transport mechanisms and the concentration gradient that exists between the tubular and the peritubular capillaries.

The proximal tubule is responsible for bulk resorption. The brush border of the proximal tubule has a large resorptive capacity, and it transports many substances through the tubular wall into the surrounding interstitium and back into the blood via the peritubular capillaries. Glucose is completely resorbed in the proximal tubule; it appears in the urine only when the blood glucose level exceeds 180 mg per 100 ml. Approximately 85 percent of electrolytes are resorbed in the proximal tubule. Urea, the chief waste product of protein catabolism, is a passively transported substance. A large portion of filtered urea is resorbed in the proximal tubule because of its tubular permeability.

The descending limb regulates the fine adjustment of sodium and chloride. The descending limb and the ascending limb are surrounded by the interstitium of the medulla. The interstitial fluid has a progressively higher concentration of sodium and urea from cortex to papilla. The descending limb is fully permeable to water. As fluid travels down the descending limb, the osmotic pressure created by the sodium and urea gradient causes water in the descending limb to move out into the interstitium. The remaining fluid enters the ascending limb, which is impermeable to fluid. Sodium ions flow from the ascending limb into the interstitium of the medulla.

Countercurrent Mechanism

The kidneys have a mechanism for concentrating urine called the countercurrent mechanism (Fig. 32-5). That mechanism depends on the anatomical arrangement of the loops of Henle of the juxtamedullary nephrons and of the vasa recta loops, which supply blood to the medulla. The osmolality of the interstitial fluid in the outer medulla and papilla is hyperosmotic to arterial blood as the glomerular filtrate enters the proximal tubule; its normal osmolality is about 300 mOsmol per liter. Since the osmolality of the interstitial fluid of the medulla of the kidney becomes progressively greater deeper into the medulla, there is an increase from 300 mOsmol per liter in the cortex to 1200 mOsmol per liter at the pelvic tip of the medulla. The osmolality is about four times that of plasma. The increase is due to the sodium ions that are trapped in the medulla. As fluid returns through the ascending limb, there is a reversal in the osmolality. Fluid entering the distal tubule is hypotonic (100 mOsmol/L) as compared to the fluid in the proximal tubule (300 mOsmol/L).

It is theorized that as the small volume of fluids travels through the ascending limb, sodium chloride is actively pumped out of the tubular lumen. Since the ascending limb is impermeable to water (heavy lines, Fig. 32-5), water does not follow the sodium chloride; therefore the fluid becomes hypotonic relative to the fluid in the papilla. The osmolality is raised by the sodium ions that are pumped into the interstitium; they cause water to leave the water-permeable descending limb (thin lines, Fig. 32-5). Fluid that descends the loop becomes progressively more concentrated. Fluid that started out at 300 mOsmol per liter at the outer medullary junction increases to 1200 mOsmol per liter at the tip, only to fall to 100 mOsmol as it leaves the ascending limb. From there the ascending thick-limb urine passes to

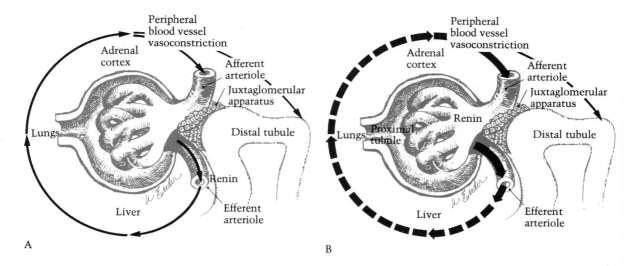

A

B

Figure 32-6

Effects of the enzyme renin on the renal blood flow. A. Normal renal blood flow. B. Low renal blood flow, increased renin secretion.

the distal convoluted tubules, where active sodium transport continues. Antidiuretic hormone (ADH) from the pituitary controls the permeability of the distal tubule to water. Excretion of potassium occurs there. Although approximately 85 percent of water resorption has occurred as it passed from the proximal to the distal tubule, ADH increases water resorption in the distal tubule and collecting duct. Aldosterone aids in sodium resorption in the distal tubules. Cortisols, which are salt-regulating hormones, also help in sodium resorption and decrease potassium resorption at this point.

Distal tubule fluid then enters the collecting ducts in the medulla, where concentration and fine adjustments of sodium, chloride, potassium, and acid-base occur. At this point aldosterone accelerates sodium resorption and is matched by passive chloride resorption; thus potassium and hydrogen are exchanged.

Fluid in the collecting ducts is also exposed to the osmotic forces from the cortex to the medulla, as previously discussed. Water permeability in the collecting ducts, which is also controlled by ADH, causes water to move by osmosis into the medullary interstitium.

The collecting ducts filter the fluids, which are converted into urine, the end product of kidney function. Urine flows from the collecting tubules to the pelvis of the kidney. From there the urine goes via the ureters to the urinary bladder.

Urine is composed of organic wastes (urea, creatinine, uric acid, ammonia, inorganic salts, chloride, sulfate, phosphorus, sodium, potassium, and magnesium). Urine is normally acidic; its pH is 5.5 to 6.5 and its specific gravity is 1.010 to 1.025. It should be clear yellow and test negatively for sugar, acetone, and albumin.

Regulatory Mechanisms

The regulatory mechanisms by which the kidneys adapt to the body's changing needs are renin, aldosterone, and ADH. Despite the widely varying arterial pressure, the blood flow through the kidneys and the glomerular filtration rate remain almost constant.

RENIN

When the renal blood flow is low, the macula densa juxtaglomerular complex causes afferent arteriolar vasoconstriction. These cells are near the afferent arteriole that supplies the glomerulus with blood.

The juxtaglomerular apparatus, an important structure in the distal tubule, is a specialized part of the afferent arteriole. It contains specific granulated cells and the macula densa, a part of the distal tubule (Fig. 32-6A). The macula densa (or dense spot) is so named

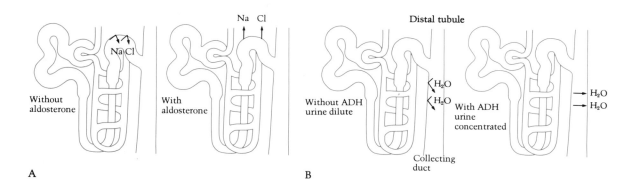

Figure 32-7
A. Effect of aldosterone on the kidney. B. Effect of antidiuretic hormone (ADH) on the kidney.

because of the closeness of its cell nuclei. In the macula densa, the distal tubular cells have a different morphology. The basement membrane outside the macula densa disappears, bringing the macula densa and the afferent arteriole into close contact. The close relationship between the distal tubule and the afferent arteriole appears to be the basis for the following feedback mechanism, which controls the blood flow through the afferent arteriole [17] (Fig. 32-6B). When the blood pressure is low, the juxtaglomerular cells secrete renin, which converts angiotensin, a plasma protein produced by the liver, into angiotensin I. Angiotensin I is converted to angiotensin II by an enzyme found in pulmonary tissue. Angiotensin II, a vasoconstrictor, causes the systematic arterioles to constrict. It stimulates the adrenal cortex to secrete aldosterone. The aldosterone causes increased sodium resorption and thus increased extracellular fluid. As the sodium level rises, the macula densa slows the secretion of renin. The amount of angiotensin II in the body also reflects the amount of circulating renin. Thus as the renal blood flow is decreased, the renin secretion increases. When the renal blood flow increases, the renin secretion is decreased.

Aldosterone and ADH

Aldosterone and ADH are important in regulating fluid volume (see Chap. 27, Acute Adrenal Insufficiency, for details). Aldosterone regulates primarily the ions in the extracellular fluid, whereas ADH regulates water excretion.

Aldosterone causes an increased retention of sodium and of water and thus elevates the arterial blood pressure by increasing the extracellular fluid volume (Fig. 32-7A). The process occurs mostly in the distal convoluted tubules, where the sodium chloride and potassium levels are regulated.

The osmotic changes in plasma result in the hypothalamic release of ADH from the posterior pituitary. ADH acts primarily on the distal tubule cells and the collecting ducts (Fig. 32-7B). If the extracellular fluid is concentrated, ADH causes water to be resorbed and results in concentrated urine. If the extracellular fluid is diluted, ADH is not released; extracellular volume is decreased, and diluted urine results.

Most circulatory reflexes play a role in the regulation of blood volume. The baroreceptor reflexes respond to low arterial pressure, causing afferent arteriolar constriction in the kidney and thus a retention in the extracellular fluid. The volume receptors located in the walls of the atria and the great veins respond to excess filling of those structures and send renal reflexes to elicit an increase in the urine excretion. Also, those signals are sent to the hypothalamus to cause a reduced ADH output and thus an increased excretion of urine by the kidneys.

Osmolality refers to the total number of particles concentrated in a solution. The osmolality of urine has a wide range. The patient's clinical condition determines what his urine osmolality is. Plasma osmolality is the main regulator of ADH. The osmolality of the plasma is the same as that in the other body compartments because water moves freely between the cells, the blood, and the interstitial fluid. The normal average serum osmolality is 290 ± 10 mOsm per kilogram, and it is constant.

The plasma osmolality is determined mainly by the concentration of the serum sodium; the serum osmolality is always high when serum sodium is high. However, the serum sodium may be low and the plasma osmolality normal or high when plasma is expanded by other agents, notably glucose and urea nitrogen. If a person drinks excessive amounts of water, the osmolality decreases. The urine becomes more dilute because the release of ADH is blocked. If a person does not drink enough water, the osmolality rises. The rise stimulates the release of ADH, thereby causing the kidneys to conserve water and excrete a more concentrated urine. With a maximum water load and ADH suppression, the kidneys are able to dilute urine to 50 mOsm per kilogram. With water restriction, the kidneys can concentrate urine to 1200 mOsm per kilogram.

In a given situation, the kidneys can conserve water by concentrating urine or they can eliminate water by diluting urine. Hypertonic urine is dependent on high blood levels of ADH. ADH makes the distal tubules and collecting ducts highly permeable to water. But hypotonic urine occurs when there is a low blood level of ADH, which causes the distal tubules' permeability to water to be low. The amount of sodium resorbed by the distal tubule determines the dilution of the urine. The water permeability of the distal tubule depends on the circulating ADH blood levels. Therefore, the more dilute urine is produced by "waterloaded" people.

Renal Control of Water

Three basic processes are involved in the renal control of water: (1) delivery of the filtrate to the ascending limb of the loop of Henle, (2) separation of water from electrolytes in the ascending limb, and (3) controlled resorption of water from the collecting duct under the influence of ADH.

Acid-Base Balance

Acids are formed continuously by the metabolic processes of the body. Each day, the healthy person eats food that contains proteins. The breakdown of the proteins produces hydrogen ions that contain sulphur and phosphorus, which form acids. Organic acids that are not metabolized by the body are also produced.

In order to maintain a normal acid-base balance, the lungs and kidneys constantly regulate the hydrogen ion concentration in the body fluids. The lungs act in minutes to eliminate carbonic acid. The kidneys can also directly excrete hydrogen ions. However, the correction of acid-base imbalances by the kidneys is a matter of hours or days, not minutes.

Maintenance of the acid-base balance implies the regulation of the hydrogen ion concentration in the body fluids. If the hydrogen ion concentration is great, the fluids are acidic; if the hydrogen ion concentration is low, the fluids are basic.

The mechanisms for maintaining the acid-base balance by the kidneys may be described as follows. Hydrogen ions are removed from the extracellular fluids when the hydrogen ion concentration becomes too great. Sodium and bicarbonate ions are removed when the hydrogen ion concentration becomes too low. For example, if the pH of extracellular fluid is alkaline, the urine pH also becomes alkaline owing to the loss of alkaline substances from the body fluids. If the pH of the extracellular fluid becomes acidic, the urine pH also becomes acidic owing to the loss of large amounts of acidic substances from the body fluids. In either situation, the pH is returned toward normal because of the loss of alkaline or acid substances.

Hydrogen ions are continually secreted into the tubular fluid by the distal tubule epithelium. Weak acids are formed when the hydrogen ions combine with the sodium salts contained in the tubular fluid and thus free the sodium ions bound in the salts. The sodium is then able to be resorbed through the tubular wall to return to the extracellular fluid. The hydrogen ion concentration is decreased by the loss of hydrogen ions from the extracellular fluid and sodium ion resorption. Thus a net exchange of hydrogen for sodium ions occurs owing to the hydrogen ions' being excreted into the urine and the sodium ions' being resorbed. The process helps keep the fluid more basic and helps control the continuous formation of acid by the normal daily metabolic processes.

The hydrogen ion secretion into the distal tubules is determined by the carbon dioxide concentration in the extracellular fluid. An excess of carbon dioxide in the extracellular fluid is usually associated with increased carbonic acid and hydrogen ion concentrations, which indicate acidosis. When fluids are acidic, the hydrogen ion secretion is greater; thus the kidneys attempt to eliminate the excess acid.

In alkalosis, alkaline substances combine with carbonic acid, forming bicarbonate salts; thus the extracellular bicarbonate ion concentration is increased. As the bicarbonate ion concentration increases, the ions are excreted into the urine in the form of sodium bicarbonate. The excretion causes the loss of alkaline substances by the body, thus correcting the alkalosis.

Acute Renal Failure

Acute renal failure can occur in any clinical setting. Typically, a rapid decrease in renal function accompanied by progressive azotemia with or without oliguria is seen [5, 36]. The accumulation of nitrogen waste is referred to as azotemia. In progressive azotemia the blood urea nitrogen (BUN) and creatinine levels become elevated over several days (about 20–30 mg/100 ml/day and 1–2 mg/100 ml/day, respectively). The BUN and creatinine levels rise as a result of a decrease in urea clearance by the kidney. The normal ratio of BUN to creatinine is 10:1, and the ratio of elevation is maintained in a stepwise fashion. Disproportionate elevations are observed closely in the differential diagnosis of acute renal failure. The progressive elevations of plasma BUN and creatinine levels over several days with or without oliguria are an indication of acute renal failure. Oliguria implies that the urinary output is less than 400 ml per day. Although the clinical course of acute renal failure can be dramatic, it is one of the few kinds of organ failure that are completely reversible.

Causative and Precipitating Factors in Acute Renal Failure

Acute renal failure may occur in hypovolemia of any cause, in altered peripheral resistance, and in decreased cardiac output. Hypovolemia is frequently caused by surgical procedures, diarrhea, vomiting, excessive sweating, pancreatitis, peritonitis, and burns. Altered peripheral vascular resistance is most frequently caused by anaphylactic reactions, drug overdoses, metabolic acidosis, or gram-negative septicemia. The most commonly occurring causes of decreased cardiac output are acute congestive heart failure, acute myocardial infarction with cardiac dysrhythmias, and cardiac tamponade.

The important precipitating factors in acute renal failure are shock, trauma, septicemia, mismatched blood transfusions, allergic disorders, dehydration, and nephrotoxic drugs. The common causes of those precipitating factors are crushing injuries, surgery, and bacteremic shock. Following cardiovascular surgery, especially surgery of the great vessels, aorta, or heart, the renal circulation is interrupted and some degree of acute renal failure can be expected if the period of decreased circulation is long. Nephrotoxic drugs may be ingested, inhaled accidentally in a confined space, given therapeutically, or taken in a suicide attempt. The therapeutic drugs that are commonly associated with acute nephrotoxicity are the aminoglycosides (streptomycin, neomycin, kanamycin, tobramycin, and gentamicin). Antibiotics are among the nephrotoxic drugs commonly given in the hospital setting [4, 5, 6, 28]. Subtle drug interactions, rather than an easily recognized nephrotoxin, may become increasingly important in potentiating acute renal failure. One must remember that all drugs are potentially toxic [4, 5]. In the anephric patient, certain drugs require dosage reduction (Table 32-1).

Categories of Acute Renal Failure

Acute renal failure is divided into the categories prerenal, intrarenal, and postrenal [11, 17, 18, 32, 34]. Table 32-2 gives the causes of each type. Treatment is aimed at identifying the category and managing the difficult manifestations of the acute event.

PRERENAL

The prerenal causes of acute renal failure (see Table 32-2) are the abnormalities in which not enough blood perfuses the kidney to produce enough urine. The term prerenal azotemia is used in this situation and refers to a decreased circulatory volume with poor renal perfusion and a decreased glomerular filtration rate. The urine sodium is usually less than 20 mEq per liter. A favorable response of the patient to volume expanders or salt suggests a prerenal mechanism.

INTRARENAL

The intrarenal causes of acute renal failure are (1) a change in the interstitium, the site of resorption in the kidneys, and (2) diseases that involve the nephron. When the cause is intrarenal, the kidneys are no longer able to excrete the nitrogen waste produced by protein metabolism. The tubules are damaged and cannot concentrate urine. (A type of acute renal failure frequently seen in the critical care unit, acute tubular necrosis, falls in this category and is due to an intrarenal dysfunction.)

Table 32-2
Major Causes of Acute Renal Failure

	Manifestations
Prerenal causes	
Hypovolemia	Skin losses (through sweating, burns), gastrointestinal losses (through diarrhea, vomiting), renal losses (caused by diuretics, osmotic diuresis in diabetes mellitus), hemorrhage, sequestration (in burns, peritonitis)
Cardiovascular failure	
Myocardial failure	Infarction, tamponade, dysrhythmias
Vascular pooling	Sepsis, septic abortion, anaphylaxis, extreme acidosis
Intrarenal causes	
Postischemic	All the conditions that cause prerenal failure (see Prerenal causes)
Heme pigments	
Intravascular hemolysis	Transfusion reactions, hemolysis due to toxins or to immunological damage, malaria
Rhabdomyolysis	Trauma, muscle disease, prolonged coma, seizures, heat stroke, severe exercise
Nephrotoxins	
Pregnancy-related causes	Toxic abortifacients, septic abortion, uterine hemorrhage
Postrenal causes	
Obstruction	Calculi, neoplasms of the bladder and the pelvic organs, prostatism, surgical accidents, ureteral instrumentation
Rupture of bladder	
Other causes	
Glomerulitis	Poststreptococcal conditions, lupus erythematosus
Vasculitis	Periarteritis, hypersensitivity angiitis
Malignant hypertension	
Acute diffuse pyelonephritis, papillary necrosis	
Severe hypercalcemia	
Intratubular precipitation	Myeloma, presence of urates after use of cytotoxic drugs, sulfonamides
Hepatorenal syndrome	
Pregnancy-related causes	Eclampsia, postpartum renal failure
Vascular obstruction	
Arterial	Thrombosis, embolism, aneurysm
Venous	Thrombosis, vena caval obstruction, diffuse small vein thrombosis in amyloidosis

Adapted from Brenner, B. M., and Rector, F. C. *The Kidney.* Philadelphia: Saunders, 1976.

POSTRENAL

The postrenal causes of acute renal failure are obstructions of any type. The hallmarks are a sudden decrease or increase in the urine output. An output that varies from day to day when the intakes are stable increases the suspicion that a bladder outlet obstruction is present. In postrenal states, the kidney functions properly but the urine does not leave the bladder. The obstructions occur below the level of the collecting ducts, anywhere from the pelvis of the kidney to the external urethral orifice. The obstructions are either functional or anatomical. Functional obstructions can follow the use of drugs that interrupt the autonomic supply to the urinary passages or the bladder (e.g., antihistamines and ganglionic blocking drugs). Anatomical obstructions may be caused by the encroachment of adjacent abdominal or pelvic organs on the bladder or by tumors, stones, or strictures.

Pathology of Acute Renal Failure

Acute renal failure is classified as either oliguric or nonoliguric. It is a sudden and almost complete loss of kidney function [10, 11, 13] caused by glomerular or tubular damage or failure of the renal circulation. Substances that are normally eliminated in the urine (uric acids, urea, and creatinine) accumulate in the body fluids. When hypovolemia, altered peripheral resistance, or decreased cardiac output is severe enough, the glomerular filtration rate falls. Fluid then automatically travels through the tubules at a slower rate, increasing the water and sodium resorption and decreasing the urinary output.

Differential Diagnosis

When a patient has an abrupt fall in urinary output and rapidly progressive azotemia, the physician must decide what diagnostic features must be managed [14, 19, 23]. Prenatal, intrarenal, or postrenal mechanisms must be identified. The following laboratory and radiographic investigations are done in patients suspected of having or known to have acute renal failure.

LABORATORY STUDIES

Laboratory studies include determinations of the serum sodium, chloride, potassium, bicarbonate, creatinine, uric acid, and BUN levels and of the osmolality. If there is no extensive muscle damage, the serum creatinine level is less sensitive than the BUN level to prenatal and to other catabolic factors, and, therefore, it reflects renal function more closely.

Determinations of the hemoglobin, hematocrit, and the white blood cell count should be done, and a blood smear should be evaluated. Because it has become more widely known that disseminated intravascular coagulation (DIC) can cause acute renal failure, coagulation studies are often done, depending on the clinical setting. The coagulation studies include determinations of the prothrombin time, clotting time, bleeding time, partial thromboplastin time, platelet count, and the fibrinogen level. If DIC is detected, the early administration of heparin could prevent permanent renal damage.

Urinalysis

A few studies of the renal function and of the urine can show whether the renal function is normal or abnormal and if it is abnormal, to what degree. Urine specimens should be obtained before the patient is given diuretics; only then are the sodium determinations reliable. Urine specimens are studied to analyze

Table 32-3
Urinalysis Findings in Acute Renal Failure

Proteinuria is common but the amount is generally less than 1 gm/24 hr

Red blood cells (if present) are usually microscopic

White blood cells usually occur in small numbers

Bacteria are often present in the later phases

The casts vary in amount; they may increase in the diuretic phase

Sugar may be present

The urine sodium level is > 30 mEq/L

A urine urea–plasma urea ratio of < 5:1 is usually only supportive evidence of acute renal failure

The urine osmolality approaches the plasma osmolality

The myoglobin level should be checked

the urea nitrogen, sodium concentration, heme pigment, specific gravity or osmolality, and formed elements.

The urinalysis may give valuable information (Table 32-3). Examination of the urine sediment is of value in the differential diagnosis of acute renal failure. The patient's urine sediment is evaluated closely for tubular cells, known pigmented granular casts, and renal tubular cell casts. Those cells are strong evidence of intrarenal rather than prenatal or postrenal causes of acute renal failure.

Specific Gravity and Osmolality of Urine. In prenatal azotemia, the urine usually has a high specific gravity (higher than 1.015–1.020). With intrarenal mechanisms, the specific gravity usually becomes fixed at 1.010 because the diseased kidneys are unable to form concentrated urine. Normally, the specific gravity of urine can go from 1.001 to 1.030, depending on the patient's water balance. Concentrated urine shows a water deficit, and dilute urine shows a water excess.

With prenatal mechanisms, the tubules are functioning and are able to resorb sodium. Therefore the urine sodium levels are low, and the urine osmolality is high. A low urinary sodium level usually suggests a prenatal category. In the intrarenal category, the tubules are damaged and cannot resorb sodium or concentrate urine. The amount of urine may be excessive, and the urine is dilute, with a low specific gravity and a low osmolality. Because of the lack of normal sodium resorption, the urine sodium content tends to be high. The urine-plasma osmolality ratio is a valuable determinant in acute renal failure. Since in intrarenal states the kidneys are unable to concentrate urine, a urine osmolality that is higher than the plasma osmolality suggests a prerenal category. The test results that are most helpful in the diagnosis of acute renal failure are a urine-plasma osmolality ratio of 1 : 1, a urine urea nitrogen–blood urea nitrogen ratio of less than 10 : 1, and an elevated urinary sodium level (usually one that is higher than 20–30 mEq/L).

Creatinine Clearance. The creatinine clearance test measures renal excretory function. Creatinine, a by-product of muscle metabolism, is excreted in the urine because of glomerular filtration. Therefore, it is indicative of the glomerular filtration rate. The creatinine clearance can be determined in the following manner:

U = urine creatinine (mg/100 ml)
V = urine volume (ml/min)
P = plasma creatinine concentration (mg/100 ml)

$$\text{Creatinine clearance} = \frac{UV}{P}$$

The normal serum values are about 0.6 to 1 mg/100 ml in women and 0.8 to 1.3 mg/100 ml in men. Throughout the day and from day to day, the plasma creatinine level varies little. Since the plasma creatinine concentration remains constant in persons with stable renal function, creatinine clearance can be determined by obtaining a 24-hour urine sample (or some other "timed" urine sample), determining the urine volume and the urine creatinine concentration, and obtaining a blood sample to determine the plasma creatinine concentration. To obtain accurate values, the urine sample must be a complete one.

When the kidneys are damaged by a disease, the creatinine clearance decreases and the serum creatinine concentration rises. In acute renal failure the serum creatinine concentration is an adequate index of renal dysfunction. The urine creatinine clearance is often difficult to determine in a state of oliguria or anuria.

Electrocardiogram

An ECG is obtained for baseline information and to assess the cardiac rhythm and any ectopy. During the phases of acute renal failure, the ECG can also serve as in immediate index of the serum potassium concentration (Fig. 32-8).

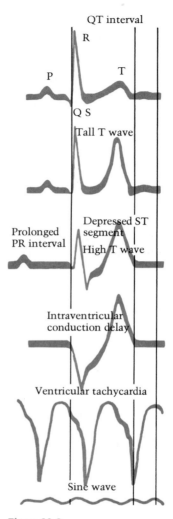

Figure 32-8
Electrocardiographic patterns associated with elevated serum potassium levels.

X rays

The routine x-ray studies are a chest x ray and a plain abdominal x ray. The plain abdominal x ray may be useful in determining the cause of acute renal failure. In acute renal failure, the kidneys are usually normal or may be enlarged. Radiologic evidence that the kidneys are small is a clue to chronic renal failure. Calcific densities indicate possible obstruction. In some patients, retrograde studies and ultrasound may be needed to gather further evidence of an obstruction. In some situations, a renal scan may give information about the return of renal function. When the scan indicates the presence of blood flow, a significant degree of renal function usually returns [2, 7].

RENAL BIOPSY

Rarely, a renal biopsy may be indicated for unexplained acute oliguric renal failure. The kidney biopsy is an invasive procedure, but it may be needed to arrive at a prognosis and to manage the patient. It should be done only by the experienced physician, and some type of localization method should be used. A renal biopsy carries the risk of bleeding and hematuria. In some medical centers, ultrasonic guidance for renal biopsy is the method of choice [27].

Awareness of the Events That Cause Acute Renal Failure

Since acute renal failure can develop slowly, awareness of the clinical circumstances in which it can occur is essential to early diagnosis [26]. The methods used to detect it are not routinely used during the normal postoperative period or in the emergency room. If a patient is suspected of having acute renal failure, he must be closely monitored early. His hourly urine outputs should be followed carefully. The clinical course of acute nonoliguric renal failure has been shown to be similar to that of acute oliguric renal failure. The incidence of acute nonoliguric renal failure is difficult to estimate since often it goes unrecognized because the patient seems to have an adequate volume of urine.

Clinical Picture and Course of Acute Nonoliguric Renal Failure

Acute nonoliguric renal failure usually occurs as a complication of surgery, shock, trauma, nephrotoxic drugs, and infection. If it is diagnosed early, it can be managed easily and conservatively. It is usually not fatal [3, 29, 32, 35].

The patient who has acute nonoliguric renal failure has progressive azotemia without oliguria. He usually voids from one to several liters of urine per day. Typically he has increasing azotemia for 10 to 12 days and

a return toward normal for the next 10 to 12 days. During the peak period of azotemia, his urine volumes also peak and then slowly return to normal. His electrolyte and BUN levels must be observed closely so that the physician can regulate the patient's electrolyte management according to his daily urine output. Even when a patient's urine output is normal, fluid overloads can still occur and precipitate pulmonary edema. Dialysis is often not required in acute nonoliguric renal failure. The complications of the condition are similar to those of acute oliguric renal failure, but electrolyte, fluid, and nutritional problems are more easily managed. Infection, overhydration, dehydration, and hyperkalemia are the most frequently occurring complications, and they are managed as they are in acute oliguric renal failure.

Clinical Picture and Course of Acute Oliguric Renal Failure

Acute oliguric renal failure typically has three phases: oliguria, diuresis, and recovery [5, 12, 19, 36]. Some patients go through all three phases, but some do not have a diuretic phase. However, it is necessary to watch for complications that can occur if the patient does enter the diuretic phase.

OLIGURIC PHASE

During the oliguric phase, the patient's urine output varies from 50 to 400 ml/24 hr. The oliguria usually lasts 10 to 14 days, but it may last only a few days or as long as six to eight weeks. If the oliguric phase follows a typical course, the BUN level rises to 20 to 30 mg/100 ml/day and the creatinine rises to 1 to 2 mg/100 ml/day. The degree of tissue necrosis and the rate of endogenous protein catabolism determine the rate at which the BUN level rises.

Complications During Oliguric Phase
The most commonly occurring complications during the oliguric phase are infection, heart failure due to overhydration, pulmonary edema, hyperkalemia, acidosis, and gastrointestinal bleeding from stress.

Treatment is aimed at preventing complications. If complications occur, they must be carefully managed. In some situations, furosemide and/or mannitol may be given in an attempt to reestablish a normal urine flow early in the oliguric phase. The evidence that those diuretics are clinically beneficial is not conclusive, especially when they are used after a nephrotoxic insult [19].

Infection

Infection is the most frequent cause of death in acute renal failure [6]. The hospital organisms found most often in the patient with acute renal failure are *Staphylococci* and *Pseudomonas*. Close attention must be paid to healing surgical wounds, to Foley catheters and to the changing of sterile dressings. All are possible sources of infection. If infection occurs despite preventive measures, antibiotic therapy should be used only after the specific infection has been identified, and, if possible, after information about specific sensitivity has been obtained.

To prevent tissue necrosis, special attention must be paid to the patient's mouth and skin. Drying of the buccal and pharyngeal mucosa is frequently seen in patients who mouth-breathe. The patients must be given extremely good mouth care to prevent parotitis and stomatitis, which is produced by the bacterial production of ammonia from urea. The nurse should give careful range-of-motion exercises to the patient's extremities if he must remain at bedrest. If possible, the patient should be encouraged to walk. He should also be encouraged to cough, deep breathe, and change his position at least every hour to prevent atelectasis. When the patient is too ill to move, cough, and deep breathe on his own, he must receive assistance to accomplish these maneuvers.

Fluid Overload

Fluid management must be carefully monitored to prevent circulatory overload [7]. The patient's daily weight is a strong indication of adequacy of fluid replacement. The patient must be weighed consistently on quality scales, i.e., on the same scales and at the same time each day. Since these patients are catabolic, they will lose 0.5 to 1.0 kg of body weight per day. This normal weight loss must be considered in fluid replacement. (One kg of weight is equal to 1 liter or 2.2 lbs of fluid retained.) Appropriate fluid replacement is based on daily loss of body weight.

Sodium and potassium are given only to replace losses. In those patients who develop heart failure, dialysis is the only effective treatment. Fluid intake is restricted to the volume required to replace urinary and extrarenal losses. If the patient has a fever and has excessive losses in the form of perspiration, these losses must be closely observed and charted for adequate replacement.

Avoidance of Negative Nitrogen Balance

To avoid negative nitrogen balance, a certain amount of protein of high biological activity must be taken in for tissue maintenance and repair. The best sources of essential amino acids (listed in order of their utilization) are eggs, milk, meat, fish, and poultry. The recommended daily quantity of protein for a healthy person is one gm of protein per kg of body weight. The patient in acute renal failure may be limited to 20 to 40 gm of protein depending on the severity of his state. Carbohydrates are also necessary to save the protein from being used as a caloric source. Carbohydrates are needed daily in order to slow protein catabolism and to reduce azotemia, metabolic acidosis, and hyperkalemia. Such diets provide about 1700 calories a day, depending on the content of essential amino acids and carbohydrates [1, 6]. That amount provides the best protection against the catabolism of lean tissue but it cannot prevent it. In the presence of nausea or vomiting, oral feedings should not be given. If the patient is unable to take the needed amount of essential amino acids orally, parenteral alimentation may be necessary [1]. It has been suggested that the infusion of hypertonic glucose containing essential amino acids increases the patient's chances of survival and an accelerated return of renal function [1]. Since the hypertonic solution is irritating to the vessel wall, large central veins, such as the superior vena cava, should be used. The procedure should be used in selected cases because of the high added risk of infection [6].

Hyperkalemia

Frequently, the ECG changes indicate possible hyperkalemic cardiac arrest. The nurse must watch for increased changes in T-wave height and shape, a widened QRS interval (greater than .09), and no atrial activity (loss of P wave) changing to ventricular tachycardia and sine wave (Fig. 32-8).

Because hyperkalemia has significant effects on the cardiac conduction system, the serial ECG results must be carefully evaluated; the plasma potassium levels do not always correlate with the ECG results. Dysrhythmias occur often. Probably they are most often caused by an electrolyte imbalance and a fluid overload, but they can be caused by hyperkalemia. Digitalis intoxication is also a cause of dysrhythmias

Table 32-4
Degrees of Hyperkalemia in Acute Renal Failure

Types	Plasma Potassium Levels	ECG Findings	Treatments
Minimal hyper-kalemia	5.5–6.5 mEq/L	Normal	Cation exchange resins Oral route Kayexalate (15–20 gm 3 or 4 times daily) in combination with sorbitol (20 ml of a 70% solution) By enema Kayexalate (50 gm) in a mixture of sorbitol (50 ml of a 70% solution) and tap water (100 ml)
Moderate hyper-kalemia	6.5–7.5 mEq/L	Peaked T waves	Hypertonic glucose infusion Regular insulin Sodium bicarbonate (2 or 3 ampules) for acidotic patients
Severe hyper-kalemia	7.5 mEq/L or greater	Disappearance of P wave, slurred and broad QRS complex, ventricular dysrhythmias	Calcium gluconate (10–30 ml infused at 2 ml/min) with continuous ECG monitoring Dialysis

in those patients with electrolyte imbalance [5]. It has been suggested that hyperkalemia can be classified as minimal, moderate, and severe [6] (Table 32-4). Hyperkalemia can be treated by several different methods, depending on the degree of hyperkalemia. Potassium can be removed from the body by ion exchangers (e.g., Kayexalate) in minimal hyperkalemic states. If Kayexalate is used, for every milliequivalent of potassium removed one milliequivalent of sodium is put in as the exchange. If a patient is in cardiac failure, the physician must be careful not to overload him with sodium. If the patient cannot take an oral medication, the cation exchange resin may be administered by a retention enema. Sorbitol may be given in conjunction with Kayexalate; it acts to prevent fecal impaction and to help remove sodium freed from the resin in loose stools [6]. Kayexalate should not be given in fruit juices because the potassium in the fruit juices would bind with the resin and so render Kayexalate ineffective.

In moderate hyperkalemic states, potassium can be shifted from the extracellular to the intracellular fluid by the infusion of hypertonic glucose and insulin. That treatment can be effective within 30 minutes [6]. If the patient is acidotic and not fluid overloaded, sodium bicarbonate may be added to the infusion.

In severe hyperkalemia, the most effective treatment for cardiac intoxication is calcium infusion.

Cardiac intoxication may be antagonized by raising the serum calcium concentration without altering the serum potassium concentration. That treatment has an effect in five minutes. Since the effect is of short duration, it should be followed by the intravenous administration of glucose and bicarbonate. Hyperkalemia increases the neuromuscular excitability by lowering the resting potential toward the threshold level, and hypercalcemia opposes that state by decreasing the threshold level [6]. It is usually necessary to begin dialysis for patients who have moderate-to-severe hyperkalemia because the measures just discussed have only transient effects.

Acidosis
In acute renal failure, the normal acids of metabolism are not excreted by the kidneys. Since protein restriction to minimize the azotemia usually diminishes the acids of metabolism, specific therapy for acidosis is usually not required. If acidosis is a clinical problem, it may be corrected by the administration of sodium bicarbonate. In situations of increasing acidosis, dialysis may be necessary.

Gastrointestinal Bleeding from Stress
Gastrointestinal bleeding from stress that occurs as a complication of acute renal failure is managed like gastrointestinal bleeding from any other cause, except

varices. The physician directs his treatment toward four specific areas: the cause of the bleeding, the amount of blood lost, the rate of bleeding, and the location of the bleeding.

A nasogastric tube is inserted, and the stomach is lavaged. An evaluation of the location and cause of bleeding is based first on the history and physical examination. After the patient's blood volume has been assessed and vital signs are stabilized, further diagnostic studies are done. The evaluation and therapy depend on the patient and on the situation. Collaboration of the internist, nephrologist, and gastroenterologist is usually indicated.

Anemia

Anemia is a complication that usually occurs during the first week of oliguria. It is caused by a mild increase in the erythrocyte destruction and a deficiency in the red blood cell production [20]. Both erythropoiesis and red cell survival are diminished in acute renal failure. The predominant mechanism varies with the type and the acuteness of the renal disease [6]. Blood replacement is usually not required. If it is required, it should be given in the form of packed red blood cells to avoid serious overexpansion of the plasma volume.

Neurological Manifestations

The neurological manifestations that may occur during the oliguric period are convulsions and coma. The precipitating events may be rapid changes in body fluid composition.

Early in the course of acute renal failure, hyponatremia may cause seizures or somnolence. Hypertonic saline infusion can correct the electrolyte imbalance. If hypertonic saline is used, extreme care must be taken to avoid the complication of heart failure with overhydration.

During the oliguric phase of acute renal failure, the patient may require dialysis. Ideally, the patient is dialyzed long before his condition deteriorates into a state of severe uremia [10]. The term *uremia* has no pathophysiological implication; it refers to the symptom complex that is associated with a severe impairment of renal function, regardless of the cause [6]. Some of the symptoms that may occur are fatigue, loss of appetite, decreased urinary output, apathy or mental dullness, elevated blood pressure, edema of the face and feet, itching, restlessness, and seizures. Those symptoms vary widely. They may develop over

a period of several days when acute renal failure occurs.

The patient's underlying illness and related complications usually determine the outcome when early and continued dialysis is provided. The type of dialysis used is determined by the physician's close examination of the patient's history, clinical course, and laboratory reports.

Peritoneal Dialysis Versus Hemodialysis During Oliguria

Uncontrolled hyperkalemia, severe fluid overload, severe acidosis, and uremic symptoms are the chief indications for dialysis in acute renal failure [6]. A complicated clinical picture, in which early and severe manifestations of uremia can be expected, often leads to early and repeated dialysis, before the overt signs and symptoms of uremia occur. Hemodialysis is usually highly preferable; it is a highly developed technology in centers where it is routinely used. The patient who requires dialysis must be assessed individually to determine whether he needs peritoneal dialysis or hemodialysis. Peritoneal dialysis has the advantage that it can be done in virtually any hospital. The advantage of hemodialysis is that it can be done in a shorter period of time on patients who are not candidates for peritoneal dialysis, with the same goals being achieved (Table 32-5).

Peritoneal Dialysis

If the patient with acute renal failure requires peritoneal dialysis, his physician should explain the procedure to him and tell him why it is being done (Table 32-6). Before the nurse has the patient sign the consent form for the procedure, she should again explain the procedure to the patient and his family and answer any questions they might have. It is extremely important that during the entire procedure the nurse pay attention to the patient and his needs—and not only to the technical aspects of the dialysis. The nurse can ask the patient to help at certain points and thus make him feel important and involved.

Peritoneal dialysis involves a combination of three basic mechanisms: osmosis, diffusion, and filtration. Waste products are removed, and the fluid and electrolyte balance is reestablished. The patient's peritoneum is used as the dialyzing membrane to replace the damaged kidneys via a closed drainage system (Fig. 32-9). The peritoneum approximates the surface area of the glomerular capillaries.

Table 32-5
Comparison of Peritoneal Dialysis and Hemodialysis

Factors to Be Compared	Peritoneal Dialysis	Hemodialysis
Personnel needed	Skilled nurses	Specialized nurses
Length of each treatment	24–72 hr	4–10 hr
Supplies needed	Usually available	Complex
Equipment needed	Sterile, simple	Nonsterile and sterile, complex
Drugs	Only small amounts of heparin, if any, required	Heparinization required
Site	Patient must not recently have undergone surgery involving the retroperitoneum	Good vessels needed for shunt or fistula
Side effects	Peritonitis Protein loss Disequilibrium syndrome (rapid fluid and electrolyte changes)	Disequilibrium syndrome (rapid fluid and electrolyte changes) Heparinization, bleeding

Table 32-6
Indications for and Contraindications of Peritoneal Dialysis

Indications	Contraindications
Refractory hyperkalemia	Presence of abdominal drains or surgery that involves the retroperitoneum
Metabolic acidosis when alkali cannot be administered	Undiagnosed acute abdomen
Circulatory overload	Adhesions
Acute renal failure	Prosthetic material in abdomen
Chronic renal failure	Colostomy Impending kidney transplant

During the controlled dwell time (the time the dialysate is left in the peritoneum), a specific concentration of glucose (usually two liters of a 1.5% glucose solution) is instilled into the peritoneal cavity through a peritoneal catheter and then drained in a siphon effect through the catheter. If the patient is retaining fluid, a 4.25% glucose solution can be used to enhance the osmotic removal of water. Depending on the patient's serum potassium level, various concentrations of potassium may be ordered.

The dwell time in the abdomen is usually 15 to 30 minutes. The fluid remains in the abdomen because the peritoneal catheter is clamped. The most important part of the dwell time is the first 5 to 10 minutes, during which time a maximum concentration gradient occurs. If the blood and the dialysate are kept in the abdomen longer, they begin to equal each other, the glucose molecules are absorbed, and the urea clearance drops drastically. The dialysate is diffused into the patient's bloodstream, and the possible complication of fluid overload can occur.

The peritoneal catheter is unclamped, and the fluid is collected in bottles or a urinary bag using a closed drainage system. The returned fluid must be accurately measured. If 2 liters of fluid are infused and not all of it is returned, the patient is "plus fluid"; if more fluid than was infused is returned, the patient is "minus fluid." The goal of peritoneal dialysis is a negative balance. A negative balance helps the patient to lose fluid as well as the toxic waste products that have accumulated in his blood because his kidneys are functioning poorly. The nurse must remember that before each dialysis the dialysate should be warmed to body temperature [15]. A dialysate that approximates the body temperature increases the urea clearance, prevents the patient from losing body heat, and causes less discomfort.

Nursing care during peritoneal dialysis requires astute observations because of the complications that can occur [30]. Hypoventilation is a common complication. The patient undergoing peritoneal dialysis has a tendency to hypoventilate owing to the presence of the dialysate in his abdomen. He is prone to atelectasis and pneumonia, and so he must be encouraged

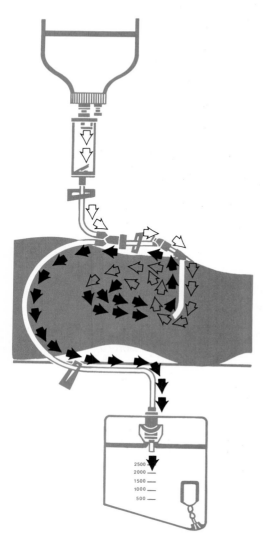

Figure 32-9
Insertion of the catheter for peritoneal dialysis.

is mandatory if the complications of peritonitis are to be avoided. A break in aseptic technique when the dialysate setup is changed is one of the most frequent causes of contamination of the dialysate. It is suggested that the use of a millipore filter for peritoneal dialysis can drastically reduce the incidence of peritonitis [31]. Peritoneal dialysis is usually done for 48 to 72 hours. When the dialysis is discontinued, a sample of the returned fluid and the tip of the catheter that was in the patient's abdomen are sent to the laboratory for culture. Peritoneal dialysis that lasts longer than 72 hours carries a high risk of infection. Other complications are perforation of the bowel, bladder, or blood vessels by the peritoneal catheter and an inability to drain the abdomen of the dialysate.

Hemodialysis
The principles of peritoneal dialysis apply to hemodialysis also (Table 32-7). In hemodialysis, the semipermeable membrane is a thin porous plate of cellophane. There are several different types of membranes, all of which are subject to the same laws. Water and low-molecular-weight substances move freely across the membrane. Plasma, proteins, bacteria, and blood cells are too large to pass through the membrane. The blood flows from the patient to the hemodialysis machine through catheters from the patient that are connected to the machine. The patient's blood is one compartment, and the dialysate is another compartment. A concentration gradient is achieved by the difference in the concentration of substances in each compartment. Over a period of 4 to 12 hours (the time depends on the patient's condition and what needs to be achieved clinically), toxic substances pass from the patient's blood into the dialysate. The dialysate varies with each patient's needs. In certain situations electrolyte levels (e.g., sodium, potassium, phosphorus, bicarbonate, and magnesium levels) are corrected as needed during the procedure [16].

Access to the patient's circulation in an emergency or for short-term hemodialysis is usually achieved by means of an arteriovenous (A-V) shunt [16]. Placement of the A-V shunt is carried out under local anesthesia in the operating room (Fig. 32-10). The procedure consists of the placement of two soft Silastic cannulas. One is inserted into an artery and the other into a vein. They are usually inserted into the patient's nondominant forearm. If chronic dialysis is anticipated, the legs can be used; thus the vasculature of the arms is reserved for fistulas. When the A-V

to cough and to deep breathe. Elevation of the head of the patient's bed also helps the patient to be comfortable, and it increases his ease of breathing.

When the patient who is receiving hypotonic fluids is obtunded, the nurse must check his serum glucose and electrolyte levels as ordered to look for signs of hyperglycemia and hypernatremia. If the patient is a known diabetic, his serum glucose levels must be checked more often.

Sterile technique in performing peritoneal dialysis

Table 32-7
Indications for and Contraindications of Hemodialysis

Indications	Contraindications
Refractory hyperkalemia	Patient actively bleeding
Circulatory overload	
Acute renal failure	
Chronic renal failure	
Need for rapid reversal of specific drug intoxication	

shunt is not in use, a hard plastic connector is inserted into the Silastic cannulas to allow blood to flow freely between the artery and the vein. For a dialysis procedure, those two tubes are clamped and disconnected. The hard plastic connector is removed, and the two tubes are then connected to the tubing of the artificial kidney and unclamped, allowing blood to flow in the anticipated manner. The arterial line allows blood to flow from the patient to the artificial kidney, while the venous line returns purified blood to the patient. The shunt life is dependent on cleanliness, proper alignment of the cannulas, gentle handling, and frequent observation to prevent clotting and infection.

Access to the patient's circulation can also be gained by creating an A-V fistula in a surgical procedure that anastomoses an artery and a vein. An A-V fistula in the wrist arteriolizes the superficial veins of the forearm. The veins are prominent, and a good blood flow is achieved in two to four weeks. Dialysis should be attempted at the site only after that length of time so that the surgical wound will be firm. For dialysis, two 14- or 16-gauge needles are inserted into the fistula, one into the arterial side of the fistula, which removes blood from the patient, and one into the venous side, which returns blood to the patient. There is now a machine that uses only one needle to (alternately) remove and infuse the blood.

Femoral catheters, bovine grafts, and synthetic grafts can also be used for acute dialysis to gain access to the patient's circulation. Shaldon catheters (Teflon cannulas) can be used for percutaneous access to the femoral veins for inflow and outflow of blood from the artificial kidney. Femoral catheters are used if a new shunt or fistula is not ready for use and the patient needs dialysis immediately [16]. Fistulas, bovine grafts, and synthetic grafts are seldom used in acute renal failure. They may be used for the patient undergoing chronic dialysis.

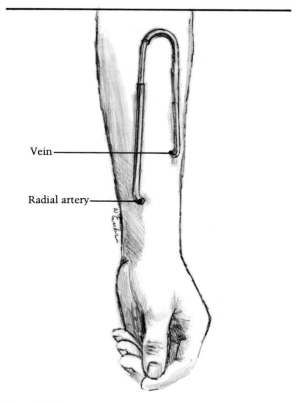

Vein

Radial artery

Figure 32-10
Arteriovenous shunt for hemodialysis.

Nursing care during hemodialysis also requires astute observations because of the complications that can occur [16, 21]. Hypovolemia can occur owing to a rapid volume depletion during dialysis caused by excessive fluid removal. Or the hypovolemia may have been present before hemodialysis, or it may occur because of an overload of fluids during hemodialysis. Hypotension may be caused by excessive ultrafiltration or existing states of hypovolemia. When hypertension occurs, it is usually the result of anxiety or of fluid overload.

The neurological manifestations that can occur during hemodialysis and peritoneal dialysis are referred to as the dysequilibrium syndrome. The dysequilibrium syndrome is most commonly caused by too rapid dialysis and by ultrafiltration [6]. The symptoms are nausea, vomiting, irritability, headaches, muscle twitching, cramps, and convulsions. They can be corrected by sedatives and the reduction of the blood flow rate. If the symptoms become worse, the dialysis may be discontinued and hypertonic solutions (e.g., hypertonic saline and albumin) given. Laboratory values help regulate the electrolyte disturbances that often occur during dialysis.

DIURETIC PHASE

The diuretic phase of acute renal failure follows the oliguric phase. During the diuretic phase, an increase in the urine volume occurs that normally doubles each day for several days until the output is about 1 to 2 liters. The increase indicates that renal function has started; it does not indicate that the renal function is normal. During this phase there are still degrees of renal function impairment, such as in concentrating ability and in the tubular transport system. This is clinically evident because early in the diuretic phase the BUN and creatinine levels are elevated, phenomena that indicate a continued reduction of the glomerular filtration rate.

The use of dialysis early in the oliguric phase has reduced the massive diuresis noted in earlier reports. Regular dialysis prevents severe azotemia, which causes osmotic diuresis due to the excretion of retained urea. Overhydration is more consistently limited now than was possible prior to the early use of dialysis [6]. Although massive polyuria is rarely a problem, precautions must be taken during this period because complications can occur. During the early diuretic phase, infection, heart failure, hyperkalemia, gastrointestinal bleeding, and convulsions may continue. If any of those complications occur, the treatment is the same as in the oliguric phase.

Treatment
Treatment during the diuretic phase involves trying to avoid complications. If the patient is volume overloaded and his urinary output is several liters a day, sodium wasting can cause electrolyte depletion. During the diuretic phase, the patient is usually able to take oral feedings and fluids in amounts sufficient to prevent the potential deficiencies. The intake of fluid and electrolytes should be increased to counter fluid and electrolyte losses.

If the patient is unconscious, elevations of the sodium and chloride levels are common during the diuretic phase when the water replacement is inadequate. If the urinary potassium excretion exceeds the potassium intake, the serum potassium level can fall below normal. It must be corrected.

RECOVERY PHASE

The last phase of acute renal failure is recovery. During that phase, renal function continues to improve for 3 to 12 months. The majority of patients who survive are able to achieve normal functioning and maintain it indefinitely although they may have subtle functional defects.

Treatment
Treatment during the recovery phase consists of patient education. The patient must be educated about the need for follow-up medical care. If he is to be on a special diet or to take a certain medication after he is discharged, he should be given written information about the details and assessed in regard to what he and his family understand about his care.

Nursing Orders
Problem/Diagnosis

The patient has acute renal failure.

OBJECTIVE NO. 1

During the oliguric phase of acute renal failure, the patient should be assessed in regard to his clinical manifestations and the severity of his condition.

To achieve the objective, the nurse should:

1. Reverse the circulatory failure that has initiated the ischemic episode of the kidneys. She should:
   a. Be aware that if overhydration occurs, pulmonary edema may also occur.
   b. Closely observe the patient's blood pressure, pulse, temperature, urinary output, urine specific gravity, and cardiac rhythm.
2. Assess the patient's level of anxiety. Explain all procedures to him. Include the patient's family when appropriate. Evaluate the patient's level of understanding.
3. Maintain fluid and electrolyte balance. (During the oliguric phase, the urinary loss is usually less than 400 ml/day. Insensible losses average 600 ml/day, which are free of electrolytes.) The nurse should:
   a. Keep an accurate flow sheet that shows the intake and output.
   b. Know that fluid replacement should average 600 ml per day in addition to the replacement of other measured fluid losses. (The amount

depends on the patient's size, his temperature, and the room temperature.) If the patient is alert and can participate, let him help make up the schedule for his 24-hour oral fluid intake.

c. Weigh the patient daily (on the same scale). The patient's weight is a reliable index of his fluid balance. He should lose 0.5 to 1 lb a day as a result of consuming his own fat and protein. One kg of weight gain is equal to 1 liter (2.2 lb) of fluid retained.

d. Assess the following parameters closely to determine whether the patient has hypervolemia or hypovolemia.

centration. If potassium intoxication occurs, give potassium-exchange sulfonic resin as ordered by physician. Kayexalate, which is given by mouth or in an enema, usually reduces an elevated serum potassium level by 1 or 2 mEq every 24 to 48 hours. If Kayexalate is given in an enema, the patient should retain the enema for 30 to 60 minutes so that the potassium can be removed. It is preferable to give Kayexalate by mouth because the oral route allows the resin to come in direct contact with more of the gastrointestinal tract and thus pick up more potassium. Kayexalate should not be

Phenomena to Assess	Hypervolemia	Hypovolemia
Temperature	May or may not be significant	Usually not elevated
Pulse	Full, rapid	Rapid, thready, weak
Respirations	Rapid dyspnea, moist rales	Shallow, rapid
Blood pressure	Normal to high	Small pulse pressure, orthostatic hypotension, low
Thirst (depends on tonicity, except with acute hypovolemia)	May or may not be significant	Present, sometimes is acute
Saliva	Frothy, excessive	Scanty, thick
Tongue	Moist	Coated, fissured
Face	Periorbital edema	Sunken eyes
Subcutaneous tissues and skin	Pitting edema over bony prominences, moist, warm, wrinkled skin from pressure of clothing and linens	Loss of elasticity, dry
Weight	Gain	Loss

Adapted from Hudak, C., Lohr, T., and Gallo, B. *Critical Care Nursing* (2nd ed.). Philadelphia: Lippincott, 1977.

e. Monitor the fluid intake and output (include perspiration, gastric suction, drainage, stools, and urine).

f. Give 100 to 150 gm of carbohydrate daily to reduce the protein breakdown.

g. Match the potassium and sodium intakes to the potassium and sodium losses.

h. If nausea and vomiting are present, avoid oral feedings. If nausea prevents oral intake and acidosis from renal failure threatens, alkalinization solution (usually in the form of sodium bicarbonate) may be given intravenously; calcium may be added if hypocalcemia is present.

i. Monitor the cardiac rhythm and use it as immediate index of the serum potassium con-

mixed in fruit juices. Sorbital may be given with Kayexalate to cause osmotic diarrhea and thus help excrete potassium and prevent constipation. Infusions of hypertonic glucose solution with insulin have a transient effect like that of Kayexalate. The infusions help shift extracellular potassium to intracellular pools. Hyperkalemia associated with acidosis may be brought under control by the administration of intravenous sodium bicarbonate. If the hyperkalemia cannot be controlled and if cardiac dysrhythmias are present, hemodialysis is indicated.

j. Using the information in the tabular material that follows, assess the patient for the common fluid and electrolyte imbalances.

Electrolyte Abnormalities	Major Symptoms	Physical Signs	Causes
Hypokalemia	Weakness	ECG changes (T waves and prominent U waves), paralytic ileus, paralysis	Vomiting, diarrhea, diuretics, excessive use of laxatives
Hyperkalemia	Weakness	ECG changes (spiked T waves and widening of the QRS complex), paralysis	Excessive potassium replacement, decreased renal excretion, acidosis
Normal sodium and decreased water	Thirst	Often those found in decreased sodium and water (or no findings)	Excessive sweating, fever, lack of water, diabetes insipidus
Increased sodium and water	Dyspnea	Rales, edema, anasarca	Fluid retention from renal failure, congestive failure, liver disease
Decreased sodium and water	Lethargy, thirst	Dry mouth, decreased skin turgor, postural hypotension, tachycardia, sunken eyes	Renal disease, use of diuretics without replacement, diarrhea, vomiting, excessive sweating, Addison's disease
Decreased sodium, normal water	Psychological changes, headaches	Pathological reflexes, hyperreflexia, convulsions, coma	Excessive ADH, water given without sodium replacement
Acidosis	Lethargy	Kussmaul's respiration	Diabetic acidosis, renal disease, use of certain intoxicants, poor tissue perfusion
Hypermagnesemia	Weakness	Flushing, hypotension, hypoventilation, weak muscles	Renal disease with antacids

Adapted from Hudak, C., Lohr, T., and Gallo, B. *Critical Care Nursing* (2nd ed.). Philadelphia: Lippincott, 1977.

4. Help restore adequate blood flow to the kidneys. Give intravenous fluids as ordered, paying close attention to the rate of administration of the total intake. The nurse should give mannitol or furosemide as ordered to improve renal plasma flow, to increase the blood flow to the renal cortex, and to decrease the intrarenal vascular resistance. When electrolyte studies are ordered, the nurse should see that they are done before the patient is given diuretics.

5. Be alert to the importance of a good diet and of protein balance. The nurse should:
   a. Reduce the blood nitrogen levels by restricting the protein intake.
   b. Give essential amino acids as ordered. (If the patient is limited to 10 to 20 gm of protein per day, in planning his diet the nurse should consider the fact that milk and eggs are the best sources of protein.)
   c. Explain to the patient the reason for the special diet.
   d. Learn the patient's food preferences. The nurse should plan his diet with the dietitian.
   e. Check the patient's food tray to see whether he has been served the food he wanted and whether he ate his meal. (About 20 gm of essential amino acids is needed each day for tissue maintenance.)
   f. Know the causes of increased protein catabolism and try to prevent or correct them when they occur. The causes are:
      (1) Fever
      (2) Traumatized cells
      (3) Steroids
      (4) Internal bleeding
      (5) Immobilization
      (6) Tissue necrosis
      (7) Infection

6. Prepare the patient for diagnostic blood work and the procedures the physician orders to help diagnose (rule out) and treat acute renal failure. The nurse should:
   a. Obtain the results of the diagnostic blood studies, the urinalysis, and the ECG.
   b. Obtain the results of the plain x ray of the abdomen.
   c. Obtain a cystoscopy, retrograde pyelogram, or sonography (those procedures are ordered when an obstruction is suspected) [2, 6].
   d. Obtain a renal arteriogram radioactive scan (sometimes ordered when the cause is not clear).
7. Obtain further serum electrolyte levels every 6 to 12 hours as ordered. Report any abnormalities to the physician.
8. Anticipate the complications of renal failure during the oliguric phase. The nurse should:
   a. Be aware of the signs of heart failure. Observe and assess the patient's clinical status, which indicates whether or not excess fluid is present. The signs to look for are dyspnea, tachycardia, gallop rhythm, peripheral edema, pulmonary edema, and distended neck veins. Give a low-salt diet, diuretics, digitoxin, and antihypertensive medication as ordered to control water retention and hypertension.
   b. Prevent infection and reduce any fever.
   c. Remove the Foley catheter as soon as possible. Catheterize the patient only once in 24 to 48 hours, using careful aseptic technique. If the Foley catheter must remain, give meticulous closed-seal catheter care.
   d. Encourage deep breathing and coughing to prevent atelectasis.
   e. Give careful mouth care to prevent crusting and ulceration. The patient whose oral intake is curtailed is prone to stomatitis and parotitis due to the breakdown of urea by bacteria. The ammonia that results is irritating to the mucous membranes of the mouth.
   f. Be prepared for cardiac arrest if hyperkalemia persists and has caused lethal cardiac dysrhythmias.
9. Be prepared to help with peritoneal dialysis or hemodialysis when indicated. The nurse should:
   a. Reinforce the explanation of the procedure the physician gave the patient.
   b. Answer the questions asked by the patient and his family.
   c. Have the patient sign the consent form for the procedure (if the patient is unable to sign it, a member of his family may sign it).
   d. Weigh the patient before the procedure and every 24 hours after it.
   e. Record the patient's temperature, pulse, respiration, and blood pressure.
   f. Have the patient urinate (if he can) before the procedure to avoid perforating his bladder.
   g. Record the patient's tolerance to peritoneal catheter insertion.
10. During the procedure, keep accurate records of the following:
   a. The exact time the infusion was started
   b. The amount and concentration of the infusion
   c. The medications added to the infusion
   d. The exact time the infusion was finished
   e. The exact time the drainage was started
   f. The color of the outflow (usually it is straw-colored)
   g. The exact time the drainage was finished
   h. The exact amount of fluid drained from or retained by the patient. Retention of fluid will create a positive balance and fluid loss will be a negative balance. The goal is a negative balance.
   i. Any leakage around the peritoneal catheter
11. Make astute observations to avoid or recognize the complications. The nurse should:
   a. Check the patient's vital signs every 15 minutes during the first exchange, and then every four hours unless otherwise indicated.
   b. Note any increases in the pulse rate or any drops in the blood pressure. (They may be signs of early shock.) If the vital signs do not return quickly to a normal range, clamp the drainage tube and contact the physician.
   c. Use careful aseptic technique with each peritoneal dialysis infusion to avoid peritonitis. Assess the patient's pain: If the pain continues, the nurse should:
      (1) Change the patient's position.
      (2) Decrease the dialysate volume temporarily.
      (3) Give analgesics as ordered if the pain persists.
      (4) Contact the physician if the pain or respiratory distress increases.
   d. Record and report any elevated temperature. (It may be a sign of infection.)

e. Note any cloudiness of the outflow. (It may be a sign that bacteria are present.)
f. Note any bleeding. (The first few exchanges of dialysate may be blood-tinged because of subcutaneous bleeding. After that blood-tinged exchanges may be a sign of abdominal bleeding.)
g. Record the fluid intake and output (include urine, emesis, and diarrhea). Diarrhea that occurs after the first infusion must be evaluated; it may be a sign of bowel perforation. The output of urine-colored return after the first infusion must also be evaluated; it may be a sign of bladder perforation. The infusion must be stopped and the physician notified.
h. Watch for leakage around the peritoneal catheter.
i. If the dressing is changed, weigh it while it is wet and record the weight (1 gm = 1 ml).
12. If hemodialysis is indicated, have the patient sign the consent form for the procedure after the physician explains the procedure to him. (Hemodialysis is a complex procedure. The staff nurse should refresh her knowledge of it by consulting a textbook or the hospital teaching plan before sending the patient for hemodialysis.) The nurse should weigh the patient before the procedure is begun and record his weight, check and record his vital signs, and keep accurate records during the procedure.
13. Make astute observations during the hemodialysis to avoid or to recognize its most commonly occurring complications:
a. Hypovolemia
b. Hypervolemia
c. Hypotension
d. Hypertension
e. The dysequilibrium syndrome
f. Electrolyte imbalance
g. Dysrhythmias
h. Bleeding
i. Technical problems with the equipment

OBJECTIVE NO. 2

During the diuretic phase of acute renal failure, the patient should be continuously assessed to avoid complications.

To achieve the objective, the nurse should:

1. Avoid dehydration and salt depletion.

2. Determine the daily serum sodium and potassium levels when ordered.
3. Sustain the diuresis by replacing the fluids lost in the preceding 24 hours.
4. Weigh the patient daily and record his weight.
5. Be aware that when the patient's azotemia improves, he may take in larger amounts of protein. (When the BUN level falls below 80 mg/100 ml, more protein is allowed; the body can use the protein to replete the lost tissue stores of protein.)

OBJECTIVE NO. 3

During the recovery phase of acute renal failure, the patient should show a restoration of his renal functioning.

To achieve the objective, the nurse should:

1. Educate the patient about his need for follow-up care and encourage him to get it.
2. Encourage the patient to gradually increase the amount of exercise he gets.
3. If the patient is on a special diet or medication schedule, give him written information about the details and evaluate his and his family's understanding of the diet and the schedule.

Summary

Acute renal failure is the condition in which the renal excretory function is severely compromised. Acute renal failure may be due to hypovolemia, a decreased cardiac output, an altered peripheral resistance, renal tubular degeneration from renal ischemia, toxic drugs, obstructions, or stricture. Acute renal failure has an abrupt onset and three clinical phases. The first phase is oliguria (a urine output of less than 400 ml/24 hr), which usually lasts 10 to 14 days. The aim of treatment during the oliguric phase is to maintain the fluid and electrolyte balance and to avoid the complications of a negative nitrogen balance and fluid and electrolyte imbalances, which usually result in overhydration, hyperkalemia, and infection. The second phase is the diuretic phase. In that phase the patient begins to show a progressive return of his normal urine output. The nurse must make astute observations during the diuretic phase if dehydration, salt depletion, and a second period of oliguria are to be avoided. This phase usually lasts for 7 to 14 days. The third phase is the recovery phase, which lasts from 3 to 12 months. During the recovery phase, the patient must be educated about his diet, medications, and follow-up medical care.

Study Problems

1. What are the most common clinical manifestations of acute renal failure?
2. What complications of acute renal failure does the nurse anticipate and try to prevent?
3. Why is furosemide given along with intravenous fluids in the oliguric phase of acute renal failure?
4. What are the three most common causes of reduced renal perfusion?
5. In the hospitalized patient, what is the most common group of nephrotoxic drugs that causes acute renal failure?
6. What three categories of azotemia must be diagnosed by the physician?
7. What phases of acute renal failure must the nurse and physician be aware of in order to anticipate and prevent complications?

Answers

1. Nausea, lethargy, and a reduced urine output.
2. Potassium intoxication, infection, hypertension, acidosis, congestive heart failure, and/or pulmonary edema.
3. To improve renal plasma flow, to increase blood flow to the renal cortex, and to decrease intrarenal vascular resistance.
4. Hypovolemia, a decreased cardiac output, and an altered peripheral vascular resistance.
5. Antibiotics.
6. Prerenal azotemia, intrarenal azotemia, and postrenal azotemia.
7. The oliguric phase, the diuretic phase, and the recovery phase.

References

1. Abel, R. M., Beck, C. H., Jr., Abbott, W. M., et al. Improved survival from acute renal failure after treatment with intravenous essential L-amino acids and glucose. Results of a prospective, double-blind study. *N. Engl. J. Med.* 288:695, 1973.
2. Barnett, E., and Morley, P. Diagnostic ultrasound in renal disease. *Br. Med. Bull.* 28:196, 1972.
3. Baxter, C. R., Zedlitz, W. H., and Shire, G. T. High

output acute renal failure complicating traumatic injury. *J. Trauma* 4:567, 1964.
4. Bennett, W. M., Singer, I., and Coggins, C. H. Guide to drug usage in adult patients with impaired renal function: A supplement. *J.A.M.A.* 233:991, 1973.
5. Bobrow, S. N., Jaffe, E., and Young, R. C. Anuria and acute tubular necrosis associated with gentamicin and cephalothin. *J.A.M.A.* 222:1546, 1972.
6. Brenner, B. M., and Rector, F. C. *The Kidney*. Philadelphia: Saunders, 1976. Vols. I and II.
7. Cattell, W. R., McIntosh, C. S., Moseley, I. F., et al. Excretion urography in acute renal failure. *Br. Med. J.* 2:575, 1973.
8. Clark, J. E., and Caldo, R. E. Fluid and electrolyte management in renal failure. *Prac. Ther.* 5:125, 1972.
9. Dudrick, S. J., Steiger, E., and Long, J. M. Renal failure in surgical patients: Treatment with essential amino acids and hypertonic glucose. *Surgery* 68:180, 1970.
10. Dunea, G. Peritoneal dialysis and hemodialysis. *Med. Clin. North Am.* 55:155, 1971.
11. Epstein, F. H. Acute Renal Failure. In T. R. Harrison et al. (eds.), *Principles of Internal Medicine* (7th ed.). New York: McGraw-Hill, 1974.
12. Fay, F. C. Pulling a patient through acute renal failure. *RN* 11:61, 1978.
13. Flamenbaum, W. Pathophysiology of acute renal failure. *Arch. Intern. Med.* 131:911, 1973.
14. Freedman, P., and Smith, E. Acute renal failure. *Heart Lung* 4:873, 1975.
15. Gross, M., and McDonald, H. P., Jr. Effect of dialysate temperature and flow rate on peritoneal clearance. *J.A.M.A.* 202:215, 1967.
16. Gutch, C. F., and Stoner, M. H. *Review of Hemodialysis for Nurses and Dialysis Personnel* (2nd ed.). St. Louis: Mosby, 1975.
17. Guyton, A. *Textbook of Medical Physiology* (4th ed.). Philadelphia: Saunders, 1971.
18. Hall, J. W., et al. Immediate and long term prognosis in acute renal failure. *Ann. Intern. Med.* 73:515, 1970.
19. Harrington, J. T., and Cohen, J. J. Acute oliguria. *N. Engl. J. Med.* 292:89, 1975.
20. Harrison, T. R., et al. *Principles of Internal Medicine* (7th ed.). New York: McGraw-Hill, 1974.
21. Jennrich, J. Some aspects of the nursing care for patients on hemodialysis. *Heart Lung* 4:855, 1975.
22. Kemp, G., and Kemp, D. Diuretics. *Am. J. Nurs.* 6:1006, 1978.
23. Kennedy, A. C., Burton, J. A., Luke, R. G., et al. Factors affecting the prognosis in acute renal failure. *Br. Med. J.* 42:73, 1973.
24. Lancour, J. ADH and aldosterone: How to recognize their effects. *Nurs. '78* 9:36, 1978.
25. Lewers, D. T., et al. Long-term followup of renal function and histology after acute tubular necrosis. *Ann. Intern. Med.* 73:523, 1970.
26. McMurray, S. D., Luft, F. C., and Kleit, S. A. Iatrogenic

factors in acute renal failure. *Postgrad. Med.* 73:523, 1978.

27. Mailloux, L. U., Mossey, R. T., McVicar, M. M., et al.   Ultrasonic guidance for renal biopsy. *Arch. Intern. Med.* 138:438, 1978.

28. Muth, R. G.   Furosemide in severe renal insufficiency. *Postgrad. Med.* 47:21, 1971.

29. Powers, S. R.   Maintenance of renal function following massive trauma. *Trauma* 10:554, 1970.

30. Richard, C.   Nursing implications in prevention of complications in peritoneal dialysis. *Heart Lung* 4:890, 1975.

31. Sarles, H. E., Lindley, J. D., Fish, J. C., et al.   Peritoneal dialysis utilizing a millipore filter. *Kidney Int.* 9:54, 1976.

32. Shires, G. T., Carrico, J., and Canizaro, P. C.   *Shock.* Philadelphia: Saunders, 1973.

33. Siegler, R., and Boomer, H. A.   Acute renal failure with prolonged oliguria. *J.A.M.A.* 225:133, 1973.

34. Smith, E. C., and Freedman, P.   Dialysis—current status and future trends. *Heart Lung* 4:879, 1975.

35. Stahl, W. M., and Stone, A. M.   Effect of ethacrynic acid and furosemide on renal function in hypovolemia. *Ann. Surg.* 174:1, 1971.

36. Thomson, G. E.   Acute renal failure. *Med. Clin. North Am.* 57:6, 1973.

Renal Transplantation

Carolyn Rea Atkins

The advent of renal transplantation as an accepted mode of therapy for patients with end-stage renal disease (ESRD) opened up a new and challenging field of nursing concepts and care. The field is an ever changing one, and its many different facets are being explored.

The first renal transplant was performed by Varonay in 1936 [13], but renal transplantation as a tool for treating humans was essentially unexplored until 1956, when Merrill, Hume, and Murray successfully transplanted a kidney from one identical twin to another. Three years later, the same group did the first nontwin transplant [6].

Many difficulties have been encountered since those early days. The immunological problems (acute and chronic rejection) are the greatest threat to successful organ transplantation, and immunosuppression is perhaps the greatest threat to the patient's survival [6].

The refinements of renal transplantation have proceeded in three directions: (1) the development of more specific forms of immunosuppressive drugs and of their dosages, (2) the investigation and identification of more specific antigens that might permit better selection of donors and recipients [6], and (3) the development of techniques to preserve cadaver kidneys for longer periods of time [1].

33

Objective

This chapter aims to give an overview of renal transplantation and the nursing care needed by patients involved in renal transplantation.

Achieving the Objective

To develop an approach to nursing care of the patient involved in renal transplantation, the nurse should:

1. Be aware of the indications, implications, and immunological aspects of renal transplantation.
2. Know thoroughly the preoperative and postoperative care of the patient.
3. Understand the psychological impact on the patient, his family, and the hospital staff.

Because society is more mobile than it used to be and because a greater number of transplants will be performed, it is reasonable to assume that more nurses will come in contact with transplant patients and their families.

Case History

Ms. C. B., a 25-year-old white woman with chronic glomerulonephritis, had been undergoing chronic hemodialysis in a limited care dialysis center for 22 months. She was married, and she had a 3-year-old child. Shortly after she was placed on chronic hemodialysis, she was evaluated for a renal transplant and accepted as a transplant candidate. Unfortunately, Ms. B. had no family member who could be the kidney donor. She was an only child, and her parents were elderly and had numerous medical problems. Ms. B.'s name was put on a computer list of patients awaiting cadaver transplantation.

Ms. B.'s dialysis treatment was complicated by severe and refractory anemia that required intravenous iron therapy, intermittent packed cell transfusions, and anabolic steroids. The side effects of anabolic steroid therapy, hirsutism and a deepening of Ms. B.'s voice, began to cause her anxiety because of loss of body image. Her only other major problem was hypertension, which was controlled with apresoline and propranolol. At the time she was notified about the possible transplant, Ms. B. had resumed her former full-time job as a secretary.

Ms. B. was at home when the call came about the potential cadaver kidney. She was excited, but she managed to tell the calling physician that she did not have a recent febrile illness, skin infection, or cold—all conditions that would prevent her from undergoing surgery. She was told to report to the transplant unit as soon as she could without breaking the speed limit!

On Ms. B.'s arrival at the hospital, she underwent the usual hectic preoperative evaluation. It began with (1) an extensive explanation of the risks of transplantation (including death) and statistics on patient and graft survival, and (2) an explanation of the medications (azathioprine and prednisolone) needed to prevent rejection, including their side effects. Time was given to answer the questions Ms. B. and her family had.

It was also explained to Ms. B. that the transplant surgery would be cancelled if any abnormalities were uncovered by the laboratory work, chest x ray, ECG, or physical examination. If the results of those tests were negative, another test would be done—a crossmatch, which involved testing Ms. B.'s serum and the donor's lymphocytes for compatibility. If Ms. B.'s serum reacted against the donor's lymphocytes, it would indicate that her body would reject the kidney immediately. Ms. B. was told that the crossmatch would take about three hours to perform and that while it was being done, her workup for surgery would continue.

Ms. B. was anxious, a normal reaction for a potential kidney recipient, but she seemed willing to accept the challenge and risk of transplantation. Her family seemed to support her decision. (But in our experience, potential kidney recipients do not really listen to or fully understand the information given them during the evaluation because they are so eager to "get a transplant" and "get off dialysis." Thus it is extremely important to repeat the explanations throughout the evaluation period.)

After the initial discussion period, Ms. B. was admitted to the unit. She was weighed, and routine laboratory tests were done. Baseline cultures were obtained of her blood, nasal secretions, sputum, and urine. An ECG and chest x ray were made; they were normal. A voiding cystourethrogram (VCUG) was normal. Ms. B.'s physical examination was essentially normal; her blood pressure was 140/90 and her pulse was 70. She had no fever, and she said that she had not had a fever during the past month. Her chest and cardiac examinations were normal, and her extremities were free of edema. She had a functioning arteriovenous fistula in her left arm; it was free of infection.

After her physical examination, Ms. B. was given saline enemas until the return was clear, and then betadine scrub showers. Members of the transplant team were available to answer Ms. B.'s questions, repeat the explanations, and give reassurance and support.

After the preparations had been completed the operative procedure, patient and graft survival rates, and risks of transplantation were again explained to Ms. B. and her family. They were allowed time to ask questions and receive answers. Their decision remained to go ahead with the surgery as planned. The informed consent and operative forms were then signed and witnessed.

The medications needed to prolong the survival of the graft (azathioprine and prednisolone) were given to Ms. B. in a milligram per kilogram of body weight dosage. Then the results of the crossmatch were awaited. Ms. B. used the waiting period as a time of reflection. She knew from experience about hemodialysis, its problems and possible outcomes, but to enter the world of transplantation was to enter the unknown. She had been told that cadaver kidneys often do not begin to function immediately and that if hers did not she would undergo dialysis until the kidney began to function. She had also been told that she could have a severe rejection episode which could cause her to lose the kidney.

Finally, the waiting period was over—the crossmatch test was negative and she was on her way to surgery.

The surgery took about five hours. It was basically uneventful. In the recovery room, her blood pressure was measured at 200/110. There was only about 5 ml of urine in the urimeter. She was arousable and she asked whether the kidney was working. She was given a fluid challenge of 300 ml of normal saline solution in combination with intravenous furosemide (Lasix, 100 mg) to see whether the kidney would respond. During the next hour, the urinary output picked up briskly to 400 ml per hour. Fluid replacement therapy was instituted, using the following formula: fluids amounting to 75 percent of the previous hour's urinary output were given for the next hour in the ratio of two parts normal saline solution to one part 5% dextrose in water solution (200 ml of normal saline solution and 100 ml of a 5% dextrose in water solution). That schedule continued for the next 24 hours.

After an hour and a half, Ms. B. was transferred to the transplant unit, where she was to remain in reverse isolation for five days. The next 24 hours were busy ones for her. Her urinary output and fluid replacement measurements and her vital signs were checked hourly. She was turned, and she was encouraged to deep breathe and cough every two hours. It was not a restful night for her or her family, who stayed nearby in case they were needed.

Ms. B.'s serum creatinine level, which had been 14.2 mg per 100 ml preoperatively (normal is 0.5–1.2 mg/100 ml), fell over the next three days to 2.3 mg per 100 ml, and then slowly declined to 1.5 mg per 100 ml (by the fifth postoperative day). On the sixth postoperative day, Ms. B.'s creatinine level rose slightly (to 1.7 mg/100 ml), her urine protein excretion, blood pressure, and weight increased, and her temperature rose to 101°F. She had tenderness in the upper pole of the transplanted kidney. A Glofil-125 clearance test ([125I]) and a simultaneous creatinine clearance test showed a marked drop from the clearance values that had been determined on the day of surgery and on the third postoperative day (Fig. 33-1).

Rejection, "that feared word," was diagnosed. After cultures of her blood and wound were obtained Ms. B. was begun on acute rejection therapy consisting of the administration of 1 gm of intravenous methylprednisolone every other day for a total of 4 gm. After the initiation of rejection therapy, decreases were seen in her weight, proteinuria, and serum creatinine level over a period of eight days. Simultaneous Glofil-125 and creatinine clearance tests that were repeated nine days after the initiation of the rejection therapy showed an increase in values that indicated that the kidney had responded to therapy (Fig. 33-1).

Except for Ms. B.'s one rejection episode, her early hospital stay was uneventful medically. But it was a trying time emotionally. Laboratory tests were done every morning, and Ms. B. waited eagerly to find out her serum creatinine level. She continually wondered whether her urinary output was adequate. It was again pointed out to her that there was no "normal" urinary output for a transplant patient and that each patient reaches a level that is normal for him. As long as Ms. B.'s creatinine level was falling, everything was fine; she could tolerate almost anything. However, when the level began to rise, Ms. B.'s fear of losing the kidney grew and her ability to cope with even slight annoyances declined. The nurses reassured her by answering her numerous questions as honestly as possible while pointing out to her that not all patients had the same course and that the word *rejection* did not necessarily mean losing the kidney. When she was on dialysis, Ms. B. had heard stories from patients who had lost kidneys because of rejection and it was difficult for her to sort out facts from fiction.

Ms. B.'s discharge preparations were begun early in her hospital stay. She was taught the names, dosages, and side effects of her medications, as well as the signs and symptoms of rejection and what to do if they appeared. At home, she was to continue to weigh herself daily, measure her fluid intake and output, and monitor her temperature. She was given the telephone numbers of people she could call 24 hours a day if she had a question or otherwise needed help.

Sixteen days after the transplantation, Ms. B. was discharged from the hospital to be followed in the transplant clinic. Her wound had healed well and without any sign of infection, her blood pressure and her renal functioning were stable, and her anemia had begun to improve. Her discharge medications were:

Azathioprine:	125 mg	orally daily
Prednisolone:	95 mg	orally daily, decreasing by 5 mg per day
Ferrous sulfate:	300 mg	orally three times a day
Propranolol:	40 mg	orally three times a day
Furosemide:	40 mg	daily
Maalox:	30 ml	four times a day

Ms. B. made an appointment to visit the clinic three days after her discharge. During that visit she was found to have a purulent drainage from her wound, a 1.5 kg increase in weight, 2+ pitting edema of her lower legs extending from her knees to her ankles, and presacral edema. Her temperature was 99.6°F. Her laboratory values were normal, except

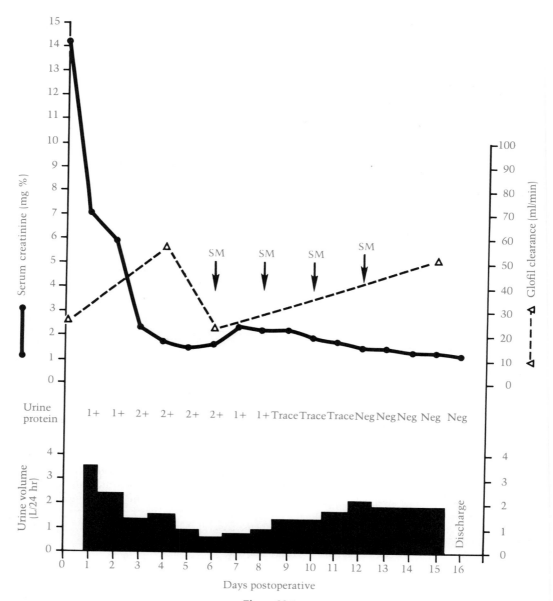

Figure 33-1

Initial postoperative functioning of a kidney after a kidney transplantation. Correlation of serum creatinine, Glofil (^{125}I) clearance, urine protein, and 24-hour urine output values with acute rejection. The arrows represent the treatment of a rejection episode with methylprednisolone (Solu-Medrol; *SM*) 1 gm intravenously, with subsequent response of renal function to therapy.

for her white blood cell count, which was 4×10^3 (normal is $5-10 \times 10^3$).

Second Admission

Ms. B. was readmitted to the hospital for drainage of a superficial wound abscess. After cultures were obtained, she was initially placed on intravenous methicillin (1 gm every six hours). After five days the medication was changed to cloxacillin (750 mg orally every six hours). Ms. B.'s fever disappeared after she had been on that regimen for four days. The intravenous pyelogram (IVP) and the abdominal sonogram results were negative for perinephric abscess.

Ms. B. was discharged in a week. Her medications at home were to be:

Azathioprine:	50 mg	orally daily (the dosage was decreased because her white blood cell count had dropped to 4.0
Prednisolone:	60 mg	orally daily, decreasing by 5 mg every other day to a level of 40 mg daily
Ferrous sulfate:	300 mg	three times a day
Propranolol:	40 mg	orally daily
Furosemide:	80 mg	orally daily
Cloxacillin:	500 mg	every six hours
Maalox:	30 ml	three times a day

Ms. B. was told to monitor her temperature closely. If she developed a fever of 99.6°F or higher, she was to notify the clinic or the transplant unit. She returned to the clinic the next day because her temperature was 100°F, but no other abnormalities were found. The wound was probed, but no purulent material was found. Three days later, she again returned to the clinic because she had a temperature of 101°F; she was readmitted to the hospital for an evaluation of her febrile illness.

Third Admission

Ms. B.'s admission physical examination was negative, except for a mild tenderness in the upper pole of the transplanted kidney. Her wound was healing, and it showed no evidence of infection. A repeat IVP and a sonogram were negative, as were the urine, blood, sputum, and wound cultures. Ms. B.'s cloxacillin therapy was discontinued on the second day of her admission. Her temperature continued to spike (to 102°F–103°F) for three days after her admission.

On the fourth day, there was an increase in Ms. B.'s serum creatinine level, proteinuria, blood pressure, and weight, along with a decrease in her urine output to less than 1000 ml per 24 hours. Simultaneous Glofil-125 and creatinine clearance tests were done; the results showed a 30 percent decrease in her renal function. Because of those findings, Ms.

B. was given methylprednisolone antirejection therapy (1 gm every other day for a total of 4 gm). Her oral prednisolone dosage was increased to 100 mg daily. The simultaneous Glofil-125 and creatinine clearance tests were repeated on the eleventh renal hospital day, after the end of therapy; the results showed that her renal function had returned to her previous high level of 65 ml per minute (Fig. 33-2).

Ms. B. was then discharged again on tapering doses of prednisolone and because her white blood cell count had returned to normal levels, she was again given her original dose of azathioprine (125 mg daily).

During the next week, Ms. B. came to the clinic every other day. She had a low-grade fever, but no clinical signs of infection or rejection. She was anxious about her condition: she thought that by this time she should be "normal."

Fourth Admission

Eight days after Ms. B.'s third hospitalization, she was again admitted to the hospital for evaluation of a temperature fluctuating between 99.8°F and 101°F. Multiple cultures of blood, urine, wound, and sputum were negative, as were a chest x ray, an IVP, a sonogram, an upper GI series, a small bowel series, and an oral cholecystogram. A spinal tap was done. It was normal; the fluid cultures were negative. Gallium scans that were done at 6, 24, and 48 hours to look for abscess formation were negative.

Serologic studies (to look for febrile agglutinins, mononucleosis, herpes zoster, herpes simplex, rubella, and cytomegalovirus [CMV]) were done. The studies were negative, except for the CMV titers, which showed a significant titer at a dilution of 1:32. (Ms. B.'s previous titers had been less than 1:8.) Ms. B. was discharged after two and one-half weeks; the probable diagnosis was that a CMV infection had caused her fever.

Ms. B. continued to do well after her last admission. She was seen in the transplant clinic once a week. At first, she called almost every day to ask a question or two, but actually she was seeking reassurance that she could handle being at home with the new transplant. Three months after the transplantation, she returned to work on a part-time basis and soon after on a full-time basis.

Five years later the nursing staff observed that Ms. B. was still anxious about her transplanted kidney. Her anxiety was apparent when she visited the clinic every three months. She was mildly hypertensive, had tachycardia, and was extremely apprehensive. The anxiety is typical of transplant recipients, who are afraid that something wrong will be found when they come to the clinic for their follow-up visits. When the clinic visit is over and they have been found to be well, they are visibly relieved.

Ms. B. no longer monitors her fluid intake and output closely, but she continues to weigh herself daily and she calls occasionally to ask a question or two about something that bothers her. Her long-term prognosis is good and she has returned to everyday life with all its inherent problems.

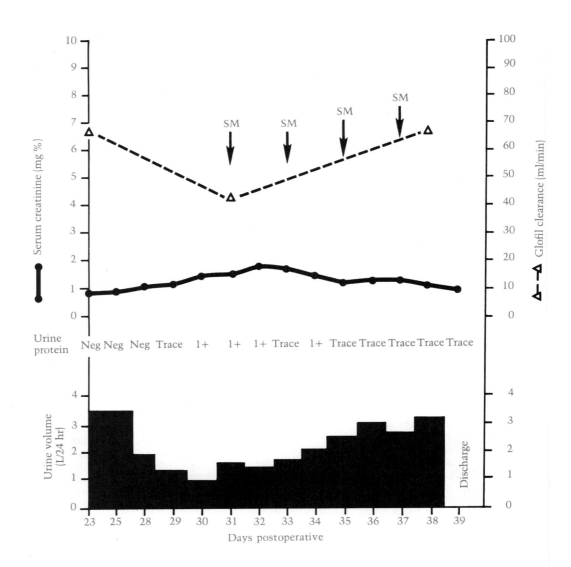

Figure 33-2
Third hospitalization. The treatment of a second rejection episode, with the same correlations as those shown in Figure 33-1.

Reflections

Transplant nursing is relatively new as a specialized area of nursing. It is challenging and changing, and it encompasses all phases of nursing and medicine. It combines surgery, medicine, psychology, public health, pediatrics, social work, and patient education.

In transplant nursing as in other types of nursing, one cannot simply take care of the needs of the diseased or transplanted organ. The disease entity—in this case, renal failure—truly affects the body-mind-spirit of the patient and of his family. Some disease processes are "curable"; renal failure is "controlla-

ble." It can be controlled by hemodialysis and/or renal transplantation, but neither mode of therapy offers an absolute, long-term cure.

The patient knows that, but he uses many types of denial to try to live a normal life. Many patients adjust well to the changes in life-style brought about by renal failure, but some do not. Some patients cannot adjust to being controlled by a machine (as in hemodialysis) or by medications (as in transplantation).

Both hemodialysis and transplantation have risks, but perhaps transplantation has the greater risks. Most patients, particularly younger patients, view dialysis as a form of prison from which they hope to escape. They do not realize that the escape (transplantation) will return them not to a paradise but to their former lives. After renal transplantation, there are still rules and regulations to observe, body changes to adjust to, and medical problems to replace the problems of dialysis. Some patients are surprised to find that they still have the same problems at home, work, and school and with their families that they had before renal failure.

In working with the patient who has had a transplant, the team must look at him as a whole, considering the outside pressures and influences on him. They should know, for example, that a patient may stop his medication because he develops cushingoid features, gains weight, and develops acne—or because he looks on medication as a sign of illness and he just does not want to be ill. It has been estimated that about 4 percent of patients stop their immunosuppressive medications for those reasons.

When a patient stops his medication, the staff's first reaction is anger. But despite their anger, the staff must continue to work with the patient. They must try to promote his self-esteem while they emphasize his need to continue the medication.

The patient who is a chronic complainer or questioner is asking for reassurance that he is doing the right thing and he is telling the staff that he is afraid. It is important to listen not only to what the patient and his family *are* saying but also to what they are *not* saying. Useful information can be obtained by that kind of listening.

The staff must be aware of their own feelings of happiness, anger, frustration, sympathy, friendship, and involvement if they are to help care for and rehabilitate the transplant recipient. They must be able to work out those feelings if they are to be objective and are to give "total patient" care.

Total patient care is what the nurse should give, regardless of her area of interest. The nurse should also be committed to her speciality. The better the nurse understands how body processes are affected by the underlying disease and its treatment, the better able she is to help the patient recognize and handle his problems. Also, the nurse should learn as much as possible about the patient and his ability to function under stress. That knowledge is acquired not in a short period of time, but through continued association with the patient.

The following discussion of renal transplantation aims to give the reader an insight into what the patient and his family undergo before and after transplantation.

Immunology

Through the work of Dausset, Van Rood, Amos, Terasaki, Payne, and others, the main human histocompatibility antigens (the HLA antigens) were identified [6]. For years, the typing of red blood cell antigens (the ABO system) made blood transfusions possible [4]. The antigens of the ABO system are important in organ transplantation also, and they must be matched. But human red blood cells do not carry the HLA antigens; therefore blood lymphocytes are used for HLA typing.

The HLA region is found on the sixth human chromosome. It is known to contain at least four genetic loci: HLA-A, B, C, and D. Each person inherits a set of those four HLA antigens (called a haplotype) from both parents (Fig. 33-3). In everyday practice, typing is frequently limited to HLA-A and HLA-B antigens, every person then having four antigens (although it is not always possible to identify each of the four). Because the antigens of the HLA region are inherited together, siblings who have the same HLA-A and HLA-B antigens usually also have the same HLA-D antigens [7].

A parent is always one haplotype identical with his child, but it is possible for the siblings each to inherit a different haplotype from each of the parents, and thus be a complete mismatch with each other (Fig. 33-3). For that reason, when a transplant candidate is being tissue typed, it is important for as many family members as possible to be typed so all the antigens can be clearly identified and the most suitable donor found [4, 6].

To date, about 30 HLA antigens have been identified with an estimated 10 percent left to be identified. There are 7000 to 8000 possible combinations of the known antigens. Also, the distribution of HLA antigens varies significantly among the Caucasian, Negro, and Oriental races [4, 6]. The field of immunology is constantly changing, resulting in discovery of new antigens and their influence on the outcome of graft survival.

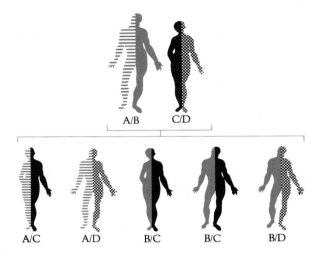

A/B   C/D

A/C   A/D   B/C   B/C   B/D

Figure 33-3
Interpretation of HLA matching antigens. How haplotypes are acquired from parents; how siblings are matched. (Courtesy of Pedro Stastny, M.D.)

Cytotoxic Antibodies

Because of the possibility that the transplant candidate may have developed serum cytotoxic antibodies against the donor's antigens (through prior exposure to leukocytes and platelets in blood transfusions, in a pregnancy, or in a previous renal transplant), a crossmatch test is done immediately before transplantation. The test is done by incubating the transplant candidate's serum with lymphocytes from the donor. If the donor lymphocytes are killed by the candidate's serum, it would indicate that the candidate has antibodies against that particular donor kidney, and performing the transplant could result in a hyperacute rejection of the transplanted kidney at the time of surgery. A positive crossmatch test is an absolute contraindication (the only one) to surgery [4].

In an attempt to make the crossmatch as sensitive as possible, serum samples are obtained from all potential transplant recipients every two months. An attempt is also made to collect serum samples approximately 7 to 10 days after a blood transfusion since this is the peak time of antibody formation. These serum samples are kept frozen until a kidney becomes available. At that time, *all* the sera are crossmatched (in addition to a freshly drawn one) with the donor lymphocytes. If *any* of the sera (no matter how long ago it was drawn and stored) is positive, it is a contraindication to proceeding with the transplant.

Recipient Selection

The patient being considered for renal transplantation involving a living, related donor or a cadaver usually has irreversible ESRD. Factors considered favorable in patient selection are (1) age of the recipient (it appears the most successful transplants occur in patients between the ages of 10 and 40 years [4]), (2) a normal lower urinary tract outflow, (3) the recipient's underlying renal disease, (4) the absence of any major associated diseases (coronary artery disease, malignancy, infection, and pulmonary obstructive disease), and (5) the absence of a peptic ulcer or a history of peptic ulcer [6].

The transplant candidate goes through a thorough evaluation to prepare him for transplantation. The evaluation includes laboratory tests, a complete review of the body systems, a VCUG, a psychological evaluation, and an immunological evaluation (Table 33-1). The advantages, disadvantages, risks, benefits, and survival rates of the patient and transplanted kidney are discussed with the patient and his family by his physician and members of the transplant team. The information is given to the patient gradually, after his condition has been stabilized by hemodialysis. The patient makes the decision for a transplant or for hemodialysis, or he may refuse both treatments and elect to die.

If, while the patient is undergoing the screening, an abnormality is found (e.g., a ureteral reflux as shown by the VCUG), additional surgery (e.g., a nephroureterectomy, removal of the kidney and ureter) should be done before the transplantation to avoid an infection from refluxing urine. There are other reasons for performing a nephroureterectomy before the transplantation surgery. They are: (1) the patient has uncontrolled hypertension, (2) the patient has an infection from pyelonephritis, polycystic kidneys, or stones, and (3) the patient's diseased kidneys may act as a potential pathogenic agent in the recurrence of the primary renal disease in the transplanted kidney [15].

When the preliminary evaluation is completed, the patient is ready for the transplantation.

Types of Transplants

There are two donor source of kidneys for transplantation. A relative may donate one of his kidneys, or if there is no suitable donor among the patient's rela-

Table 33-1
Evaluation of Candidate for Renal Transplantation

Tests	Reasons for Tests
Immunological tests	
ABO and HLA typing	To determine the patient's blood group and to identify his HLA antigens
Antibody screening	To determine the presence of cytotoxic antibodies and the percentage of reactivity, which allows one to predict with some accuracy whether the transplant recipient will ever be able to accept a kidney
History taking and physical examination	To determine the patient's past and present status. His past medical history is extremely important, especially any history of peptic ulcer disease or symptoms, cardiac disease, kidney stones, malignancy, and hypertension. The physical examination of a woman patient always includes a pelvic examination and a Pap smear
Psychological evaluation	To determine the patient's emotional maturity, motivation, cooperativeness, and ability to learn about his medications and to take instructions. To determine any underlying psychopathology. The information gathered enables the transplant team to know what support the patient and his family need.
Laboratory tests	
Complete blood count and platelet, partial thromboplastin time, and prothrombin time studies	To obtain baseline information
Liver function tests (total protein, albumin, globulin, total bilirubin, serum glutamic oxaloacetic transaminase, and alkaline phosphatase studies)	To screen for liver abnormalities, which would delay transplantation until further work was done to pinpoint the cause of the abnormalities (congestion due to fluid overload and acute or chronic hepatitis)
Australian antigen test	To screen for Australian antigen positivity, which would not necessarily rule out transplantation but would identify the patient as a carrier
Calcium, phosphorus, alkaline phosphatase studies	To evaluate hyperparathyroidism
Blood urea nitrogen and creatinine studies	To obtain baseline information
Electrolyte studies (of Na, K+, Cl, and CO_2)	To obtain baseline information
Fasting glucose test	To screen for an unsuspected tendency toward glucose intolerance (some patients develop steroid-induced diabetes after the transplant)
VDRL test	To screen for venereal disease
Amylase study	To screen for active pancreatitis
Renal evaluation	
Voiding cystourethrogram	To detect any ureteral reflux, urethral stricture, or bladder abnormality (inability to empty the bladder completely or a diverticulum). If any abnormality is present, corrective procedures are done prior to the transplantation
Kidney, ureter, bladder studies	To screen for kidney stones
Urine cultures	To screen for a urinary tract infection. If the patient has had a number of urinary tract infections, bilateral nephrectomy is done to eliminate a potential source of infection after the transplantation
Cystometrogram (CMG)	To evaluate the bladder's ability to empty completely. A CMG is not done routinely; it is done only if it is suspected that the patient has a neurogenic bladder (e.g., a diabetic patient) or if the patient has been shown by x ray to have residual urine
Cardiopulmonary evaluation	
ECG	To obtain a baseline tracing and to evaluate cardiac status
Evaluation for infection	To detect any infections (infections are the leading post-operative complication) and thus prevent doing a transplantation in someone who has an active infection
Fungal skin tests	
Viral titers	
Cultures of blood, sputum, nose, and skin	

tives, a cadaver kidney may be obtained. Nonrelated, living donor kidneys were used in the past. They are no longer used because: (1) statistically there is no difference in the survival of a cadaver kidney and a nonrelated, living donor kidney [15], (2) there is some risk to a person who donates the kidney, and (3) there are now improved ways to preserve cadaver kidneys until a suitable recipient can be found [4]. It is better to receive a kidney from a relative, because the patient and the graft survival rates are better than they are when a cadaver kidney is used [15].

Living Related Donor Kidneys

In living related donor transplantation, the recipient or some other family member asks the patient's family about donating a kidney. Initial ABO and HLA typing are done on the family members who are willing. The same categories apply to ABO compatibility in transplantation as in blood transfusions; that is, type AB is the universal recipient, and type O is the universal donor. (Crossing those blood barriers results in a hyperacute rejection of the kidney at the time of surgery.) A donor is then selected on the basis of the results of the ABO and HLA typing and his willingness to be a donor [15].

If the potential donor is willing and compatible, he must undergo an extensive evaluation. First, he is seen by the physician, who explains the short-term and long-term risks of kidney donation. The overall risk, including death, of donation in an otherwise healthy donor has been estimated at 0.05 percent [15], but the actual results are better than the risk indicates. The long-term risk has been estimated at 0.07 percent, which takes into account that the donor might lose his remaining kidney from trauma or cancer. The combined total risk to the donor is about 0.1 to 0.2 percent [6]. Risk aside, the donor experiences pain and anxiety, and he loses time from work and home during the evaluation and surgery.

A family member may be willing to donate a kidney for one or more of a number of reasons. He may feel that it is his duty to donate a kidney. He may feel guilty about the fact that his refusal might mean that the patient would die. He may wish to repay the patient for something the patient has done for him. Or he may wish to gain or regain his family's approval [4].

Whatever their reasons, most donors seem to make the decision to donate or not donate immediately.

The rewards the donor receives are his satisfaction in seeing the recipient improve and an increase in his self-esteem that is long lasting, even when the transplantation is not successful [5].

The nurse should be aware of the psychological aspects of donation. It is reasonable to think that a potential donor is or has been subjected to family pressures to donate or not to donate [16]. A sibling may be reluctant to donate because of past conflicts and rivalries with the candidate. Society expects a parent to donate a kidney to his child [4]. The potential donor must be told that if at any time during the evaluation he changes his mind, he should not go through with the donation. If the potential donor changes his mind, he can be "given" a medical reason that eliminates him as a donor. The potential donor can offer the medical reason to the family and thus, it is hoped, avoid family conflicts. If, during the evaluation, the members of the transplant team think that the potential donor is unstable or immature and so would not be able to withstand the pressures of donation, the physician will rule him unacceptable as a donor on medical grounds [6].

The donor should be evaluated in steps to minimize the time he loses from work and home. The least invasive procedures are done first; if everything is normal the evaluation culminates in a renal arteriogram, the most invasive procedure of the evaluation. At each step, the donor is in contact with a member of the team who can answer questions and explain how the evaluation progresses and why each test is important. If even a slight abnormality is found during the evaluation, the evaluation is stopped until the abnormality is corrected. (The donor evaluation is outlined in Table 33-2.)

After the evaluation is completed and after the potential donor has been repeatedly briefed about the risks for him and the chances of success for the recipient, he is asked to decide about donating and to give his informed consent in writing [5].

If a suitable family donor is not found, the recipient's name is placed on a computer list of people awaiting a cadaver kidney. Unfortunately, the wait for a cadaver kidney sometimes is long and often is frustrating for the patient.

Cadaver Donor Kidneys

Because most patients with renal failure do not have a suitable living, related donor, most transplant pro-

Table 33-2

Evaluation of a Living Related Donor

Tests	Reasons for Tests
ABO and HLA typing	To determine whether donor and recipient are compatible
History taking and physical examination	To make an extensive review of all systems: previous illnesses, past family history, previous surgeries. Any abnormalities found are investigated further before any invasive tests connected with donation are done
Laboratory tests	
Complete blood count and platelet, partial thromboplastin time, and prothrombin time studies	To assess the hematological system
Liver function tests (total protein, albumin, globulin, total bilirubin, serum glutamic oxaloacetic transaminase, and alkaline phosphatase studies)	To determine whether donor has a liver abnormality or dysfunction
Australian antigen test	To determine whether donor has a liver abnormality or dysfunction
Blood urea nitrogen and creatinine studies	Preliminary assessment of renal function
Electrolyte studies (of Na, K+, Cl, and CO_2)	To screen for abnormalities
Fasting glucose test	To screen for diabetes
VDRL test	To screen for venereal disease
Viral titers	To screen for active viral infections
Calcium, phosphorus, uric acid	To screen for abnormalities
Cardiopulmonary evaluation	
ECG	To determine the patient's cardiac status
Chest x ray	To determine the presence or absence of pulmonary disease and to evaluate cardiac status
Psychological evaluation	To assess the donor's motivation; to examine and evaluate the intensity of any family pressures on him to donate; to determine that the donation will not be detrimental to the donor; to give the donor an opportunity to express himself more fully than he might to the physician; to help the staff work with the donor and his family preoperatively and postoperatively
Renal function studies	
Routine urinalysis	To screen for renal disease or abnormal findings (glycosuria, proteinuria, and abnormal sediment) (microscopic examination should be done by the examining physician)
Urine culture	To determine the presence or absence of active urinary tract infection
Two 24-hour urinalyses for the assessment of the protein and creatinine levels	To assess the amount of protein excreted in a 24-hour period. If an abnormality is found, an orthostatic protein test is done. If those results are normal, the donor is considered to be normal in regard to protein. Urine creatinine levels are determined for clearance studies and to ensure that the 24-hour urine output is an adequate one
Timed Glofil-125 (^{125}I) and/or timed creatinine clearance study	To assess the actual renal function or the glomerular filtration rate
Intravenous pyelogram	To screen for renal abnormalities. To determine that the potential donor has two kidneys that are normal anatomically and in regard to their excretory function
Renal arteriogram	To determine the status of the donor's renal arteries and renal vasculature bilaterally. A small percentage of the population have multiple renal arteries. It is preferable to use a kidney that has only one renal artery. The arteriogram shows any renal lesions and any abnormalities of the vessels, such as stenosis or fibromuscular hyperplasia, which would rule out the person as a donor. The arteriogram is done last and only if the rest of the evaluation was normal (the arteriogram is the most invasive procedure, and it has a slight risk for the potential donor)

grams rely on the use of cadaver kidneys. It has been estimated that 15,000 kidneys are needed each year in the United States to treat patients with end-stage renal disease. If the kidneys of only 5 percent of the 60,000 people who die in automobile accidents and the 60,000 people who die in other accidents were donated, there would probably be enough kidneys for the patients waiting for them [2].

CADAVER DONOR SELECTION

Factors considered favorable in donor selection are: (1) a donor who is 2 to 65 years old, (2) the absence of a history of renal disease or diabetes, (3) the absence of a history of hypertension, (4) the absence of evidence of generalized infection, (5) the absence of a history of malignancy (except primary brain tumors, which do not metastasize), and (6) a donor who died in the hospital after having been under observation [2, 15].

The potential donor of a cadaver kidney is cared for by a physician who has no connection with the transplant team. The decision of when death occurs is a clinical one. It is made after a period of observation and it is based primarily on the clinical criteria of irreversible brain damage. Those criteria are: (1) the person has fixed and dilated pupils, (2) he is unresponsive to external stimuli, (3) he is unable to maintain his vital signs (heartbeat, blood pressure, respirations) without artificial support, (4) he has no corneal or pharyngeal reflexes, (5) he is unreactive to tracheal suctioning, (6) he has no deep reflexes or plantar reflexes, (7) he shows hypotonia, (8) his EEG is flat and (9) there is radiologic evidence that there is no blood flow to his brain [15, 16]. (The criteria may differ slightly in different transplant centers.)

Management of the potential cadaver donor has two aspects: (1) he is treated for his specific injury without regard for his status as a kidney donor and (2) after his brain death has been determined and permission has been obtained from his family, his treatment is directed toward maintaining adequate renal function [2].

When a potential donor of a cadaver kidney becomes available, he is typed for ABO and HLA antigens. The criteria for an acceptable antigen match are different in different transplant centers. Some centers use only kidneys of donors whose antigens closely match the recipient's antigens (three out of four or better), while other centers use ABO typing only (and thus unmatched grafts).

Cadaver kidneys are "shared" among transplant centers. That is, if when a kidney becomes available the center does not have a suitable recipient, the kidney is sent to a center that does have a suitable recipient. New methods of storing kidneys have made the sharing program possible.

Preservation of Cadaver Kidneys

Two methods are used to preserve cadaver kidneys: (1) simple hypothermic storage and (2) continuous pulsatile perfusion [1].

In simple hypothermic storage, after nephrectomy the kidneys are flushed out with a cooling solution, then placed in a cold solution in a sterile environment, and kept there at 2°C to 4°C until they are needed for transplantation. That type of storage is relatively inexpensive and simple. Its disadvantage is that the kidneys cannot usually be kept for a long period of time [1].

Continuous pulsatile perfusion machines have been in use since 1967. They provide continuous perfusion of the kidney with a perfusate that contains albumin and lipids as well as keep them cold and oxygenated. After nephrectomy, the kidneys are flushed with a cooling solution, the renal artery of each kidney is cannulated, and the kidney is attached to the machine. The method allows more time for doing necessary tests and for finding a suitable recipient, and it thus makes cadaver transplantation a semielective procedure [1].

The second advantage of continuous pulsatile perfusion is that the viability of the kidney can be tested while it is being perfused. Flow rates through the cannulated renal artery of the kidney, as well as the diastolic pressure, can be measured. Low flow rates (less than 100 ml/min) and an elevated diastolic pressure indicate vasospasm in the kidney. Pulsatile perfusion characteristics, as well as the information obtained about the medical treatment and care of the donor, are used as indicators of the viability of the kidney. The disadvantage of continuous pulsatile perfusion is the cost of the machine and of the people to operate it [1].

Many studies have been done to determine the advantage of one method over another. In the simple hypothermic method, different solutions have been used to store the kidneys, with varying results [12]. Studies are also being done of methods, such as freezing of the kidney [1], that permit longer storage periods.

The donor kidney, regardless of its source, has to be helped to survive in its new environment. In all transplant recipients, except identical twins, the help takes the form of immunosuppressive drugs.

Immunosuppression

It is well known that the body recognizes a foreign substance and produces antibodies to fight it. Immunosuppressive therapy in renal transplantation involves the use of a number of methods to block or decrease the intensity of the body's immune response to the graft. Most transplant centers use a combination of agents, but the two drugs that most if not all transplant recipients must take for the life of the graft are azathioprine and a steroid (prednisolone or prednisone). Azathioprine and steroids came into general use as immunosuppressive drugs for humans in 1962 [4], and now they are generally utilized as the standard immunosuppressive drugs [15].

Azathioprine

Azathioprine (Imuran) and its products of metabolism depress the production of antibodies against the transplanted organ by interfering with the proliferation of leukocytes. The drug is rapidly absorbed; a significant amount of it appears in the blood within 15 minutes of its oral administration [4, 6]. It is eliminated in the urine and, by metabolic degradation, in the liver [20]. Because it is excreted in the urine, there are differing opinions as to whether the drug should be discontinued or its dosage decreased in the presence of anuria [6, 15, 20].

The dosage of azathioprine is different in different transplant centers; usually it is about 2 to 5 mg per kilogram of body weight. However, most patients can only tolerate a dosage of 2 mg per kilogram. It is usually given orally, but it can be given intravenously if the patient cannot tolerate oral fluids.

The most common toxic side effect of azathioprine is bone marrow depression resulting in leukopenia. When the white blood cell count falls below 3000, the dosage is decreased or discontinued until an upward trend in the white blood cell count is seen. The dosage level at which bone marrow depression occurs

varies from patient to patient and it seems to be independent of the patient's size and weight. When the correct dosage is established for a particular patient, he generally remains on it for the life of the graft. Other side effects of azathioprine are liver disease, nausea, stomatitis, skin rash, and an increase in the incidence of malignant diseases, especially lymphoreticular tumors [4, 20].

Steroids

Corticosteroids (prednisone, prednisolone, and methylprednisolone) are almost always used in conjunction with azathioprine to potentiate the immunosuppressive effects [6]. Steroids have a number of effects on the body's immunological and inflammatory systems. Even though the exact mechanisms by which they exert their immunological effects are poorly understood, it is thought that they have a major inhibitory effect on inflammation and on the influx of granulocytes and (perhaps) other cells into the transplanted organ [20]. Steroids also have the following effects in the immune process: lympholytic effects, general inhibitory effects on protein synthesis, and effects on phagocytosis and complement activity, as well as a stabilizing effect on lysosomes when sensitized lymphocytes make contact with the target tissue [14, 20].

The clinical use of steroids varies. Most transplant centers use steroids prophylactically, beginning a few days before the transplantation. However, some transplant centers do not use steroid therapy until the onset of a rejection episode [15]. The initial dose of oral prednisone also varies from center to center; e.g., 60 mg daily at one center or 2 mg per kilogram of body weight at another. The initial high oral dose is tapered rapidly in the two weeks after the transplantation and then more slowly until the patient reaches a daily maintenance dose of 0.25 mg to 0.5 mg per kilogram of body weight [6]. For example, a person who weighs 70 kg would take 17 mg of prednisone daily as a maintenance dose. The oral dose is usually increased at the onset of a new rejection episode.

The side effects of long-term steroid therapy are numerous. They include cushingoid changes (acne, purpura, striae, hirsutism, and changes in the fat distribution), an increased incidence of peptic ulcers, psychosis, hyperglycemia, impaired wound healing, cataracts, aseptic necrosis of the head of the femur, a predisposition to infections [20], obesity, pancreatitis, and arrested bone growth (in children).

Antilymphocyte Globulin

Antilymphocyte globulin (ALG) was first used in humans by Starzel in 1966, when he became disillusioned with graft survival when only azathioprine and prednisone were used [15]. Today, ALG is used in conjunction with the main immunosuppressive drugs in the transplant centers that manufacture it.

ALG is manufactured by injecting lymphocytes or purer cell forms from human lymph nodes and thoracic duct, spleen, thymus, and human cells in tissue culture into horses, rabbits, goats, and other animals. There are always a number of variables in the production of ALG because presently each center that uses it manufactures its own. Among the variables are (1) the number of lymphocyte cells obtained, (2) the number and frequency of injections in the animal, (3) the time interval between the injection and the harvesting of antibodies from the injected animal, and (4) the animal's response to the antigenic stimulus.

Because the methods of production are unstandardized and the assay for potency is unsatisfactory, how ALG works in humans as an immunosuppressive agent is not clearly understood [20]. It is generally thought that intravenous ALG acts on thymus-derived recirculating lymphocytes by adsorbing to and coating the outside of the lymphocytes in the circulating pool. Complement is then fixed by the antibody, resulting in cell lysis and phagocytosis by the reticuloendothelial system, especially the liver [20]. The thymus-derived lymphocytes are thought to be vulnerable to ALG because of (1) their rapid recirculation, which exposes them to ALG in the circulating blood and (2) their sensitivity to ALG and other immunosuppressive drugs [6].

ALG can be given intramuscularly, but it is usually given intravenously. The dosage, frequency, and number of treatments given vary among the transplant centers that use it. It is administered to the recipient of a living, related donor kidney from several days to two weeks before the transplantation, and it may be continued for up to three months following surgery. In cadaver kidney transplantations, the initial doses are usually higher since one must move quickly when a cadaver kidney becomes available. The dosage of ALG is usually calculated in terms of mg of ALG per kilogram of body weight [15].

Like all immunosuppressive drugs, ALG has adverse side effects. They include a local reaction (pain, swelling, erythema, and induration) when given intramuscularly, a febrile reaction, severe thrombocytopenia and anemia, an anaphylactic reaction, and (probably) a slight increase in the number of fungal, viral, and protozoan infections [9].

Local Graft Irradiation

Local graft irradiation is also used in conjunction with other immunosuppressive agents. It may prolong graft survival in some cases although there is not conclusive evidence that it does. Low doses of radiation destroy the thymus-derived lymphocytes (T-lymphocytes), which are responsible for cell-mediated reaction on the graft. Irradiation also acts as an anti-inflammatory agent by indirectly slowing leukocyte migration and thus allowing fewer cells to reach the graft [20].

Irradiation is used either immediately after surgery or at the onset of a rejection episode. The dosage is 100 to 150 rads per treatment every other day, for a total of 600 to 800 rads per series. If needed, the procedure may be repeated later, for a combined total dose of 1500 rads. Radiation doses below 1500 rads may produce functional changes in the kidney, but the disease known as radiation nephritis does not occur at that level [20].

Although there is no conclusive evidence that local irradiation of the graft reduces the number or the severity of rejection episodes, irradiation seems to be the only immunosuppressive agent that presents a low risk to the patient and his kidney [20].

Rejection

As discussed, immunosuppressive agents are used in renal transplantation to prevent rejection and thus prolong the life of the graft. The body's immune system is able to recognize foreign substances (antigens), to isolate them, and by producing antibodies to destroy them in preparation for their removal by other cells [4]. When immunologically competent cells recognize a foreign antigen, they enlarge, multiply, and produce sensitized lymphocytes (involving thymus-dependent cells or T-lymphocytes)—this is called *cell-mediated immune response*. Those immunologically competent cells also produce specific antibody-secreting plasma cells developed in the lymph nodes and the spleen (B-lymphocytes) in a process called *humoral immune response*. These two types of immune responses work together to attack and destroy any foreign substance or graft, including a transplanted organ if it is untreated [4, 10].

In all transplants, except those between patients whose antigenic makeup is identical (identical twins), the immune response is aimed at rejecting the newly transplanted kidney (or other organ). The rejection process has three different stages of intensity: hyperacute, acute, and chronic.

Hyperacute Rejection

Hyperacute rejection can occur at the time blood flow to the transplanted kidney is established or up to several hours after the surgery is completed. Hyperacute rejection is usually caused by preformed circulating antibodies that attack the new graft violently. Because of its time of onset it is a humoral response. Hyperacute rejection also occurs when there is an ABO incompatibility between the donor and the recipient. There is no treatment for that type of rejection, and the kidney must be removed as soon as the diagnosis is made. On microscopic examination, leukocytes are seen in the glomerular capillaries, and intravascular renal thrombosis is present [15, 20].

Acute Rejection

Acute rejection may occur soon after or long after the transplantation. An acute rejection episode that occurs in the early postoperative period (two days to two weeks after the operation) is primarily a cellular immune response, while an acute rejection that occurs later is a combination of a humoral immune response and a cellular immune response. Treatment of an acute rejection consists of the administration of high-dose steroids either orally (up to 300 mg daily) or intravenously (1–3 gm of methylprednisolone daily or on alternate days). In some transplant centers, a combination of high-dose oral prednisone and intravenous methylprednisolone is used daily. That dose continues from 5 to 10 days, or until renal function has stabilized or improved. Recovery from an acute rejection episode usually occurs in a week to 10 days. If there is no response to treatment, the daily dose is slowly tapered to maintenance levels, and the pa-

Table 33-3
The Signs and Symptoms of Acute Rejection

Clinical signs
  Fever (without an accompanying infection)
  Weight gain (more than two pounds in a 24-hour period)
  Malaise
  Enlargement of the graft with upper pole tenderness
  Hypertension
  Decreased urinary output
  Edema, especially periorbital edema and edema of the legs
  Anorexia
Laboratory signs
  Leukocytosis (may also be due to high-dose steroids or to infection)
  Increased blood urea nitrogen levels
  Increased serum creatinine levels
  Increased proteinuria
  Decreased Glofil-125 and/or creatinine clearance values
  Decreased urine sodium level
Radiological evidence
  An enlarged kidney (as shown by a comparison of a flat-plate x ray of the abdomen with one done earlier)
  A renal scan may show poor flow through the kidney due to edema
  A sulfur colloid study may show a positive uptake of sulfur colloid in the transplanted kidney
  An arteriogram may show vessel changes, with irregularity and loss of smaller vessels, a prolonged circulation time, and a poor nephrogram

tient's renal function is watched closely for any further deterioration. The treatment of acute rejection varies considerably from center to center and from patient to patient [20].

Functional changes induced by acute rejection seem to be reversible in many cases, making the prompt recognition and treatment of each rejection episode important. If acute rejection goes untreated for a long time, severe and irreversible renal damage occurs [15]. (The signs and symptoms of acute rejection are listed in Table 33-3.)

Chronic Rejection

Chronic rejection is the most difficult type of rejection to diagnose because it has few clinical signs and symptoms. The laboratory values may show a gradual decline in the patient's renal function over a period of months that often is noticed only when the patient returns for a routine follow-up appointment. Usually a course of treatment like that used for acute rejection is tried. If there is no response, the patient is kept on

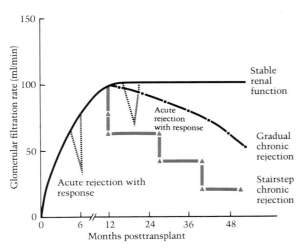

Figure 33-4
Stages of chronic rejection. The different pathways chronic rejection may take: gradual and stairstep.

his maintenance dose of immunosuppressive drugs until his renal function deteriorates further. When the deterioration occurs, it must be decided when to bring the attempts to save the kidney to a halt. At the same time, a long-range plan about a return to dialysis and a future transplantation is discussed with the patient. As long as the patient's condition is stable and he shows no signs or symptoms of uremia and has adequate renal function, the kidney is not removed [20]. Chronic rejection occurs over an indefinite period of time, and it can occur gradually or in a stairstep fashion (Fig. 33-4).

Surgical Considerations

Donor Surgery

In renal transplantation, it is preferable to use the left kidney of a living, related donor because the renal vein is normally longer on the left side. Careful dissection of the renal artery, vein, and ureter is carried out through a flank incision. It is extremely important that the ureter not be stripped clean because it derives its blood supply from the perinephric fat. To prevent clotting within the kidney, systemic heparin is given before the kidney is removed. The heparin is counteracted systemically after the kidney has been removed by giving the patient protamine. Close observation is made of the patient's vital signs, urine

output, and fluid status during the procedure and afterward to maintain an adequate urine output and to prevent damage to the remaining kidney [15].

In the immediate postoperative period, there may be a transient rise in blood pressure and a transient fall in creatinine clearance with subsequent small rise in the blood urea nitrogen and serum creatinine levels. These phenomena abate after several days with the creatinine clearance returning to 70 percent of the predonation levels, where it remains. The compensatory response occurs rapidly in renal donors. Long-term follow-up studies show that the donor's health and life expectancy are not affected by the donation [15].

As soon as the kidney is removed from the donor, it is put in a sterile basin that contains iced Ringer's lactate solution with procaine to ease intrarenal vessel spasm and heparin to prevent small thrombi from forming. The solution not only cools the kidney rapidly, preventing damage from warm ischemia, but it is also used to remove blood from the kidney. The kidney is flushed with the iced solution until the fluid coming from the renal vein is clear. The kidney is kept in the iced solution until it is ready to be placed in the recipient [15].

Recipient Surgery

While the kidney is being removed from the donor, a team in an adjoining operating room is preparing the recipient. The donor kidney is usually placed in the recipient's right iliac fossa (Fig. 33-5). That site is used because the right common iliac artery and external iliac veins are more superficial—and therefore more accessible—than are those on the left side. However, the left iliac fossa can be used if the right iliac fossa was used in a previous operation [15].

The renal artery of the donor kidney is generally anastomosed end to end to the recipient's hypogastric artery. The donor renal vein is anastomosed end to side, using the recipient's external iliac vein. Usually urine can be seen coming from the ureter a few minutes after the vascular clamps have been released. It is important that the recipient not become hypovolemic at that point because hypovolemia interferes with kidney perfusion and the resumption of renal function [15].

There are several ways to restore the continuity of the upper urinary tract. The most common way is to make a tunnel incision through the trigone area of the

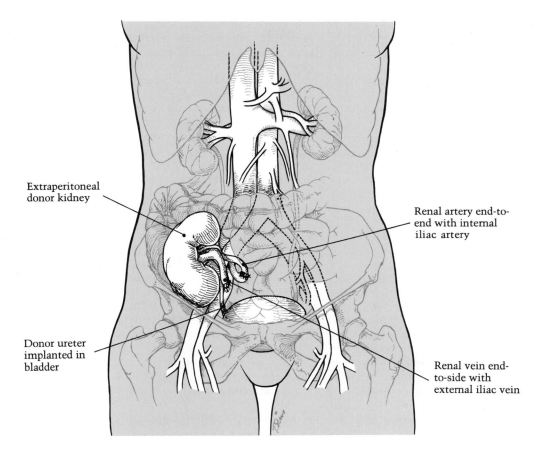

Extraperitoneal
donor kidney

Renal artery end-to-
end with internal
iliac artery

Donor ureter
implanted in
bladder

Renal vein end-
to-side with
external iliac vein

Figure 33-5
Anatomical placement of the transplanted kidney. The placement of the transplanted kidney in relationship to the other organs.

bladder and insert a catheter through the tunnel and then through the lateroposterior bladder wall. The ureter is pulled through the tunnel tract and sutured to the mucosal wall. The bladder is closed. A Foley catheter is kept in the bladder to facilitate urinary drainage and to keep the bladder decompressed, thereby reducing the incidence of urinary leaks from the ureteral anastomosis [15]. In our experience the catheter has been removed after 24 hours with no increase in leakage and with fewer urinary tract infections.

Because the iliac fossa seems to be ideally formed to receive a kidney, it is not necessary to suture the new kidney in place unless the blood flow appears to be obstructed due to kinking of the vessels [15]. In most transplant centers, metal clips are placed on the upper and lower poles of the kidney as well as along the medial aspect of the kidney. Those clips help to determine the size and location of the kidney by x ray.

Physiology of the Transplanted Kidney

In almost all recipients of living, related donor kidneys and in some recipients of cadaver kidneys, the urinary output begins immediately and is of high volume. The urinary output can reach a volume of 5 to 10 ml per minute during the first hours and then (depending on the patient's fluid intake) gradually return to a normal volume in 48 to 72 hours. The electrolyte levels in the initial urine are abnormal: the sodium level is high (100–125 mEq/L), the chloride level is low (49–100 mEq/L), and the potassium level is significant (14–27 mEq/L), as is the urine osmolality (the average is 352 mOsmol/L) [6].

The phenomenon of postoperative polyuria probably represents osmotic diuresis in association with a diminished resorption in the proximal tubules. The driving force of this diuresis can be attributed to the following: (1) the recipient's serum is hyperosmolar because of the increase in blood urea and other substances, (2) there is some degree of salt and water retention despite adequate hemodialysis, and (3) lesions that affect tubular resorption may be caused by the ischemia resulting from cooling of the kidney at the time of the transplant [6].

Close attention must be paid to the fluid and electrolyte balance in the immediate postoperative period to avoid the complications of dehydration and/or hypokalemia. Enough fluids should be given to prevent dehydration but not enough to prolong the polyuric phase. Usually replacement fluids consist of half normal saline solution and 5% dextrose and water solution. The proportion of each solution the patient receives differs from center to center. If urinary output is 200 ml per hour or less, replacement is usually 100 percent, but if the output exceeds 200 ml per hour, replacement therapy is reduced to a percentage of the previous hour's output. The immediate reestablishment of renal function and the polyuria often result in the lowering of the blood urea nitrogen and serum creatinine levels to nearly normal by the third postoperative day [6].

Proteinuria is also often present in the immediate postoperative period. It is due to hematuria and/or ischemic changes in the renal tubules. In most cases, the proteinuria diminishes or disappears within a few days. A reappearance signifies that a different process is occurring [6], such as rejection, recurrent disease, or renal vein thrombosis.

Complications

Receiving a renal transplant does not signify the end of the patient's problems. Instead, the transplantation can and usually does produce many more problems. Some patients are fortunate in that they have few if any short-term or long-term complications of the transplant, but most patients are not so fortunate. Rejection, the most frequent complication, has been discussed. The other complications are discussed in the following pages.

Infection is the leading cause of death in all transplant recipients. Infection poses a great threat in the immediate postoperative period (when bacterial organisms are the most common causes of infection) and also in the long run (when fungal and viral organisms are the most common causes of infection). The reason is that the patient must continue to take immunosuppressive drugs to prevent rejection. That immunosuppression of defense mechanisms makes him the perfect target for opportunistic organisms [20].

Several defects that are known to be present in the immunosuppressed patient allow infections to become lethal. The defects are [20]:

1. Alteration of local (skin and mucosal) defenses. Postoperative hematomas, foreign objects, and obstruction of normal drainage tracts combine to offer a significant risk factor in the immediate postoperative period. Long-term high-dose steroid therapy impairs wound healing and collagen synthesis and enhances skin breakdown.
2. Alteration of the acute inflammatory system. To deal with pathogenic organisms, normal granulocytes, which have phagocytic and bactericidal activities, must migrate to the infected area. The normal migration is altered by steroids and azathioprine.
3. Alterations of cellular immunity. Steroids cause depression of the cellular immune response. The depression either enhances the cell's susceptibility to intracellular pathogens or it activates latent viral infections. These types of infections are usually more common after treatment of an acute rejection episode with high-dose steroids.
4. Alteration of the humoral immune response. The immunosuppressive agents combine to depress the formation of antibodies in response to antigens. The depression in antibody formation increases the incidence and the severity of bacterial infections.

The occurrence of other complications can usually be divided into: (1) the immediate postoperative period (they are usually surgical complications), (2) 5 to 30 days postoperatively, and (3) long term.

The Immediate Postoperative Period

In the immediate postoperative period, different processes may adversely affect the transplanted kidney.

Table 33-4
Causes of Postoperative Oliguria and Anuria

Causes	Observations
Prerenal causes	
Hypovolemia	Assure adequate volume expansion by monitoring pulse, blood pressure, and skin turgor
Poor cardiac status	Assess cardiac status, observe for congestive failure, and institute appropriate treatment
Renal artery lesion	Monitor blood pressure; observe for sudden pain in the abdomen, a bruit, an increase in blood pressure, and a decrease in urinary output
Renal causes	
Rejection	Small volumes of urine are obtained that have a low sodium content and a high osmolality. An increase in blood pressure and pain around the upper pole of the graft caused by the size increase are noted
Acute tubular necrosis (ATN)	ATN results in small quantities of urine that have a high sodium content. Review the data about the condition of the donor before his kidney was removed. Difficulty with the arterial anastomosis at the time of surgery can also contribute to ATN
Postrenal causes	
Catheter obstruction	Check the catheter for patency, kinking, and clots. Gently irrigate the catheter if necessary
Ureteral leak	A sudden increase of fluid from the drain site, a feeling of fullness in the abdomen
Ureteral obstruction	If the urine is extremely bloody and contains many clots, the ureter may be obstructed by clots
Renal vein obstruction	The graft will become larger; massive proteinuria is present; venograms are essential to the diagnosis

Everyone involved is happy when urine is seen to move steadily through the catheter and closed drainage system. But early oliguria and anuria can occur. They can be caused by many different factors, each of which must be checked out systematically (Table 33-4). Those factors are:

1. Obstruction of the urinary flow. The catheter should be checked for patency. Something as simple as a kink in the catheter or tubing can obstruct the flow of urine. If the urine is bloody and contains clots, the catheter needs to be irrigated gently, using sterile technique. A bigger catheter may be needed. If clots have caused the decrease in urinary flow, the urinary output should increase 10 to 15 minutes after the catheter has been irrigated [15].

2. Hypovolemia. Hypovolemia may be due to blood loss during surgery or postoperatively. Serial decreasing hematocrit levels, displacement of intraperitoneal organs (shown by abdominal x ray), and a graft that cannot be palpated suggest a hematoma. Or the patient may simply need more fluids. If he does, a bolus of intravenous fluids will increase his urinary output [15].

3. Thrombosis or stenosis of the renal artery or the renal vein. Complete thrombosis of the renal artery, a rare condition, is usually seen in patients who have atherosclerotic disease involving the iliac vessels. Partial obstruction of the renal artery can occur from torsion or kinking of the vessels. The best diagnostic sign is a sudden decrease in urinary output that (often) is associated with an increase in blood pressure. The only accurate diagnostic approach is a renal flow scan followed by a renal arteriogram, which would demonstrate an arterial stricture or occlusion. If an occlusion or a significant stricture is present, the patient is returned immediately to surgery for corrective procedures [15].

Venous occlusion is an even rarer occurrence in the immediate postoperative period, but a partial venous thrombosis can occur later in the course of the transplant. If a venous thrombosis is suggested by the arteriogram, venography should be done [15].

4. Acute tubular necrosis. Acute tubular necrosis (ATN) is rare in transplants of living, related donor kidneys because the ischemia time of the kidney is not prolonged. ATN is seen more often in cadaver transplants, in which both the warm and cold ischemia times are prolonged. Also, the donor may have been hypotensive for a period of time before the nephrectomy, resulting in hypoperfusion of the kidneys. When ATN occurs, intermittent hemodialysis is required until the kidney function returns. Hemodialysis at this stage can lead to other complications, such as hypovolemia or a hematoma in the wound caused by the use of heparin. The hematoma may become infected and cause serious problems [2].

5. Ureteral leaks. At one time ureteral leaks were the

most common complication of renal transplantation. The leaks are due to distal ureteral necrosis from ischemia. The most common cause of the ischemia is the stripping of the perihilar and periureteral fat, which disturbs the blood supply of the ureter [2]. It is less common in surgical procedures in which a ureteronecocystostomy (a tunneling of the ureter into the bladder) is used rather than a ureteroureterostomy (anastomosis of the transplanted ureter into the patient's ureter) or a pyeloureterostomy (anastomosis of the patient's ureter into the pelvis of the transplanted kidney). The leak can usually be seen readily on an IVP. Even though ureteral leaks usually occur in the first week after the transplant, cases have been reported to occur more than one month after the transplant [2, 15].

The leak must be treated immediately. It is a potentially serious complication that could lead to infection and even death. Depending on the location and size of the leak, surgery may be necessary, with reimplantation of the ureter into the bladder; nephrostomy, or pyleoureterostomy to the host ureter, may be required. Rarely, necrosis of the ureter extends into the pelvis of the kidney resulting in nephrectomy of the transplanted kidney [15]. If the leak is small, a urethral (Foley) catheter can be inserted to provide adequate drainage until the site is healed, and thereby to avoid surgical intervention. However, use of the catheter can be associated with a significant increase in infections.

The Postoperative Period

The obvious postoperative complications of kidney transplantations (and of all types of surgery) are pneumonia and wound infections. Scrupulous pulmonary hygiene is mandatory after the transplantation to prevent atelectasis and pneumonia. Strict aseptic techniques are observed in changing dressings and giving wound care to decrease the incidence of wound infections and cross contamination of patients.

Bacterial infections that end in septicemia have a high mortality among people who have had organ transplants. The infections seem to occur more often in recipients of cadaver kidneys than in recipients of a living related donor kidney, perhaps because the recipient of a cadaver kidney has been on hemodialysis longer and has had more complications. Recipients of

cadaver kidneys also seem to have more episodes of rejection and ATN and so receive higher doses of steroids for longer periods of time.

Infections around the graft usually are manifested within a month after the transplantation, but in some rare cases they are dormant for several months. The use of prophylactic antibiotics just before and during surgery seems to decrease the incidence of wound infections after the transplantation [20].

Bacterial infections of the central nervous system occur infrequently. Often they are masked in their early stages by the anti-inflammatory actions of the steroids. The mortality among patients with central nervous system involvement is high [20].

Some workers find gram-negative organisms the most common cause of bacterial infections (in 75% of cases), with *Pseudomonas* infections being the most common; but we have found *Escherichia coli* infections to be the most common ones. The most common gram-positive organism is *Staphylococcus* (in 10–15% of cases); it is usually found in A-V fistulas, shunts, and wounds [20].

The most common site of infection is the urinary tract, and urinary tract infections have the lowest mortality. A urological workup is done to rule out an anatomical cause (e.g., reflux or partial obstruction), and the patient is taught double voiding and good personal hygiene in an effort to eliminate the sources of infection. If urinary tract infections recur often, the patient is placed on long-term immunosuppressive therapy, which seems to have no adverse side effects [20].

Pulmonary infections are the second most common infection, and they have a high mortality. Pulmonary infections may be fungal or viral, alone or combined with bacterial organisms. Since bacterial organisms are easily cultured from the sputum, it is the one treated with antimicrobial therapy. But it may not be the causative organism, since fungal and protozoan organisms are not easily cultured from the sputum and tracheal aspirates. If no response to treatment is shown clinically or by serial chest x rays, it may be necessary to obtain a tissue diagnosis by a brush biopsy, a needle biopsy, or an open biopsy of the lung [15, 20].

About 20 percent of pulmonary infections that occur in people who have undergone transplantation are due to fungi, *Nocardia*, and *Mycobacterium*. *Candida* infections are the most common fungal infections. The causative organism is usually found in the urinary tract and oral cavity, and it disseminates to the esophagus and lungs. When dissemination occurs, systemic antifungal therapy is required in addition to topical therapy [20].

Long-Term Complications

All the complications of long-term renal transplantation stem from the patient's state of immunosuppression and from the use of immunosuppressive drugs (Table 33-5).

CUSHING'S DISEASE

The most visible complication of renal transplantation is Cushing's disease, which results from the use of high-dose steroids. The severity of the disease depends on the daily dose of steroids and the number of rejection episodes the patient has had. The visual changes in the patient's body include [15]:

1. A round, puffy face.
2. Redistribution of the body fat from the extremities to the trunk and face.
3. Acne over the face, arms, and trunk.
4. An increase in the growth of hair on the face, arms, and trunk.
5. Changes in the skin texture (caused by the breakdown of protein and the diversion of amino acids) that result in thinning, striae, and bruises.

STEROID-INDUCED DIABETES

Steroid-induced diabetes is said to be a result of long-term steroid therapy [15], but we have found the onset to occur within one to two months after the transplantation. Even though steroid-induced diabetes is not reported to be a frequent complication, its onset is insidious; often the patient presents in a diabetic acidosis state without having shown any signs or having had a history of diabetes. Steroid-induced diabetes is usually mild and easily controlled, although some patients may require insulin rather than oral agents.

OCULAR COMPLICATIONS

The most common ocular complication of transplantation is cataracts, which occur as a result of the steroid therapy, and (apparently) regardless of the dose. The problems are minimal, but the cataracts do mean

Table 33-5
Long-term Complications of Renal Transplantation

Pulmonary complications
  Embolism
  Fungal infection
  Viral infection
Gastrointestinal complications
  Gastric ulcer
  Pancreatitis
  Hepatitis
  Esophageal varices
Hematological complications
  Leukopenia
  Polycythemia
Musculoskeletal complications
  Hyperparathyroidism
  Avascular (aseptic) necrosis of the bone
  Osteoporosis
Endocrine complications
  Cushing's disease
  Steroid-induced diabetes mellitus
Neurological complications
  Stroke
  Fungal and viral infections of the central nervous system
Ophthalmological complications
  Cataracts
  Viral infections
Cardiac complications
  Myocardial infarction
  Coronary artery thrombosis

another operation for the patient. An advance in cataract surgery is cryoextraction, a procedure in which a cryoprobe that has been cooled to −40°F adheres to the cataract and pulls it out through the incision. Phacoemulsion, an even newer procedure, utilizes a pencil tip–sized probe that is inserted through a small incision in the anterior chamber. Ultrasonic waves break up the cataract into small pieces, which are then removed by a suction needle through the same incision [3]. In our experience, phacoemulsion has lessened the trauma of cataract surgery. Patients treated by phacoemulsion are not limited in their activities after surgery and their hospital stay is usually only one day.

Other ocular complications of renal transplantation are bilateral depigmentation of the retinal pigment epithelium, elevated intraocular tension, and CMV retinitis, which can result in blindness [11].

The patient should have his eyes examined often to detect any abnormalities as early as possible.

ASEPTIC NECROSIS

Aseptic necrosis of the heads of the femur probably occurs as a result of the steroid dosage and the alterations in lipid metabolism that are caused by the fluctuations in the steroid dosage. The underlying bone disease that occurs in most patients who have chronic renal failure probably also contributes to the disease. The patient usually has symptoms of hip pain several months before radiographic evidence. Initially the treatment is symptomatic, but progressive bone destruction or continued pain requires surgical intervention in the form of total hip replacement [15]. In our experience, only a small percentage of the transplant population had aseptic necrosis. Total hip replacement was done in all patients without any postoperative complications.

MALIGNANCY

Malignancy occurs as a result of long-term immunosuppressive therapy. Lymphoma occurs 35 times more often, skin and lip cancers occur 4 times more often, and other types of cancer occur 2½ times more often in the transplant population, than in the normal population [18, 20]. It is not clear whether the increased incidence is due to oversuppression, to the immune response alone, or to a combined effect added to continued antigenic stimulation from the foreign graft.

LIVER DISEASE

Hepatic dysfunction in the transplant recipient is postulated to have a number of causes: azathioprine intoxication, a CMV infection, the hepatitis B antigen, or an unidentified virus. The incidence of hepatitis, the severity of the disease, and the progression to massive hepatic necrosis or postnecrotic cirrhosis are different in different reports. It appears that hepatic dysfunction can be classified into three types: (1) acute reversible, (2) acute fulminant progressing to death, and (3) chronic liver disease [21].

About 33 percent of our transplant recipients have some form of liver disease, and only 2 to 3 percent show Australian antigen positivity. The other patients have acute reversible or chronic liver disease. Two patients died from fulminant hepatitis within six months after the transplantation and about two weeks after the onset of the liver abnormalities. Our patients who have chronic liver disease seem to fall into two groups: (1) those who have chronic liver disease and no progression (as shown by serial biopsies) and (2) those who have progressive chronic liver disease (also as shown by biopsy). Many approaches have been taken to reverse or stabilize the progression of the chronic disease, ranging from substituting cyclophosphamide for azathioprine to withdrawing all immunosuppressive agents—but to no avail. One of the most frustrating things about progressive liver disease in the transplant patient is that the staff caring for the patient feels helpless. All our patients who died from liver disease had a functioning transplanted kidney.

OTHER COMPLICATIONS

Even the transplant recipient who survives five years or more with a functioning transplanted kidney remains at risk. The causes of death in one group of patients (they are probably the same in every group of transplant recipients) were: pneumonitis, disseminated CMV infection, chronic aggressive (progressive) hepatitis, vascular occlusions of the mesenteric and coronary arteries, and suicide either by voluntarily discontinuing medications or by refusing hemodialysis and treatment when the transplanted kidney failed. Most of the deaths occurred in patients who had functioning transplanted kidneys and who were taking maintenance doses of immunosuppressive drugs [17].

Another complication—a social complication—is the high divorce rate among transplant recipients. Among our patients, the divorce rate seems to be higher among those who receive transplants than it is among those being treated by dialysis. A possible explanation for the difference is that it is not socially acceptable to divorce someone who is chronically ill (i.e., someone who depends on a machine for his life), whereas it is acceptable to divorce someone who has a kidney transplant and who is viewed, even by himself, as normal. The pressures on the spouse of a transplant recipient and the recipient's move toward independence also seem to affect the divorce rates.

Fever

Fever, alone, is not actually a complication of transplantation, nor is it a disease process. However, it is extremely important to the patient to attempt to determine the source of any fever. Its significance is due, in part, to the antipyretic action of steroids (steroids often mask a fever). Because fever is an indicator of rejection as well as infection, there are several factors to consider when a transplant patient presents with fever. Among these factors are [20]:

1. Infection occurs at some time in almost 80 percent of transplant recipients. Bacterial infections are the most common type of infection in the first three months after the transplantation.
2. In the immediate postoperative period the most common sites of infection are wound sites, the urinary tract, and the lungs.
3. In the long-term transplant recipient, opportunistic fungal, viral, and protozoan infections should be ruled out.
4. It must be remembered that bacterial and fungal septicemias do not necessarily have initially recognizable foci.
5. The source of the fever may be a viremia from CMV, herpes, or another adenovirus.
6. The source of the fever may never be discovered.

Regardless of its cause, a fever should be extensively evaluated before it is treated and it should be considered septic until proved otherwise. The evaluation should include a detailed history obtained from the patient or his family, a white blood cell count with a differential count, an examination of the urine sediment, and cultures of the blood, sputum, cerebrospinal fluid, urine, and wound (if there is a wound). The laboratory tests that should be done are those of the blood urea nitrogen, creatinine, and electrolyte levels, liver function, viral titers, fungal titers, and febrile agglutinins. The chest and abdominal x rays should be reviewed [20]. The unexpected causes of fever should be considered but the common causes should not be neglected.

Depending on the test results, further diagnostic studies may be indicated. Every effort should be made to identify the causative agent before the patient is treated. Unless the patient is obviously septic, the use of nonspecific antibiotics could allow the overgrowth of resistant organisms, especially fungi. If broad-spectrum antibiotics must be used, the necessary cultures should be done before antibiotic therapy is begun [20].

Advantages of Transplantation

The patient who has had a successful renal transplant is soon on his way to rehabilitation. He gradu-

ally regains strength as the different body systems that were affected by uremia return to normal. The cardiovascular system improves with the reduction in heart size and the correction of the fluid overload [4].

Hypertension usually resolves unless the patient has stenosis of the transplanted artery, a delay in the recovery of renal functioning or a poorly functioning graft. In some instances, in patients with normally functioning grafts, hypertension is traceable to the original kidneys and removal of those kidneys can bring the blood pressure back to normal [6]. In many cases that result can be predicted by renin studies of the renal vein or from a history of increased blood pressure when the patient was on dialysis.

The anemia seen in the dialyzed patient disappears because the transplanted kidney secretes erythropoietin. In uncomplicated cases the anemia is corrected in one to two months after the transplantation [6].

Uremic neuropathy, which is manifested by itching, burning, and muscular weakness, usually disappears rapidly after transplantation. Peripheral neuropathy, which is manifested by a disturbance in gait and in nerve conduction velocity, is slower to disappear, but it resolves completely in most patients so affected [6].

Gradually the patient who has had a successful transplant begins to adapt to his new condition as his stress is decreased and he begins to feel well and not sick. Tensions in the family seem to decrease, at least to the level that existed before the renal failure, as the patient resumes his role in the family and the financial burdens are lessened. The immediate fear of death decreases [16] even though it readily surfaces when another transplant patient dies. When that happens, the patient needs to be assured that people are different and they respond differently, even to the same disease.

After transplantation, sexual feelings and functioning and fertility return to normal. Menstruation usually returns in two to eight months after the transplantation. Men report an improvement in their potency [4].

Pregnancy After Transplantation

There have been successful pregnancies among transplant recipients, but the patient who is considering pregnancy should be counseled about the risks to her and to the fetus. In the largest series of well-followed transplant recipients, it was found that the children of male transplant recipients were at less risk than were the children of female transplant recipients. Among the 39 pregnancies involving male transplant recipients, there were two abortions and one child who had severe congenital defects [8]. Among the female transplant recipients, there were only 22 live births out of 31 pregnancies. The other pregnancies resulted in one stillborn baby, one ectopic pregnancy, and seven abortions (one was spontaneous, and six were done at the patient's request). Of the 22 newborns, nine had an uncomplicated neonatal course. The remaining 13 newborns had one or more complications, including respiratory distress syndrome, adrenocortical insufficiency, septicemia, seizures, congenital abnormalities, and prematurity [8].

In our experience, transplant recipients have had 24 pregnancies; 11 pregnancies involved 5 male transplant recipients and 13 pregnancies involved 12 female transplant recipients. Five abortions occurred among the female transplant recipients, four at the patient's request and one as a result of hyperbilirubinemia. The other eight babies of the female transplant recipients were normal and had no neonatal complications. All the female transplant recipients who carried their babies to term became hypertensive (even though they were admitted to a high-risk pregnancy care unit four to six weeks before their due date) and were delivered by cesarean section. All 11 infants of the male transplant recipients were delivered at term, and they had no prenatal or postnatal complications.

Teaching Aids

Renal transplant recipients make up a cross section of the population. Not all patients have the benefit of an education or, as in the case of the diabetic transplant recipient who is blind, the benefit of sight. Yet those patients too can and must learn about their disease, how to care for the new kidney, and how to take the medications and learn to feel that they are at least partly responsible for their own care.

Patient education must be related to subjects that the patients understand. For instance, the action of azathioprine on white blood cells (and the reason for taking azathioprine) can be compared to a battle. Azathioprine is given to "kill the bad group of the white cells that attack the kidney, but azathioprine also kills some of the good group of white cells" and so leaves the patient susceptible to infections. Most

patients can understand the "good guy, bad guy" explanation; it helps them to understand why they are required to take their medications and why they have to be careful of infections.

A blind recipient must have a relative or friend help with his care, but he can take some responsibility for his care. He can learn to identify his medications from rubber bands put around the medication bottles: for example, one rubber band could indicate azathioprine, two rubber bands could indicate prednisolone, and three rubber bands could indicate the antihypertensive medication.

Even transplant recipients who are illiterate can learn to take care of themselves. We have had several illiterate patients and each one was a challenge in regard to nursing. One patient who could not read, write, or count was also color blind. But he was eager to learn. Besides the immunosuppressive drugs, he was taking several antihypertensive drugs and a diuretic. To make sure that he took his medications correctly, each pill was taped to the top of an index card and circles were drawn on the card that corresponded to the size of the pill and the number of pills to be taken. At his medication times, his medications were brought to him in their respective bottles. He then took a pill from its bottle, matched it to a pill on the index card, and then placed a pill in each circle until all were filled. He did that with each medication until he had taken all his medications. If a dosage was increased or decreased, a circle was added or deleted. Gradually, the patient learned the names of the medications and what they were for: "kidney" pills (azathioprine and prednisolone), the "high blood" pill (the antihypertensive), and the "water" pill (the diuretic). The patient was an eager pupil, and he was very proud of his accomplishment. Also, he learned how to monitor his kidney function, and he called when he noticed anything wrong. Unfortunately, even though he was cautioned about avoiding people who had infections, we neglected to mention common childhood diseases in particular (he was 49 years of age). The patient died one year after transplantation from varicella pneumonia, which he caught from his six-year-old daughter. His transplanted kidney was functioning at the time of his death.

Our center has drawn up a *Letter to the Patient*, a pamphlet that explains the transplantation surgery and the events surrounding it. The pamphlet has proved useful in providing the dialysis patient basic information about renal transplantation. At the time of his discharge, the patient is also given written instructions so that he has something tangible to refer to if he has any questions. The instructions list the signs and symptoms of rejection and also give the patient general advice about monitoring fluid intake and output and weighing himself every day.

Medication cards should be given to the patient at the time of his discharge. In the excitement of leaving the hospital, patients have been known to forget to take their medicines. The medication cards are a reminder to the patient of the dosages, and they also lessen confusion about later increases or decreases in dosages.

Follow-Up Care

The transplant recipient is usually discharged two to three weeks after surgery if he has had no major complications. He is then checked twice a week on an outpatient basis. The number of clinic visits decreases as the patient's condition becomes more stable, and over a period of four months the visits are gradually reduced to one a month. If the patient's condition remains stable, his routine clinic visits occur once every four to six months, and laboratory checks are done between visits. If the patient becomes ill—develops leukopenia, liver disease, or acute or chronic rejection—his clinic visits once again become more frequent.

Acute rejection episodes are usually treated on an outpatient basis unless the patient's renal function has deteriorated rapidly. With every acute rejection episode, an IVP or a sonogram is done to rule out a partial ureteral obstruction, and a renal scan is done to try to rule out an arterial lesion.

Continuity of care is provided for the transplant recipient as an outpatient in the sense that the clinic staff is familiar with his hospital course and problems. Similarly, the transplant unit staff is kept informed of any problems the transplant recipient has as an outpatient. The transplant recipient is given telephone numbers of people to call 24 hours a day if a problem arises.

The outpatient checkup includes a complete blood count; blood urea nitrogen, serum creatinine, liver function, and Australian antigen tests; 24-hour urine tests to check the protein and creatinine concentrations; a urinalysis; a physical examination; and weight and blood pressure checks. The patient is encouraged to continue to weigh himself daily and to report any sudden increase in weight accompanied by

edema of the legs. A dietitian is available for consultation at every clinic visit.

Most patients return to work six to eight weeks postoperatively. Children are encouraged to continue their schoolwork with a "homebound" teacher until they are able to return to school.

Trends in Transplantation

In the early years of transplantation, most transplanted kidneys were taken from living, related donors. Since 1973, most transplanted kidney have come from cadaver donors. As the era of transplantation has progressed, there has been a decrease in the recipient mortality and a stabilization of the rate of "functional" success (of transplanted kidneys that are functioning after one year). The improvement reflects the trend to remove a poorly functioning transplanted kidney early (and return the patient to hemodialysis) rather than to bombard the patient with immunosuppressive agents, which do little to restore renal function and which make the patient more susceptible to infections and death [18, 19].

Even the transplant recipient who survives five years or more with a functioning graft remains at risk. The causes of death in one group studied were: pneumonitis, disseminated CMV infections, chronic aggressive hepatitis, and vascular occlusions of the mesenteric and coronary arteries. Most of the deaths occurred in patients who had functioning grafts and who were taking maintenance doses of immunosuppressive drugs [17].

Advances in transplantation depend on further research in more effective treatment modalities such as Cyclosporin-A, donor-specific blood transfusions, and radiation of the lymphatic system. The hope is that more specific immunosuppression would result in less severe side effects. Until this is accomplished, infection remains the greatest threat, often resulting in the death of a patient with a functioning kidney.

Nursing Orders

Problem/Diagnosis

Renal transplantation.

OBJECTIVE NO. 1

The patient should receive preoperative teaching and observation.

To achieve the objective, the nurse should:

1. Assess the patient. She should:
   a. Assess the patient's knowledge of renal transplantation and reinforce the physician's explanation to the patient of the procedure and its risks, benefits, and possible outcomes. The nurse should remember that although the patient may think that he understands renal transplantation, much of his information has come from rumor.
   b. Discuss with the patient and his family the preoperative procedures and why they are done.
   c. Begin to teach the patient about his medications: their names, dosages, side effects, why they have been prescribed, and the consequences of discontinuing them.
   d. If the patient cannot read or is blind or for some other reason is not able to administer his medications himself, include another family member in the teaching session. If that is not possible, the nurse should draw up a discharge plan that includes information about outside help for the patient, such as that given by a visiting nurse.
   e. In the teaching program, discuss the possibility that a rejection episode might occur after transplantation, emphasizing that such an episode does not necessarily mean the patient will lose his kidney. The nurse should prepare the patient for the possibility that hemodialysis might be needed postoperatively, especially if he is to receive a cadaver kidney.
   f. Realize that the psychological preparation of the patient is important. The nurse should answer the questions of the patient and his family honestly but without terrifying them.
   g. Involve the patient in his daily care, giving him responsibilities that make him feel a part of the process (e.g., recording his fluid intake and output and weighing himself daily).
   h. Explain the isolation procedures (if any) that will be followed after the transplantation, telling the patient the reason for the isolation and how long it will last and assuring him that he will not be completely alone.
   i. Anticipate the questions the patient wants to ask but does not because he is embarrassed or thinks that the questions seem "silly." For example, assure a patient that if he receives a kidney from a member of the opposite sex, it will not affect his sexual ability or characteristics. Many people worry about that, but few have the courage to ask about it.

2. Do a physical examination and a laboratory assessment. The nurse should:
   a. Observe, monitor, and record the patient's temperature, blood pressure, and pulse every four hours. The source of any fever should be determined. A fever rules out surgery.
   b. Weigh the patient daily. It is important to obtain baseline information about the patient's weight and to make sure the patient does not become volume overloaded before surgery.
   c. Know that the patient's daily fluid intake and output give some indication of his fluid balance. The 24-hour urine output is important before transplantation as baseline information, and it could be helpful in assessing renal function after the transplantation. (For example, a 1000 ml per 24 hours output before the transplantation would make a 50 ml per hour output after the transplantation actually only 10 ml per hour, which would be a major concern.) The importance of the fluid intake and output should be explained to the patient before he assumes the responsibility of recording it.
   d. Have baseline cultures done of the blood, urine, throat, sputum, nose, and groin area. It is important to identify potential sources of infection before surgery.
   e. Have baseline laboratory tests done before including a complete blood count; platelet, prothrombin time, electrolyte, blood urea nitrogen, creatinine, liver function, amylase, calcium, phosphorus, uric acid, VDRL, and Australian antigen studies; and viral titers.
   f. Every day have a complete blood count and platelet, electrolyte, blood urea nitrogen, and creatinine studies done. The white blood cell count is extremely important in determining the daily azathioprine dose. It is equally important to monitor the serum potassium level and to report and treat any abnormal levels.
   g. Have a chest x ray done to evaluate the patient's cardiopulmonary status.
   h. Have a baseline ECG done to rule out any abnormalities.
   i. Check the patient's skin for excoriation, pustules, and rashes, especially in the area of the hemodialysis access (the Scribner shunt or the A-V fistula).

j. Instruct the patient in the use and importance of the intermittent positive pressure breathing machine and/or the incentive spirometer. Have him practice using the equipment before surgery so that he is familiar with it.

OBJECTIVE NO. 2

The patient should be prepared for the anticipated surgery.
To achieve the objective, the nurse should:

1. Be aware that in most instances, the patient is dialyzed the day before surgery to bring him to the best physiological state.
2. Begin administering azathioprine and prednisolone as ordered.
3. The day before surgery, in the samples for the daily morning blood work include serum for crossmatching with donor lymphocytes as well as blood for typing and crossmatching for blood transfusions.
4. To minimize the bulk content, give the patient liquid meals the day before surgery.
5. With the physician, again tell the patient about the transplantation procedure, risks, benefits, and graft and patient survival. Have the informed consent and the operative forms signed in the presence of witnesses.
6. To prevent bowel complications postoperatively, give the patient saline enemas until the return is clear.
7. Have the patient take Betadine scrub showers to decrease the number of endogenous bacteria.
8. Talk with the patient and his donor (if a living, related donor kidney is used) and with their families, giving them a chance to ask questions. Give them reassurance and support.

OBJECTIVE NO. 3

On the day of surgery, everything should be scrutinized to be sure the patient is ready for surgery.
To achieve the objective, the nurse should:

1. Check the laboratory results immediately before surgery for any abnormalities, especially an elevated potassium level. Notify the physician immediately if an abnormality is present. Record the values on the chart.
2. Give immunosuppressive medications before sur-

gery. They may be given intravenously in same dosage as ordered for their oral administration.
3. Encourage the patient to verbalize his feelings. *Be a good listener.*
4. Check the patient's vital signs to be sure there are no marked abnormalities, especially a fever.
5. Weigh the patient before surgery to help evaluate his fluid status postoperatively.
6. Administer preoperative medication as prescribed by the anesthesiologist.
7. Give supportive care to the family and keep them informed about the progress of the surgery.

OBJECTIVE NO. 4

The transplant recipient should be closely observed in the immediate postoperative period.
To achieve the objective, the nurse should:

1. Assess the patient. She should:
   a. Maintain an adequate airway and evaluate the patient's respiratory function. If the patient is intubated, keep his airway free of secretions.
   b. Assess the patient's readiness to be extubated by evaluating his alertness, strength, and respiratory state. Notify the anesthesiologist and help with the extubation. Have suctioning equipment available.
   c. Observe the patient closely after the extubation for respiratory difficulties. (A respiratory arrest can occur after the extubation.)
   d. Provide the patient with heated oxygen mist.
   e. Check the patient's vital signs carefully. If his temperature is below normal, put warm blankets on him. If the patient is extremely cold (as he often is in the operating room), his peripheral vessels constrict. The patient's blood pressure can be an accurate index to his fluid status. If the blood pressure is abnormally high or low for the particular patient, report that fact to the physician immediately. Any change in the pulse rate could indicate loss of blood, pain, or hypovolemia. Monitor the patient's vital signs every 15 minutes until they are stable, and then every 30 minutes. Gradually decrease the monitoring to every hour if the patient's condition remains stable.
   f. Determine the patient's actual fluid status by finding out (from the anesthesia and operative records) the estimated blood loss and the amount of fluid or packed cells given. Check

how much urine was obtained in the operating room. When massive diuresis occurs, the vascular system is extremely sensitive to volume changes.

g. Auscultate the patient's chest for signs of pulmonary congestion.

h. Order a chest x ray to evaluate the patient's pulmonary and cardiac status and a flat plate of the abdomen to obtain baseline information about the placement of the transplanted kidney.

i. Check the hemodialysis access (the A-V fistula and/or the Scribner shunt) for patency. The access must be kept functioning because hemodialysis might be needed postoperatively. If the patient has an A-V fistula, the application of warm towels to the area helps to increase the flow. If there is no flow in the fistula (and if she has been trained to do so), the nurse should massage the fistula, beginning on the arterial side and moving to the venous side. If a shunt is present, the nurse should observe it for low flow or clotting. If the shunt or the fistula stops functioning, the nurse should notify the physician immediately. The nurse should continue to check for patency frequently. Patients become upset if the shunt or the fistula stops functioning because they look on them as their lifelines, at least until they feel sure that the kidney is functioning.

2. Assess the patient's renal function. The nurse should:

a. Make sure the indwelling catheter is connected to a closed drainage system, that there are no kinks in the catheter, and that the drainage tubing and bag are properly connected to the bed, with no tension on the catheter.

b. Empty the urimeter and drainage bag and measure the amount of urine on the patient's arrival in the recovery room. Begin the hourly collections of urine.

c. Check the urine for blood or blood clots. The urine will be slightly bloody for some time because of the bladder surgery. If it suddenly becomes grossly bloody, the physician should be notified immediately.

d. If there are many blood clots, check frequently for obstruction of the catheter. If obstruction by clots occurs, irrigate the catheter *gently*, using sterile technique.

e. Check the intravenous line and fluid. Change the fluids to normal saline solution and 5% dextrose in water solution. That combination usually replaces the electrolytes that were lost through the urine. Begin replacement therapy using the output during the previous hours as a guide to the amount of intravenous fluids that should be given during the following hour. For example, if the patient's urinary output from 7 P.M. to 8 P.M. was 240 ml, from 8 P.M. to 9 P.M. the patient should receive 160 ml of normal saline solution and 80 ml of a 5% dextrose and water solution (the ratio is two parts normal saline solution to one part 5% dextrose and water solution). The urinary output from 8 P.M. to 9 P.M. determines the amount of fluid to be given from 9 P.M. to 10 P.M., and so on throughout the day.

f. Have a complete blood count, prothrombin time, blood urea nitrogen, creatinine, and electrolyte studies done to use as baseline information in the recovery room. The nurse should be sure to check the results, especially the serum potassium and carbon dioxide levels. Any abnormalities should be corrected with medications as ordered by the physician. If the kidney is functioning well, there will be a progressive drop in the serum creatinine level.

g. If the patient's condition is stable and his urinary output is adequate, begin a urine collection to use in assessing the patient's glomerular filtration rate (GFR) by doing a timed creatinine clearance and/or a Glofil-125 (^{125}I) clearance study. We have found timed clearances to be the most accurate index of renal functioning. The clearance should be repeated in two days for comparison and to document any improved renal functioning.

3. Assess the surgical site. The nurse should:

a. Check the dressings for drainage. If drains are used, the nurse should be sure that the drain site is dressed separately from the incision site.

b. If the drainage suddenly increases or becomes bloody, notify the physician immediately. The increased drainage could indicate a ureteral leak. The sudden appearance of blood from the incision site might indicate a small bleeder or an arterial leak. Be sure to distinguish between bloody drainage and serosanguinous drainage.

c. If the dressing is dry, leave it on. It is better to

leave it in place until the wound seals itself. If the dressing must be changed, it should be changed with strict sterile technique.

OBJECTIVE NO. 5

The patient's vital signs and renal function must be observed continuously and closely in the immediate postoperative period to determine as soon as possible whether an abnormality is present.

To achieve the objective, the nurse should:

1. Watch for a sudden change in blood pressure. If the blood pressure suddenly falls, the cause may be volume depletion or bleeding. The rate of fluid infusion should be increased immediately. Hypotension results in low perfusion to the transplanted kidney, as well as an obvious danger to the patient. If the blood pressure suddenly increases, the patient may be suffering from hyperacute rejection or compression of the renal artery, especially if the increase is associated with a sudden decrease in the urinary output, or it could indicate fluid overload.
2. Be aware that a decrease in urinary output may be a result of: (a) hypovolemia, which can be corrected by the administration of fluids, (b) an obstruction of the catheter by clots or kinks that can be corrected by irrigating or straightening the tubing, (c) an obstruction of the ureter by clots (it is not common), or (d) compression of the renal artery, as shown by a renal scan or renal arteriogram. If the artery is partially occluded, surgical intervention is necessary immediately to restore blood flow and prevent damage to the kidney (Table 33-4).

OBJECTIVE NO. 6

Measures should be taken to reduce the incidence of infection in the immediate postoperative period.

To achieve the objective, the nurse should remember that infection is the leading cause of complications in the transplant recipient. For that reason, the following precautions are taken during the postoperative period to decrease the incidence of infection:

1. Isolation precautions can be used during the first postoperative days. The isolation rules prevent unauthorized personnel from entering the room. Staff members with skin infections or colds should not take care of the patient.
2. Thorough hand-washing techniques must be used to prevent cross contamination of the patients.
3. Sterile technique should be observed in changing the wound dressing. If drainage is present, it should be cultured routinely. When changing the dressing, the nurse should look for the signs of infection: fullness, erythema around the incision, purulent drainage, and tenderness.
4. Good pulmonary hygiene should be maintained through the use of intermittent positive pressure breathing, coughing, and deep breathing every two hours to prevent postoperative atelectasis and pneumonia.
5. The urinary catheter should be removed after 24 hours. If it has to remain longer, care should be taken to keep the system a closed one. A urine culture should be made when the catheter is removed. We have found that the longer after 18 to 24 hours the catheter is left in place, the higher is the incidence of urinary tract infections.
6. The site of the intravenous line should be observed closely for signs of infiltration or infection. If an intravenous line is needed for more than 24 hours, more than one site should be used.

OBJECTIVE NO. 7

The patient should be assessed closely during the rest of his hospital stay; his laboratory values, renal functioning, and rehabilitation should be monitored.

To achieve the objective, the nurse should:

1. Assess the patient. She should:
   a. Be aware that the urinary catheter and intravenous lines are usually removed in 24 to 48 hours. She should encourage early ambulation in order to decrease the incidence of the postoperative complications of thrombophlebitis, pulmonary embolism, and pneumonia.
   b. Resume weighing the patient daily. Initially the patient should lose weight as the kidney removes excess fluid. An increase in weight could be a sign of early rejection or fluid retention.
   c. Monitor the patient's vital signs every four hours. If his temperature rises above 100°F, blood cultures should be done. Any dramatic change in the patient's blood pressure or pulse

should be reported to the physician, because it may indicate the onset of an acute rejection episode.

d. Remember that monitoring the patient's fluid intake and output is an essential part of his care. Both intake and output are measured at 8-hour intervals, and the 24-hour total is recorded on the patient's chart. A downward trend in the output (particularily the overnight output) suggests an impending rejection episode. An abrupt decrease in output should be evaluated as to its cause: hypovolemia, rejection, ureteral leak or obstruction, or arterial obstruction. The nurse should encourage the patient to measure and record his intake and output. To do so gives him a sense of responsibility for his own care.

e. Listen carefully to the patient's complaints of pain and, with the patient's help, differentiate between incisional pain and tenderness in the upper pole of the kidney caused by the swelling of the kidney due to rejection. The kidney is easily palpated, and any change in its size or any tenderness should be assessed, recorded, and reported to the physician.

f. Continue to give the immunosuppressive medications as ordered. Encourage the patient to describe his medication and dosage. Tell the patient how to identify his medications.

g. Observe for the presence of edema in the legs or the periorbital region. If edema occurs in conjunction with an increase in daily weight, the patient may have to be placed on fluid and sodium restriction.

h. Encourage the patient to observe good hygiene and eating habits.

2. Assess the patient's laboratory values. The nurse should:

a. Be aware that a complete blood cell count and platelet, blood urea nitrogen, creatinine, and electrolyte studies continue to be done daily to assess the patient's renal function. Liver function tests, and calcium, phosphorus, and viral titers, are done weekly to observe for any abnormalities.

b. Check the white blood cell count daily before administering azathioprine. If the white blood cell count decreases to 4000, check with the physician before giving the drug. When the white blood cell count falls below 3000, the dosage may be decreased or discontinued until the count shows an upward trend. At levels below 3000 the patient has a greater risk of infection.

c. If the hemoglobin and hematocrit suddenly decrease, test the patient's stool for occult blood. Gastrointestinal bleeding may be associated with the use of high-dose steroids, stress, or preexisting uremia. In most transplant centers, vigorous antacid therapy is used as a precaution in the postoperative period.

d. Check the serum creatinine levels daily. The levels should be almost normal by the third postoperative day if the patient's transplant is functioning properly and there is no evidence of ATN or rejection. If the downward trend in the serum creatinine level slows or stops, it must be carefully investigated.

e. Be aware that usually the potassium level is not a problem postoperatively unless the kidney is not functioning properly or there is a very high intake of potassium.

f. Check the patient's daily urine protein levels. The urine protein test should be negative by four days after surgery, provided there is no hematuria. Once the test is negative, reappearance of urine protein indicates acute rejection, renal vein thrombosis (rarely), or recurrence of the original disease.

g. See that (as in our transplant center) a Glofil-125 and/or a creatinine clearance test is performed at specified intervals (two to three days) postoperatively. The values measured at that point should be higher than the values measured immediately postoperatively in the recovery room. Values that have changed only slightly could be an early indication of impending rejection, even though the serum creatinine level might not reflect it.

OBJECTIVE NO. 8

The patient should be taught about all aspects of renal transplantation.

To achieve the objective, the nurse should:

1. Instruct the patient about the following signs and symptoms of rejection (Table 33-3), which he can monitor himself: malaise, fever, tenderness in the

upper pole of the transplanted kidney, peripheral and periorbital edema, an increase in weight, a decrease in urinary output, and an increase in the urine protein level. Suspected rejection can be documented by laboratory tests that show an increase in the serum creatinine level and/or a decrease in the Glofil-125 and creatinine clearance values.

2. Instruct the patient about the following signs and symptoms of impending wound infection: pain, fever, redness, and swelling around or drainage from the incision.

3. If the patient has had a wound infection and is to be discharged with an open wound, begin to teach him and a member of his family about sterile technique and wound care. Let them change the dressings in the hospital under close observation.

4. Instruct the patient about the following signs and symptoms of urinary tract infection: burning, frequency, and a change in the color or odor of the urine. Teach him about hygienic care of the perianal area.

5. Warn the patient about being around people who have contagious diseases, especially childhood diseases such as chickenpox and measles. The patient cannot live in a sterile environment when he is discharged, but he should take some precautions because of his depressed immune system. Instruct the patient about notifying the transplant center if he has been exposed to a contagious disease.

6. Encourage the patient to have good eating habits. After transplantation, the patient usually has no dietary restrictions. Because they have been deprived so long, transplant recipients tend to want to eat everything in sight. Steroids are known to increase appetite and the patient should be warned about that.

7. Give the patient medication cards that contain the names and dosages and frequency of his medications. Make changes on his card as his steroid dosage changes. Have the patient count each set of pills, name each type of pill, and tell its purpose and importance. The patient must assume responsibility for taking his medications before he is discharged. It is important that he be able to recognize each medication in case he should be given an incorrect prescription.

8. Before the patient is discharged, make sure he or a member of his family has a thermometer and *can read* it.

OBJECTIVE NO. 9

The patient, physicians, and nurse should know that communication is the best teaching tool.

To achieve the objective, the nurse should:

1. Remember that in transplantation, as in all phases of medicine, the line of communication must be kept open between the patient, the physician, and the nurses to ensure comprehensive patient care. The medical personnel must depend on the patient to tell them how he feels, what problems he has, and what changes he notices in his renal function.

2. Remember that accurate reporting and record keeping are essential in the care of renal transplant recipients, which involves many different facets of medicine.

3. Provide emotional support and reassurance not only to the patient but also to his family. The nurse should remember that the time is a stressful one for everyone. Nurses (and other personnel) tend to forget that usually it is the patient's first time to experience a transplant. Because nurses are so used to the procedures, they accept them as routine, whereas all things are new and unique to the transplant recipient.

4. Be aware that open, honest communication about the transplant's functioning and expectations is essential. The patient can better tolerate untoward events that he has been prepared for or (if they have arisen suddenly) that are explained to him immediately and in detail.

5. Realize that thorough explanations of the procedures are necessary. It often falls to the nurse to reinforce the physician's explanation of the procedures and to provide the reassurance and support the patient needs.

6. Realize that all staff members and patients will not always get along. That fact should be recognized and dealt with so as not to compromise patient care.

Summary

The risks of transplantation are great. They lead one to ask why a patient with ESRD chooses transplantation rather than hemodialysis. The explanation is not a concrete one; it has to do with "the quality of life" concept, which has a different meaning to each patient. Many patients are willing to take the risks so that they can return to a more normal life, one that is not controlled by machines.

Even though a conscious or an unconscious fear of rejection persists regardless of how many years the patient has had the transplanted kidney, most patients are able to adapt to their new condition. But they are bothered by the fact that they are dependent on medications, which reminds them of their vulnerability.

An interdisciplinary team approach should be used in caring for the transplant recipient. The problems encountered should be dealt with openly by the nephrologists, surgeons, and nursing staff, as well as other disciplines. The patient benefits from the team approach. Each member of the team should contribute to the care of the patient and should share his observations with the other members of the team.

The nurse's ability to participate in the care of the transplant recipient is based on her understanding of all aspects of the transplantation process: anatomy and physiology, immunology, immunosuppression, statistics, and the psychological stress on the patient and his family. If the nurse has that basic knowledge, her experience will bring her further growth and understanding.

References

1. Belzer, F. O. Renal preservation. *N. Engl. J. Med.* 291:402, 1974.
2. Belzer, F. O., and Salvatierra, O. Renal Transplantation: Organ Procurement, Preservation, and Surgical Management. In B. M. Brenner and F. C. Rector (eds.), *The Kidney.* Philadelphia: Saunders, 1976. Vol. 2.
3. Boyd-Monk, H. Cataract surgery. *Nurs. '77* 7:56, 1977.
4. Brundage, D. J. *Nursing Management of Renal Problems.* St. Louis: Mosby, 1976.
5. Fellner, C. H. Selection of living kidney donors and the problem of informed consent. *Semin. Psychiatry* 3:79, 1971.
6. Hamburger, J., Crosnier, J., Dormont, J., et al. *Renal Transplantation: Theory and Practice.* Baltimore: Williams & Wilkins, 1972.
7. Dessmeyer-Nielson, F. (ed.). *Histocompatibility Testing.* Copenhagen: Munksgard, 1975.
8. Makowski, E. L., and Penn, I. Parenthood Following Renal Transplantation. In deAlvarez (ed.), *The Kidney in Pregnancy.* New York: Wiley, 1976.
9. Monaco, A. P. Circumventing Graft Rejection: Antilymphocyte Serum. In J. S. Najarian and R. L. Simmons (eds.), *Transplantation.* Philadelphia: Lea & Febiger, 1972.
10. Najarian, J. S., Howard, R. J., Foker, J. E., et al. Renal Transplantation: Criteria for Selection and Evaluation of Patients and Immunological Aspects of Transplantation. In B. M. Brenner and F. C. Rector (eds.), *The Kidney.* Philadelphia: Saunders, 1976. Vol. 2.
11. Oberman, A. E., and Chatterjee, S. N. Ocular complications in renal transplant recipients. *West. J. Med.* 123:184, 1975.
12. Opelz, G., and Terasaki, P. I. Kidney preservation: Perfusion versus cold storage—1975. *Transplant. Proc.* 8:121, 1976.
13. Russo, V., and Marks, C. Renal transplantation: An analysis of operative complications. *Am. Surg.* 42:153, 1976.
14. Santos, G. W. Circumventing Graft Rejection: Chemical Immunosuppression. In J. S. Najarian and R. L. Simmons (eds.), *Transplantation.* Philadelphia: Lea & Febiger, 1972.
15. Simmons, R. L., Kjellstrand, C. M., and Najarian, J. S. Kidney: Technique, Complications and Results. In J. S. Najarian and R. L. Simmons (eds.), *Transplantation.* Philadelphia: Lea & Febiger, 1972.
16. Simmons, R. G., and Simmons, R. L. Sociological and Psychological Aspects of Transplantation. In J. S. Najarian and R. L. Simmons (eds.), *Transplantation.* Philadelphia: Lea & Febiger, 1972.
17. Starzel, T. E., Weil, R., and Putnam, C. W. Modern trends in kidney transplantation. *Transplant. Proc.* 9:1, 1977.
18. The 13th Report of the Human Transplant Registry, Advisory Committee to the Renal Transplant Registry. *Transplant. Proc.* 9:9, 1977.
19. The 12th Report of the Human Renal Transplant Registry, Advisory Committee to the Renal Transplant Registry. *J.A.M.A.* 233:787, 1975.
20. Thier, S. D., Henderson, L. W., and Root, R. K. Renal Transplantation: Medical Management of the Transplant Recipient. In B. M. Brenner and F. C. Rector (eds.), *The Kidney.* Philadelphia: Saunders, 1976. Vol. 2.
21. Ware, A. J., Luby, J. P., Eigenbrodt, E. H., et al. Spectrum of liver disease in renal transplant recipients. *Gastroenterology* 68:755, 1975..

X. Special Considerations in Critical Care Nursing

The "new therapies"—relaxation techniques, meditation exercises, biofeedback regimens—are being applied to patient care in increasingly wider circles. With an understanding of body-mind-spirit concepts, these new techniques begin to make sense to the nurse who employs them. Without this understanding, they can be bewildering.

Are critical care areas ready for body-mind-spirit concepts? There will be personal exceptions, but generally the answer at this point is "No."

Unless we want to play catch-up, we must begin now. Beginning unfamiliar endeavors is hard work, and dealing with what seem to be incomprehensible concepts can be frightening. *But we must make a beginning.*

> Nature is rude and incomprehensible at first,
> Be not discouraged, keep on, there are divine things well envelop'd,
> I swear to you there are divine things more beautiful than words can tell. . . .

Walt Whitman
"Song of the Open Road"

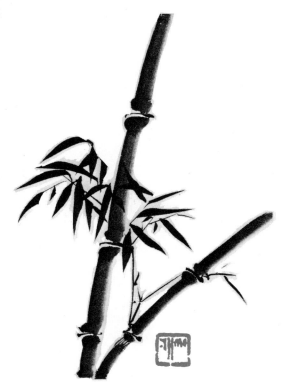

Multisystem Trauma

Cornelia Vanderstaay Kenner
Kathleen MacKay White

Because trauma nursing involves many of the traditional nursing roles, nurses need education and clinical experience in a variety of different settings: the emergency room, the operating room, the critical care unit, the intermediate care unit, the convalescent unit, the rehabilitative unit, and community health agencies. Trauma nurses working in any of those areas need to be cognizant of their own role on the health team and to develop expertise in their particular clinical focuses.

Trauma has become a great problem in health care delivery. Statistically, trauma is the fourth leading cause of death for people of all ages and the leading cause of death for those under the age of 38 [55]. Approximately 150,000 people die each year from trauma. If two or more organ systems are involved, the patient's chances of survival decrease. Disability and readjustment are of paramount importance since 20 percent of seriously injured patients have some degree of disability. Many of the people afflicted are in the prime of life, and most of them are young, between the ages of 20 and 40.

Objective

After synthesizing and analyzing the information in this chapter, the reader should be able to collect the appropriate information about the patient who has

34

had trauma, assess his injuries, make the nursing diagnoses, plan interventions for him, implement the plan, and evaluate his response to care.

Achieving the Objective

To achieve the objective, the nurse should be able to:

1. Identify the physiological mechanisms of shock.
2. Compare and contrast the low flow state due to pump failure with the low flow state due to hypovolemia.
3. Determine the priorities for a patient who is in clinical shock, make the nursing diagnosis, plan interventions for him, and evaluate his response to care.
4. Write a paragraph describing the changes that take place in blood while it is stored.
5. Assess the extent of injury of a patient who has had a gunshot wound.
6. Compare and contrast abdominal paracentesis and peritoneal lavage.
7. Compare and contrast the initial findings and the patient's clinical course in regard to the type of abdominal injury.
8. Assess and monitor a fractured extremity in a person who has had an associated nerve injury and in a person who has not.
9. Monitor preoperatively and postoperatively the patient who has a vascular injury.

How to Proceed

To develop an approach to multisystem trauma, the nurse should:

1. Read and analyze the material that follows.
2. Read the references for added information.
3. Analyze the case example. The nurse should:
   a. Outline the steps for assessing and managing the patient at the accident site, in the emergency room, and in the critical care unit.
   b. List the problems to be anticipated.
4. Gain clinical skills in all areas of trauma nursing.
5. While continuing to focus on direct observation of the patient himself, develop psychomotor skills in working with measurement techniques and treatment devices.
6. Participate in trauma patient rounds.
7. Assess areas of weakness. To gain knowledge in

trauma nursing, the nurse should select pertinent modules and audiovisual materials from the libraries of the hospital, the school of nursing, the American College of Surgeons, Emergency Department Nurses' Association, Society of Critical Care Medicine, and/or the American Association of Critical Care Nurses.
8. Perform clinical practice under direct supervision of a role model.

Case Study

Mr. T., a 28-year-old man, was admitted to the emergency room on an ambulance stretcher. He had been rabbit hunting, and while he was climbing over a fence, his .22-caliber rifle had discharged. The bullet struck his right thigh. During the trip to the hospital, the ambulance driver lost control of the vehicle, and the ambulance was in an accident.

According to Mr. T.'s wife, prior to the accidents, Mr. T. was in excellent health. He had not been drinking, nor had he taken any medications for 12 hours before his injury. She further said that after the ambulance accident, Mr. T. had complained of severe pain in his right thigh and moderate pain in his abdomen. She said that Mr. T. had no known allergies and that he had had his last tetanus booster about five years ago. Mrs. T. seemed to be a reliable informant.

The paramedics who had attended Mr. T. at the scene of the accident noted that he was pale, his skin was cool, his blood pressure was 90/60 mm Hg, his pulse was 120 and faint, and his respirations were 24 and nonlabored. Mr. T. was restless, and he complained of thirst and abdominal pain. Abdominal palpation revealed guarding. He had a profuse hematoma of his right thigh, a gaping wound on the lateral aspect of his right thigh, moderate, nonpulsatile bleeding, and obvious debris in the wound. Crepitation was noted over his right femur as an incidental finding, and the position and angulation of the thigh seemed abnormal. Mr. T. was oriented in regard to time, place, and person; he answered questions appropriately but somewhat irritably.

The paramedics treated Mr. T. immediately for shock, giving him Ringer's lactate solution. Before moving Mr. T., the paramedics stopped the bleeding in his thigh wound by direct pressure and a compression bandage. Stability of the femur was achieved by splinting the leg with minimal manipulation.

During his trip to the hospital, Mr. T. became apathetic. He complained of feeling exhausted and chilly, and then he became difficult to arouse. An oral airway was inserted during the trip.

Emergency Room Examination

The following observations were made during the emergency room examination:

1. General appearance: a well-developed, well-nourished man admitted on a stretcher.

2. Respiratory system: spontaneous breathing with an airway in place. Rate 28 and depth increased. Chest excursions symmetrical bilaterally. Breath sounds normal with no rales or wheezes.
3. Cardiovascular system: carotid pulse thready, regular, and 120. Radial and femoral pulses not palpable. Systolic blood pressure 80 (diastolic pressure was not obtainable). Capillary refill in nailbeds slow. Big toe was cool to touch. ECG showed sinus tachycardia but no dysrhythmias.
4. Neurological system: patient extremely difficult to arouse by verbal command. Pupils equal in size; reacted briskly with consensual response. Eye movements spontaneous and random. Painful stimuli applied to sternum evoked prompt avoidance response. No pathological reflexes present. Tendon reflexes 2+ in all extremities, except the right, which was deferred.
5. Gastrointestinal system: no penetrating injuries to abdomen. No abdominal distention. Bowel sounds absent. Gastric contents, obtained via nasogastric tube, negative for blood.
6. Integument and musculoskeletal system: skin cold, ashen to cyanotic; circulation response to pressure blanching very sluggish. Peripheral pulses imperceptible. Right thigh swollen; tissue about the open wound appeared crushed and nonviable. Wound grossly contaminated with cloth and dirt. Compound fracture of the femur in midportion of diaphysis.
7. Genitourinary system: genitalia appeared normal. Catheterization and urinalysis showed no hematuria.

Emergency Room Management

An oral airway remained in place. Mr. T. was appraised as being in hypovolemic shock. A large-bore (16-gauge) catheter was inserted into his right arm. The intravenous infusion into his left antecubital vein was continued. Blood samples were obtained for a complete blood count, electrolyte, glucose, urea, and amylase studies, and typing and crossmatching. A radial artery puncture was performed for arterial blood gas analysis.

Fluids were given rapidly (2 L of Ringer's lactate solution given in 45 minutes). Following the rapid infusion of fluids Mr. T. showed a transient improvement, as indicated by his improved sensorium (he responded to his name and to commands), a rise in blood pressure (to 100/60 mm Hg), and a decrease in pulse (to 100). No urine was obtained. During the improvement in Mr. T.'s hemodynamic state, the intactness of circulation to the right lower extremity was verified. His pedal pulses could be heard with the Doppler relative flow ultrasonic amplifier.

The results of bilateral peritoneal flank taps were negative for nonclotting blood. Consequently, a peritoneal lavage of 1 liter of Ringer's lactate solution was begun. The results were negative.

Mr. T.'s thigh wound was irrigated repeatedly with several liters of normal saline solution. Exploration of the wound,

ligation of vessels, and removal of foreign materials were postponed until the wound could be adequately inspected during surgery. Packing the wound with sterile gauze and applying hand pressure brought the bleeding under control. A Thomas splint was used to stabilize the femur during Mr. T.'s trip to the operating room.

As prophylaxis, Mr. T. was given 0.5 ml of tetanus toxoid booster and started on 2 gm of cephalothin sodium (to be given intravenously 6 times an hour). A Levine tube was placed.

Continued monitoring showed no urinary output. Mr. T.'s abdomen was not distended, and his bladder was not palpable. A new catheter was inserted, but urine was not recovered from his bladder. An intravenous pyelogram showed no excretion of contrast media from either kidney. Angiography confirmed the presence of bilateral renal artery thrombus secondary to disruption of the intima of the renal arteries.

Surgery

Exploratory surgery was carried out. It revealed bilateral renal artery thrombosis with no pulsations in the artery distal to the point of trauma. The area of intimal injury in the right renal artery was resected, and the renal artery was anastomosed. Pulsatile flow through the arterial tree was good. The traumatized area in the left renal artery was resected, and an incontinuity vein graft was inserted to bridge the defect. Pulsatile arterial flow was reestablished.

The thigh wound was incised and debrided widely, and the necrotic tissue was removed. Muscle tissue that was considered nonviable was also removed. Foreign material and blood clots were removed by irrigation to avoid a nidus for infection. The wound was left open to drain.

A Steinmann pin was inserted under strict aseptic conditions. Balanced surgical traction using a Thomas splint with a Pearson attachment and 25 pounds of weight was to be employed postoperatively to stabilize the fractured femur.

When Mr. T. arrived in the critical care unit, his vital signs were T97, P98, R18. His respirations were easy and even. He was awake, and his responses were appropriate. The arterial pressure monitor registered his blood pressure at 100/68. Analysis of an arterial blood sample taken from the radial artery catheter site showed PO_2 97 mm Hg, pH 7.41, PCO_2 39 mm Hg, and delta base +1. Mr. T.'s peripheral pulses were strong, and his urine was pink. He was receiving 1000 ml of Ringer's lactate solution and his fifth unit of whole blood was running (see assessment sheet).

Clinical Presentation of Case Study

Mr. T. remained in the critical care unit seven days, and then he was transferred to the orthopedic floor. He had no complications. His vital signs remained stable, he was alert, and his urinary output was normal. He began to eat and drink. Supplemental alimentation had been discussed, but it was not needed because his protein and calorie intake was satisfactory. Sepsis was identified as a potential problem, and the

Critical Care Nursing Admission Assessment
Major Systems Approach

PATIENT'S NAME: _Mr. J._   DATE: _8/16_   TIME: _4 p.m._

DIAGNOSIS: _Fractured femur_   Repair bilateral artery 2° thrombosis following MVA   T: _97_   A.P.: _98_   R.P.: _98_   R.: _18_
   2° MVA and gunshot wound

B.P.: _100/68_   E.C.G. RHYTHM: _NSR_   ECTOPY: ____   WT: _72 kg._   HT: _6'1"_

ADMITTED VIA: _stretcher_   INFORMANT: _patient/wife_   LAST MEAL: _8 am_

I. CHIEF COMPLAINT: _"Shot myself in the leg while hunting + ambulance had accident on the way to hospital"_

II. PATIENT PROFILE:
1. Age _28_   2. Sex _male_
3. Marital Status (M) W D S
4. Race _W_   5. Religion _Protestant_
6. Occupation _Farmer_
7. Availability of Family _Live on outskirts of city, transportation available_
8. Dietary _deferred_
9. Sleeping _deferred_
10. Activities of Daily Living _deferred_

III. HISTORY OF PRESENT ILLNESS: _Initial therapy for shock + injuries in E.R. Bilateral renal artery thrombosis noted on angiography. Taken to O.R. for resection + repair. Insertion of Steinmann pin to permit traction for fractured femur._

IV. PAST MEDICAL HISTORY:
1. Pediatric & Adult Illnesses _usual children's illnesses_
2. Cardiac
3. Hypertension
4. Respiratory _negative_
5. Diabetes Mellitus
6. Renal
7. Jaundice
8. Infections
9. Other
10. Hospitalizations & Surgeries _none_

11. Current Medication _none_

12. Allergies _none_

13. Habits _former smoker, 1 pack/d. for 5 yrs., stopped 2 yrs. ago_

V. FAMILY HISTORY: _Mother 58, Father 60 alive + well. One sister 30, alive + well_

VI. PSYCHOSOCIAL:
1. Behavior During Assessment _still not completely awake; cooperative_

2. Specific Problems _anxiety_

VII. PHYSICAL EXAMINATION:
1. General _well-developed man, balanced skeletal traction_

2. Respiratory System ____
Airway _patent_
Inspection _no abnormalities noted_

Rate _18_
Rhythm _regular in amplitude_
Chest Wall _intact_

Palpation _deferred_

Percussion _deferred_

Auscultation
Voice Sounds *no increased transmission*
Breath Sounds _____
Normal _____ Increased _____ Decreased *LLL* lobes
Adventitious Sounds *rales both bases*

3. Cardiovascular System
A.P. *98* R.P. *98*
B.P. Supine R _____ L *100/68*
P.M.I. *5th ICS* *MCL*
Heart Sounds *Normal S_1, S_2, Physiologic*
split of S_2 during inspiration
Thrills *none*
Peripheral Pulses *2^+*

4. Neurological System
Level of Consciousness *alert*

Respiratory Pattern *regular*

Cranial Nerves *deferred*

Eyes _____
(1) Pupils   OD   OS
Size *4 mm*   *4 mm*
Shape *round*   *round*
Light *react*   *react*
Consensual *react*   *react*
Accommodation *react*   *react*
(2) Ocular Movements *full movement*
range
Motor *R leg deferred, moves rest*
of body
Sensory *deferred*
Coordination *grossly assessed and*
intact
Reflexes *2^+ R patellar, Achilles and*
patellar deferred

5. Gastrointestinal System
Nose & Mouth *Levine tube in place*

Stomach *no bleeding*

Abdomen *deferred*

Bowel Sounds *hypoactive*
Liver *deferred*
Spleen *deferred*

6. Renal & Genitourinary Systems
I. _____ O. *30 ml/hr.*
Urinary Bladder & Urethra *deferred*

Kidneys *deferred*

7. Musculoskeletal System
Spine *no tenderness*
Extremities *R femur in skeletal*
traction

Sacral Edema *none*
Masses *none*

8. Hematologic System
Petechiae ⎫
Ecchymosis ⎬ *negative*
Gingiva ⎭

9. Endocrine System
Breath ⎫ *negative*
Skin ⎭

VIII. LABORATORY:
1. Hematology
HGB *15 gm. %* HCT *45 %*
W.B.C. *8400 / cu. mm.*
2. Chemistry
Na *142*   K *3.8*
CO_2 *24*   CL *100*
Blood Sugar *200* Amylase *< 320*
BUN *14*   Cr *0.8*
3. Urinalysis *to laboratory*

4. Electrocardiogram
Rate *98* Rhythm *NSR*
P-R *0.18* QRS *0.08* ST *0.12*
Interpretation *normal sinus Rhythm*
5. Chest x-ray *normal*

IX. PROBLEM LIST:
ACTIVE   INACTIVE
1. *Incomplete data base*
2. *Bilateral renal artery*
thrombosis $2°$ MVA
8/16 → resection + repair
bilateral renal arteries
3. *Fractured femur + soft tissue injury*
$2°$ GSW and MVA
→ insertion Steinmann pin + application
of balanced skeletal traction
4. *anxiety over hospitalization*

5. *Immobility*
6. *Pain*

NURSE'S SIGNATURE
Cornelia Kenner RN, CCRN

medical team gave meticulous wound care and was alert to the environmental factors that could produce wound contamination. Mr. T. was given the same attentive care on the orthopedic unit. Mr. T. and his family were receptive to all teaching programs, and they helped with several volunteer projects. Mr. T. was discharged six weeks after his injury.

Reflections

At the weekly trauma team conference, the possible dehumanization of the trauma patient was discussed. Particularly obvious to most participants was the depersonalization of care given in the emergency critical care setting. The emphasis was seen to be on action—action directed toward the patient's malfunctioning or damaged body parts or systems. Most nurses thought that the "action" approach was necessary because the situation was urgent. But there seemed to be a flagrant disregard for the patient's psychological needs. It was asked at the conference, does the obtunded or comatose patient have psychological needs?

Several of the nurses commented that all trauma patients were not obtunded, and all of the nurses could recall patients who had shown fear or even terror in the critical care setting. What effect, it was asked, does the behavior of the medical team have on the patient's physiological responses to trauma? For example, how are fear and anxiety translated into cardiovascular responses? Would it not be wiser, asked one nurse, if members of the trauma team substituted their banter and casual remarks for a manner that was more in keeping with the patient's anxieties? Could the patient's anxiety be decreased by the nurses' being aware of the effects of their behavior, including the way they touched their patients and the tone of voice they used with the patients? A view of the patient as more than a traumatized body gradually emerged from the conference.

A corollary was also realized. Many nurses came to see that their behavior was an expression of their own anxiety and that their feelings frequently mirrored the patient's feelings. Often, the more desperate the patient's situation, the more casual and flippant the nurses' behavior becomes. The nurses acknowledged that they had emotional reactions to emergencies and that they participated emotionally in the patients' crises. It was apparent that the nurses were not neutral participants in critical events despite the stereotype of the professional as a calm, detached, and dis-

passionate person. The nurses' feelings seemed to be a function of the patient's situation, just as the patient's response was a function of the nurses' collective professional skills.

The participants in the conference agreed that the critical care nurse must, above all, react immediately and skillfully to the patient's physical problems. But they began to see the interplay of action and feeling in the critical care setting as a complex mosaic in which more factors than those involved in technical skill were operative.

Hemorrhagic Shock

A succinct description of shock is difficult since so many factors interact in shock. One very good description is also a very simple one: shock is a low flow state with poor tissue perfusion. More specifically, shock is a clinical syndrome caused by an insufficient flow of blood to organs and tissues when the cardiac output is inadequate to maintain the volume of blood in the arterial vasculature under sufficient pressure to meet the body's demands [55]. Too little blood reaches the microvasculature, the circulatory system becomes less effective, and the low flow state results.

Classification

Basically, shock results from a defect in one or more of the following: the pump, the fluid pumped, the arterial vessels, and the venous bed capacity. The following classification of shock is based on the hemodynamic changes that occur in shock, and it is commonly used in clinical practice [53]:

1. Cardiogenic shock
   a. Pump failure
      (1) Coronary thrombosis
      (2) Cardiac dysrhythmias
      (3) Severe valvular disease
   b. Decreased venous inflow (decreased preload)
      (1) Mediastinal shift
      (2) Cardiac tamponade
      (3) Vena caval embolism or ligation
2. Volume decrease
   a. Whole blood loss
   b. Plasma volume loss
   c. Extracellular fluid loss

3. Changes in resistance of vessels
   a. Decrease in resistance
      (1) Spinal anesthesia
      (2) Neurogenic reflexes
      (3) Preterminal event in hypovolemic shock
   b. Septic shock
      (1) Change in peripheral resistance
      (2) Change in venous capacitance

The etiologic classification is extremely practical, because the patient may have a number of problems, and the principal cause of his shock may not be the most obvious problem (Table 34-1). For example, the patient who has been injured in a motor vehicle accident may be in shock not only from blood loss and inadequate volume but also from cardiac failure caused by tamponade.

Shock from volume decrease, or hypovolemia, may be caused by the body's loss of blood, plasma, or water. Blood loss may be external, as in a severe laceration, or internal, as in a pelvic fracture or a ruptured spleen. Plasma loss may be internal and external, as in a thermal injury, or internal, as in peritonitis. Water loss may be from water deprivation, in which electrolytes become concentrated in a decreased amount of body water or from the actual loss of water and electrolytes from the body, as in vomiting and diarrhea [53].

Hemorrhagic shock is a type of hypovolemic shock. It results from external or internal blood loss. External blood loss is a visible loss, and it can be measured. Common causes of external blood loss are severe lacerations, gunshot wounds, and stab wounds. Internal blood loss is a hidden loss, and it is difficult to quantitate. Common causes of internal blood loss are fractures, crushing injuries, and a ruptured spleen, liver, or vena cava. In an internal blood loss, serial assessments of the significant body parts and physiological parameters must be made so that a gross estimate of bleeding may be made.

Hemodynamics

In hemorrhagic shock, the volume of circulating blood is decreased to the extent that adequate tissue perfusion and oxygenation are no longer possible. Also, with insufficient intravascular volume to fill the heart, not enough blood leaves the heart. Cardiac output remains decreased since output depends in part on volume.

In essence, cardiac output and peripheral vascular resistance produce the arterial blood pressure. Thus the blood pressure is one indicator of cardiac output and peripheral vascular resistance. If cardiac output decreases, compensatory mechanisms raise peripheral vascular resistance so that the blood pressure remains normal. With hypotension and inadequate volume, the heart rate must increase in order to pump the same amount of blood. Stimulation of pressure receptors in the great vessels activates the autonomic nervous system and the adrenal medulla. The peripheral vasculature constricts, thus altering peripheral vascular resistance in such a way that the flow of blood containing oxygen and nutrients is increased to vital areas, such as the heart and brain.

Increased afterload, along with arteriolar and venular constriction, produces tachycardia, decreased venous capacitance, and increased ventricular contractility. Those secondary effects attempt to increase cardiac output. But if the cardiac output does not increase, the response is detrimental, and tissue ischemia and shock continue.

Multiorgan system failure occurs. First kidney failure occurs and last cerebral and cardiac failure occurs. Stagnation and hypoxia at the tissue level transform aerobic metabolic pathways to anaerobic ones. Increasing quantities of lactic acid are produced, the base bicarbonate level falls, acidosis progresses, and the serum potassium level increases to the point of diastolic cardiac arrest.

STAGES OF SHOCK

Hemodynamic changes produce several levels, or stages, of shock, namely, early, middle, and late shock (Table 34-2). During the early stage of shock, arterial blood pressure and cardiac output decrease,

Table 34-1
Clinical Picture Exhibited by Patient in Shock

	Pump Failure	Volume Decrease	Change in Resistance
Urinary output	↓	↓	Normal to ↓
Blood pressure	↓	↓	↓
Cardiac output	↓	↓	Normal to ↓ (early ↑)
Central venous pressure	↑	↓	Normal to ↓
Temperature	Normal	↓	↑ or ↓
Peripheral vascular resistance	↑	↑	↓

Table 34-2
Clinical Picture Exhibited by Patient According to Degree of Shock

	Early	Middle	Late
Sensorium	Oriented to time, place, person	Remains oriented; words slurred	Disoriented
Pulse	Rate, 110–120 Quality, full to decreased	Rate, 120–150 Quality, decreased and variable	Rate, greater than 150 Quality, weak
Blood pressure	Normal to low (10–20% decrease but may be slightly increased as compensatory mechanism)	Decreased 40–50 mm Hg below normal (20–40% decrease)	Systolic less than 80 Diastolic may not be heard
Urinary output	35–50 ml/hr	20–35 ml/hr	Less than 20 ml/hr
Color	Pale	Pale	Mottled
Capillary refill	Circulation return slightly slowed	Circulation return slowed	Circulation return very slowed; skin pale both before and after Large differences between rectal and big toe temperature

but they are restored to normal by the body's compensatory mechanisms. The early stage of shock is characterized by increased cardiac activity. In the middle stage of shock, the compensatory mechanisms are no longer effective, and extrinsic support must be given. The middle stage is characterized by increased cardiac activity that tends to progress to a stage in which myocardial contractile function is depressed. In the late (sometimes called irreversible) stage, compensatory mechanisms are nonexistent, and total failure of the body systems is imminent.

Early cardiac failure is manifested by the development of a decreased mean arterial pressure without a change in cardiac output in the face of an elevated central venous pressure. Failure of the cardiovascular system produces low cardiac output, peripheral pooling of blood, minimal tissue perfusion, the translocation of protein into the extracellular extravascular spaces, and metabolic alterations.

Mechanism of Fluid Change

The work of Shires and his associates [56] on resuscitation with Ringer's lactate solution has revolutionized the treatment of hemorrhagic shock. Initially, their research recognized that despite blood replacement, many people in clinical shock died and that many of those who lived had damaged kidneys

and even renal failure. Investigations were made of several aspects of the extracellular fluid (ECF) and the actual mechanism operating at the cellular level.

Early in their studies, Shires and his associates noted that the extracellular fluid volume loss was greater than anticipated. They postulated that the mechanism for the extracellular fluid loss included a tremendous shift of sodium and water into the intracellular compartment. In such a shift, the cell membrane loses its integrity in that the membrane potential decreases markedly and the sodium pump is no longer efficient [62]. Normal concentrations of sodium and potassium are altered, and significant increases occur in the intracellular sodium and extracellular potassium levels. In essence, the cell becomes leaky, and protein moves into the cell, resulting in increased oncotic pressure and intracellular swelling. The water in the intracellular compartment rises, but the total body water remains the same. An internal shift redistributes, or translocates, extracellular fluid into the intracellular compartment.

Later, the results of successful studies were utilized in the management of patients who were transferred to the trauma facility in hemorrhagic shock. Their treatment centered on the administration of Ringer's lactate solution as well as of whole blood. The use of a balanced salt solution and blood returned the extravascular space to normal and significantly decreased the incidence of renal failure.

Deficiency of Adenosine Triphosphate

Since the breakthrough of Shires and his associates, many other researchers have sought to explain the complex systemic interrelationships. Cellular alterations are varied, interrelated, and progressive. In tissues that are not well perfused with oxygen and are without adequate substrates, changes occur in the energy pathways. Intracellular and extracellular levels of lactate rise since not enough oxygen is present to oxidize lactate to carbon dioxide and water. Rather, anaerobic pathways produce large quantities of lactic acid and little adenosine triphosphate (ATP).

The work of Baue and his associates [9, 10] with the experimental shock model in the awake, bled rat demonstrated a deficiency of ATP within the cell and the reversal of mortality in hemorrhagic shock with the administration of ATP. Treatment seemed to correct the intracellular accumulation of sodium and water. Significantly, the fact that intracellular concentrations of ATP may be brought to levels three times greater than normal shows that ATP does cross the cell membrane.

A mechanism that begins with alteration at the cellular membrane and a decrease in the membrane potential has been proposed. The sequence is as follows: intracellular sodium and extracellular potassium rise, sodium and potassium ATPase is activated, ATP is utilized, and stimulation of the mitochondria is followed by a decrease in cyclic adenosine monophosphate (AMP). Concomitant with the decrease in cyclic AMP are (1) a change in the insulin response, (2) changes in the end results of many hormones, (3) a further decrease in metabolic capability, (4) a decreased production of ATP, and (5) the breakdown of lysosomes [34]. Eventually, as the process continues, sodium enters the mitochondria, the ATP levels are reduced, and swelling occurs in the mitochondria, endoplasmic reticulum, and the cell in general.

Fluid and Electrolyte Abnormalities

Predictably, fluid and electrolyte abnormalities persist for extended periods of time. Randall [43] measured total mean body mass in hemorrhagic shocked dogs and showed increases in sodium and water with decreases in potassium intracellularly for five-day periods and longer. In severely stressed patients who had undergone elective surgery, sodium and water levels in the intracellular spaces were shown by muscle biopsy to be increased for 10 to 20 days after surgery [22].

Antidiuretic hormone (ADH) acts to increase the retention of free water by the kidney. The actual mechanism by which ADH increases permeability to water in the distal convoluted tubule and collecting ducts is not understood. One theory is that ADH increases the diameter and/or the number of pores in an area of the cell membrane (not in the total area available for diffusion). By osmosis, the water flows through the pores and into the extracellular fluid of the renal medulla that is hypertonic because of the countercurrent mechanism active in the loop of Henle. Thus the intratubular fluid is no longer as hypotonic as it was following the active transport of solute out of the ascending limb of the loop, but it has the same osmotic concentration as the extracellular space. Systemic absorption is completed by the blood's flowing through the vasa recta. The stimuli primarily responsible for ADH secretion are decreased vascular volume and increased plasma osmolarity. When the effective vascular volume diminishes, decreases in arterial pressure or central venous pressure stimulate receptors, which, in turn, transmit impulses to the central nervous system and produce the release of ADH. Further loss of volume in the urine is prevented by the increased water absorption produced by ADH. When the osmolarity or concentration of solute in the plasma is increased by even a small percentage, osmoreceptors near the supraoptic nuclei induce the release of ADH. The free water resorbed decreases the osmolarity (dilutes the solutes in the plasma). In both processes, inhibition is by a feedback system.

The corticosteroids also play a part in the retention of sodium and water. The most important mineralocorticoid is aldosterone. Resorption of sodium into the extracellular fluid is stimulated. The process is governed to a large extent by angiotensin II, which stimulates the zona glomerulosa of the adrenal gland to synthesize and release aldosterone. Although the effects of aldosterone appear relatively slowly and do not peak for several hours, a fine control is exerted over extracellular fluid volume and potassium secretion. Every resorbing epithelium in the body responds to the hormone. Because sodium, accompanied by water and anions, is resorbed and not lost, extracellular osmolality and hence volume are maintained. Acid-base balance and potassium metabolism are affected by the hormone in the distal tubule. The magnitude of potassium secretion depends on sodium resorption since potassium moves passively into the tubular fluid according to the electrochemical potential gradient. When large amounts of aldosterone are present, sodium resorption in the distal tubule is stimulated and potassium is excreted. Partially through exchange of potassium and hydrogen ions in the tubule, sodium is retained, resulting in decreased serum levels of potassium and hydrogen. Logically, urinary sodium levels decrease and urinary potassium and hydrogen ion levels increase (Chap. 32). Those changes produce a change—the decrease in the ratio of urinary sodium to urinary potassium—that is often used as a clinical indicator. The process leads to metabolic alkalosis since increased acidification of the urine results from both hypokalemia and a specific but unidentified effect of aldosterone on the tubular acidification mechanisms [38].

Assessment and Management

The presence of the low flow state is evidenced by decreased mentation and urinary output, increased pulse, peripheral vasoconstriction, cool clammy skin, decreased cardiac output and blood pressure, and metabolic acidosis. The administration of Ringer's lactate solution, besides being a therapeutic measure, is a clinical means to assess the preexisting degree of blood loss [56]. The solution is administered at a rapid rate so that in a period of 30 min 1000 to 2000 ml has been given intravenously.

Three classical responses to Ringer's lactate infusion have been described [53]. With less than 10% volume loss without continued loss, the blood pressure returns to normal after 1 to 2 liters, and it stabilizes even if the patient initially had marked hypotension. If correlated with measurements of the blood volume, the degree of preexisting blood loss would be shown to be relatively minimal. With severe blood loss and continuing hemorrhage, the response in vital signs (with elevation of blood pressure and decrease in pulse) following rapid intravenous infusion is transient. Whole blood that has been typed and crossmatched is administered. With patients who do not respond to the initial 1 to 2 liters of Ringer's lactate solution, uncrossmatched type O, Rh negative or type-specific blood is administered. In that group of

patients, the prognosis is poor unless immediate surgical intervention can correct the problem.

Intravenous infusions should be started in at least two extremities with large-bore catheters or needles. Shires [55] warns that in the presence of an abdominal vascular injury, fluids given in the legs may enter the peritoneal cavity and so would not be available to increase the circulating blood volume. Additional volume support may be gained by elevating the legs at a 45-degree angle. (The deep Trendelenburg position is not recommended because it interferes with respiratory exchange; it is beneficial only in neurogenic shock.)

Because the composition of Ringer's lactate solution is close to that of the extracellular fluid, it is called a balanced salt solution or an extracellular fluid mimic. The ratio of lactate to chloride is 28:109. More bicarbonate need not be administered since the lactate is rapidly converted to bicarbonate [54]. There is a slight difference in the sodium concentration; the sodium in Ringer's lactate solution is 130 mEq per liter and the sodium in the extracellular fluid is 140 mEq per liter. The concentrations of potassium and calcium are the same (potassium is 4 mEq/L, and calcium is 3 mEq/L).

After the initial period, accurate monitoring of oxygenation, organ perfusion, and hemodynamic status is imperative in order to determine trends and assess the patient's changing status. (The monitoring is described in Chapter 36.)

Blood Replacement

Replacement of the blood that was lost may be life saving. Although whole blood is often needed, fractionalization or component therapy is used for specific purposes, and it is standard practice in trauma centers. Transfusions may take any of the following common forms: whole blood, packed red cells, platelet concentrates, cryoprecipitate, single-donor fresh or fresh-frozen plasma, single-donor aged plasma, and leukocyte preparations (leukocyte-poor red cells or leukocyte-rich preparations).

The main purpose of administering whole blood is to increase oxygen delivery at the tissue level, particularly in the patient who is hemorrhaging massively. Since the oxygen content of arterial blood depends on the hemoglobin concentration, increasing the hemoglobin is vastly superior to administering oxygen in regard to transporting oxygen to the tissue level. Tissue function is closer to normal when the hematocrit is kept above 35 percent. A marked increase in blood loss and defective coagulation at the operative site have occurred in patients whose hematocrits are below 20 percent.

The use of blood filters to remove particulate matter is an accepted practice in the critical care unit. Blood contains several hundred thousand microaggregates of various sizes that could obstruct the microcirculation and impair the functioning of the heart, kidneys, liver, brain, and lungs. (Although microaggregates have been commonly considered causative factors in the adult respiratory distress syndrome, that idea is being questioned.) The nylon mesh filter seems the most effective one [58]. When it is used (one filter may be used for one to three pints of whole blood), aggregates of 8 μm to 50 μm in size are filtered without an alteration in perfusion pressure.

STORED BLOOD

Potassium levels increase proportionately with the age of the blood (30–40 mEq/L in 3-week-old blood), making hyperkalemia a potential problem. In an acidotic patient who has renal impairment, the potassium increase could lead to a fatal dysrhythmia. In rare instances, rapid transfusion into an acidotic patient may require alkalinization.

Many authorities recommend the use of calcium for counteracting the effect of the citrate used in bank blood. (The reduced calcium, bound by the citrate, augments the effects of hyperkalemia on the myocardium.) Other authorities think that citrate intoxication does not occur at transfusion rates below 1 unit of blood every 5 minutes in an adult whose circulation is intact and whose liver is functioning.

In patients who have hepatic insufficiency, the ammonia increase in aged blood may precipitate hepatic coma. In those patients, the administration of aged blood must be avoided.

Platelets are significantly affected by storage. If blood is transfused within 6 hours of donation, the platelets are viable. But the platelets' function is severely impaired after only a few minutes of refrigeration. From 6 to 48 hours after donation, the blood may be used in thrombocytopenia associated with massive transfusions (a single transfusion of more than 2500 ml or a number of transfusions that total 5000 ml or more in a 24-hour period), but the use of platelet concentrates is the preferred approach. In general, the greater the amount of whole blood transfused, the greater the platelet deficit in both function and quantity. In the traumatized patient, two other factors that affect the platelets are present. Tissue trauma and shock increase the platelet consumption and, in the hemorrhaging patient, massive transfusions may produce a dilutional thrombocytopenia.

LEFT SHIFT OF THE OXYHEMOGLOBIN DISSOCIATION CURVE

A shift of the oxygen dissociation curve to the left is particularly significant in decreasing the oxygen available at the tissue level. In such a shift, the transfusion of stored blood is a primary culprit (see Chaps. 17 and 36).

The ability of the red blood cells to accept and release oxygen is controlled by 2,3-diphosphoglycerate (2,3-DPG), a glycolytic intermediate and the most abundant phosphate in the cell. Reduced hemoglobin preferentially binds 2,3-DPG and so markedly lowers its own affinity for oxygen. The red cell glycolytic rate, the concentrations of 2,3-DPG and ATP, red cell survival, and the delivery of oxygen are interdependent.

Blood stored in an acid medium has red blood cells that are low in 2,3-DPG. The transfusion of large volumes of those cells into the patient significantly increases the affinity of hemoglobin for oxygen. For that reason, the recommended preservative for blood is citrate-phosphate-dextrose (CPD), not acid-citrate-dextrose (ACD). The pH of blood stored in ACD is 7; in approximately 21 days it decreases to 6.6. By the end of only one day, the levels of 2,3-DPG have decreased by 50% and by the end of five days they have dropped to insignificant amounts. The pH of blood stored in CPD is 7.2 (since the amount of citrate is lower); in approximately 28 days it decreases to 6.8. The levels of 2,3-DPG are considered satisfactory for oxygen delivery at the tissue level for about seven days.

Although the initial pH is higher and deterioration is slower in CPD-stored blood, the levels of 2,3-DPG diminish and produce a left shift in transfused patients. Nine-day-old blood is considered deficient in 2,3-DPG. When it is used for transfusions, correction of the cellular deficiency takes 24 hours. Thus in the hemorrhaging patient, a ratio of 1:2 is preferred; that is, for every two pints of blood that are older than nine days, one pint that is less than two days old should be transfused.

BLEEDING DIATHESIS

Multiple clotting defects induced by massive transfusions, trauma, and complications may produce an uncontrollable bleeding. The danger increases with each unit of blood administered. In particular, a bleeding diathesis may be produced when platelets and clotting factors are reduced by 70 percent or after the replacement of approximately 5 liters of blood.

Intravascular hemolysis, a life-threatening complication of blood transfusions, usually results from incompatibilities involving the ABO blood-group system. Since the hemolyzed donor red blood cells release hemoglobin into the plasma, the plasma is tinted a reddish pink. Haptoglobin, a plasma protein of the albumin type, is able to bind 125 to 150 mg of free hemoglobin per 100 ml of plasma. Bound hemoglobin is not filtered into the urine. However, if large amounts of hemoglobin are released as a result of the hemolysis of many red blood cells, the hemoglobin-binding capacity of haptoglobin is exceeded, and free hemoglobin is filtered into the urine, turning the urine red or pink. If the urine is acid or if the hemoglobin has been in the plasma for longer than 24 hours, the iron in the hemoglobin is oxidized from the ferrous state to the ferric state, or, in other words, from hemoglobin to methemoglobin. Since methemoglobin is brown, the urine is a brownish color.

Ballistics

Patients who have been critically injured by gunshot wounds present special challenges in assessment and management. Evaluating the extent of the injury can be very difficult. Some wounds are small, punctate, clean, and nonbleeding, and others are large, gaping, grossly contaminated, and hemorrhagic. Some look relatively benign on the outside although the internal damage is extensive. Others look extensive on the outside but in fact affect only the superficial tissues and a small amount of muscle mass. A number of factors, including the missile ballistics, tissue characteristics, type of weapon used, distance from the weapon at time of wounding, and characteristics of the injuring missile, determine the extent of injury. The nurse who understands those factors is better equipped to evaluate the extent of injury, understand the treatment, and anticipate the patient's problems.

Mechanisms

The extent to which a missile creates injury depends on the occurrence of any combination of three wounding mechanisms [14]:

1. Laceration
2. Tissue disruption (cavity formation by mechanical shock waves)
3. Muzzle blast (tissue and bone destruction by burning and expanding gases)

LACERATION

Laceration is the result of penetration and the severance of tissue by a sharp, moving object. The severity of the damage is related to what structures have been transected. Impairment of major blood vessels and spinal cord transection are examples of lethal injuries that can result from laceration. Another complication is that damage occurs in more than just one structure. The organs and vessels that lie in the missile's path are affected by forward movement of the missile as it cuts its path. Figure 34-1 illustrates the many injuries that can result from only one missile.

TISSUE DISRUPTION

Another mechanism of missile injury is the tissue disruption that results from the missile's kinetic energy. Research done during World War II found that the severity of a gunshot wound is directly related to the amount of kinetic energy expended by the bullet in the tissue. The greater the kinetic energy lost by the bullet in the tissue, the greater the amount of tissue damaged. That phenomenon of transmission of energy from the missile to the tissue can best be illustrated by observing a propelled object striking a stationary object. An example is what happens when a billiard cue ball (a missile) that has been set in motion by a cue stick (a weapon) hits an eight ball (a tissue). The cue ball stops, and the eight ball, having received the cue ball's kinetic energy, is set in motion. That is what happens mechanically to tissue when the kinetic energy of a missile is transmitted: the tissue is set in motion.

Experiments performed with blocks of gelatin used

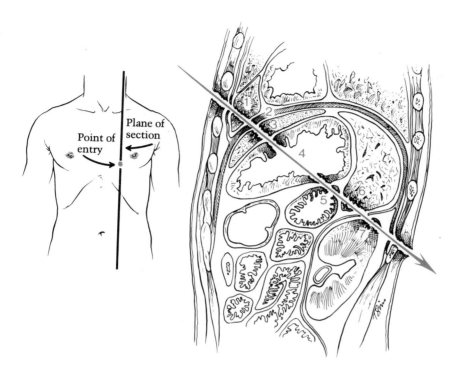

Figure 34-1
Left parasagittal section showing a multiorgan injury produced by one bullet. (1) Lung, (2) diaphragm, (3) liver, (4) stomach, (5) jejunum, (6) spleen, (7) kidney.

to simulate human tissue have shown how kinetic energy affects the surrounding tissue. As the missile penetrates, it produces a permanent wound tract and temporary displacement of the tissue away from the tract. The phenomenon has often been described as a shock wave that surrounds the missile path and radiates from it. A temporary cavity is created that may be much larger than the missile's path; the size depends on how much kinetic energy the missile had to begin with and how much of it was transmitted to the tissue [28]. The volume of the temporary cavity may be as much as 30 times the volume of the missile, and the pressure exerted against the walls of the cavity may be as much as 100 times atmospheric pressure. Although the lifetime of the cavity is only 5 to 10 msec, the rapid, forceful expansion of the cavity can damage muscle, injure nerves, rupture blood vessels, and fracture bone, even when those structures

may have been in a position outside the direct path of the bullet. Furthermore, the pressure of the cavity itself is subatmospheric, allowing air and any contaminants in the air to be drawn into the depths of the cavity and finally contaminate the whole of the missile tract.

Kinetic Energy
Since the amount of cavitation is directly related to the amount of kinetic energy transmitted to the tissue, the extent of injury can be assessed by estimating the amount of kinetic energy expended by the wounding missile. The kinetic energy (KE) is defined as

$$KE = \frac{1}{2} mv^2$$

where KE is kinetic energy
     m is mass
      v is velocity

Thus the kinetic energy of a missile is proportional to the product of its mass and the square of its velocity. As the energy formula shows, velocity is the more important determinant of kinetic energy. Thus if two missiles have the same velocity but one has twice the mass of the other, the more massive missile has twice as much kinetic energy. But if two missiles have the same mass but one has twice the velocity of the other, the faster missile has four times more kinetic energy.

The energy formula is illustrated by the following example for the .22 short bullet (the .22 short is the smallest handgun bullet made and is fired from a .22 caliber gun, the barrel of which is .22 inch in diameter).

Given:

1. $\text{Mass} = \dfrac{\text{weight (lb)}}{\text{acceleration of gravity (ft/sec}^2)}$

2. 1 lb = 7000 grains
3. Acceleration of gravity = 32.2 ft/sec²
4. Weight of .22 short = 29 grains
5. Velocity of .22 short = 1045 ft/sec

Therefore:

The mass of a .22 short is

$$= \frac{29 \text{ grains}}{7000 \text{ grains}} \times \frac{1}{32.2 \text{ ft/sec}^2}$$

$$= 1.2866 \times 10^{-4} \text{ lb/ft/sec}^2$$

The kinetic energy of a .22 short is

$$KE = \tfrac{1}{2} \, MV^2$$

$$= \tfrac{1}{2} \, (1.2866 \times 10^{-4} \frac{\text{lb-sec}^2}{\text{ft}})(1045)^2$$

$$= \tfrac{1}{2} \, (1.286 \times 10^{-4}) \, (1.09203 \times 10^6)$$

$$= 70 \text{ ft-lb}$$

The principle of energy transmission from missile to tissue also accounts for the variety of bullet designs. A bullet that merely passes through and through, only severing as it goes, transmits very little energy to the tissue. To be able to transmit its energy and thus inflict greater damage, the missile must slow down dramatically or stop in the tissue. Various bullet designs have been made with that end in mind. For example, bullets with a hollow-point nose expand in a mushroom effect while passing through the tissues. This flattening out of the bullet causes it to slow down in the tissue and give up greater amounts of its kinetic energy to the tissue. Soft-nosed and flat-nosed bullets undergo a similar effect when passing through the tissues.

Besides the mushrooming effect some bullets have, two other factors tend to slow down and/or stop a missile in the tissue, thus causing an increased loss of energy and greater damage due to cavity formation:

1. The bullet's angle of yaw at the time it hits the body. Yaw is the deviation or deflection of the nose of the bullet from its straight, "nose first" line of flight. Instead of striking the body nose first, the bullet strikes the body at an angle. The greater the angle of yaw, the more the bullet is retarded and the more kinetic energy is lost to the tissue.
2. The density of the tissue. The greater the density of the tissue the bullet passes through, the more the bullet is retarded and the more kinetic energy is lost to the tissue. The size of the temporary cavity depends on the specific gravity of the tissue and its cohesiveness and elasticity. Those two properties tend to counteract the expansion of the wound tract. Thus tissues that are more cohesive and more elastic have greater resistance to injury. For example, although the energy absorbed by both the liver and muscle tissue may be essentially identical, the temporary cavity and the resultant permanent wound tract are larger in the liver than in the muscle tissue [35].

The principle of greater speed for greater injury is the basis of the magnum handguns [15]. The .357 and the .44 magnum bullet have essentially the same caliber as the .38 special bullet and the .45 automatic bullet, respectively. The difference is in the kinetic energy. The magnum bullet contains much more gunpowder, which propels the bullet at a much greater speed, thus capitalizing on the velocity advantage shown in the kinetic energy formula. (The kinetic energy of various types of handguns is shown in Table 34-3.) Cavity formation and tissue destruction by a magnum bullet are obviously greater than those inflicted by the regular .38 or .45 bullet.

To better understand the effect of a high-speed bullet, one should look at injuries produced by a high-powered rifle instead of those produced by hand-

Table 34-3
Kinetic Energy of Selected Handgun and Rifle Bullets

Bullet	Weight (grains)	Muzzle Velocity (ft/sec)	Muzzle Energy (ft-lb)
Handgun			
.22 short	29	1,045	70
.25 automatic	50	810	73
.357 magnum	158	1,410	695
.38 special	158	855	256
.44 magnum	240	1,470	1,150
.45 ACP	230	850	370
Rifle			
222 Remington	55	3,020	1,114
243 Remington	100	2,960	1,945
30-30 Winchester	150	2,390	1,902
30-06 Springfield	150	2,920	2,839
308 Winchester	150	2,820	2,648

guns [68]. Although magnums cause greater injury because of their greater bullet speed, the increase over other handguns is very small compared to the relative speed of high-powered rifles. The dramatic difference between the speed and kinetic energy of handgun bullets and the speed and kinetic energy of high-powered rifle bullets can be seen in Table 34-3.

The size of the temporary cavity produced by a high-velocity missile can be grasped if one considers the destruction caused by a 150-grain bullet. A bullet with an impact velocity of 2500 ft per sec perforates an 8-inch thigh and exits at a velocity of 1500 ft per sec. During its travel through the tissue, the bullet will have expended 1331 foot pounds of energy ($.5 [150/7000] \times 1/32.2 [2500^2 - 1500^2] = 1331$ ft-lb), creating a temporary cavity with a maximum diameter of 12 to 15 in. That explains why nerves, vessels, and bones that are distant from the bullet's path may be injured. In fact, a many-times-lethal injury may occur even to structures that are remote to the bullet's path [16].

High-velocity missile wounds of the head are often extremely destructive owing to the pressure that develops in the skull when a temporary cavity forms. The skull is a closed, rigid structure, and it cannot yield to the large, expanding temporary cavity. The high pressures produced by the cavity are relieved only by the skull's giving up its bony continuity.

MUZZLE BLAST

A third mechanism of wounding is muzzle blast, the cloud of hot gas and burning powder present at the muzzle immediately after firing and extending outward 1 to 3 feet. Although muzzle blast is a factor in tissue injury only when the gun is in physical contact with the skin, massive and lethal injury can be produced after the gas enters the wound made by a shotgun. Once inside the body, the gas and powder continue to expand and burn, causing a severe injury by "internal explosion." If the shotgun wound is to the head, a wound similar to the massive bursting open characteristic of high-powered rifle injuries results, not from the cavity formation but from the combustion of the powder inside the rigid skull and the rapid, forceful expansion of the gases. Most of the victims of that type of injury are not taken to the hospital because the wound is instantly fatal. Internal combustion does not occur in contact wounds inflicted by handguns because the amount of gas is less, and the wound is too small to permit entry. Instead, the gas is trapped between the bone and skin, and it expands making the skin balloon out away from the bone. If the elasticity of the skin is exceeded, a stellate tear of the skin is produced.

When the contact wound is not over bone, the subcutaneous tissues are able to yield sufficiently and a stellate tear does not occur.

Shotguns

Shotguns have characteristics that distinguish them from handguns and rifles. Although shotgun shells, like handgun bullets, are fired at a relatively low velocity, the shotgun "bullet" is actually a shell containing many round lead pellets instead of a single slug. Those pellets are designed to form a dense pattern to greatly enhance the hunter's chance of hitting small game with one firing. The pellets (Fig. 34-2) usually range in size from .08 in. in diameter (for the No. 9 shot) to .33 in. (for the 00 buckshot). The shell may contain anywhere from 200 small pellets to nine pellets (in 00 buckshot); the number depends on the size of the pellets and the gauge of the gun. An obvious danger of a shotgun blast is that one shell contains many pellets, or many individual missiles. It has been observed that being shot once with a shotgun that takes 00 shot can be the same as being shot nine times with a .32 caliber handgun.

Besides the pellets, the shell contains gunpowder and a plastic or paper wad that separates the powder from the pellets. When the shotgun is fired, the powder does not explode or detonate; rather it burns with

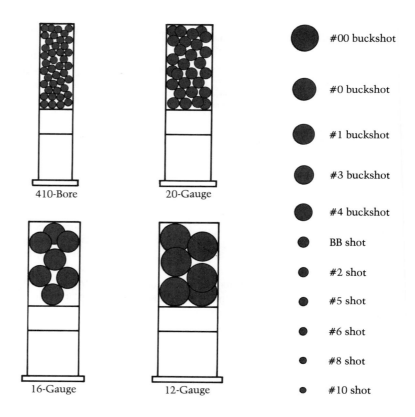

Figure 34-2

Structure of shotgun shells with various gauge and pellet loads. The gauge of a shotgun is determined by how many barrel-sized lead balls it takes to make a pound. For example, it takes 20 balls the size of a 20-gauge shotgun barrel to weigh a pound. Similarly, it takes only 12 balls the size of a 12-gauge shotgun to weigh a pound.

great speed, creating an expanding volume of hot gas to drive the wad and pellets forward (without the wad, the hot gases would melt and deform the pellets). Since the wad is heavy and flat, it quickly loses momentum in the air and falls to the ground about 6 ft from the end of the shotgun barrel. The pellets, meanwhile, are ejected out the end of the barrel in a pattern that initially is dense but that gradually widens the farther the pellets travel from the gun.

The extent of injury produced by shotgun pellets depends in large part on the distance from the weapon at the time of wounding [45]. At less than 6 ft, all combinations of shotgun shells and gauges produce a tight, dense pattern. Damage is extensive, with pulverizing and crushing of the tissues, since the pellets hit the body almost like a single mass. At 3 to 6 feet, the single entrance wound is 1.5 to 2 in. in diameter, and it shows "scalloping" of the edges. At distances closer than 12 in. and with contact wounds, the single round entrance wound is 0.75 to 2 in. in diameter. Extensive contamination occurs because shotgun wadding, bits of clothing, skin, hair, and burning and un-

burnt powder are driven into the wound. Not until the distance is greater than 8 to 10 yd do the pellets separate from the main mass and produce the characteristic speckled appearance of a shotgun wound. The damage that occurs then is more the result of the mass and velocity of each individual pellet. Since the pellets are round, they are not particularly efficient in retaining speed and energy over extended ranges. At 40 yd, the shot has lost more than 50 percent of its original energy. The greater the distance, the less likely it is that any one pellet will do extensive damage by itself [17].

If the distance is close, the wad may contribute to the wounding. In contact wounds, the wad is propelled into the body through the large single entrance wound. If the distance is more than 10 to 15 ft, the wad will have separated from the pellets and will not enter the body. But it may mark the body or leave an impression on the skin before it falls to the ground.

Assessment

Nurses who understand the mechanisms of missile wounding and the variables that determine the extent of injury are better equipped to assess the patients' wounds. The following approach indicates the direction of and the priorities in the assessment.

If possible, it should be determined what type of weapon was used. If a high-velocity hunting rifle was used, the internal injury is much more extensive than if a handgun has been used. A person wounded by a .45 caliber bullet that has a hollow-point design probably has a more extensive internal wound than does the person injured by the lower-powered, solid-point .22 caliber handgun, the type commonly used in domestic arguments [23].

Injury to major vessels by any missile, large or small, slow or fast, may produce profound levels of shock due to blood loss. The patient's blood pressure should be determined immediately. Systolic pressures of less than 80 that do not respond to the rapid administration of 2000 ml of blood indicate that 30% of the total blood volume has been lost and that immediate operative intervention is required [27].

If possible, the examiner should locate both the entrance and the exit wounds and plot mentally the structures that lie between those two points. That will indicate the complications to be anticipated and the steps that may be taken by the physician. If there is no obvious exit wound, the examiner should palpate for the missile. Often it is found to lie subcutaneously, having spent its energy before exiting. The examiner should beware of wounds that have no exit; those wounds have received all the energy the missile could transmit.

To assess the degree of neurovascular involvement in wounds of the extremities, the examiner should test for neurovascular deficits distal to the injury. Damage to the peripheral nerves is indicated by sensory loss (failure to respond to a pinprick stimulus) and by motor loss (inability to move the extremities on command). Injury to specific nerves may be determined by localizing the areas of sensory and motor loss.

Vascular compromise in a wounded extremity may be assessed by a number of methods. The examiner should:

1. Observe the extremity closely for cyanosis or mottling.
2. Feel the extremity for coolness, especially compared to the uninjured extremity.
3. Palpate the extremity for the major pulses, noting their quality and force.
4. Test the capillary refill by pinching the nailbed and noting any delay in the return of color.
5. Test for loss of sensation.

Abdominal Trauma

Trauma to the structures in the abdomen can occur in car accidents, gunshot and knife wounds, falls, or forceful types of physical contact (e.g., in sports or in fist fights). The wounds are managed according to their general category, that is, whether they are blunt wounds or penetrating wounds. The reason for the distinction is that blunt trauma is often accompanied by associated injuries that may complicate both making the diagnosis and (because the abdominal wall is intact) identifying what organs are involved.

In blunt trauma, an exploratory laparotomy and search for the injured organ seems the simple solution. But exploratory laparotomy, which is relatively safe for a healthy person, may be extremely risky for the patient who has multiple injuries [26]. If abdominal trauma is suspected in such a patient, the physician carefully weighs the risks of operating against the risks of not operating. The patient should not be subjected routinely to the risks of operating.

With penetrating injuries there are usually no associated head or chest injuries and therefore few or no decisions to be made about operating. Laparotomy is generally the treatment of choice. With stab wounds, the situation is different. Because the results of an exploratory laparotomy done routinely in stab wounds are often negative, the patient is carefully and thoroughly assessed before surgery is performed.

The nurse who has cared for a patient who had multiple abdominal injuries and who then developed complications probably knows how frustrating those injuries can be in regard to nursing care and the patient's recovery. Probably the most notable feature of abdominal trauma is that it can be extremely difficult to detect, identify, and manage [18]. The reasons are multiple:

1. Injuries to the abdominal structures subject the patient not only to hemorrhage and/or organ death but also to the release into the peritoneal cavity of potent digestive enzymes which produce additional injury by digesting the neighboring organs.
2. The virulent bacterial contents of the bowel may be spilled into the peritoneal cavity, thus subjecting even the uninjured structures to bacterial invasion and cell death. Sepsis is a particular danger when that occurs [67].
3. The release of some organ excretions, even ones that are not enzymatic, may result in collections of fluid that provide excellent culture media for the development of abcesses.
4. Abdominal trauma involves the loss of the patient's digestive functions and, depending on the severity, may result in prolonged starvation and delayed wound healing due to malnutrition and/or a continued catabolic state.

Some abdominal organs are more likely than others to be injured; the frequency depends largely on how the injury was produced and on the location of the injured organ. A series by Griswold and Colliet [33] has determined the following incidence of organ injury in abdominal trauma:

Spleen	26.0%
Kidneys	24.0%
Intestines	16.0%
Liver	15.0%
Pancreas	1.4%
Diaphragm	1.1%

The spleen, kidney, intestines, and liver are injured more often because they are close to the abdominal wall. The pancreas is well protected by the stomach, intestines, and diaphragm, and so it is injured much less often. The intestines may be injured by blunt injury; for example, in an automobile accident the steering wheel may compress the bowel against the vertebral column with the result that a loop of intestine is first closed off and then ruptured by the forceful, continued compression. Sudden elevation of the intraperitoneal pressure due to fixation of the lower half of the torso with a lap seat belt may contribute to the mechanism just described [12].

Indriven fractures are also notorious for injuring certain organs, with the spleen vulnerable to a left lower rib fracture, the liver to a right lower rib fracture, the kidney to a posterior floating rib fracture, and the bladder to a pelvic fracture. A patient who has one or more of those fractures should be carefully evaluated; a force strong enough to produce a fracture is strong enough to produce an intraabdominal injury.

Deceleration forces, particularly in motor vehicle accidents and falls, may tear organs from their points of fixation. For example, the liver may be torn from the diaphragm and the inferior vena cava, the bladder from the bladder neck, and the kidney from the renal artery and vein.

Blunt trauma tends to injure solid viscera (e.g., the spleen, kidney, liver, and pancreas). Hollow viscera (e.g., the intestines and the bladder), however, are also vulnerable to blunt trauma when they are distended. In penetrating injuries, particularly stab wounds, the bowel may escape penetration by the knife blade because of the bowel's ability to "slide out of the way." Fixed organs are more vulnerable to knife wounds.

Assessment

The initial assessment and management of the patient who possibly has an abdominal trauma always consider the emergency priorities: first, establishing the airway, breathing, and circulation, then assessing the respiratory, cardiac, and circulatory systems. The abdominal trauma is not assessed until those systems are assessed and/or supported and the patient's condition is stabilized. Identification of intraabdominal injury depends essentially on frequent abdominal examination, peritoneal lavage, laboratory studies, and the x-ray procedures that may be indicated.

The assessment of an intraabdominal injury begins with obtaining an adequate history of the injury. Once a description of the accident has been obtained, the next step is evaluation of the patient for the following signs and symptoms of peritoneal irritation:

1. Generalized pain and/or tenderness
2. Rebound tenderness
3. Pain on movement or coughing
4. A localizing point of maximum tenderness
5. Abdominal wall rigidity
6. Splinting of the abdominal muscles and thoracic breathing
7. Abdominal distention

8. Guarding
9. Decreased or absent bowel sounds

The first four symptoms are usually regarded as evidence of intraperitoneal lesion until proved otherwise [60]. All the signs and symptoms are the result of irritation of the peritoneal membranes by spilling bowel contents, digestive enzymes, urine, bile, or blood into the peritoneal cavity. The onset of peritonitis may be insidious because blood does not always irritate the peritoneum and because small bowel lacerations may be nearly painless if the leakage is minimal. Therefore, continuous, careful assessment must be carried out so that occult injuries are detected as soon as possible.

The evaluation of intraabdominal injury is based on (1) the history of the injury and (2) the description of the pain, both of which require an alert, verbal, oriented, and cooperative patient. It is apparent why blunt abdominal trauma carries a higher mortality than penetrating trauma. A patient who has sustained a blunt abdominal trauma usually has an associated injury. If the patient has an associated head injury, he is unable to give a history of the injury or to describe the pain. If he has an associated chest injury, pain and irritation of the diaphragm caused by a hemothorax may produce peritonitis-like abdominal rigidity and guarding. The pain of fractures of the lower ribs or pelvis may mask the signs of peritonitis. The patient may be unconscious as a result of shock or alcohol intoxication. Finally, a patient who has a spinal cord injury at the thoracic level or above may have a flaccid abdominal wall and sensory loss, and he has no abdominal pain, even in the presence of an intraabdominal injury.

How often abdominal injury is accompanied by other injuries is indicated by a survey by Tovee [60]. He found that 70 percent of patients who had abdominal trauma had one or more lesions of the head, chest, or extremity. The mortality rate of each group of patients greatly increased according to the number of associated injuries:

Abdominal injury alone	13.4%	mortality
Associated abdominal and chest injuries	40%	mortality
Associated abdominal, chest, and head injuries	87%	mortality

Obviously, the overall condition of the patient who has multisystem trauma equals more than the sum of his individual injuries. It also is apparent that setting the right priorities, making an assessment that does not miss subtle but important signs, and designing a plan of care that is expeditious and as specific as possible can be a complex task.

PARACENTESIS AND PERITONEAL LAVAGE

Two diagnostic tools that have been of great help to the physician in detecting intraabdominal injury are paracentesis and peritoneal lavage. In paracentesis, an 18-gauge short-bevel spinal needle is attached to a syringe and inserted through the abdominal wall, which has been prepared and anesthetized (locally). Figure 34-3 shows where the needle is inserted. An attempt is then made to aspirate any free intraperitoneal blood that may be present as a result of intraabdominal injury. (Because four quadrants are aspirated, the procedure is often called a "four-quadrant tap.") The aspiration of even a small amount of nonclotting blood is considered a positive tap and evidence of an intraabdominal injury that requires an exploratory laparotomy. A paracentesis that fails to aspirate blood is not definitive; that is, it does not indicate that the patient's abdomen has not been injured [59]. Other diagnostic procedures must be used to prove that there is not an injury.

The following problems are associated with paracentesis and must be considered whenever the procedure is undertaken:

1. An intraabdominal blood vessel may inadvertently be entered. If it is, the aspirated blood does clot, which differentiates it from blood from the peritoneum, which does not clot.
2. An accidental puncture of the intestine may occur. However, it happens rarely, and when it does happen it is relatively harmless because the hole made by the 18-gauge needle is small, seals off quickly, and usually does not allow the bowel contents to leak.
3. Accidental puncture of the rectus abdominis sheath may produce a large hematoma of that muscle [49].
4. Free intraperitoneal blood that settles in the posterior aspects of the abdomen may not be accessible to the needle, thus resulting in a false-negative result. Overall, 5 percent to 40 percent of patients who undergo paracentesis have false-negative results.

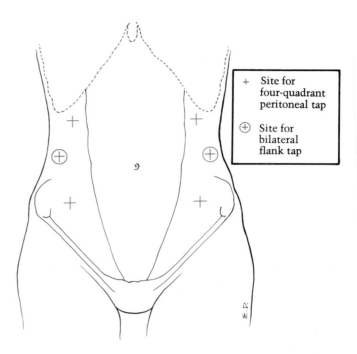

+ Site for
four-quadrant
peritoneal tap

⊕ Site for
bilateral
flank tap

Figure 34-3
Anatomical sites for paracentesis.

If the following precautions are taken, the problems of paracentesis may be minimized:

1. Peritoneal taps should be avoided in the patient whose bowel is markedly distended.
2. Peritoneal taps should be avoided in areas of scar, where the bowel may be fixed to the abdominal wall.
3. Care should be taken to insert the needle at the proper site, namely, lateral to the rectus abdominis sheath.
4. If the tap in one quadrant is negative, it is repeated in the other quadrants. If the taps in the four quadrants are negative, taps of the flanks may be done.

Peritoneal Lavage
Peritoneal lavage is more accurate (96%) than paracentesis and gives fewer false-negative results [41, 59]. Peritoneal lavage is also being performed on victims of stab wounds who are stable and have a nontender abdomen in order to rule out intraabdominal injury and avoid laparotomy. In peritoneal lavage, a peritoneal dialysis catheter is inserted and advanced into the peritoneal cavity (Fig. 34-4). If no blood or fluid is aspirated, 1 liter of a balanced saline solution

is rapidly infused into the peritoneal cavity (in children, 15 ml/kg). The patient is turned from side to side (except the patient who has a pelvic fracture or who for some other reason cannot be turned), the empty intravenous bottle or bag is positioned below the patient's abdomen, and the fluid is siphoned out of the peritoneal cavity. The fluid that is collected is evaluated for the presence of red and white blood cells, amylase, bacteria, and bile. The criteria for positive peritoneal lavage [59] are gross blood in the lavage fluid or one or more of the following:

1. More than 100,000 red blood cells per cu mm
2. More than 500 white blood cells per cu mm
3. An elevated amylase level
4. The presence of bacteria or bile

Like paracentesis, peritoneal lavage has some disadvantages. Accidental puncture of intraabdominal structures may occur. Injuries to the retroperitoneal space cannot be evaluated since the space does not communicate with the peritoneal cavity and hence is inaccessible to the lavage fluid. Sometimes the insertion of the peritoneal catheter may cause enough abdominal bleeding to produce false-positive results. That problem can be prevented by using a local anesthetic preparation that contains epinephrine (to constrict the locally traumatized vessels). Lavage is contraindicated in the following patients:

1. Patients who have a history of many operations, because adhesions increase the likelihood that the bowel will be penetrated and that the lavage fluid will be trapped, making its return difficult
2. Women patients who are pregnant (because of possible danger to the fetus)
3. Patients who have missile injuries of the abdomen

MONITORING BLOOD PRESSURE

Continuous assessment of patients who have occult abdominal injuries is crucial to early detection of those injuries. Besides the continuous monitoring of the patient for peritoneal signs, serial measurements of the patient's blood pressure can be used to provide very useful information. Many patients who have multiple injuries are admitted to the hospital in varying degrees of shock.

Patients whose hypotension is the result of mild volume losses or of neurogenic causes usually respond promptly to the rapid infusion of 500 to 1000 ml of Ringer's lactate solution. But patients who have multisystem injuries, and whose blood pressure responds for a moment to vigorous fluid resuscitation therapy and then returns to hypotensive levels, are strongly suspected of having continued occult bleeding. When the source of bleeding is not visible the most likely cause is progressive hemoperitoneum. For that reason—and also because slow bleeding that progresses to ever deepening shock is always a danger in the normotensive patient—serial measurement of blood pressure is a valuable part of the assessment approach.

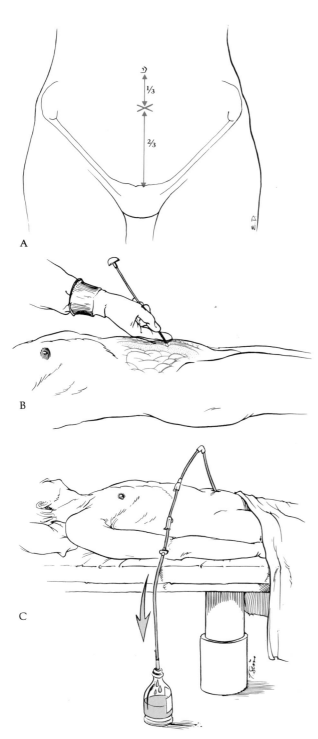

A

B

C

Figure 34-4
Peritoneal lavage. A. Anatomical site for the percutaneous insertion of a lavage catheter. B. After penetration of the peritoneum and removal of the trocar, the lavage catheter is inserted. C. After lavage, the solution is infused into the peritoneal cavity and the patient is moved from one side to the other; the lavage fluid is siphoned out of the peritoneal cavity.

LABORATORY TESTS

Besides the analysis of the peritoneal lavage fluid, several other laboratory tests are helpful in gathering evidence of the presence and the location of intraabdominal injuries. A blood leukocyte count of more than 15,000 per cu mm suggests that a solid viscus has been ruptured. White blood cell counts of more than 25,000 per cu mm may occur in rupture of the spleen and (occasionally) in rupture of the liver.

The hemoglobin and hematocrit levels give little information about an acute blood loss, but they do show a decline 6 to 8 hours after the acute episode [52]. Because of the fluid shifts that occur after the trauma, the hemoglobin and hematocrit levels are difficult to interpret, and they are not generally used as the only guide to fluid and blood replacement.

The serum amylase level may become elevated whenever amylase leaks into the peritoneal cavity, where it is freely absorbed into the blood. That spill of amylase may result from direct pancreatic trauma or from injury to the upper small bowel and duodenum (where the pancreatic enzyme is secreted into the bowel by way of the pancreatic duct) with leakage of amylase-containing fluid from the injured bowel into the peritoneal cavity. Hyperamylasemia that occurs immediately after trauma may thus also indicate a second injury: small bowel perforation. A rise in the amylase level caused by a significant and direct pancreatic injury may not occur until 12 to 24 hours after the injury [40]. Therefore a rising or a persistently elevated serum amylase level suggests a pancreatic injury rather than a small bowel injury.

Splenic Injury

The spleen is injured more often than any other abdominal organ; it is involved in more than 25 percent of all intraabdominal injuries. Located in the left upper quadrant, near the abdominal wall and under the diaphragm, the spleen is partly protected by the left lower ribs but it is also vulnerable to the ribs when they are fractured. Twenty-five percent of the patients who have a splenic injury have a fracture of the left lower rib. Splenic injuries are to be suspected in any type of blunt trauma, particularly after motor vehicle accidents, falls, bicycle accidents, and blows received in vigorous contact sports.

The danger of splenic injury is directly related to the spleen's high vascularity. The spleen is the most vascular organ in the body; it is perfused by more than 350 liters of blood per day. Small splenic tears, lacerations, and ruptured splenic hematomas are notorious sources of persistent and profuse bleeding into the peritoneal cavity. Massive amounts of blood may be lost into the peritoneal spaces, resulting in severe and sometimes fatal hypovolemic shock. Evidence of such bleeding depends on the amount of blood lost and the extent of peritoneal contamination.

Types of Splenic Injury

Two types of injury occur following blunt trauma: splenic rupture and subcapsular hematoma. Rupture of the splenic parenchyma is the more common injury (occurring 85% to 90% of the time), and it is an emergency. Subcapsular hematoma occurs in 10% to 15% of the cases; it involves trauma to the splenic tissue with subsequent local bleeding that is arrested by the thick (1-to-2 mm) capsule surrounding the spleen. The result is the formation of a hematoma between the spleen and the capsule. The hematoma prevents immediate intraperitoneal bleeding, but it is only temporarily benign. Eventually, the capsule yields to the expanding hematoma, and the spleen ruptures. When delayed rupture occurs, it usually has not been anticipated, and the blood loss may be great before the diagnosis is made. The rupture may not occur for as long as a week to 10 days, during which time few if any symptoms occur.

Assessment

Splenic bleeding may be detected by several assessment parameters. A history of injury, however slight, to the left upper quadrant (LUQ) followed by pain in the LUQ should raise the staff's index of suspicion. Varying degrees of hypovolemia may be present, with such signs as tachycardia, hypotension, and syncope. The patient may have difficulty breathing as intraperitoneal blood collects under the diaphragm and irritates it. In 50 percent of the patients, Kerr's sign is present (i.e., pain that is referred to the left shoulder tip because blood is irritating the diaphragm). Occasionally the patient may have to be placed in a Trendelenburg position for Kerr's sign to be elicited. Muscular rigidity and guarding in the LUQ may occur in association with the LUQ pain.

Other parameters are important in assessing

splenic injury. Peritoneal lavage is helpful in documenting the presence of intraperitoneal blood. X rays may show such positive diagnostic signs as an elevated left hemidiaphragm, an enlarged spleen, gastric displacement, or hemorrhage into the gastrosplenic ligament, which separates the spleen and stomach. Leukocytosis of 15,000 to 25,000 per cu mm is common, as are declining hematocrit and hemoglobin values, shown by serial determinations. When the history of injury strongly suggests splenic trauma but other assessments have nebulous results, angiography may be performed through the splenic artery to identify any discontinuity in the vascular system of the spleen [19]. In any event, a history that suggests splenic trauma followed by serial assessments of the patient's condition is a prerequisite to diagnosing both acute and delayed splenic trauma.

Management

Splenic injuries are usually treated by total splenectomy. Because of the delicate vascular nature of the spleen, suture repair results in rebleeding and an increased mortality (25%–50%). Total splenectomy carries less chance of rebleeding (2.8%) and results in a much reduced mortality (5%–15% in blunt trauma; 1% in penetrating trauma). The mortality, however, may increase from 15 to 40 percent if other serious injuries are present. If splenectomy is not performed, the mortality is 90 to 95 percent [60].

When splenectomy is performed, drains may be placed in the splenic bed and kept there 3 to 5 days. The drains:

1. Remove fluid collections that could lead to abscess formation in the splenic bed.
2. Prevent the collection of pancreatic enzymes that may have been released as a result of operative trauma.
3. Make it possible to recognize postoperative rebleeding.

A phenomenon called splenic fever may occur postoperatively in the patient who has had a splenectomy. It is characterized by fever, an elevated white blood cell count, and an elevated serum amylase level. The signs are those of a traumatic pancreatitis that usually resolves spontaneously in 3 to 4 days.

Abscess formation and/or infection are postoperative complications in 4 percent of patients following

splenectomy. Immediate or delayed rebleeding occurs in 2.8 percent of patients.

The incidence of thrombus formation is 3.7% [33]. Thrombus formation is the result of a rebound elevation of the thrombocytes, which sometimes reach levels three to five times normal. The increase in thrombocytes may stimulate the formation of thrombi, which can circulate to the pulmonary vasculature and cause pulmonary embolism. Thus, it is important postoperatively to take steps to prevent or reduce the amount of thrombus formation, including the use of antiembolism stockings and early ambulation. Care is taken to prevent injuries that could precipitate clot formation.

Renal Injury

An injury to the kidney or other genitourinary structure is usually accompanied by an injury to another abdominal organ. Consequently, the sign of an injury to the other organ often masks the renal injury and delays or prevents its detection. Because the incidence of renal injuries is second only to the incidence of splenic injuries, the staff must have a high index of suspicion of renal trauma and must diligently assess all patients who have abdominal trauma [36].

Renal Pedicle Injury

Because of the magnitude of blood flow into and out of the kidney, an injury to the renal pedicle (artery and vein) must be diagnosed and treated immediately if the patient's kidney (and sometimes his life) is to be saved. Pedicle injuries are caused five times more often by the penetrating trauma of stab wounds and gunshot wounds than by a blunt, decelerating force [50].

In a high-speed motor vehicle accident, the sudden halt in rapid forward motion exerts a shearing force on the vessels of the renal pedicle [29]. The layers (intima, media, adventitia) of the vessels' wall may be sheared, torn, or even completely avulsed from the kidney (which is relatively mobile) as the kidney continues its forward motion away from the more stationary aorta. Renal arteries that are torn or damaged can easily thrombose, resulting in rapid ischemia and/or death of the kidney [63]. A laceration or avulsion of the renal pedicle is life threatening in that it may involve the loss of massive amounts of blood.

Most of the blood is often lost into the retroperitoneal spaces, and so the blood loss is not detected by the usual physical examination of the abdomen.

A history of deceleration accompanied by signs of massive blood loss is strong evidence of a laceration of an intraabdominal vessel, and particularly of the renal pedicle. Since profound hemorrhagic shock usually accompanies an injury to the renal pedicle, the diagnostic procedures done right before the operative repair are greatly limited. Flank mass and pain are rare, and hematuria may be absent. If the systolic blood pressure is greater than 90, an emergency intravenous pyelogram (IVP) may be performed with minimal difficulty to define the injury more clearly. A preoperative IVP also gives vital information about the functioning of the uninjured kidney when removal of the injured kidney is seriously considered. Although an arteriogram would permit a more accurate diagnosis, the patient's unstable condition usually does not allow time for it to be done.

Intimal damage of the renal artery that results in renal artery thrombosis poses special problems in the early assessment period. Since the total renal functioning can be assumed by the ininjured kidney, few (or no) symptoms of the thrombosis and renal ischemia may be present immediately after the injury. Flank pain, along with a history of injury, may make up the whole clinical picture. More often, the injury is found days, weeks, even months later, when the patient returns to the physician with symptoms of hypertension. Renal artery thrombosis followed by the release of renin and angiotensin with secondary hypertension occurs in a small percentage of those patients [63]. Nephrectomy is often required to eliminate the source of the angiotensin release and to relieve the hypertension.

Kidney Injury

Unlike renal pedicle injury, injury to the kidney itself is more often (75% of cases) caused by a blunt rather than a penetrating injury. Like the spleen, the kidney responds to blunt trauma with contusion, hematoma, stellate tears, lacerations, fracture and avulsion of either pole, or diffuse rupture and fragmentation (Fig. 34-5). Also, like the spleen, the kidney is covered by a capsule that may arrest bleeding and so cause the formation of a subcapsular hematoma. Those hematomas, however, tend not to expand but to tamponade and in a matter of weeks to resolve spontane-

ously. Delayed rupture, therefore, is not as great a danger in blunt injury to the kidney as it is in blunt injury to the spleen.

High-velocity gunshot wounds of the kidney deserve special mention because of the complications that can occur postoperatively. The temporary cavity formed by a high-velocity missile produces crushing trauma to renal tissue several centimeters from the wound tract. The crushed renal tissue may seem viable at the time of operative repair, but later may deteriorate due to microthrombosis formation, internal elastic tissue breakdown, hemorrhage, acute inflammation, thrombotic occlusion of the small vessels, and (eventually) anoxia, necrosis, or bleeding. Profuse hematuria and delayed bleeding, evidenced by falling serial hematocrit and hemoglobin levels, signal the presence of that type of delayed development. Nephrectomy may be needed to stop the bleeding [1].

ASSESSMENT

In blunt injury, the presence of a renal injury may be heralded by pain at the costovertebral angle (CVA tenderness) and hematuria. Flank mass is rare. The signs of blood loss vary according to the extent of the injury. Bowel sounds may be absent because of a reflex ileus. Fractures of the lumbar vertebrae or lower ribs may also be associated with kidney injury.

The presence of hematuria is helpful in detecting renal injury, but its absence does not mean that the kidney is free of injury. In 20 to 29 percent of patients who have a renal injury, the urine is free of red blood cells [50]. Furthermore, urine that seems on visual inspection to be free of blood may actually contain blood. Urine does not look pink until it contains more than 500 red blood cells per cu mm (gross hematuria). Detection of red blood cells in quantities less than 500 per cu mm (microscopic hematuria) requires microscopic examination. The presence of as few as 10 red blood cells per cu mm of urine is considered abnormal.

The presence of gross or microscopic hematuria necessitates further investigation. With an IVP, dye that has been injected into the peripheral vein circulates to the kidney, where it can be shown by x ray to be concentrated by the kidney and excreted into the collecting system. Dye that is concentrated in the uninjured areas of the kidney will cause those parts of the kidney to visualize on x ray. Areas of kidney that are injured will not be able to concentrate the dye and

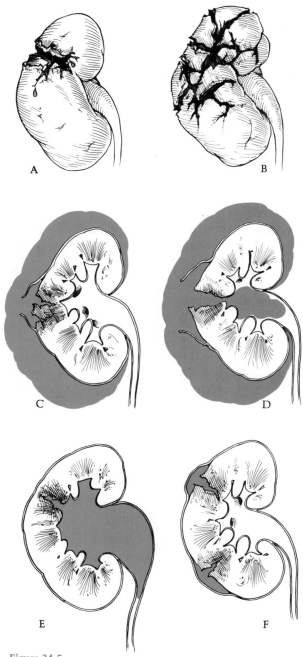

cannot therefore be visualized on the x ray. Furthermore, if the collecting system has been violated, the concentrated dye can be seen to leak (extravasate) from the injured area. X rays are taken at intervals of 5, 10, and 15 min after the injection of the dye in order to record the egress of the concentrated and excreted dye into the calyces, ureters, and bladder. Injury in any of those areas will be shown by dye extravasation or by obstruction of the dye's progress through the system.

MANAGEMENT

The management of the renal injury, the type of surgical repair (if any) needed, and the complications to be anticipated postoperatively depend on the type and degree of the injury. Most patients (80%) do not require surgery. Bedrest, forced fluids, monitoring of vital signs, and blood tests are usually the therapeutic measures needed and are followed by clearing of the hematuria and loss of the flank pain.

Tears or lacerations in the outer parenchyma that do not invade the collecting system (the calyx) usually cause minimal bleeding and can be treated with suture repair and/or Penrose drainage. Once the collecting system has been invaded, however, extravasation of urine into the peritoneal spaces or around the kidney provides an excellent environment for bacterial growth and invites infection and abscess formation. Suture repair of the renal parenchyma or of the collecting system and ample Penrose drainage of extravasated urine are necessary. If there is extensive damage to the upper collecting system (the calyx or the upper ureter), a nephrostomy tube may be inserted to drain urine from the calyx until the edema subsides and healing has begun. In that way the perils of an obstructive nephropathy may be avoided. Localized rupture of either pole of the kidney is frequently managed by heminephrectomy [64].

It is important for the nurse to watch postoperatively for rebleeding and abscess formation because localized urinary extravasation has occurred. Diffuse rupture of the kidney involving both poles and the midportion results in extensive blood loss and urinary leakage. The damage is usually beyond repair. It is best treated by total nephrectomy.

Ureteral Injury

Injuries to the ureter are rare, and they are hard to detect early in their course [13]. Sometimes they are

Figure 34-5
Examples of renal injuries. A. Capsular rupture. B. Fragmentation. C. Hematoma from cortical laceration. D. Hematoma from cortical laceration with renal pelvis laceration. E. Renal pelvis hematoma. F. Subcapsular hematomas from cortical laceration.

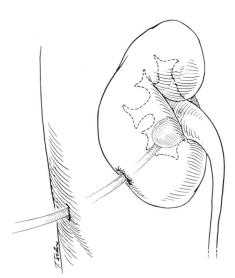

Figure 34-6
Placement of nephrostomy tube frequently seen after renal surgery.

discovered during a diagnostic work-up for another injury (usually during an IVP), but more often they are not recognized until flank pain, fever, and infection develop. When a ureteral injury is diagnosed, reconstructive repair must be carried out to prevent hydronephrosis from ureteral stricture and to drain the intraabdominal collections of extravasated urine. Ureteral repair and reanastomosis is a difficult type of operation because postoperative stricture can occur easily. After surgery the patient usually has (1) a ureterostomy tube that serves as a stent to the ureter to prevent stricture and (2) a nephrostomy tube to insure adequate drainage of the urine until the anastomosis has healed (Fig. 34-6). The stent may be kept in place as long as 10 to 14 days and the nephrostomy tube as long as 4 to 6 weeks to insure adequate drainage of the urine while the ureter heals [20].

On rare occasions, patients who have suffered extensive trauma will have lost large segments of the ureter. In those patients, complicated reconstructive surgery involving anastomosis of the viable end of the ureter to the other ureter (ureteroureterostomy), reimplantation of the ureter into the bladder (ureteroneocystostomy), or mobilization of the kidney with its short viable ureter closer to the bladder for reimplantation may be undertaken.

Besides the other aspects of nursing management, careful aseptic management and maintenance of the patency of all drainage tubes are very important postoperatively to insure the success of these, as well as the more common, ureteral repairs.

Bladder Injury

Most bladder injuries are the result of blunt trauma of considerable force, usually from automobile accidents. Twenty percent of bladder injuries are intraperitoneal and 80% are extraperitoneal. Typically, intraperitoneal rupture occurs when the bladder is distended and full and a substantial blow is delivered to the lower abdomen. The pressure of the blow is transmitted to the dome of the bladder, structurally the weakest portion of the bladder wall. Rupture in that location allows urine to escape into the peritoneal cavity, and it may produce a fatal peritonitis. Besides intraperitoneal rupture, the bladder is vulnerable to extraperitoneal rupture when torn by indriven fragments of a fractured pelvis (usually the symphysis pubis and/or the superior or inferior rami). Although that type of injury is not attended by the perils of peritoneal contamination, it may be attended by significant blood loss.

Signs and symptoms of bladder rupture include lower abdominal pain, inability or difficulty in voiding, and hematuria. Occasionally extraperitoneal rupture permits urine to dissect along the fascial planes and enter the thighs or ascend into the abdominal wall. In intraperitoneal rupture, signs of peritonitis develop within 24 hours (sooner if the urine is infected).

When bladder rupture is suspected, a retrograde cystogram, which allows dye to fill the bladder, is ordered to determine the location of bladder tears. Since urine leaks continuously from the tear, operative repair must be carried out as soon as possible. After the bladder wall is repaired, a suprapubic cystostomy tube, along with a urethral catheter and Penrose drains, is placed to insure continuous drainage of urine and to prevent the accumulation of urine, which might interfere with the healing of the wound. The suprapubic tube may be kept in place up to two weeks, and urethral catheterization continued until the suprapubic wound is closed.

Small Bowel Injury

Small bowel injuries can be caused by both penetrating and blunt trauma. Typically in blunt trauma that occurs in an automobile accident, a sudden, forceful blow to the midabdomen by a steering wheel forces the bowel against the vertebral column. When the bowel is compressed suddenly, the intraluminal pressure rises quickly. If the loop of bowel is pinched closed by the vertebral column or other structures, rupture results. Lap seat belts have also been known to cause a similar injury when rapid deceleration forces the abdomen against the restraining belt [12].

Assessment and Management

Signs of peritoneal irritation can be surprisingly few following rupture of the ileum or jejunum. The pH of the bowel contents at that point is neutral to the peritoneal cavity and the small bowel fluid is relatively sterile. Rupture of the duodenum, however, can cause fulminant signs and symptoms of peritoneal irritation because the pH of the duodenal contents is highly alkaline to the peritoneal membranes. Irritating substances, such as bile and pancreatic enzymes, are also highly concentrated in the duodenal contents. Despite the irritating nature of the duodenal contents, however, duodenal injuries may produce minimal signs and symptoms when the blunt injury produces a retroperitoneal injury. In such a case, the retroperitoneal and not the intraperitoneal spaces are contaminated by the duodenal secretion, and the classic signs of intraabdominal injury may be absent.

The detection of small bowel injury depends heavily on a history of severe blunt injury, abdominal pain located in the periumbilical areas or radiating to the shoulder tips, peritoneal lavage, and x ray. An abdominal x ray that reveals free intraabdominal air is the strongest evidence of small bowel rupture.

Treatment of small bowel injuries consists chiefly of simple suture repair. But when perforation, rupture, thrombosis, or necrosis is extensive, small bowel resection and reanastomosis must be undertaken. Postoperatively the patient has a number of gastrointestinal tubes—nasogastric, gastrostomy, or jejunostomy—which are designed to decompress the bowel, reduce tension on the suture lines, and drain the small bowel secretions, enzymes, blood, and bile. Ample Penrose drainage is also included to insure the removal of fluid collections and prevent abscess formation.

Complications that occur postoperatively can cost a great deal in terms of time, morbidity, and patient morale and comfort. Immediately postoperatively,

large extracellular volume deficits may occur as the result of edema and translocation of fluid into a nonfunctional "third space" in the injured bowel wall and irritated peritoneum. Electrolyte imbalances can be severe when gastrointestinal suction and decompression are prolonged. If large amounts of the small bowel have been removed, malabsorption syndromes may result, making adequate nutrition difficult to achieve. Finally, poor blood supply to the repaired bowel, infection, tension on the suture lines, or distal obstruction can cause fistulas to form in the small bowel, peritoneal cavity, and/or drain tracts. When that occurs, the mortality increases to 50% since leakage of the small bowel contents into the peritoneal cavity increases the probability of sepsis.

The treatment of small bowel fistulas requires sump drainage and suction through the drain tracts and decompression through the gastrointestinal tubes to insure evacuation of small bowel leakage, to promote collapse and healing of the fistulous tract, to keep irritating drainage off the skin, and to help estimate fluid and electrolyte losses. Furthermore, nutrition is provided through a feeding jejunostomy tube and/or parenteral nutritional therapy. Occasionally, secretions suctioned from the gastrostomy or duodenostomy tubes are reinfused through the feeding jejunostomy so that fluids and electrolytes are not lost from the body.

Liver Injury

Trauma to the liver may result in three types of injury:

1. The liver capsule may rupture. That is the most common type of liver injury, and it results in the loss of blood and bile into the peritoneal cavity and in immediate evidence of peritoneal contamination.
2. A subcapsular hematoma may form. Like a hematoma of the spleen, it may be essentially undetectable on the patient's admission to the hospital, only to rupture spontaneously several days later. Bleeding from the delayed rupture can be fatal [31].
3. An intrahepatic hematoma may form. That too is an occult injury that can cause major complications later, with extensive tissue necrosis, abscess formation, and erosion of hepatic vessels with bleeding into the bile ducts (hemobilia). When that

occurs, large amounts of blood can be lost through the bile ducts where they drain into the duodenum, producing massive and sometimes fatal gastrointestinal bleeding.

Most of the liver injuries (60%) require only suture repair and drainage. It is extremely important that the physician drain the fluid collections near the wound, because the environment is so favorable for abscess formation. Patients who have had liver repair will have several large Penrose drains in place postoperatively. Many patients (30%) need only Penrose drainage and no suture repair because their liver is not bleeding at the time of surgery and it is better not to traumatize the organ by suture repair.

A number of patients who have liver trauma (10%) have such extensive wounds (usually stellate tears and ruptures from gunshot wounds) that partial hepatic resection is needed to control the bleeding. Those patients can do well as long as at least 20 percent of the liver remains and as long as ample drainage is provided. Those patients also have a T tube in place to drain the common bile duct, because blood can accumulate in the duct and can clot, causing biliary obstruction.

Assessment

The overall mortality in liver trauma (11%) is attributable to massive intraabdominal bleeding that occurs immediately after the injury as well as to the late complications of delayed rupture, gastrointestinal bleeding, and sepsis [60]. To reduce the morbidity and mortality in liver trauma it is extremely important to make careful, serial assessments of the patient's condition. The early signs and symptoms of complications may thus be assessed and treatment started as soon as possible. Patients who have blunt trauma to the right upper quadrant and who have no immediate problems should be watched for several days for delayed rupture [42]. It is important to watch for the signs and symptoms of peritoneal irritation, because blood or bile may collect. In the patient who has had liver repair, drainage from the Penrose tubes should be evaluated carefully for evidence of blood or purulence. If biliary drainage continues in copious amounts, a biliary fistula should be suspected. Patients who complain of acute, colicky type abdominal pain of sudden onset coupled with sudden hypotension should be evaluated for the pos-

sibility of hemobilia and resulting gastrointestinal bleeding.

Liver Failure

When there is extensive damage, such as from high-velocity gunshot wounds, severe liver edema with necrosis and fibrosis formation may occur, followed by liver dysfunction and eventually liver failure. The edema, necrosis, and fibrosis interfere with the important complex functions of the liver by obstructing its two vascular systems, the portal system and its own blood supply system. (Together those systems circulate 1500 ml of blood per minute.) The obstruction not only compromises the function of individual liver cells, it also produces mechanical obstruction of blood flow through the portal system, resulting in a cascade of complications for the liver as well as the entire body.

Venous blood that leaves the abdominal organs (intestines, esophagus, stomach, and spleen) circulates through the portal system into the liver, where it undergoes complex metabolic changes. The most important of those processes are as follows:

1. Carbohydrate metabolism, including gluconeogenesis and glycogen storage
2. Protein metabolism, including the manufacture of most of the plasma proteins and detoxification of ammonia to form urea for excretion
3. Fat metabolism, including the formation of lipoproteins and phospholipids
4. The manufacture of important clotting factors, including fibrinogen, prothrombin, and factor VII
5. The removal by the reticuloendothelial system (Kupffer's cells) of 99 percent of the bacteria that entered the portal system from the gut
6. The formation of lymph
7. The breakdown and disposition of bilirubin
8. The manufacture of bile, which is necessary for digestion

In an extensive injury, all the functions just listed are affected. Blood flow through the hepatic vasculature is reduced, causing death to the liver cells. Carbohydrate metabolism is reduced, ammonia and bilirubin accumulate in the blood, and the manufacture of clotting factors, plasma proteins, lymph, and bile is severely impaired. Also, blood flow through the portal system is obstructed, resulting in portal hypertension. Bacteria accumulate and grow in the portal system as phagocytosis via the Kupffer cells is impaired. Increasing pressure in the portal system (from a normal of 8–30 mm Hg) causes fluid to shift from the vasculature into the interstitial and abdominal spaces (resulting in ascites). The fluid that transudates is almost pure plasma; it contains 80% to 90% as much protein as does normal plasma. The transudation, in addition to the reduced production of plasma proteins by the damaged liver, produces a profound loss of normal plasma oncotic pressure followed by severe hypovolemia as fluid is lost (as edema) to the interstitial spaces. The increasing pressure in the portal system eventually causes passive congestion of the organs it drains (the spleen, intestines, and esophagus). The pressure causes dysfunction of those organs just as it does of the liver.

In the later stages of liver failure, the patient shows:

1. Jaundice, from the loss of the liver's ability to break down bilirubin.
2. Edema, from the loss of plasma proteins.
3. Volume depletion, from the loss of the plasma oncotic pressure.
4. Hemorrhagic tendencies, from the loss of the liver's ability to manufacture clotting factors.
5. Anemia, leukocytopenia, and thrombocytopenia from hypersplenism.
6. Fever and sepsis from bacterial invasion via the unguarded portal system.

Colon Injury

Injuries to the colon can be more serious than injuries to the small bowel because the contents of the colon are more virulent and its blood supply is less abundant. Until World War II, colon injuries carried a very high mortality, but with antibiotic therapy, reduction of time between injury and treatment, and the increased use of colostomy as a means of treatment, the mortality has been greatly reduced.

The colon may be injured by both blunt and penetrating mechanisms, but penetrating injuries are more frequent. The signs of intraabdominal contamination and peritoneal irritation develop very rapidly. Peritoneal lavage reveals the presence of blood and fecal material. Rectal examination may also demonstrate the presence of blood. X rays are an important diagnostic tool in detecting free intraperitoneal air that has escaped through perforations or tears of the colon.

Because of the virulence of the spilled contents of the colon, it is extremely important that intravenous antibiotics be administered as soon as possible.

The operative repair has changed from primary closure to diverting colostomy and delayed closure. In that way, the virulent colonic contents are diverted from the wound so that the anastomosis may be protected and decompression assured. The movement of fecal material is thus under control and the danger of leakage, peritoneal contamination, and stress on the repaired segment of bowel is minimized.

A diverting colostomy has two stomas (double barreled); one is located proximal to the wound to divert fecal material from the wound and the other represents an exteriorization of the area of wounded colon. Depending on the extent of damaged bowel, the colostomy may be closed as early as 2 to 3 weeks after the injury or as late as one year after the injury.

Postoperative complications are usually related to continued fecal soiling of the peritoneal cavity. Also, abscess formation, small bowel obstructions, bowel ischemia, gangrene, and stenosis can all result from the continued inflammatory process. In those cases, another operation for abscess drainage, relief of obstruction, resection of more bowel, colostomy revision, and intraabdominal irrigation with antibiotic solutions may be necessary. The postoperative care requires careful fluid and electrolyte replacement and nutritional supplementation with tube feedings or parenteral nutritional therapy.

Pancreatic Injury

Because of its rather protected, retroperitoneal location, the pancreas is not often injured. Penetrating trauma is the most frequent cause of pancreatic injury, accounting for 70% to 80% of all cases. Although the overall mortality is low (20% at most), the morbidity for pancreatic injuries can be very high, owing to the chemical peritonitis that follows the leakage of potent pancreatic enzymes into the peritoneal cavity. The mortality, however, increases when there are associated injuries (usually of the spleen, vena cava, or stomach, which are in close proximity to the pancreas). In those cases, the mortality may be as high as 60%.

Pancreatic injury due to penetrating trauma is treated with immediate exploration and operative repair. Treatment of pancreatic injury due to blunt mechanisms, however, is much more difficult to plan. Actual injury to the pancreas can be severely occult, producing the first physical signs and symptoms as late as 12 to 24 hours after the initial injury. The pancreas is particularly vulnerable to decelerating accidents because its retroperitoneal location and immobility make the pancreas unable to withstand decelerating, shearing stresses. As digestive enzymes are leaked by the injured pancreas into the peritoneal cavity, the signs and symptoms of peritonitis begin to occur; they are pain, tenderness, guarding, fever, and paralytic ileus. The injury can be detected before the actual signs and symptoms occur through the use of abdominal paracentesis or peritoneal lavage. Those procedures may reveal the presence of amylase. Also, a serum amylase level that is elevated immediately after injury and that stays elevated as shown by serial determinations strongly suggests pancreatic injury and malfunction.

The operative procedure used to treat pancreatic injury depends on the type of injury; it ranges from simple drainage for laceration to a Roux-en-Y pancreaticojejunostomy for pancreatic transection. In all cases, however, the single most important factor in promoting recovery is adequate drainage of the leaking enzymes. Drainage is usually done with the placement of Penrose drains and a sump tube connected to 100-mm Hg suction. The drainage usually continues 2 to 4 weeks.

Although the initial mortality in penetrating trauma is higher than that in blunt trauma, the complication rate is higher in blunt trauma because greater organ disruption usually occurs. The major problems are delayed hemorrhage, infection, pancreatitis, fistula, and pseudocyst.

A pancreatic fistula results when a disrupted pancreatic duct does not heal and continues to pour enzymes into a fistulous tract that communicates with the peritoneal cavity and, sometimes, even with the abdominal wall. Treatment is conservative; it involves supportive care, including bedrest, fluid replacement, and continued suctioning to remove the secretions so that the skin and tissues will not be damaged. In some instances, atropine sulfate is administered every 4 hr to decrease the amount of secretions produced.

A pancreatic pseudocyst is a collection of pancreatic secretions surrounded by a fibrous wall. Not only is the collection of fluid an excellent medium for bacterial growth and abscess formation, it also produces an obstruction to the flow of enzymes through the ductal system. The signs and symptoms of pseudocysts are apparent approximately 14 to 21 days after the injury; they are pain, fever, ileus, nausea, vomiting, and anorexia. An abdominal mass may be palpated. Treatment for pseudocyst and abscess formation consists of surgical drainage to prevent rupture and spillage of the contents into the peritoneal cavity.

Under normal circumstances, pancreatic secretions are inactive; they have no proteolytic activity until they are activated in the duodenum. A direct vascular injury, however, can activate trypsin and other substances that in turn activate the pancreatic enzymes. Activation of the pancreatic enzymes results in autodigestion of the pancreas and surrounding tissues and varying degrees of edema, hemorrhage, coagulation necrosis, and fat necrosis. If the blood flow to the pancreas is reduced 40 to 60 percent, the resulting ischemia can convert edematous pancreatitis into hemorrhagic pancreatic necrosis. In both cases, large amounts of fluid may be lost, as either transudation from the swollen, edematous pancreas or as actual blood lost from a hemorrhagic pancreatitis. Enough fluid may be lost to produce even a shock state. A particularly disastrous result of the low flow state is renal failure, in which the mortality approaches 80 to 90 percent.

Pelvic Fractures

Pelvic fractures are potentially lethal. A great deal of soft tissue injury as well as bone injury from the fractured pelvic ring (the pubic rami and ischium, acetabulum, ilium, sacrum, pubic symphysis and sacroiliac joints) can be present. If the ilium is fractured, the internal iliac vein can be torn, with resulting extensive retroperitoneal hemorrhage. Massive blood loss may require replacement of as many as 12 to 20 units of blood, and it is usually the underlying cause of profound shock. But many pelvic fractures are mild and have relatively benign courses. Often the fractures are difficult to detect by x ray since the bones move very little and only a crack can be seen.

Because many urological structures are in the pelvic area, any abnormality makes an intravenous pyelogram, a retrograde cystourethrogram, and a urological evaluation imperative. The key assessment parameter is blood in the urine. If the patient voids urine that is not bloody, his chances of having a urological injury are greatly reduced. Potential problems exist with the diaphragm, the viscera, and/or the bladder [47]. The anteroinferior surface of the bladder is contiguous with the pubic bones, and is not covered with peritoneum. The triangular ligament, or urogenital diaphragm, is stretched across the pubic arch, through which the membranous urethra passes. Any fracture of the symphysis is likely to injure the bladder and/or the urethra. As a matter of fact, 10 percent of patients who have pelvic fractures have an associated bladder injury. If blood is found in the urine, rupture of the bladder must be considered. Also, because the various structures are so close, hematuria is common even when a significant injury has not occurred. Also (and obviously), a full bladder is more susceptible to injury than an empty one.

Rectal injuries are less common; they are most likely to be caused by a fracture of the ischium. On rectal examination by the physician, the presence of rectal bleeding is suggestive of injury and the palpation of a bony spicule is diagnostic of injury.

For the purposes of management, Trunkey and his associates [61] have divided pelvic fractures following crushing, blunt trauma into unstable fractures and stable fractures (Fig 34-7). The most serious type of pelvic injury is the comminuted, or crushing, fracture. It is classified as a type I injury, and it involves three or more structures of the pelvic ring. Usually such a fracture is unstable, and it involves extensive soft tissue injury and hemorrhage. The patient is treated with bedrest and perhaps a pelvic sling.

Another kind of unstable fracture, a type II injury, has four variants, all requiring immobilization or traction to reduce hemorrhage and/or to maintain the position of the weight-bearing portions of the pelvis: (1) fracture characterized by actual or potential displacement of the hemipelvis toward the head; (2) undisplaced diametric fracture (a diametric fracture is one in which the fracture extends anteriorly through the rami or symphysis and posteriorly through the sacrum, sacroiliac joint, or ilium, resulting in displacement of the hemipelvis); (3) the sprung pelvis, or the "open book"; the posterior structures are intact (like the spine of a bound book), while the anterior structures are fractured and opened (like the pages of a book); and (4) a fracture of the acetabulum; such a fracture may be further complicated by dislocation of the head of the femur, and in some instances it may require internal fixation.

A type III injury is a stable fracture, and it usually brings little danger of hemorrhage. Limited immobilization is necessary, and early weight bearing is encouraged. Type III injuries are usually isolated fractures; they include isolated fractures of the pubic

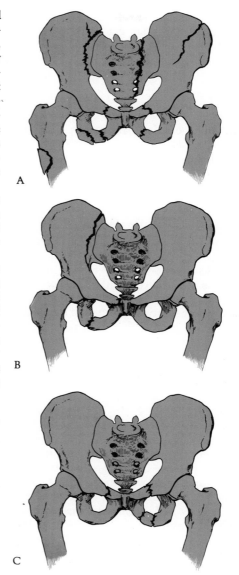

A

B

C

Figure 34-7

Unstable and stable pelvic fractures. A. Type 1 injury. Unstable fracture involving three or more structures of the pelvic ring. B. Type 2 injury. C. Type 3 injury. Stable fracture.

rami. The patients are often elderly. They are treated with bedrest and then they are gradually mobilized until they are able to bear weight.

Extremity Trauma

Musculoskeletal injuries involve any combination of the following: bone, cartilage, ligaments, muscles, soft tissues, blood vessels, nerves and, sometimes, the skin. Associated peripheral nerves are usually involved in some manner.

Fractures

A fracture of the bone occurs when either direct or indirect forces placed on the bone exceed its elasticity and thus cause deformation (Fig. 34-8). The normal continuity of bone or cartilage is interrupted with an associated soft tissue injury. A direct force commonly is a blow or a crushing injury and results in fracture(s) and soft tissue injury. If more than two fractures are present, the fracture is comminuted. Indirect forces, on the other hand, are transmitted through the bone, and fractures occur in an area of weakness. Also, the direction taken by the line of force or breakage produces a transverse, oblique, or spiral fracture. A transverse fracture usually results from simple angulatory forces, with the long axis of the bone at a right angle to the fracture surface. A spiral fracture usually results from torsion, and the fracture itself is spiral. An oblique fracture is one in which the fracture forms an oblique angle with the long axis of the bone. If only part of the thickness of the bone is broken, the fracture is termed incomplete; that is, it is a buckle, greenstick, fissure, or depressed fracture [44].

Fractures are closed or open wounds. In a closed (simple) fracture, there is no communication between the fracture and the skin (although wounds are sometimes in close proximity to the fracture). In an open fracture, the skin or mucosa associated with the fracture is broken, and the fracture site is in contact with the outside environment. If a dark hematoma extrudes from the wound, and especially if fat globules are mixed with the blood, the fracture is probably an open one. Open fractures are not probed in the emergency room. Examination and debridement are done in the operating room [30].

Also it must be kept in mind that injuries often involve arteries, veins, nerves, and tendons. In many in-

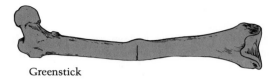
Greenstick

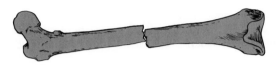
Transverse

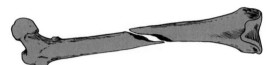
Spiral

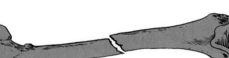
Oblique

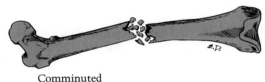
Comminuted

Figure 34-8
Common types of fractures.

stances those structures lie in close proximity, and one or all may be damaged. Shock may result from hemorrhage and pain.

After the fracture, skeletal stability is lost, and soft tissue is injured. Bleeding and, in some instances, even hemorrhage into the injured area originate from the ends of the bone as well as the torn muscles and/or damaged blood vessels of the soft tissue. Immediately after the fracture, the surrounding muscles are flaccid for 10 to 40 minutes and then go into a spasm. Possibly, the spasm interferes with the circulation of the blood and lymph; in any event, it is painful, and it increases the deformity by pulling the bone fragments further out of alignment. Deformity, swelling, ecchymosis, crepitus, localized tenderness and abnormal motion are classic signs of fracture.

HEALING

Once the extravasated blood around the end of the bone clots, healing begins (Fig. 34-9). An aseptic inflammatory response is soon apparent with blood vessel dilatation, resulting in a hyperemia and a local increase in the temperature. Increased capillary permeability permits protein and granulocytes to leak out into the tissue and produces edema. Both ecchymosis and swelling result. Organization of the blood clot is rapid (36–48 hr) in that the conversion of fibrinogen to fibrin forms a meshwork of fibers that later collects albumin, globulin, fibrinogen, and other extravasated cells. Granulation tissue thus invades the clot, and reticuloendothelial cells remove the debris. The pH of the tissue fluid around the bone fragments decreases so that some of the calcium goes into solution. New capillaries grow into the blood clot, and fibroblasts follow the pattern established by the fibrin meshwork. The torn edges of periosteum, endosteum, and bone marrow produce cells that help form new bone.

After 2 weeks, the alkaline phosphatase concentration increases around the bone fragments, and the pH of the tissue rises. Since calcium is then no longer soluble, calcium salts precipitate in the meshwork. Osteoid tissue is produced by the bone-forming cells, collagen is formed from fibroblasts, ground substance is formed from myxoplasts, and cartilage is formed from chondroblasts. Calcium salts and ground substance are deposited onto and around the collagen meshwork. The process takes place both around the bone fragments and at a distance. Thus an irregular bridge or callus is built from one bone fragment to another. At first, the callus is composed of fiber bone, but later it is absorbed and remodeled with osteal bone according to the stresses and strains that have occurred.

OPEN FRACTURES

Open fractures are an entity unto themselves. A primary objective of care of open fractures is the prevention of infection and the encouragement of bone union. The causes of open fractures range from a laceration to a crushing injury. By definition, open fractures communicate with the external environment and thus are

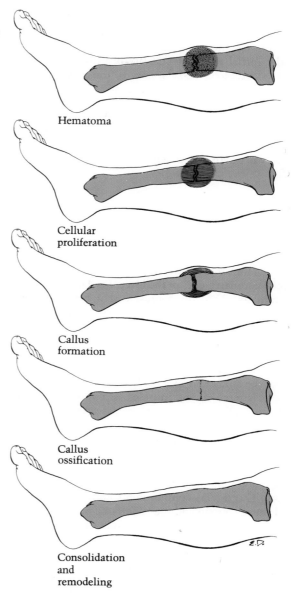

Hematoma

Cellular proliferation

Callus formation

Callus ossification

Consolidation and remodeling

Figure 34-9
Progression of fracture healing.

contaminated with microorganisms, have soft tissue injury, and possibly contain a foreign body. As in all forms of trauma, the greatest variable is the severity of the initial accident and the resulting damage to bone, skin, blood vessels, nerves, muscles, and tendons [5]. Added to the problems of the initial injury are the possible complications of decreased circulation, infection, osteomyelitis, delayed union, and nonunion. Every fracture is carefully assessed as to whether it is open or closed. If any doubt exists, it usually is treated as an open fracture.

Lower Extremity Compartment Syndrome

Transverse or comminuted fractures, whether from a direct blow or motor vehicle accident, often have considerable soft tissue contusion. Any of the four fascial compartments of the lower leg (Fig. 34-10) may contain tightly swollen muscle that becomes compressed and ischemic. Also, pieces of torn muscle can act with fascial tears as a ball valve and close an already swollen compartment.

Anterior compartment compression is most common. The deep peroneal nerve controlling dorsiflexion of the ankle and toes could be affected. Pain with passive stretch of the muscles is a cardinal sign of ischemia. The parameters to be assessed are the patient's ability to dorsiflex his toes and to feel sensation in the dorsal web space between his first and second toes. As in all compression syndromes, the surgical treatment is opening of the compartment.

Compression of the lateral compartment is unusual. The lateral compartment contains the peroneal muscle group and the superficial peroneal nerve. The assessment parameters include the loss of eversion power and sensory loss of the dorsum.

Compression in the posterior compartment is even rarer. The assessment parameters include the functioning of the soleus and the gastrocnemius muscles.

In the deep posterior compartment are the posterior tibial nerve, artery, and vein, the tibialis posterior muscle, and the long toe flexors. The assessment parameters include the tone of the toe flexors and plantar sensation.

Often, all four fascial compartments require decompression. The measurement of intracompartmental pressures is advocated by some orthopedic surgeons to determine if patients need decompression by fibulectomy and/or fasciotomy. In fasciotomy, each of

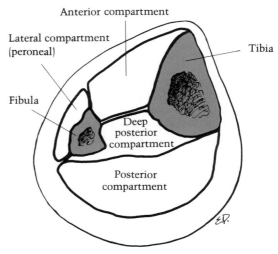

Figure 34-10
Cross section of compartments in the middle third of the leg.

the four fascial compartments of the leg is opened widely. Wound healing occurs usually by second intention while the patient is immobilized in a long leg cast. An alternate treatment is several days of elevation of the leg followed by delayed primary suturing and skin grafting.

Arterial Injury

Traumatic damage of a large artery that supplies blood to an extremity most often results from a penetrating injury. The vascular injury is frequently complicated by an associated fracture or dislocation. Surgical exploration is performed when there are many penetrating wounds in the vicinity of a major artery. Angiograms are routinely used to determine what patients are candidates for surgery. If a major artery in an extremity is injured, direct repair or reconstruction of the artery is usually needed to prevent the loss of function or amputation. Ligation and amputation are no longer accepted procedures under normal circumstances.

Vascular injuries are particular problems for the general surgeon. If possible, a vascular surgeon is consulted. The nurse is in a position to assist in the initial assessment and to monitor the patient carefully.

Vascular injuries are suspected when the patient demonstrates any of the following: (1) a diminished or absent distal pulse, (2) a persistent arterial bleeding, (3) a large hematoma that increases in size, (4) wounds that are close to a major vessel, (5) an aberration in functioning of a nerve that is in close anatomical position to the vessel, (6) a bruit from partial thrombosis or A–V fistula, and (7) shock [55]. The presence of a normal distal pulse does not mean that an artery has not been damaged. Because of collateral circulation, a normal pulse may be palpated. Most likely, a "soft clot" has formed through which pulsations but not blood may pass. Angiography is considered to be 95 percent accurate, and it is particularly useful in patients who have associated skeletal injuries and scattered bullet wounds of the extremities.

Blood loss is also not necessarily a determinant of the severity of the injury. Hemorrhage from an arterial tear may be profuse, whereas a transected artery may clamp down to stop blood loss.

Emergency care entails, first, the use of simple digital pressure. Then with the patient under anesthesia, devitalized tissue is debrided and an incision is made to allow proximal and distal visualization of the injured vessel.

Some surgeons may use surgical sympathectomy, sympathetic blockade, or mechanical dilatation and the application of magnesium sulfate to prevent arterial spasm. During the procedure, the proximal and distal segments are injected with about 10 ml of a balanced salt solution containing 1:10 solution of heparin to prevent thrombosis. (Some surgeons use systemic heparinization.) If a clot is present in the segment, a balloon-type (Fogarty) catheter or a small suction catheter is used to dislodge and retrieve the clot and establish flow.

The type of repair depends on the extent and type of injury. It may be a lateral repair, an end-to-end anastomosis, or a graft. Because the wound is contaminated, a greater saphenous vein graft rather than a synthetic graft is generally used.

Besides the usual monitoring done in a critical care unit, the patient must be monitored in regard to his blood pressure (every 15 min), temperature and color of the skin, and his distal pulses. The Doppler is an invaluable aid.

Peripheral Nerve Injury

A frequent concomitant of trauma is an injury to one or more peripheral nerves. Open fractures are described in the literature as the classic predisposing problem but the cause may as well be a closed fracture, or a crush, blunt, or penetrating injury.

Injuries may be caused directly or indirectly. For example, a sharp object (e.g., a knife or the end of a splintered bone) may damage a nerve directly. An injury may occur from edema or hemorrhage, resulting in ischemia or nerve compression. Later, the injury may become apparent because of neural entrapment in scar tissue or callus formation during bone healing.

A high-velocity projectile missile has a destructive effect over a considerable distance from the missile's path. Damage results from the release of large amounts of energy in the tissues. The injuries to the nerves are often unrecognized, and the nerve deficit is not identified. Nerve bundles suffer varying degrees of damage, ranging from a loss of conductivity to complete severance and paralysis. Such concussion to the nerve may cause sensory loss and paralysis that lasts just a few days. If the return of function is fast, the injury has been a concussive one from the pressure transmitted by the blast effect. But the return of functioning can be delayed for weeks. If the nerve is completely severed, complete paralysis and a sharply defined loss of deep sensitivity are present.

Essentially, hundreds of axis cylinders enclosed in endoneural tubes comprise a peripheral nerve. The axis cylinder in the center of the axon is continuous with the nerve cell itself, and a thin membrane covers both. Myelin envelops the cylinder and, in turn, is surrounded by a sheath of Schwann cells, which are essential for regeneration. The endoneurium, a loose, fibrous tissue, separates one fiber from another, and the perineurium (a thin, strong connective tissue sheath) encases groups of fibers (fascicles). The fascicle is usually composed of both motor and sensory axons. The epineurium is the outer covering of the nerve.

Nerve injuries are classified according to the damage and the recovery time. A first-degree injury is usually the result of a contusion or prolonged compression. Functioning returns in 1 week to 4 months. Although no actual break in continuity is present, the conductivity of the axis cylinders is decreased or blocked. Structurally, the axon is intact although segmental damage can be present. The return of sensation is first noted, and is followed by the return of motor power.

In a second-degree injury, several of the axis cylinders are severed and degenerate. Recovery is preceded by Wallerian nerve degeneration of the distal segment. Because the proximal end of the nerve degenerates to the nearest node of Ranvier, the axon in the distal segment is not in contact with the nerve cell itself. Thus for 3 to 7 days after the injury, the distal segment degenerates into fragments and the myelin sheath is digested by the Schwann cells. As part of the process, Schwann cells proliferate and nerve regeneration is initiated by growth of the proximal axon down the Schwann cell encasement at the rate of 1 to 2 mm a day, or about 1 in. per month. The Schwann cells layer fresh myelin around the nerves, and the distal nerve segment swells to about twice its original size. The entire process takes about 30 days. Generally, sensation returns before motor functioning does. Sensation returns first in the area proximal to injury, but the sensation is not normal at first. For example, tingling sensations or paresthesias are common responses to stimulation. Those responses tend to travel down the length of the nerve as growth proceeds (Tinel's sign). Physical therapy and some type of splinting are important to maintain the paralyzed area during the regeneration process so that permanent functional abnormalities do not ensue.

In a third-degree injury, the internal structure of the nerve is disorganized. The endoneural tube around the cylinder remains intact even though all the tubes are no longer intact.

In a fourth-degree injury, the continuity of the epineurium is disrupted and the nerve shrinks to a slender thread.

In a fifth-degree injury, the nerve is completely severed. Since there is no continuity of the epineurium, there is nothing to guide regeneration. The involved muscles are totally paralyzed. Surgical repair is mandatory. It may be done immediately, or it may be delayed for 2 to 6 weeks. If the wound is not excessively contaminated and if the nerve ends can be satisfactorily approximated, repair at the initial wound closure is often the treatment of choice. Some surgeons decide on delayed repair because in time the extent of damage is clearly demarcated and the supporting axon structures (the perineurium and the epineurium) have thickened and increased the tensile strength. Interfascicular suture is attempted. The return of functioning is problematic because the undulating, twisting growth of nerve fibers from one fascicle to another forms various new plexuses throughout the length of the nerve. Factors that play a significant role in the quality and the quantity of regeneration are the type of injury, the age of the patient, the level of injury, the duration of the injury, the alignment of

nerve ends, a tension-free anastamosis, and any associated injuries.

An alternate classification of peripheral nerve injuries entails descriptions of neuropraxia, axonotmesis, and neurotmesis [51]. In neuropraxia, the axon is structurally intact with no anatomical disruption of the nerve fiber, but transmission is decreased. In some areas of the axon there may be demyelination. In axonotmesis, the axon is disrupted, but the supporting structures (e.g., the epineurium, the perineurium, and the Schwann cell tubes) are intact. In neurotmesis, nerve fibers and their sheaths of connective tissue are transected.

Injuries of the brachial plexus and of the nerve trunks proximal in the extremities (e.g., the ulnar and the sciatic nerve) usually have a poor prognosis. Movements that require fine muscle control are often not recoverable. Sensation such as proprioception in small joints and two-point discrimination are slow to recover and often they remain abnormal. Light touch and proprioception are frequently maintained, even though a small number of sensory fibers are present.

Nerve lesions may be complete or incomplete. Overall functioning can be decreased, or one type of conduction deficit can be more apparent than another (e.g., there may be more motor loss than sensory loss). In general, motor dysfunction is more common than sensory dysfunction. The patient may not be able to move a body part yet feel pain in that part. Motor nerves seem to be damaged more easily than sensory nerves because they are larger and conduct impulses more rapidly. An analagous phenomenon is present in the sensory nerves in regard to touch and pain; that is, the patient may lose the sense of light touch yet retain the sense of pain.

Nerve fibers are different in size. The motor nerve fibers are the largest and most heavily myelinated ones. The fibers concerned with proprioception and cutaneous sensation are next in size, and the pain fibers and the fibers of the autonomic nervous system are small. The large, heavily myelinated fibers conduct impulses at a faster rate.

In the upper extremities, there are five major nerves: the median, ulnar, radial, circumflex (axillary), and musculocutaneous nerves. The areas of the dorsal aspect of the hand supplied by the median, ulnar, and radial nerves are shown in Figure 34-11. Involvement of the median nerve results in both motor loss and sensory loss; namely, motor loss of wrist and finger flexion, loss of forearm pronation and fin-

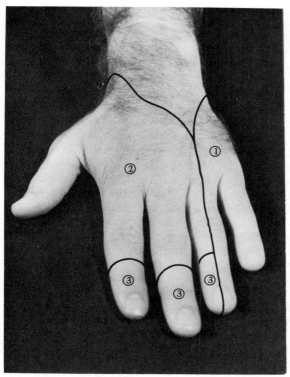

Figure 34-11
Dorsal view of the hand, with the areas supplied by the ulnar (1), radial (2), and median (3) nerves outlined.

ger-thumb opposition, and sensory loss in the palmar aspects, including the thumb, index finger, middle finger, and radial half of the ring finger. Assessment is made of the patient's ability to oppose his thumb and little finger and to flex his wrist. Involvement of the ulnar nerve results in motor and sensory loss over the ulnar border of the hand, the ulnar side of the ring finger, and the little finger. Assessment is made of the patient's ability to abduct those fingers. The involvement of the radial nerve is mainly a motor loss. Most of the extensor muscles of the elbow, forearm, and hand are innervated by the radial nerve, and the involvement results in wrist drop. Sensory loss includes the dorsal web space between the thumb and index finger. Assessment is made of the patient's ability to hyperextend his wrist and fingers. Involvement of the circumflex nerve results in a sensory loss in the skin over the deltoid muscle and in a

motor loss of the deltoid muscle. Assessment entails abduction of the arm at the shoulder. Involvement of the musculocutaneous nerve results in a sensory loss on the radial side of the forearm and a motor loss of the biceps brachii, brachialis, and coracobrachialis muscles. Assessment is made of the patient's ability to flex his arm at the elbow.

Involvement of the peroneal nerve results in foot drop since the anterior tibial peroneal and toe extensor groups are not innervated [65]. Assessment entails the patient's ability to dorsiflex his foot. Involvement of the tibial nerve is assessed by asking the patient to plantarflex his ankle and noting if he is able to flex and extend his toes.

Assessment and Management

After the initial trauma assessment and the treatment of such conditions as upper airway obstruction, hemorrhage, shock, and neurological injuries, the injured extremity is assessed [8]. First, the neurovascular functioning is evaluated in regard to circulation, sensation, and motor power. People who have gunshot wounds and open fractures are particularly likely to have problems. Then the local skin trauma and soft tissue injury are evaluated, noting whether the injury is open or closed, the degree of bleeding, the degree of contamination, and the extent of injury. Finally the bone injury is evaluated.

The patient's circulation is assessed by palpating his distal pulses and evaluating his capillary refill, color, and temperature. Clinical signs that suggest arterial injury are looked for. In general, a penetrating injury in the region of a major blood vessel or nerve is explored by the surgeon. If the ischemia is severe enough, an excruciating pain or (sometimes) a glovelike anesthesia is present. Sensation in the injured area is assessed by touch and pinprick. Motor power is assessed as good, poor, or absent. Movement or hand grip is a satisfactory indicator for the arms and dorsiflexion is a satisfactory indicator for the feet.

The amount of blood loss depends on the structures in the particular bone and on the type of fracture. Also, blood flow to the fractured extremity is increased after an injury. Assessment of the site itself entails comparison of the injured side to the uninjured side in regard to appearance and size. When measured with an accurate tape measure, the circumference of the injured extremity can be used as an indicator of blood loss; each 1-in. increase in circumference indicates a one unit loss of blood.

Bone with Closed Fracture	Possible Hidden Blood Loss
Tibia or fibula	500 ml–1000 ml
Femur	500 ml–2000 + ml
Radius and/or ulna	50 ml–750 ml

Assessment parameters for the fracture are instability, pain, deformity, shortening, rotation, ecchymosis, swelling, and crepitus. The site should not be palpated for crepitus, but crepitus should be recorded if it is present. With positive fracture signs, further evaluation includes two plane x rays at the fracture site taken perpendicular to each other. To determine the particular nerve involved, the paralyzed muscles and the area of anesthesia are described. Important data are history of the accident, location of the nerve, and a comparison of both sides of the body.

The classic clinical parameters for extremity injury are known as the five Ps: pain, pulselessness, pallor, paralysis, and paresthesia.

The patient must be considered as an entity, and his whole body should be checked systematically. For example, an injury to the shoulder might be accompanied by an injury of the brachial plexus or of the radial nerve and artery. An injury of the shaft of the humerus can injure the radial nerve [7]. A fractured elbow can cause problems with the radial artery and median nerve. In a crushing injury of the forearm, both hand and forearm functioning must be assessed.

Injuries of the lower extremities are frequently associated with significant problems. At particular risk is the elderly woman who has a fractured hip and many associated geriatric problems [39]. Fractures about the knee may be accompanied by significant popliteal artery damage. Evaluation of the pulse and an arteriogram are important, because many patients who have injured arteries have satisfactory distal pulses. Dislocations of the knee are notorious for being associated with damaged popliteal arteries, and the surgeon routinely orders an arteriogram following reduction of the dislocation. Injuries of the tibial plateau are associated with the anterior compartment syndrome. Bleeding results in tightness and tenseness, which produces paralysis. Initially, the syndrome is manifested by decreased sensation to light touch on the dorsum of the foot. Any findings that

suggest anterior compartment syndrome must be referred to the orthopedic surgeon immediately. The situation must be treated as an emergency if the patient is to retain function [6].

WOUND CARE

The principles of wound management must be followed. The fracture site is covered with a sterile dressing and splinted until it can be shaved and debrided through an extension of the wound. Cold is applied, the extremity is elevated to reduce swelling, and any exposed tendons are covered with a wet saline dressing. Intravenous fluid is never infused into the fractured extremity. Antibiotics (commonly Keflin, 1–2 gm intravenously every 6 hr) are administered. In some instances, cultures are done before and after debridement. Treatment is instituted within 6 hr of the injury under optimal surgical conditions.

Maintaining anatomical position, the extremity is splinted above and below the fracture to align the fracture and to immobilize the bone fragments. To temporarily stabilize a fracture distal to and including the knee or elbow, an air splint may be used. The splint is inflated to an internal pressure of 30 mm Hg or to the point where external pressure compresses the splint 0.5 in. For a fracture of the humerus or shoulder, a sling is used. For a fracture of the femur, a traction splint (e.g., a Thomas splint) is used to overcome muscle spasms. For a closed fracture, preparations are made for the application of a cast. For an open fracture, preparations are made for immediate wound debridement and skeletal traction.

In severe wounds and extensive soft tissue injury, the wound is usually kept open. If the dressing is dry and the wound is not draining, a delayed primary closure is performed in 5 to 7 days. In particular, most physicians will keep open an injury caused by a rotary lawn mower or gunshot and an injury that is questionable. To avoid further damage to the blood supply, early metal fixation is usually not utilized. Rather, the wound is again debrided in 4 to 5 days, and the bone is stabilized. For the same reason, intramedullary rods are usually not used early after injury, because the blood supply is in the medulla [21].

Each patient must be treated as an individual. The decision about treatment is made after assessing the patient's fractured bone, foreign material, and damaged tissue. The nurse must be prepared to assist with whatever treatment approach the physician chooses and she should be able to answer the patient's and the family's questions. The possible treatment approaches are:

1. Primary closure or cover by suture or split-thickness skin graft
2. Delayed primary closure or cover by suture or split-thickness skin graft
3. Secondary closure or cover by suture or split-thickness skin graft
4. Healing by granulation or secondary intention

Tetanus Immunization

Immunization against tetanus is determined according to the following recommendations of the Committee on Trauma of the American College of Surgeons [2, 11, 66]:

1. Previous immunization
   a. Active immunization in the past 10 years. For a patient whose injuries are more than 24 hours old or who has severe injuries, give 0.5 ml of adsorbed tetanus toxoid (unless he has had a booster in the last year).
   b. Active immunization more than 10 years ago
      (1) For a patient whose injuries are more than 24 hours old or who has a severe injury, give:
         (a) 0.5 ml of adsorbed tetanus toxoid.
         (b) 250 units of human tetanus immune globulin. The administration of penicillin or tetracycline should be considered.
      (2) For other patients, give 0.5 ml of adsorbed tetanus toxoid.
2. No previous immunization
   a. With clean minor wounds when tetanus is highly unlikely, give the initial immunizing dose of 0.5 ml of adsorbed tetanus toxoid. Give the same dose again in 4 to 6 weeks and again in 6 to 12 months.
   b. For all other patients, give the same dose listed in 2a plus 250 units of human tetanus immune globin. The administration of penicillin or tetracycline should be considered.

Nursing Orders

The initial assessment and management of the injured patient is dependent on a systematic evaluation by a well-educated team whose roles are defined and who have planned for all contingencies [4].

Of first importance is care at the accident site. Speed alone is not the primary consideration. Identification of the problem and appropriate and immediate care prior to and during transit will bring a viable patient to a well-equipped, well-staffed hospital for definitive care. Appropriate on-site care increases the chances that the patient's life can be saved. The fate of the injured person to a large extent depends on his initial care. Emergency medical care is being taken out of the realm of the haphazard and inexperienced and is moving toward organized and sophisticated systems of care. The essential components of emergency medical care include communications, evacuation and transportation by ground and air ambulance, categorization of hospitals, education of and practice for personnel (e.g., lay groups, emergency medical technicians and paramedics, firemen, policemen, physicians, nurses, and respiratory therapists) and program evaluation. Prehospital emergency care takes a multifaceted approach: (1) system design, (2) selection of personnel, (3) provision for a rapid response to emergencies through good distribution of equipment and personnel, (4) safe transportation to the hospital by well-trained personnel, good equipment, and enough vehicles, and (5) standardized algorithms for therapy [3].

On the patient's arrival in the emergency room, it is suggested that the following protocol be observed:

1. Open airway.
2. Ensure breathing.
3. Maintain circulation.
4. Carry out definitive therapy.
5. Apply pressure to hemorrhaging sites. External hemorrhage is best controlled by putting direct finger pressure on the bleeding wound or vessel. Application of pressure to major pressure points may also be used. A tourniquet is used only when too few medical personnel are available to institute higher priority measures. If the exposed vessel is accessible, it can be ligated. Wounds should not be probed, because probing may dislodge a clot. An external injuring instrument, such as a knife, should not be removed from the patient since it may be acting as a tamponade. The surgeon will examine the wound and remove the instrument under optimal surgical conditions [70].

Internal hemorrhaging requires surgical intervention. The nurse should observe the nasogastric and Foley drainage and measure the girth of neck, abdomen, and thighs as indicated to watch for an increase in size.

6. Perform a rapid assessment to determine presence of critical injuries and to establish priorities [54]. The following should be differentiated:
   a. Injuries or conditions that interfere with vital physiological functions and thus are an immediate threat to life (e.g., an obstructed airway).
   b. Injuries that are not an immediate threat to survival (e.g., some gunshot wounds, stab wounds, or blunt trauma to the chest or abdomen in which the vital signs remain stable).
   c. Injuries that produce occult damage (chiefly, blunt trauma to the abdomen where the exact nature of the injury is not apparent). In such injuries, there is time for extensive laboratory studies, x rays, and a general physical examination because surgery may be delayed or may not be necessary.

7. Assess the patient for a spinal fracture. All patients should be treated as though they had a spinal fracture until proved otherwise.

8. Restore an adequate circulating volume by crystalloid and blood therapy [24, 32, 37, 55, 69]. Ringer's lactate solution is given initially in amounts up to 2 liters and then continued at the rate of 10 to 15 ml/kg/hr. Blood is replaced as indicated by the degree of loss. A large-bore (14–16 gauge) catheter is placed in each arm. If possible, the subclavian route is not used because of complications associated with its use. Within the first 24 hours after the trauma, all the intravenous sites that were used at first are changed.

9. Place a Foley catheter unless blood is present at the meatus or a perineal or scrotal hematoma is present.

10. Place a nasogastric catheter unless the base of the patient's neck has been traumatized and a vascular injury might be present. Administer antacids as ordered.

11. Send samples to the laboratory for a complete blood count, serum amylase and arterial blood gas determinations, and a urinalysis.

12. Have a clot sent to the blood bank for typing and cross matching for 6 to 8 units of whole blood.

13. Perform a physical examination.

14. Cover any open wounds.

15. Splint any fractures.

16. Obtain a history. The nurse should:
    a. Begin the history even before the patient arrives at the hospital, using the radio report from the emergency medical technicians or the telephone report from the medical team or transferring facility.
    b. Obtain the history as soon as is feasible. The major points are gathered while the physical examination is being performed.
    c. Be aware that a history is difficult to obtain from a severely injured person.
    d. Persevere in the history taking, even when the patient is severely injured, and combine a systematic examination with careful, meaningful questions.
    e. Obtain information from bystanders, friends, and family.
    f. Record information about the circumstances surrounding the injury in an orderly fashion. Get the details of the accident, including when the accident occurred, the patient's position at the time of the accident, any subsequent displacement, and whether the patient struck, or was struck by, an object.
    g. Record information about any treatment administered before the patient arrived in the emergency room.
    h. Record the time of the patient's last meal.
    i. Record information about: preexisting disease (e.g., cardiovascular, pulmonary, renal, metabolic, or neurological disorders), the use of drugs, alcohol, and/or narcotics (in detail), tetanus immunization, medications, allergies, and drug sensitivities.

17. Use adjunct assessment parameters (e.g., chest x ray, spinal x ray, ECG, angiogram, intravenous pyelogram, and voiding cystogram) as ordered by the physician.

18. Set new priorities.

19. Administer tetanus prophylaxis as ordered.

Problem/Diagnosis

Respiratory dysfunction due to an obstructed airway secondary to trauma.

OBJECTIVE

The patient should maintain a patent airway. To achieve the objective, the nurse should know that an obstructed airway is a grave danger to the traumatized patient. It probably causes more deaths than does any other malfunction.

The nurse should:

1. Know the information about basic airway management given in Chapter 18.
2. Use tonsil suction to rapidly remove blood, debris, and broken pieces of teeth.
3. Place an esophageal airway if needed.
4. If necessary, keep the airway open with an endotracheal tube. Endotracheal intubation is frequently lifesaving, and the Committee on Trauma of the American College of Surgeons recommends that nurses working in emergency rooms acquire the skill. Like all skills, the technique of endotracheal intubation must be practiced. If it is not, dexterity decreases. Thus the nurse who is not able to acquire and keep up her proficiency must develop methods for emergency care appropriate and specific for that setting. In regard to endotracheal intubation, the nurse should:
   a. Know that endotracheal intubation is necessary if a patient cannot maintain his airway, handle his secretions, or ventilate himself adequately. If there is any question of spinal cord damage, the nasotracheal route rather than the oral route should be selected.
   b. Be sure endotracheal tube is inserted into the trachea to allow a direct means to improve the respiratory status. The laryngoscope consists of two parts, the handle and a straight or a curved blade (the blade retracts the tongue and permits visualization of the vocal cords as the tube is inserted).
   c. Know that a stylet may be used to ease the insertion of the tube. The stylet is a malleable wire that has a blunt end. It is placed in the endotracheal tube to make it stiffer. The stylet must be kept at least one inch back from the tip of the tube. If it is not, the stylet may perforate the trachea or bronchus, resulting in mediastinitis.
   d. Use a tube of the proper size; usually a 7.5-mm tube is used for adult females and an 8.5-mm tube is used for adult males. All tubes have the standard 15-mm adapter.
   e. Before insertion, check the tube to make sure it will inflate easily, hold air, expand evenly, and deflate completely.
   f. If desired, lubricate the tip of the tube with a water-soluble or a 5% xylocaine jelly (the jelly should not get inside the tube).
   g. Before intubation, position the patient with his neck flexed forward and his head hyperextended. Use a roll under his neck and shoulder to help keep the head in alignment.
   h. Ascertain that a suction apparatus is available.
   i. If possible, administer 100% oxygen for 3 to 5 minutes to increase alveolar oxygen concentration. Oxygen is supplied at a flow rate greater than minute volume so that nitrogen is replaced by oxygen. Thus during intubation, when the patient's air exchange is not adequate, any decrease in the arterial oxygen tension will not be as significant.
   j. Perform intubation with the person's head hyperextended.
   k. Use the left hand to hold the laryngoscope and the little finger of the left hand to move the tip.
   l. Use the right hand to manipulate the patient's head.
   m. As the blade is inserted into the right side of the mouth to visualize the larynx, see that the tongue is pushed to the left and held out of the way by the ridge on the blade (Fig. 34-12).
   n. Use different techniques with straight and curved blades. With the curved-blade technique, the epiglottis is visualized and the blade is placed in the vallecula, between the base of the tongue and the epiglottis. With the straight-blade technique, the epiglottis is not visualized. The blade should be placed all the way to the posterior wall of the pharynx below the epiglottis so that the epiglottis will be out of the line of vision.
   o. Exert traction on the handle of the laryngoscope in an upward direction to expose the glottic opening. Be careful to lift the blade and not use a levering motion with the wrist, because it is easy to break the patient's front teeth.
   p. Insert the endotracheal tube along the right side of the patient's mouth (not down the blade).
   q. Continue to visualize as the tube goes between the vocal cords above the arytenoid cartilages.
   r. When the tube has been placed so that the cuff is 1 in. beyond the vocal cords, remove the scope, inflate the cuff, and ventilate.
   s. Assess the placement of tube. Use a positive pressure device immediately and note the adequacy of chest expansion and breath sounds bilaterally. If the tube goes into the right

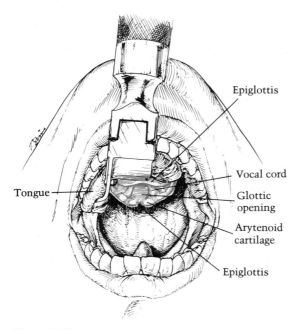

Figure 34-12
Endotracheal intubation.

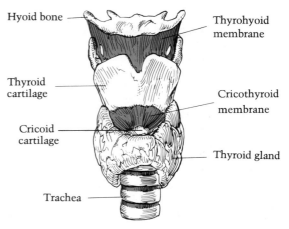

Figure 34-13
Cricothyroid membrane.

mainstem bronchus, the left lung is perfused but not ventilated.

   t. Mark the endotracheal tube at the level of the patient's lips.

   u. Keep the tube in place with a bite block and adhesive tape.

5. If necessary and if other appropriate measures have failed, perform transtracheal catheter ventilation.

   a. Insert a 14-gauge plastic intravenous catheter with needle attached to a syringe through the cricothyroid membrane (Fig. 34-13). The cricothyroid membrane may be identified by two methods of palpating the transverse indentation between the thyroid and cricoid cartilage: (1) palpate the larynx and the first tracheal ring (the membrane between the two is the cricothyroid membrane) and (2) place the index finger at the sternal angle and slide it up until the first definite palpable ridge is encountered. Slightly further (approximately 1 cm), the finger will fall into a notchlike indentation. It is the cricothyroid membrane. If the larynx is palpated, the finger has gone too far.

   b. Ascertain return of free air.

   c. Advance the catheter and remove the needle.

   d. Use flexible tubing to attach to a hand-operated valve connected to an oxygen source.

   e. Open the valve for inspiration. Observe for chest expansion and auscultate breath sounds.

   f. Close valve for expiration (ratio 1 : 2).

   g. Repeat as needed.

6. If the preceding measures have failed, perform a cricothyroid stab (cricothyreotomy or coniotomy).

   a. Palpate the cricothyroid membrane.

   b. Make an incision through the cricothyroid membrane with a knife. Usually the incision is 0.5 in. long, and it may be vertical or horizontal.

   c. Put something in the opening to act as an artificial airway (because the membrane tends to close).

   d. Observe the patient for bleeding. (There should be little bleeding since the area is relatively avascular.)

Problem/Diagnosis

Shock secondary to trauma.

OBJECTIVE NO. 1

The patient should demonstrate a stable physiologic response and any alteration in status will be identified.

To achieve the objective, the nurse should:

1. Assess the patient's mental status every hour.
2. Monitor his hourly urinary output. Notify the physician if it is less than 0.5 to 1 ml per kilogram per hour.
3. Monitor his temperature, apical and radial pulses, respirations, and blood pressure as indicated.
4. Monitor his apical heart beat for rate and heart sounds every 30 minutes.
5. Assess his respiratory system, including rate, rhythm, breath sounds, and presence of adventitious sounds every hour.
6. Connect the ECG monitor and set the alarm for 30 beats above and 30 beats below the baseline rates. Notify the physician of abnormalities.
7. Obtain a 12-lead ECG as indicated.
8. Note arterial pressure measurement on the monitor every 30 min. Check the pressure with a cuff every 2 hr. If an arterial line is not present, check the arterial pressure with a cuff every 30 to 60 min as indicated. Notify the physician of a systolic pressure less than 90 mm Hg.
9. If ordered, draw arterial blood gas samples from the arterial line every 4 hr. Monitor oxygenation.
10. Observe for any signs of peripheral vasoconstriction every hour.
11. Once the patient's condition is stable, the MAST trousers may be systematically and sequentially deflated over a period of 15 to 30 min as ordered.
    a. When they are applied the trousers essentially provide an autotransfusion of the equivalent of two units of blood; the reverse is true when they are removed.
    b. Before removing the trousers, have two intravenous infusions running.
    c. Obtain baseline vital signs.
    d. Deflate the abdominal portion of the trousers.
    e. Monitor the vital signs for 5 to 10 min. If the patient's pulse increases and his blood pressure decreases, administer 100 to 200 ml of intravenous fluid until the vital signs stabilize (about 10 min).
    f. Deflate one leg of the trousers. Monitor the vital signs for 5 to 10 minutes. If the patient's pulse increases and his blood pressure decreases, administer intravenous fluid until his pulse decreases and his blood pressure increases.
    g. Deflate the other leg of the trousers. Monitor the vital signs for 30 min.

12. Measure pulmonary artery and central venous pressures every hour.
13. If ordered, measure the pulmonary capillary wedge pressure and cardiac output via thermodilution technique.
14. Every 15 minutes, check for bleeding from orifices or dressings. Mark dressings.
15. If a vascular injury is present, note the color and pulse in distal extremity every 15 minutes. Use the Doppler.
16. If possibility of injury exists, perform serial assessments of neck, abdomen and/or extremities with tape measure. (A tape measure that does not stretch when it is wet should be used.)
17. Monitor and assess the trends in the laboratory parameters (e.g., hemoglobin, hematocrit, serum amylase level, and the white blood cell count).
18. Weigh the patient daily.
19. Determine the patient's temperature during surgery. Postoperative rise in temperature is often related to the drop in temperature during surgery. (The temperature should be taken about every 2 hr.)

OBJECTIVE NO. 2

The patient should maintain an adequate oxygen-carrying capability by means of blood transfusion.

To achieve the objective, the nurse should:

1. In the emergent situation, initiate therapy with Ringer's lactate solution and have blood typed and crossmatched. If the patient does not respond, use type-specific blood rather than low-titer O negative blood. The blood group determination takes 5 min and the crossmatch procedure takes 45 min. The whole blood is typed but not crossmatched.
2. Not obtain blood from bank until it is needed, and infuse it within 2 hr. If the blood is warmed, administer it immediately.
3. Check the blood type against the patient's name and blood type according to the established protocol.
4. In rapid administration, use a heat exchanger or a warming apparatus or place the tubing in a pan of warm water. Under no circumstances should cold blood be administered through a central line; cardiac dysrhythmias begin to occur when the body temperature is below 92°F.

5. Use a nylon mesh filter. Change it after every third pint.

6. Use a pressure cuff as needed for rapid transfusion. Do not squeeze the bag.

7. For rapid administration as ordered by the physician, packed red blood cells may be reconstituted with saline solution to a 500-ml volume. Observe the patient's clinical and laboratory findings; hypofibrinogenemia and hypoalbuminemia have been noted during massive transfusions with packed red blood cells diluted with saline solution [25].

8. Obtain baseline information about the vital signs and observe the patient continuously during the first 50 ml of blood transfusion. Administer blood at no more than 50 drops per min for the first 2 min. Observe and monitor the vital signs every 30 min during the transfusion and for two hours after it. Reactions may take place at the beginning of the transfusion or during or after it.

9. At any untoward sign, stop the transfusion, change the tubing, start the saline solution and notify the physician.

10. Observe for the following reactions:
    a. A pyrexial reaction, which is the most common one but which cannot be distinguished from early hemolytic reaction. The cause of a pyrexial reaction is usually not known, but it may be related to the components of the donor's blood, such as the white blood cells or the platelets. Observe for chills, a rise in temperature, nausea, vomiting, headache, and muscle pain.
    b. Allergic reactions occur in 2% to 3% of patients who receive transfusion. Observe for hives, rash, and itching. If ordered by the physician, administer an antihistamine and continue the transfusion.
    c. Bacterial reactions are now extremely rare. Observe for fever, chills, pain, hypotension, and shock. Anticipate treatment for septic shock.
    d. Incompatibility reactions occur once in every 15,000 to 20,000 transfusions. The nurse should:
       (1) Observe for (1) an inappropriately severe aching pain, particularly in the flank, shoulders, back and/or hamstrings, a burning pain in the infusion arm or a constricting pain in the chest, (2) a very tense or anxious feeling, (3) nausea and vomit-

ing, (4) hemoglobinuria, (5) an increase in temperature, pulse, and respirations, (6) headache and chills, and (7) oliguria.
       (2) Monitor vital signs every 15 min.
       (3) Save all the transfusion equipment and return it to the laboratory.
       (4) Save the urine.
       (5) Monitor the fluid intake and output hourly.
       (6) As ordered by the physician, administer fluid therapy at sufficient volume to maintain the urinary flow at 50 ml per hour. The fluid ordered is usually Ringer's lactate solution. Sodium bicarbonate is ordered to alkalinize the urine and to prevent precipitation of hemoglobin in the tubules. Mannitol is often administered to maintain the urinary flow.

11. In the case of multiple transfusions, for every 2 pints of blood 9 days old or more, if possible give 1 pint that is less than 48 hr old.

12. Verify the following protocol with the physician: For every 10 units of packed red blood cells transfused acutely and rapidly, administer 2 to 3 units of platelets and 2 units of fresh, frozen plasma (which contains all the protein constituents of plasma and all the active labile clotting factors).

13. If ordered, administer 10 ml of calcium gluconate (or 44 mEq of calcium chloride) for every 3 units of blood administered rapidly. Do not add calcium to the blood. Monitor the patient for dysrhythmias with an ECG. If the patient needs 10 to 20 units of blood, call the physician before administering calcium to avoid excessive calcium therapy.

14. If old blood is given, monitor for the signs of hyperkalemia. If hyperkalemia occurs, the treatment includes the use of insulin and glucose to drive the potassium intracellularly: Hyperkalemia is not anticipated unless renal functioning is impaired or unless the blood is given at a rate greater than 100 to 150 ml per min.

15. Know that the patient may exhibit a transitory jaundice after multiple transfusions. If the production of bilirubin is greater than 500 to 900 mg per day, the normal liver cannot excrete all the pigment load. Both the indirect and direct serum bilirubin levels are elevated. In the 24 hr following transfusion, approximately 10% of the transfused blood undergoes hemolysis. Thus

with multiple transfusions, the pigment load is often exceeded and the bilirubin level increases. Also, particularly after retroperitoneal hemorrhage, the breakdown of blood produces the same sequence, and the patient exhibits jaundice.

16. Monitor for pulmonary edema and thrombophlebitis.
17. Observe for signs of hepatitis after about 6 weeks. Although the testing protocol for hepatitis antigen has decreased the incidence of hepatitis, the risk remains.

OBJECTIVE NO. 3

The patient should demonstrate an adequate respiratory status.

To achieve the objective, the nurse should:

1. Administer 40% to 50% oxygen for approximately 6 hr after the procedure. Temporary hypoxemia is present due to general anesthetic, loss of surfactant, airway closure, microatelectasis, and shunting.
2. Explain the following procedures to the patient and have him carry them out:
   a. Deep breathing once every hour. Have the patient inhale slowly and evenly, hold his breath for 3 sec, and exhale normally. Repeat five times.
   b. Coughing once every hour. The patient should take several deep breaths and then cough. Splint his abdomen with his hands or pillow. (Check the tubes and the connections.)
3. Use the incentive spirometer.
4. Turn the patient every 1 to 2 hr.
5. Assess the patient's recent smoking history.

OBJECTIVE NO. 4

The patient should show signs of returned gastrointestinal functioning.

To achieve the objective the nurse should:

1. Explain to the patient the purpose and procedure of gastric intubation.
2. Maintain the patency of the nasogastric tube. Check the functioning of the suction machine, check the nasogastric tube for kinks or obstruction, and check the connections. Pin the tube to the bed sheet. Irrigate the nasogastric tube with 20 to 30 ml of saline solution every 2 hr.
3. Record and check the drainage (amount, type, consistency, and odor).
4. Observe for and report any nausea or vomiting. To ameliorate any symptoms the nurse should:
   a. Avoid a sudden change in position.
   b. Maintain the patency of the nasogastric catheter.
   c. Keep the room well ventilated.
   d. Keep odors to a minimum.
   e. Apply an ice collar to the patient's neck.
   f. Administer antiemetic medications as ordered. In a calm voice, tell the patient how the medicine will help him. Plan a rest period for the patient after the injection.
   g. If vomiting occurs, the nurse should:
      (1) Turn the patient's head to the side and downward.
      (2) Support his forehead.
      (3) Have an emesis basin available.
      (4) Have a suctioning machine available.
   h. Following emesis:
      (1) Remove the vomitus.
      (2) Help the patient freshen up with a cool, wet washcloth and give mouth care.
      (3) If necessary, change the bed linens.
      (4) Provide a period of rest.
      (5) Remember that often the best relief for nausea is vomiting.
5. Give mouth care every 2 hr. Have the patient use mouthwash and apply a Chap Stick or mentholatum to his lips.
6. Lubricate his nares with a water-soluble lubricant to prevent dryness and irritation.
7. Change the tape daily.
8. Auscultate for bowel sounds.
9. Check the patient's abdomen for distention.
10. Report the passage of flatus.
11. Check dressings hourly; report any drainage.

OBJECTIVE NO. 5

The patient should not exhibit inordinate discomfort.
   To achieve the objective, the nurse should:

1. Administer analgesics if needed. In the low flow state, absorption is irregular, and analgesics should be administered intravenously in small doses. The time interval may be by continuous titrated drip or be from 30 min to 3 hr, depending on the quantity of the last dose, the patient's size, and the degree of pain.

2. Assess for pain and check the time of the patient's previous analgesic injection.
3. Perform additional comfort measures, such as giving a back rub, changing the patient's position, and giving him clean bed linens.
4. Speak in a calm voice and work efficiently and carefully.
5. Use relaxation techniques.

Problem/Diagnosis

Abdominal injury secondary to trauma.

OBJECTIVE NO. 1

The patient should be observed for further complications.
  To achieve the objective, the nurse should:

1. Observe for a localized area of pain or tenderness, generalized pain, pain on movement or coughing, abdominal distention or rigidity, decreased or absent bowel sounds, rebound tenderness, increased abdominal size.
2. Not palpate or percuss the spleen because it may be fragile and might rupture.
3. Observe for indications of liver trauma, including an elevated white blood cell count, elevated serum glutamic-oxaloacetic transaminase (SGOT) and serum glutamic-pyruvic transaminase (SGPT) levels (several hours after trauma) and an increased serum bilirubin level (3 to 5 days after the trauma).
4. Observe for pancreatitis by noting any nausea, vomiting, increased temperature, severe abdominal pain, and rigid abdomen.
5. Observe for hematobilia by noting any colicky pain, melena, hematemesis, and mild to severe jaundice.
6. Observe, record and report any of the following signs of infection: fever, liver pain, an enlarged and tender liver, chills, anorexia, nausea, vomiting, diaphoresis, an increased alkaline phosphatase level, and an elevated white blood count (18,000–20,000/cu mm).
7. Measure all drainage every 8 hr. Record and report any abnormal amounts.
8. In an injury of the spleen, observe closely for an occult liver injury. Twenty-five to 30 percent of patients who have injuries of the spleen from blunt trauma have an associated liver injury.

9. Note the presence of respiratory depression associated with pain. Relieve the pain as much as possible. The usual protocol is (1) the administration of small amounts of intravenous analgesics titrated against the patient's respiratory rate and depth and (2) nursing comfort measure. If those measures are not successful, the anesthesiologist may be consulted about performing a nerve block.
10. Note the drains and tubes and know the purpose of each one. Protect the patient's skin from drainage and maintain sterility.
11. Remember that sutures are removed when enough collagen has been laid in the wound. The time of removal varies according to the patient and his injury. Also, the rate of healing varies in different people, in different parts of the body, and under different conditions. The tensile strength is at near normal levels at the end of the first month, and it very slowly increases during the next 2 years.

OBJECTIVE NO. 2

The patient should establish a functioning bowel if the bowel has been temporarily exteriorized.
  To achieve the objective, the nurse should:

1. Explain to the patient and his family the purpose of the colostomy and how it works. The patient should be told that the colostomy is temporary.
2. Observe and record the first passage of flatus and drainage from the temporary colostomy. Auscultate for bowel sounds.
3. Determine which stoma is from the proximal loop and which from the distal loop.
4. Consult with the physician about the coverage for the stoma in the early postoperative period. The dressings are usually impregnated with petroleum jelly or an antibiotic, such as neomycin or gentamicin.
5. Keep the stoma and the surrounding skin clean. Wash the skin with soap and water as it is soiled and keep it dry.
6. Determine whether the skin needs an adhesive or a protective preparation.
7. Order colostomy bags, preferably ones with a karaya seal. Keep an extra bag on hand, and change the bag as needed.
8. Apply Stomadhesive wafers to the surrounding skin to protect it. Bags and/or dressings will adhere to the adhesive rather than to the skin.

9. Be aware that single-use bags may be used if the drainage is minimal and infrequent. Change the bag as needed.
10. Know that drainable bags are used if the drainage is profuse and frequent.
11. If the stoma is too large for the bag, cut a larger opening in the bag. If the stoma is still too large, use a colostomy belt.
12. With the patient or a member of his family, select foods from the bland, low-fiber menu. Add new foods one at a time to determine whether they cause flatulence.
13. Observe the patient to see when he wants to participate in his colostomy care.
14. Secure the dressings before the patient begins ambulation. Assure the patient that his dressings will be secure during ambulation.

OBJECTIVE NO. 3

The patient should demonstrate psychological acceptance of his present condition.
    To achieve the objective, the nurse should:

1. Visit the patient frequently. Include his family.
2. Establish a rapport with him.
3. Ask him open-ended questions during conversations with him.
4. Show an interest in his welfare.
5. Take time to listen; do not seem rushed.
6. Be alert for clues that he is anxious.
7. Encourage him to participate actively in his plan of care. Be aware of what activities he cannot perform for himself (e.g., personal care or ambulation) and help him with them. Keep articles within his reach.
8. Respond to his requests as soon as possible.
9. Encourage him to ventilate his feelings about his condition.
10. Listen—attentively.
11. Maintain eye contact with him when conversing with him.
12. Answer his questions directly.
13. Provide for periods of uninterrupted rest.

OBJECTIVE NO. 4

The patient should maintain hepatic stability following a liver resection.
    To achieve the objective, the nurse should:

1. Assess the patient. The following are considered normal findings:

a. A normal blood ammonia level.
b. A normal prothrombin time.
c. An increased transaminase level.
d. An increased alkaline phosphatase level.
e. Mild, transient jaundice.
2. Monitor carefully if the physician orders analgesics, major tranquilizers, or hypnotics that are normally detoxified by the liver. (Paraldehyde and phenobarbitol are commonly ordered instead.)
3. Administer albumin if ordered. (The usual amount is 25 to 50 gm daily for 6 to 12 days, to maintain the serum albumin level above 3 gm.)
4. If the prothrombin time is abnormal, administer vitamin K as ordered. Notify the physician when the prothrombin time is normal.
5. Administer whole blood or platelets if they are ordered.
6. Increase the patient's calorie and protein intake. Observe the intravenous site (a 10% dextrose in water solution may prove irritating to the blood vessel). Encourage the patient to take nourishment by mouth.
7. If hepatic failure is a threat, take steps to (1) prevent hyperammonemia, (2) control active bleeding, (3) remove blood from the gastrointestinal tract, and (4) decrease bacterial flora in the gastrointestinal tract. The cause of the encephalopathy seems to be the failure of the diseased liver to detoxify and/or remove the metabolic products of dietary protein. The nurse should:
a. Anticipate that the patient will have an endotracheal tube inserted and will be placed on mechanical ventilation. In hepatic failure with hypoxia and hypercapnia, the cerebral blood flow does not increase reflexly. In the presence of alkalosis, the nondiffusible ammonium ion is converted to toxic diffusible free ammonia. Thus even small derangements in the arterial oxygen and carbon dioxide levels must be corrected.
b. Administer pitressin for active bleeding if ordered.
c. Perform gastric lavage if ordered.
d. Administer magnesium sulfate (15 ml) for catharsis if ordered.
e. Give tap water enemas twice daily if ordered.
f. Administer neomycin, kanamycin, chloramphenicol, or tetracycline as ordered. The usual therapy is neomycin sulfate (1 gm every 4 hr).
g. Administer diuretic therapy as ordered.
h. Administer potassium salts with diuretic therapy as ordered (the increase in blood ammonia

accompanying diuretic therapy is thought to be associated with hypokalemia). Remember that the patient is abnormally sensitive to central nervous system depression.

i. Decrease the patient's protein intake to 50 gm per day or less as ordered.

j. Encourage the patient to eat carbohydrates, because glucose inhibits the bacterial production of ammonia.

k. With the dietitian, plan frequent small feedings. Teach the patient to eat slowly and chew thoroughly.

l. Use an ice collar for nausea.

m. Give mouth care before meals. If the patient's gums bleed easily, use a soft toothbrush or swabs or a gauze pad. Use extreme care, and do not agitate the patient.

n. Plan rest periods for the patient.

o. Record the patient's fluid intake and output.

p. Weigh the patient daily.

q. Use padded side rails and keep them in the up position.

r. Protect the patient from infection.

s. Assess the patient's clinical degree of jaundice daily.

t. Observe the stool for consistency and for the presence of blood.

u. Prevent pressure areas by turning the patient every hour, by using an alternating pressure mattress, and by putting foam rubber or sheepskin protectors under the pressure areas.

v. Use small-gauge needles for injections. Apply pressure to the injection site for 5 min after injecting the medication.

w. Shave male patients daily and with extreme care.

x. Elevate edematous extremities, keeping each distal part higher than the proximal part.

y. If the patient complains of pruritus, bathe him with sodium bicarbonate or cornstarch (no soap) and use a soothing lotion. Keep his fingernails short.

z. If ordered, administer medications, such as L-dopa or lactulose. Lactulose is administered in doses of 25 to 30 ml three times a day to achieve a stool pH of 5.5 or less. In all likelihood, the colon bacteria convert the lactulose into lactic acid and acetic acid. In the presence of acid, the free ammonia diffusing into the gut is converted into the nondiffusible ammonium ion and excreted. A mild diarrhea is produced.

Problem/Diagnosis

Fracture secondary to trauma.

OBJECTIVE NO. 1

The patient should demonstrate healing with no untoward signs.

To achieve the objective, the nurse should:

1. Prepare the patient preoperatively. She should:
   a. Clean the operative site by sudsing it repeatedly. Leave the suds on 5 to 10 min.
   b. Cleanse the site for 10 to 30 min.
   c. Remove hair from the site (if possible with a depilatory).
   d. Cover the site with a sterile dressing.
2. Prevent the complications of immobilization. The nurse should:
   a. Keep the patient as active mentally and physically as possible.
   b. Change his position and have him cough and deep breathe every 2 hr with assistance. Use an incentive spirometer.
   c. Help the patient do active exercises of unaffected areas every 2 hr with assistance (e.g., gluteal setting exercises, knee bends, straight leg-raising exercises, and ankle flexion exercises). Give him a specific number of times to perform each exercise.
   d. Observe for signs of thrombophlebitis (tenderness, swelling, pain on dorsiflexion of the foot), especially in the calf.
   e. Following a conference with the physician, encourage isometric exercises of the affected area.
   f. Encourage the patient to take fluids (up to 3000 ml/day). Find out what the patient likes to drink and set up a "beverage schedule" with him. It should be specific: for example, orange juice, 120 ml at 9 A.M.
   g. Encourage the patient to eat a well-balanced diet.
   h. If ordered, administer prophylactic "minidose" heparin (5000 units subcutaneously every 12 hr to prevent thrombophlebitis).
   i. Apply antiembolic stockings. Have two pairs. Rotate them daily and keep one pair washed.
   j. Keep all pressure off the calf and the heel or possible pressure areas.
   k. Not routinely raise the knee gatch. A small amount of elevation that does not place pres-

sure on or decrease the blood flow in the lower extremity is satisfactory.

l. Refrain from dangling the patient's legs.

m. Following a consultation with physician, encourage the patient to get out of bed as soon as possible and encourage early ambulation. Plan his schedule carefully and slowly increase his activity level each day. For example, the first day the patient may take 3 steps, the next day 6 steps, and the next day 10 steps. Evaluate his pulse and tolerance so that the activity level can be decreased if necessary.

OBJECTIVE NO. 2

The patient who has a fractured mandible should maintain a patent airway and he should heal optimally.

To achieve the objective the nurse should:

1. Observe carefully for signs of airway obstruction or nausea and vomiting.
2. Keep wire cutters and a hemostat at the head of the patient's bed (to be used in case of aspiration). If the patient vomits, assess the situation carefully since most patients are able to expectorate vomitus and do not require cutting of wires.
3. Monitor vital signs (1) four times every 30 min, (2) then four times every hour, (3) then six times every 2 hr, and (4) then once every 4 hr or as deemed appropriate after physiologic assessment.
4. Keep the patient in full view of the staff and the staff in full view of the patient.
5. Explain the situation fully to the patient so that he understands it and feels secure.
6. Keep a call bell within the patient's reach.
7. Visit the patient frequently. Use a pencil and paper or a Magic Slate as needed to improve communication.
8. Assist the patient as needed with his liquid diet.
9. Provide mouth care before and after meals, using half-strength hydrogen peroxide (lemon and glycerine swabs tend to be drying).

OBJECTIVE NO. 3

The patient should demonstrate proper healing while he is in a cast.

To achieve the objective, the nurse should:

1. Perform neurovascular check every hour for 48 hr and then every 8 hr. Observe the patient's pulse, color, temperature, sensation, active and passive mobility, and edema. The physician should be notified of any abnormalities. If bleeding occurs, mark the cast and monitor the patient.
2. Use care when moving patient (have sufficient help).
3. While plaster is wet, use the palms of her hands when moving. The cast should be kept uncovered, and the entire cast should be elevated on firm pillows (but plastic-covered pillows should not be used).
4. Notify the physician of any painful areas under the cast that are still present when the cast is elevated.
5. Teach the patient isometric exercises and help him to do them every 2 hr.
6. Pad the edges of cast to make the patient comfortable.
7. If the cast is in the perineal area, use plastic to protect it.

OBJECTIVE NO. 4

The patient should maintain skin traction.

To achieve the objective, the nurse should:

1. Apply tincture of benzoin to the skin first, then moleskin, and then the traction device. The device should be secured with an elastic bandage wrap.
2. Support the foot or the hand to avoid a position of extreme flexion or extension.
3. Use no more than 8 to 10 lb of weight as ordered.
4. Support the lower leg with a pillow.
5. If the patient tends to slip down to bottom of bed, elevate the lower portion of bed one foot.
6. Avoid putting pressure on the peroneal nerve over the head of the fibula.
7. On walking rounds at change of shift, inspect the area about the Achilles tendon.

OBJECTIVE NO. 5

The patient should maintain skeletal traction (1) to reduce fractures by the application of force, (2) to stabilize the muscle and to minimize muscle spasm, (3) to provide immobilization, and (4) to prevent or correct contractures and joint problems.

To achieve the objective, the nurse should:

1. Before setting up traction, make sure that all clamps are functional, lubricate the pulleys, and make sure that the ropes are not frayed.

2. Use a firm mattress and a fracture bed.
3. Position the patient so that the ropes and pulleys maintain an appropriate pull on the long axis of the bone.
4. Keep the ropes unobstructed and the weights hanging free. Secure and wrap the knots with adhesive tape.
5. After traction is set up, take a Polaroid picture of the apparatus and put the picture at the head of the bed.
6. Compare the injured extremity with the normal one in regard to size, color, temperature, blanching, numbness, and motor activity (1) eight times every hour, (2) then four times every 2 hr, and (3) then once every 4 hr.
7. Explain the traction apparatus to the patient and his family, using pictures and diagrams. Educate the patient about what movements are permitted and what ones are restricted. The patient's questions should be answered and the answers reinforced.
8. Keep the patient's shoulders and hips in alignment.
9. In an affected extremity, maintain a neutral position with a trochanter roll, sandbags, and/or a footboard.
10. Maintain the integrity of the patient's skin by massaging the bony prominences every 8 hr, turning him every 2 hr if possible (with assistance), and using a sheepskin, an air pressure mattress, a flotation pad, or an egg crate mattress.
11. Observe for pressure areas, particularly areas at the edges of the splint and under the splint. Use a mirror attached to a long handle to inspect the body parts that are not immediately visible.
12. Keep the popliteal space, tibial tuberosity, malleolar areas and the head of fibula free of pressure.
13. Keep the bed dry and wrinkle free.
14. Use analgesics and comfort measures to relieve pain.
15. Perform range-of-motion exercises of the hand or foot three times a day.
16. Inspect and clean the pin site every 8 hr. Use hydrogen peroxide and then Betadine. Instruct the patient in care of the pin when he is able to take the responsibility.

Problem/Diagnosis

Feelings of depersonalization secondary to response of being in critical care unit.

OBJECTIVE NO. 1

The patient should feel secure in the critical care unit, and his environmental stresses should be minimized.
    To achieve the objective, the nurse should:

1. Familiarize the patient with the environment and the protocols. She should tell the patient about:
    a. The staff members.
    b. The nurses' call bell.
    c. The monitoring equipment.
    d. The hospital routine.
    e. The treatments and medications.
    f. The visiting hours.
2. Provide care in an interested, knowledgeable manner.
3. Assess the patient's pain and use comfort measures as well as analgesics to alleviate any pain.
4. Provide the patient with a clock and a calendar.
5. Relieve the monotony.
6. If possible, increase the patient's mobility.
7. Plan nursing procedures to allow the patient uninterrupted periods of sleep.
8. Use reality orientation principles.
9. Have the patient's family bring in familiar objects from home.
10. Assess the patient's knowledge and anxiety levels and give (and reinforce) the information he needs about the critical care unit.
11. Keep noises to a minimum and provide pleasing sounds, such as music and soft voices.

OBJECTIVE NO. 2

The patient should be treated as an individual.
    To achieve the objective, the nurse should:

1. Provide individualized nursing care. She should:
    a. Assess the patient for psychological as well as physical problems using an assessment tool as an outline.
    b. Use the data she collects to plan and evaluate care.
    c. Coordinate care and communicate information to the staff of the unit to which the patient is transferred.
2. Demonstrate respect for the patient by addressing him properly and by including him in conversations, particularly on rounds.

3. Be sensitive to the patient's feelings and take time to assess his behavior.
4. Help the nurses to get in touch with their own feelings.
5. Have the same staff care for the patient as much as possible.
6. Have respect for the patient's privacy, shielding him as necessary. (Acknowledge his territorial imperative.)
7. If the patient's scheduled activities must be changed, ask him to confirm the changes.
8. Provide uninterrupted periods for talking with the patient, and talk with him while caring for him.
9. Listen to what the patient says.
10. Use eye-to-eye contact when talking with the patient.
11. Use good communication techniques with the patient (e.g., open-ended statements, simple and truthful answers, and reassuring voice tones and touches).
12. Encourage communication.

OBJECTIVE NO. 3

The patient should be included in his own care.
To achieve the objective, the nurse should:

1. If the patient is not too ill, have him plan his care with the nurse.
2. Let the patient have as many responsibilities as he can handle (e.g., for doing gluteal setting exercises).
3. Teach the patient the value of self-care.
4. Allow the patient to know when painful procedures may be carried out and include regular rest periods.
5. Assist the patient in making menu selections.

OBJECTIVE NO. 4

The patient's family should be included in the health team.
To achieve the objective, the nurse should:

1. Familiarize the family with the surroundings and the protocols.
2. Assess the family's dynamics and ability to cope.
3. Answer the family's questions and refer them to people who can help them.
4. Help the family during their visits to the critical care unit.

5. In conjunction with the trauma team, institute family education classes.

References

1. Ahoniemi, P. J., Fisher, R. G., and Rulfs, D. M. Delayed multifocal intrarenal bleeding: A complication of high velocity trauma. *J. Urol.* 110:625, 1973.
2. Altemeier, W. A., and Hummel, K. P. Treatment of tetanus. *Surgery* 60:495, 1966.
3. Atkins, J. M., Roberts, B. G., and Thal, E. R. Emergency Medical Systems. In A. H. Giesecke (ed.), *Anesthesia for the Surgery of Trauma.* Philadelphia: Davis, 1976.
4. Beitz, D. Algorithm for critically injured patients. *J. Trauma* 17:55, 1977.
5. Burkhalter, W. E. Open injuries of the lower extremity. *Surg. Clin. North Am.* 53:1439, 1973.
6. Burkhalter, W. E., and Protzman, R. The tibial shaft fracture. *J. Trauma* 15:785, 1975.
7. Callahan, J. J. Fractures of the proximal portion of the humerus. *Orthop. Rev.* 4:35, 1975.
8. Chan, D., Kraus, J. F., and Riggins, R. S. Patterns of multiple fracture in accidental injury. *J. Trauma* 13:107, 1973.
9. Chaudry, I. H., Sayeed, M. M., and Baue, A. E. Depletion and restoration of tissue ATP in hemorrhagic shock. *Arch. Surg.* 108:208, 1974.
10. Chaudry, I. H., Sayeed, M. M., and Baue, A. E. Effect of adenosine triphosphate–magnesium chloride administration in shock. *Surgery* 75:220, 1974.
11. Committee on Trauma, American College of Surgeons. A guide to prophylaxis against tetanus in wound management. *Bull. Am. Coll. Surgeons* December, 1972.
12. Dardik, H., Warren, A., and Dardik, I. Diaphragmatic, visceral, and somatic injuries following rear lap seat belt trauma. *N.Y. State J. Med.* February 15, p. 577, 1973.
13. Del Villar, R. G., Ireland, G. W., and Cass, A. S. Ureteral injury owing to external trauma. *J. Urol.* 107:29, 1972.
14. DeMuth, W. E. The mechanisms of shotgun wounds. *J. Trauma* 11:219, 1971.
15. DeMuth, W. E. Ballistic characteristics of "magnum" sidearm bullets. *J. Trauma* 14:227, 1974.
16. DiMaio, V. J. M. Wounding ballistics. *Forensic Sci. Gazette* 3:2, 1972.
17. DiMaio, V. J. M., Jones, J. A., and Petty, C. S. Ammunition for police: A comparison of the wounding effects of commercially available cartridges. *J. Police Sci. Admin.* 1:269, 1973.
18. Durphy, J. E., and Way, L. W. *Current Surgical Diagnosis and Treatment* (2nd ed.). Los Altos, Calif.: Lange, 1975.
19. Gold, R. E., and Redman, H. C. Splenic trauma: As-

sessment of problems in diagnosis. *Am. J. Roentgenol. Radium Ther. Nucl. Med.* 116:413, 1972.

20. Gregory, C. F., and Paradies, L. H. Principles in Fracture Management. In G. T. Shires (ed.), *Care of the Trauma Patient.* New York: McGraw-Hill, 1966.

21. Guerrierco, W. G., Carlton, C. E., and Jordan, G. L. Management of combined injury of the pancreas and upper urinary tract. *J. Urol.* 110:622, 1973.

22. Gump, F. E., Kinney, J. M., and Long, C. L. Interrelationships between total body sodium, potassium and water in patients postoperatively. *Surg. Forum* 19:374, 1968.

23. Hayman, W. B. The point is hollow. *Emergency* 8:28, 1976.

24. Holcroft, J. W., and Trunkey, D. D. Extravascular lung water following hemorrhagic shock in the baboon: Comparison between resuscitation with Ringer's lactate and plasmanate. *Ann. Surg.* 180:408, 1974.

25. Howland, W. C., Schweizer, O., Fleisher, M., et al. Fibrinogen and albumin deficiencies associated with packed red blood cell transfusions. *Anesth. Analg.* 54:87, 1975.

26. Karaharju, E. O. Blunt abdominal trauma in patients with multiple injuries. *Injury: Br. J. Accident Surg.* 4:307, 1973.

27. Kranik, A. D., and Kelly, M. The emergency management of gunshot wounds. *Emergency* 8:14, 1976.

28. Krauss, M. Studies in wound ballistics: Temporary cavity effects in soft tissue. *Milit. Med.* 121:221, 1957.

29. Kulowski, J. *Crash Injuries.* Springfield: Thomas, 1960.

30. Larmon, W. A. Disorders of the Musculoskeletal System. In D. Sabiston (ed.), *Textbook of Surgery.* Philadelphia: Saunders, 1972.

31. Longmire, W. P., and McArthur, M. S. Occult injuries of the liver, bile duct, and pancreas after blunt abdominal trauma. *Am. J. Surg.* 125:661, 1973.

32. Lucas, C. E. Resuscitation of the injured patient: The three phases of treatment. *Surg. Clin. North Am.* 57:3, 1977.

33. Martin, J. D. Massive Abdominal Injury in Civilian Practice. In J. P. Hardy (ed.), *Critical Surgical Illness.* Philadelphia: Saunders, 1971.

34. McArdle, A. H., Chiu, C. J., and Hinchey, E. J. Cyclic AMP response to epinephrine and shock. *Arch. Surg.* 110:316, 1975.

35. Moffat, W. C. Missile wounds in limited war and civil aid. *Proc. R. Soc. Med.* 66:291, 1973.

36. Morse, T. S. Renal injuries. *Pediatr. Clin. North Am.* 22:379, 1975.

37. Moss, G. S. An argument in favor of electrolyte solution for early resuscitation. *Surg. Clin. North Am.* 52:3, 1972.

38. Mountcastle, U. B. *Medical Physiology.* St. Louis: Mosby, 1974.

39. Nerubay, J., Glancz, G., and Katznelson, A. Fractures of the acetabulum. *J. Trauma* 13:1050, 1973.

40. Olsen, W. R. The serum amylase in blunt abdominal trauma. *J. Trauma* 13:200, 1973.

41. Olsen, W. R., Redman, H. C., and Hildreth, D. H. Quantitative peritoneal lavage in blunt abdominal trauma. *Arch. Surg.* 104:536, 1972.

42. Price, J. B. Hepatic disease in an intensive care unit. *Med. Clin. North Am.* 55:1285, 1971.

43. Randall, H. T. Fluid, electrolyte and acid-base balance. *Surg. Clin. North Am.* 56:1019, 1976.

44. Raney, R. B., Brashear, H. R., and Shands, A. R. *Handbook of Orthopedic Surgery.* St. Louis: Mosby, 1971.

45. Remington Arms Co., Inc. *1976 Sporting Firearms and Ammunition.*

46. Reul, G. J., Solis, R. T., Greenberg, S. D., et al. Experience with autotransfusion in the surgical management of trauma. *Surgery* 76:546, 1974.

47. Reynolds, B. M., Balsano, N. A., and Reynolds, F. X. Pelvic fractures. *J. Trauma* 13:1011.

48. Sabiston, D. C., Jr. (ed.). *Davis-Christopher Textbook of Surgery* (10th ed.). Philadelphia: Saunders, 1972.

49. Sasmaz, O., Petridis, I., and Alican, F. Hematoma of the rectus abdominis muscle. *Arch. Surg.* 100:8, 1970.

50. Scott, R., Carlton, C. E., and Goldman, M. Penetrating injuries of the kidney: An analysis of 181 patients. *J. Urol.* 101:247, 1969.

51. Seddon, H. J. Peripheral Nerve Injuries. In *Medical Research Counsel.* London: Her Majesty's Stationery Office, 1954.

52. Sherman, R. T. Some pitfalls in the management of abdominal trauma. *Ariz. Med.* p. 152, 1969.

53. Shires, G. T., and Carrico, C. J. Current Status of the Shock Problem. *Current Problems in Surgery.* Chicago: Year Book, 1966.

54. Shires, G. T., and Jones, R. Initial management of the severely injured patient. *J. Am. Med. Assoc.* 213:1872, 1970.

55. Shires, G. T., Jones, R. C., Perry, M. O., et al. Trauma. In S. S. Schwartz (ed.), *Principles of Surgery.* New York: McGraw-Hill, 1979.

56. Shires, G. T., Williams, J., and Brown, F. Simultaneous measurement of plasma volume, extracellular fluid volume, and red blood cell mass in man utilizing I^{131}, $S^{35} O_4$, and Cr^{51}. *J. Lab. Clin. Med.* 55:776, 1960.

57. Shires, G. T., Williams, J., and Brown, F. Acute changes in extracellular fluids associated with major surgical procedures. *Ann. Surg.* 154:803, 1961.

58. Soeter, J. R., Suehiro, G. T., Ferrin, S., et al. Comparison of filtering efficiency of four new in-line blood transfusion filters. *Ann. Surg.* 181:114, 1975.

59. Thal, E. R., and Shires, G. T. Peritoneal lavage in blunt trauma. *Am. J. Surg.* 125:64, 1973.

60. Tovee, E. B. Blunt abdominal trauma. *J. Trauma* 10:72, 1970.

61. Trunkey, D. D., Chapman, M. W., Lim, R. C., et al. Management of pelvic fractures in blunt trauma injury. *J. Trauma* 14:912, 1974.

62. Trunkey, D. D., Illner, H., Wagner, I. Y., et al. The effect of hemorrhagic shock on intracellular muscle action potentials in the primate. *Surgery* 74:241, 1973.

63. Unger, J., Bare, C., and Haight, J. Traumatic bilateral renal artery thrombosis. *J. Trauma* 17:64, 1977.

64. Waterhouse, K., and Gross, M. Trauma to the genitourinary tract. *J. Urol.* 101:241, 1969.

65. Webb, K. J. Early assessment of orthopedic injuries. *Am. J. Nurs.* 74:1048, 1974.

66. Weinstein, L. Tetanus. *N. Engl. J. Med.* 289:1293, 1973.

67. Williams, L. F. The acute abdomen. *Am. J. Nurs.* 71:299, 1971.

68. Winchester Western Co. *1976 Sporting Arms, Ammunition and Reloading Components.*

69. Wright, C. J. Regional effects of hypovolemia and resuscitation with whole blood, saline or plasma. *J. Surg. Res.* 18:9, 1975.

70. Zuidema, G. D., and Weldon, C. Initial Evaluation and Treatment of the Injured Patient. In W. F. Ballinger, R. B. Rutherford, and G. Zuidema (eds.), *The Management of Trauma.* Philadelphia: Saunders, 1973.

Burn Injury

Cornelia Vanderstaay Kenner

Many persons who have experienced burn trauma are treated in emergency rooms and critical care units. Although theoretically accidents are preventable, their numbers are increasing. Prevention of injury thus becomes an ever increasing responsibility of each burn team member.

Burn care is being regionalized to a large extent. The person who has a moderate or a major injury first receives emergency care in his local hospital and then, under the supervision of a medical team, is taken by ground or air ambulance to a burn facility or a burn center. This chapter discusses the care given in both the resuscitation and acute care phases of burn injuries.

Objective

After assimilating the material in this chapter, the nurse should be able to identify the important aspects of the care of a patient who has had a burn injury and to begin to care for the patient.

Achieving the Objective

To achieve the objective, the nurse should be able to:

1. Quickly obtain the pertinent historical details of the accident and the patient's medical history.

35

2. List the important facts surrounding the accident.
3. Systematically assess the patient's injuries.
4. According to the Rule of Nines and the Berkow formula, calculate the extent of injury.
5. Calculate fluid resuscitation therapy according to the crystalloid formula.
6. Identify the clinical and laboratory criteria that show adequate resuscitation from burn shock.
7. According to appearance, differentiate first-degree, partial-thickness, deep partial-thickness, and full-thickness burns.
8. Describe the types of hospitals in which burn patients with various areas, depth, and extent of injury can be treated successfully.
9. Correlate burn wound sepsis with the results of surface cultures, biopsy reports, and therapy.
10. Compare and contrast the effectiveness of five topical antimicrobial drugs.
11. Identify the important aspects of patient care after the application of heterograft.
12. Write a paragraph describing positioning and exercises needed for a patient who has limited range of motion in his hand.

How To Proceed

To develop an approach to burn injury, the nurse should:

1. Study the material that follows until she has attained all the cognitive objectives.
2. In the learning laboratory—and working with a fellow learner—construct five patient situations and role play the systematic assessment and management of each patient.
3. Observe how the burn team functions during the initial care and later, when the patient is in the critical care unit.
4. Plan for herself clinical experiences with the clinical burn specialist. The nurse should reach an agreement with an experienced nurse who will act as a nurse preceptor. The nurse should begin by caring for patients who have minor to moderate injuries and progress to caring for patients who have severe injuries.
5. Attend the staff development classes.

Case Study

Mr. H. S. was admitted to the critical care burn unit with a 65 percent total body surface area (TBSA) burn and a possible inhalation injury. He had been burned at the local community center while he was cleaning a shower stall with gasoline. The fumes had ignited, trapping him in the enclosed space for a short period of time. He did not become unconscious. When he got out of the building, he rolled in the grass to put out the fire. He was transferred to the regional burn center in a ground ambulance, arriving at 3 P.M., one hour after he was burned.

Mr. S.'s assessment for airway involvement and life-threatening trauma was negative. His vital signs were T 97.2°F, P 140, R 28, and BP 100/70. His burn was calculated as a 65 percent TBSA partial-thickness and full-thickness injury that covered his face, upper chest, arms, and parts of his legs and back. Based on the extent of his burn and his weight (77 kg), his fluid resuscitation was calculated to be 20,000 ml for the 24-hour period after the injury. Fifty percent of that amount (10,000 ml) was to be infused in the next 6 hours and 45 minutes, 25 percent (5000 ml) in the second 8-hour period, and 25 percent in the third 8-hour period.

Blood samples were drawn for arterial blood gases, serum electrolytes, SMA-12, complete blood count, and typing and crossmatching. A Foley catheter and a nasogastric catheter were placed.

Mr. S.'s history indicated that he did not have a preexisting disease. On physical examination, he was noted to have singed nasal hairs, red and swollen mucous membranes, and soot in his sputum. His carboxyhemoglobin level was 6%. His arm burns were circumferential, and they were clinically classified as full-thickness injuries. His radial pulses had decreased to 1+. His bowel sounds were absent.

On 40% oxygen, Mr. S.'s arterial blood gas measurements were PO_2 138, pH was 7.63, PCO_2 was 15, bicarbonate level was 24.5, and delta base was −3. His blood review showed hemoglobin 13.3 gm/100 ml, hematocrit 39.6%, red blood cells 5.1×10^6 cu mm, and mean corpuscular volume 78 (see assessment sheet).

Clinical Presentation of Case Study

4:00 P.M. Mr. S. was alert and oriented, with a urinary output of 50 ml per hour. His vital signs were T 99.2°F, P 130, R 22, BP 100/70, and CVP 3 cm H_2O. His cardiorespiratory assessment showed an adequate airway, a normal sinus rhythm, a productive cough, and no rales or wheezes. The bronchoscopic examination showed no mucosal exudate, ulceration, or erythema. Oxygen therapy continued to be 10 L, administered through a face tent. Positive pressure breathing was ordered to be given every six hours. External heat was maintained by a heat shield. Preventive antacid therapy was given every two hours, with Amphojel and Maalox alternating (30–60 ml). A gastrointestinal assessment showed Mr. S. to have a dark-brown drainage in his nasogastric tube and abdominal distention. His right and left radial pulses were palpated at 1+, and they were heard with the Doppler. A clinical examination revealed no numbness, tingling, or decreased motor activity. Ringer's lactate solutions (Nos. 3 and 4) were given in the right arm and the left leg, respectively.

The ophthalmologist reported that Mr. S.'s left eye was normal but that in his right eye the pupil reacted to light and accommodation, vision was blurred, there was a superficial partial-thickness burn on his eyelids with singed eyelids, and his upper corneal epithelium was stained (apparently because of a superficial injury). His right eye was to be patched continuously and gentamicin ophthalmic drops were to be put in the eye every three hours.

5:00 P.M. Morphine sulfate (10 mg intravenously) was administered before wound care was begun. Explanations were given before the treatment was started. During tubbing, Mr. S. complained of numbness in his hands; his pulses were barely palpable. After the tubbing and elevation of his extremities, his pulses were palpated at 1+.

6:00 P.M. Mr. S. was alert, with a urinary output of 60 ml per hour and clearing of the hematuria. His vital signs were T 101°F, P 130, R 28, BP 100 with the Doppler, and CVP 3 cm H_2O). Ringer's lactate solutions (Nos. 7 and 8) were given. Mr. S. complained of numbness in both hands that was decreased somewhat following exercise. His pulses were not palpable, but they were heard with the Doppler. During the family's visit, the nurse stayed at his bedside.

7:00 P.M. Mr. S. was alert, with a urinary output of 50 ml per hour. His vital signs were T 101.4°F, P 110, R 28, BP 90 with the Doppler, and CVP 4 cm H_2O. His urine was light pink. He complained of discomfort in his hands, and his motor activity had decreased.

8:00 P.M. Mr. S. was alert, with a urine output of 70 ml per hour. His vital signs were T 101.8°F, P 130, R 26, BP 100 with the Doppler, CVP 4 cm H_2O. He had a normal sinus rhythm. A urine test for sugar and acetone was neg/neg. Ringer's lactate solutions (Nos. 9 and 10) were given. Examination of his arms revealed decreased sensation, increased discomfort in his hands, and an occasional skipped radial pulsation with the Doppler. Silver sulfadiazine was reapplied to Mr. S.'s open wounds.

9:00 P.M. Mr. S. was alert, with a urinary output of 60 ml per hour. His vital signs were P 156, R 32, BP 96 with the Doppler, and CVP 4 cm H_2O. Arterial blood gas measurements on 40% O_2 were PO_2 108, pH 7.41, PCO_2 33 and delta base −2. Evaluation of Mr. S.'s arms showed decreased motor activity and a deep, aching pain. With the use of the Doppler, the flow was detectable for five or six

seconds and then undetectable for two or three seconds. Bilateral escharotomies of his forearms and distal upper arms were performed. Bleeding was controlled by using pressure and a sterile microcrystalline collagen hemostat. The bulging underlying edematous tissue was covered with silver sulfadiazine, and, to maintain elevation, the patient's arms were wrapped with fine mesh gauze and a flexible, expandable meshlike dressing.

10:00 P.M. Mr. S. was alert, with a urinary output of 60 ml per hour. His vital signs were T 102°F, P 140, R 24, BP 90 with a Doppler. His urine was dark yellow. Bowel sounds were present. Ringer's lactate solutions (Nos. 11 and 12) were given, and the rate was recalculated at 625 ml per hour.

MIDNIGHT Mr. S. was alert, with a urinary output of 50 ml per hour. His vital signs were T 101°F, P 110, R 24, BP 82 with a Doppler, and CVP 3 cm H_2O. Morphine sulfate (10 mg intravenously) was administered for pain.

2/9
(1st post-
burn day)

2:00 A.M. Mr. S. was alert, with a urinary output of 40 ml per hour. His vital signs were P 120, R 24, BP 90 with a Doppler, and CVP 4 cm H_2O. He slept for long periods.

6:00 A.M. Mr. S. was alert, with a urinary output of 60 ml per hour. His vital signs were T 101°F, P 100, R 24, BP 90 with a Doppler, and CVP 5 cm H_2O. Mild hoarseness was noted. His arterial blood gas measurements on 40% O_2 were PO_2 110, pH 7.38, PCO_2 33, delta base −2. The blood test results were RBC 6.72 × 10^6 cu mm, Hgb 21.2 gm/100 ml, Hct 60.5%, WBC 18,900, glucose 164 mg/100 ml, Na 140 mEq/L, K 4 mEq/L, Cl 105 mEq/L. Ringer's lactate solutions (Nos. 16 and 17) were given. Ice chips were taken orally. Mr. S.'s escharotomies were oozing, and a collagen hemostat was reapplied, and the dressings were changed. The ophthalmologist noted that the epithelium of Mr. S.'s right eye had improved and that his eyelids, although swollen, were only mildly involved; it appeared that a tarsorrhaphy would not be needed.

10:00 A.M. Mr. S. was alert, with a urinary output of 50 ml per hour. His vital signs were T 101.2°F, P 116, R 20, BP 94 with the Doppler, and CVP 5 cm H_2O. His hoarseness had not increased. His arterial blood gas measurements on 40% O_2 were PO_2 114, pH 7.53, PCO_2 27.2, and delta base −4. Mr. S.'s wounds were wet and weeping. Morphine sulfate (10 mg intravenously) was administered before wound care was given by the bedbath procedure. The open method of therapy was main-

Critical Care Nursing Admission Assessment
Major Systems Approach

PATIENT'S NAME: _Mr. H.S._   DATE: _2/8_   TIME: _4 pm_

DIAGNOSIS: _65% TBSA burn c̄ possible inhalation injury_   T: _99.²_   A.P.: _130_   R.P.: _130_   R. _22_

B.P.: _100/70_   E.C.G. RHYTHM: _NSR_   ECTOPY: _—_   WT: _77 kg._   HT: _6'_

ADMITTED VIA: _stretcher_   INFORMANT: _patient_   LAST MEAL: _11³⁰ a.m._

I. CHIEF COMPLAINT: _"while cleaning a shower stall c̄ gasoline, the fumes ignited burning me."_

II. PATIENT PROFILE:
  1. Age _28_   2. Sex _M_
  3. Marital Status (M) W D S
  4. Race _W_   5. Religion _Prot._
  6. Occupation _policeman_
  7. Availability of Family _in waiting room, wife + parents live in city_
  8. Dietary _deferred_
  9. Sleeping _deferred_
  10. Activities of Daily Living _deferred_

III. HISTORY OF PRESENT ILLNESS: _trapped in closed space for short period of time, brought immediately to hospital, wounds covered during transport with Helafoam_

IV. PAST MEDICAL HISTORY:
  1. Pediatric & Adult Illnesses _usual childhood illnesses_
  2. Cardiac
  3. Hypertension
  4. Respiratory
  5. Diabetes Mellitus
  6. Renal _negative_
  7. Jaundice
  8. Infections
  9. Other
  10. Hospitalizations & Surgeries _fractured arm, age 15 healed without complication_

11. Current Medication _none_

12. Allergies _none_

13. Habits _does not drink or smoke_

V. FAMILY HISTORY: _Mother and father, a+w. 1 brother, age 32,_

VI. PSYCHOSOCIAL:
  1. Behavior During Assessment _Asks questions about hospital; answers all questions completely; anxious_

  2. Specific Problems _anxiety pain_

VII. PHYSICAL EXAMINATION:
  1. General _Partial & full thickness burn to face, upper chest, portions of back and legs and circumferential both legs_

  2. Respiratory System
  Airway _patent_
  Inspection _singed nasal hairs, red swollen mucous membranes, soot in sputum, cough_
  Rate _18_
  Rhythm _regular amplitude_
  Chest Wall _intact_

  Palpation _tenderness noted in burned areas, no increased fremitus_
  Percussion _no dullness or hyperresonance_

Auscultation
Voice Sounds _normal_
Breath Sounds _____
　Normal ✓ Increased____ Decreased ____
Adventitious Sounds: _no rales or_
_____ _rhonchi_

3. Cardiovascular System
　A.P. _130_ R.P. _130_
　B.P. Supine　R _100/70_　L _____
　P.M.I. _5th ICS mcL_
　Heart Sounds _normal $S_1 S_2$_

　Thrills _____
　Peripheral Pulses _R and L radial 1+, rest 2+_

4. Neurological System
　Level of Consciousness _____
　_____ _alert_
　Respiratory Pattern _regular_

　Cranial Nerves _II - XII grossly intact_

　Eyes _____
　(1) Pupils　　　OD　　　OS
　　　Size _4mm_ _4mm_
　　　Shape _round_ _round_
　　　Light _react_ _react_
　　　Consensual _react_ _react_
　　　Accommodation _react_ _react_
　(2) Ocular Movements _EOMs intact_

　Motor _moves all extremities_

　Sensory _intact R+L arms, no numbness_
　Coordination _intact_

　Reflexes _2+_

5. Gastrointestinal System
　Nose & Mouth _Levine tube_

　Stomach _no bleeding_

　Abdomen _deferred_

　Bowel Sounds _absent_
　Liver _deferred_
　Spleen _deferred_

6. Renal & Genitourinary Systems
　I. _____ O. _50 ml/hr._
　Urinary Bladder & Urethra _____
　_____ _deferred_
　Kidneys _deferred_

7. Musculoskeletal System
　Spine _no tenderness_
　Extremities _cool_

　Sacral Edema _none_
　Masses _none_

8. Hematologic System
　Petechiae _____
　Ecchymosis _____ | _negative_
　Gingiva _____

9. Endocrine System
　Breath _____
　Skin _____

VIII. LABORATORY:
1. Hematology
　HGB _13.3 gm/100 ml_ HCT _39.6 %_
　W.B.C. _31.5 /cu. cm._
2. Chemistry
　Na _139_ K _4.2_
　CO_2 _20_ CL _102_
　Blood Sugar _215_ Amylase _< 320_
　BUN _20_ Cr _0.9_
3. Urinalysis _cath, hemoglobin present_
　_pH 5.0, sp. gr. 1.013_
4. Electrocardiogram
　Rate _130_ Rhythm _NSR_
　P-R _0.18_ QRS _0.08_ ST _0.12_
　Interpretation _normal sinus rhythm_
5. Chest x-ray _normal_

IX.　PROBLEM LIST:
　　　　ACTIVE　　　　INACTIVE
　1. incomplete data base　8. Fx arm
　2. 65% burn to face,　　　age 15
　　upper chest, both arms,
　　+ portions of back + legs
　3. history of closed space
　　c̄ soot in sputum
　4. pain
　5. circumferential full
　　thickness burns of R+L arms
　6. anxiety
　7. impaired mobility
　　　　NURSE'S SIGNATURE
　Cornelia Kenner, RN, CCRN

821

tained, with a slight modification—light mesh dressings were applied over the silver sulfadiazine.

NOON Mr. S.'s plasma volume was 3789 ml and his hematocrit was 46%. Administration of 8 units of plasma was anticipated.

2:00 P.M. Mr. S.'s mental status and urinary output were unchanged. His vital signs were T 101.2°F, P 140, R 24, BP 94 with the Doppler, and CVP 8 cm H_2O. His hoarseness had increased slightly. He complained of thirst and was given ice chips. His resuscitation therapy with 20,000 ml of Ringer's lactate solution was completed, and resuscitation therapy for the fourth eight-hour period was begun with aged plasma. The blood test results were RBC 5.35 × 10⁶/cu mm, Hgb 17 gm/100 ml, Hct 47.9%, WBC 8100/cu mm, and platelets 215,000/cu mm.

4:00 P.M. Wound care given.

6:00 P.M. Mr S. was alert; his improved spirits were indicated by the spontaneous comments he made to his family and the staff. The questions he asked about patient care procedures showed that he understood the previous explanations. He asked whether his family could remain with him for a short time after visiting hours. He said that he was very tired and that it was painful for him to move. Mr. S.'s wife later told the staff that Mr. S. feared for his life but felt he was going to live.

8:00 P.M. Mr. S.'s urinary output was 64 ml per hour. His vital signs were: T 100°F, P 116, R 24, BP 130/90, and CVP 7–9 cm H_2O. Productive cough and hoarseness were increased, and a few rales were heard in the left lower lobe. His arterial blood gas measurements on 40% oxygen were PO₂ 94, pH 7.44, PCO₂ 31, and delta base −2. The blood test results were Hgb 15.2 gm/100 ml, Hct 47.1%, Na 132 mEq/L, potassium 4.5 mEq/L, glucose 225 mg/100 ml, blood urea nitrogen 16 mg/100 ml, and calcium 6.4 mg/100 ml. Mr. S. complained of being cold, and his over-the-bed heater was turned up. He took clear liquids in small amounts. His total body edema had increased as anticipated, and his joint movement was minimal because of the edema.

10:00 P.M. Wound care given. The unit's nighttime procedures were again explained to Mr. S. and he was prepared for sleep.

2/10
(2nd post-
burn day)

MIDNIGHT Mr. S.'s vital signs and general condition re-
−8:00 A.M. mained stable. He slept for long periods, and he was given pain medication once.

8:00 A.M. Mr. S. was alert, with a urinary output of 68 ml per hour. His vital signs were T 100°F, P 148, R 22, BP 116/92, and CVP 7 cm H_2O. On cardiores-

piratory examination, a loud S_4, wheezes, and a normal sinus rhythm on ECG were noted. The bowel sounds were active, and his nasogastric tube was removed. He was able to take a clear liquid diet without nausea.

10:00 A.M. Mr. S. was bathed in the hydrotherapy tub. He was not submerged in the water but was placed horizontally on a plinth over the tub. He was then gently sprayed with filtered tap water and gently washed with Betadine.

NOON Mr. S.'s vital signs were T 100°F, P 140, R 24, BP 100/94, and CVP 10 cm H_2O. His arterial blood gas measurements on 40% O_2 were PO₂ 123, pH 7.47, PCO₂ 29, and delta base −1. Mr. S.'s wife helped him with his liquid diet.

4:00 P.M. Wound care was given.

6:00 P.M. Mr. S. was alert, with a urinary output of 40 ml per hour. His vital signs were T 100°F, P 140, R 26, BP 130/60, and CVP 13 cm H_2O. His arterial blood gas measurements on 40% O_2 were PO₂ 90, pH 7.59, PCO₂ 28, and delta base +7. His Hgb was 17.4 gm/100 ml, and his Hct was 51.6%. Two units of aged plasma were given.

10:00 P.M. Mr. S. was given an analgesic intravenously before his dressings were changed.

2/11   Mr. S. was alert, with a urinary output of 35 to 70
(3rd post-   ml per hour. His vital signs were normal. His
burn day)   lungs were clear, and his abdomen was slightly distended, with active bowel sounds. Mr. S. was able to see without difficulty. Positioning splints applied to both hands for 24-hour wear. The invasive devices (e.g., intravenous lines and monitoring devices) removed. Betadine was ordered for topical therapy.

2/12   Mr. S.'s vital signs were stable. No respiratory in-
(4th post-   volvement was noted. His arterial blood gas mea-
burn day)   surements were essentially unchanged, and his cornea was clear. Serum sodium level had decreased to 129 mEq/L and so his water intake was restricted to 1000 ml daily. His daily nutritional needs were calculated to be 4800 calories and 180 gm of protein. Following a nutritional assessment, his diet was planned. A small nasogastric feeding tube was placed so that he could be given high-protein calorie supplements.

2/13–2/17   Excisional therapy was scheduled for the fifth
(5th–9th   postburn day and then cancelled because Mr. S.
postburn   showed clinical signs of possible sepsis: an in-
days)   creased respiratory rate and disorientation. On 2/16, biopsies of his wounds showed *Pseudomonas aeruginosa* 10⁴ (100,000/gm of tissue). He had a second episode of disorientation and an increased respiratory rate that was accompanied by ileus and a decreased urinary output. He responded to intravenous fluid administration. His antibiotic therapy was changed, and his topical therapy was changed to Sulfamylon. His

gastrointestinal tract was functioning; his calorie intake averaged 2800, and his protein intake averaged 85 gm. His arms were placed in abduction.

2/18–2/22 (10th–14th postburn days) Parenteral nutritional therapy was started, and it was increased in small steps. On 2/22, Mr. S. had an episode of hyperosmolar coma; his blood sugar level was higher than 900 mg/100 ml and his electrolyte levels were Na 162 mEq/L, K 5.9 mEq/L, and Cl 126 mEq/L. He was treated with water and insulin. Six hours later the blood test results were sugar 310 mg/100 ml, Na 149 mEq/L, K 5.4 mEq/L, and Cl 117 mEq/L. His topical therapy was changed to cerium nitrate and silver sulfadiazine. To prevent deep venous thrombosis from immobilization, low-dose heparin therapy (5000 units every 12 hours) was started.

2/23–2/27 (15th–19th postburn days) Mr. S. had improved from his hyperosmolar state, receiving 3 liters of a 5% dextrose in water solution for 24-hour periods and maintaining a 60 to 100 ml hourly urinary output. He was well oriented, and he was again given parenteral nutrition (2/27); he was able to eat, but he was observed carefully for nausea and ileus because his bowel sounds were hypoactive. His hemoglobin was 10.4 gm/100 ml, and his hematocrit was 33%, and so he was given two units of packed cells. The areas of partial-thickness injury to his face, arms, and legs were beginning to granulate. His topical therapy was changed to silver sulfadiazine. Full range of motion was maintained, and his arms were abducted on shoulder boards.

2/28–3/4 (20th–24th postburn days) Until 3/1, Mr. S.'s antibiotic therapy was intravenous carbenicillin and gentamicin (250 mg in 250 ml half normal saline solution) given via subeschar clysis. On 3/1, Mr. S. had an episode of low temperature (95.6°F rectally), increased pulse and decreased urinary output. His white blood count was 4500/cu mm, with a segmented to nonsegmented ratio of 15 to 54. Blood cultures were done; the results were negative. The sensitivity reports from the tissue biopsy studies showed *Pseudomonas* to be sensitive to tobramycin, and *Citrobacter* to be sensitive to colistin. Mr. S. was started on those antibiotics. The gentamicin subeschar clysis therapy and the intravenous carbenicillin therapy were discontinued. His topical therapy was changed to Betadine for his back and Sulfamylon for his other burned areas. On 3/4, a second episode of impending hyperosmolar coma was recognized when Mr. S.'s blood sugar level reached 618 gm/100 ml; the condition was successfully treated with water and insulin.

3/5–3/9 (25th–29th postburn days) The areas of second-degree injury were almost healed and areas of full-thickness injury were debrided daily as the eschar separated. Since Mr. S.'s hemoglobin and hematocrit had decreased, he received two units of packed cells. He understood how important eating was to his general welfare; his average protein intake was 50 gm and his average calorie intake was 2500. Mr. S. had a great deal of pain that was relieved only slightly by the administration of a narcotic and by relaxation. At times Mr. S. expressed feelings of depression, and he wondered whether he would leave the critical care unit alive. Mr. S. participated in all aspects of his physical therapy program, but he found it increasingly difficult to maintain full range of motion and to feed himself.

3/10–3/14 (30th–34th postburn days) Daily wound care was continued to remove areas of eschar; heterograft and wet to dry dressings were used in the debridement process. In several places, the heterograft adhered to the underlying tissue. Mr. S.'s daily protein and calorie requirements were met by the combination of enteral and parenteral therapy. The biopsy reports showed no bacterial growth, and the antibiotic therapy was discontinued. The routine chest x ray that was done after a change of the subclavian catheter showed a pneumothorax. A chest tube was inserted and attached to a water-sealed chest bottle system.

3/15–3/19 (35th–39th postburn days) A urine culture showed *Escherichia coli* and *Klebsiella*, and antibiotic therapy with colistin was started. To prepare Mr. S. for surgery (on 3/19), he was given one unit of packed cells because his Hgb was 11.5 gm/100 ml and his Hct was 36.3%. The surgical procedures consisted of the application of split-thickness skin grafts to his chest, arms, and legs. Occlusive dressings and straight elbow splints were used to immobilize the grafted areas.

3/20–3/29 (40th–49th postburn days) Mr. S. was moved to the intermediate care unit. His dressings were removed on the fifth postoperative day. The graft take was 85%. Homografts were applied to areas where the graft did not take. The antibiotic therapy and the catheter feeding were discontinued. Mr. S.'s spirits were very much better. He could visit for longer periods with his family, and he began to talk more and more about going home. He visited with other patients frequently, and he was a source of encouragement to others. He attended patient and family education classes and offered to teach one of the classes.

3/30–4/11 (50th–62nd postburn days) Mr. S.'s remaining open burned areas were grafted in two procedures. The second procedure, a short and minor one, was for spot grafting. Mr. S. began to spend most of his day in the physical medicine department, exercising and rebuilding his muscle tone. He went home on a pass for two weekends, and soon after that he was discharged from the acute care setting. His rehabilitation care had only begun; besides his home care, he came to the physical medicine department for therapy every day for a month, and then he came three times a week and, later, two times a week for three-month periods. He was then seen in the clinic once a week for two months. He must still undergo many short surgical procedures for contracture release and many plastic surgical procedures.

Fully realizing that the effects of burn injury may last for a lifetime, Mr. S. acted maturely, and he expressed a desire to help others in a similar predicament. He became a founding member of the local chapter of Burns Recovered, an organization to help burn patients and their families adjust to the aftermath of burn injury.

Reflections

Pain is a common denominator in the critical care unit. It is a daily companion of the patient, the family, and the staff. Everyone who has had even a small burn remembers the pain associated with it. If a small burn can cause a great deal of pain, what must be the pain caused by a burn over a large part of the body?

The patient's pain varies according to the depth and extent of his injury, the type of therapeutic measures used, his response to pain, and his anxieties and fears. For the family, the waiting, their feeling of helplessness, and their sorrow in watching their loved one suffer often make their pain unbearable. To the staff, the patient's pain brings many anxieties. In their skilled hands lie many techniques to help relieve the discomfort. But what of the pain they must inflict on the patient during such procedures as bathing him and debriding his wounds? Even in the most skilled hands, those procedures bring anguish. Some patients cannot tolerate the pain, and they attack the staff verbally, calling them unkind and inflictors of pain, and thus bring more distress to the staff.

Pain increases the stress level in the critical care unit. There is no easy solution to the problem of pain. Skilled nursing care, patient and family education, staff development classes, patient rounds, and group sharing sessions are helps. A good nurse–patient relationship and the nurse's empathic care of the patient also help.

Pain is a complex physiological phenomenon that is perceived peripherally and transmitted to the brain centers. The psychological impact of pain can be mild (e.g., in cases of moderate and short-lived pain) or it can be devastating (e.g., the chronic, agonizing pain of patients who have intractable trigeminal neuralgia often drives them to suicide).

The critical care nurse should view pain as an ini-

tial physical insult that finally has spiritual repercussions. Those repercussions vary. They range from temporary ego dissolution ("I am so small and my pain is so large") to psychosis if the pain is severe and unrelenting and if the patient sees no hope of escape from it ("The only escape from my overwhelmingly real pain is to leave reality"). Pain diminishes the sufferer's sense of worth. It forces on him dependence and helplessness—and with a vengeance. Not only is he rendered helpless, as in a major body burn, he is in agony while he is helpless.

The loss of consciousness that often occurs in severe pain has long occupied the attention of investigators. Has the mind tired of the onslaught of pain and temporarily protected itself by "shutting down"? Are the coma, hallucinosis, psychosis, and delusional mental states that are often seen in patients who have severe pain simply protective mechanisms against pain that has overwhelmed reason?

Also interesting is the mind's ability to forget pain. Pain is not remembered in its original intensity. Is that phenomenon simply a matter of the mind's forgetting an unpleasant event, or is it something more?

And what of the individual variations in pain "tolerance"? For example, what of the soldier who during battle permits his leg to be amputated without anesthesia and feels no pain? Examples like that are plentiful. And what of the voluntary control of pain some devotees of certain religious sects have achieved? And how has acupuncture affected the Western idea of the physiology of pain?

There are more questions than answers about pain. The research underway is promising. The study of endorphins, endogenous chemicals important in pain mediation, may lead to breakthroughs in the understanding of pain.

It is demeaning to patients in pain to be judged by others as "tolerant" or "intolerant" of pain or as "unable to cope with pain" or as "liking their morphine" or as being "infantile" in handling pain. Nurses (and others) know too little about the physiology of pain to be judgmental. A proper approach is to regard pain as an existential experience that has physiological roots—as an example of the body-mind-spirit continuum.

Categorization

A burn injury is the most complex form of trauma. In general, the patient with a major burn suffers the same alterations in body functioning that other trauma patients do, but he exhibits the most extreme response. In a burn injury every body system is likely to go awry.

It is estimated that there are more than 2,000,000 burn injuries in the United States every year. More than 250,000 people are hospitalized every year for burn injuries, and the mortality is 12,000 a year. Many of those who survive have debilitating problems. The rehabilitation period is seven times as long as the hospitalization period—and the person may never be able to return to his former life-style.

Not every hospital has facilities to care for massively burned patients. In order to determine the seriousness of the patient's injury and his need for clinical care facilities, the American Burn Association has developed the categorization discussed in the following paragraphs.

1. Patients who have major burn injuries should be cared for in a burn unit or a burn center. A major burn injury is (a) a partial-thickness injury of more than 25 percent TBSA in adults or 20 percent TBSA in children, (b) a full-thickness injury of 10 percent TBSA or more, (c) a burn involving the hands, face, eyes, ears, feet, and perineum, (d) an inhalation injury, (e) an electrical injury, and (f) a burn associated with extenuating problems, such as a soft tissue injury, fractures, other trauma, or significant preexisting health problems.
2. Patients who have moderate, uncomplicated burn injuries should be cared for in a hospital with special facilities for and people specially trained in burn care or in a burn unit or a burn center. A moderate, uncomplicated burn injury is a partial-thickness injury of 15 to 25 percent TBSA in adults or 10 to 20 percent TBSA in children or a full-thickness injury of less than 10 percent TBSA that is not associated with the complications listed in item #1.
3. Patients who have minor burn injuries may be cared for in a hospital emergency room that has complete facilities and after that they should be treated as outpatients. A minor burn injury is a partial-thickness injury of less than 15 percent TBSA in adults or 10 percent TBSA in children or a full-thickness injury of less than 2 percent TBSA that is not associated with any complications.

Fluid Changes

Burn Shock

The burn shock, or low-flow, state is characterized by a decreased cardiac output. The cardiac output plummets after a burn injury. Before any decrease in blood or plasma volume can be measured (in the animal model), cardiac output must approach 50 percent of the baseline levels. Then as the plasma volume declines, the cardiac output continues to decrease until, in surviving animals, it reaches 20 percent of baseline levels [66]. All the compensatory hemodynamics occur at the expense of adequate perfusion. In order to maintain arterial pressure and venous return, the splanchnic bed constricts and blood flow to the kidneys, liver, and intestines decreases. The decreased blood flow causes decreased oxygenation. Cellular hypoxia results in cellular changes and metabolic acidosis. The magnitude of the response is proportional to the extent and depth of the injury and the patient's physiological status at the time of the injury.

Two responses to the decrease in cardiac output are pertinent: the early response and the response associated with the volume decrease. Since resuscitation is based on the response to the volume decrease, that response is discussed first.

VOLUME DECREASE

The most significant physiological change that follows burn injury is the sequestration of fluid into the injured area, which results in a decrease in the volume of available fluid. Soon after the injury, large amounts of isotonic fluid are translocated from a functional space into a nonfunctional one. The volume decrease (translocation) continues for 18 to 24 hours, and it is greatest during the first 12 hours after the injury [13].

Measurement of the fluid spaces using isotopes show that the decrease in the extracellular fluid volume is even greater than the decrease in the plasma volume. Within 18 hours after a 40 percent full-thickness scald or flame injury in primates, the extracellular fluid volume has decreased a mean of 44 percent [9].

Normally, the capillary and venular walls are permeable only to electrolytes and water. However, after a burn injury, the vasculature is permeable also to plasma proteins. Another phenomenon connected with the increased permeability is that the colloid osmotic pressure is no longer effective in maintaining the fluid compartment equilibrium. Although the increased permeability is found primarily in the burned area, it is present all over the body [10].

With the use of electrophoresis, the protein concentration of burn wound edema fluid has been determined to be remarkably similar to the protein concentration of plasma. Molecules of high molecular weight have been found in the edema fluid. The leaking of large molecules is demonstrated by the fact that the edema fluid contains proportionately as much globulin as albumin. Fibrinogen has been found at levels of 3 gm per 100 ml. Interestingly, despite the use of every resuscitative method, the increased permeability persists until sealing occurs, approximately 18 to 30 hours [7].

Aldosterone is released from the adrenal cortex; it produces maximal sodium resorption with a decrease in the urinary sodium level. Antidiuretic hormone is released from the posterior pituitary; it produces maximal water resorption in the distal renal tubules. The result is oliguria, with an increased urine concentration and a decreased sodium concentration.

Also, a process similar to that seen in hemorrhagic shock is present. The transmembrane potential is decreased so that water and sodium enter normal skeletal muscle cells in 30 to 60 minutes after the burn [10].

MYOCARDIAL DEPRESSANT FACTOR

Investigators have attributed the direct effect on the cardiac output to a circulating myocardial depressant factor (MDF). MDF has been described in studies, but its cause is not known nor has it been classified. Quite probably, the amount of MDF released or formed is related to the degree of injury. In patients with burns greater than 65 percent TBSA, the MDF may be the primary limiting factor in response to fluid therapy [52].

Late Phase of Edema Formation

Clinically, edema can be observed to slowly increase for two to two and one-half days after the burn. Baxter [9] suggests the following explanations of that late phase of edema, when deeper tissues that have not been damaged contain the greatest portion of the sequestered fluid: (1) the edema of surrounding tissues may result from the effects of histamine, bradykinins, and/or other amines released in response to the injury and (2) because of nonproteolytic changes in collagen, those deeper areas have an increased affinity for sodium and water and essentially act like a sponge.

Edema following a burn injury is different from other kinds of edema in that it is viscous, or gellike. It is thought that that kind of edema is due to its high concentration of fibrinogen. Because of the gellike state, local lymphatics and venules are occluded, and draining of the damaged area is occluded, resulting in extension of the edema both in depth and laterally.

Beginning approximately 36 hours after the burn, potassium is excreted in large amounts in the urine because of respiratory alkalosis, high aldosterone levels, and a high urinary output. Although serum potassium levels may remain in the normal to low normal range, the intracellular deficit may be quite high. As a matter of fact, as much as 80 to 200 mEq of potassium must be administered daily to maintain the total body potassium levels.

The mobilization of burn edema begins after the second day. The time varies, but usually the edema is mobilized by the tenth to fourteenth day after the burn.

Evaporative Water Loss

When the vapor barrier of the skin is removed in burning, the amount of water lost through evaporation increases from 4 to 15 times normal. If the burn wound is covered with a piece of plastic, drops of condensed water vapor are visible in a few minutes. The mean loss is estimated at 1.5 ml/kg/TBSA and may be as high as 3.5 ml/kg/TBSA. The increased loss of water from partial-thickness injuries is as significant as that from deeper injuries, and it is proportional to the TBSA [35].

Hematological Problems

Following a major burn injury, the patient demonstrates changes in his red blood cell mass, white blood cells, platelets, and fibrinogen.

In the early postburn period in patients who have injuries greater than 40 percent TBSA, the hematocrit usually reaches 50 to 70 percent and remains elevated until the plasma volume is restored. Thus an elevated hematocrit is an expected finding. Serial increases in the hematocrit are used in some burn units as one of the indicators of inadequate fluid resuscitation.

The initial red blood cell destruction (of 3–15% of the red blood cell mass) is produced by the insult and followed by a progressive anemia (3–9% daily loss of the red blood cell mass for about two weeks). Previously, mobilization of burn wound edema was thought to expand the blood volumes so that the hemoglobin concentrations only appeared to be low. The concept is not true; in actuality, a profound anemia exists. The severity of the anemia directly correlates with the extent and severity of the injury. Loebl and his associates [36] postulated that the anemia is caused by a microangiopathic condition probably produced by an unidentified plasma factor. In the study, red blood cells from burn patients that were transfused into normal men had a normal half-life, whereas red blood cells from normal men transfused into burned patients showed a significantly reduced half-life. Thus the anemia probably is not intrinsic, nor is it caused by the injury; it is probably produced by a circulating factor or an environmental problem producing a defect in the red cell membrane (possibly due to the altered metabolic response). In any event, the injured patient needs frequent transfusions of packed red cells to correct the anemia and maintain his hematocrit between 35 and 40 percent.

White blood cell adhesiveness and entrapment in edema fluid may produce an early leukopenia, which tends to be a poor prognostic sign [10, 38]. Neutrophil function is particularly important since as function decreases, the number of bacteria in the eschar increases. By the third postburn day, the oxygen consumption of white blood cells decreases by 50 percent unless ascorbic acid is administered and the patient's nutritional needs are met.

Through the first five postburn days, the patient exhibits accelerated platelet destruction and a progressive thrombocytopenia. Platelet counts then rise to normal or elevated levels. Platelet adhesiveness, hypercoagulability, and increased blood viscosity are present. Platelets and leukocytes aggregate and produce a progressive vascular thrombosis. Thrombin times are prolonged, but prothrombin times and partial thromboplastin times are variable.

Initially, plasma levels of fibrinogen decrease largely because of sequestration within the burn wound [24]. During the first six postburn hours, fibrinogen concentrations in burn wound edema reach levels of 28 percent of the plasma concentration. By 36 to 48 hours after the burn, the plasma fibrinogen measurements are at nearly normal levels and then they rapidly rise to elevated levels [18]. Elevations in fibrin split products (FSP) accompany the changes in the fibrinogen levels, with elevated levels of fibrin split products first seen in the edema fluid and later in the plasma. Curreri

and his associates [21] have suggested that FSP elevations in the first 10 to 14 postburn days are secondary to coagulation in the extracellular edema fluid rather than secondary to abnormal intravascular coagulation.

Clotting factors V and VIII are elevated four to eight times normal, and they remain elevated for two to three months.

Respiratory Problems

After injury, the initial stability of the pulmonary blood volume is followed by a change in the venous pulmonary vasculature. Pulmonary engorgement occurs as a result of increased pulmonary blood volume and vascular resistance.

A decreased arterial oxygenation is often seen before resuscitation is initiated. The reason for the decrease is not known, but restoration of the cardiac output improves the oxygenation. Serial determinations of arterial oxygen that show decreasing oxygen levels indicate a pulmonary tract injury or a declining left heart output [44].

Often the patient has been trapped in a burning building and has inhaled a significant amount of carbon monoxide. He arrived at the hospital disoriented, possibly even maniacal, and with elevated carboxyhemoglobin levels. Thus carbon monoxide poisoning is always suspected in a patient who is hypoxic, restless, and confused, even though several hours have passed since the accident.

Upper-airway obstruction may proceed to total-airway obstruction. The immediate cause of respiratory distress is often laryngeal edema or spasm and accumulation of mucus. The signs of obstruction are not apparent for several hours. Suctioning helps to clear the mucus and evaluate the extent of involvement. The edema may continue to develop for 72 hours; endotracheal intubation or tracheotomy is often needed.

Circumferential full-thickness burns of the chest limit the movements of the thorax (Fig. 35-1). The patient shows increasing symptoms of respiratory distress since the tight eschar prevents adequate movement of the chest and proper oxygenation. An escharotomy allows the chest to expand, and it alleviates the symptoms.

Lower-airway obstruction arising from a respiratory tract burn or inhalation injury impairs the pulmonary functioning by increasing the resistance to breathing,

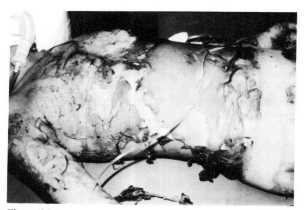

Figure 35-1

Circumferential full-thickness burn of the chest.

lowering the distribution of inspired air, and decreasing the diffusion of gases across the alveolar membrane [26, 81]. Both the central and the peripheral airways are affected. Usually, the lower respiratory tract injury is not directly attributable to the burn since rapid vaporization results in cooling that protects the pulmonary tree [55]. Inhalation of steam results in a true burn of the lower respiratory tract. Most commonly, especially in closed-space injuries, inhalation of the products of incomplete combustion leads to chemical pneumonitis [82, 83]. First the pulmonary tree is irritated, then it becomes edematous, and the pneumonitis occurs. Inflammatory changes occur during the first 24 hours after the injury, but they are not clinically apparent until the second 24 hours [3]. Pulmonary edema may occur any time from the first few hours to seven days after the injury. The treatment involves respiratory support and assisted ventilation, and bronchodilators.

Bronchopneumonia may be superimposed on other respiratory problems at any time, and it may be hematogenous or airborne [61, 63]. Hematogenous pneumonia (miliary pneumonia) begins as a bacterial abscess secondary to another septic source, most likely the burn wound. The time of onset is usually more than two weeks after the injury. Airborne pneumonia (bronchopneumonia) is the more common (65% of cases) and is contracted from an external source. The onset tends to occur soon after the injury, and often it is associated with a lower-airway injury or with aspiration.

Metabolic Problems

The metabolic response to burn injury has three facets: hypermetabolism, severe protein wasting, and weight loss [77]. Apparently mediated by the secretion of catecholamines, the metabolic rate is characterized by a rapid increase from its normal value to a peak (hypermetabolic) rate and then a gradual decrease as the wound is closed. The peak rate is reached between the sixth and tenth postburn days. The amplitude of the response is proportional to the size of the injury, with a maximum reached at 40 to 50 percent TBSA. Oxygen consumption returns to normal when the wound is closed [76]. The amount of protein in the body decreases, mainly, it is thought, from the catabolism of skeletal muscle. Amino acids are converted to glucose, and nitrogen and other intracellular constituents are lost. Weight loss greater than 20 percent of the preburn weight may be expected in patients who have an injury greater than 40 percent TBSA, unless attention is given to caloric support [19]. The problem is related to sex, body build, preburn nutritional status, severity of injury, and complicating factors [18]. If the patient has a loss in body weight greater than 10 percent of his preburn weight and a loss of body water, his ability to perform work is decreased. If he loses one-fourth to one-third of his protein mass or 40 to 50 percent of his body weight, he is likely to die [27]. Increases in body protein and in body weight do not usually occur until wound closure.

Curreri et al. [20] showed that a caloric intake of 6000 calories per day in burned injured patients stabilizes the condition of the red blood cell so that a normal concentration of intracellular sodium is maintained. They suggested that *thermal* burn injury either inhibits the active transport mechanism of red blood cells or produces a defect in the red blood cell membrane and that the inhibition or defect may be reversed by the maintenance of a positive energy balance. The functioning of the red blood cells may reflect the functioning of the other body cells, and thus intracellular sodium concentrations may reflect the effectiveness of nutritional support.

Wilmore et al. [78] demonstrated that blood flow to a burned extremity is increased, and furthermore the increased blood flow is not related to the extremity's aerobic metabolic demands. In the body's response to injury, the healing wound has top priority. Although the uninjured extremity does not utilize glucose, the healing wound does. The hyperdynamic systemic response appears essential to maintain the circulatory and metabolic needs of the healing wound. Underlying the patient's metabolic response to the burn injury is his response to stress [77]. Physiologically, sympathetic stimulation, adrenergic activity, and energy needs are increased so that the body fuels are used rather than stored. Many different mechanisms figure in the stress phenomenon, but the same response seems to occur. The greater the stress, the greater the response. It is theorized that in the burn injured patient, first nervous or hormonal stimuli alter the central nervous system functioning. Next, a reset phenomenon occurs in the hypothalamus that causes increased adernergic stimulation. The result is increased catecholamine and glucagon levels and decreased insulin levels. The change in the normal glucagon-insulin ratio directly affects the cell in a way that alters substrate flow. Increased levels of glucagon are consistent with catabolism: glycogenolysis, gluconeogenesis, and ureagenesis rather than the synthesis of protein. Once support levels of protein and calories are attained, the insulin flow increases and reverses the glucagon-insulin ratio. Protein synthesis and anabolism are then possible. Substrate flow is affected, and the negative nitrogen balance and weight loss are decreased. Hypermetabolism continues until wound closure.

Formerly, it was accepted that the hypermetabolic response was due to the increased caloric expenditure needed to provide for the evaporation of water [25]. Further definitive work has identified other important factors. Zawacki et al. [80] proved that a raised metabolic rate in burn patients was not the direct result of water evaporation. They showed that prevention of the evaporative water loss by covering the injured area with an impermeable piece of plastic film for periods up to 12 hours did not significantly reduce the patient's oxygen consumption. Studies by Wilmore [77, 79] demonstrated that the evaporative water loss is not primary in the metabolic response but that the increased energy production is related to the reset of the metabolic activity. The thermally injured person produces great quantities of heat as a consequence of his injury, and he is internally warm, not externally cold. Increased water loss is a means to transfer the heat generated.

Gastroduodenal Problems

Almost every person who sustains an injury of over 20 percent TBSA initially develops gastric dilatation and paralytic ileus. Also, sepsis is frequently accompanied by gastric distention and paralytic ileus. The danger of vomiting and subsequent aspiration is significant.

Two important causes of bright red and coffee-ground hematemesis are hemorrhagic gastritis and Curling's ulcer. The uncommon causes are peptic ulcer disease, disseminated intravascular coagulation, and gastric erosion from a Levin tube.

Hematemesis of small amounts of coffee-ground material in the first 48 hours after a burn injury is characteristic of hemorrhagic gastritis. Congested gastric capillaries rupture and produce the emesis. The congestion and irritation may set the stage for further acute gastroduodenal disease.

Acute Gastroduodenal Disease

Curling's ulcer has been seen at autopsy in about 25 percent of all burn patients [51]. Its presence may be heralded by a massive hematemesis of bright red blood or the passage of tarry stools [41]. However, its presence may also be identified on investigation of mild abdominal discomfort or even as an incidental finding in an asymptomatic patient. Perforation is the initial symptom in 10 percent of patients [52]. With the advent of cimetidine therapy and prophylaxis with antacids, the syndrome is rarely seen today.

The cause of Curling's ulcer is unknown; early ischemia and adrenal hormone secretion appear to play a significant role. Hyperacidity and preexisting ulcer disease do not seem to be causative factors. According to Moncrief and Pruitt [54], the part sepsis plays in Curling's ulcer is not completely understood, but it is known that sepsis is an added stress. In one two-year period, 77 percent of patients had sepsis at the time Curling's ulcer was diagnosed. Other possible causative factors are: (1) elevated steroid levels, (2) decreased gastroduodenal blood flow (hemoconcentration, elevated catecholamine levels, and hypovolemia), (3) the lytic effect of regurgitated chyme, and (4) a quantitative or qualitative change in mucus.

In an effort to determine the incidence and natural history of acute gastroduodenal disease, Czaja and his associates [22] performed early and serial gastroduodenoscopes in 32 patients who had a thermal injury. In areas of intense superficial mucosal injury, after the first 72 postburn hours, 22 percent of patients had a gastric ulcer and 28 percent had a duodenal ulcer. Prophylactic antacid therapy has significantly decreased the incidence of bleeding [43].

Stress

The burned patient undergoes many severe physiological and psychological stresses. The injury itself produces fear and pain, and the victim has numerous anxieties. Powerlessness, depersonalization, fear of the unknown, pain, dependency, change in body image, disfigurement, loss of function, and even death are possibilities that may confront the patient day by day [4, 68].

Often during the period of hospitalization, the pain and stress alter the patient's defenses for an indefinite period of time [42]. Regression and denial are often present; they seem to be protective mechanisms. The stages of grief are frequently seen, and the denial stage tends to be prolonged. A commonplace occurrence is that the patient does not seem to realize the extent of his injury. Denial may be an adaptive mechanism the patient employs because he is not ready to cope with his problems.

Patients respond individually to burn injuries, and it is difficult to talk of personality characteristics. In general, after the acute stage the patient is like he was before he was burned. If he was well adjusted before the injury, he tends to be well adjusted after the injury [45].

Sepsis

In sepsis, the most significant complication in the acute phase of injury, one or more of the following problems may be found: burn wound sepsis, pneumonia, suppurative thrombophlebitis, closed-space infection, urinary tract infection, prostatitis, and/or infection in any part of the body. The use of invasive procedures and monitoring devices increases the likelihood of infection and requires strict adherence to the aseptic protocols (see Chap. 36).

The Burn Wound

The burn wound is the most frequent source of infection. Loss of the skin is the loss of the body's first line of defense against microorganisms. The destroyed tissue is an excellent culture medium, and bacteria proliferate [65]. If infection is not controlled in the areas of a partial-thickness injury, a progressive tissue necrosis converts the wound to a full-thickness injury.

In a series of investigations in the animal model,

Order and his associates [59] demonstrated the vascular characteristics of the burn wound. In partial-thickness injury, the body's ability to elicit an inflammatory response is maintained beneath the eschar. Underlying blood vessels begin to form new canals approximately two days after the injury, and the process is completed at approximately seven days. A full-thickness injury is characterized by arterial occlusion and the absence of an inflammatory response. Coagulation necrosis is manifested clinically as thrombosed blood vessels. The tissue under the destroyed eschar remains without a blood supply until granulation tissue develops, a process that begins approximately 14 days after the injury and is completed approximately 21 days after the injury. The established capillary network in mature granulation tissue enables the phagocytic cells to conjugate at the site of infection, producing a resistance to infection.

Colonization of the burn wound usually occurs between the fifth and twenty-fifth day after the injury, but it may occur in 24 hours. Three types of colonization have been described: supraeschar, intraeschar, and intrafollicular [73]. Supraeschar colonization is defined as bacterial growth on the wound, intraeschar colonization is defined as growth within the wound, and intrafollicular colonization is defined as growth within the hair follicles. Intrafollicular colonization emanates from bacteria trapped at the time of the burn injury.

Infection in the burn wound can be caused by a variety of organisms. Early after the injury, the organisms are likely to be gram positive, and later, even in the first week, the organisms are likely to be gram negative (*Pseudomonas, Klebsiella, Enterobacter, Escherichia coli,* and *Serratia*). Transferable resistance to antibiotics has been reported with several gram-negative organisms [46]. Other opportunistic organisms, such as *Candida, Phycomycetes, Aspergillus,* and viruses, may cause significant problems.

Host Defense Mechanisms

Burn trauma is accompanied by marked abnormalities in the host's defense system. The altered inflammatory response and the defect in the intracellular capacity of neutrophils to kill bacteria seem to be more significant than the humoral defects.

After the injury, the injured cells release membrane-active substances that produce a generalized body response and vascular permeability [33].

Neutrophils are trapped in capillary beds and unable to reach the infection. The chemotactic index that measures the attraction of white blood cells has been found to be depressed [74]. After the initial period, the membrane-active substances provide the impetus for the development of granulation tissue [1].

Significant abnormalities are present in neutrophil functioning. The cyclic variation in neutrophil functioning that exists in a normal person is accentuated and negatively affected after a burn injury. Burn wound sepsis occurs when the ability of phagocytic cells to kill ingested bacteria is depressed [2]. Preliminary studies have shown that preceding and accompanying the septic process is a reduction in the results of the nitroblue tetrazolium test, which measures the intracellular capacity of neutrophils to kill bacteria [17].

The complement levels are not restored until the second week after the injury, and they play an unknown role in the etiology of early sepsis. However, the levels are restored, and no relationship has been found between sepsis and total complement or component complement levels [23]. Accordingly, the immunoglobulins IgE and IgA are temporarily decreased after burn trauma but that does not seem to be significant [28]. Synthesis and catabolism of the gammaglobulins appear to be balanced, and the body's ability to synthesize a specific antibody remains intact [1]. Depression of cellular immunity is manifested by the longer survival time of biological dressings [16, 58].

Bacterial Monitoring

After bacterial colonization of the wound and invasion of the adjacent subcutaneous tissues, the infectious process reaches systemic proportions. The proliferation and active invasion of the burn wound by 100,000 or more microorganisms per gram of tissue is commonly defined as burn wound sepsis. The definition is based on the work of Teplitz and his associates [73] with the animal model, using *Pseudomonas aeruginosa* as a prototype. Supraeschar and intrafollicular colonization was followed by intraeschar colonization. Invasion of the nonviable-viable interface was followed by invasion of viable tissue and systemic spread via the lymphatics and blood.

Sepsis is time and dose related. A patient who has a 15 percent TBSA injury and biopsy counts of 10^6 bacteria per gram of tissue does not harbor as many bacteria as does a patient who has an 80 percent TBSA injury with biopsy counts of 10^5 bacteria per gram of tissue. The person usually cannot survive if his bacterial concentrations remain higher than 10^6 or 10^7 bacteria per gram of tissue for more than 12 days or if more than one organism is present in concentrations higher than 10^{10} bacteria per gram of tissue. But, if the base is healthy granulation tissue, the patient can survive bacterial concentrations of up to 10^7 per gram of tissue [12].

Early in the course of the infection, the appearance of the wound may not change, and the patient may not have any clinical signs of sepsis. For that reason sampling methods for monitoring bacterial growth have been developed.

Full-thickness wound biopsy [37] is the method most authorities use to quantitate bacterial colonization and to determine the predominant organism(s) and antibiotic sensitivities. A small piece of the entire thickness of eschar and underlying tissue is excised, and the number of organisms per gram of tissues is determined. Since the laboratory determinations require 24 hours for completion, a patient with a biopsy culture of 10^4 per gram of tissue is usually treated for sepsis; the assumption is that bacteria have continued to proliferate and are at invasive levels by the time the laboratory reports are received. The wound biopsy thus can be used to evaluate the progression or regression of bacterial growth and thus the effectiveness of therapy.

Monitoring by surface culture techniques alone is not satisfactory; the correlation between surface colonization and deep tissue colonization is poor. Contact plates help predict what organism is likely to cause problems, but contact plates have several disadvantages: (1) a contact plate is likely to identify a variety of organisms, (2) topical antimicrobial therapy changes the surface flora, and (3) bathing may increase the bacterial count since mechanical agitation breaks up the colonies. Similar problems are present with the capillary gauze and swab techniques.

Blood cultures have limited usefulness in the early diagnosis of sepsis. Blood cultures are positive only a small portion of the time the patient is septic; however, when the cultures are made of a terminally ill patient, a high percentage are positive. The study of Marvin et al. [40] demonstrated positive blood cultures in only 4 percent of patients although 13 percent died with sepsis; 19 percent demonstrated clinical signs, and 27 percent had burn wound biopsy cultures that had more than 10^4 organisms per gram of tissue.

Contractures

Contractures are caused by the scar, or cicatrix, as well as by problems in the joint or bone. Scarring of the skin and deeper structures follows most burn injuries. The surrounding normal tissue is drawn toward the scar, and the blood flow to distal areas is hampered. The scar is deep and dense, and the surface tends to be avascular and thus to injure easily. Blood vessels cannot get to the top, and so ulcerations and blisters form. The skin is thin and healing is slow, after even minor trauma.

Flexion contractures are common; they involve primarily the skin although deeper structures are also involved. Positions of flexion tend to be positions of comfort; thus positions of comfort tend to be positions of contracture. Infections also contribute to flexion contractures since healing is delayed. The delayed healing results in greater amounts of red, moist, vascular granulation tissue, which in turn results in greater contracture. In addition, muscles shorten and joint capsules fibrose, phenomena that lead to contracture.

Proper positioning, including avoiding positions of comfort and pressure areas, early in the course of the burn injury maintains functional range of motion and proper body alignment, decreases edema, and prevents deformities and decubitus ulcers [34]. Potential problems are maceration of tissue, refractory edema, and soft tissue calcification, which results in ankylosis of the joints, tendon exposure, heterotrophic bone, and peripheral neuropathies.

Current therapy is based on information gathered from studies of granulation tissue [75]. It has been noted from tissue biopsy reports that if whirlpools of collagen are present they grow and evolve into swirls of nodular collagen. (Swirls that are visible are called hypertrophic scars.) If the fibers of collagen develop parallel to the direction of stress, the nodular swirls are not as likely to form. Thus therapy aims to maintain extension and to parallel fibers of collagen by proper positioning, splinting, exercising, and using traction. However, it must be emphasized that although prevention is the best therapy, because of the nature of the burn injury, not all deformities are preventable. Care must always be individualized for the patient [15].

Management

Resuscitation Phase

The primary goal of initial fluid therapy is the rapid and complete restoration of the cardiac output. Many different techniques of calculating fluid therapy are described in the literature; the one described in this chapter uses the crystalloid resuscitation formula (also known as the Parkland formula, the Dallas formula, and the Baxter formula) [9, 47, 52]. The formula has been derived from a series of studies. It is designed to restore the extravascular extracellular fluid compartment deficit and the intravascular plasma volume deficit.

Replacement of fluid sequestered as a result of burn injury is the most important part of the initial therapy. Achieving the best physiological response depends ultimately on the ability of various solutions to restore the intravascular and extracellular fluid volumes and to effect a rapid and complete cardiovascular response. Fluid replacement is dependent on the rate of fluid loss, the total quantity of fluid sequestered, and the composition of the burn edema [14].

Clinically, burn shock seems to be helped by all the fluid resuscitation regimens. The crucial point is prompt institution of therapy [6, 51]. In general, parenteral treatment is mandatory for all patients who have an injury of over 20 percent TBSA, except for elderly patients and for children who have injuries of less than 20 percent TBSA. What formula is used for fluid resuscitation does not significantly affect the survival of patients who have an injury of less than 40 percent TBSA. But the survival of those burned over 40 percent TBSA does depend on the careful selection and evaluation of fluid therapy [9].

CRYSTALLOID FLUID THERAPY

According to the crystalloid resuscitation formula, fluids are administered in four time periods of eight hours each. In the first three eight-hour periods (24 hours), Ringer's lactate solution (RL) (Hartmann's solution) is administered according to the following formula (Fig. 35-2):

4 ml RL × wt (kg) × % TBSA burned =
ml RL for the first 24 hr

One-half the total amount calculated is given in the first eight hours after the injury. (The time is calculated from the time of the injury, not from the time

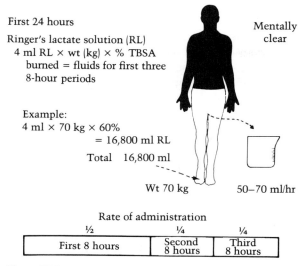

First 24 hours

Ringer's lactate solution (RL)
  4 ml RL × wt (kg) × % TBSA
    burned = fluids for first three
    8-hour periods

Example:
  4 ml × 70 kg × 60%
      = 16,800 ml RL
    Total 16,800 ml

Wt 70 kg   50–70 ml/hr

Mentally clear

Rate of administration

½	¼	¼
First 8 hours	Second 8 hours	Third 8 hours

Figure 35-2
Fluid resuscitation according to the crystalloid formula for the first three 8-hour periods postburn.

Second 24 hours

Plasma
  0.35–0.5 ml plasma × wt (kg)
    × % of TBSA burned = plasma
    for the fourth 8-hour period

Example:
  0.4 ml × 70 kg × 60%
    = 1680 ml plasma

Dextrose in water:
  5% solution
  2000–6000 ml for 24–48 hours

Hematocrit within normal range
Serum sodium level maintained
  at 140 mEq/L

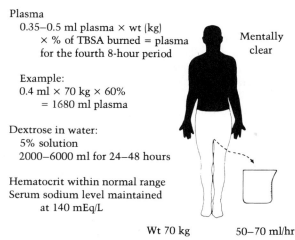

Mentally clear

Wt 70 kg   50–70 ml/hr

Figure 35-3
Fluid resuscitation according to the crystalloid formula for the second day postburn.

therapy is initiated.) In the second eight-hour period, one-fourth the total amount of calculated Ringer's lactate solution is given, and in the third eight-hour period, the remaining one-fourth is given. Although the formula is remarkably accurate, individual patient differences must be assessed and the fluid rate altered if necessary. In the fourth eight-hour period, plasma is administered (0.3–0.5 ml × kg × % TBSA burned) (Fig. 35-3).

The formula was systematically derived from studies of serial changes in plasma and extracellular fluid volumes, cardiac output, and acid base equilibrium. Fluid translocation occurs by 24 hours postburn. It is greatest in the first eight hours, and so the intravenous replacement of fluid is done at a rapid rate that is consistent with the ongoing pathophysiological mechanism.

Crystalloid therapy rapidly restores the functional extracellular fluid compartment deficit to within 10 percent of baseline volumes (the normal volume of extracellular fluid is 20% of body weight). *No further decrease in extracellular fluid volume occurs.* Cardiac output is restored in 12 to 24 hours to 3 liters per minute per square meter. The transmembrane potential is restored, resulting in decreased cell size and decreased intracellular sodium and water. With the restoration of membrane potential and cell integrity, extracellular fluid is kept "pumped" out of the cell, and it accumulates around the cell. Thus the fluid is available for translocation during the late phase of burn edema.

As expected, plasma volume levels are not adequately restored by crystalloid therapy. However, because of the capillary permeability, colloid therapy also has a minimal effect on the plasma volume. Once the capillary permeability significantly decreases (about 24 hours [± 6 hours] after the burn), the plasma volume increases by the amount of plasma administered to the patient. The plasma volume measurements, if available, may be used to calculate the deficit. The hematocrit may be used to evaluate the adequacy of plasma restoration; however the hematocrit is not a useful tool for judging plasma restoration after 48 hours.

Previously, the mortality for the first 48 postburn hours approached 75 percent, and death was due largely to the ravages of the low-flow state. Significantly, renal failure was prominent among the terminal conditions. Today it is well established that the "early" renal failure was a result of decreased cardiac output and renal perfusion. Maintenance of urinary output in normal limits (50–70 ml/hr) is a sign of adequate renal perfusion. Without adequate volume therapy, the urinary output is minimal or nonexistent. As volume is replaced, the renal blood flow improves and the urinary volume increases. Hemoglobinuria is indicative of a deep burn; it clears within the first 300 to 400 ml of urinary output without the need for osmotic diuretics. Complications in renal function are usually the result of inadequate fluid and electrolyte replacement. Baxter [7] states that low urinary sodium concentrations (below 20 mg per liter) indicates inadequate volume replacement.

The most common reason burn patients have a decreased urinary output is that the calculated amount of fluid is behind schedule. The second most common reason is that the extent of the burn has been underestimated, especially in children. Recalculating the extent of the burn after the initial care has been given helps avoid that error. Other causes of a decreased urinary output are associated injuries, respiratory injury, disseminated intravascular coagulation, myocardial depression, delayed resuscitation, and renal failure.

After the fourth eight-hour period, the fluid administered is a 5% dextrose in water solution. It is administered in amounts that will maintain a normal serum sodium range, usually 2000 to 6000 ml [8].

The amount of fluid required by each burn patient cannot be determined exactly; frequent laboratory assessments are needed to ascertain the patient's status. In general, 3 to 5 liters of water per day are needed to replace the evaporative water losses. That amount is significantly affected by the amount of burn surface exposed to the air, by the wound care, and by the environmental air currents. On the other hand, giving too much water quickly leads to water intoxication. The following formula can be used to approximate the patient's water needs:

Square meters × (% TBSA burned + 25) =
                  evaporative water loss per hour

Acute Phase

Following the initial period of burn shock, the goal is closure of the wound. Not until the eschar is removed and the wound is covered by an autograft or not until a partial-thickness wound is reepithelialized are the severe derangements resulting from the open wound reversed. There are two main approaches to wound closure: the conservative approach and the aggressive approach.

In the conservative approach (the more common one), the wound is covered with a topical antimicrobial agent to prevent and control burn wound sepsis [50, 53]. Hydrotherapy is employed and debridement is done daily until the areas of partial-thickness injury heal and the areas of full-thickness injury develop granulation tissue. Homografts and/or heterografts are used as temporary biological coverings to restore the water vapor barrier, decrease the protein loss from the wound, protect the site from infection, relieve pain, allow active joint functioning, help debride dermal debris, stimulate the growth of epithelium and graulation tissue, and act as a test material prior to autografting [67].

Aggressive therapy means surgery or excisional therapy. The removal of eschar is followed by autografting or the application of a homograft as a temporary biological covering. Traditionally, excisional therapy has been limited to patients with a burn injury of less than 15 percent TBSA. Today staged excisions are performed on patients with large injuries in an attempt to effectively decrease the extent of the burn. For elderly patients in particular, small staged excisions done as limited procedures are beneficial because the patients' inelastic cardiovascular systems cannot tolerate the more extensive procedures. Homografts must be available. Excision is first performed five days or less after the injury and before significant bacterial colonization has occurred. The specific criteria for selecting and further evaluating patients undergoing excisional therapy are being developed. Candidates for excisional therapy are evaluated in regard to their age, the extent, depth, and location of the injury, the presence of associated injuries or illnesses, their cardiopulmonary status, bacterial colonization, their ability to fight infection (as determined by their white blood cell count and by other laboratory procedures), their clotting factors, and their general physiological status.

Primary excisional therapy entails removal of the full-thickness injury with a scalpel, electrosurgical cautery, a carbon dioxide laser, or a dermatome. The area is then covered with a biological dressing or autograft [39]. Tangential excision, another form of excisional therapy, is used to increase mobility and hypertrophic scarring. Debridement is done to the point of active capillary bleeding. The eschar is shaved away layer by layer until active bleeding and viable tissue are reached. The shaving does not usually go deep enough to remove all the skin elements, and so regeneration of the epithelium can occur [31, 32]. A biological dressing such as heterograft or homograft is then applied to protect the wound from infection until it heals or until an autograft is done.

AUTOGRAFTING

In both the conservative and aggressive approaches, areas of full-thickness injury require the use of an autograft for coverage. Skin grafts can be taken from any area of the body that is not burned and applied to the clean, red vascular bed.

The graft's blood supply is established by both vascular anastomoses and new vascular growth from the graft bed into the graft. During the first day after the grafting, a fibrin layer is produced that provides contact but not fixation between the graft and the graft bed. During the second day, the fibrin reticulum organizes and advances, and the granulation tissue contains immature fibroblasts and a few open spaces with erythrocytes. Three days after the grafting, the granulation tissue is so organized that it is difficult to differentiate the graft from the graft bed by microscopic study. The percentage of graft take is high if the wound has been carefully prepared, infection does not intervene, and pressure does not disrupt the graft.

Different types of skin grafts are used. Each patient's care must be individualized because coverage of his burned area is dependent on where he has been burned and what areas remain to be used as donor sites for autografting. If the injury is extensive, the first consideration is to closing as large an area as possible. The order of priority is (1) face, (2) hands, (3) feet, (4) neck and other joint areas, (5) genitalia and perineum, and (6) other areas, such as the back.

Various depths of skin are used. A full-thickness graft uses the entire depth of skin. It is used for specific areas, such as the eyelids, the tip of the nose, or the hands. Split-thickness grafts are most commonly used; they are transferred to the wound bed in a continuous sheet if enough donor sites are available. If they are not available, a mesh skin graft is used [72]. Using the Tanner-Vandeput mesh dermatome, a number of slits are cut so that the skin expands to an area three to nine times the size of the donor site. Unless very large areas must be covered, the skin is not expanded to a ratio greater than 3:1 (Fig. 35-4). The meshed skin is applied to the clean wound and covered with a moist dressing. Tissue fluid drains from the wound and eliminates the problem of fluid

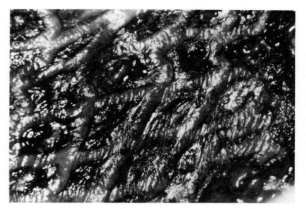

Figure 35-4
Meshed autograft five days postgrafting.

collecting under the graft. Skin then grows outward from the outline or rows of graft and closes the interstices. Unfortunately, a number of portals of entry for infection are present and the healed meshed area has more scarring than does a sheet graft. If possible, the use of the mesh dermatome is limited to areas where appearance is less important, such as the back, the abdomen, and the thighs.

Nursing Orders

Nursing care is directed not only toward the patient's current problems but also toward his potential problems. The prevention of complications is a primary responsibility of everyone on the health team. The following is a list of the most common complications of burn injury.

Fear	Evaporative water loss
Pain	Fever
Powerlessness	Oliguric renal failure
Depersonalization	High-output renal failure
Sleep deprivation	Acute gastroduodenal
Sensory deprivation and	disease
sensory overstimulation	Gastrointestinal bleeding
Burn shock	Fluid and electrolyte imbalance
Myocardial depressant factor	Liver failure
Resuscitation failure	Stroke
Dysrhythmias	Altered level of consciousness
Hypertension	Loss of function

Carbon monoxide poisoning
Upper-airway obstruction
Lower-airway obstruction
Death
Pneumonia
Adult respiratory distress syndrome
Pulmonary embolism
Hypermetabolism, protein loss, and weight loss

Sepsis
Suppurative thrombophlebitis
Disseminated intravascular coagulation
Organ necrosis
Allergy
Postoperative complications
Multisystem organ failure
Contractures
Disfigurement
Amputations
Peripheral neuropathy

Problem/Diagnosis

Burn injury.

OBJECTIVE NO. 1

The patient with a burn injury should receive initial care according to the established protocol and from a well-functioning team.

ACHIEVING THE OBJECTIVE

To achieve the objective, the nurse should:

1. Maintain a patent airway.
2. Assess and manage any associated life-threatening injuries according to the trauma protocol.
3. Wash areas of chemical injury with copious amounts of water.
4. Initiate fluid therapy according to the crystalloid resuscitation formula as ordered. Use a peripheral site for administration, even though it may be one in the burn wound. Monitor for signs of adequate resuscitation.
5. Obtain the results of baseline laboratory tests (arterial blood gas measurements, a complete blood count, serum electrolyte, blood urea nitrogen, glucose, sickle cell tests, and typing and crossmatching).
6. Monitor for signs of carbon monoxide poisoning, upper-airway obstruction and/or inhalation injury.
7. Place nasogastric and urethral catheters.
8. Monitor all areas of circumferential full-thickness burn in regard to the need for escharotomy.
9. Cover the burn with a clean sheet to decrease the contact with air currents and to promote comfort. Limited areas may be covered with sterile, moist, light dressings.
10. Calculate the burn area and weigh the patient.
11. Take a history of the accident: Did the burning occur in a closed space? Did the patient inhale excessive amounts of smoke? Did he lose consciousness? What type of agent caused the burn? What were the other relevant circumstances of the accident? The nurse should find out also about:
    a. Any preexisting disease, especially cardiovascular, pulmonary, renal, metabolic, and neurological disorders.
    b. The patient's past health history including any medications and allergies and the date of his last tetanus immunization.
    c. The patient's immunizations and his use of alcohol and/or narcotics.
12. Initiate intravenous penicillin for beta-hemolytic streptococcal prophylaxis if ordered.
13. Administer tetanus prophylaxis as ordered.
14. If the patient responds adequately to fluid therapy, administer an intravenous analgesic as ordered.
15. Assess the patient's status in regard to the hospital's facilities. If necessary, have a staff member make arrangements to transfer the patient elsewhere for treatment.
16. Clean and debride the wound using aseptic technique.
17. Apply topical antimicrobial dressings. (If the patient has a tar burn, apply neopolycin dressing. Two applications may be needed to remove the tar.)
18. Apply porcine heterografts to areas of partial-thickness injury as ordered.
19. Elevate burned extremities above the level of the heart [56].
20. Monitor the urinary sugar and acetone levels every four hours to look for pseudodiabetes.

OBJECTIVE NO. 2

The patient should demonstrate the restoration of normal hemodynamics and of his fluid and electrolyte balance.

ACHIEVING THE OBJECTIVE

To achieve the objective, the nurse should:

1. Administer Ringer's lactate solution (RL) according to the following formula as ordered:

$$4 \text{ ml RL} \times \text{wt (kg)} \times \% \text{ TBSA burned} = \text{ml RL for the first 24 hr}$$

(One-half the total amount should be given in the first eight hours after the injury, one-fourth should be given in the second eight hours after the injury, and one-fourth should be given in the third eight hours after the injury.)
2. Monitor every 30 to 60 minutes for the signs of adequate resuscitation: a clear lucid sensorium, a urinary output of 50 to 70 ml per hour, a pulse that is < 120, the return of bowel sounds, a normal to slightly alkalotic acid-base status, a pulmonary capillary wedge pressure that is normal (or a central venous pressure that is < 5 cm H_2O), and a normal to slightly elevated cardiac output.
3. Calculate the extent of injury. The nurse should:
   a. Use the Rule of Nines for triage and before initiating fluid therapy to approximate fluid therapy. Each arm and the head (including the neck) represents 9 percent TBSA burned. Each leg and the anterior and posterior trunk represents 18 percent TBSA burned. The perineal area represents 1 percent TBSA burned.
   b. Determine the extent of injury to calculate fluid therapy before cleansing the wound—use the Berkow formula (or the Lund and Browder burn chart).
   c. After cleansing the wound, make a more accurate calculation of the burned area. Calculate the percentage of unburned area, add that figure to the calculation of the percentage of burned area, and make sure that the addition equals 100 percent of the total body surface area. Then recalculate the fluid therapy using the crystalloid formula.
4. Weigh the patient on a metabolic scale.
5. If the urinary output is decreased, determine whether the fluids are behind schedule and recalculate the fluid therapy. If the urinary output is less than 35 ml for two hours, the physician should be notified. The nurse should monitor renal functioning.

6. Prepare for plasma restoration during the fourth eight-hour period. Usually the amount of plasma administered is 0.3 to 0.5 ml × kg × % body surface area burned. Plasma volumes may be measured or their adequacy assessed according to the signs of adequate resuscitation and to the hematocrit.
7. Administer a 5% dextrose in water solution (2000–6000 ml) in the second 24 hours as ordered (the amount is determined by the patient's serum sodium level).
8. Refer to Chapter 36, which discusses how to assess changes in the fluid and electrolyte balance.
9. Administer potassium as ordered. If more than 40 mEq of potassium is to be added to a single intravenous infusion, it should be administered by a controlled infusion device or the hourly quota should be placed in a volutrol.
10. Administer magnesium, calcium, zinc, and other medications as ordered.

OBJECTIVE NO. 3

The patient should demonstrate adequate respiratory functioning.

ACHIEVING THE OBJECTIVE

To achieve the objective the nurse should:

1. Assess for signs of hypoxemia (Chap. 36). Patients with hypoxemia are often wrongly thought to be showing signs of pain.
2. Assess for upper-airway obstruction. The nurse should look for:
   a. Singed nasal hairs.
   b. Dry, red mucosa.
   c. Soot in the sputum.
   d. Dyspnea.
   e. Drooling.
   f. An inability to handle secretions.
   g. Increasing hoarseness (to evaluate, the nurse should ask the patient the same question every 15 minutes).
3. Assess for inhalation injury. The nurse should determine whether the patient:
   a. Has a closed-space injury.
   b. Has inhaled smoke or a noxious gas.
   c. Has lost consciousness during the fire.

d. Showed signs of inhalation injury on his admission physical examination and chest x ray.
e. Has carbonaceous sputum.
f. Has a carboxyhemoglobin level that is greater than 15%.
g. Is hoarse.
h. Has a brassy cough.
i. Has dyspnea.
j. Has a burned face, lips, or nose or has burned mucosa.
k. Has increased secretions and rales, bronchi, or wheezes.
l. Has an arterial oxygen pressure of less than 60 mm Hg.

The nurse should consult the physician about positive findings from the bronchoscopic examination (mucosal blisters, massive nasal edema, or erythema, and mucosal hemorrhage and ulceration in the upper airway) [30], a positive ^{133}xenon lung scan (unequal scintillation density, a clearance time of greater than 90 sec, and an impairment in ventilatory function with marked airway obstruction) [57], alterations shown by spirometry, flow-volume loops, and the single-breath nitrogen test, and alterations in the residual volume.

4. Monitor the patient in regard to his respiratory rate and rhythm, cough, findings on auscultation, increased work of breathing, arterial blood gas measurements, and spirometric findings. The physician should be notified of significant trends.
5. Administer humidified oxygen as ordered.
6. Have the patient cough and deep breathe and turn him every one to two hours as indicated by his pulmonary status. Encourage inspiratory maneuvers.
7. Maintain pulmonary hygiene.
8. Administer bronchodilators and other medications if ordered.
9. Be prepared for endotracheal intubation and ventilatory assistance [71].

OBJECTIVE NO. 4

The patient should not suffer pain unnecessarily.

ACHIEVING THE OBJECTIVE

To achieve the objective, the nurse should:

1. Assess the patient's pain history, anxiety level (when appropriate, use the trait-state test), and response to pain.

2. Educate the patient about painful procedures and about the techniques used to decrease pain. Plan approaches to relieve pain; evaluate and document their effectiveness.
3. Be gentle and efficient as well as thorough in performing all nursing care procedures.
4. If silver sulfadiazine is ordered, keep the patient's wounds covered.
5. When a heterograft is ordered, apply it immediately.
6. Administer the analgesic ordered either before hydrotherapy and debridement or after those procedures (when relaxation is possible).
7. Make sure that the patient has enough rest and sleep.
8. Meet the patient's calculated nutritional needs.
9. Make minor alterations in technique to help the patient maintain proper body alignment and positioning. For example, when abduction boards are used for the arms, remind the patient to move his arms from supination to pronation and back to supination three times every 15 minutes. With hyperextension of the neck, place a small pillow under the patient's head for five minutes out of every hour.
10. Use environmental comfort measures, such as the use of clean dressings and a calm speaking voice.
11. Consult with the staff psychologist.
12. Keep the patient warm and keep him from shivering.
13. Investigate and use mind-body-spirit relaxation techniques.

OBJECTIVE NO. 5

The patient should maintain adequate circulation in all areas of a circumferential full-thickness burn.

ACHIEVING THE OBJECTIVE

To achieve the objective, the nurse should:

1. Assess the depth of the wound. Although the exact depth cannot be determined for several days, clinical assessment may be used early to identify areas of full-thickness injury. The injuries are usually not entirely full thickness or partial thickness; they are of different depths. The thickness of the skin varies with the site of the injury and with the patient's age. With similar exposure, an area on the back of the hand

might well be full thickness whereas an area on the back might be partial thickness.

2. Identify a first-degree burn by its characteristics:
   a. The burn occurs after brief contact with heat, such as exposure to the sun.
   b. The burn involves the epidermis.
   c. Erythema is present.
   d. The burn is painful.
   e. Minor vasodilatation and chilling are present.
   f. The burn heals in approximately one week.

3. Identify a superficial second-degree (partial-thickness) burn by its characteristics:
   a. The burn occurs after a flash explosion or a brief exposure to hot liquids, hot objects, or chemicals.
   b. The burn involves the epidermis and dermis.
   c. Blisters may be formed.
   d. The burn is moist.
   e. The burn is pink or mottled red.
   f. The burn is painful.
   g. The burn heals in 10 to 14 days.

4. Identify a deep second-degree (partial-thickness) burn by its characteristics (Fig. 35-5):
   a. The burn is often clinically indistinguishable from a full-thickness injury.
   b. The burn appears drier than a superficial partial-thickness injury, is mottled and may contain waxy, white areas.
   c. The burn heals in 30 to 60 or so days by reepithelialization from elements in the hair follicles.

5. Identify a third-degree (full-thickness) burn by its characteristics (Fig. 35-6):
   a. The burn occurs after contact with flame or electricity or after prolonged contact with hot water, hot objects, or chemicals.
   b. The elasticity of the skin in the burned area is destroyed.
   c. The burned area is insensitive to a pinprick.
   d. The burn is white, cherry-red, or black.
   e. Marked edema is present (blisters may be trapped in the dermis).
   f. Thrombosed blood vessels may be present.
   g. The burn may have a dry, hard, leathery appearance.
   h. The burn needs skin grafts.

6. Elevate any burned extremities above the level of the heart. Encourage active exercise for five minutes out of every hour.

7. Monitor all patients with circumferential full-thickness burns of the chest for:

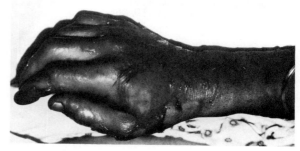

Figure 35-5
Partial-thickness burn injury.

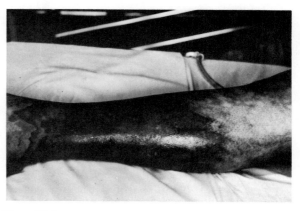

Figure 35-6
Full-thickness burn injury. (Photographer—Brian Anderson)

   a. Increased work of breathing.
   b. Rapid, shallow breathing.
   c. Respiratory distress.

8. Monitor the patient with full-thickness burns of the extremities for the signs of impaired circulation. Notify the physician about:
   a. Irregular to absent pulses measured with the Doppler (pulses may no longer be palpable but the circulation may still be intact).
   b. Numbness.
   c. Decreased sensation.
   d. Decreased motor activity.
   e. Decreased capillary refill.
   f. Cyanosis.
   g. Deep, aching pain.

9. If the patient's circulation is severely impaired, prepare for escharotomy (the incision will be

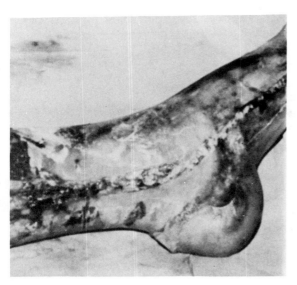

Figure 35-7
Escharotomy site.

made through the entire thickness of the eschar) (Fig. 35-7). The nurse should have at hand:

  a. Scalpels, gauze sponges, iodophor solution.
  b. Sterile gloves.
  c. A collagen hemostat.
  d. Gauze dressings, fine mesh gauze, and Kling wrap.
  e. Silver sulfadiazine.

10. Control bleeding by direct pressure and the application of a collagen hemostat.
11. Following escharotomy, monitor circulation, maintain hemostasis, and prevent infection. Keep a topical antimicrobial agent and light dressings over the site. Change the dressing every eight hours.

OBJECTIVE NO. 6

The patient's calculated nutritional needs should be met.

ACHIEVING THE OBJECTIVE

To achieve the objective, the nurse should:

1. Refer to Chapter 36 for the protocol. (One gram of nitrogen is needed for each 150 calories.)
2. Institute nutritional support by the third day for patients who have large burns and by the fifth day for patients who have 20 to 40 percent TBSA burns.
3. Administer vitamins (three times the normal dosage) and ascorbic acid (2 gm/day) as ordered.

OBJECTIVE NO. 7

The patient should receive prophylaxis for acute gastroduodenal syndrome.

ACHIEVING THE OBJECTIVE

To achieve the objective, the nurse should refer to the pertinent information in the Nursing Orders section of Chapter 36.

OBJECTIVE NO. 8

The patient should not demonstrate signs of systemic infection resulting from burn wound sepsis.

ACHIEVING THE OBJECTIVE

To achieve the objective, the nurse should:

1. Maintain an aseptic environment.
2. Follow the protocols established by the infection control committee.
3. Keep the burned area covered with a topical antimicrobial agent (and remove it before giving wound care).
4. Cleanse the wound aseptically two to three times a day using the bedbath, tub, or shower procedure. (Some units, however, do not wash the patient's wound. They remove the old topical antimicrobial agent and apply the new agent.)

   a. Assess the cardiopulmonary status, fluid status, bacterial count, and site of infection.
   b. Explain the cleansing procedure to the patient.
   c. Give pain medication (15 to 30 minutes before cleansing the wound if given by intramuscular injection or immediately prior to cleansing if given by intravenous injection).
   d. Give perineal care.
   e. Remove the dressings and the topical antimicrobial agent (a tongue blade may be used—gently).
   f. Clamp the Foley catheter but maintain a closed drainage system.
   g. Weigh the patient on a metabolic scale.
   h. Monitor the patient continuously.
   i. Use heat shields.

j. Help patient get on and off the stretcher by using transfer techniques.

k. Keep the water temperature comfortable.

l. Keep the environment clean.

m. If the patient has many open wounds, do not submerge him. Have him lie on a plinth and gently spray him with water.

n. Use sterile gloves and use a fresh iodophor sponge for each part of the body burned.

o. Shave the hair in the burned area and the areas around it.

p. Limit the patient's time in the tub to 20 min.

q. If possible, debride the wounds while cleansing them.

r. Apply the topical antimicrobial agent.

s. Evaluate the patient's cardiopulmonary status, wounds, temperature, and comfort after his return to bed.

5. Pay particular attention to the body folds (e.g., the axilla, breasts, and perineum).

6. Cover the sites of invasive devices in the wound with iodophor gauze dressings. Change the dressings every eight hours.

7. Prevent cross contamination among patients.

a. Maintain reverse isolation.

b. Use thorough hand-washing techniques.

c. Give one-to-one nursing care (one nurse to one patient). If the patient is critically ill he needs two nurses (determination of acuity and hours of nursing care is based on patient needs).

d. Wear a plastic apron over the scrub dress.

e. Maintain a clean scrub dress; change her scrub dress whenever it is soiled.

f. If she is to attend to another patient, wear a plastic apron and/or change her scrub dress.

g. When turning the patient, try to avoid contamination of her upper arms and/or scrub dress. She should change to clean clothes as needed.

h. Monitor the technique of the other staff members.

i. Clean the equipment each time it is used.

j. Elect nurses to the infection control committee. Establish appropriate policies. Determine the feasibility of laminar air flow units and establish protocols about their use.

8. Obtain burn wound biopsies three times a week.

a. Assess the wound in regard to distribution, presence and character of eschar (color, consistency, distribution, depth, and odor) and exudate.

b. Select areas for tissue biopsy (1) that are representative, (2) that contain eschar (especially if the eschar is darkening or changing in character or re-forming), and (3) that will be excised during surgical therapy.

c. Do not take tissue for biopsy from the face, hands, or feet.

d. Using aseptic technique, clean the area with saline-soaked gauze pads and alcohol swabs. Allow it to dry.

e. Using sterile technique and a scalpel, make two parallel incisions approximately 1.5 cm apart and 1 to 2 cm in length through the entire thickness of the eschar.

f. Grasp some tissue for biopsy with forceps and remove it by making a horizontal cut at the level of viable tissue; make sure that a small portion of unburned underlying fat is included.

g. Transfer the sample to a sterile culture tube.

h. Apply pressure and/or a collagen hemostat to the area to stop the bleeding.

9. Obtain burn wound culture plate three times a week.

a. Assess the wound for exudate, purulent drainage, and foul odor.

b. Select areas for culture that are representative of the wound. In particular, select the following areas: thin eschar, purulent exudate, an area covered by a purulent biological dressing or a biological dressing that has not adhered, granulating surfaces, a rejected graft, areas to be operated on, and the hands, face, and feet.

c. Remove the topical antimicrobial agent or biological dressing and wipe the area with a dry gauze pad.

d. Press the plate firmly to the area prepared.

e. Reapply the topical antimicrobial agent.

10. Monitor for positive bacteriological cultures. Notify the physician of any.

11. Do not allow patients whose ears are burned to use a pillow under their heads. Observe them for signs of inflammation (chondritis): tenderness, swelling, or change in color. Notify the physician of any.

12. Monitor for the clinical signs of sepsis: an altered sensorium, an increased respiratory rate, glycosuria, and a decreasing platelet count.

13. Maintain all supportive measures in order to achieve optimal resistance to infection. The nurse should:

a. See that the patient's nutritional requirements are met.

b. Keep him warm.

c. Prevent respiratory infections.
d. Administer blood as ordered [68].
e. Reduce stress.
f. Encourage mobility.
14. Monitor for sepsis (Chap. 36).

OBJECTIVE NO. 9

The patient should demonstrate adequate wound debridement.

ACHIEVING THE OBJECTIVE

To achieve the objective, the nurse should:

1. Assess the patient's need for an analgesic.
2. Clean and debride the burn wound initially. The nurse should:
   a. Make sure the room is clean.
   b. Wear a gown, mask, and gloves.
   c. Wash the wound gently with iodophor solution.
   d. Remove the loose epidermis with a gauze pad, using slight pressure. If necessary, use scissors.
   e. Not use scrub brushes.
   f. Shave the hair from the burned area and the adjacent unburned area.
   g. Leave the blisters on the palms and soles intact.
3. Have another staff member present to help the patient focus on other thoughts or surroundings during the treatment.
4. Identify areas of subeschar suppuration by applying gentle pressure to the wound with a gloved hand.
5. Unroof and remove the eschar that has been lysed by bacterial suppuration. In doing so, the nurse should:
   a. Use sterile scissors and forceps (Fig. 35-8).
   b. Be gentle.
   c. Allow 30 minutes three times a day for debridement.
   d. Stop the procedure for a few minutes if the patient requests it.
6. Control the bleeding with direct pressure.
7. To remove the remnants of eschar and dermal debris, use wet to dry dressings (Fig. 35-9). The nurse should:
   a. Apply large-pore expandable dressings (Kerlex) that have been wet with saline solution or triple antibiotic solution.
   b. Allow them to dry (approximately three to four hours).

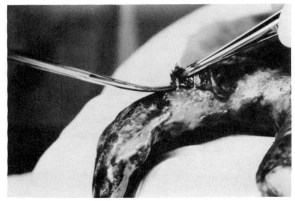

Figure 35-8
Burn wound debridement. (Photographer—Brian Anderson)

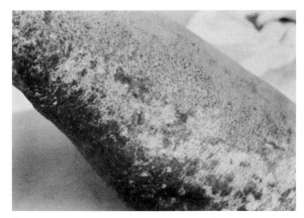

Figure 35-9
Typical burn wound that would benefit from the use of wet to dry dressings.

   c. Assess the patient's need for pain medication.
   d. Remove the dry dressing.
   e. Use a steady motion (the removal is painful).
   f. Reapply the dressing.
8. If Travase (an enzymatic debriding agent) is ordered, be aware that:
   a. Travase may be used during the first 24 postburn hours.
   b. Travase is used when the quantitative biopsy reports list less than 10^4 bacteria per gram of tissue.
   c. The patient must be monitored for sepsis [29].

d. Cross-hatching may be needed to allow maximum penetration of the eschar.

e. Cultures and biopsies should be done three times a week.

f. Travase should not be used on the face, hands, feet, or ankles or over the tendons.

g. Fluid loss may occur after the application of Travase. If Travase is used 48 to 72 hours after the burn, the fluid loss will be greater than the normal bleeding. Monitor fluid balance.

h. The patient's temperature may rise to 102 to 103°F, but it should return to baseline in a few hours.

i. The patient may feel pain when Travase is applied to a partial-thickness wound, and he may require an analgesic.

j. Transient dermatitis may be noted. It disappears once the wound is clean and Travase therapy is discontinued.

k. Daily wound care is needed. It consists of:

(1) A bedbath or hydrotherapy. The nurse should be sure that all the iodophor is rinsed off before Travase is applied.

(2) The application of Travase to clean wound. (The gauze should not be impregnated with Travase.)

(3) The application of silver sulfadiazine-impregnated gauze over the Travase.

(4) Covering the wound with a Kling bandage and wrapping it with Kerlex. The procedure should be repeated twice a day until the wound is relatively clean (rarely longer than six days).

OBJECTIVE NO. 10

The patient should demonstrate bacteriological control of the septic process in the burn wound and healing of partial-thickness wounds.

ACHIEVING THE OBJECTIVE

To achieve the objective, the nurse should:

1. Apply silver sulfadiazine (1%) as ordered. The nurse should:
   a. Assess for an allergy to sulfa.
   b. Use aseptic technique.
   c. Apply the drug three times a day; between applications, keep the wounds white with cream.
   d. Use a nonocclusive dressing if desired.

e. Educate the patient about applying the agent himself.

f. Remember that silver sulfadiazine is effective against a wide range of gram-positive and gram-negative organisms as well as against *Candida albicans*. Unfortunately, it has several disadvantages: (1) resistant strains of *Pseudomonas* often appear, (2) a few cases of leukopenia have been reported, and (3) occasionally a patient exhibits a hypersensitivity reaction. The drug has many advantages. It need not be used with dressings (although a thin, dry dressing may be applied). That "open" method of treatment, combined with a softened eschar, allows the patient increased joint mobility. Since the agent is poorly absorbed, no systemic metabolic derangements occur. Sensitive areas are protected from air currents, and the patient feels relatively comfortable.

2. Apply mafenide acetate (Sulfamylon) (11%) as ordered. The nurse should:

a. Assess for an allergy to sulfa.

b. Apply a thin layer (⅛ in.), no more than once every 12 hours.

c. Assess the patient's pain when the drug is applied to partial-thickness wounds to determine his need for an analgesic.

d. Monitor for metabolic acidosis and tachypnea.

Mafenide has a water-soluble base, and it diffuses through the entire avascular eschar. It is thus the agent of choice for patients who have electrical injuries. Mafenide ("burn butter") was developed specifically to combat *Pseudomonas*, but it is effective against a wide range of gram-positive and gram-negative organisms. It is not effective against fungi and some strains of gram-negative rods. On body areas where it has been the only topical agent used, resistant organisms such as *Providencia stuartii* have proliferated. Mafenide is an excellent agent. Like silver sulfadiazine, it can be used with the open method of therapy. Bulky dressings are not needed, and the patient has greater mobility. Unfortunately, its use may result in metabolic acidosis for two reasons. First, the end product of the breakdown of mafenide is an acid salt that increases the hydrogen ions in the body's buffer system. Second, an alkaline urine is produced by the inhibition of carbonic anhydrase. The body compensates by tachypnea. If pulmonary complications arise, compensatory mechanisms are altered, and the physician temporarily discontinues the agent. A hypersensitivity reaction also occurs in 5 percent of patients. It is characterized by a maculopapular rash. The drug is discontinued only if the rash is severe.

3. Apply povidone ointment (Betadine) as ordered. The nurse should:
   a. Assess for an allergy to iodine.
   b. Apply the agent quickly and wrap the body with light dressing (unless the agent has been applied in preparation for excisional therapy).
   c. Encourage the patient to be mobile.

   This relatively new agent in burn therapy is being evaluated. Iodine has been long known for its germicidal properties, but the directions for its use in the care of burn injury cannot be described until the evaluation has been completed. At body temperature, the agent changes from a semisolid ointment to a liquid, and so a light dressing must be used over the drug. The dressing, combined with a hardened eschar, makes decreased mobility a distinct possibility. Quantitative burn wound biopsies are not completely satisfactory for monitoring bacterial growth while povidone ointment is used. The tissue specimen may contain iodine concentrations that inhibit bacterial growth during the laboratory test even while infection might be increasing in the patient. Besides its antibacterial activity, it has two major advantages. It makes the wound translucent, and so the depth of injury can be more easily determined. Also, it can be used preoperatively to harden the eschar.

4. Apply cerium nitrate as ordered. The nurse should:
   a. Use aseptic technique.
   b. Monitor for gram-positive infections. She should consult with the physician about adding silver sulfadiazine to the therapy.
   c. Monitor for methemoglobinuria.

   Cerium nitrate, a new agent, is being evaluated. It may be used as a cream or in aqueous solution [48]. In its early trials, it significantly reduced infections with gram-negative and fungal organisms. Since gram-positive flora have predominated and have been associated with the septic process, simultaneous treatment with silver sulfadiazine has been instituted. Although not enough time has elapsed to assess its effectiveness and the parameters for care, the early reports are promising.

5. Apply silver nitrate (0.5%) if ordered. The nurse should:
   a. Before applying silver nitrate, make sure there is no bacterial colonization.
   b. Apply thick (5-cm) dressings.
   c. Saturate the dressings every 4 hours with warm solution, and change them every 12 hours.
   d. Cover the body with a light blanket to decrease evaporation and retain heat.
   e. Conduct active debridement.
   f. Monitor clinically for signs of hyponatremia, hypokalemia, hypocalcemia, and the syndrome associated with decreased serum levels of chloride.

   Silver nitrate is used as a solution, and it is applied as a continuous wet soak in large bulky dressings. It is quite effective against *Staphylococcus*, *Streptococcus*, and *Pseudomonas*, but it is ineffective against *Enterobacter*, *Klebsiella*, and *Aerobacter*. The dressings must be put on the wound three to five days before bacterial colonization occurs because silver nitrate does not penetrate the eschar and is not effective after colonization. Active debridement to remove the eschar must accompany the drug therapy so that the drug can penetrate to the infection. The silver ion is inactivated and precipitated once it is combined with tissue fluid. A crust results. It must be frequently removed by debridement beause bacteria proliferate under it. The dressing should be kept saturated with a warm solution because if dried, the high concentration of silver would be toxic to the tissues. Silver nitrate has several major disadvantages. First, it is a hypotonic drug, and it causes significant losses of sodium, potassium, calcium, and chloride. The burn wound acts as a semipermeable membrane, and all four electrolytes diffuse quickly into the dressings. Methemoglobinemia is a potential complication, because nitrate may be oxidized to nitrite in the wound and be absorbed. A bulky occlusive dressing must be used, and limits mobility and thus increases the possibility of contractures. Last, but not least, silver nitrate stains black everything with which it comes in contact.

6. Rotate the topical agents as indicated by how effective each one is.

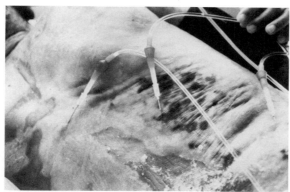

Figure 35-10
Subeschar clysis. (Photographer—Richard Schmitt)

7. Administer an antibiotic via subeschar clysis as ordered (Fig. 35-10). The nurse should:
   a. Use hypodermoclysis technique.
   b. Know that the carrier fluid ordered is normal saline solution or half normal saline solution.
   c. Use the gravity drip or the injection technique.
   d. Divide the amount of antibiotic solution ordered into 100-ml aliquots.
   e. Insert a 22-gauge needle at a 45-degree angle into the subeschar space.
   f. Allow 25 ml of solution to infuse the area (that amount covers an area that is approximately 8 cm in diameter).
   g. Change the needle and repeat the procedure in a site that is 15 cm away.
   h. Cover the entire wound with serial systematic infusions.
   i. Apply a topical antimicrobial agent.
   j. Remember that subeschar antibiotic therapy is used as an adjunct to topical therapy in clinical burn wound sepsis, as prophylaxis for bacterial colonization in the amount of 10^4 per gram of tissue, for patients whose hospital admission was delayed and who have infections, and for patients who have severe allergies.
8. Administer systemic antibiotics if ordered.
   Systemic antibiotics cannot reach the viable–nonviable interface and granulation tissue in concentrations high enough to prevent bacterial growth. The systemic route is generally used when specific evidence of infection is present; in a very few burn centers prophylactic antibiotics are used.

OBJECTIVE NO. 11

The patient should demonstrate the ability to cope psychologically with his illness.

ACHIEVING THE OBJECTIVE

To achieve the objective, the nurse should:

1. Gather information about the patient's background, personality, and level of coping from his family, friends, and from him (as appropriate).
2. In administering care, remember Maslow's hierarchy of needs (see Chap. 5); the patient with a severe injury usually focuses first on his physiological needs.
3. Offer the patient a simple explanation of the body's response to injury and treatment (e.g., "the swelling will go down in a few days"); do not overwhelm him with information.
4. Explain all nursing care procedures to the patient and his family.
5. Maintain a warm, human manner and perform nursing care duties efficiently and competently.
6. Decrease the patient's pain and provide him with as much comfort as possible.
7. Do not attempt to hurry the patient through the stage of denial. Look for behavioral signs that he is ready to deal with his problems.
8. Refer to Chapters 13 and 36.
9. Assist patient and his family to adapt to a prolonged stay in the critical care unit. Establish short-term goals and point out ways in which the patient is better from week to week. If necessary, set limits on the patient's behavior.

OBJECTIVE NO. 12

The patient should maintain wound coverage after a homograft or heterograft has been applied (Fig. 35-11).

ACHIEVING THE OBJECTIVE

To achieve the objective, the nurse should:

1. Maintain aseptic technique.
2. Remove the topical agent and cleanse the wound with iodophor solution.
3. Apply a biological dressing in single pieces, with the shiny side next to the wound.
4. Smooth the skin and remove any air pockets with a sterile gloved hand or with forceps.

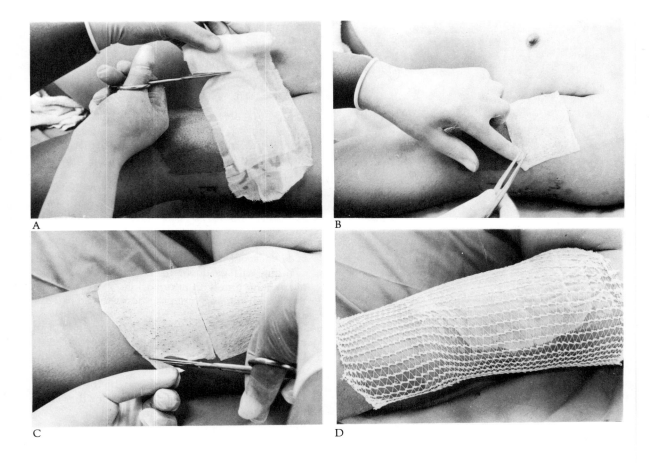

A

B

C

D

5. Trim the dressing with scissors so that the skin covers the wound and does not overlap it.
6. Repeat the procedure until the wound is covered.
7. Cover the dressing with gauze impregnated with antibiotic ointment or cover it first with a fine mesh gauze and then a light dressing.
8. Monitor the patient's vital signs for 24 hours after the dressing has been applied (his temperature may be mildly elevated because the wound is covered).
9. Observe the wound for small accumulations of serous drainage under the biological dressing. Gently pierce the dressing with a sterile needle to drain the serous accumulation and thus enable the dressing to adhere to the wound.
10. Observe the wound for suppurative drainage or large areas of nonadherent dressing. If any are present, notify the physician, remove the dressing, cleanse the wound, and reapply the dressing.

Figure 35-11
Heterograft application. A. Apply the dressing, putting its shiny side next to the burn wound and using aseptic technique. B. Smooth the skin and remove any air pockets. C. Trim the skin in accordance with the wound margin; avoid overlapping. D. Secure the dressing with the expandable, netlike material. (Photographer—Brian Anderson)

11. Monitor for tissue rejection phenomena. She should look for:
    a. Spotty, raised, edematous granulation tissue.
    b. Increased temperature and pulse.
    c. Irritability.
    d. Anxiety.
    e. Gastrointestinal malfunctioning.

OBJECTIVE NO. 13

The patient should maintain range of motion.

ACHIEVING THE OBJECTIVE

To achieve the objective, the nurse should:

1. Elevate the patient's burned extremities above the level of his heart for approximately 72 hours. She should:
   a. After covering the topical antimicrobial agent with a light dressing and flexible, netlike material, suspend patient's arms from intravenous poles or a substitute means.
   b. Every hour, discontinue the suspension and encourage active exercise.
   c. Elevate the foot of the patient's bed.
2. Consult with the physical medicine department about the need for splints. The most common splint is a static splint constructed from thermoplastic material that holds the wrist in 30-degree extension, the mid-interphalangeal joints in 65-degree flexion, and the proximal and distal interphalangeal joints in full extension.
3. Consult with the physical medicine department about an exercise program for the patient. As a rule of thumb, each burned area is taken through full range of motion five times, at least four times a day.
4. Encourage active exercise and include the activities of daily living. Perform passive exercise gently and do not go past the patient's point of pain.
5. With burns of the neck, after 48 to 72 hours maintain neck hyperextension by having the patient lie on a pediatric mattress that has been put on top of a regular hospital mattress. The patient should rest his head on the regular mattress. The patient's position should be changed every hour. Several times a day, a small roll should be placed under the patient's head for short periods.
6. Remember that flexion and contracture tend to be positions of comfort.
7. Keep the patient's shoulders and arms abducted—on abduction boards. His elbows, wrists, hands, and (supinated) forearm and palms should be extended. The distal portion of his arms should not be dependent.
8. Keep the patient's hips straight and elevated, knees extended, and legs in slight abduction. The nurse should:
   a. Prevent the patient's knees from falling into the frog-leg position. A trochanter roll and footboard should be used.
   b. Use foam rubber to relieve pressure and prevent tissue breakdown under the patient's heels and buttocks and/or along the sides of his feet.
9. Place a small roll lengthwise against the patient's spine to allow his shoulders to move backward into alignment.
10. Turn the patient every two hours when he is awake. A circuloelectric bed or another type of bed should be used as needed.
11. Assess the patient's ability to get out of bed. The nurse should consider:
    a. The severity of the patient's injury.
    b. The presence of any complications.
    c. His vital signs.
    d. His metabolic status.
    e. His volume status.
    f. The infectious process.
    g. His respiratory status.
12. Observe the patient for any exposed tendons. If they are present, exercise should be discontinued, the physiatrist should be notified, the tendons should be covered with a moist gauze dressing or pigskin, and the area should be immobilized.
13. Encourage the patient to exercise (in bed) non-burned areas, such as his buttocks (by gluteal tightening).

OBJECTIVE NO. 14

The patient should demonstrate vascularization of his autograft and the healing of donor sites.

ACHIEVING THE OBJECTIVE

To achieve the objective, the nurse should:

1. Educate the patient and his family about preoperative, intraoperative, and postoperative care.
2. Consult with the surgeon and the occupational therapist about any special splints or positioning devices that will be needed at the time of surgery. Plan their use with the operating room nurse.
3. Immobilize the graft site following the surgery. If large bulk dressings have been applied to immobilize the graft, ask the operating room nurse about special precautions the surgeon may have given.
   a. Do not permit the graft to be disrupted by the application of external devices or by movement. Investigate use of the Air Flow Bed.

b. Use a bed cradle.

c. Keep the patient comfortable.

d. Keep the skin intact in areas of prolonged pressure while the patient is immobilized.

e. Keep articles the patient may want within his reach.

f. If necessary and appropriate, change the family visiting hours so that the patient's family may remain with him.

g. Discontinue physical therapy and hydrotherapy for five days. Consult with the surgeon and the physiatrist about when the patient should resume activities.

h. When the patient is prone, use established positioning techniques to maintain his comfort; for example, elevate the waist and hips and allow the feet to be positioned over the edge of the mattress.

i. Apply elastic bandages to grafts of the legs before permitting the legs to become dependent. New grafts should be wrapped first with Adaptic or antibiotic gauze.

4. Determine whether the dressing used on the donor site is gauze, heterograft (a frozen lyophilized one or a fresh one that has been placed in hot water), homograft, collagen dressing, or another therapy.

5. In regard to the gauze dressing:

a. Observe it for bleeding.

b. Do not remove the single layer of gauze next to the donor site.

c. Leave the dressing open to the air.

d. Use a heat lamp at a distance of 12 to 18 inches for 24 to 48 hours.

e. Keep the patient comfortable.

f. Monitor the donor site for a purulent, infected appearance. If any, the physician should be notified.

g. Resume exercise 24 to 72 hours after surgery.

h. Trim the raised, dry areas of gauze as healing occurs and as the gauze separates.

References

1. Alexander, J. W. Immunologic Consideration and the Role of Vaccination in Burn Injury. In H. Polk and H. H. Stone (eds.), *Contemporary Burn Management*. Boston: Little, Brown, 1971. Pp. 265–280.

2. Alexander, J.W., Diongi, R., and Meakins, J. L. Periodic variation in the antibacterial function of human neutro-phils and its relationship to sepsis. *Ann. Surg.* 173:206, 1971.

3. Ambiavager, M. B., Chalon, J., and Zargham, I. Tracheobronchial cytolic changes following lower airway thermal injury. *J. Trauma* 14:280, 1974.

4. Andreasen, N. J. C., Noyes, R., Hartford, C. E., et al. Management of emotional reactions in seriously burned adults. *N. Engl. J. Med.* 286:65, 1972.

5. Artz, C. P., and Moncrief, J. A. *The Treatment of Burns*. Philadelphia: Saunders, 1969.

6. Baxter, C. R. Evaluation of the Burned Patient. In *Current Diagnosis* (2nd ed.). Philadelphia: Saunders, 1967. Pp. 915–919.

7. Baxter, C. R. Crystalloid Resuscitation of Burn Shock. In H. Polk and H. H. Stone (eds.), *Contemporary Burn Management*. Boston: Little, Brown, 1971. Pp. 7–32.

8. Baxter, C. R. Response to Initial Fluid and Electrolyte Therapy of Burn Shock. In J. B. Lynch and S. R. Lewis (eds.), *Symposium on the Treatment of Burns*. St. Louis: Mosby, 1973. Pp. 42–48, vol. 5.

9. Baxter, C. R. Fluid volume and electrolyte changes of the early postburn period. *Clin. Plast. Surg.* 1:673, 1974.

10. Baxter, C. R. Pathophysiology and Treatment of Burns and Cold Injury. *Rhoads Textbook of Surgery*. Philadelphia: Lippincott, 1977.

11. Baxter, C. R. Burns. In G. Tom Shires (ed.), *Care of the Trauma Patient*. New York: McGraw-Hill, 1966. Pp. 197–222.

12. Baxter, C. R., Curreri, P. W., and Marvin, J. A. The control of burn wound sepsis by the use of quantitative bacteriologic studies and subeschar clysis with antibiotics. *Surg. Clin. North Am.* 53:1509, 1975.

13. Baxter, C. R., Curreri, P. W., and Marvin, J. A. Fluid and electrolyte therapy of burn shock. *Heart Lung* 2:707, 1973.

14. Baxter, C. R., Marvin, J. A., and Curreri, P. W. Early management of thermal burns. *Postgrad. Med.* 55:131, 1974.

15. Boswick, J. The management of fresh burns of the hand and deformities resulting from burn injuries. *Clin. Plast. Surg.* 1:620, 1974.

16. Burke, J. F., Quinby, W. C., Bondoc, C. C., et al. Immunosuppression and temporary skin transplantation in the treatment of massive third degree burns. *Ann. Surg.* 182:183, 1975.

17. Curreri, P. W., Heck, E., Browne, L., et al. Stimulated nitroblue tetrazolium test to assess neutrophil antibacterial function: Prediction of wound sepsis in burn patients. *Surgery* 74:6, 1973.

18. Curreri, P. W., Rayfield, D. L., Vaught, M., et al. Extravascular fibrinogen degradation in experimental burn wounds: A source of fibrin split products. *Surgery* 77:86, 1975.

19. Curreri, P. W., Richmond, D., Marvin, J. A., et al. Di-

etary requirements of patients with major burns. *J. Am. Diet. Assoc.* 65:415, 1974.

20. Curreri, P. W., Wilmore, D., Mason, A., et al. Intracellular cation alterations following major trauma: Effect of supranormal caloric intake. *J. Trauma* 2:390, 1971.

21. Curreri, P. W., Wilterdink, M. E., and Baxter, C. R. Characterization of elevated fibrin split products following thermal injury. *Ann. Surg.* 181:157, 1975.

22. Czaja, A., McAlbany, J. C., and Pruitt, B. A., Jr. Acute gastroduodenal disease after thermal injury. *N. Engl. J. Med.* 291:925, 1974.

23. Daniels, J., Larson, D., Aleston, A., et al. Serum protein profiles in thermal burns. II: Protease, inhibitors, complement factors, and C-r protein. *J. Trauma* 14:153, 1974.

24. Davies, J. W. L. The Metabolism of Fibrinogen in Burn Patients. In A. B. Wallace and A. W. Wilkinson (eds.), *Research in Burns*. Edinburgh: Livingstone, 1966.

25. Davies, J. W. L., and Liljedahl, S. O. Metabolic Consequences of an Extensive Burn. In H. Polk and H. H. Stone (eds.), *Contemporary Burn Management*. Boston: Little, Brown, 1971. Pp. 151–169.

26. DiVincenti, F. C., Pruitt, B. A., Jr., and Reckler, J. M. Inhalation injuries. *J. Trauma* 2:109, 1971.

27. Gump, F., Martin, P., and Kinney, J. Oxygen consumption and caloric expenditure in surgical patients. *Surg. Gynecol. Obstet.* 134:489, 1973.

28. Howard, R. J., and Simmons, R. L. Acquired immunologic deficiencies after trauma and surgical procedures. *Surg. Gynecol. Obstet.* 139:771, 1974.

29. Hummel, R. P., Kautz, P. D., MacMillan, B. G., et al. The continuing problem of sepsis following enzymatic debridement of burns. *J. Trauma* 14:572, 1974.

30. Hunt, J. L., Agee, R. N., and Pruitt, B. A., Jr. Fiberoptic bronchoscopy in acute inhalation injury. *J. Trauma* 15:641, 1975.

31. Janzekovic, Z. A new concept in the early excision and immediate grafting of burns. *J. Trauma* 10:1103, 1970.

32. Janzekovic, Z. The burn wound from the surgical point of view. *J. Trauma* 15:42, 1975.

33. Jelenko, C., Jennings, W., O'Kelly, W., et al. Threshold burning effects in distant microcirculation. *Arch. Surg.* 102:617, 1971.

34. Koepke, G. H. The role of physical medicine in the treatment of burns. *Surg. Clin. North Am.* 50:1385, 1970.

35. Leape, L. Initial changes in burn tissue in burned and unburned skin of rhesus monkeys. *J. Trauma* 10:450, 1970.

36. Loebl, E. C., Baxter, C. R., and Curreri, P. W. The mechanism of erythrocyte destruction in the early post burn period. *Ann. Surg.* 178:681, 1975.

37. Loebl, E. C., et al. The use of quantitative biopsy cultures in bacteriologic monitoring of burn patients. *J. Surg. Res.* 16:1, 1974.

38. Lowenthal, R. M. Granulocyte transfusions in treatment of infections in patients with acute leukemia and aplastic anemia. *Lancet* 1:353, 1975.

39. MacMillan, B. C. Deep Excision and Early Grafting. In H. Polk and H. H. Stone (eds.), *Contemporary Burn Management*. Boston: Little, Brown, 1971. Pp. 357–365.

40. Marvin, J. A., Heck, E. L., Loebl, E. C., et al. Usefulness of blood cultures in confirming septic complications in burn patients: Evaluation of a new culture method. *J. Trauma* 15:657, 1975.

41. Mason, A. D., and Pruitt, B. A., Jr. Curling's Ulcer. In J. B. Lynch and S. R. Lewis (eds.), *Symposium on the Treatment of Burns*. St. Louis: Mosby, 1973. Pp. 79–81, vol. 5.

42. Mattsson, E. I. Psychological aspects of severe physical injury and its treatment. *J. Trauma* 15:217, 1975.

43. McAlhany, J. C., Czaja, A. J., and Pruitt, B. A., Jr. Antacid control of complications from acute gastroduodenal disease after burns. *J. Trauma* 16:645, 1976.

44. McCann, R. The oxyhemoglobin dissociation curve in acute disease. *Surg. Clin. North Am.* 55:637, 1975.

45. McDaniel, J. W. *Physical Disability and Human Behavior*. New York: Pergamon, 1969. P. 138.

46. Minshew, B., Holmes, R., Sanford, J., et al. Transferable resistance to tobramycin in *Klebsiella pneumoniae* and *Enterobacter cloacae* associated with enzymatic acetylation of tobramycin. *Antimicrob. Agents Chemother.* 6:492, 1974.

47. Monafo, W. W. The treatment of burn shock by the intravenous and oral administration of hypertonic lactated saline solution. *J. Trauma* 10:575, 1970.

48. Monafo, W. W., Tandon, S. N., Ayvazian, V. H., et al. Cerium nitrate: A new topical antiseptic for extensive burns. *Surgery* 80:465, 1976.

49. Moncrief, J. A. Burns of specific areas. *J. Trauma* 5:278, 1965.

50. Moncrief, J. A. Topical therapy. *Surg. Clin. North Am.* 50:1301, 1970.

51. Moncrief, J. A. Medical progress. *N. Engl. J. Med.* 288:444, 1973.

52. Moncrief, J. A. Burns. In T. Seymour and T. Schwartz (eds.), *Principles of Surgery*. New York: McGraw-Hill, 1974. Pp. 253–274.

53. Moncrief, J. A., Lindberg, R. B., Switzer, W. E., et al. Use of topical antibacterial therapy in the treatment of the burn wound. *Arch. Surg.* 92:558, 1966.

54. Moncrief, J. A., and Pruitt, B. A., Jr. The Massive Burn with Sepsis and Curling's Ulcer. In J. P. Hardy (ed.), *Critical Surgical Illness*. Philadelphia: Saunders, 1971.

55. Moritz, A. R., Henriques, F. C., and McLean, R. The effects of inhaled heat on the air passages and lungs: An experimental investigation. *Am. J. Pathol.* 21:311, 1945.

56. Moylan, J. A., Wellford, W. I., and Pruitt, B. A., Jr. Circulatory changes following circumferential extrem-

ity burns evaluated by the ultrasonic flow-meter: An analysis of 60 thermally injured limbs. *J. Trauma* 11:763, 1971.

57. Moylan, J., Wilmore, D., Mouton, D., et al. Early diagnosis of inhalation injury using [133]xenon lung scan. *Ann. Surg.* 176:477, 1972.

58. Munster, A. M., Eurenius, K., Katz, R. M., et al. Cell-mediated immunity after thermal injury. *Ann. Surg.* 177:139, 1973.

59. Order, S. E., Mason, A. D., Jr., Switzer, W. E., et al. Arterial vascular occlusion and devitalization of burn wounds. *Ann. Surg.* 161:502, 1965.

60. Proctor, H. J., Fry, J, and Lennon, D. Pharmacologic increases in erythrocyte 2,3-diphosphoglycerate for therapeutic benefit. *J. Trauma* 14:127, 1974.

61. Pruitt, B. A., Jr. Progressive pulmonary insufficiency and other pulmonary complications of thermal injury. *J. Trauma* 15:369, 1975.

62. Pruitt, B. A., Jr., and Curreri, P. W. The Use of Homograft and Heterograft Skin. In H. Polk and H. H. Stone (eds.), *Contemporary Burn Management.* Boston: Little, Brown, 1971. Pp. 397–418.

63. Pruitt, B. A., Jr., DiVincenti, F. C., Mason, A. D., Jr., et al. The occurrence and significance of pneumonia and other pulmonary complications in burned patients: Comparison of conventional and topical treatments. *J. Trauma* 10:519, 1970.

64. Pruitt, B. A., Jr., Foley, F. D., and Moncrief, J. A. Curling's ulcer: A clinical pathology study of 323 cases. *Ann. Surg.* 172:523, 1970.

65. Pruitt, B. A., Jr., and Moncrief, J. A. Current trends in burn research. *J. Surg. Res.* 7:280, 1967.

66. Shires, C. T., Carrico, C. J., Baxter, C. R., et al. Early Resuscitation of Patients with Burns. In C. Welch (ed.), *Advances in Surgery.* Chicago: Year Book, 1970. Vol. 4.

67. Shuck, J., Pruitt, B. A., Jr., and Moncrief, J. A. Homograft skin in wound coverage. *Arch. Surg.* 98:472, 1969.

68. Steiner, H., and Clark, W. Psychiatric complication of burned adults: A classification. *J. Trauma* 17:134, 1977.

69. Stone, H. H. Management of Respiratory Injury According to Clinical Phase. In H. Polk and H. H. Stone (eds.), *Contemporary Burn Management.* Boston: Little, Brown, 1971. Pp. 111–123.

70. Stone, H. H., Graber, C. D., and Martin, J. D. Evaluation of gamma globulin for prophylaxis against burn sepsis. *Surgery* 58:810, 1965.

71. Suter, P. M., Fairly, H. B., and Isenburg, M. D. Optimum end-expiratory airway pressure in patients with acute pulmonary failure. *N. Engl. J. Med.* 292:284, 1975.

72. Tanner, J. C., Vandeput, J., and Olley, J. F. The mesh skin graft. *Plast. Reconstr. Surg.* 34:287, 1964.

73. Teplitz, C., Davis, D., Mason, A. D., Jr., et al. *Pseudomonas* burn wound sepsis. I: Pathogenesis of experimental *Pseudomonas* burn wound sepsis. *J. Surg. Res.* 4:200, 1964.

74. Warden, G, Mason, A.D., Jr., and Pruitt, B. A., Jr. Evaluation of leukocyte chemotaxis in vitro in thermally injured patients. *J. Clin. Invest.* 54:1001, 1974.

75. Willis, B., Larson, D., and Abston, A. Positioning and splinting the burned patient. *Heart Lung* 2:696, 1973.

76. Wilmore, D. W. Energy Requirements of Seriously Burned Patients and the Influence of Caloric Intake on Their Metabolic Rate. In G. Cowan and W. Scheetz (eds.), *Intravenous Hyperalimentation.* Philadelphia: Lea & Febiger, 1972. Pp. 97–108.

77. Wilmore, D. W. Nutrition and metabolism following thermal injury. *Clin. Plast. Surg.* 1:603, 1974.

78. Wilmore, D. W., Aulick, L. H., Mason, A. D., and Pruitt, B. A., Jr. Influence of the burn wound on local and systemic responses to injury. *Ann. Surg.* 186:444, 1977.

79. Wilmore, D. W., Long, J. M., Mason, A. D., et al. Catecholamines: Mediator of the hypermetabolic response to thermal injury. *Ann. Surg.* 180:653, 1974.

80. Zawacki, B. E., Spitzer, K. W., Mason, A. P., et al. Does increased evaporative water loss cause hypermetabolism in burn patients? *Ann. Surg.* 171:236, 1970.

81. Zawacki, B. E., Jung, R. C., Joyce, J., et al. Smoke, burns and the natural history of inhalation injury in fire victims: A correlation of experimental and clinical data. *Ann. Surg.* 185:100, 1977.

82. Zikria, B. A., Budd, D. C., Flock, H. F., et al. What is chemical smoke poisoning? *Ann. Surg.* 181:151, 1975.

83. Zikria, B. A., Ferrer, J. M., and Flock, H. F. The chemical factors contributing to pulmonary damage in smoke poisoning. *Surgery* 71:704, 1971.

Multisystem Failure

Cornelia Vanderstaay Kenner

The complications seen in any critically ill patient may be multifaceted. The initial problem(s) itself is significant, and any complication imposed on the patient makes the patient's condition even more precarious. Every patient is liable to have complications, but the patient who has suffered multisystem trauma is one of the most likely to have complications.

Once one complication is present, there is an increased likelihood of having two or more complications. Sequential multisystem failure may be seen.

The nursing care administered must be expert. Only the most knowledgeable, skilled, and experienced nurses should care for patients who have complications. The time spent in the critical care unit is long, and it is physically and emotionally draining for the patient, his family, and the staff.

Objective

The nurse should be able to use the nursing process to coordinate and attend to the many aspects of care required by the patient who has complications.

Achieving the Objective

To achieve the objective, the nurse should be able to:

1. Assess and monitor the patient who has hypoxemia.

36

2. Taking into consideration the body's altered metabolic response, modify all nursing procedures to minimize stress and provide for adequate rest while maintaining the patient's mobility.

3. In consultation with the patient and other members of the health team, assess the patient's nutritional needs and develop an appropriate plan for meeting those needs. If parenteral nutritional therapy is added to the regimen, the nurse should use meticulous technique.

4. Adhere to a rigorous schedule to prevent gastrointestinal bleeding. If bleeding ensues, determine the nursing diagnosis and prepare for the various modes of therapy the physician might choose.

5. Utilize all principles of nursing care to prevent sepsis.

6. To prevent further deterioration of the septic patient's condition, pay close attention to "total-patient" support.

7. Describe the clinical syndrome of disseminated intravascular coagulation and write a plan of care for a patient who has that syndrome.

8. Monitor the physiological and psychological parameters in order to titrate therapy accurately.

How to Proceed

To develop an approach to the patient with multisystem failure, the nurse should:

1. Study the material that follows and read the articles listed in the references.

2. Engage in further educational endeavors by taking a course in critical care nursing.

3. Seek employment in a critical care unit that offers an orientation program and an extensive ongoing staff-development program.

4. In association with a clinical specialist, develop a series of educational goals and plan experiences to meet those goals by working with a nurse preceptor.

5. Administer patient care under supervision and slowly assume independence at an individual rate. Gain the necessary psychomotor skills. The nurse should not hesitate to ask questions and to ask for clarification.

6. Since each patient often needs two or even three nurses over an eight-hour period, clarify the division of duties with the primary care nurse and plan the patient's care with her so that the care is complete and not fragmented.

7. Always treat the patient and his family with dignity.

8. Participate in organizations that foster community educational programs. The nurse might join in safety campaigns as follows:
   a. Encourage safety advertising.
   b. Encourage the use of seat belts in motor vehicles.
   c. Write her congressmen about legislation requiring (1) that motor vehicles have air bags, safer front-end designs, and other safety features and (2) that highways be made safer by the use of innovations such as the placement of large cylinders at highway divisions.
   d. Identify high-risk groups of people, such as those who are suicidal or alcoholic, or those with repeated traffic violations; plan programs to increase their awareness.

Case Study

Mr. T. H., a 22-year-old carpenter, was admitted to the community hospital emergency room with multiple injuries. He had been hit by a car while he was riding his motorcycle. He was noted to be in profound shock and to have the following injuries: a bilateral pneumothorax, a lacerated spleen, a ruptured stomach, a fractured pelvis, an open fracture of the left tibia, and a fracture of the distal radius. Following placement of chest tubes, immediate surgical procedures were splenectomy, partial gastrectomy, and debridement of the open fracture. He was given 5 units of blood. He was started on carbenicillin (10 gm every 8 hours) and gentamicin (80 mg every 8 hours).

Subsequently, during the next 24 hours, Mr. H. remained hypotensive and his urinary output was less than 15 ml per hour. On his second postoperative day, he returned to the operating suite for a tracheotomy, and he was given 3 units of blood. His intravenous fluids were increased in an effort to increase his urinary output, but it remained minimal. He had no response to the administration of furosemide (120 mg). His blood urea nitrogen level rose to 138 mg/100 ml and his creatinine level rose to 5.3 mg/100 ml. On the second postoperative day, he had bleeding and massive swelling in his left pelvic area and, that evening, he had a tonic-clonic seizure. His total intake for the three days was 25,500 ml, and his total output was 3000 ml. On the fourth day, he was transferred by air ambulance to the regional trauma center.

Mr. H.'s wife and parents were very distressed during this period but they understood the explanations given them and they were able to make decisions. They described Mr. H. as an outgoing, active, sports-loving person who had never had any serious health problems.

On his arrival at the trauma center, Mr. H.'s vital signs

were T 99°F (rectally), P 120, R 16, and BP 120/70. He was maintained on the volume ventilator, his chest tubes were patent, and bloody mucus was obtained on suctioning. His arterial blood gas measurements on 40% FIO_2 were PO_2 159, pH 7.43, PCO_2 29, and delta base −11. His laboratory test results were hemoglobin 8 gm/100 ml, white blood count 20,000 per mm³, platelets 75,000 per mm³, prothrombin time 15 sec (control time was 12), partial thromboplastin time (PTT) 45 sec, fibrinogen 320 mg/100 ml, sodium 141 mEq/L, potassium 4.8 mEq/L, carbon dioxide combining power 24 mEq/L, chlorides 91 mEq/L, creatinine 5.4 mg/100 ml, blood urea nitrogen 152 mg/100 ml, and serum amylase more than 320 Somogyi units. His chest x ray showed bilateral lung infiltrates. His renal arteriogram showed normal arteries with a decreased flow ro the right renal superior pole and a delayed right renal vein flow. A cystogram and a retrograde pyelogram showed a moderate-sized bladder, no tears, and bloody urine from both orifices.

Mr. H.'s initial care included (1) the administration of three units of packed cells, one unit of fresh frozen plasma, vitamin K, prophylactic antacids, and parenteral nutrition, (2) the discontinuance of carbenicillin and gentamicin, and (3) the institution of monitoring parameters.

After the initial interval, the primary care nurse assessed Mr. H.'s immediate problems (see assessment sheet) and planned his nursing care. In collaboration with the clinical specialist (and as part of the in-depth nursing care plan), she requested consultations with the renal clinical specialist and nurse epidemiologist. A patient staffing conference was planned for the next morning with the other members of the team.

Clinical Presentation of Case Study

2/13 1:00 P.M.   Mr. H. remained on the volume ventilator at an 1100-ml tidal volume and a 1300-ml sigh. His arterial blood gas measurements on 40% FIO_2 were PO_2 88, pH 7.40, PCO_2 35, and delta base −2. His arterial oxygen tension on 100% O_2 was 450 mm/Hg. His chest x ray showed basilar infiltrates.

Neurologically, Mr. H. was confused and gave inconsistent responses to verbal commands. His pupils were equal and round, and they reacted to light and accommodation; his disks were flat with no papilledema. Full doll's eye movements were present. On his right side, Mr. H. exhibited continuous rhythmical seizure activity that seemed myoclonic. It was treated with intravenous dilantin (500 mg).

Mr. H. exhibited a small degree of bleeding from his tracheostomy site. His hemoglobin was 10.1 gm/100 ml, platelets 50,000 mm³, prothrombin time 15.5 sec (control time was 11.5 sec), PTT time 45 sec, and fibrinogen 300 mg/100 ml. His blood urea nitrogen

level rose to 180 mg/100 ml, and his creatinine level rose to 5.6 mg/100 ml. Platelet packs, fresh frozen plasma, and vitamin K were administered.

A Scribner shunt was placed in Mr. H.'s right leg with venous access through a right saphenous cutdown at midthigh. He underwent hemodialysis for three hours, and he was put on a dialysis schedule of every other day. His fluid intake was restricted to 10 ml per hour and his hyperalimentation fluids were decreased to 500 ml every 12 hours.

2:00 P.M.   Mr. H. responded to verbal commands; focal motor activity was absent in his left arm. His jaw and limb reflexes were + 3½; no posturing was present. Maintenance administration of intravenous dilantin was ordered (100 mg three times a day).

7:30 P.M.   He was placed on PEEP, 5 cm H_2O, for pulmonary edema.

2/14   T 100.8°F (rectally), P 128, R 10, BP 114/70. Mr. H.'s continuing fluid overload was shown by tachycardia (no murmurs or gallops). The following were noted: central venous pressure of 16 cm H_2O, basilar rales, basilar opacification on chest x ray, and pitting dependent edema.

His arterial blood gas measurements on 40% oxygen with a PEEP of 5 were PO_2 80, pH 7.37, and PCO_2 40. His lung compliance was 29. Digitalization was begun (0.5 mg at first and then 0.25 mg a day). The exact dosage was to be determined by his serial blood measurements.

His total volume was decreased to 1000 ml, his sigh decreased to 1200, and his respiratory rate decreased to 8. His electrolyte levels were: sodium 140 mEq/L, potassium 4.8 mEq/L, carbon dioxide 25 mEq/L, and chlorides 88 mEq/L. For several hours, his urinary output was 4 to 6 ml per hour.

Mr. H.'s coagulopathy was resolving. The oozing previously noted during dressing changes stopped but bloody mucus was still suctioned from the tracheostomy. His hematocrit was 37%, prothrombin time 12.5 sec (the control time was 11 sec) with 79.5% activity. Heparin administration was discontinued. The cause of the coagulopathy could not be determined because the parameters were nondiagnostic. The coagulopathy was thought to be secondary to trauma, a washout coagulopathy, and/or a carbenicillin platelet dysfunction.

Mr. H.'s left lower leg was markedly

Critical Care Nursing Admission Assessment
Major Systems Approach

PATIENT'S NAME: _Mr. J.H._ DATE: _2/13_ TIME: _12^N_

DIAGNOSIS: _multiple injuries 2° MVA $\bar{c}$_ _acute renal failure_ T: _99^R_ A.P.: _120_ R.P.: _120_ R.: _16_

B.P.: _120/70_ E.C.G. RHYTHM: _tachycardia_ ECTOPY: _−_ WT: _62 kg_ HT: _5'7"_

ADMITTED VIA: _air/ground ambul._ INFORMANT: _flight nurse + wife_ LAST MEAL: _−_

I. CHIEF COMPLAINT: _hit by car while riding motorcycle on 2/9_

II. PATIENT PROFILE:
1. Age _22_ 2. Sex _M_
3. Marital Status Ⓜ W D S
4. Race _W_ 5. Religion _Baptist_
6. Occupation _Carpenter_
7. Availability of Family _staying in family room_
8. Dietary _previously 3 well balanced meals/d._
9. Sleeping _8 hrs/night, usually 10pm – 6 am_
10. Activities of Daily Living _arose, showered, breakfasted and worked from 8-4³⁰. Dinner usually about 6³⁰. Attended church every Sunday + Wednesday night_

III. HISTORY OF PRESENT ILLNESS: _Thoracoabdominal injuries and fractures required surgery. Acute respiratory failure required tracheostomy on 2nd post-trauma day. Transferred $\bar{c}$ acute renal failure_

IV. PAST MEDICAL HISTORY:
1. Pediatric & Adult Illnesses _____
2. Cardiac _____
3. Hypertension _____
4. Respiratory _negative_
5. Diabetes Mellitus _____
6. Renal _____
7. Jaundice _____
8. Infections _____
9. Other _____
10. Hospitalizations & Surgeries _none_

11. Current Medication _none_

12. Allergies _NKA_

13. Habits _tobacco ½ pk/day occasional beer_

V. FAMILY HISTORY: _parents A&W no siblings_

VI. PSYCHOSOCIAL:
1. Behavior During Assessment _confused and not able to communicate_

2. Specific Problems _family having to make arrangements to live away from home_

VII. PHYSICAL EXAMINATION:
1. General _well-developed young man in previous good health $\bar{c}$ multiple injuries_ ABG: PO_2 _159_, pH _7.43_

2. Respiratory System pCO_2 _29_, Δ base _−11_
Airway _tracheotomy_
Inspection _bruise on ℞ chest. Bloody mucus on suctioning_
Rate _16_
Rhythm _on ventilator $\bar{c}$ F_1O_2 40%_
Chest Wall _chest tubes patent²_

Palpation _deferred_

Percussion _deferred_

Auscultation
Voice Sounds _____
Breath Sounds _____
Normal_____ Increased_____ Decreased ✓
Adventitious Sounds _____
_____ rales both bases _____

3. Cardiovascular System .
A.P. _120_ R.P. _120_
B.P. Supine R _120/70_ L _—_
P.M.I. _5th ICS___MCL_
Heart Sounds _Tachycardia_

Thrills _____none_____
Peripheral Pulses _____2+_____
4. Neurological System
Level of Consciousness _Confused c̄ inconsistent_
responses to verbal commands
Respiratory Pattern _on Ventilator_

Cranial Nerves _deferred_
_____
_____

Eyes _____
(1) Pupils   OD   OS
Size _____4mm_____ _4mm_
Shape _round_ _round_
Light _react_ _react_
Consensual _react_ _react_
Accommodation _react_ _react_
(2) Ocular Movements _full dolls eye_
present
Motor _on ®️ continuous_
rhythmical seizure activity
Sensory _____deferred_____
Coordination _____deferred_____

Reflexes _____3+_____

5. Gastrointestinal System
Nose & Mouth _Levine tube in place_
_____ pH >7 _____
Stomach_ no bleeding _

Abdomen _____deferred_____

Bowel Sounds _____present_____
Liver _____deferred_____
Spleen _____deferred_____

6. Renal & Genitourinary Systems
I._3000_ O. _500_
Urinary Bladder & Urethra _____
_____ deferred _____
Kidneys _____deferred_____

7. Musculoskeletal System
Spine _____no tenderness_____
Extremities _Fx Ⓛ tibia_
Fx ®️ distal radius

Sacral Edema _____none_____
Masses _____none_____
8. Hematologic System
Petechiae _____—_____
Ecchymosis _Ⓛ thigh, Ⓛ buttock_
Gingiva _oozing, bloody mucus_
on suctioning

9. Endocrine System
Breath _____—_____
Skin _____—_____
VIII. LABORATORY:
1. Hematology
HGB _8 gm %_ HCT _29%_
W.B.C. _20,000/cu.mm_ platelets 75k
2. Chemistry
Na _141_ K _4.8_
CO₂ _24_ CL _91_
Blood Sugar _120_ Amylase _>320_
BUN _152_ Cr _5.4_
3. Urinalysis _____to laboratory_____

4. Electrocardiogram
Rate _120_ Rhythm _NSR_
P-R _0.12_ QRS _0.05_ ST _0.08_
Interpretation _____tachycardia_____
5. Chest x-ray _bilateral lung infiltrates_

IX. PROBLEM LIST:
2/13   ACTIVE   INACTIVE
1. Incomplete data base | 6. ↓ platelets c̄ gingival
2. Bilateral pneumothorax 2° oozing
trauma ²⅓ chest tubes→Resp. 7. Impairment of skin
Failure ²⅓ Tracheostomy | integrity c̄ pre-existing
3. Lacerated spleen ruptured conditions for sepsis
liver ²⅓ Partial gastrectomy 8. Altered metabolism c̄
and splenectomy | nutritional deficit
4. multiple Gx: pelvis /®️ distal 9. Altered state of
radius + open fx. Ⓛ tibia consciousness
5. acute renal failure | 10. Impaired mobility
11. Total self-care deficit

NURSE'S SIGNATURE #4
Cornelia Kenner, RN, CCRN

855

swollen, and the anterior portion of the wound was necrotic. His distal pulses remained palpable. Two kinds of gram-negative rods were cultured from the site. His white blood count rose to 21,800/mm³, with a shift to the left. The wound was debrided and irrigated with hydrogen peroxide. Systemic antibiotics were given: intravenous tobramycin (80 mg) and aqueous penicillin (2.5 million units followed by 1 million units every 4 hours). His serum amylase level was greater than 640 units.

Mr. H. remained lethargic and responsive to verbal commands. His treatments were explained to him in simple terms, and he tried to help turn himself. His family remained at the hospital during the day and went to a nearby motel at night. During Mr. H.'s visits from his family, the nurse remained at his bedside.

2/15   T 101.8°F (rectally), P 120, R 8, BP 104/68. Mr. H. rested for short periods through the night; he was unable to rest for long periods.

On auscultation, a gallop and basilar rales were heard. Mr. H.'s arterial blood gas measurements were PO₂ 66, pH 7.38, PCO₂ 40.6, and delta base −1. On chest x ray, apical clearing was seen, but basilar infiltrates remained. Mr. H. remained on PEEP of 5 cm H_2O, and pancuronium (2–4 mg given by intravenous push) was ordered every hour as needed to treat respiratory agitation. Mr. H.'s chest tubes were removed.

For several hours, Mr. H.'s urinary output was 3 to 4 ml per hour. Hemodialysis to remove excess fluid and improve his pulmonary status was done daily. Mr. H.'s electrolyte levels were sodium 135 mEq/L, potassium 4.6 mEq/L, carbon dioxide 26.5 mEq/L, and chlorides 90 mEq/L; his fluid intake was 3955 ml and his output was 1668 ml.

The blood work showed a hemoglobin of 11.9 gm/100 ml, a hematocrit of 34.2%, and a white blood count of 22,300 mm³. His prothrombin time was 14.5 sec (the control time was 11.5 sec), and his PTT was 23 sec.

At the base of the wound over Mr. H.'s tibia, foul drainage and necrotic tissue were noted. The wound was debrided and irrigated.

Under Bier block anesthesia, a closed reduction of a Salter II fracture of Mr. H.'s distal radius was carried out. Postreduction films were made, and a splint was applied to Mr. H.'s right arm.

5:00 P.M.   Insertion of a Swan-Ganz catheter resulted

2/16   in a 25% left pneumothorax. A chest tube was inserted in the left anterior axillary line in the second intercostal space.

T 102.4°F, P 120, R 10, BP 124/80. On auscultation, a grade I holosystolic murmur that was similar to a pericardial rub and basilar rales were heard. Arterial blood gas measurement showed no further deterioration in Mr. H.'s condition. Infiltrates seen on the portable chest x ray were thought to be pneumonia. Mr. H. continued to respond to verbal commands, and no focal neurological signs were seen. His parenteral nutritional therapy was increased to 2000 ml per day.

2/17–2/18   T 102.6°, P 114, R 10, BP 102/64. Mr. H.'s respiratory status was maintained by the volume ventilator, respiratory paralysis, an FiO₂ of 50%, and a PEEP of 10 cm H_2O. Arterial blood gas measurements were PO₂ 76, pH 7.41, PCO₂ 25, and delta base −3. Mr. H.'s lung compliance curve was plotted from the following data.

Tidal Volume (ml)	Peak Airway Pressure (cm H_2O)	Static Pressure (cm H_2O)	Static Compliance
900	46	36	25
1000	53	43	23.26
800	40	30	26.7
700	36	27	25.9

Based on those data, a tidal volume of 800 ml was selected. Mr. H.'s pulmonary capillary wedge pressure was 6. On 2/17, his cardiac output was 4.4 liters per minute (Lpm) with a PEEP of 10 cm H_2O and 5.5 Lpm with no PEEP; and on 2/18 his cardiac output was measured at 9.6 Lpm. Mr. H. remained in the oliguric phase of acute renal failure, and he underwent dialysis on an every-other-day schedule. His platelet count fell to 17,500/mm³. His serum amylase level was higher than 800 units, and the results of an abdominal sonogram were negative.

2/19–2/20   Mr. H. remained lethargic; his exact level of consciousness was impossible to determine because of his metabolic status and the medications he was taking. His dilantin dosage was increased to 400 mg per day because the neurosurgeon noted that his dilantin levels were 2 to 3 μg/ml (therapeutic levels are 10 to 20 μg/ml).

Mr. H.'s sputum culture was positive for a gram-negative bacillus, and his white blood cell count increased to 25,000/mm^3. His arterial oxygen was 83, and his arteriovenous (A-V) oxygen difference was 3.22. A chest x ray showed that a small pneumothorax persisted. Mr. H.'s primary care physician consulted with members of the departments of infectious disease and pulmonary medicine. His sputum, urine, and blood were recultured, and they were specifically labeled for *Candida*. Mr. H. was given methicillin (6 gm daily) and tobramycin (1.5 mg/kg) after every dialysis. His urinary output approached 200 ml for a 24-hour period.

2/21–2/22   Mr. H.'s urine and sputum cultures were reported positive for *Pseudomonas*, which was sensitive to tobramycin. Following peritoneal lavage, the fluid obtained was blood tinged, straw colored, and not odorous. The laboratory analysis was as follows: serum amylase level 377, white blood cell count 27,000/mm^3, lymphocytes 24%, polymorphonucleocytes 71%, and red blood cell count 10,800/mm^3. Since his serum glucose levels remained at 300 to 400 mg/100 ml despite increased amounts of insulin, his hyperalimentation fluids were decreased to 2000 ml per day. His platelet count increased to 43,000/mm^3.

2/23–2/24   Weight: 60.5 kg. Mr. H.'s family was acutely aware of his physiological and psychological traumas, and they sought ways to function within the stressful situation. They assessed their own family situation, and they established priorities. A schedule was made so that a family member would always be at the hospital, except during their sleeping hours. The time away from the hospital was used to run errands and to take care of important business. They were careful to eat well and otherwise take care of themselves so that they would not become ill.

Mr. H. remained on the ventilator. On a PEEP of 10 cm H_2O and an FiO_2 of 50%, his arterial gas measurements were PO_2 73, pH 7.33, PCO_2 37, and delta base −6, and his mixed venous blood gas measurements were PO_2 46, pH 7.30, PCO_2 41, and delta base −6. His pulmonary capillary wedge pressure was 8 to 9, and his cardiac output was 6 to 8 Lpm. His electrolyte levels were sodium 135 mEq/L, potassium 4.3 mEq/L, carbon dioxide 21 mEq/L, and chlorides 90 mEq/L, with an anion gap of 24.

Mr. H. was found to have suppurative

thrombophlebitis in his right saphenous vein. On sonography, a sonolucent fluid collection was noted in the right upper quadrant; it measured 8 × 5 cm.

2/24–2/25   Abdominal surgery was performed because Mr. H. showed further signs of infection (a white blood cell count of 30,000 to 40,000/mm^3 and a KUB film suggestive of an intraabdominal infection). He was found to have pancreatitis with soaparification of the lesser sac and tail of the pancreas and an abscess around the tail of the pancreas. Mr. H.'s pancreas was drained to the left upper quadrant with six one-inch drains, and a jejunostomy tube was placed. Mr. H.'s highest temperature after surgery was 99°F.

The following day Mr. H.'s arterial blood gas measurements were PO_2 68, pH 7.36, and PCO_2 40. His carbon dioxide retention was attributed to the severity of acute respiratory distress syndrome and a marked increase in physiologic dead space. Mr. H.'s lung compliance curve was plotted from the following data.

Tidal Volume	Static Pressure
600 ml	42 cm H_2O
800 ml	50 cm H_2O
1000 ml	58 cm H_2O
1100 ml	70 cm H_2O

Since optimal pulmonary management was then considered to be the tidal volume at the peak of the compliance curve with a rapid rate, Mr. H.'s optimal tidal volume was 1000 ml. The physician left an order that he could have a lower tidal volume with a faster rate if his PCO_2 became difficult to control.

2/26–2/27   Positive pressure ventilation was continued, with arterial blood gas measurements of PO_2 63, pH 7.30, PCO_2 41.8, and mixed venous blood gas measurements of PO_2 35, pH 7.26, and PCO_2 50.4. Amber fluid drained through the chest catheter. The examination of the chest x ray by the radiologist indicated that the subclavian catheter was probably in the chest. The catheter was replaced by a new central line.

Mr. H.'s bacteriologic cultures were negative for gram-positive organisms, but his sputum cultures were positive for *Pseudomonas aeruginosa*, and his urine cultures were positive for *Enterobacter cloacae*.

Colistin (1.5 mg/kg) (after dialysis) was ordered because the *Enterobacter* was sensitive to tobramycin only at a dosage of 16 units per milliliter, but it was sensitive to colistin and amikacin at 8 units per milliliter. On the recommendation of the nurse epidemiologist, isolation procedures were instituted.

2/28–3/1   T 103.4°F, P 130, R 8, BP 100/70. Mr. H. demonstrated increasing response to verbal commands and limited spontaneous response on the left side. His urinary output was measured at 375 to 400 ml over a 24-hour period. His creatinine level was 3.8 mg/100 ml, but his blood urea nitrogen level remained markedly elevated, reflecting his marked catabolic state. Because of the acute respiratory distress syndrome, the intravenous administration of fluid was not increased, and a wedge pressure of 7 was maintained. Even though recovery from acute renal failure was slowed by limited fluid administration, no lasting deleterious effect on Mr. H.'s renal functioning was anticipated. An increased anion gap secondary to renal failure and parenteral nutritional therapy was treated with sodium bicarbonate. The hemodialysis was complicated by mild hypertension, but the hypertension was successfully treated with salt-poor human albumin, blood, and saline.

3/2–3/3   The FIO_2 was decreased to 40% without deterioration of the arterial blood gases. Wound cultures from the right tibia showed *Enterobacter*, and the colistin dosage was increased.

3/4–3/7   Temperatures of 102°F to 103°F continued. Mr. H.'s cardiac output was measured at 14.5 Lpm, and his arterial venous oxygen difference was 3.1 to 5.2. His urine cultures were sterile, but *Pseudomonas* continued to be reported from the sputum cultures. The tobramycin therapy was discontinued.

3/8–3/11   Mr. H.'s daily urinary output increased to 500 to 700 ml, with a minimal response to the furosemide challenge. The nephrologist assessed that Mr. H. was slowly entering the diuretic phase, and he decided to continue hemodialysis on an every-other-day basis as long as the predialysis blood urea nitrogen level was greater than 100 or the urinary output was less than two liters per day.

Yellow serous drainage from the tibial wound was noted. Areas of new granulation tissue were present. Colistin therapy was discontinued, and amikacin therapy was begun. (In renal insufficiency, the recommended dosage of amikacin after dialysis is 7.5 mg/kg. For the patient who is off dialysis, the recommended dosage is 7.5 mg/kg at intervals calculated by multiplying the serum creatinine level by every 9 hours.)

3/12–3/15   The PEEP was lowered to 3 cm H_2O, and the arterial oxygen tension remained above 80. The caloric intake utilizing both jejunostomy feedings and parenteral therapy was estimated to be 3500 to 3750 calories per day. Hemodialysis was discontinued.

3/15–3/18   Following extensive debridement of the tibial wound, Mr. H.'s temperature spiked to 104.5°F, he had a rash over most of his body, and his serum potassium level rose to above 6 mEq/L. Kayexalate was used to lower the serum potassium level, and a new Scribner shunt was placed. A fungus thought to be *Mucor* was isolated from the tibial wound. Antibiotics and parenteral therapy were discontinued, and intravenous catheters were replaced. Amphotericin therapy was considered but not begun.

Mr. H. became abusive and seemed to be psychotic. Since the staff was unable to protect him from himself, restraints were applied.

3/19–3/22   The fungemia was resolved clinically; the culture reports pointed to *Candida* rather than *Mucor*. Mr. H. had severe diarrhea, which was thought to be secondary to the use of Kayexalate and sorbitol. His volume depletion was particularly apparent from a tachycardia of 180. Normal saline solution was administered at a rate of 50 ml per hour, and paregoric was begun.

Mr. H.'s respiratory rate decreased to 15, and his FIO_2 was decreased to 40%. His arterial blood gas measurements on 40% oxygen were PO_2 80, pH 7.37, PCO_2 33.5; on 100% oxygen, they were PO_2 375, pH 7.35, and PCO_2 37.

Mr. H. slept for only short periods during the night and took infrequent naps during the day. He cried easily (he felt best during his visits with his family). He had no memories of his early stay in the critical care unit.

3/23–3/26   Mr. H.'s respiratory status continued to improve, and intermittent mandatory ventilation was started. Jejunostomy feedings were begun again, and they were slowly increased. At rest, Mr. H. maintained a position of medial and ulnar denervation, and so a volar positioning splint was applied.

3/27–3/30 Mr. H. felt better day by day, and he slept for long periods during the night. He asked few questions; he seemed to understand the explanations given. His family rearranged their schedules to give them more time away from the hospital so that they could attend to family affairs.

After dialysis, Mr. H.'s blood urea nitrogen level was 24 and his creatinine level was 1.6. Although his blood cultures remained negative, multiple cultures revealed many sites of sepsis. Sputum reports indicated a light growth of *Providentia stuartii* and a heavy growth of *Pseudomonas aeruginosa*, both of which were sensitive to tobramycin. The urinalyses indicated the presence of *Enterococcus* and yeast. The wound cultures from the jejunostomy site indicated the presence of *Bacteroides*, and the cultures from the tibia indicated the presence of *Serratia marcescens*.

Mr. H.'s lung compliance increased slowly. The dead space volume was determined from a Douglas bag collection of expired gas using a Searle respirator and 35% oxygen. The dead space volume was 46.7%—two standard deviations from normal.

A dorsiflexion positioning splint was made for Mr. H.'s left lower leg to relieve pressure on his calcaneus.

3/31–4/6 Mr. H. continued to feel better each day, and he became more and more involved in his care. His family visited him for longer periods, and they offered help to the families of other patients.

The process of weaning Mr. H. from the respirator was begun. His caloric intake was 3000 to 4000; the calories came mainly from feedings. Blood culture reports were positive for *Enterococcus*, which was sensitive to ampicillin and tobramycin.

4/7–4/13 Arterial blood gas values measured by the T-bar were PO_2 88, pH 7.28, and PCO_2 28. The blood, sputum, and urine cultures remained positive.

4/14–4/30 Before Mr. H.'s transfer to the general unit, many of the staff came to the unit to meet him. His primary care nurse conducted nursing rounds and outlined the plan of care. His respiratory condition stabilized, and his cultures were negative.

Mr. H. went to the physical therapy department daily, and his strength gradually increased. He began to eat well, and he gained weight. Final discharge planning was done by the health team at a staff conference. Since both patient and family education had been an important part of nursing care during his stay in the critical care unit, Mr. H. and his family were well informed and understood much of his rehabilitative care. Mr. H. returned home feeling very fortunate and knowing that he had to make outpatient follow-up visits often and over a long period of time.

Reflections

Many factors affect the consciousness of the patient who has sustained system failure. Changes in his thoughts and feelings are part of the trauma. The mind as well as the body is affected: to traumatize the body is to traumatize the mind (Fig. 36-1).

A person cannot be bombarded with stimuli for long periods of time and maintain his functional integrity. The person may become overwhelmingly tired and irritable. Seemingly minor incidents or aspects of care may seem to him insurmountable problems. His hopelessness may be complete.

Etiology

The critically ill patient may have many complications. Any organ system affected may exhibit significant alterations and in turn, other organ systems may be affected. The complications discussed in this chapter are hypoxemia, fat embolism, the body's metabolic response to injury, acute gastroduodenal stress ulceration, disseminated intravascular coagulation, and sepsis and septic shock. (The adult respiratory distress syndrome is discussed in Chapter 17, and acute renal failure is discussed in Chapter 32.)

Hypoxemia

Arterial hypoxemia is a decrease in the total arterial oxygen content of the blood. A lowered arterial oxygen results in tissue hypoxia. Since all four mechanisms of hypoxemia (hypoventilation, diffusion defects, ventilation-perfusion imbalance, and left to right shunting) involve a ventilation-perfusion imbalance, a discussion of alveolar ventilation and

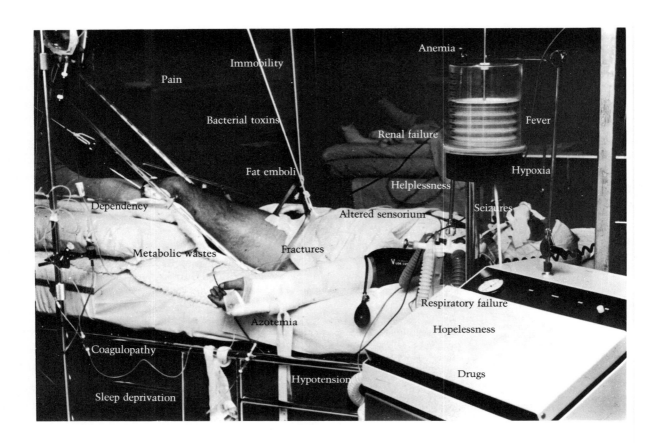

Pain
Immobility
Anemia
Bacterial toxins
Fever
Renal failure
Fat emboli
Hypoxia
Helplessness
Dependency
Altered sensorium
Seizures
Metabolic wastes
Fractures
Azotemia
Respiratory failure
Hopelessness
Coagulopathy
Hypotension
Drugs
Sleep deprivation

oxygenation must precede the discussion of the mechanisms.

Figure 36-1

Multiple stresses encountered by the patient. (Photographer—Brian Anderson)

Ventilation

The amount of inspired air that reaches perfused alveoli is referred to as the alveolar ventilation. The inspired volume that does not go to perfused alveoli is referred to as the dead space ventilation. In regard to only a single breath, the dead space volume (V_D) is subtracted from the tidal volume (TV) to give the alveolar ventilation (V_A).

$$V_A = TV - V_D$$

The minute ventilation is the total amount of gas exhaled by the patient per minute; it is the sum of the dead space ventilation and the alveolar ventilation. Use of the minute volume and the alveolar ventila-

tion is particularly helpful in determining the dead space ventilation for patients who are on respirators. The following calculations are frequently done:

$$\text{Alveolar ventilation} = \left(\frac{\substack{\text{carbon dioxide tension} \\ \text{in venous blood to} \\ \text{determine carbon} \\ \text{dioxide production}}}{\substack{\text{carbon dioxide tension} \\ \text{in arterial blood}}}\right) 0.863$$

A more accurate method of determining alveolar ventilation consists of collecting air samples of expired air and measuring the percentage of carbon dioxide and oxygen in the expired air. The following formula is used:

$$V_A = \frac{(VCO_2)(0.863)}{(PaCO_2)}$$

Dead space ventilation/min = minute ventilation
$\qquad\qquad\qquad\qquad\qquad$ − alveolar ventilation/min

Dead space per breath = $\dfrac{\text{dead space ventilation}}{\text{respiratory rate}}$/min

When the air taken in during inspiration arrives in the alveoli, gas exchange takes place. Oxygen diffuses into the pulmonary capillary bed, and carbon dioxide diffuses into the alveolus. The exchange is effected by pressure differences. As carbon dioxide enters the alveolus, oxygen leaves the alveolus. Carbon dioxide is not present in the inspired air. Thus it does not exert any pressure and it diffuses 20 times as fast as oxygen does. After gas exchange has taken place in the alveolus, the pressure of the oxygen and the pressure of the carbon dioxide are equal to the pressure that was exerted by the oxygen alone.

The partial pressure of a gas is determined by multiplying the total pressure times the concentration of gas. For example, at sea level the barometric pressure is 760 mm Hg, and the concentration of oxygen in the air is 0.21. Thus the pressure of oxygen in the air is 160 mm Hg. Two important phenomena must be mentioned. First, air contains water vapor. The pressure exerted by water vapor is used as the standard measurement 47 mm Hg. Second, since barometric pressure is different in different parts of the United States, the local standard pressure must be used. For example, if the barometric pressure is 747 mm Hg, then the pressure of oxygen in the air is (747−47) (0.21), or 147 mm Hg.

The respiratory quotient must also be understood. Since there is essentially no carbon dioxide in the inspired air, the amount of carbon dioxide leaving the body is usually less than the amount of oxygen consumed. The relationship of oxygen consumption divided by carbon dioxide production is commonly expressed as a decimal. The value varies: 0.8 is the average value. The alveolar air equation is as follows:

$$
\begin{pmatrix}\text{Alveolar}\\\text{oxygen}\\\text{pressure}\end{pmatrix} = \begin{pmatrix}\text{barometric}\\\text{pressure} -\\\text{water vapor}\\\text{pressure}\end{pmatrix}\begin{pmatrix}\text{inspired}\\\text{oxygen}\\\text{concen-}\\\text{tration}\end{pmatrix} - \begin{pmatrix}\dfrac{\begin{array}{c}\text{arterial}\\\text{plasma}\\\text{pressure}\\\text{of carbon}\\\text{dioxide}\end{array}}{\begin{array}{c}\text{respiratory}\\\text{quotient}\end{array}}\end{pmatrix}
$$

Under normal circumstances, the mean alveolar oxygen pressure is higher than the peripheral arterial oxygen pressure. The reasons are that fully oxygenated blood from well-ventilated alveoli mixes with less-well-oxygenated blood from poorly ventilated alveoli, and that a small amount of venous blood mixes with arterial blood from direct communications between the pulmonary artery and pulmonary vein and from the thebesian veins draining into the left heart. The difference between the mean alveolar oxygen pressure and the arterial oxygen pressure is referred to as the alveolar-arterial oxygen gradient (the A-a gradient, or difference). Approximately 3% to 6% of the normal cardiac output may bypass ventilated lung. Normally, the A-a gradient is 15 mm Hg or less on room air and 50 mm Hg or less on air that has high percentages of oxygen [54]. To calculate the A-a gradient, the alveolar oxygen pressure is determined (using the alveolar air equation) and the arterial oxygen pressure is subtracted from the alveolar oxygen pressure.

Example

The patient is in Dallas, Texas, breathing room air (0.21). His arterial oxygen partial pressure is 90 mm Hg and arterial carbon dioxide pressure is 40 mm Hg.

$$
\begin{aligned}
\text{Alveolar oxygen pressure} &= (747 - 47)(0.21) - \frac{40}{0.8}\\
&= 147 - 50\\
&= 97 \text{ mm Hg}
\end{aligned}
$$

$$
\begin{aligned}
\text{A-a oxygen gradient} &= \begin{pmatrix}\text{alveolar}\\\text{oxygen}\\\text{pressure}\end{pmatrix} - \begin{pmatrix}\text{arterial}\\\text{oxygen}\\\text{pressure}\end{pmatrix}\\
&= 97 - 90\\
&= 7 \text{ mm Hg}
\end{aligned}
$$

Oxygenation

Determination of the adequacy of tissue oxygenation is an important part of assessment. The normal oxygen uptake and the normal carbon dioxide elimination are maintained by the ventilation-perfusion balance. The transportation of oxygen from the alveolus to the peripheral tissues depends on many factors: the oxygen concentration, the partial pressure oxygen in the inspired air, the alveolar ventilation, the ventilation-perfusion relationship, the blood volume, the cardiac output, and the hemoglobin saturation.

Blood carries oxygen in two states: (1) physically dissolved in plasma and (2) chemically combined with hemoglobin. The number of milliliters of oxygen per 100 ml of blood can be calculated if the PaO_2, percent of saturation, and hemoglobin are known. Knowing the number of milliliters of oxygen per 100 ml of blood allows a more accurate determination to be made of the adequacy of oxygenation than is afforded by the PaO_2 and percent of saturation alone. The number of milliliters of oxygen contributed by oxygen that is physically dissolved in the blood is a small portion of the total. The major part of the total oxygen content is combined with hemoglobin. The number of milliliters contributed by dissolved oxygen is calculated by multiplying the PaO_2 by 0.003 ml/mm Hg. The number of milliliters contributed by oxygen that is combined with hemoglobin is calculated by multiplying the hemoglobin concentration by the percent of saturation by 1.39 ml/% saturation. For example, assume that a patient has the following values: hemoglobin 15, PaO_2 90, percent saturation 96. The total content would be 20.30 ml/100 ml blood, with 0.27 ml/100 ml contributed by dissolved oxygen and 20.03 ml/100 ml blood contributed by oxygen that is bound to hemoglobin.

When the data are plotted on a graph, the relationship between the amount of oxygen combined with hemoglobin and the amount of oxygen dissolved in the arterial system is not shown to be a linear (or a straight-line) relationship. Rather the relationship between arterial oxygen and percent saturation is depicted by an S-curve. (That curve, which is called the oxygen dissociation curve, is shown in Fig. 17-7.) A change in the position of the curve to the right or left reflects the affinity of hemoglobin for oxygen and the transfer of oxygen from the hemoglobin to tissue cells.

Study of the graph verifies several important points. It should be noted first that at an oxygenation of 100 mm Hg, hemoglobin is 97.5% saturated. Since the hemoglobin is almost saturated, it can accept little more oxygen. Even if the arterial oxygen pressure is raised above 100 mm Hg, the total oxygen content increases only slightly since oxygen may only be added to the blood in the form of dissolved oxygen. Since the oxygen-carrying capacity of the blood is virtually dependent on the amount of hemoglobin present and on the percent saturation, maintenance of the hemoglobin levels is essential for adequate oxygenation.

It should next be noted that the curve is relatively flat between 70 and 100 mm Hg. At 70 mm Hg, the hemoglobin is 93% saturated, which means that even a severe drop in arterial oxygen pressure (say to 70 mm Hg) produces only a minimal change in the oxy-

gen content of the blood because the hemoglobin saturation, the major determinant of the oxygen content, changes by only a small amount. However, below 60 to 70 mm Hg, the downward slope of the S-shaped curve is encountered. In that part of the curve, small changes in dissolved oxygen produce large changes in the percent saturation and total content. The curve is particularly steep between 10 and 40 mm Hg. Since small changes in arterial oxygen tension cause large changes in percent saturation in that part of the curve, one can produce large changes in total content simply by increasing the arterial oxygen level a small amount. In other words, because of the chemical characteristics of arterial oxygen and hemoglobin, values of arterial oxygen tension below 60 mm Hg produce a rapid decrease in the amount of hemoglobin saturated and the total oxygen content—and thus in the total tissue delivery.

The oxyhemoglobin dissociation curve is not a single curve but a series of curves. The shape of the curve changes with the hydrogen ion concentration, the partial pressure of arterial carbon dioxide, the temperature, 2,3-diphosphoglycerate (DPG) and the electrolyte levels. The effect the carbon dioxide tension and the hydrogen ion concentration have on the affinity of oxygen for hemoglobin is called the Bohr effect. An increase in any of the parameters just mentioned produces the release of oxygen by hemoglobin at a lower PaO_2. In other words, acidosis or an increased level of 2,3-DPG causes the dissociation curve to shift to the right. With a shift to the right, the hemoglobin binds oxygen less avidly, and the amount of oxygen given up to the tissues is increased.

The opposite is true for *decreases* in the hydrogen ion concentration, the arterial carbon dioxide tension, the 2,3 DPG level, the temperature, and the electrolyte levels. With decreases, the curve is shifted to the left. At a given level of arterial oxygen tension, the percentage of oxyhemoglobin is greater and less oxygen is given up to the tissues. Clinically, the patient's tissues may be oxygen deprived because the affinity of oxygen for hemoglobin is greater, and the amount of oxygen released is reduced.

P_{50}

Assessment of the many influences on the position of the oxyhemoglobin dissociation curves is difficult because the means of measurement are still being developed. The most important question is the effect at the level of the peripheral capillary. There is no clinically applicable method of directly assessing the adequacy of tissue oxygenation. The net effect of the many factors that may affect the oxyhemoglobin curve can be assessed using the P_{50}. The P_{50} is the partial pressure of arterial oxygen at which 50 percent of the available hemoglobin is saturated.

Two means of determining the P_{50} are commonly used:

1. Several blood gas calculators have been modified to determine the P_{50} value from the measured oxygen tension and saturation using a sample of venous blood. Corrections are included for any deviations in pH, base excess, or temperature.
2. Canizaro and his associates [55] have developed a nomogram for estimating the P_{50} from the oxygen tension and saturation of a sample of venous blood. Accurate measurement of the sample is essential, because a small error would cause a large error in the derived P_{50} value. Ideally, for determination of the P_{50}, the oxygen saturation in the venous blood sample should be between 40% and 75%.

OXYGEN DELIVERY

The amount of oxygen being delivered to the tissues is the important factor. Oxygen delivery is equal to the cardiac output multiplied by the oxygen content expressed in volumes per 100 ml. The A-V oxygen difference (the $C[a\text{-}v]O_2$) is the arterial oxygen content minus the venous oxygen content. Since the arteriovenous oxygen content difference increases in low cardiac output states, it can be used to assess changes in cardiac output at times when therapy is being titrated (e.g., initiation or increase of respiratory support). A problem in oxygen delivery (or cardiac output) is determined by an increasing or widening difference and thus alerts one to decrease respiratory intervention and to increase circulation. The actual oxygen extraction may be determined by multiplying the A-V oxygen difference by the cardiac output. Since the advent of the Swan-Ganz catheter and the availability of mixed venous blood samples, that measurement can be determined accurately.

The oxygen extraction ratio or the utilization coefficient $(CaO_2 - C\bar{v}O_2 / CaO_2)$ defines the amount of delivered oxygen that is used (normal value approximates 0.25). If the ratio is high, the need for oxygen is greater than that available; thus the oxygen delivery is inadequate. If the ratio is low, the delivery is mal-distributed (e.g., suprahigh cardiac output or shunting).

Mechanisms of Hypoxemia

The degrees of severity of hypoxemia are classically described in terms of arterial desaturation when the patient is breathing room air (0.21). In mild hypoxemia, the arterial oxygen is less than 75 mm Hg and more than 60 mm Hg. In moderate hypoxemia, the arterial oxygen is less than 60 mm Hg and more than 40 mm Hg. In severe hypoxemia, arterial oxygen is less than 40 mm Hg.

The four mechanisms of hypoxemia are discussed in the following pages. They are hypoventilation, diffusion defects, ventilation-perfusion imbalances, and shunting.

HYPOVENTILATION

In hypoventilation, the arterial carbon dioxide levels are always elevated because the lungs cannot maintain an alveolar ventilation that will eliminate the carbon dioxide produced by the body. The nitrogen equilibrium is not altered, and, as the alveolar carbon dioxide level rises, the alveolar oxygen level falls. A review of the alveolar air equation shows that an increase in the carbon dioxide levels will make the number to be subtracted a larger pressure and the resulting alveolar oxygen pressure smaller. If no other mechanism of hypoxemia is present, the A-a gradient will remain within normal limits at any fractional concentration of inspired oxygen.

If the patient does not have a respiratory disorder, the hypoventilation itself is corrected by his breathing normal volumes of room air. For example, if the patient's tidal volume has decreased because of an overdose of analgesics, his effective alveolar ventilation has decreased and produced the syndrome.

If the patient has a respiratory disorder and a defect in alveolar oxygenation from hypoventilation, a small increase in the oxygen concentration in the inspired gas will increase the oxygen pressure in the alveolus. If oxygen is administered via a nasal cannula at 3 liters per minute, the oxygen is increased from about 21% (150 mm Hg) to 28% (200 mm Hg). Because of the corresponding increase, the alveolar oxygen tension increases by 50 mm Hg.

Frequently the decision must be made about discontinuing oxygen when the patient has respiratory failure and when hypoventilation is the only mechanism of hypoxemia present. The anticipated alveolar oxygen pressure may be predicted by using the patient's values for arterial carbon dioxide tension and the concentration of oxygen for room air in the alveolar air equation.

DIFFUSION DEFECTS

The overall diffusion capacity involves physical diffusion through the alveolar pulmonary capillary membrane and capillary plasma and diffusion within the red blood cell. The discussion here is limited to diffusion through the alveolar pulmonary capillary membrane. The diffusion pathway includes the layer of pulmonary surfactant, the alveolar epithelium, the alveolar basement membrane, the interstitial fluid, and the pulmonary capillary endothelium. The rate of diffusion is dependent on the pressure gradient, the thickness of membrane, the surface area available for diffusion, the membrane permeability characteristics, and the gas diffusion characteristics.

The best measure of the diffusion process is the diffusion capacity, the total amount of gas transferred per minute across the alveolar membrane per millimeter difference in the pressure of the gas on the two sides of the membrane. In regard to the noncritically ill patient, a technician from the pulmonary function laboratory determines the diffusion capacity for carbon monoxide and using that measurement, calculates the values for oxygen (normal is 20–30 ml carbon monoxide/min/mm Hg). In the critically ill patient, determination is made using the clinical and laboratory findings. Clinically the patient has symptoms that are consistent with alveolar capillary block. Other mechanisms of hypoxemia are usually present. If only a diffusion defect is present, the arterial carbon dioxide levels are below 40 mm Hg and the A-a oxygen gradient at rest is 15 to 20 mm Hg. Any conditions that produce an increased cardiac output produce an increased A-a oxygen gradient. In the critical care situation, diffusion defects have minimal clinical relevance since they cannot be defined at the bedside and differentiated from ventilation-perfusion imbalances and shunts unless the diffusion defect is enormous; that is, most of the lung is destroyed.

Alveolar pulmonary capillary block is associated with thickening of the diffusion pathway. Diffusion defects are seen in patients who have diffuse pulmonary fibrosis or increased edema. The defect is not seen in the resting condition until the disease process is advanced. It results from a block to the entrance of oxygen into the blood through the alveolar capillary diffusion pathway. For example, in a patient who has pulmonary edema, the thickened pulmonary capillary membrane interferes with oxygen diffusion across the membrane. That is true even with adequate alveolar ventilation. As the pulmonary edema worsens, fluid in the alveolus increases and the presence of either a film or a bubbling fluid interferes with oxygen diffusion.

VENTILATION-PERFUSION IMBALANCE

An imbalance or a mismatch in the ventilation-perfusion ratio is the most common mechanism of arterial hypoxemia. In the usual clinical situation, the extent of arterial desaturation due to hypoventilation and shunt is determined, and all otherwise unexplained hypoxemia is attributed to an uneven distribution of the lung functioning. Actually all the mechanisms are alterations of the ventilation-perfusion ratio, but they are not so categorized.

Under normal circumstances, the pattern of air ventilation does not follow the pattern of blood perfusion in all regions of the lung. For example, the volume of air ventilating the lung apices is less than that ventilating the other lung regions. The amount of blood perfusing the apices is comparatively small. On the other hand, the amount of blood perfusing the apices is even less than the amount of air ventilating the apices. A different condition is found in the lung bases. There proportionally more blood is perfused than air is ventilated.

Because of gravity, changes in position produce changes in ventilation and perfusion. For example, in dependent lung areas, blood flow per unit volume increases more rapidly than does ventilation. Since the changes are not uniform, a multitude of inequalities are produced.

There are four possible ventilation-perfusion combinations in scattered groups of alveoli: (1) well-ventilated and well-perfused alveoli, (2) poorly ventilated and well-perfused alveoli, (3) well-ventilated and poorly perfused alveoli, and (4) poorly ventilated and poorly perfused alveoli. In the poorly ventilated, well-perfused alveolus, the alveolar hypoxia produces vasoconstriction. For example, in atelectasis, because the alveolar oxygen pressure is decreased in the unventilated portion, the blood flow (perfusion) is redistributed to the parts of the lung that are better ventilated. In the well-ventilated, poorly perfused alveolus, gas exchange cannot take place and the physiologic dead space is increased.

The best measure of a ventilation-perfusion imbalance is a large or a widened A-a oxygen gradient on room air at rest that is corrected when high concentrations of oxygen are given. The hypoxemia is relieved by breathing oxygen. In patients who have chronic obstructive lung disease, ventilation-perfusion imbalance is the most common reason for hypoxemia. Unless the lung disease is complicated by pneumonia or atelectasis, the hypoxemia is corrected by making small increases in inspired oxygen.

RIGHT-TO-LEFT SHUNT

Hypoxemia (a fall in arterial saturation) results when venous blood that has not come in contact with ventilated lung mixes with arterial blood that has come in contact with ventilated lung. The phenomenon is referred to as a right-to-left shunt or a venous admixture. As previously discussed, a certain degree of mixing normally occurs. The expected shunting in patients who have chronic obstructive lung disease is slightly increased. It is 6% to 12% of the cardiac output. Abnormal mixing occurs with perfusion of non-ventilated lung, an A-V fistula within the lung, a communication between the right and left sides of the myocardium, and an anastomosis between the systemic venous system and the pulmonary venous system.

The best measure of the presence of a shunt is an increased A-a oxygen gradient, even with the administration of high concentrations of oxygen. The administration of 100% oxygen is the means to evaluate if the patient has a ventilation-perfusion imbalance or a right-to-left shunt. Any existing ventilation-perfusion imbalance is negated by the administration of 100% oxygen, because the partial pressure of oxygen is equalized in all ventilated alveoli. In shunting, the hypoxemia and A-a gradient remain, because the anatomical shunts remain. The arterial oxygen increases but not to the levels to be expected from the elevated alveolar oxygen pressure. The oxygen needed to saturate the hemoglobin is provided from the increased gas physically dissolved in the plasma. Arterial oxygen pressure levels must fall to approximately 100 mm Hg before significant desaturation of the hemoglobin occurs and the shunt produces a rapid decrease in the arterial oxygen.

Calculation of the Right-to-Left Shunt
To calculate the right-to-left shunt, the nurse should:

1. Administer 100% oxygen (for about 3 to 30 minutes). (Currently, there exists some disagreement about the amount of time the patient may safely be repeatedly placed on 100% oxygen. Also, some believe that pure oxygen increases the calculated shunt and that FIO_2 values of 30 to 60% are more effective in determining venous admixture. A nitrogen analyzer is sometimes used to determine when less than 1% nitrogen remains.)
2. Draw samples for arterial blood gas measurements.
3. Using the alveolar air equation, calculate the alveolar oxygen pressure.
4. If there is a significant difference between the calculated alveolar value and the measured arterial value, know that a right-to-left shunt is present. (For every 100 mm Hg difference, the shunt is 6%. For example, when the difference is 300 mm Hg, the shunt is 18%.)
5. Using peripheral arterial and mixed venous blood from the Swan-Ganz catheter for a more exact estimation of the shunt, use the following equation to calculate the shunt.

$$\text{Shunt} = \frac{\text{arterial oxygen deficit}}{\text{arteriovenous oxygen difference}}$$

$$= \frac{\left(\begin{array}{c}\text{oxygen content}\\\text{of pulmonary}\\\text{capillary}\end{array}\right) - \left(\begin{array}{c}\text{oxygen content}\\\text{of arterial blood}\end{array}\right)}{\left(\begin{array}{c}\text{oxygen content}\\\text{of pulmonary}\\\text{capillary}\end{array}\right) - \left(\begin{array}{c}\text{oxygen content}\\\text{of mixed}\\\text{venous blood}\end{array}\right)}$$

Since the oxygen content of the pulmonary end capillary blood cannot be measured directly, the calculation is based on an important assumption. During the inspiration of 100% oxygen, the amount of alveolar oxygen is more than enough for total saturation of hemoglobin, and so the pulmonary capillary partial pressure of oxygen is essentially equal to the alveolar partial pressure of oxygen. The following calculation is made:

$$\begin{array}{c}\text{Oxygen}\\\text{content of}\\\text{pulmonary}\\\text{capillary}\end{array} = \text{Hgb} \times \%\text{ saturation} \times 1.39 + \left(\begin{array}{c}\text{alveolar}\\\text{oxygen}\\\text{partial}\\\text{pressure}\end{array}\right)0.0031$$

(oxygen chemically bound to hemoglobin)   (oxygen physically in solution)

If the arterial oxygen content is not reported by the laboratory, the value may be calculated by substituting the arterial oxygen partial pressure in the preceding equation. The different calculations for venous admixture used in critical care units across the country are all variations of that equation. The variations have been derived by changing the form of the equation so that the measurements available in the particular critical care unit may be used directly in the equation, thus decreasing the work required for the calculations.

6. The following is a modified shunt equation commonly used for patients who have an arterial oxygen pressure of more than 150 mm Hg [52]:

$$\text{Shunt} = \frac{\left(\begin{array}{c}\text{partial pressure of}\\\text{alveolar oxygen}\end{array}\right) - \left(\begin{array}{c}\text{partial pressure of}\\\text{arterial oxygen}\end{array}\right) 0.0031}{\left(\begin{array}{c}\text{arterial}\\\text{oxygen}\\\text{content}\end{array} - \begin{array}{c}\text{mixed}\\\text{venous}\\\text{oxygen}\\\text{content}\end{array}\right) + \left(\begin{array}{c}\text{partial}\\\text{pressure}\\\text{of alveolar}\\\text{oxygen}\end{array} - \begin{array}{c}\text{partial}\\\text{pressure}\\\text{of arterial}\\\text{oxygen}\end{array}\right) 0.0031}$$

7. Shunt calculation.

Example

Patient on ventilator with a tidal volume of 800 cc and a rate of 12 breaths per minute.

4:00 P.M.
  Objective Data
    ABG: FIO_2 = 40%
          PaO_2 = 56
          $PaCO_2$ = 51
          pH   = 7.32

    Assessment: Hypoxemia from hypoventilation with acute carbon dioxide retention and other unidentified mechanisms.

    Plan: Ventilation. Increase tidal volume to 1000 cc and rate to 16 per minute.

6:00 P.M.
  Objective Data
    ABG: FIO_2 = 40%
          PaO_2 = 64
          $PaCO_2$ = 38
          pH   = 7.41

  Assessment
    $PaO_2 = (747 - 47)(.4) - 38/1$ (In clinical situa-
          $= 280 - 38$ tions, to facilitate
          $= 242$ mm Hg   computation 1 is
                                      used for the respi-
                                      ratory quotient.)

Hypoxemia continues because of a ventilation-perfusion imbalance or a right-to-left shunt. A diffusion defect is not likely because of an improvement in PaO_2. The arterial oxygen pressure should be in the range of 220 to 240 mm Hg.

Plan: Differentiate a ventilation-perfusion mismatch from a right-to-left shunt. On 100% O_2, the oxygen tension is uniform in all the alveoli so that any difference is due to shunting. Increase the oxygen to 100% for 30 minutes.

6:45 P.M.
  Objective Data
    ABG: FIO_2 = 100%
          PaO_2 = 280
          $PaCO_2$ = 26
          pH   = 7.43

Assessment: Right-to-left shunt.

Predicted value
    $PAO_2 = (747 - 47) 1 - 26/1$
          $= 700 - 26$
          $= 674$ mm Hg

A-a O_2 gradient $= 674 - 280$
                  $= 394$

Shunt $= \dfrac{394}{100} \times 6$
      $= 4 \times 6$
      $= 24\%$

Fat Embolism

Fat embolism most commonly occurs 12 to 48 hours after a fracture of a long bone. Although the condition may occur in people of any age, it occurs most commonly in people aged 20 to 30 (among whom the tibia and the femur are the long bones most commonly fractured) and in people aged 70 to 80 (among whom the hip is the long bone most commonly fractured). Fat embolism also occurs with extensive trauma, burns, and infection that develops after cardiac resuscitation, bypass procedures, and renal transplantations, and in diabetes and alcoholism.

The etiology of fat embolism is not fully known, but two theories are popular. The first theory focuses on alterations in the blood lipids. In nontraumatic conditions, embolic fat chemically resembles blood lipids rather than either fat from the marrow or depot fat. The action of lipase in the lung and the hydrolysis of neutral fat emboli result in the release of free fatty acids. Those in turn result in a capillary leak from the pulmonary endothelium damage and microatelectasis from the decreased secretion of surfactant from the alveolar type II cells. Chemical pneumonitis and the formation of platelet thrombi in the pulmonary capillaries follow.

The second theory is more commonly accepted. It associates the mechanical event of trauma with fat in the bloodstream. Following trauma, pressure in the long bones that have a high fat content is increased. Since the veins within the bone are prevented from collapsing because they adhere to the bony framework, fat droplets are forced into the bloodstream.

The lung is the primary filter, and embolism results in parenchymal damage as well as increased pulmonary vascular resistance that affects the patient's cardiac status [65]. Embolism is also interpreted as a neurological alteration and as petechiae in the skin. The symptoms depend on the body system affected.

Disseminated Intravascular Coagulation

Many pathological conditions may activate the clotting system and produce the syndrome known as disseminated intravascular coagulation (DIC). A partial list of those conditions includes trauma, burns, prolonged hypotension, renal transplant rejection, malignancy, snake bites, abruptio placentae, transfusion reactions, and heat stroke. A partial list of causative factors following trauma include shock, sepsis, ischemia, ischemia followed by the recirculation of blood, hypoxia, tissue thromboplastin, proteolytic enzymes, azotemia, intravascular hemolysis, transfusions of stored blood and particulate matter, endotoxins, and the severance of the vessels of the microcirculation.

It is generally accepted that DIC is an intermediary mechanism of disease that complicates the preexisting condition. Pathological activation of blood coagulation and fibrinolysis results in a clinical syndrome (Fig. 36-2). The primary problem is the generation of excess thrombin with resultant fibrin formation, ischemic tissue damage, and utilization of clotting factors and platelets. Once DIC occurs, consumption of platelets and clotting factors, plus the anticoagulant properties of fibrin split products (FSPs), creates a potential bleeding problem. The deposition of fibrin in small vessels blocks the capillary flow to organs, resulting in ischemic tissue injury. Following the initial clotting and the resultant fibrinolysis, the repolymerization of fibrin and FSPs (paracoagulation) produces a secondary fibrin mesh in the small vessels. Red blood cells are mechanically damaged while they travel through the meshwork, resulting in schistocyte formation and a microangiopathic hemolytic anemia [72].

Excess Thrombin

Excess thrombin and clinical intravascular clotting may be produced in three ways: (1) the endothelial wall may be injured by such factors as bacterial toxins and activation of the intrinsic clotting system, complement system, or plasmin and the kinin system, (2) tissue injury causes the release of tissue thromboplastin, activating the extrinsic pathway, (3) a combination of intrinsic and extrinsic system activation may be operational, as in hemolytic transfusion reactions, where phospholipids released by the red blood cells indirectly set both pathways in motion. Following the formation of excess thrombin, clotting factors are consumed and fibrin deposition occurs. The thrombi are particularly damaging to the microcirculation, and they may result in a consumptive coagulopathy.

Fibrin Formation

As a normal mechanism, the production of thrombin is essential in the conversion of fibrinogen to fibrin. Fibrinogen is composed of three paired chains, called alpha, beta, and gamma chains. Thrombin (1) cleaves the alpha chain and then the beta chain, releasing fibrinopeptides (A and B), (2) activates factor XIII, and (3) aggregates the platelets. What is left of the fibrinogen is named the fibrin monomer (a molecule of low molecular weight). The monomer combines with itself (or polymerizes) to form a gel. The gel is stabilized by factor XIII, forming cross links between the gamma chains and the alpha chains. The end result is a stable fibrin clot [50].

As an immediate consequence of intravascular clotting, fibrinogen, platelets, and other coagulation factors are utilized, and fibrin is formed as small strands and clots. Vascular thrombosis and occlusion may occur at sites of localized trauma and/or resting sites of emboli. In particular, since circulating fibrin is phagocytized and cleared by reticuloendothelial

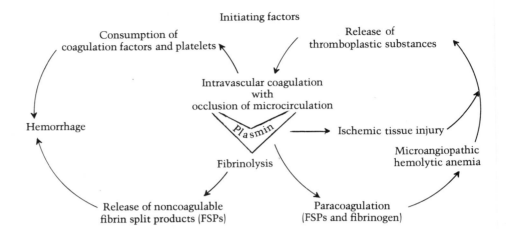

Figure 36-2

Disseminated intravascular coagulation. (Courtesy of James Smith, M.D.)

cells in the liver and spleen, impairment of those cells may allow fibrin deposition in the microcirculation. Ischemic damage is probably seen in the kidney, adrenal glands, lung, liver, and skin.

Secondary Fibrinolysis

Following intravascular clotting and fibrin formation, local fibrinolysis is evoked as a homeostatic compensatory mechanism in order to maintain the patency of the microcirculation. Such secondary fibrinolysis elaborates fibrinogen-fibrin degradation and FSPs, whose anticoagulant actions contribute to the severe hemorrhagic diathesis.

Activators act directly on plasminogen or they act on a proactivator in the plasma that in turn acts on plasminogen to produce plasmin (fibrinolysin), a proteolytic enzyme. Many substances that seem to be activators have been isolated from bacteria (streptokinase), urine (urokinase), and tissues, such as the prostate, pancreas, uterus, and, particularly, endothelial cells. Since plasmin is incorporated into the fibrin clot, it can digest the fibrin. Circulating plasmin can digest fibrinogen. Plasmin digests the same proteins that thrombin activates, and it causes fibrinolysis by enzymatically breaking fibrin into FSPs. Initially, plasmin cleaves the alpha and beta chains of the fibrinogen molecule and later the gamma chains. The fragments (polypeptides) liberated are termed FSPs, and they are named X, Y, D, and E. Fibrinogen reacts with FSPs to form webs of abnormal FSPs and fibrin, which cause the hemolytic phase of the disorder.

Since FSPs are present, any one of several things

may happen. The fibrin monomer may react with fibrinogen to form a soluble gel able to be stabilized by factor XIII. Or the fibrin monomer may polymerize in the presence of some FSPs (fragments D and E), forming an unstable, abnormal, weak web, and it may react with other FSPs (fragments X and Y), forming unclottable complexes. Plasmin carries on digestion continuously; the products formed vary in size and in characteristics—from slowly clottable fragments to nonclottable fragments. Initially, fragment X is formed, which clots more slowly than fibrinogen but clots completely; further degradation of fragment X produces two nonclottable fragments, Y and D. Fragment Y inhibits the action of thrombin on fibrinogen, while degradation of fragment Y produces more D and E fragments, which inhibit the early stages of clotting.

The anticoagulant action of FSPs has been called antithrombin VI. Interference with hemostasis involves the following mechanisms:

1. Thrombin action is inhibited.
2. Fibrin polymerization is inhibited.
3. Abnormal polymers with a diminished tensile strength are formed.
4. Fibrinogen-fibrin monomer-FSP complexes are formed.
5. Thromboplastin generation is inhibited.
6. Platelet functioning is inhibited.

Hematological Abnormalities

Since red blood cells cannot travel through thrombosed vessels, secondary and imperfect fibrin strands from the combination of fibrin and FSPs must be formed before passage. During their movement through the fibrin meshwork, the red blood cells are mechanically injured. The result is a microangiopathic hemolytic anemia characterized by evidence of intravascular hemolysis and by the presence of fragmented red blood cells.

Depression of the platelet count may be caused by platelet utilization in the fibrin meshwork, adhesion at sites of damaged endothelial surfaces, and aggregation from the effects of endotoxin, thrombin, antigen-antibody complexes, particulate matter, and loose FSP complexes. Coagulation factors are depleted by the continuous formation of thrombi and fibrin. The syndrome is further complicated by anoxic tissue damage to the liver, which impairs synthesis of new factors.

Assessment

DIC may be difficult to assess, or it may be apparent from the clinical situation. Many patients have disturbances in their clotting mechanisms, but they do not bleed unless they are operated on or unless their underlying disease worsens and so precipitates the bleeding state. When they bleed, the bleeding is often obvious and dramatic. Many sites are involved, and usually the patients seem to bleed "all over." Bleeding may be noted following injections in the skin, from the wound, from the gastrointestinal and/or urinary systems, and from old puncture wounds.

LABORATORY TESTS

The most common combination of laboratory aids selected as a clotting profile are the platelet count, peripheral smear, fibrinogen level, prothrombin time, partial thromboplastin time, thrombin time, and various tests for the presence of FSPs. There is no pathognomonic test.

Thrombocytopenia is almost always present when the platelet count averages 50,000 per cubic millimeter or less. The presence of large platelets in the peripheral smear may reflect rapid utilization. Red cell fragments may be seen; they are indicative of damage inflicted on the cells while they traveled through secondary and abnormal soluble fibrin web. The absence of fragmented red cells in the peripheral smear may make the physician hesitant about the diagnosis.

A progressive decrease in fibrinogen levels occurs. If the levels have been elevated previously, a level within the normal range is considered positive.

The prothrombin time is elevated (normal values are determined for each laboratory). The extrinsic pathway is evaluated by the prothrombin time test.

The partial thromboplastin time is prolonged.

The thrombin time reflects the interaction of thrombin with fibrinogen. It is measured by the time needed to clot after thrombin has been added to the patient's serum. If the thrombin time is prolonged, the test plasma is diluted 1:1 with normal plasma, and the test is repeated to determine whether the problem is due to low fibrinogen levels or to the presence of circulating anticoagulants (e.g., FSPs or heparin). If the thrombin time remains prolonged, that indicates the presence of FSPs that inhibit the action of thrombin and slowly produce an unstable fibrin clot.

The presence of FSPs reflects secondary fibrinolysis. Paracoagulation tests, such as the *ethanol gelation* and *protamine sulfate* tests, are relatively simple to perform, and they are screening tests in that they measure precipitable nonclottable complexes of degradation. When protamine sulfate and fibrin monomer–fragment X complexes react, the fibrin monomer is freed and able to polymerize. The measurement is expressed in terms of the degree of translucency of the resulting solution. Other tests are more specific, but they take more time. Thrombin may be added to the patient's plasma and the resulting serum examined for substances antigenic to fibrinogen. In the *staphylococcal clumping* test, bacteria clump in the presence of fibrinogen, fragment X, and fragment Y. A factor associated with the bacterial wall causes the clumping. The test is not as sensitive with fragments D and E. The *tanned red cell hemagglutination inhibition immunoassay* (the Mersky method) detects early and late degradation products and soluble fibrin monomer. Since red cells treated with tannic acid are conjugated to fibrinogen, antifibrinogen antiserum will produce agglutination. However, if FSPs were already present in the antiserum, the antiserum is neutralized, and it will not produce hemagglutination. The *Fi test* is similar in sensitivity to the Mersky method. Latex particles are coated with fibrinogen antibodies so that agglutination occurs if serum-containing fibrinogen fragments are added.

Management

Since DIC is an intermediary mechanism resulting from some underlying disease, treatment of the underlying disease (if it can be treated) abolishes the coagulopathy. Thus the primary treatment of DIC is first aimed at the underlying disease.

In the bleeding patient, heparin therapy may be used [18]. Heparin and a plasma cofactor act together to inhibit the action of thrombin so that the conversion of fibrinogen to fibrin and the platelet aggregation (induced by thrombin) are retarded. Therapeutic success is signaled by a decrease in the bleeding and an improvement in the clotting parameters. Warfarin is not used because it does not completely block the action of thrombin and because it takes about two days to work.

The next type of therapy (one that is rarely needed) is replacement therapy to restore the coagulation factors and/or the platelets to hemostatic levels. Patients normally first are heparinized, because the addition of procoagulants will allow consumption and fibrin deposition to proceed. The amount of platelets administered is determined by the patient's blood volume and weight. For example, a 70-kg man whose blood volume is 5000 ml would need 10 units of platelets to raise his platelet count to 50,000 per cubic millimeter.

Acute Gastroduodenal Ulceration

The syndrome known as acute gastroduodenal ulceration may occur in patients following multisystem trauma, fractures, burns, shock, sepsis, jaundice, respiratory and renal failure, elective surgeries, DIC, central nervous system trauma, and/or any severe illness. In particular, the syndrome is seen frequently in patients who have multiple intraabdominal organ trauma [55]. In the severely ill, the mortality is greater than 50% [45]. Day [22] has stated that in the patient who has a severe, multisystem injury, the gastrointestinal tract is the secondary victim of total-body economy.

Since fiberoptic endoscopy has become widely used clinically, more patients have been studied and stress ulceration has been better defined. The lesions develop following an initial episode of gastritis. They are acute erosions that generally extend no deeper than the muscularis mucosa. However, the ulcers may also range from deep craters to full-thickness necrosis of the gastric wall (gastromalacia). The most common initial lesion is in the fundus of the stomach, with lesions in the antrum and duodenum following later. The amount of bleeding ranges from occult blood in the stool to massive hemorrhage.

Mechanism

The actual etiology of the syndrome has not been defined. The syndrome is probably the result of a chain of events that involve many factors. The most plausible explanation is based on the concept that a severe stress may cause ischemia of the gastroduodenal mucosa. Since autonomic nervous system activity and circulating catecholamines may open submucosal shunts, the capillary bed of the mucosa would not then receive an adequate blood supply [38]. The resultant mucosal ischemia may be prolonged for hours to days. Increased mucosal permeability results, permitting acid back diffusion to occur. (Hydrogen ions move into and out of the gastric lumen; the movement outward is named acid back diffusion.) Increased back diffusion of gastric acid through the gastroduodenal mucosa may contribute to the further disruption of the gastric mucosal barrier (and it may also be one of the reasons for the low initial net acid output). Recent work has shown that actively secreting mucosa is able to withstand the back diffusion of hydrogen ions better than can ischemic mucosa [51]. Further mucosal membrane damage may be produced by serotonin and histamine, vasoactive amines released from the degranulation of mast cells. Ischemia leads to hypoxia and to a plasma protein leak in the stomach. Regenerative ability in the mucosal cells decreases and focal necrosis results. Leonard [38] has postulated that, following the initial period, there may be a period of increased parasympathetic stimulation that produces a relative hypersecretion of gastric acid caused by stimulation of the parietal cells. Most important, the submucosal shunts close and more blood flows through the capillaries of the gastroduodenal mucosa. Engorgement produces even more mucosal injury and necrosis. The result may be ulceration, bleeding, or perforation.

The adrenal corticosteroids were formerly thought to play a primary role, but now their role is a matter of controversy. It is not clear whether the secretion of gastric mucus is altered qualitatively or quantitatively (or both) by stress [61]. Formerly it was thought that adrenocorticotropic hormone stimulated the hypersecretion of endogenous corticosteroids, which in turn altered mucous chemistry and glycoprotein. The result was loss of the mucous barrier. Factors such as hydrochloric acid and protein enzymes were then more easily able to injure the damaged mucosa.

The mechanism may differ in DIC. In DIC, ulceration may be the end result of acute thrombosis within the blood vessels of the gastric mucosa.

The mechanism does differ following central nervous system trauma. Patients with central nervous system trauma secrete excessive amounts of gastric acid. Since the hypersecretion is blocked by the administration of anticholinergic medication, the cause is probably parasympathetic stimulation. It is thought that increased intracranial pressure stimulates the vagal nuclei [59].

Assessment

Clinically, the problem is often difficult to identify. Usually the patient's presenting signs are hematemesis (the vomiting of gross blood) and/or melena (the passage of black tarry stools that contain digested blood). Although usually reddish in color, the hematemesis may be dark because hemoglobin has been converted to hematin by hydrochloric acid.

The bleeding may be from any site. Besides stress ulcers, the following lesions may also bleed: chronic peptic ulcers, esophageal varices, and the lesions of Mallory-Weiss syndrome and of esophagitis [46]. Frequently, the cause of the bleeding is a peptic ulcer of the stomach or duodenum. Arterial bleeding is usual; however, bleeding may also result from congested vessels or granulation tissue around the ulcer or small veins. Since the condition is chronic, a carefully taken history should alert the staff to the potential complication. The use of drugs such as alcohol, salicylates, and/or steroids may disrupt the gastroduodenal mucosal barrier. Esophageal varices are accompanied by portal hypertension and are seen 50% to 75% of the time in patients who have advanced cirrhosis. The friable vessels near the cardiac sphincter may produce massive bleeding. The mortality for the initial bleeding approaches 50%; and once a patient has bled, another bleeding is anticipated. Esophageal tamponade may be ordered by the physician, and surgery may be performed when the patient's condition is such that he has a better chance of surviving surgery. In the Mallory-Weiss syndrome, continued vomiting produces tears in the cardiac mucosa. That syndrome is usually associated with such factors as the ingestion of alcohol or poison. Esophagitis may result from prolonged intubation or repeated vomiting. In many instances, massive bleeding is prevented by the early identification of the problem.

Management

Prophylaxis is the most important aspect of management. In the haste of the initial emergency, the patient and his family may fail to answer correctly questions about gastrointestinal symptoms. The primary care nurse must elicit pertinent historical information and notify the physician if any gastrointestinal symptoms are discovered.

In stress ulceration, antacid and cimetidine therapy are the mainstays of prophylaxis [44]. In animal studies, acute gastric lesions do not occur in the absence of hydrogen ions in the gastric juice. Buffering the gastric contents to a pH of 5 or greater is the simplest and most effective prophylaxis. Initial sampling and treatment identify each patient's baseline acidity and outline the protocol specific for that patient. Litmus paper sensitive to pH is used. The recommended pH values are 3.5 to 7. Cimetidine, a gastric acid inhibitor, is frequently administered intravenously to suppress gastric acid secretion.

Extremely important is the prevention of other problems, such as sepsis, nutritional depletion, and respiratory complication; patients suffering those complications have a higher incidence of stress ulceration. Avoiding the recumbent position, promoting inspiration, and coughing thus have more than one purpose.

Once the patient's bleeding is significant, any one of several measures may be taken. Endoscopy is used by the physician to identify the source of the bleeding. Antacid therapy may be continued. Iced lavages with large amounts of saline solution given through a large lumen gastric tube (e.g., an Ewald tube) may be used to rid the stomach of clots and to allow vasoconstriction. A topical vasoconstrictor (e.g., neosynephrine or norepinephrine) may be added. Blood replacement and four to six platelet packs may be used. Parenteral anticholinergic drugs may be given to decrease the levels of gastric acid and pepsin and to shunt blood from the bleeding mucosa by opening gastric submucosal shunts.

If the bleeding continues, the physician must decide between operative and nonoperative therapy. In nonoperative therapy a vascular catheter may be used in two ways to stop the bleeding. If the patient is critically ill, intraarterial infusion may be used to ameliorate the situation; it is a successful alternative to surgery. A splanchnic vasoconstrictive drug (e.g., epinephrine or vasopressin) is infused through the catheter into the artery or a proximal artery. Localized vasoconstriction decreases the blood flow and a clot forms. Usually, the intraarterial infusion is preceded by an angiogram initiated from an injection site of the celiac, superior mesenteric, or left gastric artery. That procedure is more successful in a patient who has a single bleeding site than in a patient who has many bleeding sites. Since about 50 percent of patients have a single bleeding site, the procedure has potential value for a large segment of the patient population. Infusions of vasopressin may be continued for one to two weeks, but usually they are recommended for no more than three to five days. When the procedure just described is not effective because of poor clotting factors, another useful procedure is embolic occlusion of the bleeding artery, the medical equivalent of surgical ligation.

If more conservative measures (e.g., iced saline lavage and vasoconstrictor infusion) have failed, surgery is indicated. The type of surgery to be chosen is controversial; it ranges from vagotomy and pyloroplasty to total gastrectomy. Many surgeons consider vagotomy and partial gastrectomy the procedure of choice. Since even that procedure carries an overall mortality as high as 50 percent in the critically ill patient, surgery must always be weighed against a "good" chance of controlling the bleeding. The patient is always considered individually.

Metabolic Response

The body's metabolic response to injury reflects the effects of undernutrition and injury. Although the mechanisms underlying the body's metabolic response to injury have not been fully elucidated, many studies have identified significant alterations. Because of differences in people, site and severity of trauma, the kind of injury, treatment, and complications, the response varies. In all likelihood, alternate patterns of endocrine-metabolic response characterize different sequences [47].

An imbalance between anabolism and catabolism is generally considered central to the problem. Injury

accentuates the use of body protein and increases gluconeogenesis for unknown reasons. Increases in nitrogen excretion tend to parallel increases in resting metabolic expenditure. Without nutritional supplements injured people lose weight to an extent that is roughly proportional to the severity of the metabolic insult.

Moore [47] has described the metabolic response as having four phases: (1) the catabolic phase (also called the initial phase, the adrenergic-corticoid phase, and the negative nitrogen balance phase), (2) the early anabolic phase (also called the turning point and the corticoid withdrawal phase), (3) the anabolic phase, and (4) the late anabolic, or convalescent, phase.

The intensity of the changes in and the length of each phase vary considerably. In the patient who has a minor injury, the catabolic phase results in minimal changes and may last only two to four days, whereas in the patient who has a multisystem injury, the same phase may produce extensive changes and may last for weeks.

In the catabolic phase, the patient's energy requirements are increased, and the hormone levels (e.g., the adrenergic and adrenal corticoid hormone levels) are elevated. Since the normal eating pattern is altered in most patients, those patients must get their nourishment from body processes, exogenous alimentation, and the food they are able to eat.

The transition from the catabolic phase to the anabolic phase is called the early anabolic phase; it lasts for one or two days. The potassium balance becomes positive, and the nitrogen losses decrease.

In the anabolic phase, which lasts two to five weeks, the body is in positive nitrogen balance and body proteins are synthesized. The patient feels much better, begins to eat well, and gains weight.

In the late anabolic phase, the positive nitrogen balance becomes normal and the person returns to his normal weight. The late anabolic phase lasts several months.

Starvation

The trauma state is superimposed on the starvation state. During the first two days of food deprivation, body processes continue, and the person still requires carbohydrates, proteins, fats, vitamins, and minerals. Calories are derived mainly from fats and proteins. Most of the small amounts of carbohydrate stored as glycogen in the liver and the muscles are quickly depleted the first day. The body's glucose requirements must be met by the formation of glucose (gluconeogenesis). The breakdown of tissue protein is the main source of the substrates.

Since glucose cannot be synthesized from fatty acids, glycerol and the glucogenic amino acids are converted into glucose in the liver. Proteolysis and increased gluconeogenesis characterize the response [13].

It is extremely important that the body's protein be in a dynamic state and not stored. Each molecule of protein has an essential purpose; that is, as part of an enzyme, an organ, a skeletal muscle, an oncotic molecule, and so on. Thus loss of protein means loss of function [23]. The breakdown products of protein catabolism are excreted in the urine as urea and ammonia, measuring 10 to 15 gm of urinary nitrogen (the amount of nitrogen excreted is multiplied by 6.25 to give the number of grams of protein oxidized). The amount of urinary nitrogen is a good indicator of this process. However, for the purposes of careful research studies of nitrogen balance, urinary nitrogen measurements are not enough. For one reason, much of the nitrogen in the urine originates from the portion of dietary protein not used as amino acids for the synthesis of protein. For another reason, nitrogen is excreted by other routes. Thus all nitrogen going into and out of the patient must be measured.

In particular, skeletal muscle and liver proteins are catabolized, the synthesis of proteins decreases, and amino acid release to the systemic circulation falls. (The chief amino acids released from the muscle bed for transportation to the liver are alanine and glutamine.)

Although most of the body uses fatty acids and ketoacids, the brain, renal medulla, bone marrow, erythrocytes, and leukocytes must have glucose. The brain converts the glucose to carbon dioxide and water, and the other elements that require glucose convert glucose to lactate and pyruvate. Resynthesis of those substances into glucose (via the Cori cycle) takes place in the liver. Therefore, the only sources of glucose are glucogenic amino acids, glycerol, lactate and pyruvate, and whatever liver glycogen has been spared.

The blood levels of glucose and insulin fall, and the blood levels of glucagon rise. Insulin release is associated with a rapid reduction in the plasma levels of all amino acids by enhancing their deposition and/or reducing their release from muscle. The release of glucagon from the alpha cells is stimulated by hypo-

glycemia and by the rise in the levels of plasma amino acids, and it is associated with glycogenolysis, gluconeogenesis, muscle proteolysis, and the elevation of serum free fatty acids and triglycerides. A high insulin-to-glucagon ratio enhances synthesis and anabolism, and a low insulin-to-glucagon ratio enhances catabolism.

With the administration of 140 to 150 gm of glucose during starvation, the nitrogen loss in the urine is reduced to about 4 gm daily. That phenomenon has been called the nitrogen-sparing effect. The current theory is that glucose's chief benefit is that it stimulates the beta cells to release insulin. Since insulin inhibits the release of amino acids from muscle, the amino acids are not available for extraction by the liver and for gluconeogenesis.

After 48 hours, the body adapts to the starvation state by sparing protein—thus enhancing the chances of survival. The total nitrogen loss is reduced to 3 to 5 gm per day. Although the mechanism of adaptation is not known, two changes seem to be important: (1) the brain converts from glucose metabolism to ketone metabolism so that the body's glucose needs are reduced by 50 percent, or 100 gm per day, and (2) the low levels of alanine seem to limit the rate of gluconeogenesis. Most of the glucose is derived from glycerol, lactate, and pyruvate, and it is produced by the kidney as well as by the liver. The metabolic rate is reduced. Fatty acids or ketones remain the primary sources of energy for skeletal muscle, the heart, the kidney cortex, and most of the rest of the body. Tissue fat supplies approximately 85 to 90 percent of the calories required, while protein supplies 10 to 15 percent. An interesting side note is that obligatory water losses are decreased because nitrogen losses are decreased.

Alanine is the principal amino acid used by the liver for gluconeogenesis; its levels decrease rapidly to less than one-third of normal [13]. In experiments the administration of small quantities of alanine rapidly produces an increase in the blood glucose levels. It is hypothesized that the overall control of gluconeogenesis in a starving person lies in the muscle and ultimately depends on the formation and release of alanine.

Trauma

In the changes that occur after trauma, the patient is hypermetabolic. The greater the trauma, the greater the catabolism. Protein is not spared. Gluconeogenesis is increased. Increases in the urinary excretion of potassium and nitrogen tend to parallel increases in the resting metabolic expenditure, but not necessarily in a cause-and-effect relationship.

Visceral protein from all over the body is utilized in the catabolic response. The use of body protein as an energy source is an extremely significant phenomenon. Enzyme systems are disturbed. Utilization of liver protein itself from the time of the trauma, coupled with therapy that produces hyperglycemia, may set the stage for deposition of fat in the liver and thus for liver failure. Importantly, the catabolism of respiratory muscles as an energy source will decrease the size of the muscle mass and may limit respiration, thus setting the stage for pneumonia. Decreases in the albumin and immunoglobulin levels and in cellular immunity set the stage for infection.

The daily measurement of the urinary excretion of urea may be used to categorize patients according to severity of their injury [10]. Patients in categories III and IV excrete more than 10 gm of nitrogen daily for long periods, or they excrete higher levels of nitrogen daily for shorter periods. Corresponding problems of people in categories III and IV are hypermetabolism, metabolic disturbances, weight loss, and disturbances in the levels of electrolytes, vitamins, and trace minerals. Protein is depleted from the body in many other ways, among them: hemorrhage, plasma- or protein-containing fluid loss (as in a major soft tissue injury), and atrophy of bone and muscle from bedrest and other conditions of immobility.

The severity of the metabolic insult is also approximately proportional to the weight loss. Patients who have major fractures may lose 10 to 25 percent of their weight. The amount and rate of loss is accentuated if fever and/or sepsis is imposed. The patient's actual weight is difficult to determine because weight is affected by his state of hydration (a large proportion of weight loss is a result of water loss). Kinney [36] observes that the water loss seems to be greater than the protein loss and the other physiological parameters that affect the amount of body water and indicate that the phenomenon should be investigated.

Although many authorities start nutritional supplementation early, a 10 percent weight loss is commonly the maximum weight loss tolerated before parenteral alimentation is started. A weight loss of 40 to 50 percent is invariably fatal, and amounts less than that result in malaise and impaired physical performance.

The hypermetabolic response is at its extreme in the thermally injured patient. The metabolic rate is characterized by a rapid increase from its normal value to a peak rate and then a gradual decrease as the wound is closed. The peak rate is reached between the sixth and tenth postburn days. The amplitude of the response is proportional to the size of injury, with a maximum reached in burns involving 40 to 50 percent of the total body surface area. The body's oxygen consumption returns to normal when the wound is closed [69].

Measurements of the oxygen consumption and the carbon dioxide production in other types of surgical patients have showed that the increase in the resting metabolic expenditure approximates the increase in urinary nitrogen level [28, 29]. In patients who have undergone uncomplicated surgical procedures, the preoperative and postoperative levels of urinary nitrogen showed no significant increases. In patients who had major fractures, the caloric expenditure increased toward 20 percent for two to three weeks. If major sepsis occurred in the postoperative clinical course, increases of 10 to 40 percent were measured. Fever superimposed on an underlying disorder raised the patient's calorie expenditure by more than the usually accepted value (a 7.2 percent increase for every Fahrenheit degree of increase in the body temperature). In general, the resting metabolic expenditure was elevated 20 to 50 percent.

Endocrine Response

Sympathicoadrenal activity is rampant during the "fight-or-flight" response, resulting in an increased energy production, the release of glycogen and its conversion to glucose, an altered organ blood flow, an increased glucagon and a decreased insulin secretion, and gluconeogenesis. The cardiac output, heart rate, and systolic blood pressure rise [66]. Because of capillary dilatation, the total peripheral resistance and the diastolic blood pressure decrease. The person feels anxious, and he is tachypneic. Intestinal peristalsis and pancreatic secretion cease. Renal blood flow decreases, as does the excretion of sodium, potassium, and chloride. In simple terms, the body has gathered all its forces and is operating at full speed in an effort to protect itself.

In another aspect of the nonspecific stress reaction, the release of corticosteroid by the adrenal cortex may be increased threefold. Glucose production increases because of (1) the diminished release of insulin, (2) the production of more glucose from amino acids, (3) hepatic glycogenolysis, and (4) the suppression of fat metabolism from carbohydrates. Protein synthesis is inhibited, and protein catabolism is enhanced. Also, the movement of water into the cell is retarded.

The hyperglycemia is an expected response to trauma; the blood sugar returns to normal in a few hours in people who have only minor trauma. (Patients whose blood sugar levels become subnormal are probably close to death.) If the stress persists, the elevations persist. In most people, the blood glucose level is elevated for varying periods of time so that the substrate is ready for utilization. In others, excess glucose accumulates for a prolonged period and they demonstrate a diabetes-like syndrome (called the diabetes of trauma, or pseudodiabetes).

Insulin probably plays a central role in regulating the metabolic response. The initiation and suppression of metabolic processes are regulated by the insulin-glucagon ratio. It is hypothesized that insulin reacts with the cell membrane to dispatch a second messenger inside the cell. Thus insulin alters the metabolic response of the cell by the amount of second messenger dispatched. Muscle proteolysis is suppressed by the second messenger. In order to counteract whatever mechanism or factor produces the accelerated muscle catabolism, the insulin concentrations must increase [29].

On the other hand, studies of burn patients have suggested that the persistent hyperglycemia is the result of increased hepatic gluconeogenesis, hyperglycogenemia, and elevated catecholamine levels [70]. Glucagon and catecholamines stimulated cyclic adenosine monophosphate in the liver and were of primary importance in regulating the hepatic production of glucose. Fasting insulin levels and insulin response were not reduced during the second postburn week. The insulin response was normal in the face of hypermetabolism and a negative nitrogen balance. After that, the insulin response decreased as the time after the injury increased. During convalescence, phenomena like those that occur in starvation were noted; namely, loss of weight, a decreased blood glucose concentration, and a decrease in the rate constant for glucose disappearance.

What the exact underlying causes of the hypermetabolism are is important, because therapy can be based only on a sound understanding of the pathophysiology [17, 56]. One theory is that amino acids are mobilized to heal the wounds. Protein is broken down by the body in an effort to obtain building blocks for repairing the wounds. Also, inadequate perfusion limits the delivery of oxygen to the site of the injury and glucose is required for anaerobic metabolism. The presence of lactate may induce collagen formation. Polymorphonuclear leukocytes and immature fibroblasts utilize glucose as their main source of energy; they are present in large numbers.

Another theory (a popular one) is that the body is breaking down protein to supply extra calories and fuel since the metabolic rate is increased. Opposed to that theory is the fact that relatively few calories are provided by the deamination of amino acids, and fat oxidation seems unaffected by the trauma (although overmobilization of fat may result in fat deposits in the liver). In another theory, Kinney and his associates [36] propose that the body has a specific need for carbon intermediates, which may be used for several purposes, such as synthesizing nonessential amino acids, supplying the Krebs citric acid cycle, and supplying glucose for the metabolism of the central nervous system. After the injury, the control of gluconeogenesis is modified. An interesting question about glucose during the low flow state and cellular hypoxia remains unanswered. Is the cell membrane ischemic and unable to keep glucose outside of the cell, or is glucose actually used in an oxidative process within the cell?

In another series of studies of burn-injured patients, Wilmore [71] suggests that the metabolic response is the end-product of afferent stimuli from the injured area. He thinks that stresses (e.g., exposure to cold or heat, early starvation, pain, infection, exercise, burn injury, and trauma) are able to evoke a similar set of stress responses in the body but that the responses vary with the severity of the stress. The response elicited entails increased adrenergic activity, a change in the disposition of body fuel (from storage to utilization), and an increase in the resting metabolic expenditure. Wilmore hypothesizes that nervous and hormonal stimuli travel to the central nervous system and "reset" neuroendocrine activity. The altered set of responses probably originates in the hypothalamus and directly affects cellular metabolic rate until the wound is closed. Evidence for Wilmore's thesis is found in a clinical study of patients with large burns who were given doses of alpha- and/or beta-adrenergic blockers that were followed by a consistent decrease in the metabolic rate [71]. More recently, it has been shown that following burn injury, the increased peripheral blood flow preferentially transports heat and glucose to the wound. Essentially, the injury has increased the body's energy demands, and burn patients must sustain the increased energy demand until the wound is closed. The hypermetabolism results from a reset of the central temperature mechanism in the hypothalamus. The total body systemic response is necessary to support the healing wound in its increased metabolic and circulatory needs.

Nutritional Support

The guidelines for the critically ill patient's nutritional requirements have been formulated by many researchers, but a great deal of research remains to be done before specific baseline requirements can be determined. Kinney [36] suggests a change in the calorie-nitrogen ratio from a normal of 200 to 300 calories per gram of nitrogen in the active uninjured state to 100 to 150 calories (in some circumstances, 75 to 150 calories) per gram of nitrogen in the injured state. Dudrick [24] suggests daily supplements of about 12 to 24 gm of nitrogen and 2500 to 4000 calories for people who have major illnesses. Moore [47] suggests 200 mg of nitrogen and 50 calories per kilogram of body weight daily. Wilmore [69] recommends 15 gm of nitrogen and 2000 calories per square meter per day for thermally injured patients [67]. Curreri and his associates [19] have developed the following formula for the ideal calorie intake of burn patients that considers the person's individual differences (TBSA stands for total body surface area):
25 calories × kg body weight + 40 calories × % TBSA burned = calorie intake

Example
25 calories × 70 kg + 40 calories × 60% TBSA burned =
4150 calories

After an injury, the body's nutritional needs may be met by oral means, tube, or intravenous feedings—or by a combination of those methods. Other methods have been studied and used, but they have not been as successful.

USE OF THE GASTROINTESTINAL TRACT

If the gastrointestinal tract is functioning, it is used to the maximum. Oral feedings are often combined with tube feedings. Parenteral alimentation is instituted when other methods prove ineffective.

Basic to oral feedings is an assessment of the patient's nutritional status. Eating is a habit, and critically ill people eat the foods to which they are already accustomed. The quantity of food eaten is also based on one's eating habits. People cannot eat more after they are sick than they ate before (in fact, they eat about 10% less) [19, 69]. One may anticipate that an active adolescent patient accustomed to eating vast quantities of food will be able to eat significantly more than a frail elderly patient accustomed to eating small quantities of food. Pain, analgesics, tracheostomies, facial injuries, and general malaise may also limit oral feedings.

Feedings by tube may take the form of nasogastric, gastrostomy, or jejunostomy feeding. In unconscious or obtunded patients, the nasogastric and gastrostomy feedings may lead to aspiration, and they are not recommended. The Dobhoff tube appears as if it will be a boon to nutritional therapy. A variety of diets for total feedings or supplementary feedings may be ordered, ranging from a skim-milk or whole-milk diet to a blenderized diet. Commercially prepared high-calorie, high-nitrogen diets and elemental diets may also be ordered.

Elemental diets are chemically synthesized feedings that have high biological value, are absorbable, and are free of bulk. Electrolytes, trace minerals, and both water- and fat-soluble vitamins (except vitamin K) are included. The nitrogen-carbohydrate ratio varies in the different products. Because the diet is already broken down into amino acids and simple sugars, minimal digestive secretions and only part of the small bowel are needed for absorption. Since there is no bulk, there is no residue or stool. The diarrhea frequently encountered is caused by too high a concentration, an amount, or a rate of administration.

The feedings are often ideal for patients who have such conditions as biliary or pancreatic trauma, short bowel syndrome, and fistulas. On the other hand, the high osmolality of the solutions limits the amount that can be administered in each feeding. Complications range from the extreme of hyperosmolar nonketotic coma to nausea and diarrhea in a syndrome that is very much like the postgastrectomy syndrome.

NUTRITIONAL PARENTERAL THERAPY

If feedings by mouth or tube do not meet the patient's nutritional needs, parenteral alimentation is added to his therapeutic regimen. Although 3% crystalline amino acid solutions or fat solutions can be infused through a peripheral vein, it seems likely that protein and caloric supplements given by catheterization through a vein that has a large diameter and permits a high flow will continue to be the mainstay of parenteral therapy.

The concentration and quantity of the solution are gradually increased until the desired state is attained. The same care is usually given to discontinuing the solution. Nitrogen and carbohydrate are administered simultaneously to increase the utilization of nitrogen. Wound healing, one of the primary purposes of alimentation, is associated with cell synthesis and repletion. Thus intracellular components are needed in great supply, and a deficiency in any nutrient is readily apparent.

Each solution must be administered according to the patient's individual needs, but several guidelines are pertinent for patients in general [24]. Approximately a 5% protein hydrolysate or crystalline amino acid solution and a 20% dextrose in water solution make up the basic solution. An average of 50 mEq of sodium is added to each liter of solution, depending on the patient's acid-base status. Usually sodium is added to the protein hydrolysates as sodium chloride. Another additive is necessary with the crystalline amino acids solution, because the amino acids would precipitate as a hydrochloride salt and produce acidosis. In that instance, sodium bicarbonate is the additive.

Large amounts of potassium (averaging 40 mEq/ 1000 calories) are needed to achieve a positive nitrogen balance and to restore the depleted intracellular potassium levels. The body needs up to 250 mEq of potassium per day. Initially many of the patients who have suffered trauma are potassium depleted. Their kidneys cannot conserve both potassium and sodium. Gastrointestinal losses of potassium are high. Protein deamination is associated with potassium loss. Many of the patients are alkalotic; potassium ions have been exchanged for sodium ions in their renal tubules and excreted in their urine in an attempt to conserve hydrogen ions. Although those problems are corrected before hyperalimentation is begun, hypokalemia remains a potential problem. Potassium accompanies glucose into the intracellular space and, in the presence of a preexisting hypokalemia, may produce a lethal dysrhythmia. In any event, further hypokalemia, metabolic alkalosis, and glycosuria are likely to occur. If they do, the physician's assessment of low serum potassium levels will be followed by potassium therapy, not insulin therapy.

In the past, hypophosphatemia with weakness,

paresthesias, seizures, and a decrease in adenosine triphosphate and 2,3-DPG in the red blood cell were noted. If for some reason, the base solution does not contain phosphorus, phosphorus should be added to it. Calcium is administered on the basis of the serum calcium levels, but the administration of phosphorus may produce hypocalcemia. Usually the daily allotment is 4 to 5 mEq per liter, or 300 mg. Magnesium deficiency is prevented by the administration of magnesium sulfate (10–25 mEq/day).

Trace minerals are usually supplied by the administration of plasma. Zinc deficiency is associated with poor wound healing (it is being studied by many people). Intravenous supplementation is approximately 2 to 4 mg per day. Iron therapy is usually given by the intramuscular route.

Water- and fat-soluble vitamins (a commercial preparation, such as Berroca-C) or a multivitamin infusion is given daily. The body's need for vitamin C has been long established. It is thought that the urinary excretion of water-soluble vitamins is higher following intravenous administration than it is following oral administration. Also, vitamin K and folic acid are administered intramuscularly once a week (10 mg), and vitamin B_{12} is administered intramuscularly usually once a month (250 mEq).

A 10% fat emulsion (Intralipid) supplies calories in a concentrated form (9 calories/gm). It may be administered in a peripheral vein since the solution is essentially isotonic. It can be infused for only 12 hours a day, in contrast to the usual 24-hour hyperalimentation regimen. Intralipid supplies essential fatty acids and triglycerides that are not usually available. When Intralipid is used, fatty acid intoxication is not a problem. Since the administration of glucose stimulates the release of insulin, carbohydrates must be infused with the Intralipid. The complications of parenteral therapy, which have been well described, are given in Table 36-1.

Sepsis and Septic Shock

The physiological alterations that occur with infection range from a minor local inflammatory response to septic shock and even death. Sepsis, the systemic response to invading microorganisms, has a constellation of symptoms, physical signs, and laboratory abnormalities. It usually occurs with bacteremia, but not all people who have bacteremia also have septicemia.

The establishment and spread of sepsis is described

Table 36-1
Potential Complications from Parenteral Nutrition Therapy

Air embolism
Sepsis
Pneumothorax
Hemothorax
Hydrothorax
Tension pneumothorax
Subclavian artery injury
Cardiac dysrhythmias
Catheter embolism
Catheter clotting
Central venous thrombosis
Catheter misplacement
Cardiac tamponade
Hyperosmolar nonketotic hyperglycemia
Hypophosphatemia
Hyperglycemia
Hypoglycemia
Electrolyte abnormalities
Subcutaneous emphysema
Brachial plexus injury

by the following mechanism. The invading microorganisms get a foothold in damaged tissue and establish a primary lesion there. Sepsis is the result of the interaction between the microorganism and the patient. Different species and strains of microorganisms vary in their ability to produce disease, and patients vary in their ability to resist infection. Pathogenic organisms, including some that seem to be nonpathogenic, survive and multiply in the patient, producing tissue damage and eliciting an inflammatory response. The patient's hormonal and cellular immunological capacities may be significantly impaired.

Microorganisms produce sepsis by the invasion of tissues and the elaboration of toxins. From the time organisms and their products enter the extravascular spaces and interact with damaged tissue, the body attempts to localize them by its inflammatory response. Kininogen, a hormone present in all tissues and blood, is activated into kinin, and, along with histamine, endotoxin, and other vasoactive substances, it produces a vascular response. Blood flow is slowed by vascular constriction associated with capillary and venular dilatation. Alterations in the endothelial membrane increase permeability and permit extravasation of plasma proteins into the extravascular space and diapedesis of leukocytes. Fibrinogen forms a fibrin network that traps the bacteria. At the cellular level, the A-V oxygen difference is decreased, and local hypoxia occurs. The mechanism for the hypoxia is not known; some authorities have suggested a bypass of the cell, a defect in oxygen transport, or a problem with oxidative phosphorylation [8].

The infection is spread by direct extension or along fascial planes and elongated structures, such as the ureters. From the primary lesion (or seeding source), the infection is spread systemically by the blood, and secondary lesions can occur anywhere in the body.

Sepsis produces vasodilatation and a hyperdynamic state. The blood flow and the cardiac output are increased, and the distribution or the peripheral effectiveness of the blood flow is altered. If compensatory mechanisms fail and the prearteriolar sphincters relax, the patient lapses into septic shock. The onset is not always abrupt. The blood pressure may either drift down or drop suddenly. Often problems in other systems are caused by the decreased cardiac output. Multiorgan failure is seen [9]. For example, the patient may suffer a myocardial infarction from decreased myocardial perfusion, and/or he may be confused because of the decreased cerebral perfusion. Additionally, the low-flow state may produce not only gastrointestinal problems (especially stress ulcers) but also a dead bowel secondary to venous and/or arterial thrombosis. The patient would then have distention, absence of normal bowel sounds, and bloody diarrhea.

Causative Organisms

As other antibiotics have been developed and as treatment modalities have changed, particularly resistant organisms have arisen and mutated. Before the 1940s, the greatest problem was with *Streptococcus*; in the 1950s, *Staphylococcus*; in the 1960s, *Pseudomonas*; and in the 1970s, other gram-negative bacteria and opportunistic organisms. As antibiotics have been developed for each organism, another resistant species has seemingly come to the fore. Often the new organism was one that previously was considered to be not infectious. For example, *Pseudomonas* was once classified as nonvirulent and nonpathogenic. As a matter of fact, at first some hospitals had difficulty identifying *Pseudomonas* as the invading pathogen because their laboratories considered *Pseudomonas* nonvirulent and a normal surface contaminant of laboratory cultures, and they did not report the presence of the *Pseudomonas*.

Sepsis may be produced by many different organisms. Because gram-negative infections have become more significant, emphasis has been put on them. But gram-positive organisms—as well as polymicrobial and opportunistic organisms—still cause sepsis. Besides group A *Streptococcus*, *Staphylococcus* may cause necrotizing fasciitis (necrosis of the superficial fascia). A hemolytic *Staphylococcus* and a nonhemolytic *Streptococcus* may work together to cause progressive bacterial synergistic gangrene. An anaerobic *Streptococcus* is often the cause of myositis.

GRAM-NEGATIVE ORGANISMS

Gram-negative bacteremia occurs in about one out of every 100 hospitalizations, and it has been calculated to be the cause of about 70,000 deaths each year in the United States [4]. Besides effects of the numbers of bacteria, gram-negative bacilli contain within their cell walls a lipopolysaccharide called endotoxin that rapidly has adverse effects on the body.

For purposes of identification, microorganisms are grouped according to their biochemical reactions. Families of microorganisms are broken down into genera, each of which is divided into species. Usually an organism is referred to by its genus and species names (e.g., *Escherichia coli* and *Serratia marcescens*). Although isolates in a species have the same biochemical reactions, further laboratory classification of them can be made by immunological techniques and are based on their serological differences. Usually only a few strains in a species are the common agents of sepsis.

Escherichia coli, normally found in the colon, is the most prevalent gram-negative facultative bacterium. Thirty to 40 percent of gram-negative bacteremias (particularly in the young or in those who have recently had a urinary tract infection) and 85 percent of uncomplicated urinary tract infections are traceable to *E. coli*. Strains isolated from people outside the hospital tend to be sensitive to many antibiotics, while strains isolated from people inside the hospital tend to be resistant.

Klebsiella pneumoniae causes a large proportion of the respiratory and urinary tract infections. Strains that cause nosocomial infections [2] vary in their sensitivity to antibiotics, but most tend to be resistant. Recent epidemics have occurred with gentamicin-resistant strains. Systemic infections are common. They do not respond to carbenicillin, but they usually respond to cephalothin, cephaloridine, or cephalexin.

Aerobacter species, particularly *cloacae* and *aerogenes*, are notable problems in antibiotic-resistant nosocomial infections. All strains are resistant to cephalosporins and about one-third are resistant to kanamycin. The antibiotic of choice is usually gentamicin or tobramycin.

Pseudomonas aeruginosa infections are common, and the organism is introduced readily from the environment. It has both exotoxins and endotoxins, as well as proteolytic enzymes (in some strains). It is resistant to antibiotics, except gentamicin, carbenicillin, tobramycin, colistimethate, and polymyxin B. A polyvalent vaccine that produces active immunity has been developed and tested, but it is not available for widespread use. In many areas, strains not included in the vaccine have multiplied and caused serious problems. *Pseudomonas* is considered a water contaminant, and it is found wherever water stands or collects. The list of potential reservoirs includes sinks, sink traps, faucet aerators, tracheal catheter rinse solutions, bladder irrigation solutions, disinfectants, nail brushes, dishcloths, ventilators, fluids, local anesthetics, vegetables, and flowers. It is also frequently found on the hands and clothes of hospital personnel.

Proteus species are often involved in infections of wounds of the urinary and respiratory tracts and in decubitus ulcers, and they may cause gram-negative sepsis. *Proteus* infections are difficult to treat, and antibiotic therapy is usually discussed in terms of indole-positive and indole-negative *Proteus*, that is, by the ability or inability of the *Proteus* organism to form indole from the amino acid tryptophan. Indole-positive *Proteus* organisms have an increased resistance to antibiotics; but, fortunately, most *Proteus* infections are caused by indole-negative organisms (meningitis is a notable exception). Indole-negative *Proteus* organisms are usually sensitive to ampicillin and the aminoglycosides (kanamycin and gentamicin). Also, penicillin or the cephalosporins (cephalothin and cephalexin) may be ordered by the physician. In indole-positive *Proteus* infections, the aminoglycosides are the antibiotics of choice, but carbenicillin may be effective. Also usually considered with *Proteus* infections are *Providentia* species, particularly *P. stuartii*, which is often incriminated in postoperative ward infections, pneumonia, urinary tract infections, burn wound sepsis, and septicemia. In a few instances, overgrowth of the organism after therapy with sulfamylon has caused the death of all the patients in the critical care burn unit. Some species are resistant to all antibiotics, while others are occasionally sensitive to carbenicillin and the aminoglycosides.

Serratia marcescens is a motile gram-negative bacillus that is increasingly involved in infections, especially nosocomial infections. The most frequent problems it causes are urinary tract infections, bacteremia, and pulmonary infections. *S. marcescens* also was once considered nonpathogenic. It is a water contaminant and a soil contaminant. The red-pigmented strains are the most visible ones, but most strains are colorless. Most hospital-associated strains are very resistant; they have multiple resistances, even to gentamicin.

ANAEROBIC ORGANISMS

The increasing incidence of anaerobic infections, notably those caused by *Bacteroides* and *Fusobacterium* species, warrants a discussion. Quite probably, improved techniques for collecting and processing the specimens have contributed to the increased recognition of them. In some series, *Bacteroides* has specifically been noted in patients who have tumors of the gastrointestinal tract or phlebitis. In fact, some strains may actually contribute to the phlebitis through their ability to degrade heparin and other mucopolysaccharides. Ninety percent of the anaerobic bacteria found in the large intestine are *Bacteroides*. Bacteria of both genera are found in the mouth and in the gastrointestinal, respiratory, and urogenital tracts. The drug of choice with *B. fragilis* is usually clindamycin or chloramphenicol, but *Fusobacterium* is sensitive to most antibiotics, and the use of penicillin is indicated.

OPPORTUNISTIC INFECTIONS

Opportunistic infections are most commonly found in patients whose host defense mechanisms are compromised. The infections may be severe and may even precipitate the person's demise. Infections caused by fungi and even large viruses are considered opportunistic. As with bacterial infections, individual sensitivities must be established. The most common infections are caused by *Candida*, which grows when antibiotics are used; common sites are the mouth (thrush), esophagus, and cutaneous lesions, which can

be treated with nystatin. Systemic fungal infections (which are particularly likely to occur in the kidney) are treated with amphotericin B; the serum creatinine and blood urea nitrogen levels, the urinary pH, and the kidney's ability to concentrate urine must be monitored during treatment with that drug.

Microbial Factors

Microbial patterns of infection are in part determined by microbial density, sources of seeding, microbial virulence and invasiveness, microbial competition, and microbial resistance to therapeutic drugs [37]. The number of microorganisms present is determined by considering the area available and the bacterial load in that area. For example, a patient who has a burn that covers 80% of his body and a bacterial load of 10^5 organisms per gram of tissue has more bacteria than does a patient who has a burn that covers 10% of his body area and a bacterial load of 10^6 organisms per gram of tissue.

The ability of a microorganism to produce disease varies according to its virulence and its predilection for certain body areas. The term virulence refers to the organism's power to invade, and the more virulent organisms are the ones that infect patients a greater percentage of the time. But both virulence and pathogenicity are rather nebulous terms. The microbial world is ever changing, and many organisms that were once considered nonvirulent are now considered virulent.

The use of antibiotics can alter the endogenous microbial flora. Nonpathogenic bacteria may be able to maintain their balance and compete with antibiotic-resistant pathogenic bacteria, but they may be destroyed by antibiotics that allow resistant strains to proliferate. Resistance to antibiotics is most frequently caused by an enzyme the particular bacterium synthesizes. Either the antibiotic is destroyed by the enzyme or its conformational structure is altered so that ribosomal binding is no longer possible. Resistance also occurs after mutation in a mutant that is able to synthesize drug antagonists or essential metabolites.

Different patterns of organisms are seen in different institutions as well as in different parts of the same institution. The hospital's infection control committee knows what organisms are prevalent in the hospital and what their sensitivities are. Often the patterns of medical patients are different from those of surgical patients. Another aspect of bacterial growth is its cyclic variation, which is difficult to identify. Also, emerging pathogenic bacteria are usually seen by large medical centers before they are seen by smaller institutions, since it is particularly in the larger centers that new antibiotics are tested and resistance produced.

The transfer of R factors has recently been implicated in the transfer of antibiotic resistance from one bacterium to another [60]. The resistance is inherent in extrachromosomal pieces of DNA (variously called plasmids, episomes, genetic determinants, or resistance factors). Resistance is usually acquired by the process of transduction, but it may also be acquired by actual mating (conjugation), viral transmission, or transformation (direct entry of DNA). The transfer is usually made after two suitable bacteria come in contact and extend their pili to form a bridge of cytoplasm. The plasmid is replicated in the donor cell and transferred to the recipient cell. (A plasmid consists of two factors, one for drug resistance—the R determinant—and one for transmission of the R determinant—the resistance transfer factor, or the RTF.) Both bacteria must have both factors for transfer to occur.

Predisposing Factors

Hospital areas, including critical care units, are likely places for sepsis to occur. Host defense factors are especially important in hospitalized patients because immune defense mechanisms are depressed in people who are severely ill [1]. Pathogenic organisms, particularly *Staphylococcus* and gram-negative bacteria, are endemic in the hospital, and infections easily spread from their sources to the patient. Common sources of infection are other patients, the staff, the equipment, the air, and any moist areas. Control of the environment to prevent cross-contamination is a primary nursing responsibility.

Some of the important predisposing factors in infections are alcoholism, inadequate nutrition, extremes of age, and a serious associated disease, such as a cardiac, pulmonary, liver, or renal function disease. Other important factors, ones related to an accident or to the subsequent hospitalization, are shock, a retained bullet or other foreign body, prolonged preoperative hospitalization, preoperative antibiotic therapy, a preexisting infection, and chemotherapy, such as therapy with steroids or cytotoxic drugs. The most frequent predisposing factors in systemic sepsis are instrumentation of the urinary tract, central venous catheterization, and major surgical procedures. The use of invasive monitoring or treatment devices, particularly if they are kept in the patient too long, and the use of urinary catheters without closed drainage greatly increase the incidence of infection.

Another important predisposing factor is the wound [23]. The skin or mucous membrane is the body's first line of defense against disease, and in the traumatized person that defense is weakened. Wounds are frequently grossly contaminated with pathogenic organisms. Necrotic tissue must be debrided, and injured tissue must be given every chance to survive. The patient is prone to infection if his local blood supply is severely compromised by edema or hematomas and/or dead spaces (when foreign bodies remain in the wound). If the wound is sutured, the tissues should be apposed properly to prevent infection and facilitate healing.

Assessment

The classic signs and symptoms of infection—redness, swelling, heat, and tenderness (pain to the touch)—are local responses. The wound itself may look purulent.

The systemic signs of septicemia represent the total body response to invasive infection. Objective physical signs may also be present, depending on the underlying disease. For example, in peritonitis the patient's abdomen may be board-like; his abdominal muscles are kept in a state of tonic contraction to keep the inflamed peritoneum from moving.

The principal cellular response to bacterial infection is polymorphonuclear. In general, the more severe the infection, the greater the leukocytosis. The appearance of immature granulocytes, particularly at levels above 85 percent, or more than 15 to 20 stabs in the differential count are highly indicative of infection. That decrease in the ratio of segmented neutrophils to nonsegmented neutrophils is usually termed a shift to the left. In severely ill patients or in the elderly, the white blood cell count may be normal or even low. The leukopenia probably reflects exhaustion of the leukocyte supply as well as depression of the bone marrow.

The early signs of sepsis in the trauma patient are tachypnea, respiratory alkalosis, and an altered sensorium. The later signs are subjective feelings of severe illness, fever with shaking chills (rigors), perhaps with wide swings in the temperature, tachycardia, and oliguria. Blood cultures are only positive about 30% to 50% of the time; however, appropriate cultures of the sources will identify the specific invading microorganisms and determine the antibiotic sensitivities.

The first stage of sepsis is characterized by an increase in the cardiac output and in the blood flow to certain body parts although there is shunting of blood at other sites (e.g., the kidney and brain). The first stage may progress to septic shock (the second stage), which is characterized by a low cardiac output which progresses to death.

A significant causative factor in the patient's death may be an underlying disease, in which the patient's normal host defense mechanisms may have been impaired. In such a case, the functioning of the polymorphonuclear leukocytes may be so severely diminished (because of disease or chemotherapy) that they lose their ability to kill bacteria because (1) they cannot move toward the invading microorganisms, (2) they cannot phagocytize, and/or (3) they cannot produce hydrogen peroxide. Other important causative factors are the wrong choice of antibiotic for the initial treatment of sepsis and inadequate debridement or surgical drainage.

SEPTIC SHOCK

The incidence of septic shock has increased in the last 10 years, and the mortality has approached 50 percent. The incidence is increasing for the following reasons:

1. More—and more serious—operations are being performed on elderly patients and on poor-risk patients.
2. The incidence of severe trauma has increased.
3. The use of immunosuppressive drugs is widespread.
4. The development of virulent antibiotic-resistant microorganisms has increased.

It was once thought that gram-positive and gram-negative organisms produced different clinical syndromes, but it is now recognized that the infectious process is on a continuum and the clinical picture is dependent largely on the patient's volume status. From close observation of septic patients, MacLean and his associates [40] have identified and described two hemodynamic patterns: the normovolemic pattern and the hypovolemic pattern. Essentially, the clinical status of the patient proceeds from a normal volume status and respiratory alkalosis to a decreased volume status and metabolic acidosis.

In patients who were normovolemic before the onset of sepsis or who are in early septic shock, the pattern is characteristic but assessment remains difficult unless the staff is alert. For example, nurses in the recovery rooms will recognize the pattern correctly in the postoperative state as long as they are attuned to the problem. Basically the patient's circulatory status is hyperdynamic. Peripheral vasodilatation and/or A-V shunting increases the blood flow and results in an increased cardiac output. The body's demands are great, and the circulatory system is able to respond. Because of the vasodilatation, the patient has a low peripheral resistance and warm, dry extremities, and may have hypotension. The high cardiac index shows a normal to an increased blood volume, normal to high central venous pressures, and normal to high pulmonary artery pressures. On the other hand, high cardiac outputs and depressed cardiac functioning often are present at the same time. The hyperventilation and the resulting respiratory alkalosis (PCO_2 of < 25 mm Hg) are the hallmarks of the state. An even more altered sensorium, oliguria, and an elevated arterial lactate level indicate that the cardiac output must be increased. Control of the infection with surgical drainage and appropriate antibiotic therapy is of paramount importance.

In patients who are hypovolemic, the pattern is characterized by a hypodynamic circulation and by a clinical picture normally associated with shock. The hypovolemia may be the result of sequestration of fluid in a third space loss, for example, in the bowel or in muscle tissue (owing to poor tissue perfusion). Because of the vasoconstriction, the patient has a high peripheral resistance and cold, cyanotic extremities. The cardiac index is low, with a low cardiac output, low central venous pressures, and hypotension. Pulmonary artery pressures reflect the status of the left heart. The hallmark of frank shock is metabolic acidosis, but early in shock, the patient may still exhibit alkalosis. His temperature is usually very high or very low. With hypopyrexia of 95°F to 97°F, the body cannot generate a response, and a minimal reserve remains. The urinary output may remain elevated because of glycosuria (seen in trauma patients who have infections) and/or the catabolic state (associated with high nitrogen loads). Patients receiving parenteral nutrition often change from negative/negative to 3+/negative or 4+/negative on sugar acetone determinations when sepsis begins.

Endotoxin

Because the clinical problems caused by gram-negative infections are more prevalent and more severe than those caused by gram-positive infections, much of the literature is devoted to gram-negative infections. It is difficult to decipher the findings of much of the research, because the early research was based on endotoxin. It is now known that the syndrome differs when live bacteria are involved. Also, in the early research on hemodynamics, dogs and cats were the experimental models. The dog's heart is resistant to the early effects of endotoxin, and catecholamines have an inotropic action on the cat's heart, hiding a decrease in cardiac performance.

In all likelihood, the septic shock is initiated by endotoxins from the cell walls of gram-negative bacteria. The endotoxin molecule is a large lipopolysaccharide, and it inactivates or blocks the reticuloendothelial system. The blockade occurs after ingestible particles have saturated the receptor sites in the system, and it prevents further phagocytosis. The body may then be challenged by a minute number of microorganisms and be unable to respond.

Endotoxin has its major effect on the small blood vessels that have sympathetic innervation [35]. Changes are initiated by the endotoxin's acting as a sympathomimetic agent when it combines with antibody and complement. Associated with arteriolar and venular spasm is stagnant anoxia and pooling of blood in the pulmonary, splanchnic, and renal capillaries. The phenomena described in the discussion of hemorrhagic shock occur; namely, water and sodium move into the cell, potassium moves out of the cell, aerobic metabolism decreases, and lactic acid increases. But the time sequence may be much quicker in septic shock than in hemorrhagic shock, because the decrease in the formation of adenosine triphosphate results in a decreased synthesis of proteins and immunoglobulins. At the cellular level, the local accumulation of acid produces a relaxation of the arteriolar sphincters, and blood pools in the capillary bed. Plasma leaks into the interstitial fluid because of the increased hydrostatic pressure (see diagram). The syndrome is then perpetuated by the body's attempt

to compensate: the decrease in the blood volume decreases the cardiac output, which, in turn, decreases the systolic arterial pressure and stimulates the baroreceptors.

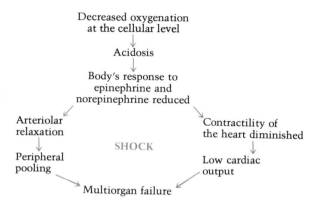

Cardiac Failure. When cardiac failure occurs is a matter of controversy. Some authorities say that cardiac failure occurs during the early or intermediate state of shock, and others say that it is terminal. In any event, the decreased arterial pressure progressively depresses the myocardium because it results in decreased coronary perfusion pressures and marginal blood flow [32]. It is recognized (1) that at some point pump failure is the chief hemodynamic problem and (2) that decreased venous return (due to the trapping of blood in the pulmonary and peripheral tissues) is not the chief hemodynamic problem.

The finding of several clinical studies of patients who did not have a preexisting cardiopulmonary disease was that as the heart failed as a pump, high cardiac output changed to low cardiac output. High central venous pressures and decreased myocardial functioning occurred when left ventricular stroke work values were low. The relationship between the two was a function of time [40, 56].

Further myocardial depression is added to poor coronary perfusion by the action of the myocardial depressant factor (MDF). Recently identified [4], MDF is present in septic shock, as well as in other forms of shock.

The findings from studies of endotoxin injected into rhesus monkey and baboon shock models [20, 26, 32, 35] suggest the following sequence. Cardiac depression begins during the early and intermediate states of shock. Within 30 minutes, pulmonary hypertension causes overloading of the right ventricle and increases in the right atrial and pulmonary artery pressures. Although the reason is not known, left ventricular changes also occur with increases in the pulmonary vein and left atrial pressures. For the next 90 minutes, the peripheral pooling increases so that the venous return and, in turn, the cardiac output decrease. During the next two to six hours, the intermediate stage of shock occurs, with the depression of pressure and stroke work. Adrenergic influences are strong; sympathetic stimulation and increases in plasma catecholamine levels occur. It follows that atrial and ventricular end-diastolic pressures are low. Thus even though cardiac performance seems normal, a heart that is only partially compensated does less work. When the model included therapeutic fluid loading in the intermediate stage, the underlying left ventricular dysfunctioning was indicated by the onset of left ventricular failure. What occurred was a rise in filling pressure that aimed to achieve a similar level of cardiac work (a shift to the right of the ventricular function curve). In one study the use of pulmonary artery wedge pressures to indicate left ventricular function, and thus avoid fluid overloading, was not useful due to concurrent conditions of left ventricular failure and hypervolemia [32]. When values predicted from pulmonary artery wedge pressures were used, the left ventricular end-diastolic pressure was greatly underestimated (by as much as 50%).

It is thought that during the next four to eight hours, as shock deepens cardiac contractility and compliance are depressed. The relationships among the right atrial pressure, left atrial pressure, left ventricular end-diastolic pressure, cardiac output, and mean arterial pressure become abnormal since the ventricular filling pressures have increased proportionately to the depressed myocardial workload. Myocardial depression is the result of decreased coronary perfusion and myocardial edema, along with diminished sympathetic influences and plasma catecholamine levels.

Modalities of Therapy

Medical patients and surgical patients are usually treated differently. Surgical patients are treated freely with antibiotics. The surgeon may not know the cause of sepsis, and often he does not have time to find the cause because the patient's condition is precarious. The aim is prevention, and if prevention is not possible, the aims are removal of the seeding source and debridement of all nonviable tissue and adequate drainage. Viable tissue is preserved for three to five days and then covered and sutured or allowed to heal by second intention.

Because antibiotics have proved effective for preventing infection, even in contaminated wounds following trauma, antibiotic therapy is begun in the emergency room preoperatively. Thus the antibiotic is present in the blood and the operative site during the operation. Alexander [3] demonstrated that the concentration of antibiotic appeared more promptly in the wound fluid when the drug was first administered by intravenous push. Sustained high therapeutic levels were achieved most easily by giving additional intramuscular injections to patients not in shock and by giving continuous intravenous infusions to hypotensive patients. Alexander also demonstrated that when early antibiotic therapy was not possible, the best antibiotics for delayed therapy were ampicillin, penicillin, the cephalosporins, and the tetracyclines.

Unless the results of cultures and sensitivity studies are available for the specific organisms, the physician often orders antibiotic coverage for both aerobic and anaerobic organisms. The combination of penicillin and gentamicin is the most common one. The choice depends on the results of previous cultures, the tissue or organ involved, the circumstances of the injury, the normal flora of the environment, and the resistance patterns. Once the results of cultures and sensitivity studies are available, the specific antibiotics are ordered.

TREATMENT FOR SEPTIC SHOCK

The treatment of septic shock centers on its early recognition, the restoration of normal hemodynamics, the identification of the septic source, the removal of the seeding source, and the appropriate antibiotic therapy.

The most meaningful physiological measurement is the cardiac output. Other physiological parameters may be altered considerably: the blood pressure is decreased, the central venous pressure may be high or low, the arterial oxygenation may be high or low, and the urinary output often remains elevated because of the associated glycosuria (however, it can also be very low). Elevated arterial lactate levels reflect poor perfusion. They may be high because circulation to the tissue buffers is compromised and buffering of the acid generated inside and outside the cell is poor.

Plasma volumes are measured, because the patient may be in hypovolemic shock from fluid sequestered in a third space.

Restoration of the Circulating Blood Volume

Restoration of an effective circulating blood volume and correction of the disturbances in the peripheral circulation are of primary importance in the treatment of the shock state. The patient may suffer from vasoconstriction or from vasodilatation, but probably he suffers from vasodilatation. His vascular tree has dilated, and the amount of circulating fluid must be increased to fill the vascular spaces. Also, the sequestration of plasma and extracellular fluid (the third space loss) that happens in peritonitis and soft tissue infections increases the patient's fluid requirements. Replacement therapy involves the use of crystalloid solutions, plasma, and blood.

Ringer's lactate solution (rather than low molecular weight dextran) is usually chosen for volume replacement therapy. In addition to the controversy revolving about crystalloid versus colloid therapy, the use of dextran carries the risk of bleeding and anaphylaxis to the trauma patient. Although it is generally agreed that once the patient has an adequate circulating volume his acid-base balance reverts to normal, that is not always the case in septic shock. In septic shock, more base, in the form of sodium bicarbonate, may have to be administered to maintain the pH at an acceptable level. The hemoglobin level is kept at 12.5 to 14 gm/100 ml for optimal oxygenation and an improved intravascular volume. Although albumin may be indicated in selected instances, the molecule is quickly connected to sugar if the patient is nutritionally depleted. Also, albumin moves into the interstitial spaces in the lung and it is followed by water, thus increasing the likelihood of respiratory failure.

Supportive Measures

Oxygen administration is often needed to keep the arterial PO_2 between 80 mm Hg and 100 mm Hg [11]. The risk of pulmonary failure is significant, and the patient may need assisted ventilation (see Chap. 17).

Diuretics are often given to promote the renal flow, but they are given at the expense of the volume status.

A digitalis drug is given for specific purposes as an inotropic agent, but it is dangerous if the patient has hypokalemia or is receiving isoproterenol. Also, the appropriate dose of digoxin is based on the patient's electrolyte levels and his acid-base balance, and the drug's peak action does not occur until one hour after its administration. The digitalizing level may be one half that normally seen, and the drug is usually administered intravenously in multiple small doses.

Steroid Administration

The use of steroids as an adjunct measure has long been highly controversial, because it has been difficult to obtain solid evidence of the beneficial effects of steroids. Most authorities use steroids in their clinical practices because the possible benefits of steroid therapy far outweigh its possible harmful effects. The double-blind randomized study by Schumer [53] has shown a significantly lower overall mortality and complication rate in the steroid-treated group than in the control group, but other workers have done identical studies in which no differences between the two groups were shown. However, Schumer's definition of septic shock, and thus his group of patients, differed from that of many authorities.

Several improvements follow administration of steroid therapy. Steroids improve the cardiac index by increasing and normalizing the cardiac output, and by decreasing the peripheral resistance. The decrease in arteriolar and venular resistance is particularly important in the lungs, kidneys, and intestines. The serum levels of lactic acid, amino acids, and phosphate are decreased, and the pH is increased. The microcirculatory flow and the tissue perfusion seem to be increased. Benefits at the cellular level include the improvement of gluconeogenesis, the acceleration of energy production, and a decrease in acidosis caused by an increase in lactic acid metabolism.

The actual mechanism of the steroid action in septic shock is not known, but several hypotheses have been offered:

1. The steroid action may be primarily immunological in that steroids interfere with the complement reaction, and the release of autocoids, histamines, and serotonin is decreased. The interaction of endotoxin and complement is the initiating factor in the production of autocoids, which essentially cause the shock syndrome by producing the third space loss. Large doses of steroids administered early at the time of diagnosis inhibit the interaction of endotoxin and complement and thus interfere with the release of autocoids. Early administration of steroids is mandatory, because

once complement and endotoxin interact, autocoids have been released and repeated doses of steroids are ineffective.

2. In sepsis and septic shock, the gluconeogenic cycle is inhibited, and steroids decrease that inhibition somewhat.
3. Steroids help prevent the release of endotoxin.
4. Steroids improve tissue perfusion by venous vasoconstriction with peripheral pooling.
5. Steroids improve cellular metabolism by assisting the impaired mitochondrial respiration.
6. Steroids prevent cellular injury (a convincing hypothesis). (Probably steroids maintain membrane integrity and prevent the release of lysosomal enzymes.)
7. Steroids (a) increase the pH gradient and correct the intracellular hypokalemia in the transfused red blood cell, (b) return low P_{50} toward normal, and (c) replenish 2,3-DPG levels.

Three basic principles of steroid therapy are [49, 53]:

1. The effects of steroid therapy in septic shock occur in the first 24 hours after administration.
2. Prolonged corticosteroid therapy has deleterious effects in that the patient's susceptibility to bacterial and fungal diseases is increased.
3. Large doses of steroids are given for short-term steroid therapy.

Vasoactive Drugs
The vasoactive drugs are extremely useful in septic shock, but all have problems in clinical use. The vasoactive drugs used initially were the vasopressor or vasoconstrictor drugs that increased pressures but not perfusion. The drugs that were used next were the vasodilators, such as isoproterenol. Unfortunately, vasodilators increase the total body perfusion, but skeletal muscle is the primary beneficiary of the increased cardiac output rather than the brain, heart, kidney, and intestines. The perfusion of vital tissues is improved by (1) the reduction of arteriolar resistance in vital organs, (2) the augmentation of perfusion pressures, (3) the increase of cardiac output, and (4) the prevention of the deleterious effects of underperfusion [39].

In patients in septic shock who have had a myocardial infarction, a balance must be maintained between the increased myocardial perfusion and the in-

creased oxygen demand in the heart. The choice of drug depends on the needs and condition of the specific patient.

Most of the drugs used act on the sympathetic nervous system or the cells innervated by the sympathetic nervous system. The baroreceptors respond to any event that lowers blood pressure for whatever reason. The sympathetic nerve centers in the hypothalamus are activated through the ninth and tenth cranial nerves. The results are increased epinephrine secretion in the adrenal medulla, increased cortisol production in the adrenal cortex, and increased norepinephrine secretion in the sympathetic norepinephrine endings. The sympathetic nervous system is an efferent motor system. It is located primarily in the thoracolumbar region, and it regulates the cardiac, smooth muscle, and exocrine functioning. Axons of the sympathetic nervous system synapse in the vertebral ganglia and collectively innervate various organs. Since they are in the ganglia, they can be activated rapidly and simultaneously. Synaptic transmission at most postganglionic terminals is carried out by norepinephrine, and so these terminals are called adrenergic. Sympathomimetic drugs may act directly on the receptor sites, or they may act indirectly by releasing norepinephrine from the adrenergic nerves. Conceptual structures (called alpha and beta receptors) are used to describe changes that occur in the precapillary and postcapillary arterioles and venules. Alpha-receptor stimulation by epinephrine and norepinephrine produces arteriolar and venular vasoconstriction that results in reduced capillary perfusion. Alpha-adrenergic responses are excitatory responses (except for intestinal inhibition), and they promote vasoconstriction and pupillary dilatation. Beta-receptor stimulation produces vasodilatation in the vasculature of striated muscle and myocardium, resulting in an increased rate and force of cardiac contraction (a positive chronotropic effect and a positive inotropic effect, respectively). The beta response mediates vasodilatation, bronchodilatation, and most metabolic responses. B_1 is the designation given to the myocardial beta receptor, and B_2 is the designation given to the vascular and bronchodilatation beta receptor.

Vasoactive drugs are used to treat (1) patients whose blood pressure is too low for perfusion of the heart and the brain and (2) patients whose blood pressure is high enough to permit cardiac and cerebral perfusion of the heart and the brain but whose blood flow to the viscera (in particular, the mesenteric and the renal vascular beds) is significantly reduced [16]. The drugs that act directly on the alpha receptors contract both arterioles and veins with little specificity. The drugs that act indirectly activate both alpha and beta receptors.

Action of Specific Drugs. Methoxamine (Vasoxyl) mainly acts directly on the alpha receptors and produces vasoconstriction. It is not useful in shock due to pump failure, because it increases both left and right atrial pressures and left ventricular work.

Metaraminol (Aramine) indirectly causes the release of norepinephrine by sympathetic nerve terminals so that action of metaraminol approximates that of norepinephrine. Patients who have an elevated cardiac output and hypotension due to decreased peripheral resistance may benefit from metaraminol since the increase in resistance and the slight increase in the cardiac output it causes may raise their blood pressure and improve their blood flow.

Norepinephrine acts as a vasoconstrictor in the peripheral circulation because of its direct action on the alpha receptors in the arteries and veins, and it acts as a cardiac stimulator because of its direct action on the B_1 receptors. The cerebral and coronary vessels dilate but the renal and the splanchnic vessels, as well as the vessels in the skin and the muscles, constrict. The potential for renal failure is significant. The drug must be given by a central venous catheter, because the local vasoconstriction it causes in an extremity is severe enough to lead to amputation. Even though the myocardium is stimulated, the cardiac output does not necessarily increase. The peripheral vasoconstriction is so intense that the heart slows reflexly and thus the cardiac output is decreased. On the other hand, if the patient is in severe shock, his blood pressure may not be increased above normal levels, but his cardiac output increases.

Epinephrine acts directly on the B_1, B_2, and alpha receptors. The myocardium is stimulated, and the vessels in the skeletal muscles and the mesentery dilate. In accordance with the response expected from alpha stimulation, the vessels in the skin and the kidney vasoconstrict. As in the fight-or-flight response, the blood flow increases, many areas of the body vasodilate, the peripheral resistance decreases, and the cardiac output increases.

Isoproterenol is a nearly pure stimulant of the beta receptors. It produces inotropic and chronotropic cardiac stimulation, vasodilatation, particularly in the blood vessels of the skeletal muscles, and bronchodilatation. The cardiac output increases while the blood pressure stays the same or diminishes slightly. Although isoproterenol has a vasodilating effect, it is not selective in the intestines and kidney. The total body vasodilatation produces a decrease in the perfusion pressure that may decrease the blood flow to these key organs at any time. The increase in the myocardial work produces an increase in the myocardial oxygen consumption that is satisfactory only as long as the increased work produces increased perfusion of the total body, including the heart. The drug may significantly improve the cardiac output of patients whose pulse is slow. Tachycardia from the drug's chronotropic effect is a distinct possibility, and the pulse must be monitored and kept below 120 to 130 beats per minute. Dysrhythmias and hypotension are also potential complications. The most effective way to administer the drug is to start with doses of 0.15 to 0.6 μgm per minute and titrate the dose up until the desired response is obtained.

Dopamine, the newest and most useful drug, produces beta stimulation of the heart, alpha stimulation of the peripheral circulation, and vasodilatation in the cerebral, coronary, mesenteric, and renal circulation. It is an endogenous catecholamine, the precursor of norepinephrine, and the metabolite of L-dopa. The drug's important selective vasodilatation effect is due to its action on the dopamine receptors. The total blood flow, as well as the cardiac output and the blood pressure, is increased. The specific action is dependent on the dose administered. In small doses (2–5 μgm/kg/min), the selective vasodilatation effect just described is called the dopaminergic effect. Cholinergic alpha and/or beta blockers do not have that effect, but phenothiazines diminish the effect. In intermediate doses (5–15 μgm/kg/min), the drug's beta-adrenergic effects are equivalent to those of norepinephrine, epinephrine, and isoproterenol. The mean arterial pressures usually stay at the same level because of the increased strength of the cardiac contractions. The cardiac output continues to increase. Tachyarrhythmias are a potential complication, but they occur infrequently since the heart rates do not usually increase. In high doses (30–40 μgm/kg/min), dopamine has an alpha receptor effect. Since the vasoconstrictive effects are most prominent, the cardiac output decreases, and the potential for tachyarrhythmias increases.

Monitoring

After the patient has been given initial care in the emergency department, he is transferred to the operating room and then to the critical care unit. (Or he may be sent directly from the emergency room to the critical care unit.) Accurate monitoring by the primary care nurse to determine trends and assess the patient's changing status is vital. Whether the patient's condition is stable, unstable, or critical, data are needed, particularly about oxygenation, organ perfusion, and hemodynamic status.

Stable Patient

If the patient's condition is stable, his vital signs are checked every 15 minutes at first and then at longer intervals. The most important indicators of the patient's condition are his sensorium and his hourly urinary output. His urinary output and renal blood flow are dependent on his cardiac output.

The presence and description of arterial pressure pulses provide a reliable parameter for assessing mechanical failure of the heart. The toe-ambient temperature gradient is likewise reliable for assessing perfusion failure. When cardiac output is reduced, the blood flow to the skin (e.g., big toe) is even more reduced. A reduction in skin temperature as related to ambient temperature suffices to ascertain the reduction in skin flow.

The sphygmomanometer can be used to make an adequate measurement of the patient's arterial pressure. A decrease in the pulse pressure and an increase in the diastolic pressure usually precede a decrease in the systolic pressure. The pulse pressure is related to stroke volume and the distensibility of the aorta, and so many authorities consider a decrease in the pulse pressure an indicator of a decrease in the stroke volume. The degree of vasoconstriction correlates with the increase in the diastolic pressure.

The amount and rate of blood flow are determined largely by mechanical properties. The difference in pressure between the proximal end and the distal end of a vessel essentially determines the blood flow. The size of the lumen is particularly important to the rate of flow in that the rate of flow in a vessel is directly proportional to the fourth power of its radius (Poiseuille's law). The amount of blood that flows through a vessel for a certain period of time is equal to the velocity of the flow multiplied by the area of the

cross-section. As the circulatory system proceeds from the aorta to the capillary beds, the area of the cross-section increases and the rate of the flow decreases. The inverse proportion ranges from an area of 2 to 5 sq cm and a rate of flow of 30 to 35 cm per second (in the aorta) to an area of 1500 to 2000 sq cm and a rate of flow of about 0.5 cm per second (in the capillary beds). Other factors are resistance, viscosity, the tone of the precapillary sphincter, and the tissue oxygenation.

Unstable Patient

If the patient's condition is not stable, monitoring of his ECG and his central venous pressure is added to the other types of monitoring. Most important is the serial measurement of his blood gases (see Chaps. 17 and 20).

The use of serial central venous pressure readings has been endorsed but then criticized by authorities. Yet the readings taken from a catheter placed in the superior vena cava or in the right atrium yield critical data about the amount of blood coming into the right heart and the ability of the right heart to pump the blood. (The right atrial pressures do not reflect the functioning of the left heart.)

One of the very best measures of perfusion failure is the arterial blood lactate. Since the degree of lactic acidosis correlates with the severity of the oxygen deficit, the arterial blood lactate level essentially quantitates the oxygen deficit (and so, the degree of shock or perfusion failure).

Critically Unstable Patients

In a patient who is critically unstable, the monitoring is altered to make use of more sensitive and accurate devices in order to titrate therapy. Unfortunately, many of the devices used are invasive, and they bring risks as well as advantages to the patient. Perfusion of the brain and kidney remains a valuable indicator. Unless other conditions are present, restlessness, confusion, and disorientation indicate a critical state, perhaps shock. The hourly urinary output should be kept within normal limits (about 50 ml/hr). Also osmolality, the sodium concentration, and the ratio of blood urea to urine urea must be monitored. A decreased urine sodium concentration and an increased urine osmolality are early indicators of shock, and a decreased urine volume is a later or a more sudden indicator of shock.

KIDNEY PERFUSION

Blood flow to the kidney and the kidney functioning are interrelated. Vasoconstriction of the renal arterioles results from a decrease in renal pressure or blood pressure and thus reduces blood flow through the glomerulus and glomerular filtrate. In shock, the juxtamedullary portions of the cortex receive more blood than the outer cortex does, but the glomerular filtration rate is even further reduced since fewer glomeruli are present in the juxtamedullary portions. The end result is a more concentrated urine since a decreased amount of filtrate reaches the renal tubules, requiring an increased uptake of sodium in the loop of Henle.

Likewise the juxtaglomerular apparatus is stimulated—by the decreased arteriolar pulse pressure (perfusion pressure) and the decreased sodium concentration in the distal tubule—to release renin, a proteolytic enzyme. Then using a glycoprotein plasma precursor (angiotensinogen), renin catalyzes the formation of angiotensin I which, in turn, is converted to angiotensin II by a substance called converting enzyme. The result is an increased production and release of aldosterone from the adrenal cortex as well as additional vasoconstriction. Aldosterone, in turn, enhances the renal retention of sodium and water.

Another response that further complicates the mechanism is the release of antidiuretic hormone (ADH) from the posterior pituitary by changes in the plasma osmolality, a decreased left atrial filling pressure, and an increased baroreceptor response. The absorption of water from the distal and collecting tubules increases.

As a general measure, the physician withholds the administration of potassium for about 24 hours after surgery. The reason is obvious if the patient is in frank renal failure, but it is not so obvious if the patient has borderline renal functioning. The glomerular blood flow and filtration rate may fall in the patient who has a volume deficit, and hyperkalemia may result. The administration of potassium to a patient who has high-output failure characterized by increased urine volumes and increased blood urea nitrogen levels may precipitate the development of hyperkalemia. Even if the patient has hypokalemia, his supplementation does not usually exceed 40 mEq of potassium chloride per hour, and the nurse must monitor carefully for the clinical and ECG signs of potassium intoxication.

Perfusion is poor, with a urine osmolality–serum osmolality ratio of greater than 1.2:1 and a urinary sodium level of less than 10 to 20 mEq per liter.

If the ratio of blood urea to urine urea is 1:20 or greater, the kidney functioning is normal. If the ratio is 1:10, the patient is considered to have prerenal or functional acute renal failure. If the ratio is 1:5 or lower, the patient has organic renal failure (unless, of course, he is in clinical shock and is being treated with vasopressors). Since determining the patient's status is of paramount importance for the patient whose ratio is 1:20 to 1:5, a challenge test with Ringer's lactate solution often is ordered by the physician. In the challenge test, 1000 ml of Ringer's lactate solution is administered in 30 to 60 minutes. If the kidneys are functioning, the response improves, but in frank renal failure, the kidneys cannot respond and the ratio is unchanged.

VITAL SIGNS

Monitoring the vital signs is important, but the information obtained must be evaluated in terms of the individual patient. The body's mechanisms for maintaining temperature may be changed, and the temperature may be very high or very low. Hypothermia blankets can be used to achieve normothermic levels.

Palpation of the pulse at the radial artery is difficult, and palpation at the carotid or femoral artery is recommended. In selected instances (and combined with other measures), the carotid and femoral sites are used to estimate the pulse volume and the mean arterial pressure.

The arterial pressure measurement obtained with the sphygmomanometer is not necessarily accurate; mean arterial pressures are often measured with an intraarterial catheter. As the stroke volume falls, the Korotkoff sounds become increasingly difficult to hear, and a wide variation in the blood pressure readings occurs. Although the great majority of patients whose Korotkoff sounds are quiet have low blood pressure, that is not necessarily the case. A Doppler ultrasonic flowmeter may be used to hear the arterial flow.

Since the mean arterial pressure is related more to blood flow than to sound, an intraarterial catheter is used to identify trends and assess changes. Usually the measurement is made with an electronic transducer and monitor, but the saline flush method may also be used. The transducer converts the mechanical pressures of the pulses to electrical impulses, which are transmitted to the bedside monitor. The pressure is seen as a waveform on the oscilloscope.

The line is generally used also to obtain samples to measure the arterial blood gases, and it is kept patent by an arterial flush system. Although the catheter may be placed in the femoral or axillary artery, the radial artery is the most common site for placement of a catheter that may remain for 48 to 72 hours.

RESPIRATORY MONITORING

The monitoring should focus on changes in the respiratory rate and, especially, changes in depth, in the alveolar ventilation, and in the arterial PCO_2. The minute ventilation increases remarkably with tachypnea and respiratory alkalosis, a nonspecific response that occurs in early shock. If shock continues, metabolic acidosis becomes the primary mechanism, and the body attempts to compensate with hyperventilation.

The serial assessment of the arterial blood gases must consider the inspired oxygen concentration, the alterations in oxygenation, the pH, the PCO_2, and calculation of base excess. It must be emphasized that raising the hemoglobin from 10 to 12 mg/100 ml does much more for total oxygenation than does raising the percentage of inspired oxygen. Assessment of the patient's respiratory status is discussed further (in Chapters 9 and 17). In general, the following parameters are monitored in the critically ill patient [11, 25]:

1. Ventilation
   a. Respiratory rate
   b. Tidal volume
   c. Vital capacity
   d. Forced expiratory volume
   e. Functional residual capacity
   f. Inspiratory force
   g. Dead space ventilation (VD-TV ratio)
   h. Lung compliance
   i. Chest x-ray results
   j. Partial pressures of oxygen and carbon dioxide in the arterial blood
2. Alveolar Capillary Gas Exchange
   a. Oxyhemoglobin saturation
   b. Partial pressure of oxygen in arterial blood
   c. Fraction of inspired oxygen (FiO_2)
   d. A-a oxygen gradient ($P[A-a]O_2$)

   e. Pulmonary venoarterial shunt
   f. Pulmonary vascular resistance (PVR)
3. Perfusion and Tissue Oxygenation
   a. Arterial oxygen content
   b. Mixed venous oxygen content
   c. A-V oxygen content difference ($C[a-v]O_2$)
   d. P_{50}
   e. Central venous pressure
   f. Mean pulmonary artery pressure
   g. Pulmonary capillary wedge pressure
   h. Cardiac output
   i. Oxygen delivery
   j. Pulmonary vascular resistance

PULMONARY ARTERY PRESSURES

Left ventricular end-diastolic pressure (LVEDP) can be estimated by the use of the Swan-Ganz catheter [63, 64]. That method of measurement has four advantages for the patient in shock: (1) it permits the measurement of the pulmonary arterial, diastolic, and wedge pressures, (2) it permits the continuous monitoring of the pulmonary arterial systolic and mean pressures, (3) it permits the sampling of mixed venous blood for the measurement of the A-V oxygen differences, and (4) it permits an estimate to be made of the cardiac output by the thermodilution method. From these measurements, numerous cardiovascular parameters may be obtained from calculations on a digital calculator (Table 36-2). Myocardial function is thus evaluated in terms of preload, contractility, and afterload.

Mitral regurgitation (commonly caused by a papillary muscle dysfunction after a myocardial infarction) may be diagnosed by the appearance of a tall, peaked V wave on the pulmonary wedge pressure tracing. A ventricular septal defect (commonly cuased by a ruptured ventricular septum following a myocardial infarction) may be diagnosed by the presence of pulmonary artery hypertension and an oxygen saturation that is higher in blood samples taken from the pulmonary artery than in samples taken from the right atrium. Cardiac tamponade is evidenced by pressures that are approximately equal in the right atrium and the pulmonary wedge positions (in contrast to the normal difference of 7 mm Hg).

PULMONARY CAPILLARY WEDGE PRESSURE

The best pressure measurement for evaluating cardiac compensation and blood volume is the LVEDP. Un-

Table 36-2

Common Parameters Measured When Monitoring Critically Ill Patients

Central venous pressure (CVP) mm Hg = CVP cm H_2O/1.36

Mean arterial pressure = arterial diastolic pressure + ⅓ (arterial systolic pressure − arterial diastolic pressure)

Mean pulmonary arterial pressure = pulmonary arterial diastolic pressure + ⅓ (pulmonary arterial systolic pressure − pulmonary arterial diastolic pressure)

Cardiac index (in Lpm/sq m) = cardiac output (CO) (in Lpm)/body surface area (BSA) (in sq m, as calculated by height and weight)

Stroke volume (SV) = CO/heart rate

Stroke index = (ml/beats/sq m) = SV/BSA

Right ventricular stroke work (RVSW) = SV × (mean pulmonary arterial pressure − CVP mm Hg) × 13.6

Left ventricular stroke work (LVSW) = SV × (mean arterial pressure − wedge pressure) × 13.6

Stroke work ratio = RVSW/LVSW

Systemic vascular resistance (SVR) = ([mean arterial pressure − CVP mm Hg]/CO) × 80

Pulmonary vascular resistance (PVR) = ([mean pulmonary arterial pressure − wedge pressure]/CO) × 80

SVR index = SVR/BSA

PVR index = PVR/BSA

Starling point (SP) (left) = LVSW/wedge pressure

SP (right) = RVSW/CVP mm Hg

SP ratio = SP left/SP right

Filling ratio = CVP mm Hg/wedge pressure

Arterial oxygen content = Hgb × percent arterial saturation × 1.39 + arterial PO_2 × 0.003

Venous oxygen content = Hgb × percent venous saturation × 1.39 + venous PO_2 × 0.003

A-V oxygen content difference = arterial content − venous content

Oxygen delivery = arterial content × 10 × CO

Oxygen consumption = A-V oxygen content difference × CO × 10

Oxygen utilization = oxygen consumption/oxygen delivery

Shunt = ([capillary content − arterial content]/[capillary content − venous content]) × 100

less the patient has mitral valve disease, his left atrial pressure (LAP) correlates significantly with his LVEDP. The pulmonary venous pressure is closely related to the LAP, and it is the primary factor in the transfer of fluid from the pulmonary venous bed into the interstitial spaces and the alveoli, as well as the primary determinant of pulmonary congestion. When the pulmonary venocapillary pressure is higher than the plasma oncotic pressure, interstitial pulmonary edema results. If the increased volume load cannot be reduced by drainage of the interstitial lymphatic system, alveolar edema results. The critical capillary pressure point is the point at which the pulmonary capillary pressure exceeds the plasma oncotic pressure and produces transudation of the interstitial fluid. In acute illnesses, pulmonary capillary wedge pressures (PCWPs) up to 14 mm Hg, and most often up to 18 mm Hg, are not associated with pulmonary edema in acute illness. In patients who have myocardial infarctions, the pulmonary capillary wedge pressures are maintained at 16 to 18 to 20 mm Hg; the upper limit in pulmonary edema is 25 mm Hg.

In most patients, the PCWP accurately reflects the LAP and the pulmonary venous pressure. If the level is below approximately 15 mm Hg, mean pulmonary capillary wedge pressure approximates the LVEDP.

The PCWP is recorded when the tip of the balloon flotation catheter wedges into a branch of the pulmonary vascular tree. Blood flow in that segment of the lung is momentarily stopped by the distended balloon. Since the column of blood is static, pressure is transmitted from the pulmonary veins, the nearest active circulatory bed [7]. An analogy may be made between that phenomenon and that of a pipe closed at both ends. If there is no flow through the pipe, the pressures at each end should be the same. The magnitude and contour of the pressure wave closely reflects the pressure in the pulmonary veins.

For a more thorough understanding of the ramifications of those measurements, attention must be paid to cardiovascular performance. Ventricular function curves for the right ventricle and left ventricle have been constructed to evaluate ventricular performance by relating the energy of contraction to the length of the end-diastolic fibers. Ventricular stroke work (SW) has been plotted against the mean atrial or end-diastolic filling pressures. As the mean atrial pressures increase, the ventricular SW rises and reaches a plateau at higher filling pressures. A shift of the curve to the right indicates a downward movement and a decrease in SW at higher filling pressures. A shift to the left indicates an upward shift of the curve and an increase in myocardial contractility. Also, in critically ill patients, the central venous pressure (the right-sided filling pressure) must be related to the right ventricular performance, and the PCWP must be related to the left ventricular performance.

Changes in the PCWP trends usually may be traced to one or more of the following phenomena: (1) poor myocardial contractility, (2) left atrial overload, (3) increased pulmonary vascular resistance, (4) airway pressure changes, (5) intrathoracic extra-airway pressure changes, and/or (6) improper placement of the intrathoracic balloon. The mean PCWP directly determines fluid transfer at the pulmonary capillary level and pulmonary congestion. Changes in the PCWP are closely related to lung changes shown on an x ray.

PULMONARY ARTERY END-DIASTOLIC PRESSURE

In patients who do not have increased pulmonary vascular resistance (PVR) and who have normal left ventricular function, the pulmonary artery end-diastolic pressure closely approximates the PCWP. Differences between the two pressures are particularly apparent in patients who have had myocardial infarctions and elevated PVRs, a too-rapid transfusion of blood, tachycardia above 120, severe hypoxemia, and pulmonary edema from noncardiac causes. The normal pulmonary vascular resistance is 200 dyne-sec cm^{-5}, and it may be calculated by subtracting the PCWP from the mean pulmonary artery pressure and dividing the answer by the cardiac output. Interestingly, the presence of an underlying pulmonary disease may be detected by determining the gradient between the PCWP and the pulmonary artery diastolic pressure. A gradient of greater than 5 mm Hg suggests the presence of pulmonary disease [11].

PULMONARY ARTERY MEAN PRESSURE

Increased mean pulmonary artery pressures are usually the result of left-to-right shunts that cause an increased pulmonary blood flow and an increased pulmonary hemocapillary or left atrial pressure. Massive thromboembolism, embolism in the smaller arterioles, atelectasis, or severe hypoxia may acutely alter the flow and elevate the mean pressure but not the PCWP.

FLOW-DIRECTED CATHETER

The catheter most often used today is a flow-directed catheter that has multiple lumens. The catheter is passed into the pulmonary artery, usually via a central vein. (Although previously recommended, the peripheral insertion site is now considered less optimal because it is more prone to changes in catheter tip location and to early thrombosis.) As in the introduction of all central catheters, the Trendelenburg position is used (1) to facilitate location of the vein by en-

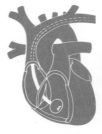
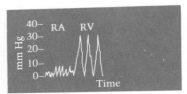

Right ventricular pressure

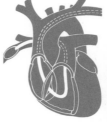
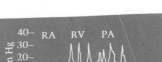

Pulmonary arterial pressure

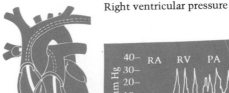
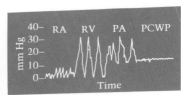

Pulmonary capillary wedge pressure

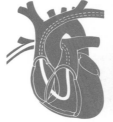
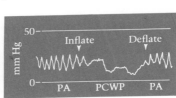

Pulmonary arterial pressure and pulmonary capillary wedge pressure

Figure 36-3
Pressure tracings with pulmonary artery catheter.

gorgement of vessels and (2) to prevent air embolism. After the insertion of a 14-gauge catheter, a guidewire is inserted four to five inches to allow removal of the catheter. An introducer is passed over the guidewire, and the inner sheath and the guidewire are removed. The Swan-Ganz catheter is then inserted through the external sheath.

The location of the catheter is verified by the pressure tracings shown on the oscilloscope (Fig. 36-3).

made of the number of 100-ml increments that passed through the peripheral tissues in that time. For example, if 4 cc of oxygen is given up by 100 ml of blood and 200 cc of oxygen is taken up in one minute, 5 liters, or 50 increments of 100 ml of blood, flowed through the peripheral tissues during that minute. An accurate determination of oxygen uptake necessarily involves an arterial blood sample, a mixed venous blood sample (preferably from the pulmonary artery), and a three-minute sample of expired air.

$$\text{Cardiac output} \atop \text{(Total flow in ml/min)} = \frac{\text{total oxygen uptake}}{\text{A-V O}_2 \text{ difference}} \times 100$$
$$\text{(or cc oxygen given up)}$$

$$\text{Cardiac output} = \frac{200}{4} \times 100$$

Indocyanine green is the dye most commonly used because (1) it does not stimulate the cardiovascular system, (2) it is rapidly removed from the circulation, and (3) its effect on the density of the blood is not affected by the hemoglobin saturation. The dye, or indicator, is rapidly injected into the right atrium or central vein, and its dilution concentration is measured using an arterial line. An indicator dilution curve can be plotted using data gathered from continuous analysis of the dilution concentration. For example, if 5 mg of dye is injected and if an average concentration of 5 mg per liter is measured in the arterial sample over a 10-sec interval, 1 liter of blood will flow by during the 10 sec. The calculated cardiac output is 5 liters per minute.

ANALYSIS OF ARTERIAL PULSE CURVE

Analysis of the central arterial pulse curve provides continuous monitoring of the cardiac output in critical care units that have a computer to perform the necessary calculations. One catheter is passed percutaneously into a central vein, and a second catheter is introduced into the radial artery and passed to the vicinity of the aortic arch. The impulses are transferred to the computer by an arterial transducer. On the oscilloscope at the patient's bedside are displayed the cardiac output, stroke volume, heart rate, duration of systole, systemic vascular resistance, and arterial blood pressure (systolic, diastolic, and mean). In studies that compared the indicator-dilution technique to the dye-dilution technique and the direct Fick calculations, the results were within 10 percent of one another [14].

Essentially, the computer multiplies the stroke volume by the pulse rate to determine the cardiac output. One measurement arrived at by the indicator-dilution techniques is needed to determine a standard (or baseline) for the calculations. Stroke volume consists of forward blood flow, and it is related to pressure and resistance, which are described by the arterial pulse curve at the central site. Forward flow occurs both during systole, with distention of the arteries, and during diastole, with contraction of the arteries. The process is based on the same concept used for the clinical determination of the cardiac output. Although among patients in critical care units the clinical determinations may vary widely, central determination using a computer has greatly increased the accuracy, and such determination is an accepted procedure.

CLINICAL ESTIMATION

In the absence of more sophisticated techniques, many authorities use a clinical estimate of the cardiac output. Stroke index is considered approximately equivalent to pulse pressure or to the volume of the radial pulse. In the pulse-pressure estimate, the pulse pressure multiplied by the heart rate gives the estimated cardiac output (± 20%–35%). In the radial-pulse estimate, a full, strong pulse beat coupled with a rate within normal limits indicates a good cardiac output. However, preliminary studies indicate that the radial-pulse estimate varies from 30% to 300% of the anticipated levels, and so the radial-pulse estimate must be used with that fact in mind. If the radial-pulse estimate is used, it should be used only in combination with an evaluation of the patient's mental status or his degree of alertness, his urinary output, and his skin color (blanching).

THERMODILUTION TECHNIQUE

The development and refinement of pulmonary artery catheterization has produced the most accepted and most accurate methods of determining the cardiac output [68]. The thermodilution method, which uses measurements obtained from heat, or a change in temperature, in the blood, produces a dilutional curve and a cardiac output determination. A calibrated thermistor located approximately 4 cm from the catheter tip records the temperature of a bolus (usually a cold bolus) that has been introduced into the circulation. Because the quantity and temperature of the bolus are known, the difference in temperature between the fluid in the bolus and the blood is the basis for the computer's calculation of the net blood flow during the time the change in temperature was measured. (A constant number that stands for the gain of heat from the tubing and thermistor is taken into consideration.) In other words, the change in temperature creates a curve, the area of which is used to calculate the cardiac output. The system is attached to an analog computer that is programmed to perform the calculation and that provides a digital readout [62].

Nursing Orders

Problem/Diagnosis

Multisystem complications secondary to traumatic insult.

OBJECTIVE NO. 1

The patient should maintain adequate respiratory functioning.

ACHIEVING THE OBJECTIVE

To achieve the objective, the nurse should:

1. Read the Nursing Orders in Chapter 17.
2. Monitor the adequacy of the oxygenation. Determine the relationship between the arterial oxygen tension and the inspired oxygen concentration. (In general, a ratio below 300 is not normal, and one between 350 and 500 is normal.)
3. Monitor the inspired oxygen concentration. Oxygen is administered in concentrations of higher than 40% to 50% only for short periods of time. A generally accepted rule of thumb is, if the arterial oxygen tension cannot be maintained at 60 mm Hg with a FIO_2 of 50%, the physician orders positive end-expiratory pressure.
4. Assess the adequacy of the respiratory status using the following criteria:
   a. An arterial oxygen tension of above 90 mm Hg on 40% oxygen.
   b. An A-a gradient of 50 to 200 mm Hg on 100% oxygen.
   c. A respiratory rate of 12 to 25 breaths per minute.
   d. A lung compliance of greater than 50 ml per cm H_2O.

   e. An arterial carbon dioxide tension of 35 to 40 mm Hg.
   f. A minute volume of less than 12 liters per minute.
5. Obtain and monitor serial arterial blood gas measurements as ordered.
   a. Via radial artery puncture. The nurse should:
      (1) Prepare ice slush and a heparinized syringe (as little heparin as possible should be left in the syringe).
      (2) Note the presence of collateral circulation by either:
         (a) Obliterating the radial and ulnar pulses. The nurse should:
            i. Have the patient open and close his hand until his palm is blanched.
            ii. To note the return of the blood flow, observe his hand while the pressure on his ulnar artery is released.
         (b) Compressing the radial artery at the wrist. The nurse should:
            i. Ask the patient to open and close his hand several times and then relax his hand.
            ii. Observe for transitory blanching of the palm followed by the return of circulation.
            iii. Use the Doppler if it is available.
            iv. If signs of ischemia persist, conclude that the circulation in the ulnar artery is inadequate.
      (3) Identify the point of maximum impulse of the radial artery.
      (4) Cleanse the site and infiltrate 0.5 ml of a 1% to 2% lidocaine solution on each side of the artery.
      (5) While palpating the artery, insert the needle with its bevel up at a 45-degree angle. (Blood will flow into the syringe when the artery has been entered.)
      (6) Expel the air, mix the blood, and put it in the ice slush.
      (7) Hold the site for five minutes.
      (8) Ascertain the presence of distal pulses.
   b. For brachial or femoral artery punctures, follow (3) to (8).
   c. Via radial, femoral, axillary, brachial or temporal arterial line. The nurse should:
      (1) Prepare a 3-ml heparinized syringe and a 5-ml syringe.
      (2) Withdraw 5 ml of blood and discard it.
      (3) Withdraw a 1-ml specimen.

OBJECTIVE NO. 5

The patient's pulmonary artery pressures should be measured without complications.

ACHIEVING THE OBJECTIVE

To achieve the objective, the nurse should:

1. If the patient has a low mean pulmonary artery pressure and a low wedge pressure, anticipate giving volume therapy.
2. For patients who have high pressures, anticipate digitalization, diuresis, and/or the use of the intraaortic balloon.
3. Know that the normal pulmonary artery pressure ranges from a systolic pressure of 16 to 19 and a diastolic pressure of 5 to 12 (the mean is 15 mm Hg). (In cardiogenic shock, the range is 16 to 20.) The physician should be notified about pulmonary artery pressures of less than 10 mm Hg and more than 22 mm Hg and wedge pressures of less than 6 mm Hg and more than 15 mm Hg.
4. Carry out the procedure. The nurse should:
   a. Explain the procedure to the patient and family. (In many units, a consent form is obtained.)
   b. Assemble a closed-pressure continuous flush system or a continuous flow system that delivers a heparinized solution. The nurse should:
      (1) Hang a 500-ml or a 1000-ml normal saline solution (with 500–2000 units of heparin added).
      (2) Connect the normal saline solution to the infusion set; a microfilter may be used in the line to remove any particles that may plug the intraflow resistance element.
      (3) Fill the tubing, put the solution in a pressure bag, and inflate the bag to 300 mm Hg (Fig. 36-5).
      (4) Connect the tubing to the input line on the intraflow element.
      (5) Open the closed valve in the intraflow element to clear the chamber of air bubbles.
      (6) Keep the system intact and free of air.
      (7) Attach the desired number of extension tubes to the transducer. Too much tubing will produce a falsely low pressure. Use high-pressure tubing from the transducer

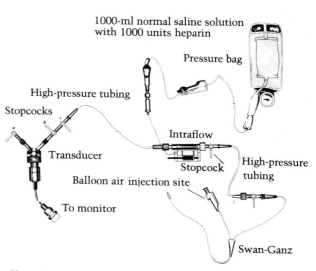

Figure 36-5
Closed-pressure continuous flush system for the measurement of pulmonary artery pressures.

to the distal port (hard to hard and soft to soft).
      (8) Attach two sterile 3-way stopcocks to the catheter connection luer. Turn the proximal stopcock toward the intraflow element. Flush the systems. Turn the distal stopcock toward the transducer but keep the proximal stopcock open.
(In the continuous flow system, the use of heparin decreases the likelihood that microthrombi will develop at the catheter tip. The assembly must include a continuous infusion pump, and provide a continuous flow of 3 ml per hour.)
   c. Observe the insertion protocol. The nurse should:
      (1) Consult with the physician about increasing the oxygen concentration to 100% during the catheter placement.
      (2) Connect the appropriate ECG equipment for continuous monitoring. Monitor for dysrhythmias.
      (3) Have a lidocaine bolus (100 mg) and a defibrillator ready for emergency use.
      (4) Before insertion, check for leaks: the balloon should be submerged in a sterile saline solution or in water and inflated

slowly to the size directed by the manufacturer. The thermistor should be tested by connecting the catheter to the cardiac output cable and making sure that the room temperature is displayed. The physician will then put his sterile, gloved finger over the tip of the catheter and make sure that an increase in temperature is displayed.

(5) While the procedure is being performed, observe the patient, note the ECG pattern and assess the wave forms. The physician should be notified of any abnormalities of the catheter site and any other abnormalities. If the catheter tip enters the thorax, the fluctuations in respiratory pressure increase.

(6) Note and record the length of catheter inserted.

(7) Note and record how much air was needed to change the wave form and the wedge pressure. The amount may differ from that recommended "outside the patient." If the wedge pressure is obtained at readings significantly less than the recommended inflation volume, the physician should be notified.

(8) After the catheter is in place, cover the site with an iodophor ointment and a sterile gauze dressing.

(9) Call the x-ray department to order a stat portable chest x ray to check the placement of the catheter (Fig. 36-6).

5. Never leave the patient unattended at any time. Massive bleeding due to an opening in the system may occur at any time.

6. Observe the site for distal pulses, temperature, color, and other signs of the circulatory status.

7. Measure the pulmonary artery pressure every hour; check the position and height of the transducer, making sure that the transducer is level with the right atrium (5 cm below the sternal angle).

8. Note catheter placement by assessing the wave form. Monitor and observe the dicrotic notch.

9. To prevent formation of microemboli at the tip of the catheter, flush the line with a heparinized saline every 15 minutes. If flushing is difficult, first check the system. If that is negative, manual irrigation with a saline solution through the proximal stopcock usually opens the system. If

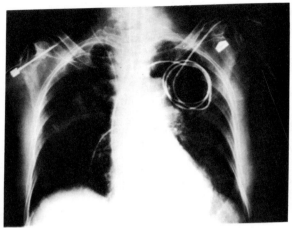

Figure 36-6
Chest x-ray verification of the position of the pulmonary arterial catheter and the absence of pneumothorax.

the system cannot be kept patent, the physician should be notified.

10. Record the serial systolic, diastolic, and mean pressures hourly as they are electrically transmitted from the scope, and observe for stability or changing trends.

11. Calibrate equipment to the scale indicated (0–40; 0–200) every four hours. The patient does not have to be recumbent.

12. As ordered, obtain the wedge pressure every four hours. The nurse should:

a. First check the catheter and the wave pattern to determine whether residual air is in the balloon tip. (The balloon should be kept deflated except when wedge pressure is being checked.) If the oscilloscope pattern or the digital reading indicates a continual wedge pressure, the physician should be notified; a permanently wedged catheter may produce pulmonary infarction and embolism.

b. Check how much air was needed previously to obtain a wedge pressure and what inflation volume was recommended by the manufacturer (0.8 ml for a #5 French catheter and 1.5 ml for a #7 French catheter).

c. Use a tuberculin or a 3-ml syringe and inflate it with the amount of air determined. Observe the pressure contour for a change in the waveform to a small fine line. Inflation is associated with a sensation of resistance.

d. After recording the pressure, remove the syringe.

13. Never use a pulmonary artery catheter to take routine blood samples or to administer medications.

14. Use the pulmonary artery site to take a mixed venous blood sample. Mixed venous samples are only representative if aspiration is slow (< 3 ml/min or 1 ml/20 sec). Rapid withdrawal is likely to aspirate blood that already has passed through the pulmonary capillaries and is oxygenated. Flush the catheter after the blood has been obtained. Guard against persistent wedging.

15. Notify the physician if blood is aspirated from the lumen of the balloon.

16. Make sure that the catheter is secured to the skin with a suture.

17. In moving the patient be particularly careful not to increase the tension and dislodge the catheter. Two people should move the patient.

18. Be sure not to use excessive amounts of tubing.

19. Change the dressing on the insertion site at least once a day. Use Betadine and an iodophor ointment covered by an occlusive dressing. Oozing from the site is to be expected, but gross redness, swelling, or foul drainage is not. At the first sign of phlebitis, the catheter should be removed. The catheter tip should be cultured on removal [5].

20. Prevent 60-cycle interference by proper grounding of the equipment.

21. Maintain a closed sterile system. Use a sterile disposable dome. The transducer is connected physically to a fluid system and electrically to a pressure amplifier and a monitor.

22. Once a day, close off the system to the patient and verify its accuracy by obtaining readings with a sphygmomanometer (see Chap. 30).

23. If there are any problems, check the patient and the entire system. (There are four parts to the system—the catheter, the transducer, the connecting lines, and the recorder—and any part may malfunction.)

24. Keep an extra cable available to test the machine (in case one cable malfunctions).

25. Know that the catheter is usually not kept in place longer than three days. Monitor the patient during and after the removal of the catheter.

OBJECTIVE NO. 6

Serial cardiac outputs should be measured using the thermodilution technique.

ACHIEVING THE OBJECTIVE

To achieve the objective, the nurse should:

1. Measure the cardiac output using the thermodilution technique every 1–4 hours. The nurse should:
   a. One hour before making the measurement, immerse the capped syringes filled with 10 ml of a 5% dextrose in water solution in an ice slush bath (unless room temperature technique is to be used). (Alcohol may be added to speed the cooling process. Be sure no air is present.)
   b. Right before making the measurement, calibrate and test the machine.
   c. Make sure the catheter is in the pulmonary artery and that the baseline temperature is stable.
   d. Decrease the infusion fluids to slow the keep-open rate.
   e. Turn off the continuous intravenous drip to the distal pulmonary artery port during the measurement.
   f. Press the start button and place syringe that contains 10 ml of a 5% dextrose in water solution (0°C) into the lumen marked for cardiac output (the right atrium).
   g. Three seconds later, when the start lamp lights and the audible start tone is heard, very rapidly inject the 10-ml bolus.
   h. Have another nurse time the injection period so that not more than 10 seconds has elapsed from the time the cold bolus is removed from the ice slush until the injection is completed. (During the half second before the audible tone first sounds, the initial or average temperature is noted by the thermistor in the pulmonary artery and stored in the computer. Changes in temperature, as well as the length of time it takes the temperature to approach the initial point and then stabilize, are measured.)
   i. Observe and record the flow in liters per minute shown on the digital display. If available on the particular machine, evaluate the cardiac output curve plotted on the graph (Fig. 36-7).
   j. Evaluate the injection by examining the shape of the curve.
   k. Know that inaccurate cardiac output measurements may be obtained when any of the following conditions are present: a serious misplacement of the catheter, a too-rapid infusion of fluids (which produces a fluctuation in temperature and changes in cardiac performance), and/or the administration of an inotropic drug.

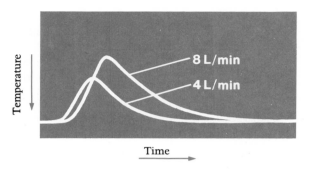

Figure 36-7
Two examples of cardiac output curves with the thermal dilution technique.

2. Monitor the patient continuously with an ECG.
3. Maintain the sterility of the system.
4. Keep the system free of air bubbles.
5. If a cold bolus is to be injected, use syringes that have air-tight caps.
6. With the physician, establish a policy for assessing measurements. For example, determine whether (1) one reading should be taken or (2) three readings should be taken (and recorded) so that an average value can be calculated.

OBJECTIVE NO. 7

The patient should demonstrate abolition of the consumptive coagulopathy.

ACHIEVING THE OBJECTIVE

To achieve the objective, the nurse should:

1. Monitor the laboratory tests for abnormal results and observe for purpura, petechiae, and bleeding from the gingiva, venipuncture sites, wounds, gastrointestinal sites, and genitourinary system. Notify physician of any abnormal findings.
2. Assist in the identification and treatment of underlying condition.
3. Monitor organ functioning in order to identify any dysfunctioning caused by thrombosis.
4. Administer heparin if ordered.
5. Administer whole blood, packed red blood cells, fresh or frozen plasma, fibrinogen, platelet concentrates or clotting factors if ordered [6, 21, 43, 58].

6. Give physical care gently to prevent bleeding.
7. Observe safety precautions to prevent bruising (e.g., pad the side rails and use an electric razor).
8. Promote rest for the patient. The nurse should:
   a. Assist with turning him.
   b. Plan rest periods for him.
   c. Administer total bath.
   d. Keep the environment quiet.
   e. Use a pillow to make him more comfortable.
   f. Assess his arterial blood gases and hemoglobin for their oxygen-carrying capacity.
9. For intramuscular injections:
   a. Use small-gauge needles.
   b. Rotate the insertion sites.
   c. Apply pressure for five minutes.
10. Administer mouth care in the morning and at night. The nurse should:
    a. Use swabs and soft gauze pads.
    b. Use a solution that is half hydrogen peroxide and half water.
    c. Apply mentholatum to the patient's lips.

OBJECTIVE NO. 8

The patient should be free of continuing gastroduodenal ulceration and hemorrhage.

ACHIEVING THE OBJECTIVE

To achieve the objective, the nurse should:

1. Monitor the gastric pH every hour. Discuss the following protocol for gastric alkalinization with physician and implement per order. If the pH falls below 7, give 60 ml of Maalox by tube. Repeat the test to make sure the pH is 7 (pepsin is not activated until the pH is 5). If the pH is below 7, repeat antacid. Decompress the stomach one hour out of four. When oral feedings are resumed and the nasogastric catheter has been removed, administer antacids in 60-ml amounts two hours after feedings, at bedtime, and at 4 A.M. (Since low levels of gastric acid may contribute to ulceration even though the primary problem is not acid secretion, constant neutralization may prevent additional mucosal damage.)
2. As ordered, administer intravenous Cimetidine (a 300-mg bolus every 6 hr). Dilute it in a 20-ml volume and inject it over a one- to two-minute period. Monitor for dizziness, rash, muscle pain,

diarrhea, and neutropenia. Notify the physician of any signs or symptoms.

3. Institute nursing measures to prevent respiratory and septic complications and to maintain nutrition.

4. Administer vitamin A if ordered. (Vitamin A is thought to increase the regeneration of gastric mucous cells and the production of protective gastric mucus.)

5. Monitor vital signs, gastric aspirate, and stool.

6. If the patient bleeds severely, initially prepare for the replacement of blood. Perform guaiac test of the nasogastric aspirate and stool. Order tests of the prothrombin time and the partial thromboplastin time, and a platelet count per physician order. Support the patient and help the physician during endoscopic and sigmoidoscopic examinations. (If alkalinization therapy is continued, cold Maalox may be ordered.)

7. Be aware that if the bleeding is from a stress ulcer, the medical treatment will probably entail the use of an iced saline lavage. If three units of blood need to be administered for replacement therapy, the specific diagnosis is usually made by an angiogram. The treatment entails the use of vasopressin or embolization and fresh blood and platelets.

8. If iced saline lavage is ordered:
   a. Explain the procedure to the patient.
   b. Obtain baseline data about the vital signs and continue to monitor for cardiac dysrhythmias.
   c. Pass a large-lumen nasogastric catheter.
   d. Position the patient comfortably in the left lateral position.
   e. Increase the patient's comfort by administering sedatives and keeping him warm.
   f. Fill 100- to 150-ml syringes from a basin full of iced saline solution, inject the solution into a large lumen catheter (e.g., an Ewald tube), and withdraw the solution. Repeat the procedure as indicated.
   g. Know that after the lavage is completed, an alkaline gastric drip may be ordered.

9. Remember that the following common techniques may be used:
   a. Gastric alkalinization.
   b. Removal of the septic source.
   c. Intragastric cooling.
   d. Intragastric levarterenol therapy.
   e. Intraperitoneal levarterenol therapy.
   f. Selective arterial vasopressin therapy.
   g. Selective arterial epinephrine and propranolol therapy.
   h. Systemic hypothermia.

10. Know the vasopressin intraarterial infusion protocol:
   a. Vasopressin (100 units) and normal saline (500 ml) are mixed. (The initial dose is usually 0.2 units/ml/min, and the infusion rate is not higher than 0.4 units/ml/min.)
   b. One baseline x ray is taken.
   c. Vasopressin is infused for 10 minutes.
   d. The radiologist injects radiopaque material, and a second x ray is taken.
   e. The two x rays are compared. The vasopressin dosage is decreased if the x ray shows severe constriction. The vasopressin dosage is maintained if the x ray shows vasoconstriction of the arteries peripheral or proximal to the infusion site, or that an infused vessel is dilated and contrast material has refluxed into the aorta (increased peripheral resistance).
   f. The infusion is continued for 12 hours; and then half the dose is infused for eight hours.
   g. The catheter is kept in place usually for three to five days. It is kept patent by continuous fluid infusion.
   h. The fluid intake and output are monitored.
   i. The vital signs, central venous pressure, and pulmonary artery pressures are monitored.

OBJECTIVE NO. 9

The patient should be able to sleep for protracted periods of time.

ACHIEVING THE OBJECTIVE

To achieve the objective, the nurse should:

1. Assess the patient's normal sleeping pattern. She should consider:
   a. His bedtime routine.
   b. His sleeping hours.
   c. His sleeping environment.
   d. His ease in getting to sleep and in staying asleep.
   e. Factors that might help if a sleeping problem arises.

2. Include in the nursing care plan a plan for sleep and rest periods and tell the staff about the plan.

3. Offer the patient simple explanations about his care and answer his questions. Clarify any misconceptions he may have because of comments he heard made during rounds or at another patient's bedside.
4. Establish trust and encourage the patient to sleep by assuring him that the staff will monitor his condition.
5. Have a presleep routine, even if only a simple one (e.g., change the patient's gown).
6. Keep the ventilation adequate and the temperature comfortable.
7. Provide an environment that is conducive to sleep. The nurse should:
   a. Be sure the lights are dim.
   b. Keep extraneous noises to a minimum.
   c. Provide a clock in the room.
   d. Make sure that the sheets are clean and straightened.
   e. Help the patient assume a comfortable position.
   f. Give the patient a back rub.
   g. Use other measures to decrease his pain.
8. Awaken the patient only for essential treatments.
9. Monitor the patient's sleep. If he has a sleeping problem, help him as follows:
   a. Try to determine the cause of the problem (e.g., does the patient need to have someone present?).
   b. Increase his comfort by changing his position or giving him a backrub.
   c. Give him ear plugs if he wants them.
   d. Alleviate his hunger.
   e. Give him warm milk.
   f. Decrease his anxiety about getting to sleep.
   g. Administer an analgesic and/or a sedative as ordered.
10. Observe the patient for the following signs and symptoms of sleep deprivation:
    a. Fatigue.
    b. Irritability.
    c. Increased sensitivity to pain.
    d. Burning eyes.
    e. Difficulty focusing.
    f. A shortened attention span.
    g. Behavioral changes (e.g., mild euphoria or apathy).
    h. Time disorientation.
    i. Slurred speech.
    j. Decreased muscle coordination.
    k. Mild tremor.

11. Prepare the patient and his family for his transfer from the unit.
12. Communicate information about the patient's sleep patterns to other appropriate nursing staff.

OBJECTIVE NO. 10

The metabolic stress on the patient should not be increased by environmental stimuli.

ACHIEVING THE OBJECTIVE

To achieve the objective, the nurse should:

1. If possible, plan procedures with the patient and work with him in drawing up his plan of care and scheduling procedures.
2. Use analgesics as needed.
3. Provide for the longest periods of sleep possible.
4. Carry out all nursing procedures with a minimum of stress to the patient; e.g., have personnel on hand to move the patient from the bed to the stretcher and remind him to perform gluteal setting exercises every two hours.
5. Maintain the patient's muscle mass by a planned exercise program.
6. For burn patients, maintain warm environment and cover burned areas with heat shields (Fig. 36-8).

OBJECTIVE NO. 11

The patient should meet his nutritional needs by the oral intake of food.

ACHIEVING THE OBJECTIVE

To achieve the objective, the nurse should:

1. In collaboration with the nutritionist and physician, assess the patient's nutritional requirements. The nurse should:
   a. Base her estimate on the patient's height, weight, age, and skin folds.
   b. Estimate the patient's calorie needs by the following rule of thumb: multiply the number of milliliters of oxygen the patient uses per minute by the factor 7 to estimate the number of calories he uses in 24 hours. For burn patients, the formula is:

   $$25 \text{ cal} \times \text{wt (kg)} + 40 \times \% \text{ TBSA burned} = \text{calories needed each 24 hr}$$

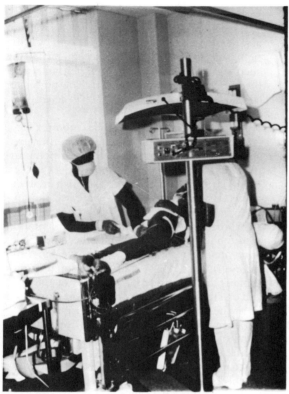

Figure 36-8
Heat shield used to maintain a warm environment for the burned patient.

2. Assess the patient's eating habits: his food preferences, his former eating habits, his traditions, his preferences about mealtimes and about the amount of food to be served.
3. Assess the patient's threshold for smells and taste.
   a. If his threshold for sweet taste is elevated, increase his sugar intake as appropriate.
   b. If beef and (occasionally) pork taste bitter to the patient, encourage him to eat poultry, fish, eggs, and cheese.
4. Consult with a nutritionist about the patient's diet during a staff conference.
5. Help select the patient's meals.
6. Involve the patient's family in selecting his food and in feeding him. If a problem arises, ask his family to bring him some of his favorite foods.
7. Make rounds during mealtimes to assess his eating.

8. Schedule laboratory tests, physical therapy, and painful procedures for times other than mealtimes.
9. If pain is a problem at mealtimes, give the patient an analgesic 30 minutes before he eats. Check him for anorexia or gastric distress after the analgesic has been given.
10. Try to make his mealtimes more social (e.g., by staying with him while he eats or having a family member present).
11. Be aware that the following drugs may depress the patient's appetite: digitalis, atropine, phenothiazine tranquilizers, antihistamines, iron and potassium salts, theophyllin, salicylates, antibiotics (especially tetracycline and erythromycin), quinidine, and procainamide.
12. Give the patient a calorie-containing beverage rather than water to take with his medications and to assuage his thirst.
13. Keep a running tabulation of the calories taken in and those still to be eaten.
14. Give mouth care every four hours and as needed. Do not use lemon and glycerine for mouth care because they are drying. Use a solution that is half hydrogen peroxide and half water. Put mentholatum on the patient's lips.
15. Give the patient liquid diet supplements. Make them more palatable by:
    a. Using various flavors.
    b. Chilling them.
    c. Making them up as ice cream, popsicles, snow cones, puddings, or sauces.
    d. Adding rum or creme de menthe to them.
16. Provide an alcoholic beverage before meals as ordered to enhance his appetite and as a calorie-containing supplement.

OBJECTIVE NO. 12

The patient should meet his nutritional needs by liquid supplementation via tube feeding.

ACHIEVING THE OBJECTIVE

To achieve the objective, the nurse should:

1. Assist in the nasogastric tube feeding (preferably by small feeding catheter or Dobhoff tube) of the patient. She should:
   a. Keep the head of the patient's bed elevated 30 degrees at all times.

b. Check the placement of the tube every eight hours or before feedings.

c. Whether the feedings are continuous or are given every hour, observe for abdominal distention, vomiting, or aspiration. Withdraw the stomach contents every four hours. If they measure more than 200 ml, stop the feedings and notify the physician.

d. Increase feedings daily by small increments to prevent diarrhea.

2. Assist in the jejunostomy feeding of the patient. The nurse should:

a. Await feeding until site is verified by x ray.

b. Observe for signs of peritonitis.

c. As ordered, begin with 200 ml of a warm feeding every two hours, on even hours.

d. If diarrhea begins, consult with the physician about the following protocol:

(1) Discontinue the feedings for 24 hours.

(2) Begin the feeding schedule from the beginning but make the increments more slowly.

(3) If the diarrhea has not abated, 30 minutes before a feeding give the patient tincture of belladonna (10 drops) or a Lomotil tablet or paregoric (5 ml) if ordered.

e. Refeed fistula drainage every two hours, on odd hours.

OBJECTIVE NO. 13

In the event the patient's calorie needs are not met by the methods outlined in objectives 11 and 12, his protein caloric needs should be met by parenteral nutritional therapy.

ACHIEVING THE OBJECTIVE

To achieve the objective, the nurse should:

1. Support and monitor patient during the insertion of the central line as follows:

a. If the line is to be inserted into the subclavian vein, have the patient lie supine in a slight (15-degree) Trendelenburg position and place a small roll between his shoulders so that his shoulders can drop and thus make the vein more accessible and enhance its filling.

b. If the needle or catheter becomes detached from the syringe or tubing, do one of three things: (1) ask the patient to hold his breath, (2) ask him to do the Valsalva maneuver, or (3) apply firm pressure to his abdomen. If an air embolism is suspected, look for the following signs: the patient becomes unconscious, his pulse is weak or absent, and a sloshing murmur is heard over the right side of his heart. The patient exhibiting such signs should be put on his left side with his feet up and his head down. The physician should be notified for emergency evacuation of air from the heart.

c. Following insertion of the tube, monitor for a possible pneumothorax. The fluid administered should be a 5% dextrose in water solution until the site is verified by a chest x ray.

d. If the chest x ray does not establish that the catheter is in the superior vena cava, innominate vein, intrathoracic subclavian vein, or right atrium, withhold the hyperalimentation solution until the physician has been notified.

e. After insertion of the tube, observe for respiratory distress, chest pain, signs of pneumothorax, tingling fingers, numbness of the arm, and/or signs of an allergic reaction (increased pulse, headache, nausea, and vomiting).

2. Maintain a continuous flow within the patient's glucose tolerance. The nurse should:

a. Check the order daily. The physician will order gradual increments until the desired amount is reached. The same procedure is normally used in discontinuing the solution, because suddenly stopping the hypertonic infusion may produce an insulin rebound and hypoglycemia.

b. Calculate the number of drops per minute and check the flow every hour. Use the following formula as an example:

$$\frac{\text{Number of ml ordered in 24 hr}}{24 \text{ hr} \times 60 \text{ min}} = \frac{x\,\text{ml (number of ml/min)}}{1 \text{ min}}$$

To calculate the number of drops administered per minute, multiply the number of millimeters per minute by the number of drops administered by the infusion set. For example, if 3000 ml is ordered in 24 hours:

$$\frac{3000 \text{ ml}}{24 \times 60} = \frac{x\,\text{ml}}{1}$$

$$1440\,x = 3000$$
$$x = 2.08 \text{ ml/min}$$

The infusion set delivers 15 drops per minute

$$2.08 \times 15 = 31 \text{ drops/min}$$

c. Attach to an electronic continuous infusion administration set.

d. Be aware that the position of patient may alter the drip rate. If the administration of the solution gets behind schedule, do not speed it up (the percentage hourly increase should be determined and carefully monitored; 10–20% increase is usual). A too rapid administration may produce hyperosmolar nonketotic coma.

e. Monitor the urine for glycosuria every six hours to make sure that the patient's glucose tolerance is not exceeded at normal rates of infusion. When the blood sugar is above 200 mg/100 ml and the glycosuria is 3^+ or greater, the renal threshold is exceeded, leading to an osmotic diuresis. However, patients who have decreased circulating volumes and a decreased renal perfusion may have extremely high levels of blood glucose and a low level of urine sugar. Water continues to be drawn into the intravascular space and excreted, resulting in hypertonic dehydration. The number of osmols in the intravascular space increases (hyperosmolar state), with increases in serum electrolytes, blood urea nitrogen, and blood sugar levels (even to more than 1000 mg/100 ml). The patient becomes progressively more lethargic and confused in a process that ends in coma and death. The treatment is insulin therapy and free water, usually given as a 5% dextrose in water solution.

f. As ordered, administer insulin for glycosuria subcutaneously or add it to the nutrient solution. As the level of endogenous insulin rises, the insulin supplementation should decrease, as the following table shows:

Glycosuria	Insulin Supplementation
1+	None
2+ (often occurs for 24–72 hours while higher insulin levels are developed)	None
3+	5 units
4+ (a blood sugar check is the accepted protocol in most critical care units)	10 units

g. Use a fresh urine specimen.

h. If the patient is receiving cephalothin, use Tes-Tape for the urine test, because false-positive results are obtained with Clinitest tablets.

i. Remember that sudden glucose intolerance with or without a fever is a cardinal sign of sepsis in the trauma patient [30].

3. Observe the physiological parameters. The nurse should:

a. Check the patient's vital signs every four hours. If the patient has a fever, the nurse should notify the physician, change the entire intravenous lines to the insertion site, change the hyperalimentation solution, and have cultures done.

b. Check the fluid intake and output every eight hours.

c. Weigh the patient daily.

d. Have the appropriate laboratory work done daily until the patient's condition has stabilized (5–7 days).

e. Check the serum electrolyte levels three times a week.

f. Check the blood sugar, blood urea nitrogen level, prothrombin time, complete blood count, platelet count, and serum calcium, phosphorus, and magnesium levels as ordered.

g. Check the serum and urine osmolality and serum protein levels as ordered.

4. Keep the solution sterile. The nurse should:

a. Inspect the bottles for cracks and the solution for a cloudy appearance.

b. Have the solution prepared under aseptic conditions, preferably under a laminar airhood and by a pharmacist. If that is not possible, the nurse should prepare the solution in a clean area of the critical care unit. She should wear a cap and a mask, and she should use strict aseptic technique (the closed transfer technique).

c. Refrigerate the bottle or bag (at 4°C) until it is used. (It should not be kept longer than 24 hours.)

d. Always clean the cap with an iodophor agent before opening the bag.

e. Never infuse a bag of hyperalimentation solution longer than 24 hours. If any solution remains at the end of a 24-hour infusion period, request a new solution from the pharmacy.

f. Not add drugs to the solution until specifically so ordered by the physician. Check the compatibility with the pharmacist.

g. Label the bag with patient's name, date, additives, preparation time, expiration time, and rate of administration.

5. Prevent infection acquired through the skin and administration lines. The nurse should:
   a. If possible, set up for catheter insertion in the treatment room or the operating room.
   b. Order enough gowns, masks, and gloves for those involved in inserting the catheter.
   c. Maintain sterile conditions during the insertion.
   d. Before insertion, determine whether the hair should be removed.
   e. Prepare the insertion site with acetone, tincture of iodine, and alcohol. For example, use a 1% iodine in 70% alcohol solution, allow it to dry 30 seconds to two minutes, then wash it off with a 70% isopropyl alcohol solution. Using friction, work from the center of the site to its periphery [27].
   f. If the patient has sensitive skin, use an iodophor skin preparation. It should not be washed off; it should be allowed to dry.
6. Monitor the insertion site. The nurse should:
   a. Inspect the site every 48 hours or whenever the dressings are changed. Observe for inflammation, phlebitis, or purulence.
   b. If the anchoring sutures become dislodged, notify the physician. With proper care, the site may be used for 30 days (even longer in selected instances). In thermally injured or septic patients, the site is changed every three days.
   c. Observe the following infection control policy: At least once every three days, clean the site with acetone to remove the tape debris, iodophor agent, and alcohol. Particular attention should be paid to the small parts of the catheter, including the plastic needle guard.
   d. Apply an antibacterial or an antifungal antibiotic ointment (e.g., a combination of bacitracin, neomycin, and polymyxin or, preferably, an iodophor ointment to the site) [42].
   e. Cover the site with an occlusive dressing. The nurse should:
      (1) Cover the site with gauze (two or three sponges).
      (2) Use benzoin on the surrounding skin.
      (3) Form an occlusive dressing with Elastoplast and adhesive tape (not paper tape).
      (4) Tape all connections.
      (5) Anchor the filter and the intravenous tubing to the dressing.
   f. Record the data on the outside of the dressing and in the nurses' notes.

7. Monitor the intravenous lines. The nurse should:
   a. Use an in-line filter between the catheter and the tubing (0.22 μ) according to the recommendations of the hospital's infection control committee.
   b. Stabilize the filter with tape so that the tubing cannot be dislodged from the filter.
   c. Change the entire administration set every 24 to 48 hours (the time is currently under investigation).
   d. Scrub the tubing and connections with an iodophor agent before and after changing the administration set.
   e. If necessary, clamp the tubing of the central venous catheter with a hemostat while changing the administration set. The patient should lie flat while the tubing is changed.
   f. Not measure the central venous pressure, administer piggyback medications, draw or give blood, or in any manner violate the line. (Research is now underway to ascertain the safety of using the hyperalimentation line for taking these measures, provided the central catheter is changed every three days.)
   g. At the first sign of infection, suspect a catheter-related sepsis.
8. Educate the patient and his family about the advantages of parenteral nutrition therapy and about the principles of asepsis.

OBJECTIVE NO. 14

The patient should show no signs and symptoms of infection.

ACHIEVING THE OBJECTIVE

To achieve the objective, the nurse should:

1. Carry out the policies of the hospital's infection control committee.
2. Wash her hands thoroughly before and after changing dressings, after any contaminating procedure and between caring for different patients.
3. Maintain aseptic conditions in the environment.
4. Use Betadine (unless the patient is allergic to it) as the major topical cleansing solution.
5. Assist with the debridement procedure.
6. Use meticulous technique in handling dressings and invasive devices (e.g., intravenous catheters and monitoring equipment). The nurse should:

a. Maintain aseptic conditions during insertion of the catheter. If aseptic conditions cannot be maintained, the catheter should be changed as soon as possible.

b. Inspect and clean the site daily. Apply either an antimicrobial ointment or a topical iodophor ointment and cover the site with a sterile dressing.

c. Clean and sterilize the transducers according to the manufacturer's instructions. Use sterile disposable domes. Maintain a closed system.

d. Not leave the indwelling intravenous cannulas in place longer than 72 hours. Change the dressing every 48 hours.

e. Use the intravenous fluid as soon as possible after opening the bag and not let it hang longer than 24 hours.

f. Use 250-ml infusion bags for keep-open intravenous administration.

g. Change the administration sets (1) after blood has been administered and (2) every 24 or 48 hours (if bacteremias are prevalent in the hospital, 24 hours is recommended).

h. Use sterile suctioning techniques when working with endotracheal tubes or tracheostomies.

i. Every day, clean the equipment used for inhalation therapy and ventilatory support (see Chap. 17) [48].

7. Use disposable equipment when possible (and not reuse it).

8. If evacuation tubes for collecting blood are re-used, to prevent back flow remove the tourniquet before the blood stops flowing.

9. Monitor for microorganisms in the ice used with invasive techniques.

10. Apply physiological dressings if ordered.

11. In accordance with the hospital's policy, have standard sputum, wound, and catheter-tip cultures done.

12. Clean all equipment thoroughly after its use and between patients.

13. Monitor the technique of the other staff members and ask them to monitor hers.

14. Separate any patient who has an infection from the other patients. Prevent cross-contamination among patients. Consult with the hospital's infection control committee about their isolation policies.

15. Monitor for signs of infection.

16. Act as a patient advocate.

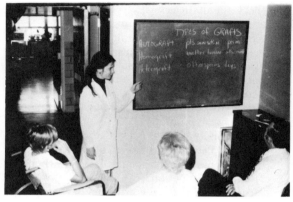

Figure 36-9
Family education is an integral aspect of nursing.

17. Educate the patient and his family concerning protocols (Fig. 36-9).

OBJECTIVE NO. 15

The patient's urine should remain sterile.

ACHIEVING THE OBJECTIVE

To achieve the objective, the nurse should:

1. Explain the purpose and the functioning of the Foley catheter to the patient.

2. Remember that catheters should only be used when necessary.

3. Insert the catheter using aseptic technique (an iodophor solution should be used for periurethral cleansing, the catheter should be the right size, and sterile drapes, sponges, gloves, and lubricant jelly should be used).

4. Maintain a closed drainage system. Do not disconnect the drainage tube and the catheter. (The efficacy of continuous three-way irrigation systems with a closed drainage system has not been established but is commonly used.)

5. Maintain the patency of the drainage system (check the tubing for kinks). Do not let the tubing hang below the level of the bag.

6. In male patients, tape the catheter to the lower abdomen to prevent tension and irritation. In female patients, tape the catheter to the thigh.

7. Keep the collecting bag below the level of the bladder at all times.

8. Check the drainage every two to three hours for color and consistency.
9. Keep the patient's perineum clean. Remove the secretions. Cleanse the area around the catheter with an antiseptic soap solution (elaborate protocols for catheter care result in irritation and an increased infection rate).
10. Report any complaints of burning or irritation to the physician promptly.
11. Not routinely change Foley catheters that have been in place less than two weeks. Change them when sediment accumulates or when the catheters malfunction.
12. If irrigation of the catheter is ordered, use sterile equipment and discard it after use.
13. Not, unless hospital policy dictates otherwise, send the catheter tips routinely for culturing; the correlation between positive catheter-tip cultures and subsequent urinary tract infections is poor.
14. If possible, not put catheterized patients in adjacent hospital beds.
15. If a urine specimen must be collected, not break the closed drainage system. The nurse should use the following protocol (or one similar to it). She should:
    a. Wash her hands.
    b. Clamp the Foley catheter until 2 to 10 ml of urine has accumulated (5–10 min).
    c. Clean the distal portion of the catheter below the Y with Betadine and/or alcohol.
    d. Using a sterile syringe, insert a 25-gauge needle bevel at a 45-degree angle to below the Y and remove the amount of urine needed.
    e. Observe for leakage.
    f. Unclamp the catheter.

OBJECTIVE NO. 16

The patient should demonstrate control and eradication of the septic source.

ACHIEVING THE OBJECTIVE

To achieve the objective, the nurse should:

1. Continue to observe all measures for prophylaxis.
2. Use strict handwashing technique before and after contact with the patient or his secretions. With resistant organisms, use gloves when performing perineal care, measuring urinary output, suctioning, changing dressings, and caring for an incontinent patient. Put soiled dressings and equipment in a waxed bag. Keep infected patients apart from one another. If possible, use one nursing staff for infected patients and another for noninfected patients (cohort nursing).
3. Before antibiotic treatment is started, obtain specimens of blood, urine, sputum, and wound exudates for bacteriological culturing and sensitivity studies. For blood cultures, obtain three blood-culture samples.
4. Administer antibiotics as ordered.
5. Assist with the debridement or drainage procedure.
6. Observe and record the parameters for monitoring an infection site (e.g., in regard to sputum, urine, or a wound).
7. Monitor the systemic parameters that indicate an escalating infection (e.g., tachypnea, an altered sensorium, respiratory alkalosis, a decreased cardiac output, an increased or significantly decreased white blood cell count, a shift to the left, and/or positive cultures).
8. Observe for other signs of infection.
9. Monitor for antibiotic effectiveness and toxicity.
10. Place a precaution notice about body discharges (sputum, urine, blood, feces, and spinal fluid) on the nursing Kardex when resistant organisms are present.
11. Monitor for signs of gram-negative septicemia. The nurse should look for the:
    a. Pulmonary signs: hyperventilation, hypoxia, respiratory alkalosis, and the acute respiratory distress syndrome.
    b. Renal signs: oliguria with or without hypotension, renal failure, and reduced renal clearance rates.
    c. Neurological signs: patient confused or obtunded (a change in orientation is a cardinal sign).
    d. Cardiac signs: chest pain, abnormal ST-T wave, normal to high cardiac output (in early sepsis), decreased cardiac output with cyanosis (in late sepsis).
    e. Metabolic signs: respiratory alkalosis, hyperglycemia and hyperlipidemia in early sepsis, and acidosis with increased blood lactate levels in late sepsis.
    f. Hepatic signs: an elevated serum glutamic oxaloacetic transaminase (SGOT) level.
    g. Gastrointestinal signs: diarrhea.
    h. Hematologic signs: leukocytosis with toxic

granulation, shift to the left, vacuolation, Döhle's bodies, leukopenia (occasionally), thrombocytopenia (in septic shock), and altered C3, C5, C6, and C9 levels.

OBJECTIVE NO. 17

The patient who is in shock associated with infection should demonstrate improvement in his septic and hemodynamic status.

ACHIEVING THE OBJECTIVE

To achieve the objective, the nurse should:

1. In conjunction with other health team members, determine the cause of the shock. They should consider:
   a. Hypovolemia.
   b. Pump failure.
   c. Anaphylaxis.
   d. Neurogenic causes.
   e. Blood flow impediments.
   f. Adrenal crisis.
   g. Sepsis.
2. Administer oxygen and/or assisted ventilation as ordered.
3. Obtain and send for culturing a minimum of two (preferably three) blood samples from separate venipuncture sites and samples from other appropriate sites.
4. Place a urethral catheter and monitor the hourly urinary output (it should be at least 50 ml/hr).
5. Administer volume expansion therapy (Ringer's lactate solution challenge) as ordered. It is often initiated at the rate of 5 to 20 ml per minute for 10 to 20 minutes unless signs of congestive heart failure are present. The pulmonary capillary wedge pressure (PCWP) or central venous pressure (CVP) is monitored. If after the first 100 ml of fluid, increases in the PCWP greater than 8 mm Hg or levels greater than 22 mm Hg (or increases in the CVP greater than 5 cm H_2O) occur, the volume expansion is discontinued. If following the fluid challenge, the PCWP does not increase 3 mm Hg or more, the volume expansion is usually repeated. Or if over a period of 10 minutes with no infusion, the PCWP decreases to the baseline pressure level or lower, the volume expansion is usually repeated. Also, in the absence of congestive heart failure, a 1000-ml infusion over a 15-minute period is ordered.

6. Anticipate that the physician may perform a paracentesis (to determine whether the patient has peritonitis) or a lumbar puncture (to determine whether a disoriented patient has meningitis) and that he may order abdominal x rays, a liver and spleen scan, and sonography.
7. Observe the data gathered from previous cultures and sensitivity studies.
8. Administer antibiotic(s) as ordered. Learn the drug characteristics, monitor for nephrotoxicity and ototoxicity as appropriate, and obtain antibiotic blood levels as ordered.
9. Monitor the arterial blood gases for decreased arterial oxygen levels and for metabolic acidosis.
10. Administer corticosteroids as ordered (may return low P_{50} and 2,3-DPG levels toward normal). The commonly used corticosteroids are (1) dexamethasone phosphate (40 mg followed by 20 mg every 4 hr until the clinical signs of shock have abated, or for 48 hr) and (2) methylprednisolone sodium succinate (200 mg initially and then 100 mg every 4 hr until the clinical signs of shock have abated, or for 48 hr).
11. Avoid chilling. (A temperature blanket may be ordered to keep the patient's temperature at normothermic levels.)
12. Administer vasoactive drugs if ordered. The nurse should know that:
    a. Dopamine hydrochloride (2–10 μgm/kg/min) is given to maintain the arterial blood pressure at near baseline levels (usually 20–30 mm Hg less than the patient's baseline level) for hypotension, chest pain, dysrhythmias, and necrosis of the digits secondary to vasoconstriction.
    b. Isoproterenol (0.2–5 μgm/min) is given after the plasma volume has expanded. (Isoproterenol is contraindicated with volume depletion.) The patient should be monitored constantly for hypotension, tachycardia, and cardiac dysrhythmias.
13. Monitor for other complications (e.g., respiratory distress syndrome, acute gastroduodenal disease, disseminated intravascular coagulation, renal failure, septic embolism, and liver failure).

References

1. Alexander, J. W. Host defense mechanisms against infection. Surg. Clin. North Am. 52:1367, 1972.

2. Alexander, J. W. Nosocomial infections. *Curr. Probl. Surg.* August, 1973.

3. Alexander, J. W., and Alexander, N. S. The influence of route of administration on wound fluid concentration of prophylactic antibiotics. *J. Trauma* 16:488, 1976.

4. Altemeier, W. A., Alexander, J. W., and Sabiston, D. C., Jr. (eds.). *Davis-Christopher Textbook of Surgery.* Philadelphia: Saunders, 1972.

5. Archer, G. and Cobb, L. A. Long term pulmonary artery pressure monitoring in the management of the critically ill. *Ann. Surg.* 180:747, 1974.

6. Barrett, J., deJongh, D. S., Miller, C., et al. Microcygregate formation in stored human packed cells: Comparison with formation in stored whole blood and a method for their removal. *Ann. Surg.* 183:109, 1976.

7. Bauly, L., Sondheimer, H., Bloom, K. R., et al. Improved technique for bedside insertion of the Swan-Ganz pulmonary artery catheter. *Ann. Thorac. Surg.* 21:460, 1976.

8. Baue, A. E. Shock and metabolism. *Surg. Gynecol. Obstet.* 134:276, 1972.

9. Baue, A. E. Multiple, progressive, or sequential systems failure. *Arch. Surg.* 110:779, 1975.

10. Blackburn, G. L., and Bistrian, B. R. Nutritional care of the·injured and/or septic patient. *Surg. Clin. North Am.* 56:1195, 1976.

11. Blaisdell, F. W., and Schlobohm, R. M. The respiratory distress syndrome: A review. *Surgery* 74:251, 1975.

12. Bole, P. V., Purdy, R. T., Munda, R. T., et al. Civilian arterial injuries. *Ann. Surg.* 183:13, 1976.

13. Cahill, G. Starvation in man. *N. Engl. J. Med.* 282:669, 1970.

14. Carey, J. S., and Hughes, R. K. Cardiac output. *Ann. Thorac. Surg.* 7:153, 1969.

15. Cervera, A., and Moss, G. Dilutional re-expansion with crystalloid after massive hemorrhage: Saline versus balanced and electrolyte solution for maintenance of normal blood volume and arterial pH. *J. Trauma* 15:498, 1975.

16. Clowes, G. H. A., Hirsch, E., Williams, L., et al. Septic lung and shock lung in man. *Ann. Surg.* 181:681, 1975.

17. Clowes, G. H. A., O'Donnell, T. F., Ryan, N. T., et al. Energy metabolism in sepsis: Treatment based on different patterns in shock and high output stage. *Ann. Surg.* 179:684, 1974.

18. Colman, R. W., Robboy, S. J., and Minna, J. D. Disseminated intravascular coagulation (DIC): An approach. *Am. J. Med.* 52:679, 1972.

19. Cushing, R. D. Antibiotics in trauma. *Surg. Clin. North Am.* 57:165, 1977.

20. Das, J., Schwartz, A. A., and Foulman, J. Clearance of endotoxin by platelets: Role in increasing the accuracy of the Limulus gelation test and in combating experimental endotoxemia. *Surgery* 74:235, 1973.

21. Davidson, I., Barrett, J. A., Miller, E., et al. Pulmonary microembolism associated with massive transfusion: I. Physiologic effects and comparison in vivo of standard and Dacron wool (Swank) blood transfusion filters in its prevention. *Ann. Surg.* 818:51, 1975.

22. Day, S., MacMillan, B., and Altemeier, W. *Curling's Ulcer: An Experiment of Nature.* Springfield: Thomas, 1972.

23. Dudrick, S. J., MacFadyen, B. V., Van Buren, C. T., et al. Parenteral hyperalimentation: Metabolic problems and solutions. *Ann. Surg.* 176:259, 1972.

24. Dhingra, O., Schauerhamer, R. L., and Wangansteen, O. H. Peripheral dissemination of bacteria in contaminated wounds; role of devitalized tissue: Evaluation of therapeutic measures. *Surgery* 80:535, 1976.

25. Ellertson, D. G., McGough, E. C., Rasmussen, B., et al. Pulmonary artery monitoring in critically ill surgical patients. *Am. J. Surg.* 128:791, 1974.

26. Garvey, J., Hagstrom, J. W. C., and Veith, F. J. Pathologic changes in hemorrhagic shock. *Ann. Surg.* 181:870, 1975.

27. Goldman, D. A., Mala, D. G., and Rhamey, F. S. Guidelines for infection control in intravenous therapy. *Ann. Intern. Med.* 79:848, 1973.

28. Gump, F., and Kinney, J. M. Caloric and fluid losses through the burn wound. *Surg. Clin. North Am.* 50:1235, 1970.

29. Gump, F. E., and Kinney, J. M. Oxygen consumption and caloric expenditure in surgical patients. *Surg. Gynecol. Obstet.* 137:199, 1973.

30. Gump, F. E., Long, C. L., Geyir, J. W., et al. The significance of altered gluconeogenesis in surgical catabolism. *J. Trauma* 15:704, 1975.

31. Gump, F. E., Long, C. L., Killian, P., et al. Studies of glucose intolerance in septic injured patients. *J. Trauma* 14:378, 1974.

32. Hinshaw, L. B. Role of the heart in the pathogenesis of endotoxin shock. *J. Surg. Res.* 17:34, 1974.

33. Holcroft, J. W., and Trunkey, D. D. Extravascular lung water following hemorrhagic shock in the baboon: Comparison between resuscitation with Ringer's lactate and plasmanate. *Ann. Surg.* 180:468, 1974.

34. Holcroft, J. W., and Trunkey, D. D. Pulmonary extravasation of albumin during and after hemorrhagic shock in baboons. *J. Surg. Res.* 18:91, 1975.

35. Hopkins, R. W., and Damewood, C. A. Septic shock: Hemodynamics of endotoxin and inflammation. *Am. J. Surg.* 127:476, 1974.

36. Kinney, J. M., Long, C. L., and Duke, J. H. Energy Demands in the Surgical Patient. In C. L. Fox and G. G. Wahas (eds.), *Body Fluid Replacement in the Surgical Patient.* New York: Grune & Stratton, 1970.

37. Krizek, T. J., and Robson, M. C. Biology of surgical infection. *Surg. Clin. North Am.* 55:1266, 1975.

38. Leonard, A., Long, D., French, L., et al. Pendular pattern in gastric secretion and blood flow following hypothalmic stimulation—origin of stress ulcer? *Surgery* 56:109, 1964.

39. Levey, M. The cardiovascular physiology of the critically ill patient. *Surg. Clin. North Am.* 55:483, 1975.

40. MacLean, L. D., Mulligan, W. S., McLean, A. P. H., et al. Patterns of septic shock in man: A detailed study of 56 patients. *Ann. Surg.* 166:543, 1967.

41. Magilligan, D. J., and Schwartz, S. E. Platelet response to regional and systemic shock. *Surgery* 77:268, 1975.

42. Maki, D. G., Goldmann, B. A., and Rhama, F. S. Infection control in intravenous therapy. *Ann. Intern. Med.* 79:663, 1975.

43. Mattox, K., Walker, L., Beall, A. C., et al. Blood availability for the trauma patient—autotransfusion. *J. Trauma* 15:663, 1976.

44. McAlhanny, J. C., Czaja, A. J., and Pruitt, B. A., Jr. Antacid control of complications from acute gastroduodenal disease after burns. *J. Trauma* 16:645, 1976.

45. McClelland, R. Acute gastroduodenal stress ulceration. In M. Sleisenger and J. Fordtran (eds.), *Gastrointestinal Disease.* Philadelphia: Saunders, 1973.

46. McKay, D. G. Trauma and disseminated intravascular coagulation. *J. Trauma* 9:646, 1969.

47. Moore, F. D. La maladie post-operative: Is there order in variety? The six stimulus-response sequences. *Surg. Clin. North Am.* 56:803, 1976.

48. Pierce, A. K., Sanford, J. P., Thomas, G. D., et al. Long term evaluation of decontamination of inhalation therapy equipment and the occurrence of necrotizing pneumonia. *N. Engl. J. Med.* 282:528, 1970.

49. Prager, R. L., Dunn, E. L., and Seaton, J. F. Increased adrenal secretion of norepinephrine and epinephrine after endotoxin and its reversal with corticosteroids. *J. Surg. Res.* 18:371, 1975.

50. Rapaport, S. J. Defibrination Syndromes. In W. J. Williams, E. Beuther, A. J. Erslow, et al. (eds.), *Hematology.* New York: McGraw-Hill, 1972.

51. Robbins, R., Idjadi, F., Stahl, W. M., et al. Studies of gastric secretion in stressed patients. *Ann. Surg.* 175:555, 1972.

52. Rushman, R. *Cardiovascular Dynamics.* Philadelphia: Saunders, 1970.

53. Schumer, W. Steroids in the treatment of clinical septic shock. *Ann. Surg.* 184:333, 1976.

54. Shapiro, A. R., Virgilio, R. W., and Peters, R. M. Interpretation of alveolar-arterial oxygen tension difference. *Surg. Gynecol. Obstet.* 144:547, 1977.

55. Shires, B. T. (ed.) *Care of the Trauma Patient.* New York: McGraw-Hill, 1978.

56. Siegel, S. H., Goldwyn, R. M., and Friedman, H. P. Patterns and process in the evolution of human septic shock. *Surgery* 70:232, 1971.

57. Skillman, J., Bushnell, L., Goldman, H., et al. Respiratory failure, hypotension, sepsis and jaundice: A clinical syndrome associated with lethal hemorrhage from acute stress ulceration of the stomach. *Am. J. Surg.* 117:525, 1969.

58. Soeter, J. R., Suehiro, G. T., Ferrin, S., et al. Comparison of filtering efficiency of four new in-line blood transfusion filters. *Ann. Surg.* 181:114, 1975.

59. Spurcer, J., Morcock, C., and Sayre, G. Lesion in the upper portion of the gastrointestinal tract associated with intracranial neoplasms. *Gastroenterology* 37:20, 1959.

60. Stossel, T. P. Phagocytosis. *N. Engl. J. Med.* 290:717, 1974.

61. Stremple, J. F., Mori, H., Lev. L., et al. The stress ulcer syndrome. *Curr. Probl. Surg.* April, 1973.

62. Sullivan, F. J., Mroz, E. A., and Miller, R. E. The precision of a special purpose analog computer in clinical cardiac output determination. *Ann. Surg.* 181:232, 1975.

63. Swan, H. J. C., Ganz, W., and Forrister, J. Catheterization of the heart in man with use of a flow-directed balloon tipped catheter. *N. Engl. J. Med.* 283:447, 1970.

64. Swan, H. J. C., and Ganz, W. Use of balloon flotation catheters in critically ill patients. *Surg. Clin. North Am.* 55:501, 1975.

65. Tachakra, S. S. Two episodes of clinical fat embolism following multiple fractures. *Injury* 8:49, 1976.

66. Tietjen, G. W., Gump, F. E., and Kinney, J. M. Cardiac output determinations in surgical patients. *Surg. Clin. North Am.* 55:521, 1975.

67. Toussaint, G. M., Burgess, J. H., and Hampson, L. G. Central venous pressure and pulmonary wedge pressure in critical surgical illness. *Arch. Surg.* 109:265, 1974.

68. Weisel, R. D., Bumer, R. L., and Hechtman, H. B. Measurement of cardiac output by thermodilution. *N. Engl. J. Med.* 2912:683, 1975.

69. Wilmore, D. Nutrition and metabolism following thermal injury. *Clin. Plast. Surg.* 1:603, 1974.

70. Wilmore, D., Mason, D., and Pruitt, B. A., Jr. Insulin response to glucose in hypermetabolic burn patients. *Ann. Surg.* 183:314, 1976.

71. Wilmore, D., Orcutt, T. W., Mason, A. R., et al. Alterations in hypothalamic function following thermal injury. *J. Trauma* 15:697, 1975.

72. Wintrobe, M. M., Lee, G. R., Boggs, D. R., et al. *Clinical Hematology.* Philadelphia: Lea & Febiger, 1974.

An Alternative Approach to Nursing Care

Barbara Giordano

37

Physiological, psychological, social and cultural forces impinge on the critically ill patient. He can be so small, and the world can be so large. The person is a unique product of his heredity, environment, past experiences, and belief and behavior systems. The nurse must view the person in such a complex perspective. The person has many complex facets, and what happens to him has many complex facets. He affects his surroundings, and his surroundings affect him.

This chapter is about a patient named Les, his hopes, his dreams, his illness (leukemia), his battles, and his future. Les is a real person—someone whom we came in contact with, someone whom we loved and cared for. The complexity of what happened to Les can scarcely be communicated by the written word. Just as clinical judgment is learned at the bedside, the patient's total clinical situation can only be transformed by the feelings and meanings within the situation. To look, to listen, to feel, to believe, to transform—those are the essence of the nurse-patient relationship.

The reader may think that there is a dichotomy between the case study and the didactic material that follows it. The dichotomy is only an apparent one. In taking care of any patient it is always easier to focus on the pathophysiology involved rather than to focus on the psychological, developmental, and sociocultural aspects. One reason for that is that pathophysiology deals with concrete, scientifically observable phenomena; hence those patient outcomes are more concrete and easier to evaluate in terms of success or failure. Another reason is the communication that nurses have with physicians and with other nurses. In a sense pathophysiological knowledge is a sign of achievement. One can argue cause and effect, and ascribe reasons for the pathology. One can cite studies to validate a point. That *is* important. Nurses must be knowledgeable care givers. However, being knowledgeable means using the "concrete" scientific data as a backdrop of care, not as the focus of care. The focus of care is the patient-person, and so nurses must not lose sight of the knowledge about which they cannot be so concrete. Knowledgeable, intelligent nursing care combines the definite knowledge with the less definite knowledge of patient care to provide wholistic and holistic care.

It is not my intent either to convert others to my philosophy or to minimize what I did to treat the physical aspects of Les's illness. It is my intent to show how I combined the pathophysiological knowledge I needed to have to care for Les's body with the more abstract knowledge I needed to care for his spirit.

I have assumed that the reader knows that Les not only had a disruption in his ability to carry out the functions of his immune system (and that "things" had to be done to prevent or minimize complications), but also had a psychological response to the events of his illness (and that "things" had to be done to prevent or minimize complications).

Objectives

The nurse should be able to (1) articulate a set of personal beliefs that can be applied to the care of the immunoincompetent patient and (2) identify the critical elements of a nursing model for a patient who has a disruption in the functioning of his immune system.

Achieving the Objectives

To achieve the objectives, the nurse should be able to:

1. Define the major elements of a nursing history.
2. Relate the relief of the anxiety state to the psychophysiological state produced by meditation.

3. Identify the major elements of the nursing and medical management of a patient who has an altered immune response.
4. Develop a framework on which to base nursing care.
5. Describe the process of imagery as a tool for communicating with the unconscious.
6. List the mechanisms of the immune response.
7. Compare and contrast nonspecific aspects and the specific aspects of the immune response.
8. Outline the three functions of the immune system.

How to Proceed

To develop an approach to a patient in isolation, the nurse should:

1. After studying this chapter, read *Mind As Healer, Mind As Slayer* [34], *The Body Is the Hero* [21], and *Getting Well Again* [37].
2. In regard to an illness she has experienced:
   a. List five ways in which she may have contributed to her illness.
   b. Discuss the feelings she has about each item.
   c. Discuss the list with someone with whom she feels comfortable doing so.
3. List five things she "got" out of her illness or (as a preventive measure) list anything that is happening now in her life that might make her wish she were sick.
4. List three-month, one-year, and five-year goals, and tell what practical steps she might take to achieve each of those goals.
5. Try the relaxation and imagery techniques on herself, using the discussion in the case study as a guide.
6. In regard to (1) a patient who is undergoing radiation therapy for cancer of the brain, (2) a leukemia patient who is undergoing chemotherapy, or (3) a patient who has cancer of the colon and who is in a remission:
   a. Practice the relaxation and imagery techniques outlined in this chapter.
   b. Draw a picture of her imagery.
   c. Describe her drawing to someone with whom she feels comfortable doing so.
   d. Evaluate her drawing using the criteria of Achterberg and Lawlis [2].
7. Develop a schedule for using the techniques to maintain her health. She should:

a. Identify the barriers or inhibitions that prevent her from beginning this schedule.

b. Identify ways to remove those barriers or inhibitions.

8. Think about two patients with whom she had a special relationship. (The special relationship may have been one in which the nurse and the patient did not get along.)

a. Identify the elements that were special.

b. Validate the principles on which she based her actions.

c. Evaluate the effectiveness of the actions and the principles that figured in the relationship.

d. Describe any changes she made or could have made to improve the relationship.

e. Tell what she learned from these two patients that helped her define her beliefs about patient care.

9. If she has worked in a critical care area or is soon to work in one, develop an orientation booklet for critical care nurses.

Case Study

The case study describes a young man who was admitted to the medical service in a teaching hospital on which I was the clinical nurse specialist.

The young man provides us with an opportunity to look at a clinical situation in which the patient demonstrates disruption of each function of the immune system in a complex fashion, not in a one-two-three sequence.

This chapter is divided into seven sections: (1) the presentation of the case history, (2) the medical framework, (3) the psychosocial framework (identifying potential problems relating to the patient), (4) the techniques of relaxation, meditation, imagery and goal setting as adjuncts to the patient's management, (5) the nursing framework on which I based my interventions, (6) the actual clinical course, and (7) the reflections on the experience.

Let me point out that the case study does not mention many of the frustrations involved in coordinating the nursing management and working with the other members of the medical team.

Nursing History

Les T., a 21-year-old college senior, was admitted to the medical service with the chief complaint of increasing weakness and fatigue of three months' duration. At first he went to the student health service, where his condition was diagnosed as iron-deficiency anemia, and he was told to take ferrous sulfate. Although his symptoms did not improve, Les continued to take the medication faithfully. He decided to consult another physician when his fatigue began to interfere with his ability to stay awake in class, the library, and the cafeteria.

Social and Family History

Les is the younger of two children in a one-parent family. His father died of a "heart attack" when Les was seven, leaving the family with a moderate income from a union pension and social security benefits.

Les's mother is 50 years old (she looks much older) and she is unemployed. Since her husband's death, she has worked off and on in a local department store. Mrs. T. volunteered the information that she never fully recovered from her husband's sudden death. She said that she felt responsible for her husband's death because the couple often argued because his work was seasonal and his income was inconsistent. She believes that her constant pressure on him to work at a number of jobs was responsible for his heart's "giving out." She describes her relationship with her children as "half good, half bad." The "half good is my Les," and "the half bad is my daughter, who doesn't pay any attention to me. She never calls me like my Leslie to find out how I'm doing."

Les's sister Tara is 30, and she works as an artist for a large advertising agency. Tara has lived in her own apartment since she graduated from college, because "my mother demands my constant attention and wants me to be home at all times. She permits us no room to breathe. She's concerned she won't be able to cope if something should happen. She's always worrying and is very pessimistic about things. She's a hypochondriac and is one big downer. She's always on Les's back about everything. She won't leave him alone. Whenever Les tries to cut the cord, something happens to her that requires Les's help. She never got over my father's death, and she just hangs on to us. Even with my own apartment she's always calling me with some concern."

Les doesn't remember much about his father's death. He describes his relationship to his father as close. "We went everywhere together." Les says that he has a less-than-ideal relationship with his mother, who "doesn't want to let me alone. She's trying to smother me. Now that I'm almost ready to graduate college, and have no firm job prospects and limited funds, I'm afraid I'll have to live with her."

Les says that he has many friends, but no close friends. He considers himself a thinker with a tendency to be a loner. He has a girlfriend, but "we're not serious."

Hobbies

Les's hobbies are reading, thinking, and talking. He has a mild interest in sports. He reads mostly political science and philosophy books. "I'm a poly sci major—but who's going to hire me? I'm not qualified to do anything. Have I wasted four years of my life? I love school and learning. I did really well in all my subjects. In fact, I'm going to graduate summa cum laude. But what does all that mean if I can't do something with it? Maybe I should go to graduate school."

Les considers himself happy-go-lucky and rarely moody. That description is not verified by his sister, who describes him as sometimes quiet, introverted, and extremely serious and sometimes friendly and gregarious.

Sleep Patterns

Recently Les has been requiring 12 hours of sleep a night. His usual pattern is six to eight hours a night. He denies that he has insomnia although he admits he often wakes up more tired than he was before he went to sleep.

Stress Patterns

Les denies that he has any major stresses aside from school, his mother, his girlfriend's pressures to get serious ("I'm not ready to commit myself") and his "questioning my life goals."

His usual response to stress is "to avoid it and, when it smacks me in the face, to deny it's really happening to me. I've been known to smoke a joint or two when the going gets rough."

Significant Other(s)

"My sister."

Physical Examination

General Appearance

Les is a tall, well-developed young man who wears a moustache. He stands with his knees locked, his shoulders slumped, and his head bent. He has shoulder-length dark-brown hair that covers his brown eyes. He has a slight downward curve to the corners of his mouth and a slight "pot belly" despite his well-developed physique. Although he is articulate when he answers questions, his speech is slow, unspontaneous, and monotoned.

Les's personal hygiene is not good. His hair is oily and not combed through. He is appropriately dressed, but his jeans and shirt show evidence of wear and tear. His nails are short but dirty, and tartar is visible on his teeth. His skin and mucous membranes are pale.

Les is 5'11" tall, he weighs 190 lbs, and his temperature is 101°F. His skin is pale, his nails are without clubbing, and he has little body hair.

Head, Eyes, Ears, Nose, and Throat

Thick, long brown hair that is evenly distributed over head (denies that he has alopecia)

Hearing intact, ear canals clear, nose patent (denies that he has sinusitis or allergies)

Vision 20/20 each eye (denies that he has diplopia, headaches, or spots before his eyes). PERRLA, EOMs intact, conjunctiva pale, visual fields normal by confrontation

Mouth without breath odor, lips dry, tongue coated, gingiva pale and friable to touch, teeth have many visible fillings, tongue midline, uvula raises on phonation, gag reflex intact. Tonsils present and enlarged, nasopharynx bright red (has complained of a sore throat "off and on for past three weeks"), lymph nodes enlarged 4 + down to cervical chain

Neck full range of motion, trachea midline, thyroid non-palpable, bilateral auxiliary nodes enlarged and nontender

RR 28, no CVA tenderness, lungs clear A-P, no adventitious sounds

BP 120/80, apical 92 and regular, no heaves and thrills, PMI fifth intercostal space, MCL, S_3 present

Abdomen

Nontender and soft

Liver: 2 FB (fingerbreadths) ↓ LCB, smooth and tender

Spleen: enlarged

Bowel sounds: heard in all four quadrants, says he has no food intolerances, has no history of diarrhea or constipation

Genitourinary System

Normal circumcised penis, descended testes, says he has no sexual dysfunction, no family history of polyuria, and no nocturia. Says he had urinary urgency and frequency the past week and difficulty in starting the stream. Says he voids in small amounts, and that his urine does not have an abnormal odor.

Blood Studies		Electrolyte Studies	
Hct	21.9%	Na	140 mEq/L
Hgb	7.3 gm	K	4.1 mEq/L
Platelets	1 million	Cl	97 mEq/L
WBC	57,500	CO_2	27 mEq/L
Differential		Creatinine	1 mg%
Neutrophils	23	Glucose	100 mg%
Lymphocytes	43	BUN	23 mg%
Monocytes	5	Iron-binding capacity 153 μg	
Eosinophils	1	Uric acid	11.3 mg
Basophils	1	SGOT	20 units
		SGPT	40 units
		LDH	22 units

Urinalysis

pH 8.3

Color: yellow

Character: cloudy

Acetone: negative

Protein: negative

Glucose: negative

Specific gravity: 1.015

Microscopic analysis

WBC 10^6 colonies/ml

RBC   2–4

Epithelial casts

Health Strengths	Health Weaknesses
Intelligent	Significant other (?)
Major organ systems: no overt evidence of pathology	Uses drugs; frequency (?)
	Immunological responses (?)
	Unhappy with present life
No allergies	No close friends and seems not to want any
Thoughtful	Urinary tract infection (?)
Denial is response to stress	Uses denial
	Poor relationship with his mother
	Depressed platelet count
	Anemia

Summary of Findings

Les is a 21-year-old, soon-to-be-graduated college senior, who is majoring in political science. His chief presenting complaints were fever and weakness and fatigue of three months' duration. The physical examination results were essentially negative. The positive laboratory results included an increased white blood cell count, a decreased platelet count, anemia, and a urinalysis that suggested a urinary tract infection. His chest x-ray results were negative.

Les is undergoing a life crisis. He is questioning the meaning and value of what he is doing in college. He has a poor relationship with his overly dependent widowed mother. His relationship with his older sister is not clear. He seems to have few close friends. He says that he has a girlfriend, but the closeness of his relationship is also not known. He says that he has only the usual life stresses and that he copes with them by denial.

Nursing Diagnosis	Medical Diagnosis
Fulminating infectious process secondary to possible altered immunological competence related to unknown cause(s)	Rule out AML (acute myelogenous leukemia)
Acute interruption in lifestyle and in developmental progress secondary to an illness	Rule out UTI (urinary tract infection)
Predisposition to bleeding and coagulation dysfunction related to a depressed platelet count	

Medical Framework

A precise definition of leukemia is elusive. Leukemia is usually considered primarily a proliferative disorder, and it may represent an abnormal proliferation of one of the white cell–forming tissues. The proliferation abnormality is really the presence of a new race of leukocytes; the basic deficit seems to be the lack of normal maturation of the leukocytes. Since leukemic cells have both a prolonged total life and a prolonged reproductive life, they not only remain immature for a longer period of time than do normal cells but they also retain their capacity to proliferate. Normally once a pluripotent hematopoietic stem cell is committed to differentiation and subsequently to maturation, the stem cell can divide only a limited number of times. But many leukemic cells may be regarded as immortal.

Normally the production of blood cells is nicely regulated, and cell production equals cell loss.

The stem cells normally produce cells both for differentiation (maturation) and for maintenance of the stem cell pool. The rate of production increases in response to trauma, exercise, or even physiological excitement or stress. Once homeostasis returns, the size of the stem cell and the maturation compartments remains virtually unchanged.

Unlike normal (self-limiting) leukocytosis, leukemia is an abnormal, generalized, self-perpetuating response to no well-defined or discernible agent [7, 8]. It has no apparent purpose, nor does it contribute to the body's general well-being. The abnormal growth process seems to be innately hardy, giving the leukemic cells an ecologic advantage over the normal cells.

However leukemia begins (i.e., whether through a failure of the immunological system to prevent a "sneak through" of the abnormal cells or because of a "bad seed" [the clonal theory] [32]), the theory accepted in this chapter is that in acute leukemia, normal and leukemic cells live together in the bone marrow as two distinct populations. (That belief is known as the two-population theory [13].) It follows then that a reasonable medical objective is to eradicate the entire leukemic population and then to restore normal marrow function. The remission statistics show that eradication is easily accomplished in acute lymphoblastic leukemia (ALL) but not in acute myelogenous leukemia (AML). Despite the strides made in the last 10 years in regard to increased survival, acute leukemia is still considered to be a highly fatal disease in both adults and children. The improvement in chemotherapeutic regimens has been responsible for an increase in complete remissions, especially in childhood ALL. Adults who have AML are treated just as aggressively as are children who have ALL, but although the number of complete remissions have increased, the overall survival time has been improved only slightly. At best, adults under 60 years of age can expect a complete remission 65 to 70% of the time, and the overall expected survival time is less than one year [26].

There seem to be two reasons that AML does not respond to chemotherapy as readily as ALL does: For one reason, there is no one cytotoxic drug that kills the leukemic myeloblasts without also being toxic to the normal hematopoietic precursors. Since those precursors are already decreased by disease, the drug therapy puts the patient at double jeopardy. He may develop and possibly succumb to an infection. For another reason, there are fewer drugs or drug combinations available that can be depended on to kill the leukemic myeloblasts rather than the lymphoblasts [13, 26]. Inducing a remission in AML is extremely hazardous.

When aggressive chemotherapeutic measures are used, excellent supportive measures must be available (e.g., a protected environment, platelet transfusions, potent bactericidal antibiotics, and, perhaps, granulocyte transfusions).

Another potentially useful form of therapy for patients who have AML is bone marrow transplantation. The process of an allogenic bone marrow transplantation involves (1) the supralethal conditioning of the patient with chemotherapy and total body irradiation and (2) the bone marrow transplantation itself.

Bone marrow transplantation may be divided into three steps:

1. The selection of a donor. As in any other type of allogenic transplantation, successful engraftment depends on ABO and HLA antigen compatibility. HLA compatibility is more difficult to establish, and it is of major importance for successful engraftment.

   HLA typing of family members involves genetic analysis of offspring who have inherited the same two haplotypes. Les and his sister must undergo chromosomal analysis of the antigens they inherited from their parents. An apparent histocompatibility can be confirmed by a mixed-lymphocyte culture, in which the leukocytes of both the donor and recipient are mixed in the same culture. An apparent genotypical compatibility can be confirmed by the nonreactivity of the leukocytes in the culture.

2. Immunosuppression. The recipient of a bone marrow graft must undergo some form of immunosuppression so that he will not reject the donor marrow graft. The patient must undergo not only immunosuppressive therapy but also therapy designed to kill all or nearly all the leukemic cells. Preparation includes a 1000-rad midline dose of total body irradiation (TBI) as well as cyclophosphamide (Cytoxan) (60 mg/kg/day) for a total of two days. TBI alone is not a potent enough immunosuppressive agent, and so cyclophosphamide is administered to increase the leukemic cell kill.

   Cyclophosphamide is one of the alkylating drugs which are the oldest type of antitumor drugs. Alkylating drugs are lethal for proliferating cells, regardless of the phase of cell cycle. Those drugs act by interfering with the chemical composition of DNA to cause cellular disorganization and disruption. Cyclophosphamide is unique in that before it affects the tumor it must be activated metabolically in the liver. Its activated metabolites reach their target site—the tumor—via the systemic circulation. The net effect of this drug is the depression of the bone marrow and a concomitant reduction of the number of leukemic cells.

   TBI completes the destruction of the bone marrow stem cells, leukemic cells and normal cells. TBI is an effective immunosuppressive agent not only because leukemic cells are extremely sensitive to irradiation but also because TBI penetrates to all the privileged sites in the body [40, 41, 45]. These sites (the central nervous system, the testes, and the skin) are more resistant to antineoplastic drugs than are the other sites.

3. Transplantation. Compared to the preceding two phases of the transplantation process, the transplantation procedure is relatively simple. The bone marrow is obtained by multiple aspirations from the donor's iliac bones, it is filtered and put in plastic bags for storage, and finally it is infused into a peripheral vein. By some unknown mechanism, the marrow migrates from the bloodstream into the marrow spaces of the bones. Successful engraftment occurs over a three- to four-week period, and in three to four months the hematological values return to normal.

Except for the risks of general anesthesia, the aspiration procedure is almost danger free for the donor. He is usually discharged the next day. He has some mild discomfort in his hip. He is given a two- to-three month supply of ferrous sulfate. (He is to take 325 mg three times a day.)

For the recipient, supportive measures are necessary before and 10 to 20 days after transplantation (until the graft begins to function), since the patient is severely aplastic. Effective supportive measures must be taken, especially since the incidence of infections is high. A supportive measure that transcends the entire transplantation process is the use of a gnotobiotic, or protected, environment. Protected-environment devices, such as the Total Body Isolator and the Laminar Air Flow room, were developed for use with patients whose resistance to infection is to be lowered by maximum bone marrow suppression. The principle underlying the use of a protected-environment is that the patient's normal body flora is potentially life threatening during times of maximum immunosuppression; therefore, he is put in a sterile environment to keep him from coming into contact with microorganisms [6]. At the same time, he undergoes prophylactic-antibiotic therapy to suppress the endogenous organisms not only on his skin but also in his gastrointestinal tract and, to a lesser extent, his urinary tract.

Although there is no definitive evidence that patients placed in a protected-environment develop infections less frequently than do those who are not in a protected environment, it was decided to give Les maximum protection during the period of maximum immunosuppression. Although the protected-environment and prophylactic-antibiotic program seems to reduce the risk of infection, major infections do develop because the infection and the number of days the infection lasts are inversely proportional to the number of circulating neutrophils [6]. When infections develop, they seem to do so during the patient's first month in the protected environment, probably because maximum reduction of the patient's microbial flora requires approximately two weeks of prophylactic antibiotic therapy and measures to decrease skin bacteria [6]. For that reason, Les's preparation was to begin while the histocompatibility studies were being done. No matter what the results of the tests were, Les was to be placed in a protected environment, a "Life Island unit."

To help Les's adjustment to the Life Island unit, it was decided to "wean" him from the world during his scrubbing (cleansing) time. The weaning would also provide time for Les and his doctors and nurses to develop relationships. Good relationships are extremely important, because once Les is in the Life Island unit

he will be dependent on the staff for his every need. Assigning one or two staff members per shift to work with Les was a key point in the organization of his nursing care. The plan for Les was to put him in a private room and to limit the number of people entering the room. After the results of the histocompatibility studies were known, Les was to be put in reverse isolation during chemotherapy and TBI. After the bone marrow transplantation, Les was to be put in the Life Island unit until the bone marrow graft took.

Psychosocial Framework

Potential Problems of the Developmental Period

Les is in a developmental and situational crisis period in which he is questioning the meaning of his life [24]. Frankl states that the basic purpose of man's striving is to determine his meaning and purpose [19, 20]. Travelbee states that since nursing is an interpersonal process, the nurse helps the person to prevent or cope with illness and suffering and to find meaning in those experiences [42]. It is not enough to help the patient deal with illness and suffering; he must also be helped to find meaning in the experience of being ill. That is not an easy task. A patient may be helped to find meaning in a situation not only by his conscience (Frankl calls it intuition), but also by the nurse who uses her educated mind and heart for the good of the person who needs her care [42].

According to Gould, a person in the 18 to 22 age group feels vulnerable and overly sensitive in regard to authority figures [24]. The major task of that period is to refute the childhood idea, "I'll always belong to my parents and believe in their world." In that period occurs the first major attempts to break the ties to childhood. One of the major false beliefs in that period is, "My parents will fall apart if I don't hold them together." That seems to be true in Les's case; his mother is overly dependent on him and is reluctant to cut the cord. Generally, by the time a person is 22, his adult consciousness is formed, and he has begun to settle into being someone [4]. Les is certainly at a vulnerable point in his life; he has not yet achieved his identity, and he is wondering who he is and where he is going.

Les has to work to find meaning in his life and to settle into an identity. The needs and potential problems for such a person are identified in the literature and confirmed by observation. Some of those needs and problems are discussed in the following paragraphs.

The Need for Approval

A person like Les needs to have authority figures acknowledge his perceptions as being right. Les might react to differences of opinion between him and his nurses with a feeling that he is unwanted or abandoned. Those feelings would have an adverse effect on Les because once he is inside the Life Island unit, he will be totally dependent on the nurses for his needs. The key to success lies in the nurse-patient relationship (Travelbee calls it the human-to-human relationship [42]), which is established and maintained by the nurse practitioner for a reason. Relatedness implies that both members of the relationship are involved. Involvement is a process that meets man's basic needs, the need to love and be loved and the need to feel worthwhile [21]. The human-to-human relationship is a reciprocal one.

The Fear of Independence

The patient may fear that if he becomes too independent, no one will love him. The patient needs to become a responsible person, a person who "is motivated to strive and perhaps endure privation to attain self-worth" [20]. Assuming responsibility for oneself underlies the ability to fulfill one's needs in a way that also allows others to fulfill their needs [19, 20, 22, 42, 43]. The patient must stop denying reality, and he must realize that he has to fulfill his needs within the established framework [22].

The nurses could help Les achieve a balance between dependence and independence by talking to him and learning about him. By sharing his opinions with the nurses, Les could test whether the nurses accept him, and he could see that his opinions matter [22, 42]. Talking with the nurses about "things" could give Les the opportunity to test people he trusts. In time Les might develop an increased sense of self-worth as he learns that people whom he trusts do not abandon him even though they might disagree with him.

Stereotyping

A third potential problem is that nurses and doctors are "nonjudgmental" and yet stereotype the patient as well as the patient's diagnosis. Les is in double trouble in that regard. He is a hippie, and he almost certainly has leukemia. There are many stereotypes about cancer—it is disfiguring, it means certain death, it is painful, it is disabling, it is dirty, it is contagious, it breaks up the person's life, it makes the patient a helpless victim (of "the big C") [33]. The staff reacted stereotypically to Les—why do anything since he's going to die anyhow? Is not the whole system of medical and nursing care based on the premise that death is the enemy? The nursing staff may also have believed time and effort were being wasted and money lost in paying attention to Les.

Les was an either–or patient; that is, either the nurses liked him or they did not like him. Those who liked him thought he was a pleasant, jovial, and intelligent young man. Those who did not like him thought he typified the things hippies stood for, that he was antiauthority (Why does he call me by first name?), and antiestablishment (Why can't he follow the rules?), and amoral (He lives with a girl, doesn't he?). Yes, Les did not bathe and wash his hair frequently, and he called everyone by first name. (But then, we called him by his first name; it seems like a double standard, does it not?) But because Les acted as he did, were those actions a reason for people to react negatively to him and to avoid treating him humanely?

The doctors' feelings about Les created no problems, but the nurses were an entirely different matter. Les was definitely not going to react well to the authoritarian structure that prevailed on the unit, since the nurses, especially the evening nurses, were not going to change.

During the last few years, primary nursing has been introduced in some hospitals to improve the quality of care provided. The essence of primary nursing is that one nurse, the primary nurse, is responsible on a 24-hour basis for planning the total patient care to a selected patient, or selected patients, throughout the entire hospitalization. The principle that underlies primary nursing is the patient and the nurse jointly plan care to avoid fragmentation of care and to provide consistency and continuity of care, thus improving the nurse-patient relationship. The primary nurse model stimulates a close nurse-patient relationship by reintroducing the idea of "my patient" and "my nurse." As with any other type of patient care assignment, primary nursing is not a solution for a problem in nursing. The effectiveness in the delivery of care depends on the nurse, her competence in the practice of nursing, and her willingness to accept increased responsibility for her decisions.

Since Les responds to me the best of all, Les will become "my" patient and I will become "his" nurse.

Denial

Les's fourth potential problem area is his use of denial as his major defense mechanism. To deny or not to deny, that is the question. Denial is often seen by health care workers. Denial helps one deal with a stress-producing situation. Generally, the function of denial is to assuage the anxiety by minimizing the perception of the threat or the anxiety-producing components of reality that comprise the threat [31, 33]. Denial as a defense mechanism may be a temporary protector of the ego, because it keeps the person from becoming overwhelmed by the anxiety of the real world. But a continued use of denial may indicate that the person has a more serious mental health problem.

The questions to be answered in regard to Les are:

1. Is Les using denial? (We all do in regard to death.) By Les's own admission, denial is his major defense mechanism.
2. Will Les's use of denial keep him from progressing toward wellness? It is difficult to predict, but if Les denies the seriousness of his illness, and if the bone marrow transplant takes (it should), he may consider himself well and he may not continue to take his medications and make follow-up clinic visits.
3. Is Les's denial permitting him to regain his control as he deals with the shock? Partly, but the question needs more exploration.
4. Why is Les using denial? I am not sure, and I will check with him about that. I believe that Les's denial gives him some control over his environment and himself. By using denial as a defense mechanism, Les bottles up his emotions; that is, no one can dislike him if he does not make any waves [31]. For what it is worth, denial is preferable to resignation and hopelessness [30]. The trick is to maintain Les's defenses yet keep him in contact with reality. I will discuss with Les the possibility of his using some form of relaxation techniques that will help him get in touch with his feelings but still allow him some control over himself.

There are so many things for the nurses to remember and to do. How can they do it all? How can they all decide on—and *all* accept—a reasonable plan of care? Whatever the nurses decide to do, Les must become an active member of the team.

Meditation, Imagery, and Goal Setting

Everyone encounters stresses in his daily life and everyone has clusters of stresses at specific points in his life, but not everyone develops cancer. The critical stresses seem to be those that rock the person's identity. The important factor seems to be not the number of the stresses or their severity, but the manner in which the person handles them (or, rather, is unable to handle them, according to the rules and regulations made early in his life) [4, 31]. Related to this is that the person under stress feels trapped and unable to alter his life [4, 30, 31]. In an effort to keep control over his world, he becomes rigid about the world. He then loses hope, and he feels that life no longer holds any meaning.

Les's life experiences seem in accordance with the model just described. His father died when Les was young. Les's college years seemed to mark the first time since his father died that Les became involved with people, learning, and life in general. College seemed to give Les an identity, friends who accepted him, and direction to his life. Now, in Les's last semester of his senior year, his identity—his life itself—seems to be ending. Les feels hopeless because he believes he is not prepared to do anything, and he does not know what to do with his life. Why does he feel let down when he has devoted so much of himself to his schooling and his friends? He seemed to be looking forward to graduation, but secretly he was dreading it. Now he is to lose his life. The process of chronic anxiety and the need to continuously adapt leave the body vulnerable [25, 34, 35, 39]. Perhaps because of changes in the body's normal balance, the body's internal environment permits abnormalities to develop [38].

How is it possible to change Les's feelings of hopelessness and helplessness? Attitude is important. Inherent in attitude is volition, or will. Volition is influenced by what one believes, a never-ending circle [25]. The key is to mobilize volition for mind-body coordination [46, 47]. The contribution of volition to one's belief system has been almost entirely ignored in modern medicine. Volition is active or passive. Passive volition (passive concentration) should be consciously developed and used.

The development of a positive self-image is especially important to someone who feels depressed and beaten [25]. That description seems to fit Les, does it not? Les's first task is to reject his old self-image and accept the possibility that by using his volition, his "freedom of will," he can learn to modify his mind-body processes [25]. Thus the will (the will to live?) is at the heart of the mind-body problem [15, 16, 17, 18, 25, 28, 34]. That is potent stuff.

But how to reverse Les's belief system? That is not an easy task. Mixed in with Les's belief system are the belief systems of his mother and sister, of others who mean something to him, and, of the doctors and nurses.

The degree to which Les is dependent on the beliefs of others is important. At the present time, he seems to be not too concerned about the attitudes of the doctors or his mother; he does seem concerned with what his sister and I believe. Thus it is important to help him to (1) redefine his stance toward life, (2) see that there are choices he can make without feeling trapped in old behaviors and attitudes, and (3) maintain a supportive and positive environment. The end result is that Les will have a new perspective on his life. He seemed almost relieved to talk about himself, and he said it was not easy for him to talk about his feelings and fears. He said he would try almost anything to help him find a direction for his life. It certainly is hard to write behavioral objectives and measurable patient objectives in such a case.

After I discussed with Les how he could alter his perspective and, secondarily, become aware of his bodily sensations, we both decided to use passive concentration (meditation and imagery) to help Les.

Meditation

Passive concentration is the end result of a number of meditation techniques (e.g., Zen, transcendental meditation [TM], Benson's relaxation response, Jacobson's progressive relaxation, and Schultz's autogenic training [AT]). In each one of those meditation techniques, the distractions of the external environment are closed out, just as though the person were in an isolation chamber. Passive concentration, or focusing the mind, may disrupt the harmful mind-body patterns [33, 35, 46, 47]. The concentration can dissipate anxiety by providing an object for attention (e.g., counting sheep or reading) [5]. Benson speculated that the concentration unlinked the thinking (cortical) system and the perceiving (limbic) system [5]. As a result, the meditator can relax deeply, remain alert, and stand apart from an angry or unhappy or frustrated self, taking on an objective attitude that is similar to the attitude of a therapist. "It has been empirically verified that the meditative process relieves nervous-system stress more efficiently than either dreaming or sleeping" [33]. Thus meditation effectively interrupts the body's physiological and psychological reaction to stress [33, 37].

The physiological state produced by meditation is counter to the state brought about by anxiety or stress. Concentrating on one thing at a time seems to have a positive effect on physiology. As the body begins to respond to a simpler event, the tension and anxiety indicators are reduced. The metabolic rate and the heart beat slow down, the blood lactate level decreases sharply, and there is a lower rate of using oxygen and producing carbon dioxide [5, 24, 30, 33].

The psychological benefits of meditation are similar to those of psychotherapy. Initially, the benefits are physical ones. The person feels a deep sense of relaxation and an unstressing of the body's muscles. The two major psychological benefits of meditation are achieving another perspective on reality and a greater efficiency and joie de vivre in everyday life [46].

Because the meditator focuses on one subject at a time, he develops what is called contemplative introspection. He adopts an attitude of self-examination and detachment as he sees in his mind's eye the interactions between the self, others, and the environment with greater clarity. Meditation removes the emotional reaction so the person can act objectively and logically. As Les begins to pay careful attention to his strengths and weaknesses during meditation, he will become concerned with his total being, including his relationships with others.

Meditation is steady work in which the meditator consistently brings himself gently back to the task at hand, concentration. The consistency strengthens the will and helps the meditator be purposeful and goal oriented, all the while minimizing distractions in accomplishing the task at hand. Thus the individual masters his environment to a degree because he can cope with individual situations and increases his sense of confidence. The person becomes more patient with himself.

Meditation is not a panacea. It is a way of being. It becomes only one part of a person's total behavior. Meditation is ". . . kind of digging the present . . . growing with the external now" [46]. When used regularly and in moderation, meditation enhances, not replaces, other aspects of a person's life.

The next issue to arise is how Les should meditate.

Since he will have some constraints on him, what he does in regard to meditation outside the Life Island unit he should be able to do while he is in the Life Island unit.

Technical Considerations

Several factors must be considered in regard to Les's meditation; namely, time, positioning, and environment. Those factors are discussed in the following paragraphs.

Les must meditate at a time when his room is quiet, and he must be without interruptions of any kind for at least 15 to 20 minutes three times a day. The position Les is to assume must also be considered. Two positions are recommended: a sitting position and a recumbent positon. Even though several types of sitting positions are favored for clinical reasons and for imaging, it was decided to use the recumbent position. (It was almost impossible to get a straightback chair into the unit, and Les needed that type of chair for maximum relaxation. For that reason, the recumbent position was chosen.) When a person is in a recumbent position, something is usually placed behind his knees so that maximum relaxation of his leg muscles can be achieved. The meditator should be aligned symmetrically, and his head should be in a comfortable position so that his neck and shoulders are not cramped or stiff. Whatever position is chosen, the important thing is that muscle tension be absent. There should be as few distractions as possible from clothing, jewelry, or glasses.

Environment is important. Watts advocates the use of incense to set the tone for meditation [46]. That is out of the question in a critical care unit, but since other natural objects can be used to set the tone, it was decided to get some plants that Les liked and put them around his room. That was perhaps the most difficult step in the preparation for meditation, because the administrator had to sign a requisition form authorizing the rental of those plants. Plants are not mandatory, of course, but they have a salutary effect in that they make a room less like a hospital room. The room that has plants is not barren; it contains living things that also must be cared for.

Mantras are used in certain types of meditation. The mantra is a word, phrase, or sentence that is to be chanted repeatedly. Chanting a mantra focuses the attention of the meditator on one thing at a time— the chanting. He is aware of the chanting and only of the chanting. Mantras are chanted not for their meaning (it is important not to chant emotionally laden words), but for their vibrational qualities, their simple tone, and their ability to accompany and slow down breathing. One of the basic mantras is OM. When OM is chanted correctly, it extends through the entire range of the voice; it symbolizes the universe [46]. A mantra is intended to give a feeling of serenity. A mantra should not be a person's name, should be somewhat unfamiliar (and therefore removed from everyday life), and, last, it should acquire special meaning to the meditator as a signal to turn inward to a peaceful state.

Once a time and a position for meditation were decided on and the environment was set, it was time to begin the meditation. Les used a modification of Jacobson's progressive relaxation, a technique advocated by Simonton and his colleagues [37].

Imagery

The second technique that was used with Les was the imaging (or visualization) process.

Imagery is used in conjunction with relaxation. The combination results in a potent instrument that can mobilize the resources of the body and mind. Imagery is a clear mental statement of what the meditator wants to happen [37]. Imagery is based on stored rather than on current information [2], and so it is a tool for communicating with the unconscious mind. The unconscious is important because it stores all the information gathered from the person, from other people, and from the environment. Anyone who wishes to modify a behavior or an attitude must look to the unconscious.

During the imagery process a person can summon and hold certain images in his mind and then explore their effects on his consciousness [34]. The person remains detached. He can focus his awareness yet remain impartial in his thoughts and emotions. In his mind's eye he can see himself in control of himself and of his environment. "By focusing upon symbolic representation of each aspect of physical and psychological functioning, the individual can achieve profound insight" [34]. In this manner the person (Les) can evaluate his beliefs and then change those beliefs as he wishes.

The conscious mind must be disciplined, not by force but by keeping it in line with the unconscious [47]. That is so because the conscious mind registers everything it sees and hears. It fails to complete anything, and it makes it impossible for the unconscious to progress toward attainment of goals [47]. Imagery thus becomes an important tool for self-discovery and for making change in our life [34, 37, 47].

The relationship between imagery and relaxation is not clear [25, 34]. What is clear is that achieving a relaxed state seems to strengthen the imagery. Benson's evaluations of responses to relaxation indicate that a person who is in a relaxed state is in a wakeful, hypometabolic state; that is, he is mentally alert but he shows evidence of hyposympathetic nervous system activity [5].

Essentially, the imagery process is a period of relaxation during which the person sees in his mind's eye his desired goal or result. Two factors necessary to successful imaging are that the directions must be in a positive framework and that only one goal (and it must not be changed in midstream) should be introduced into the unconscious mind at a time. "Induced visualization . . . used while in a state of passive concentration, i.e., meditative state, is a very powerful tool to mobilize the resources of both the mind and body" [34]. "Where the mind tends to focus, the emotions and the physiology are likely to follow" [34]. Thus the positive beliefs inherent in mental imagery are the person "visualizing his cancer, his treatment coming in and destroying it, his white blood cells attacking the cancer cells and flushing them out of the body, and finally imagining himself regaining health" [37].

The imagery process is the quickest and surest way to program the body, because its commands involve the whole person rather than only his nervous system [25]. It is not necessary that the commands be scientifically accurate. The body simply carries out the commands. So the patient visualizes what he wants to happen, and the body converts the command into action.

It is important for the person to practice the meditation and imagery process, and it is equally important that the person first draw his imagery and then describe it. The drawing and descriptions may then be rated in regard to 13 or 14 aspects [2]. Some of the aspects of Les's imagery that I included were the clarity of the cancer cell, the activity and strength of the cancer cell, the vividness of the white blood cell, the activity and strength of the white blood cell, the number and size of the cancer cells relative to the number and size of the white blood cells, the vividness and effectiveness of the medical treatment, and the concrete or symbolic nature of the imagery. Since imagery is a highly personal and symbolic language, the clinical judgment of the examiner is also involved. The outline given by Simonton and his associates of the symbols that indicate effective imagery made it easier for me to evaluate Les's drawings [37].

The outline is as follows:

1. The cancer cells are weak and confused.
2. The treatment is strong and powerful.
3. The healthy cells have no difficulty repairing any slight damage the treatment might do.
4. The army of white blood cells is vast, and it overwhelms the cancer cells.
5. The white blood cells are aggressive, eager for battle, and quick to seek out the cancer cells and destroy them.
6. The dead cancer cells are flushed from the body normally and naturally.
7. By the end of the imagery, you are healthy and free of concern.
8. You see yourself reaching your goals in life, fulfilling your life's purposes.

There are two types of imaging: active imaging and passive imaging. The type that is of interest in this clinical situation is receptive imagery. Receptive imagery is not passive; "it is a state of awareness which is receptive to whatever impression, thoughts, pictures or feelings may pass through it" [34].

Receptive imaging "is intended to promote alterations in an individual's perception of these significant others" [34]. But before Les can begin imaging his cancer, his treatment, his white blood cells, the shrinking of his cancer, the removal of the cancer from his body, his being well and full of energy, he needs to do some trial imaging. He must apply passive concentration to the imaging of other people. At first the images will be of relatively neutral people or places. Initially the images may be hazy, but with practice, they become clearer and stronger. Eventually, the images have dreamlike qualities.

Porter provided the guidelines for two imaging trials Les made [35]. Before Les began the imaging, he was taught to relax:

Now I would like you to pick a spot on the wall. Look at it comfortably and as I count back from 10, continue to stare at the spot until your eyes become very heavy: 10, 9, 8, 7, 6, 5, 4, 3, 2, 1. Now gently close your eyes, and ignore all the sounds outside the room. Just concentrate on my voice. Take some very deep breaths. Breathe slowly and deeply and let the air come in and go out. Each time you breathe out, let some of the tension leave your body. Breathe in; breathe out. Say to yourself, relax. Let that relaxed feeling spread all over your body. Now think for a moment about your feet. Let all the tension flow out of your feet. Let the muscles become very loose, very smooth, very warm. Imagine that the blood is warming your feet, making them tingle. Think for a moment about your legs, your lower legs, your calves. Let all the tension dissolve out of them, melt away, making them soft and smooth. Your upper legs, your thighs, let them become very warm. Now I would like you, at the count of 3, to be twice as relaxed as you are now. 1, 2, 3. In your mind's eye, concentrate for a moment on your hips, letting them become loose. The muscles in your abdomen, where you may be storing a lot of tension—let them go. Let the blood flow through like wind flows through wheat, carrying good oxygen to all of your body. Continue to breathe regularly and deeply. Think for a second about the many muscles in your back. Tell them to relax, to let go of all the tension and stress and anxiety that they may be holding. Imagine the tension knots in your back and in your shoulders dissolving, melting, going away. The muscles in your neck, relax them, let them become very soft, just let them go. All up and down the back of your head and the top of your head, let the tension be free to flow out. Let the tiny muscles around your eyes relax, around your jaw. Now if you still feel pain or tension in some part of your body, I'm going to pause for a moment and let you concentrate on that area.

(Pause)

Continue relaxing now for the next 10 minutes, realizing that when you do this you are participating in your own return to health. (Play the ocean sound tape for about 10 minutes.)

And now to imaging. See a familiar room which you are not now physically occupying. Be aware of all of the textures, colors, and shapes. See each object within the room. Notice the placement of decorative items. Be aware of fragrances and odors. Listen to sounds inside or outside the room. When you have seen, heard, smelled, and sensed all that you want to, return to your present location by opening your eyes.

Again, close your eyes and relax. See in your mind's eye a supermarket. Enter it and go to the produce section. See a large bin of fresh, juicy oranges. Go over to it and select an orange that meets all of your qualifications. Pick it up and hold it in your hands. Feel the weight of it. Experience the texture of the rind. Smell the fragrance. Now with your thumb break into the center of it and begin to peel the skin. Be aware of the effect of the citrus fragrance in your nose. When you have removed the skin, feel the difference in texture of the orange. Again with your thumb, break open the segments. Put a segment into your mouth and bite into it. Sense the juice flowing around in your mouth as it mixes with the saliva. Chew on the pulp. Feel the cool, refreshing juice slide down your throat. Consume each of the sections one by one, being aware of all of the sensations you experience. When the orange is gone, go to the bin where there are some fresh lemons. Select one and take time to examine it as you did the orange. When you are ready, pick up a small knife nearby and cut the lemon open. Put a slice in your mouth and suck the juice from it. Be aware of the experience your mouth is having. Smell the lemon rind. Feel the juice slip down your throat. When you have had all that you want of the lemon, return from the experience simply by opening your eyes. Gradually feel yourself in the present.

After Les feels comfortable and confident about his imaging ability, I shall use the model outlined by Simonton and his colleagues [37].

Goal Setting

Last to be used to help Les "turn it around" is goal setting. Setting goals is one way to formulate reasons for living. Goals become a statement of the patient's personal needs. Goals are a way of affirming that there are things he wants out of life and that he will make an effort to achieve. Goals state that life is worth living. The patient's will to live is stronger when he has something to live for. This is one way for him to identify the meaning of his life.

Goal setting has some additional benefits for the cancer patient. Goals are statements that (1) say he expects to recover, (2) express a confidence that he can meet his needs, (3) avow that he is taking charge of his life rather than floating along, and (4) provide a framework on which he can focus his energy and prioritize his needs and wants. At the present time, since Les has so much to adjust to, I will not ask him to write his goals just yet.

Nursing Framework

It is time to return to Les's use of denial as a major defense mechanism. Les's denial is hard for me to deal with. Just how much denial does Les need to maintain his integrity but not distort the reality of his situation? And if his denial is to be removed, what should be substituted for it? No one should be left defenseless.

Reality therapy provides some guidelines. It says that a person can give up denying the world. He can recognize not only that reality exists but also that he can fulfill his needs within its framework. That principle underlies the use of imagery and relaxation techniques. The principles of reality therapy help the nurse (or other person) achieve a completely honest, human involvement with the patient so that the patient comes to realize that the nurse accepts him as he is and will help him fulfill his needs realistically. That is what I hoped to achieve in my relationship with Les.

Communication

Talking with Les would be the primary vehicle of our relationship. In talking, Les will be able to open himself up to another person. He will be exploring his interests, hopes, fears, opinions and values, and he will find out that he can have healthy disagreements with others without his feelings of self-worth being damaged. As he argues his convictions with a trusted friend (me), he can develop a sense of self-worth. That goes hand-in-hand with meditation and imaging. Instead of confronting Les with "reality," I will use Travelbee's indirect method of symbolization. And since Les liked Tolkien's *Lord of the Rings* trilogy and *The Hobbit* very much, Les and I decided to use Tolkien's character Bilbo Baggins as a symbol of reality.

A few of the difficult aspects of nursing care are to believe that (1) cancer need not always be fatal, (2) a person may positively effect his disease process, (3) a person can change how he acts, and (4) out of a negative situation—becoming ill—something positive can occur; namely, finding meaning or direction in one's life. There are definite planned nursing interventions to assist the patient implement each of those beliefs.

Nurse-Patient Relationship

I need to spend more time thinking about how to help Les find meaning in his illness. Faced with an unavoidable or unchangeable situation, a person "is given a last chance to actualize the highest value, to fulfill the deepest meaning, the meaning of suffering" [18]. What matters in a seemingly no-win situation is the attitude the person has about his fate. Man is prepared to suffer as long as the suffering has meaning (the reason the person undergoing a particular life experience gives to the situation) [42]. Paradoxically, "the orientation of the health workers is a major barrier to accepting the concept that illness is an experience that can be self-actualizing rather than meaningless" [42].

Travelbee lists nine goals for the nurse who is trying to develop a one-to-one relationship with a patient [42]. In regard to Les and me, the important goals are to help Les (1) cope with his present problems, (2) participate in the experience of living, of which illness is a part, (3) face emerging problems realistically, and (4) test new patterns of behavior. Inherent in achieving each goal is that Les will use his problem-solving skills as I, the nurse, offer him a safe and circumscribed reality—a framework within which Les may discover his maladaptive style and create more adaptive ways to deal with the real world.

As Les fathoms the meaning of his illness, I must too. Meaning is not inherent in life experiences. The specific meaning of a person's life at a given moment must be uncovered [19, 20]. Meaning is not an abstract concept. Each person has a mission and a meaning to fulfill during his lifetime [19]. Each person must feel needed and useful. When one feels needed by someone or something, he feels significant.

The principle that a person (a patient) creates meaning applies to the stresses and events that occurred before he became ill [37]. The amount of stress and the degree to which events make the person feel hopeless and helpless—out of control—are in proportion to the meaning a person ascribes to those stresses and events [20]. Hence, he alone determines the significance of the stresses and events.

To return to Travelbee's model of nursing practice Les must first explore the beliefs that limit his responses (he must identify the problem), and then he must consider alternative ways of interpreting life events and responding to those events. As the beliefs that have blocked Les's ability to live a healthy life are discovered and dislodged, his "life energy" can begin to flow smoothly. While I help Les identify his beliefs, I will not try to uncover unconscious content or trace problems back to Les's early childhood years [41]. I am concerned with the here and now and with the future. I represent Les's real world because I acknowledge his behavior and provide feedback about its effectiveness and appropriateness. By helping Les identify his problems and his wishes for relationships with others, I will help him to give himself permission to experience life differently [37]. As Les faces reality, he will see that even though he will always have problems and stresses, he can face them with the belief that he can solve them, or, at least, he will see that he is able to make decisions that will contribute to his getting well [37]. So relaxation, meditation, and imaging help Les find meaning in his life.

Behavior

The framework developed by Simonton and his associates is to be used to help Les identify beliefs or behaviors he may want to change [37]. Les must list five major life stresses that he had in the 18 months before his illness was manifested. Les must also be helped to find other ways of responding to stress and then to find ways of eliminating stress. If Les is to do that, he must examine how he may be contributing to the stresses, and then he must consider ways of removing the stresses. Or if that is not feasible at the present time, Les must consider ways of creating other supportive or nurturing elements in his life.

In discussing the exercise with other members of the health team and with Les, I must make it clear it is not the intent of the exercise either to make Les feel guilty about his past actions or to blame him for his present condition. In this scientific era, people believe that everything has a cause. Consequently, to explain suffering and distress, people seek "blame objects" (e.g., God, bad luck, fate, relatives, punishment, and pollution). The search for a blame object is probably inherent in the ill person's attempts to find meaning in his illness or reasons for his suffering. But it is not important to *find* a blame object. What is important is that the patient and the medical personnel not remain fixed at the blame level. I could not help Les to progress beyond the blame level if I thought he was not responsible for his behavior and could not change his behavior or his destiny.

The difference between blame and participation is that blame suggests that the person consciously knew better but made the choice to behave in a self-destructive or self-damaging fashion, whereas participation suggests that the person responded to a given set of situations in the light of his unconscious beliefs and habitual behavior sanctioned by culture [37].

Under the best circumstances, it is difficult to find meaning in illness and suffering. But if the patient cannot rise above the blame level and if that behavior is reinforced by others, his situation becomes more difficult, perhaps impossible [42].

Rising above the blame level is achieved with the formation of a one-to-one relationship between the nurse and the patient. A prerequisite to developing that kind of relationship is an environment in which each person sees and accepts the other as a unique human being. The relationship develops not because of the roles each plays (the nurse role and the patient role), but because two human beings are able to transcend the barriers of role, status, and position [41].

Outcome

The outcome of the one-to-one relationship is that "the ill person will have been given the opportunity to engage in meaningful interaction with a warm, sensitive, concerned, and knowledgeable individual who is not afraid to show interest and who does not blame, condone, or express value judgements about him or his behavior. He will have been spared false reassurance, useless advice, and pep talks" [42]. More important, the patient is given the opportunity to feel accepted by a person who neither demands anything nor accepts anything in return.

One way to find meaning in an illness is for the patient to look at the secondary gains he may get from being ill. Besides causing the person much pain and suffering, in Western cultures illness is the only condition that permits a person to stop his world and engage in certain types of behavior. Illness provides the only time in a person's adult life in which he is free from responsibilities and from the pressures of achieving. He is permitted a respite without being made to feel guilty or that he needs to explain or justify his actions, needs, or wants. The ill person's body is saying he has some unmet needs, and the person is demanding attention in the only way he can. But if illness can provide a temporary halt in life and a way to fulfill needs, illness can also become a trap. A person can like being the center of attention and feeling important; therefore, he has a stake in staying sick. Whatever the person's unmet needs are, they must be met if he is to regain or maintain his health. In that point of view, illness is an opportunity for personal growth as the patient identifies what needs are being met through the illness and then finds ways to meet those needs directly, without becoming sick. So Les must be helped to find meaning in his illness to find the "why" to live so that he can endure the "how."

Clinical Course

A bone marrow test and a peripheral smear were done the day of Les's admission. The test results established that he had acute myelogenous leukemia (AML). The bone marrow had a large number of myeloblasts, few other normal precursor cells, and occasional Auer bodies. The myeloblasts were peroxidase-positive. The peripheral smear showed 79 percent blasts.

The medical team decided that Les was a candidate for a bone marrow transplant. The results of the bone marrow test and the process of the bone marrow transplant were explained to Les in detail. Les readily agreed to the transplant: "Sure. Why not? I've never been a guinea pig before. This'll be a new experience for me. My sister'll donate her bone marrow for me."

Les's sister agreed to be a potential donor. During the five-day wait for the results of the mixed-lymphocyte culture, Les was given prophylactic-antibiotic therapy and treatment to reduce his skin bacteria. The patient care objective and the nursing orders for that period were:

1. By the end of the waiting time, Les's normal body flora should have diminished, as evidenced by the culture results. The nurse should:
   a. Have cultures of the patient's mouth, throat, nares, axillae, groin, stool, and urine done before antibiotic therapy is begun.
   b. Repeat those cultures in five days.
   c. Give dental care with a soft toothbrush and warm mouthwash after meals and at bedtime.
   d. Carry out the following prophylactic antibiotic regimen:
      (1) Nonabsorbable oral drugs: polymyxin B (140 mg), vancomycin (500 mg), and paromomycin (1 gm).
      (2) Nonabsorbable antifungal drug: amphotericin B (1 gm every 8 hr).
      (3) Topical antibiotic regimens:
         (a) Spray (three times a day to the nose and throat): neomycin (900 mg/ml), vancomycin (10 mg/ml), and polymyxin B (5 mg/ml).
         (b) Ointment (three times a day to gums, ears, anterior nares, groin, and perineum): neomycin (50 mg), nystatin (25,000 units), vancomycin (5 mg), and polymyxin B (2–5 mg).
         (c) Antibiotic gel (three times a day to anus): neomycin (100 mg), nystatin (50,000 units), vancomycin (10 mg), and polymyxin B (5 mg).
   e. Have the patient take a head-to-toe Betadine shower on arising and at bedtime.
   f. Have the patient transferred to a private room and limit the number of people entering his room.
   g. Permit only those people who seem in good health to come in contact with the patient.
2. By the end of the waiting period, Les should have "hooked up" with at least one nurse on each shift. The primary nurse should:
   a. Encourage the people who want to visit Les to spend at least 15 minutes every two hours talking with him.
   b. Hold team meetings, especially at the change of shift, at which everyone can discuss their feelings about Les and their methods of handling him.

The scrubbing time moved along without any problems. During that time, Les subtly expressed some of his concerns about what was happening to him. Meanwhile, Les's sister was found to be compatible with him, and the date for the transplantation was set—seven days away.

The patient care objectives and the nursing orders for the preparatory period were as follows:

1. For the duration of the preparatory period, Les should have minimal or no signs or symptoms of the sequelae of chemotherapy. The nurse should:
   a. Know (and observe for) the gastrointestinal sequelae of chemotherapy: nausea and vomiting related to a central nervous system effect on the emesis center in the thalamus, diarrhea related to the local mucosal irritation secondary to the direct effect on the bowel, and anorexia related to a secondary reaction to the nausea and vomiting, as well as to nonspecific metabolic abnormalities. To prevent those reactions, the nurse should:
      (1) Administer Compazine (10 mg as needed) 30 min before beginning the infusion.
      (2) Give two Lomotil tablets by mouth after each loose bowel movement.
      (3) Make sure the patient is on a low-roughage diet.
   b. Know (and observe for) the symptoms of hemorrhagic cystitis related to chemical irritation of the bladder (caused by the secretion of high concentrations of the active metabolites of cyclophosphamide). The nurse should:
      (1) Force fluids to 3000 ml/24 hr.
      (2) Determine the urinary pH and check the urine for occult blood every eight hours.
      (3) Have a microscopic analysis of the urine done.
      (4) Give an intravenous infusion of 3 liters of a 5% dextrose in normal saline solution every 24 hours; add 1 ampule of sodium bicarbonate to every other infusion.
   c. Know (and observe for) the symptoms of antidiuretic hormone suppression (of unknown mechanism) in a patient receiving dosages higher than 50 mg/kg. The nurse should:
      (1) Weigh the patient every day.
      (2) Keep a record of the fluid intake and output.
      (3) Administer Lasix (40 mg) intravenously 1 hour after the infusion ends and then 7 hours later, for a total of two doses.

(4) Administer Diamox (250 mg every other day).

d. Know (and put into action) measures to reduce the patient's susceptibility to infections resulting from the immunosuppressive therapy. The nurse should:

(1) Maintain the reverse isolation procedures.

(2) Every day, cleanse the intravenous insertion site with Betadine and apply a dry, sterile dressing. Use a mask and gloves.

(3) Have a complete blood count done.

(4) Cut the patient's hair.

(5) Continue to carry out the prophylactic antibiotic regimen.

(6) Continue to have head-to-toe Betadine showers taken twice a day.

(7) Have cultures of the nose, mouth, throat, axillae, groin, stool, and urine done twice a week.

2. By the end of the preparatory period, Les should (a) have a schedule for relaxation, meditation, and imaging; (b) practice those techniques on schedule; and (c) set one-month, three-month, six-month, and one-year goals.

The first two days of the preparatory period were unremarkable. Les was eager to meditate. Imagery was not as easy for him as the meditation was. Les's imagery drawings showed that he did feel out of control and like a small fish in a big pond. During the first two days we worked hard and had long conversations about what his imagery meant. By day three (T−4) of the preparatory period, Les's imagery became more positive. He spoke of some of his fears (Les had never mentioned the fact that he had a potentially fatal disease). His biggest fear was not that he would die but that he would die without having done anything significant. In other words, he would die without having left a legacy. Since literature about the transplantation process and the Life Island unit was scarce, I suggested that Les keep a tape diary of his experiences, feelings, and concerns for the rest of his hospitalization. The tape could be transcribed, and Les could edit it and submit it for publication. I stressed the importance of such an "exposé."

Many people keep diaries. Diary keeping is valued by many cultures. Diaries have given important information about life in other periods. They have long been used in psychotherapy, so why not for Les? They are certainly a valuable help in understanding patients.

Diary keeping involves the patient in his own care and provides useful information for therapy. Since Les will be living in a fishbowl, with little or no privacy, a diary would be something that is his, something that he could share with anyone he chose and when he chose to. I think that would be important for him. It would give him some control over his environment and over himself. Rather than act out and chance retaliation from the staff, he could use it when he felt angry or out of control. Talking into a tape recorder would dissipate some of his energy. He could say anything without fear of reprisal.

Keeping a diary may help Les to see that although being ill is a negative experience, the experience can be an avenue for personal development and for reevaluation of one's life pattern and purpose. It can be a time to become reacquainted with oneself. The first question a person asks when something bad happens to him is, "Why me?" Stressing to the patient (and believing it oneself) that he can grow to the extent that he becomes aware of and accepts change is an important part of creating and maintaining a therapeutic environment. The patient's acceptance of himself as a whole is an integral part of humanistic care [1, 3]. At present, Les does not seem to accept himself. Keeping a diary would (1) help Les concentrate on the physical and other effects of therapy rather than mull over his plight, (2) help him to think carefully about his general well-being, (3) help him show his progress toward his goals and identify any obstacles to attaining those goals, and (4) help him gain insight into how his life situations may be affecting his health [3, 10, 16, 22, 27].

While we were making the physical preparation for Les's entry into the Life Island unit and transplantation, Les was also preparing. Les was cooperating with the prophylactic antibiotic therapy and Betadine scrubs. His medication-relaxation-imagery schedule was working out well. Most of the medical and nursing personnel were "nonbelievers," but they did not obstruct the process. No one interrupted Les's meditation time, and almost everyone abided by the limits that were placed on Les's behavior.

Les identified five major stresses on his life: (1) two fights he had had with his mother about his living at home after graduation, (2) his previous girlfriend leaving him for another man, (3) his failures in political science (despite his exceptionally good work in economics and history), (4) the fact that a favorite teacher of his had suddenly left teaching and the college area, and (5) his twenty-first birthday. He had a bit more trouble identifying his methods of coping. Basically, he avoided unpleasant situations at any cost. He had no trouble identifying several ways he could eliminate his stresses (e.g., change his major to economics and take a minor in history; contact his favorite teacher and his sister, who would be sources of nurturance). He had more trouble deciding how he could negotiate with his mother about his independence.

Les and I discussed what his secondary gains from his illness were. He listed the following:

1. I don't have to go find a job because by getting sick I've missed my last semester at school and was able to take an incomplete from last semester's courses.
2. If I'm in school or sick I have an excuse for not living with my mother. My mother's going to put the screws on me to come to live with her after I graduate. The awful part is that if I don't have a job and I certainly don't have any money to afford rent, then I'll be forced to live with her.
3. My sister doesn't get involved with me—but now she is.
4. I don't have to get serious with my girlfriend; she certainly would not want to marry someone as sick as I am. Not only that, but the side effects of all this therapy means I couldn't even father any kids.
5. My friends, even though they'll graduate, won't leave me if I'm sick.

Les's illness was giving him a chance to make decisions about his priorities and his life-style and to think about his future. It also gave him an escape from finding out whether he would fail to get a job, and it helped him avoid settling dependency and independency issues with his mother and his girlfriend. Finally, it gave him a chance to ask for attention and to ask for help. During the entire time Les was undergoing chemotherapy he and I worked on (1) how he should deal with his mother and his girlfriend, both of whom wanted a commitment from him, (2) how he could improve his relationship with his sister without their engulfing one another, and (3) what he should do about a career. Les was able to describe how he dealt with unpleasant situations: "by not rocking the boat, but doing anything so people don't pressure me. I guess I'm not sure of myself, so I do anything to avoid taking a stand."

Les's coping mechanisms were like those of Bilbo Baggins. Bilbo liked the easily structured existence he had led before the visit from Gandalf and the dwarves. When they came to his house to "recruit" him for their journey to resteal the gold that Smaug, the dragon, had stolen from them years ago, Bilbo was a scared and reluctant member of the team. He did not want to leave the comfort and security of his home, but he was tempted by the chance to do something different. Despite his role in the group as the burglar, neither he nor his companions believed in his capabilities. The experience that seemed to bolster Bilbo was his ability to survive separation from the dwarves and to escape from the cave by finding a special ring. After that experience and after Gandalf had left the group, Bilbo became the leader of the group. He used problem-solving skills he never used before to get the band out of trouble and to Smaug's home. After the journey was successfully completed, Bilbo returned home. Because he had been gone for such a long time, he had trouble convincing people he was alive. Bilbo was an entirely different person because of his experience. One of his tasks after returning to his home was to write memoirs of his journey.

Les could readily identify with Bilbo and his growth.

Les, too, had liked his comfortable existence despite the toll it took on his health and well-being. More important, Les, like Bilbo, was reluctant to participate in a hazardous journey and mission. Les needed to be reminded from time to time that Bilbo had what it took—and so did Les.

Concurrent with Les's attempt to find meaning in his illness came the physical preparation for his entry into and maintenance in the Life Island unit. The sterilizing of bedpans, linens, stethoscopes, thermometers, emesis basins, paper bags, clothes and special-request objects was little or no problem. A big concern was Les's nutrition. Palatability of his food was a problem since all the food was to be gamma irradiated. The dietitian was a focal person in the preparatory period, because Les's eating habits were less than ideal. Getting him to select a balanced diet, let alone to eat it, was a struggle. Les was worried that he wouldn't have any desserts. But the dietitian figured out how to sterilize cream puffs, cookies, and ice cream. It was amazing how all members of the team gave their best to him. Administration even gave permission for him to have plants in his room.

Everything progressed smoothly. Just before Les went for TBI, he set the following goals for himself:

1. Three-month goals.
   a. Return to school and change my major to economics.
   b. Call or write my sister at least once a week to share our lives with one another.
   c. Tell my mother I don't want to live with her after graduation—and do not give in to her whining and crying.
2. Six-month goals.
   a. Go to England for my last year of study.
   b. Take a creative writing class.
   c. Make one new friend who doesn't go to school with me.
3. One-year goals.
   a. Graduate from school.
   b. Make another new friend who doesn't go to school with me.
   c. Get my own apartment.

One hour after returning to his room from TBI, Les was zippered into the Life Island unit. Three hours later the bone marrow infusion began.

Les spent 32 days in the Life Island unit. His stay was relatively uneventful. Occasionally he became grouchy about the number of people who came into his room. When things did not go as smoothly as Les wished, he pouted and made threats that ranged from not washing the inside of his canopy to coming out of the Life Island unit. His behavior was hard on everyone. Since Les had trouble articulating his needs, especially his need for companionship, he made his needs known by having a tantrum. But gradually, he became better about expressing his needs, but only to some people.

The graft began to take on the thirteenth day. *Staphylococcus aureus* was consistently cultured from the inside of Les's canopy, but Les remained infection free for the duration of his stay.

Les was discharged from the hospital approximately two months after his admission to the hospital. He returned to school to attend a summer session. Arrangements were made (with difficulty) with a clinic in London for medical follow-up care. In the fall, Les went to Oxford to study economics for a year. After the year was up, he came back, rented an apartment, and got a job.

Six months after Les began his job, in the midst of a virus outbreak, he developed a viral infection that he was unable to get rid of, and he died after an illness of seven days.

Reflections

Being Les's primary care practitioner was most difficult. It was also the most rewarding experience of my nursing career. It was hard to coordinate Les's care with others, because the staff members could not understand change. It was a tooth-and-nail struggle to get anyone to go along with the idea that Les was going to die but not necessarily within the statistical six-months period. (And our efforts bore fruit; Les lived for more than two years after the diagnosis of leukemia was made.) Did the people who resented Les's behavior ever consider that attitudes are contagious, that Les's acting out behavior with them reflected the message he was receiving from them?

I learned that relaxation and imagery can work as nursing actions but they do not work for everyone. In that regard Les was an ideal patient. Other patients who used the techniques did so with various degrees of commitment. Not all people are ready, willing, or able to learn more about themselves or to take more control of their lives and themselves. That's all right, too. It seems to me (my study is not scientific and my population is skewed) that the people for whom relaxation, imaging, and goal setting worked best were the people who were the most cantankerous and who most wanted to have their questions answered—in short, not what is considered ideal patients.

I must say that Les was one of the niftiest patients I have ever had. Maybe one reason I liked him so much was that he was a first for me in many ways—the first person to undergo a bone marrow transplant in the hospital and in the city, the first person to whom I could apply Travelbee's framework (since my graduate days), the first person who did not become a six-month statistic. I do not deny that I got secondary gains from my work with Les. I do not deny that re-creating the experience on paper was hard for me because I remembered the frustrations and hard work. But what I remember best was Les's stepping out of his bubble with a huge grin on his face, opening the Dom Perignon the medical and nursing staff had bought for the occasion, and handing me the first glass. A nurse-patient interaction is never a neutral event.

References

1. Abrams, R. The patient with cancer—his changing pattern of communication. *N. Engl. J. Med.* 274:317, 1966.

2. Achterberg, J., and Lawlis, G. F. *Imagery of Cancer.* Champaign, Ill.: Institute of Personality and Ability Testing, 1978.

3. Bahnson, C. Psychologic and emotional issues in cancer: The psychotherapeutic care of the cancer patient. *Semin. Oncol.* 2:293, 1975.

4. Bahnson, M., and Bahnson, M. Ego defenses in cancer patients. *Ann. N.Y. Acad. Sci.* 164:546, 1969.

5. Benson, H., Beary, J. F., and Carol, M. P. The relaxation response. *Psychiatry* 37:37, 1974.

6. Bodey, G., and Rodrigues, V. Infections in cancer patients in a protected environment—prophylactic antibiotic program. *Am. J. Med.* 59:497, 1975.

7. Broder, S., and Waldman, T. The suppressor-cell network in cancer (Part 1). *N. Engl. J. Med.* 299:23, 1978.

8. Broder, S., and Waldman, T. The suppressor-cell network in cancer (Part 2). *N. Engl. J. Med.* 299:24, 1978.

9. Brown, H., and Kelly, M. Stages of bone marrow transplantation: A psychiatric perspective. *Psychosom. Med.* 38:439, 1976.

10. Buehler, J. What contributes to hope in the cancer patient? *Am. J. Nurs.* 75:1353, 1975.

11. Burkhalter, P., and Donley, D. *Dynamics of Oncology Nursing.* New York: Macmillan, 1978.

12. Burns, N. Cancer chemotherapy: A systematic approach. *Nurs. '78* 8 (No. 2):56, 1978.

13. Clarkson, B. Acute myelocytic leukemia in adults. *Cancer* 30:1572, 1972.

14. Creech, R. The psychologic support of the cancer patient. *Semin. Oncol.* 2:285, 1975.

15. Engel, G. The care of the patent: Art or science? *Johns Hopkins Med. J.* 140:222, 1977.

16. Frank, J. The role of hope in psychotherapy. *Int. J. Psychiatry Med.* 5:383, 1968.

17. Frank, J. Mind-body relationships in illness and healing. *J. Int. Acad. Prevent. Med.* 11:46, 1975.

18. Frank, J. The faith that heals. *Johns Hopkins Med. J.* 137:127, 1975.

19. Frankl, V. *Man's Search for Meaning.* New York: Simon & Schuster, 1959.

20. Frankl, V. *The Will to Meaning.* New York: New American Library, 1969.

21. Glasser, R. J. *The Body Is The Hero.* New York: Random House, 1976.

22. Glasser, W. *Reality Therapy.* New York: Harper & Row, 1965.

23. Glasser, R. How the body works against itself—autoimmune disease. *Nurs. '77* 7 (No. 9):38, 1977.

24. Gould, R. *Transformations: Growth and Change in Adult Life.* New York: Simon & Schuster, 1978.

25. Green, E., and Green, A. *Beyond Biofeedback.* New York: Dell, 1977.

26. Hoagland, H. C. Acute leukemia and its complications. *Mayo Clin. Proc.* 53:60, 1978.

27. Holland, J., Plumb, M., Yates, J., et al. Psychological response of patients with acute leukemia to germ-free environments. *Cancer* 40:871, 1977.

28. Jourard, S. Suicide: An invitation to die. *Am. J. Nurs.* 70:269, 1970.

29. Kellerman, J., Rigler, D., and Siegel, S. The psychological effects of isolation in protected environments. *Am. J. Psychiatry* 134:563, 1977.

30. Korner, I. Hope as a method of coping. *J. Consult. Clin. Psychol.* 34:13, 1970.

31. LeShan, L. An emotional life-history pattern associated with neoplastic disease. *Ann. N.Y. Acad. Sci.* 125:780, 1965–1966.

32. Leventhal, B., and Konior, G. Leukemia: A critical review. *Semin. Oncol.* 3:319, 1976.

33. Mastrovito, R. Cancer: Awareness and denial. *Clin. Bull.* 4:142, 1974.

34. Pelletier, K. *Mind As Healer, Mind As Slayer.* New York: Dell, 1977.

35. Porter, J. *Psychic Development.* New York: Random House, 1974.

36. Schmale, A. Relationship of separation and depression to disease: I. A report on a hospitalized medical population. *Psychosom. Med.* 20:259, 1958.

37. Simonton, O. C., Matthews-Simonton, S., and Creighton, J. *Getting Well Again.* California: Tarcher, 1978.

38. Solomon, G. Emotions, stress, the central nervous system, and immunity. *Ann. N.Y. Acad. Sci.* 164:335, 1969.

39. Surwicz, F., Brightwell, D., Weitzel, W., et al. Cancer, emotions, and mental illness: The present state of understanding. *Am. J. Psychiatry* 133:1306, 1976.

40. Thomas, E. O., Storb, R., Clift, R., et al. Bone-marrow transplantation (Part 1). *N. Engl. J. Med.* 292:832, 1975.

41. Thomas, E. O., Storb, R., Clift, R., et al. Bone-marrow transplantation (Part 2). *N. Engl. J. Med.* 292:895, 1975.

42. Travelbee, J. *Interpersonal Aspects of Nursing* (2nd ed.). Philadelphia: Davis, 1971.

43. Vaillot, M., Sr. Existentialism: A philosophy of commitment. *Am. J. Nurs.* 66:500, 1966.

44. Vaillot, M., Sr. Hope: The restoration of being. *Am. J. Nurs.* 70:268, 1970.

45. Varricchio, C. Nursing care during total body irradiation. *Am. J. Nurs.* 77:1314, 1977.

46. Watts, A. *Meditation.* California: Celestial Arts, 1974.

47. Wiehl, A. *Creative Visualization.* St. Paul: Llewellyn, 1958.

48. Williams, J. Understanding the feelings of the dying. *Nurs. '76* 2:52, 1976.

49. Zimmerman, S., Cohen, T., Diekman, R., et al. Bone marrow transplantation. *Am. J. Nurs.* 77:1311, 1977.

Epilogue

Critical care nurses may object to body-mind-spirit concepts as being unscientific or because they do not "make sense." A healthy skepticism is an admirable quality; but to persist in any belief without a thorough examination of the evidence is the worst kind of dogmatism, ill becoming the critical care nurse.

One conclusion from modern physics is that our ideas of what "makes sense" are frequently misleading. One by one, the old ideas in physics that did make sense—of space, time, mass, causation—have been replaced by newer ideas that make no sense at all.

If this concept appears wildly unscientific, we may do well to ponder a remark of the great quantum physicist, Niels Bohr. Another physicist had proposed a bizarre theory to account for some perplexing observations in atomic physics. Under severe criticism by others who were present, he turned to Bohr: "Do you think this is crazy?" Bohr considered briefly. "Yes," he said, "it is crazy but I think it is not crazy enough."*

*From an address by Dr. Joseph H. Rush before the North Texas Chapter of the Texas District Branch of the American Psychiatric Association at Dallas, Texas, January 9, 1975.

Language evolves, in general, to express what our senses tell us is true. Our words are a mirror to our senses.

Therefore, if something does not "make sense," we are unlikely to have words to express this "something." Feelings may affect us in this way. Even though we may feel something strongly, we may be speechless, wordless, in trying to express ourselves.

Artists and musicians use devices other than words to bypass this difficulty. And although skillful poets—the great poets—may use words, they know how to convey more than is said by the words themselves.

There are no problems in finding words to express case presentations. In discussing body-mind-spirit concepts, however, the situation is different. We are just beginning to develop a way of describing the interrelatedness of mind and body, as this relatedness yields more and more to scientific investigation. But as an illustration of the problem, we are still at a loss for even a name for this subject of investigation, and we are forced to depend on word combinations: "body-mind," or "psychobiological."

Because of our difficulties with words to describe the spiritual quality of man, the reader may feel adrift on a sea of confusion. The difficulties in verbally describing spiritual concepts lead one to poetry, and we have made use of this medium throughout the book. We have tried to state why it is nearly impossible to reduce spiritual concepts to words. The mystics have wrestled with the same problem in trying to express their experiences; and we say now with St. Theresa: "More than this I cannot say"; or, from the Upanishads:

There the eye goes not,
Speech goes not, nor the mind.
We know not, we understand not
How one would teach it.

The confrontation between body-mind-spirit concepts and critical care nursing is a present and immediate fact. We therefore do not believe our book is as futuristic as it might at first seem to the reader unfamiliar with these concepts. On the contrary, we believe it is present-oriented and that to delay a consideration of these issues will force critical care nursing into an unnecessarily passive position.

Critical care nurses can not only adapt these concepts to patient care but can also modify and enlarge upon them. *It is unnecessary to be defensive when we are capable of showing the way.*

Index

The interconnections of mind and body are reflected in changes of emotions and physiology. These associations may operate at conscious *and* unconscious levels. And, importantly, these interconnections are felt to be *invariable*; i.e., changes in the emotional state of the patient *always* cause changes in the physiological state, and vice versa. This body-mind relatedness is constant and always present, although the patient may not always be aware of its operation.

The psychophysiological principle, as we hypothesize it, affirms that every change in the physiological state is accompanied by an appropriate change in the mental/emotional state, conscious or unconscious, and conversely, every change in the mental/emotional state, conscious or unconscious, is accompanied by an appropriate change in the physiological state.[*]

Because of the physiological and psychological (body-mind) continuum, critical care nurses must include this consideration in their development of a personal philosophy of nursing care. Traditional definitions of health and disease, as well as attitudes toward patient care, will be changed by the idea of the patient as a psychobiological unit.

[*]Green, E., Green, A., and Walters, E. Voluntary control of internal states: Psychological and physiological. *J. Transpersonal Psychol.* 2 (1):3, 1970.

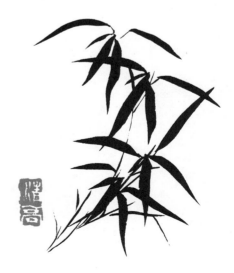

Index